Clinical Exercise Physiology

Application and Physiological Principles

Clinical Exercise Physiology

Application and Physiological Principles

Serge P. von Duvillard

Linda M. LeMura
LeMoyne College
Syracuse, New York

Serge P. von Duvillard
California State Polytechnic University
Pomona, California

LIPPINCOTT WILLIAMS & WILKINS
A **Wolters Kluwer** Company

Philadelphia • Baltimore • New York • London
Buenos Aires • Hong Kong • Sydney • Tokyo

Acquisitions Editor: Peter J. Darcy
Managing Editor: Eric Branger
Marketing Manager: Christen DeMarco
Production Editor: Jennifer D.W. Glazer
Artwork: Kim Battista
Compositor: LWW
Printer: Quebecor World

530 Walnut Street
Philadelphia, Pennsylvania 19106

351 West Camden Street
Baltimore, Maryland 21201

Printed in the United States of America

Library of Congress Cataloging-in-Publication Data

Clinical exercise physiology: application and physiological principles/[edited by] Linda
   M. LeMura, Serge P. von Duvillard
        p.; cm
   Includes bibliographical references and index.
   ISBN: 0-7817-2680-8
     1. Exercise therapy. 2. Exercise tests. 3. Physiology, Pathological. I. LeMura, Linda M.
   II. von Duvillard, Serge P.
   [DNLM: 1. Exercise—physiology. 2. Chronic Disease. WE 103 C64072 2003]
   RM725.C583 2003
   615.8'2—dc21

                                                        2003047630

The publishers have made every effort to trace the copyright holders for borrowed material. If they have inadvertently overlooked any, they will be pleased to make the necessary arrangements at the first opportunity.

To purchase additional copies of this book, call our customer service department at (800) 638-3030 or fax orders to (301) 824-7390. For other book services, including chapter reprints and large quantity sales, ask for the Special Sales department.

For all other calls originating outside of the United States, please call (301) 714-2324.

Visit Lippincott Williams & Wilkins on the Internet: http://www.LWW.com. Lippincott Williams & Wilkins customer service representatives are available from 8:30 am to 6:00 pm, EST, Monday through Friday, for telephone access.

03 04 05 06 07
1 2 3 4 5 6 7 8 9 10

This work is dedicated to my parents and siblings, for their unrelenting love and support, and to my husband Larry and our daughter Emily, for the indescribable joy they bring me each day.

Linda LeMura

To my parents and my brother for their patience, sacrifice, understanding, and love, and to my students for their perpetual thirst for knowledge, inspiration, and joy that makes teaching and research so immeasurably enjoyable.

Serge Petelin von Duvillard

Authors

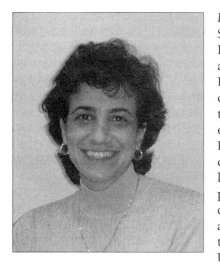

Linda M. LeMura is currently the Dean of Arts and Sciences at Le Moyne College in Syracuse, New York. Prior to her post as Dean, she was a professor of applied physiology at Bloomsburg University of Pennsylvania where she also served as the assistant chairperson of her department, and as the director of the graduate program. She obtained her doctorate in exercise physiology from Syracuse University in 1987. Her primary research interests include pediatric exercise physiology and energy metabolism; she has published extensively in these areas. She is particularly proud of the accomplishments of her graduate students who have been accepted into prestigious doctoral programs with one or more peer-reviewed publications to their credit. During her tenure at Bloomsburg University, Linda received the "Dean's Award for Excellence in Scholarship and Teaching" and was named a fellow of the American College of Sports Medicine. She has served as a reviewer for numerous journals, including *Medicine and Science in Sports and Exercise, Pediatrics, The British Journal of Sports Medicine* and *The Journal of Sports Medicine and Physical Fitness.*

A former intercollegiate athlete, Linda is married to Larry Tanner, an internationally renowned geologist. They live in Syracuse, New York, with their daughter Emily—a 9-year-old, promising musician and soccer player. Linda enjoys old movies, visiting New York City, and sports of all kinds.

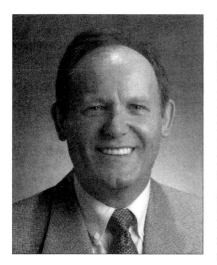

Serge P. von Duvillard is a Professor of Exercise Physiology at California State Polytechnic University in Pomona, California. His doctoral studies in exercise physiology started at the University of Southern California in Los Angeles under the mentorship of Herbert A. deVries and were completed under R. Donald Hagan at the University of North Texas in Denton, Texas. He is an Adjunct Professor of Physiology and Medicine at the University of North Dakota, in Grand Forks, and at the University of Graz in Austria, respectively. Serge is currently the chair and graduate program coordinator of the Department of Kinesiology and Health Promotion at California State Polytechnic University in Pomona, California. His research interests are energy metabolism, cardiopulmonary physiology, fat and lipoprotein metabolism, and testing of elite athletes. An author or co-author of more than 100 scientific articles and book chapters, many of his students went on to receive doctoral degrees in exercise science and exercise physiology at various distinguished institutions. Serge is fellow of the American College of Sports Medicine (ACSM) and the European College of Sport Science (ECSS). He has received several prestigious scientific awards including the Young Investigator Award, Visiting Scholar Award and the Senior Investigator Research Grant Award from ACSM. A former president of the Northland Chapter of the ACSM, Serge remains active in regional, national, and international organizations. He is a member of numerous editorial boards and continues to serve as a reviewer for many professional peer review journals including *Medicine and Science in Sports and Exercise, European Journal of Applied Physiology, British Journal of Sports Medicine, International Journal of Sports Medicine, Ergonomics,* and *Metabolism.*

A native of Germany and Slovenia, Serge is a former decathlete and alpine ski racer. He currently lives in Alta Loma, California, and is an avid sports participant. Humor and laughter are the soul of his life and so are his parents, brother, friends, colleagues, students, music, nature and animals.

Preface

We came up with the idea for this book when students at our respective universities were about to begin their capstone internship in exercise science. Our students indicated the need for one handy volume containing a comprehensive review of the physiological principles and clinical applications associated with a wide range of diseases and disabilities. Their rationale was simple: they needed a source to which they could refer in the event that a unique clinical challenge presented itself during the internship experience. To answer this need, we decided to recruit top-notch scientists and clinicians with expertise across a spectrum of diseases and disabilities to write chapters for us.

The first and second chapters that comprise the introduction include a review of exercise physiology principles and a compendium of exercise epidemiology issues, respectively. While these two chapters may not appear congruent with the intended purpose of a clinical exercise medicine volume, we decided to honor the requests of our students seeking this information. These two chapters will serve as useful summaries either independently or within the context of a clinical exercise medicine text.

Subsequent to the introduction, we divided this book into eight sections: cardiovascular, pulmonary, neuromuscular, metabolic, immunological and hematological, orthopedic, and cognitive and emotional disorders; we also included a section on aging. Each section has several specific chapters written by specialists in their respective fields. Given the scope and depth of all of the chapters, we believe that this text will be of significant value not only to students in exercise science, but also to those studying clinical exercise physiology, physical therapy, and medicine.

We organized the chapters mindful of the needs of our students. Specifically, each chapter begins with an overview of a disease or disability. In the event that a student is unfamiliar with a particular clinical situation, this overview would be a good place to start in that it provides an explanation of the etiology, prevalence, and the signs and symptoms of the disease or disability in question. In many chapters, the author(s) provide a detailed description of the genesis of the problem, which might include a discussion of its genetic basis.

A key component of this book is a description of the exercise responses specific to a given disease or disability. For instance, an individual with multiple sclerosis would respond very differently to exercise therapy than a paraplegic. These differences would be manifested during an exercise test or during routine exercise training and/or therapy. We hope that the information contained in this text will help students answer the following questions: 1) How do I interpret the information obtained from testing? and 2) How do I develop an appropriate exercise program for the individual? Other useful information includes the effects of medications on the exercise response, useful diagnostic tests, exercise limitations, and practical tips for selecting modes of exercise for individual patients or clients.

The special features found within each chapter were designed to help the students acquire important information in a "user-friendly" manner. For example, "What we know" and "What we would like to know" not only summarizes our understanding of the nature of the disease, but also provides the reader with the directions of the current research in this field. The "red flag" offers the student an important tip about what to watch for if she/he encounters a patient with that disease, and the glossary provides quick access to definitions of the key terms in the chapter. The case study with the associated questions is designed to help the student apply the material in the chapter to a clinical situation that she/he might encounter.

Although the idea for the book, the chapter template, and the special features were developed with students in mind, we did not forget about the needs of our colleagues! We included discussion questions and a list of suggested readings to augment the material presented in each chapter. It is our hope that this material will be the basis for evocative assignments and insightful discussions as you prepare your students for meaningful internship experiences and eventual professional careers.

Acknowledgments

We would like to recognize enthusiastically the many distinguished national and international scientists and scholars who have given unselfishly of their time and talents to contribute to this book. We are grateful for your dedication, enthusiasm, and your willingness to share your expertise with aspiring students, colleagues, and scientists around the world. We also wish to acknowledge each of the manuscript reviewers; we appreciate deeply your time, comments, and constructive suggestions for the improvement of this textbook.

It is impossible to convey the gratitude, affection, and respect toward the many colleagues who have influenced most profoundly our thinking and helped shape our careers. We are especially indebted to our former professors and mentors: Herbert A. de Vries, R. Donald Hagan, Roger K. Burke, Tillman J. Hall, Jürgen Stegemann, Wildor Hollmann, Alois Mader, as well as David W. Bacharach, Brenda Engbretson, Wayne Gallagher, William Green, David Hood, Hsien-Tung Liu, and Ronald Terjung.

We wish to thank our publisher, Lippincott Williams & Wilkins, specifically Susan Katz, Pete Darcy, Nancy Peterson, and Jenn Weir for supporting this project. We are particularly indebted to Eric Branger for his patience, attention to detail, and invaluable cooperation throughout the evolution of this mission. We also acknowledge Kim Battista for her meticulous work in the development of the art program.

Finally, many former and current students have directly and indirectly influenced the direction of this textbook. We appreciate your thoughts, inquisitive questions and inspiring comments. You have been our teachers.

LINDA M. LE MURA

SERGE P. VON DUVILLARD

Contributors

Paul J. Arciero, DPE, FACSM
Associate Professor
Department of Exercise Science
Skidmore College
Saratoga Springs, New York

David W. Bacharach, PhD, FACSM
Human Performance Lab
Department of Health, Physical Education,
    Recreation and Sport Science
St. Cloud State University
St. Cloud, Minnesota

Jackie Kuta Bangsberg
UW Health Sports Medicine Center
Madison, Wisconsin

Romualdo Belardinelli, MD, FESC
Cardiac Rehabilitation and Exercise
    Physiology Unit
Lancisi Heart Institute
Ancona, Italy

Ralph Beneke, MD
Department of Biological Sciences
Centre for Sports and Exercise Science
University of Essex
Colchester, England

Theresa Bianco
The University of Western Australia
School of Human Movement and Exercise
    Science
Crawley, Perth, Australia

Thomas J. Birk, PhD, MPT, FACSM
Associate Professor
Department of Physical Therapy
Department of Physical Medicine and
    Rehabilitation
School of Medicine, Wayne State University
Detroit Medical Center, Rehabilitation
    Institute of Michigan
Detroit, Michigan

Ralph S. Bovard, MD, MPH, FACSM
Occupational and Environmental Medicine
    & Orthopedics and Sports Medicine
Regions Hospital/Health Partners
St. Paul, Minnesota

William W. Briner, MD, FACSM
Lutheran General Hospital
Park Ridge, Illinois

**William W. Briner, Jr, MD, FAAFP,
FACSM**
Sports Medicine Fellowship Director
Family Practice Faculty
Advocate Lutheran General Hospital
Park Ridge, Illinois

Cathy Burt
UW Health Sports Medicine Center
Madison, Wisconsin

Kristi Cadwell
Department of Exercise and Sport
    Science
University of Wisconsin—La Crosse
La Crosse, Wisconsin

Frank W. Cerny
Department of Exercise and Nutrition
    Sciences
University at Buffalo
SUNY
Buffalo, New York

Bernard A. Clark III, MD
Acting Chairman/Director, Department of
    Medicine
Director, Non-Invasive Cardiology
Saint Francis Hospital and Medical
    Center
Associate Professor of Clinical Medicine
University of Connecticut School of
    Medicine
Hartford, Connecticut

Kerry S. Courneya, PhD
Professor and CIHR Investigator
Faculty of Physical Education
University of Alberta
Edmonton, Alberta, Canada

Stephen F. Crouse, PhD, FACSM
Professor of Kinesiology
Director, Applied Exercise Science
    Laboratory
Department of Health and Kinesiology
Texas A&M University
College Station, Texas

Diane M. Cullen, PhD
Creighton University
Osteoporosis Research Center
Omaha, Nebraska

Donald R. Dengel, PhD, FACSM
Laboratory of Physiological Hygiene and
    Exercise Science
Division of Kinesiology
University of Minnesota
Minneapolis, Minnesota

Patrick J. Devine, MD, CPT, MC, FS, USA
Department of Medicine
Walter Reed Army Medical Center
Washington, DC

Robert C. Eklund, PhD
Exercise, Health, & Sport Psychology
School of Human Movement & Exercise
    Science
The University of Western Australia
Crawley, Perth, Australia

Martin Engelhardt, MD
Städtische Kliniken Bielefeld
Klinikum Mitte
Bielefeld, Germany

Bo Fernhall, PhD
Chair, Exercise Science Department
Syracuse University
Syracuse, New York

Carl Foster, PhD
Department of Exercise and Sport Science
University of Wisconsin—La Crosse
La Crosse, Wisconsin

Christopher L. Gentile, MSc
University of Colorado—Boulder
Human Cardiovascular Research Laboratory
Department of Kinesiology and Applied
    Physiology
Boulder, Colorado

Ifigenia Giannopoulou, PhD
Lecturer
Syracuse University
Syracuse, New York

Peter Grandjean
Associate Professor
Auburn University
Auburn, Alabama

J. Robert Grove
Associate Professor
Exercise, Health, & Sport Psychology
School of Human Movement & Exercise
    Science
The University of Western Australia
Crawley, Perth, Australia

Stefanie Hatcher
Department of Exercise and Sport Science
University of Wisconsin—La Crosse
La Crosse, Wisconsin

Matthias Huetler, MD
Department of Physical Medicine and
    Rehabilitation
Haukeland University Hospital
Bergen, Norway

Kurt Jackson, PhD, MPT
Andrews University
Health Research Scientist
Dayton VA Medical Center
Dayton, Ohio

David M. Jenkinson, DO
Center for Sports Medicine and
    Orthopaedics
Chattanooga, Tennessee

Jason Johnson, MD
Sports Medicine
Lutheran General Hospital
Chicago, Illinois

Daniel A. Judelson, MA
United States Olympic Committee
Lake Placid, New York

Jill Kanaley, PhD
Professor
Syracuse University
Syracuse, New York

Arna E. Karlsdottir, PT, MS
Department of Cardiac Rehabilitation
Reykjalundur Rehabilitation Center
Mosfellsbær, Iceland

Linda LeMura, PhD, FACSM
Dean of Arts and Sciences
Le Moyne College
Syracuse, New York

David A. Lightman, MD
Ophthalmologist
Vitreoretinal Associates, PC
Evangelical Community Hospital
Lewisburg, Pennsylvania

Caroline A. Macera, PhD
Graduate School of Public Health
San Diego State University
San Diego, California

John R. Mackey, MD, FRCP(C)
Division of Medical Oncology
Department of Oncology
University of Alberta
Cross Cancer Institute
Edmonton, Alberta, Canada

Laurel T. Mackinnon, PhD, FACSM
Associate Professor
School of Human Movement Studies
The University of Queensland
Brisbane, Australia

Désirée Maltais, BSc (PT), MSc
McMaster University
Hamilton, Ontario, Canada

Robert C. Manske, MPT, MEd, SCS, ATC, CSCS
Assistant Professor
Department of Physical Therapy
College of Health Professions
Wichita State University
Wichita, Kansas

Timothy R. McConnell, PhD
Director, Faculty Development and
    Cardiac Rehabilitation
Geisinger Medical Center
Danville, Pennsylvania

Laura J. McIntosh, MD
Saint Vincent's Family Medicine Center
Erie, Pennsylvania

Katharina Meyer, PhD
Swiss Health Observatory
Espace l'Europe
Neuchatel, Switzerland

Janet A. Mulcare, PhD, FACSM
Andrews University
Health Research Scientist
Dayton VA Medical Center
Dayton, Ohio

Edward C. Nieshoff, MD
Director, Spinal Cord and Clinical
    Research
Department of Physical Medicine and
    Rehabilitation
School of Medicine
Wayne State University and
Detroit Medical Center, Rehabilitation
    Institute of Michigan
Detroit, Michigan

Bradley C. Nindl, PhD, FACSM
Research Physiologist
Military Performance Division
United States Army Research Institute of
    Environmental Medicine
Natick, Massachusetts

Patricia Painter, PhD, FACSM
Associate Adjunct Professor
University of California at San Francisco
San Francisco, California

Antonio Pelliccia, MD, FACSM
Institute of Sports Science
Italian National Olympic Committee
Rome, Italy

Kenneth H. Pitetti, PhD, FACSM
Professor
Department of Physical Therapy
College of Health Professions
Wichita State University
Wichita, Kansas

Jacques R. Poortmans
Université Libre de Bruxelles
Bruxelles, Belgium

John P. Porcari, PhD
Department of Exercise and Sport Science
University of Wisconsin—La Crosse
La Crosse, Wisconsin

Leigh Taylor Ramsey, PhD
Division of Prevention Research and
    Analytic Methods
Epidemiology Program Office
New Hampshire Department of Health and
    Human Services
Centers for Disease Control and
    Prevention
Concord, New Hampshire

Pedro Recalde
Department of Exercise and Sport Science
University of Wisconsin—La Crosse
La Crosse, Wisconsin

Iris Reuter, MD
Institute of Psychiatry
King's College Hospital
London, United Kingdom

Thomas H. Reynolds IV, PhD
Department of Exercise and Sport Sciences
School of Health Sciences and Human
    Performance
Ithaca College
Ithaca, New York

Ryan E. Rhodes, PhD
Assistant Professor
Kinesiology Program
School of Physical Education
University of Victoria
Victoria, British Columbia, Canada

David Rhude, MD
Hennepin County Medical Center
Minneapolis, Minnesota
Keith J. O'Neill Center for Healthy
    Families
Marywood University
Scranton, Pennsylvania

Thomas W. Rowland, MD
Director of Pediatric Cardiology
Baystate Medical Center
Springfield, Massachusetts

Kenneth W. Rundell, PhD, FACSM
Professor Health Science
Director Human Performance Laboratory
Keith J. O'Neill Center for Healthy
    Families
Maywood University
Scranton, Pennsylvania

Lisa Sanborn
University of Wisconsin Health Sports
    Medicine Center
Madison, Wisconsin

Andrew Schachat, MD
Karl Hagen Professor of Ophthalmology
The Wilmer Ophthalmological Institute
Baltimore, Maryland

Roy J. Shephard, MD, PhD, DPE
Faculty of Physical Education & Health and
Department of Public Health Sciences
University of Toronto
Toronto, Ontario, Canada

Ronald T. Smith, PhD
Associate Professor of Exercise Science
North Carolina Wesleyan College
Rocky Mount, North Carolina

**Ray W. Squires, PhD, FACSM,
FAACVPR, FAHA**
Director, Cardiovascular Health Clinic
Associate Professor of Medicine
Division of Cardiovascular Diseases and
    Internal Medicine
Mayo Clinic
Rochester, Minnesota

William W. Stringer, MD, FACP, FCCP
Associate Professor of Medicine
UCLA School of Medicine
Harbor–UCLA Medical Center
Torrance, California

Carla Theusch
Department of Exercise and Sport Science
University of Wisconsin—La Crosse
La Crosse, Wisconsin

Viswanath B. Unnithan, PhD, FACSM
University of San Francisco
San Francisco, California

Stacie Voelker
Department of Exercise and Sport
    Science
University of Wisconsin—La Crosse
La Crosse, Wisconsin

Ann Ward, PhD
Department of Kinesiology
University of Wisconsin—Madison
Madison, Wisconsin

Kristy F. Woods, MD, MPH
Meharry Medical College and
Vanderbilt University School of Medicine
Nashville, Tennessee

Su Zhan, MB
Department of Exercise and Nutrition
    Sciences
University at Buffalo—State University of
    New York
Buffalo, New York

Contents

SECTION IV
NEUROMUSCULAR DISEASES AND DISORDERS   205

SECTION V
METABOLIC DISEASES AND DISORDERS   301

SECTION VI
IMMUNOLOGICAL AND HEMATOLOGICAL DISEASES AND DISORDERS   385

SECTION VII
ORTHOPEDIC DISEASES AND DISORDERS   483

SECTION VIII
EXERCISE AND AGING   547

SECTION IX
COGNITIVE AND EMOTIONAL DISORDERS   583

INTRODUCTION

CHAPTER 1

Review of Exercise Physiology

David W. Bacharach

SEARCHABLE KEY TERMS

Beta-oxidation	Lactate
Bioenergetics	Lypolysis
Bohr Effect	Mitochondria
Calorimetry	Overload Principle
Catabolism	Overtraining
Economy	Oxidative Phosphorylation
Efficiency	Power
Gluconeogenesis	Steady State
Homeostasis	Work

Overview

Exercise physiology is the study of how the human body responds to physical stress under either acute or chronic conditions (1). People often use various common phrases relating human performances to machine-like actions, such as "runs like a well-oiled machine" or "just ran out of gas." The human body is in essence a machine, albeit a complex one. The body depends on a multitude of systems interacting efficiently to maintain **homeostasis**, or a **steady state**, of particular systems (1). Regardless of what the body is asked to do, multiple systems attempt to coordinate or allocate their available resources to accomplish the task. Sometimes they can do it; sometimes they cannot. The study of how the body is able to accommodate the demands we place on it in one case and not in another is the study of exercise physiology.

No single event has advanced the discipline of exercise physiology more than the establishment of the American College of Sports Medicine (ACSM). In 1954, several innovative physicians and physical educators met for the first time to discuss the role of exercise in health and medicine (2). Since that time, it has become apparent to many medical professionals that exercise has a legitimate role in prevention, treatment, diagnosis, and rehabilitation of various diseases. This chapter does not address issues of body composition, nutrition, or disease, but, rather, attempts to review the concepts important to all exercise physiologists involving the ways in which the body responds to exercise stress. These include (1) bioenergetics, (2) systemic responses to exercise, and (3) adaptations to exercise training.

Bioenergetics

Bioenergetics is defined as energy transformation in living organisms (2). We assume homeostasis to be a state in which all systems are at equilibrium during rest. When a stressor is applied to the body, the body responds automatically by first shifting out of homeostatic balance. This shift triggers what are commonly referred to as negative feedback loops. These loops involve neural and humoral entities controlled primarily by the autonomic nervous system, many of which can have far-reaching influences on the body. All major systems of the body operate under one or more of these feedback loops. For example, a rise in carbon dioxide (CO_2) detected by chemoreceptors in the circulatory system results in the stimulation of respiratory centers in the brain to increase both depth and frequency of breathing. At the same time, voluntary muscle contractions may have influenced receptors for blood pressure, venous return, blood pH, and temperature. All these systems must now be integrated into what the body perceives as an appropriate response. Sometimes, however, the response is inappropriate and leads to systemic problems. It is well known that mental stress has physical effects on the body—it can trigger sympathetic arousal loops that prepare the body for the "fight or flight" phenomenon with no one to fight or nowhere to run. This inappropriate response has been linked to almost all chronic diseases that plague Western society today. It appears, therefore, that understanding how much control we have on these feedback systems is important for determining how these influences can affect the status of each individual cell.

Several fundamental principles dictate how a cell uses energy to remain viable or to produce work. All energy released in the body is released via chemical compounds exchanging bonds or atoms between various molecules (3). Adenosine triphosphate (ATP) is the energy currency of the body. In spite of needing ATP for all energy-requiring tasks, the body stores very little ATP, and, therefore, depends on other chemical pathways to make ATP available when needed.

Energy Pathways

Figure 1.1 illustrates the three common pathways for ATP generation and shows which pathway contributes the greatest amount of ATP under various time constraints (1). Two of these pathways are anaerobic; one depends on the availability of oxygen, making it the only aerobic pathway. The first of the two anaerobic pathways involves creatine phosphate (CrP) catalyzed by an enzyme creatine kinase to produce one ATP in a single-step reaction. The advantage of CrP is that it is very fast. The disadvantage is the body's lim-

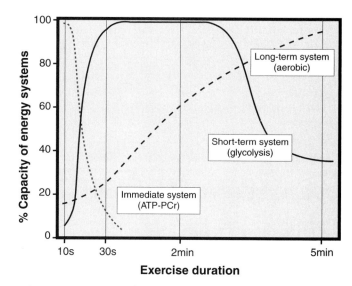

FIGURE 1.1. Energy pathways. (Modified from McArdle WD, Katch FI, Katch VL. Essentials of Exercise Physiology. 2nd Ed. Philadelphia: Lippincott Williams & Wilkins, 2000.)

ited capacity to store CrP. Most humans have enough CrP for about 6 to 10 seconds of all-out effort.

The second anaerobic pathway involves glucose or glycogen (or both)—hence its name, glycolysis. Although some energy is needed for breaking down glucose into pyruvate, the final energy yield is still two ATP. The body potentially can increase the rate of glycolysis 1,000-fold, thereby providing a substantial amount of ATP. Once again, however, protons—namely hydrogen (H^+)—generated during this process alter the cell's internal status so much that further ATP development eventually will be inhibited. Consequently, the pathway, when maximally stressed, is able to provide enough ATP for only 30 to 90 seconds of effort.

The aerobic pathway is by far the most complex of these pathways and requires the greatest time and substrate preparation. The real benefits come from its provision of the greatest amount of ATP (about 38 ATP via glucose and > 400 ATP via beta-oxidation of fat) and generation of the least obtrusive waste products (CO_2 and H_2O). Aerobic catabolism can use molecules from carbohydrate, fat, or protein, making it the most versatile pathway relative to energy substrate (Figure 1.2) (1).

As seen in Figure 1.2, nutrients also can be converted to energy in the body. This allows the body to replace important metabolic intermediates to allow each of these pathways to continue to produce ATP.

The biochemical use of oxygen takes place in the **mitochondria**, within the electron transport chain (ETC). Figure 1.3 illustrates how pyruvate from glycolysis moves into the mitochondria as acetyl CoA and is processed in Phase 1 (Krebs' cycle). Then, in Phase 2, the ETC moves protons and electrons to combine hydrogen and oxygen to form water while generating ATP. This process is called **oxidative phosphorylation**. It is interesting to note that oxygen is used in this pathway only as the final electron acceptor (1).

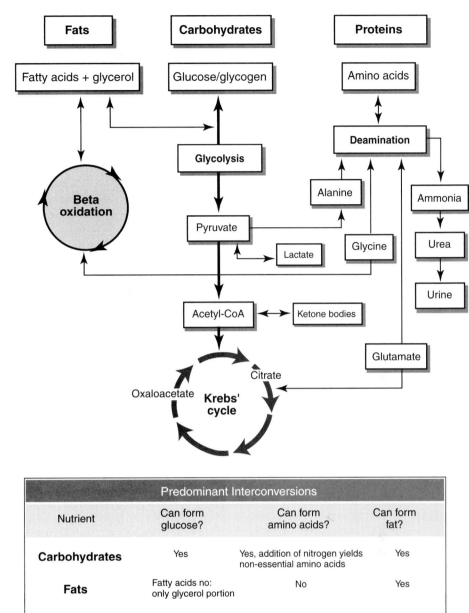

FIGURE 1.2. Metabolic mill. (Modified from McArdle WD, Katch FI, Katch VL. Essentials of Exercise Physiology. 2nd Ed. Philadelphia: Lippincott Williams & Wilkins, 2000.)

Predominant Interconversions			
Nutrient	Can form glucose?	Can form amino acids?	Can form fat?
Carbohydrates	Yes	Yes, addition of nitrogen yields non-essential amino acids	Yes
Fats	Fatty acids no: only glycerol portion	No	Yes
Proteins	Yes: glucogenic amino acids	Yes	Yes: ketogenic amino acids

Catabolism is the term used to describe the breaking down of energy-yielding substrates. When carbohydrate is broken down, it yields pyruvate (4), which can have two fates: (1) it can be converted to acetyl CoA as it is shuttled to the mitochondria for ATP production in the Krebs' cycle and ETC (see Figure 1.3), or (2) it can be reduced to **lactate** by adding 2 H$^+$ ions (see Figure 1.2). Lactate in itself does not pose a problem. In fact, the formation of lactate may actually enhance the body's ability to move usable energy substrates to other cells for ATP production. For example, resting skeletal muscle and the heart can use lactate readily as an energy source (5). However, when lactate accumulation exceeds the buffering capacity of the body, pH drops so much that the enzymes controlling glycolysis are inhibited.

When fats are broken down (**lipolysis**), they are modified via **beta-oxidation** to form acetyl CoA; then they follow the same steps shown in Figure 1.3 for carbohydrates (1). Because fats used for energy consist of a glycerol backbone and three very long carbon chains, a single fat molecule can supply an acetyl CoA molecule for the Krebs' cycle every time it cycles through beta-oxidation. It is this process that makes fat such a useful ATP producer. As long as oxygen intake is not a limiting factor, fat is the body's preferred choice of fuel for ATP production (5).

Proteins also can be catabolized; however, because the energy pathways for free fatty acids and glucose are more dominant, the liver will take up various amino acids and produce glucose or glycogen to be used by skeletal muscle, in a process called **gluconeogenesis** (2).

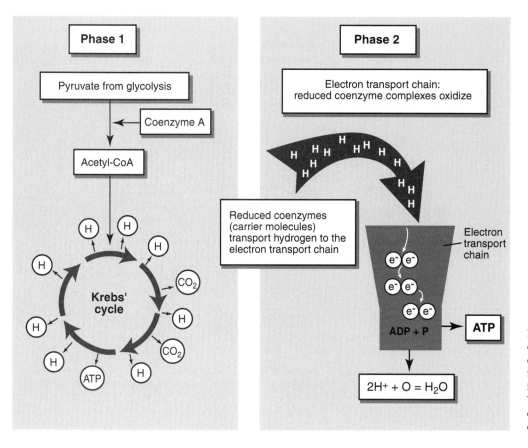

FIGURE 1.3. Pyruvate from glycolysis moves into the mitochondria as acetyl CoA and is processed in Phase 1 (Krebs' cycle). (Modified from McArdle WD, Katch FI, Katch VL. Essentials of Exercise Physiology. 2nd Ed. Philadelphia: Lippincott Williams & Wilkins, 2000.)

In essence, then, we have three energy pathways that generate ATP, with four potential energy substrates to catabolize as fuel. One pathway and substrate is CrP, offering immediate, high-intensity but short-lived energy production. A second is glycolysis, using glucose or glycogen, which makes it possible to exercise anaerobically for several minutes. This pathway usually is compromised by an increase in lactate and pH-lowering H^+ protons. In common terms, someone running an 800-meter race would slow down because the metabolic waste he or she was producing could not be removed fast enough to maintain high ATP generation from anaerobic glycolysis. Glycolysis and the ETC also can be used to exercise for extended periods—upward of several hours—before fatigue sets in due to a depletion of glycogen or glucose. A marathon runner may be reduced to a walking pace near the end of the race because all of his or her carbohydrate stores have been used up, thereby compromising aerobic glycolysis. Most of us have adequate amounts of stored fat to supply enough energy to exercise at a low intensity for several days, nonstop, provided fat is catabolized via beta-oxidation and subsequently used in oxidative phosphorylation.

Work, Power, and Calorimetry

It is important to measure the mechanical work or power required when we use energy for activity. Movement ex-

perts have developed several methods to measure work, power, and energy expenditure during movement (6). Commonly used ergometers (an ergometer is a device used to measure work) include treadmills, stationary bicycles, stair steppers, and rowing machines. To determine **work**, one needs to measure force and distance. When the amount of work is measured per unit of time, it is expressed as **power**.

A second measurement used to quantify activity is **calorimetry**. Because direct calorimetry, which measures actual heat dissipation, is difficult to manage, indirect measures are employed (4). The most common indirect method is measuring expired gases and determining the volume of oxygen ($\dot{V}O_2$) used and the volume of carbon dioxide ($\dot{V}CO_2$) being produced at the same time. Using the Haldane transformation, which assumes nitrogen is inert relative to gas exchange, one can determine volumes of O_2 and CO_2 per minute. This is particularly important because there appears to be a universal relationship between oxygen consumption and energy expenditure. For every liter of oxygen consumed, there is an expenditure of approximately 5 kcal, be they humans or elephants. Knowing how much oxygen was required for a particular task can then reveal a relative caloric expenditure for that same task.

A second element of interest to many scientists is the respiratory exchange ratio (RER) or respiratory quotient (RQ). The term RQ should be used only when calculations are based on cellular respiration alone without other potential influences on the ratio such as hyperventilation or non–steady state activity (2). The ratio $\dot{V}CO_2/\dot{V}O_2$ can be a means of estimating the proportions of fat and carbohydrate being catabolized for an activity. For example, if glucose were catabolized aerobically, it would require six O_2 molecules and it would produce six CO_2 molecules ($C_6H_{12}O_6 + 6\ O_2 \rightarrow 6CO_2 + 6\ H_2O$). This would yield a $\dot{V}CO_2/\dot{V}O_2$ ratio of 1.0. On the other hand, if fat (palmitic acid in this example) were catabolized aerobically, it would require 23 O_2 molecules while producing only 16 CO_2 molecules ($C_{16}H_{32}O_2 + 23\ O_2 \rightarrow 16\ CO_2 + 16\ H_2O$). This would yield a $\dot{V}CO_2$ ratio of 0.7. Assuming no protein is being used for ATP production, RER can be used to approximate how much energy is coming from fats and carbohydrates (1). Several conditions can alter this ratio, making it invalid. These conditions include activities that are too intense to achieve a steady-state condition, conditions that may cause hyperventilation, prolonged exercise, and measurements taken after strenuous exercise where $\dot{V}O_2$ is elevated above resting levels.

Economy and efficiency can be determined based on the measure of work and energy required to do the work. **Economy** is the energy cost of the work; **efficiency** is the relation of the mechanical energy produced to the metabolic energy used to produce the movement (4). The normal range in total body efficiency is 20 to 30%, meaning that we lose somewhere between 70 and 80% of our chemical energy in the conversion to mechanical work.

Systemic Responses to Exercise

Voluntary movements are initiated by the brain's ability to coordinate multiple systems to work together. Muscle fibers have distinct characteristics, both physical and biochemical.

Muscle Fibers and Recruitment

Although upward of six muscle fiber types currently have been identified, they can be generalized into three categories: slow-twitch or Type I oxidative fibers; intermediate or Type IIa fast-twitch oxidative-glycolytic fibers; and fast-twitch or Type IIb glycolytic fibers (1). They follow a size and recruitment pattern in which slow-twitch fibers are the smallest and the first recruited, followed by the intermediate fibers and, finally, the large Type IIb fibers (3). Each fiber type has its own advantages and disadvantages. Slow-twitch fibers do not produce much force, but are highly aerobic and, therefore, can sustain low levels of work for long periods of time. As the force requirement for the work increases, intermediate and fast-twitch fibers are recruited by the central nervous system. These fibers can generate higher force outputs, but they do so with a greater reliance on anaerobic pathways, resulting in earlier fatigue. One can readily predict which fibers will be required for certain tasks and how the metabolic pathways will

contribute to how long each task can be maintained. Clearly, a gymnast would benefit from powerful fast-twitch fibers whereas a marathoner would benefit most from lots of fatigue-resistant slow-twitch fibers.

Cardiorespiratory Capacity

Changes in ventilation and cardiac output are seen as exercise intensity progresses. The cardiorespiratory system must increase ventilation to allow for greater air exchange at the lungs, while the heart increases cardiac output to match the demands for greater blood flow to the working muscles (2). Sympathetic nervous system actions shunt blood away from internal organs and the skin to allow more blood to move to skeletal muscles. All of these actions are an effort to accommodate an increased need for ATP. During physical activity, ATP production must match ATP use, or fatigue will occur. Immediate or acute changes in skeletal muscle metabolism are dictated in part by the time demands for this energy. Time and intensity become the important factors in determining level of fitness or when fatigue will occur. Measuring maximal aerobic capacity is a common method of establishing aerobic fitness. Maximal oxygen consumption ($\dot{V}O_{2max}$) is the body's maximal rate of oxygen use during exercise. Values for $\dot{V}O_{2max}$ can be expressed in absolute terms (L/min) or relative to body mass (mL/kg/min), and they can range from less than 20 mL/kg/min in a person with a low level of fitness to more than 80 ml/kg/min in a well-trained athlete.

It is possible to chart the path of oxygen from the atmosphere to its use in the muscle. It is first necessary to consider how the respiratory system helps in this process. Before the circulatory system can deliver oxygen-rich blood to the muscle, blood must go to the lungs to receive oxygen from the inhaled air. Partial pressures of oxygen (PO_2) and carbon dioxide (PCO_2) dictate the rates of transfer in and out of the lungs and blood via diffusion. Next in importance is the oxygen-carrying capacity of the blood. Hemoglobin increases blood's oxygen-carrying capacity by a factor of 60 to 70, allowing about 200 ml of oxygen to be carried by 1 liter of blood. Figure 1.4 shows normal partial pressures and gradients for the lungs, arteries, tissue capillaries, and, finally, venous blood at rest (1). Individuals with no respiratory complications can easily load the arterial blood at a saturation level of 90% or more. This would suggest that the lungs, when operating normally, do not compromise cardiorespiratory function. That leaves the circulatory system and the skeletal muscles as the primary factors in determining exercise capacity.

A very important concept in determining aerobic fitness is the linear relationship between exercise intensity and oxygen consumption. Because of this strong relationship, exercise intensities below $\dot{V}O_{2max}$ can be expressed as a percentage of $\dot{V}O_{2max}$. Furthermore, a strong linear relationship exists between heart rate and $\dot{V}O_2$, allowing exercise inten-

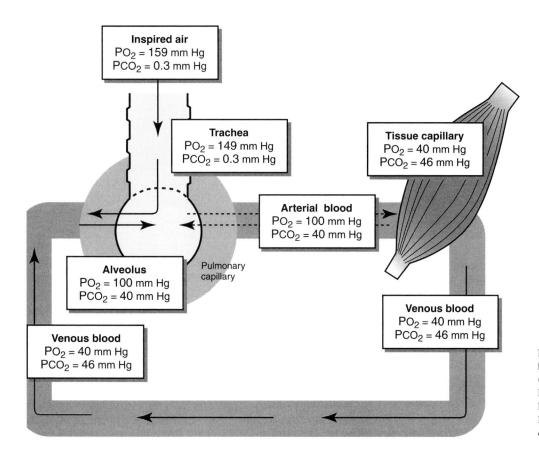

FIGURE 1.4. Pressure gradients for gas transfer in the body at rest. (Modified from McArdle WD, Katch FI, Katch VL. Essentials of Exercise Physiology. 2nd Ed. Philadelphia: Lippincott Williams & Wilkins, 2000.)

sity to be presented as a percentage of either $\dot{V}O_{2max}$ or maximal heart rate (HR_{max}). Two primary factors lead to the increase in oxygen consumption during increased exercise intensity (2) (Figure 1.5), muscle blood flow and the ability of the working tissue to extract and utilize the available oxygen. This extraction-utilization concept is set forth by the arterial-venous oxygen difference (a-vO_2 diff). Furthermore, cardiac output ($\dot{Q}$) is the most significant factor determining the circulatory system's capacity to deliver blood during exercise stress. Cardiac output is determined by quantifying heart rate and stroke volume. The Fick method often is used to calculate cardiac output using the following equation: $\dot{Q} = \dot{V}O_2 \; \beta \; a\text{-}vO_2$ diff (Figure 1.6). The average adult has a resting $\dot{Q}$ of about 5 L/min. During exercise, however, $\dot{Q}$ can increase to about 20 L/min in untrained adults and more than 35 L/min in aerobically trained athletes.

Peripheral Responses to Exercise

Delivering blood to the muscles is important; however, being able to extract and then utilize oxygen at the tissue level is equally important. Several conditions can alter how well oxygen dissociates from hemoglobin at the tissue level. The partial pressure of oxygen (PO_2) in the cell has an inverse relation to the cell's need for oxygen. When more oxy-

gen is needed by the cell, PO_2 in the cell drops, forcing hemoglobin to release more oxygen. The **Bohr effect**, as this is known, also can alter hemoglobin's binding affinity for oxygen (1). An increase in temperature or a decrease in pH increases oxygen dissociation. The decrease in pH can come from an increase in either H^+ or CO_2, both of which will cause an increase in acidity (i.e., a drop in pH). Figure 1.7 shows a normal oxyhemoglobin dissociation curve and how it can be influenced by pH or temperature.

Adaptations to Exercise Training

It is necessary for various systems to adapt under chronic conditions of exercise stress. Assuming no metabolic disorders or pulmonary complications, we must figure out how to alter the circulatory system or the muscle tissue to match the physiological demands of a given activity.

Aerobic Adaptations

From an aerobic perspective, there are two main goals for training (Figure 1.8) (1). To optimize physical activity one must be able to deliver oxygen to the muscle and then, once it is there, allow the working muscles to use it. This usually takes a long time and consistent effort. Figure 1.9 shows chronic cardiovascular adaptations to aerobic train-

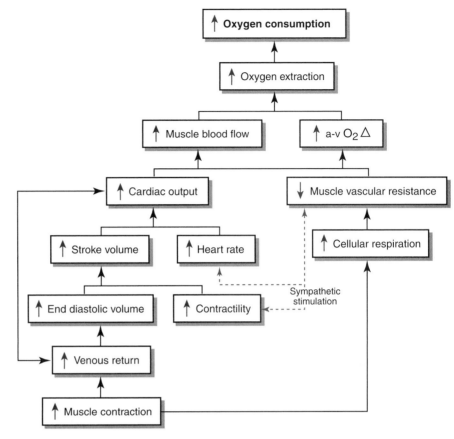

FIGURE 1.5. Exercise and cardiovascular influence on oxygen consumption. (Modified from Robergs RA, Roberts SO. Fundamental Principles of Exercise Physiology for Fitness, Performance, and Health. Boston: McGraw-Hill, 2000.)

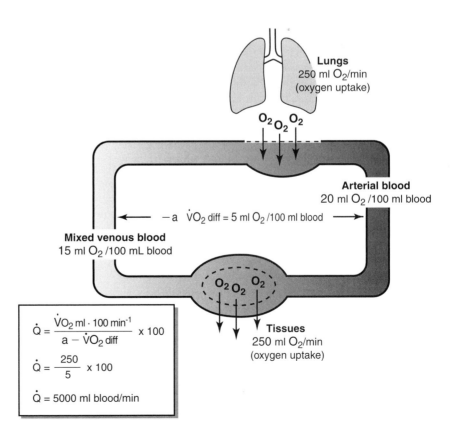

FIGURE 1.6. Fick principle and cardiac output. (Modified from McArdle WD, Katch FI, Katch VL. Essentials of Exercise Physiology. 2nd Ed. Philadelphia: Lippincott Williams & Wilkins, 2000.)

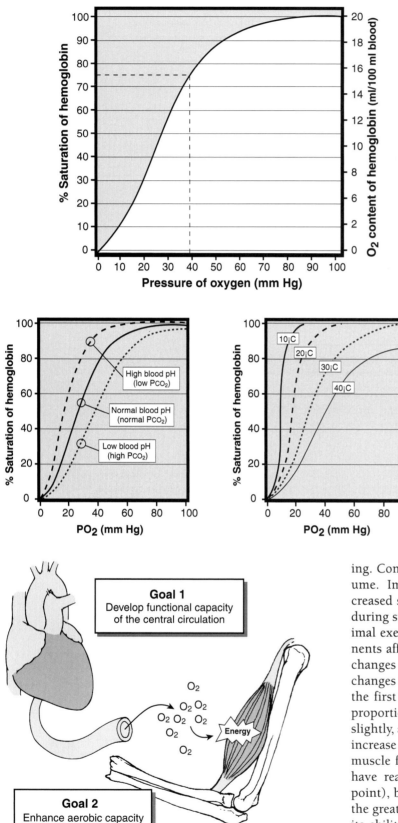

FIGURE 1.7.   Oxyhemoglobin dissociation curve and Bohr effect. (Modified from McArdle WD, Katch FI, Katch VL. Essentials of Exercise Physiology. 2nd Ed. Philadelphia: Lippincott Williams & Wilkins, 2000.)

Goal 1
Develop functional capacity of the central circulation

Goal 2
Enhance aerobic capacity of the specific muscles

FIGURE 1.8.   Goals of aerobic training. (Modified from McArdle WD, Katch FI, Katch VL. Essentials of Exercise Physiology. 2nd Ed. Philadelphia: Lippincott Williams & Wilkins, 2000.)

ing. Constituents of the blood increase, as does blood volume. Improvements in venous return resulting in increased stroke volume add to the efficiency of the system during submaximal steady-state activity as well as at maximal exercise. At the same time that these central components affecting delivery of blood are changing, peripheral changes also are taking place. Many of these peripheral changes take place with aerobic training (Figure 1.10). In the first 6 months of training, most of these changes are proportional in nature. Slow-twitch muscle fibers enlarge slightly, and $\dot{V}O_{2max}$, capillary density, and aerobic enzymes increase (1). At about 6 months with continued training, muscle fibers stop growing in size (perhaps because they have reached an optimal size for gas exchange at this point), but all other changes continue to improve. One of the greatest potential benefits of chronic aerobic activity is its ability to lower systemic blood pressure (2). This can have far-reaching implications for a prophylactic or rehabilitative prescription against hypertension. Benefits accrued via aerobic training are unfortunately lost in less time than is required to develop these benefits, suggesting

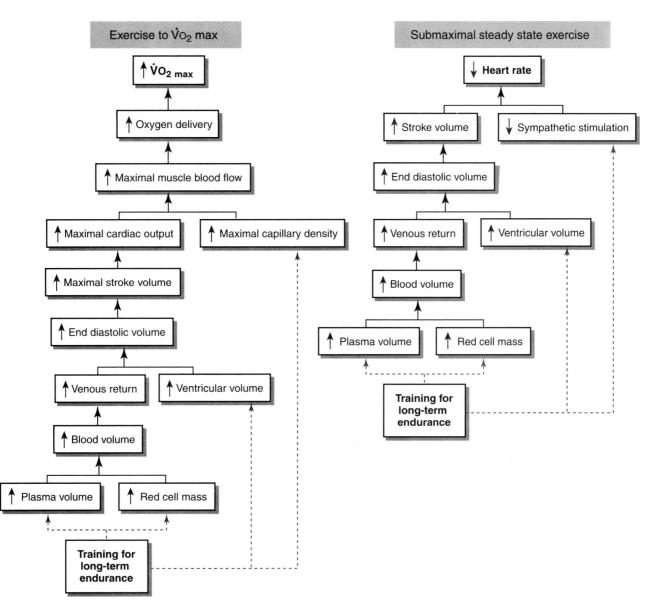

FIGURE 1.9.   Chronic cardiovascular adaptations with aerobic training.

that the common adage "use it or lose it" does have some merit relative to exercise endurance.

Skeletal Muscle Adaptations

Adaptations to resistive strength training in the cardiovascular domain are minimal in spite of having heart rates that parallel or exceed those during aerobic training (3). The requirement of having adequate strength to be able to complete aerobic training should not be discounted, however. Unfortunately, by the age of 80 years, most adults have lost about one half of their muscle mass and accompanying strength, making even standing from a seated position without the use of their arms or upper body very difficult

(3). This suggests that continued training is needed to maintain strength. Figure 1.11 outlines systemic changes with strength development. During the first several weeks of resistive strength training, gains in strength are almost exclusively neural in nature, meaning the body is learning to recruit the correct muscles in the proper sequence while inhibiting unnecessary muscle recruitment. The physiologic changes, such as an increase in contractile proteins, stored nutrients, and anaerobic enzymes, take several weeks to develop. Once the neurologic "learning" phase begins to diminish, remodeling of the muscle is beginning to take place and strength gains continue. After several years of concentrated strength training, a person will reach his or her physiologic limits, and it appears that no additional progress can be made unless it is done artificially.

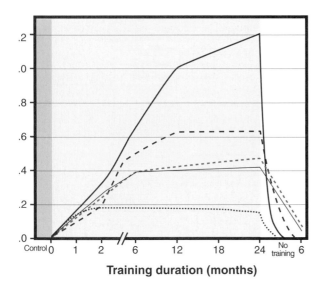

FIGURE 1.10. Peripheral adaptations of endurance training. (Modified from McArdle WD, Katch FI, Katch VL. Essentials of Exercise Physiology. 2nd Ed. Philadelphia: Lippincott Williams & Wilkins, 2000.)

General Training Principles.

Training elements consist of key factors that can affect the body in different ways, including mode, intensity, duration, and frequency of activity. Fitness training involves systematic progressions that apply the overload principle to purposeful short- and long-term goals (1). The **overload principle** states that for adaptations to occur, a threshold stress level must be exceeded. The key to quality training is providing just enough stress to elicit a positive change without using too much stress, which can cause a deterioration in fitness level. Too much training or training that is too intense can cause staleness, **overtraining**, or chronic fatigue (2). Overtraining is excessive frequency, volume, or intensity of training, resulting in fatigue.

Training also must be specific. Specific exercises produce specific adaptations, generating specific training effects. This phenomenon is known as the SAID principle—Specific Adaptation to Imposed Demands (1). One must also recognize individual differences, particularly initial levels of fitness. Once fitness levels, appropriate overloads, and specificity are understood, an optimal training program can be established for anyone.

Summary

Tolerating exercise stress is a complex task. During a 30-minute walk, the body must undergo several acute adaptations. Recruiting additional muscle fibers to match the demands of the work initiates feedback loops to match energy production to energy expenditure (4). Heart rate and stroke volume increase cardiac output. Nerves shunt blood selectively to working skeletal muscle. Ventilation begins to increase stimulated by an increase in carbon dioxide produced via oxidative phosphorylation. This increased ventilation ensures complete oxygen saturation of hemoglobin, for delivery of oxygen to muscle. Lactate produced by glycolysis in active muscle is shuttled to adjacent resting muscle fibers or the heart to be used as an energy source or to the liver for reconversion back to glucose (5). As the work continues, the body attempts to achieve a steady-state condition in which ATP production matches ATP demand. This steady-state condition can be expressed as a percentage of $\dot{V}O_{2max}$ or HR_{max}, because there is a linear relationship between work and oxygen consumption as well as oxygen consumption and heart rate. Most of this energy comes through aerobic pathways requiring an increase in oxygen consumption. With a known value of 5 kcal expended per liter of O_2, energy costs for various activities can be estimated.

With all physical activity, specificity is the key to chronic adaptations. Figure 1.12 shows how specific training can influence a variety of systems. It also is apparent from this figure that there are many interactions between systems that must be taken into account when assessing an individual's fitness level or planning a conditioning program (2). These elements have far-reaching capacities that can be tapped only with a sound understanding of acute and chronic changes with exercise.

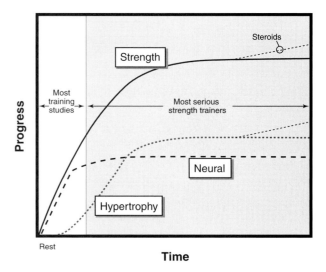

FIGURE 1.11. Progressive strength gains with resistive strength training. (Modified from McArdle WD, Katch FI, Katch VL. Essentials of Exercise Physiology. 2nd Ed. Philadelphia: Lippincott Williams & Wilkins, 2000.)

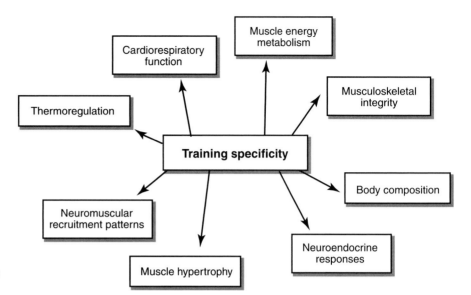

FIGURE 1.12.   Elements affected by specificity of training. (Modified from Robergs RA, Roberts SO. Fundamental Principles of Exercise Physiology for Fitness, Performance, and Health. Boston: McGraw-Hill, 2000.)

DISCUSSION QUESTIONS

 1 What are the predominant energy pathways for each of the following types of activities?
a. 3-mile walk
b. 10-km running race
c. 800-meter run
d. 100-meter sprint
e. Bench pressing 80% of maximal effort 4 to 6 times

2 How does the body attempt to achieve steady state equilibrium once exercise begins?

3 What is the biggest difference between work and power? How are they measured, and what utility does each have for determining energy expenditure and economy?

4 Describe the different types of muscle fibers found in humans and outline the process of selective muscle fiber recruitment.

5 What is $\dot{V}O_{2max}$ and how might it be useful?

6 Identify acute and chronic cardiovascular changes with aerobic activity. How might aerobic activity be used in the treatment of various diseases as well as the possible prevention of some diseases?

7 Distinguish between overload and overtraining.

REFERENCES

1. McArdle WD, Katch FI, Katch VL. Essentials of Exercise Physiology. 2nd Ed. Philadelphia: Lippincott Williams & Wilkins, 2000.
2. Robergs RA, Roberts SO. Fundamental Principles of Exercise Physiology for Fitness, Performance, and Health. Boston: McGraw-Hill, 2000.
3. Powers SK, Howley ET. Exercise Physiology: Theory and Application to Fitness and Performance. 4th Ed. Boston: McGraw-Hill, 2001.
4. Foss ML, Keteyian SJ. Fox's Physiological Basis for Exercise and Sport. 6th Ed. Boston: McGraw-Hill, 1998.
5. Brooks GA, Fahey TD, White TP, Baldwin KM. Exercise Physiology: Human Bioenergetics and Its Application. 3rd Ed. Mountain View, CA: Mayfield, 2000.
6. Kearney JT, Rundell KW, Wilber RL. Measurement of work and power in sport. In: Garrett WE, Kirkendall DT, eds. Exercise and Sport Science. Philadelphia: Lippincott Williams & Wilkins, 2000:31–52.

SUGGESTED READINGS

Hargraves M. Carbohydrate metabolism and exercise. In: Garrett WE, Kirkendall DT, eds. Exercise and Sport Science. Philadelphia: Lippincott Williams & Wilkins, 2000:1–8.
Jacobs KA, Paul DR, Sherman WM. Fat metabolism. In: Garrett WE, Kirkendall DT, eds. Exercise and Sport Science. Philadelphia: Lippincott Williams & Wilkins, 2000:9–18.
Lemon P. Protein metabolism during exercise. In: Garrett WE, Kirkendall DT, eds. Exercise and Sport Science. Philadelphia: Lippincott Williams & Wilkins, 2000:19–30.

CHAPTER 2

Epidemiology

Caroline A. Macera

Overview

In 2001, only two thirds (64.6%) of students nationwide had participated in activities that made them sweat and breathe hard for more than 20 minutes on 4 or more of the 7 days preceding that on which the survey question was asked (1). In 1998, only about 27% of adults performed sufficient physical activity to achieve health benefits (2). How do we know how much physical activity or exercise is needed for health benefits? Much of what has been learned about the way physical activity interacts with various physiologic parameters has come from carefully controlled clinical studies. However, what is known about the effect of physical activity and specific health conditions on a population basis was learned using a scientific strategy known as epidemiology. Broadly defined, epidemiology is a population-based approach to study of the causes of diseases and chronic conditions; *physical activity epidemiology* refers to the study of the relation between different types, frequencies, and intensities of physical activity and various health outcomes.

This chapter reviews some of the basic concepts of epidemiology, including study design and interpretation, and then examines several major studies that have provided a wealth of evidence regarding the effect of physical activity on the health of populations. The chapter concludes with a look at what still needs to be done and how epidemiologists will help shape the future of physical activity research.

Key Elements of Epidemiologic Research

The term *epidemiology* comes from the word *epidemic*, which is derived from the Greek *epi-* (following, or upon) plus *demos* (the people); then *logos* (study of) is added. Epidemiologic studies are characterized by large sample sizes that are representative of a defined population. Some of the basic concepts in population-based approaches have been used for centuries. For example, Ramazzini (1633–1714) was considered the father of occupational medicine because of his systematic study of diseases related to workplace exposure (3). In one study, using observational methods, he documented that nuns had higher rates of breast cancer than other women. It is now accepted that women who have not had children are at higher risk of breast cancer than women who have had children (4). In 1853 and 1854, Snow, a general practitioner in London, turned his observational skills, deductions, personal inquiries, and analytic studies to the problem of cholera. He used spot maps to identify the location of cases and public records to identify the sources of the water available via common pumps throughout the city. Using epidemiologic methodology, he was able to stop the transmission of cholera, a waterborne bacterial disease, by isolating the source of the exposure and removing the handle of the Broad Street water pump, where the people who had contracted cholera were obtaining their water (5). This work was done before the cholera bacterium was isolated; Snow was able to stop the transmission of the disease by interpretation of information achieved solely by observation.

Although much of the early work in epidemiology focused on infectious or acute illnesses, the science is now commonly used to study noninfectious or chronic diseases, such as coronary heart disease, cancer, and diabetes. Epidemiology has developed into a rich and complex science that has the potential to guide the development of interventions that prevent disease even before the exact mechanism is completely understood. For example, in 1753, long before vitamin C was identified or its relationship to scurvy understood, British sailors were protected from this disease by the provision of citrus fruits on long sea voyages (6).

The advances in technology that facilitate statistical analysis of large data sets have aided the growth of the field of epidemiology. Before computers and complex statistical software were available, analyses conducted to draw inferences about associations between health risks and outcomes were limited to calculations that could be done by hand (with calculators) or plotted by time and space.

Incidence and Prevalence

Understanding the time sequence of potential risk factors for a health outcome is a key factor in epidemiology. Two terms that distinguish the development of new cases of an **outcome** from existing cases are **incidence** and **prevalence**. These terms are used to sort out the number of new cases that develop during a period of time from existing cases. The terms *incidence rates* or *incident cases* refer to healthy people who developed the health outcome during a specific time period. *Prevalence rates* or *prevalent cases* (which includes new and existing cases) refer to all people who have the outcome during a given time period, regardless of how long they have been affected. For example, we can compute the prevalence of coronary heart disease in a population by identifying all people with evidence of coronary heart disease (including those who die) and dividing that number by the average population during that same period of time. However, to calculate an incidence rate, only new cases of coronary heart disease that developed during the time period under study would be counted in the numerator. The denominator would include all persons who did not have coronary heart disease at the start of the time period. For studies that assess the role of physical activity in reducing the risk of a particular disease, incidence data are necessary. That is, we need to know the number of people who do not have coronary heart disease to study how effective physical activity may be in preventing coronary heart disease. For surveillance and tracking purposes and for understanding the scope of the problem, however, prevalence data are useful.

Measures of Association

The most common measures of association used to quantify relationships found in epidemiology studies are the **relative risk (RR)** and the **odds ratio (OR)**. These terms refer to the strength (e.g., statistical significance) of the relationship between an **exposure** (e.g., physical activity) and an outcome (e.g., coronary heart disease). For the RR and OR, values of 1.0 signify no association; values less than 1.0 indicate an inverse (or protective) association; and values higher than 1.0 indicate a positive (or hazardous) association. To assess statistical significance, 95% confidence intervals are calculated; if the confidence interval includes 1.0 (e.g., a confidence interval that ranges from 0.8 to 1.3), then the finding is not statistically significant, because an RR of 1.0 indicates no association. Additional information on these measures of association can be found in the epidemiology or biostatistics texts listed under Suggested Readings.

Another useful statistic, **population attributable risk (PAR)**, provides an estimate of the impact on the general population of the elimination of a particular risk factor (or exposure). To calculate PAR, both the incidence of the outcome in the population and the prevalence of the risk factor are taken into consideration. For example, if the risk factor is physical inactivity, with a population prevalence of 58% and a relative risk for coronary heart disease of 1.9, the PAR is 35%—in other words, 35% of coronary heart disease deaths would not occur if everyone in the population became physically active (7). Population attributable risk is a theoretical concept, because the risk factor can never be totally eradicated. However, when the impacts of several potential risk factors are being compared, this measure can help identify which risk factor has a greater impact on the population, and may help guide prevention programs. The PAR is useful in public health because it makes it possible to compare the impact of reducing one risk factor with another. Because the PAR for physical inactivity is greater than that for the other coronary heart disease risk factors of smoking and hypertension, programs addressing physical inactivity would have a potentially greater impact than programs addressing smoking or hypertension, because the prevalence of these risk factors (about 25%) is lower than that of physical inactivity (about 58%). These measures of association and how they are calculated are shown in Box 2.1.

Study Designs

Although numerous study designs are used in epidemiology, they can be divided into two basic types: observational and experimental. Observational studies proceed by observing the natural experience of groups of people with similar characteristics, whereas in experimental studies, aspects of the natural living status or behaviors are changed in at least one of the groups. There are various designs that

can influence the interpretation of the results within both types of studies (Box 2.2).

Several types of studies have been used in building the knowledge base for the health effects of physical activity. Among those discussed here are **descriptive** studies, which include **cross-sectional** (or **prevalence**) studies, trend studies, and **ecological** studies. Studies that go beyond just describing the population and looking for cross-sectional associations also are discussed. These are the analytic studies, which include **prospective** (**cohort** or **incidence**) studies and **randomized clinical trials**. The ultimate choice of study design depends on the research question and available resources. A summary of these types of studies is found in Table 2.1. Further detail on study designs can be found in any of the epidemiology textbooks listed in the Suggested Readings section.

Descriptive studies such as **cross-sectional** or **prevalence studies** can provide basic rates (e.g., percentage of persons who are inactive) and may include a comparison of rates by subgroups (e.g., sex, education, income). In addition, these studies can be used to describe the change in rates over time (**trends**). These types of studies are useful for **surveillance** and as a starting point for **prospective** or **intervention** studies. The Surgeon General's Report on Physical Activity and Health (8) is one example of a publication that includes information obtained from all of these types of studies. These studies and others have established that the general level of physical activity among a representative sample of the population is low and has not changed over time (9). Although these studies are straightforward to conduct and analyze, they are not able to test hypotheses about the cause of the exposure/outcome relationship.

Descriptive information also can characterize the condition of a population without collecting data on individuals. Studies based on data obtained from the population level rather than the individual level are called **ecological** studies. In ecological studies, the numerator is the proportion of people in an area with a particular risk factor (e.g., smokers) and the denominator is the proportion of people in the

---

BOX 2.1. Rates and Measures of Association

Term	Description
Rate	The number of persons with the outcome (or exposure) of interest divided by the population
Ratio	A comparison of the magnitude of two rates
Relative risk (RR)	The ratio of the risk of disease in an exposed cohort over a defined time interval to the risk of disease in an unexposed cohort over the same time interval. Relative risk can be estimated from cohort studies and, for rare diseases, from case control studies. A value of 1.0 means no association.
Odds ratio (OR)	The ratio of the odds of exposure among those with the outcome divided by the odds of exposure among those without the outcome. A value of 1.0 means no association.
Population attributable risk (PAR)	A measure used to assess the public health impact of an exposure–outcome relationship that takes into account the prevalence of the exposure in the population. Usually expressed as a percentage.

BOX 2.2. Types of Studies

Observational Studies	Experimental Studies
Descriptive	Intervention
Prevalence	
Trends	Clinical or controlled trials
Ecological	Nonrandomized
Cross-sectional	Randomized
Analytic	
Prospective	
Cohort	
Case-control	

TABLE 2.1.   COMPARISON OF COMMON STUDY DESIGNS USED IN EPIDEMIOLOGY

Study Design	Measure of Association	Time Sequence for Risk Factor/Outcome	Causality
Population Level of Analysis			
Incidence studies	Rates of new cases in population at a given point in time	Time sequence known for risk factor or outcome but not both	No
Prevalence studies	Rates of existing cases in the population at a given point in time	No way to sort out time sequence	No
Trend studies	Rates over several time periods	No way to sort out time sequence	No
Ecological studies	Correlation coefficients (correlate rates of disease with average levels of exposure in an area)	No way to sort out time sequence	No
Individual Level of Analysis			
Cross-sectional	Prevalence estimates	Both measured at the same time	No
Prospective or cohort	Relative risk (or odds ratio)	Risk factor measured prior to outcome	Yes
Case control	Odds ratio	Outcome measured prior to risk factor	Sometimes
Randomized controlled trial	Relative risk	Risk factor measured prior to outcome	Yes

same area who have a particular disease (e.g., those with lung cancer). An example of an ecological study design applied to physical activity can be found in Yeager et al. (10), where linear regression models were used to compare the state-specific rates of coronary heart disease mortality to the state-specific prevalence of physical inactivity using. This study found a positive association between states with high mortality rates for coronary heart disease and states with a high prevalence of physical inactivity. Although ecological studies are efficient to conduct because they use existing data, a critical problem in interpretation is that it is not possible to determine if the individuals with low physical activity levels are the ones who are at risk of dying from coronary heart disease. Because of this problem, these studies generally are used to generate hypotheses that can be tested through other, more scientifically rigorous, methods.

Analytic observational studies are those that address a specific research question. For example, a **prospective** or **cohort study** identifies a group of individuals who are free of the outcome under study (e.g., coronary heart disease). At baseline they are assessed as to their physical activity status (e.g., active or inactive). At follow-up, the rates of new cases of coronary heart disease are compared between the groups and a measure of association, relative risk (the rate in the active group divided by the rate in the inactive group), is assessed. If the relative risk is less than 1.0 and statistically significant (i.e., the 95% confidence intervals are less than 1.0), then active people have a lower risk of developing coronary heart disease than inactive people. These studies are important for establishing the exposure and outcome time sequence.

In contrast, a **case-control** study starts by selecting individuals who have already developed the disease (e.g., breast cancer) and then identifies a comparable group of individuals who are free of disease. This study design answers the question of whether the people who have developed breast

cancer had different levels of physical activity before their diagnosis than a similar group of women (usually matched on age) without breast cancer. The measure of association for this type of study is the odds ratio (the odds of being active among those with breast cancer divided by the odds of being active among those without breast cancer), and it is interpreted in the same way as the relative risk. Because some outcomes are rare (i.e., cancer) and the **latency period** could be 20 years or more from exposure to diagnosis, it would not be effective to conduct a large cohort study with that outcome in mind. Even in large, ongoing cohort studies in which there are adequate numbers of cases, it is still more efficient to conduct a case-control study identifying both the cases and an age-matched sample of controls from the same cohort. This type of study is called a *nested case-control study* because it is "nested" within a prospective cohort study.

The strongest study design to establish a cause-and-effect relationship, a **randomized clinical trial**, also is the most difficult to conduct. In this approach, the study population is selected according to a set of criteria (e.g., subjects free of coronary heart disease and other chronic conditions and are able to exercise) and then randomly assigned to either the experimental (or intervention) group or the control group. An added difficulty for this type of study is ensuring that the participant complies with the study protocol. Because of the large amount of time and related expenses in carrying out these studies, there are very few randomized clinical trials on physical activity and health outcomes. However, there are some trials that focus on changes in intermediate markers that are associated with disease outcomes (e.g., blood pressure, cholesterol). Randomized clinical trials also have been used to assess adherence and other short-term changes associated with varying types and intensities of physical activity (12).

See Table 2.1 for an overview of the characteristics of each study design, including the appropriate measure of association derived from each and whether the study design is adequate to assess causality between the exposure and the outcomes measured.

Assessing Causality

As the science of epidemiology developed, it became clear that the criteria used to assess **causality** for infectious diseases would not be appropriate for chronic diseases because of the long latency period between exposure and disease outcome, and the likelihood of multiple interacting causes for any given chronic disease. Due to the nature of the disease process (i.e., chronic conditions that occur over a long period of time rather than acute illnesses characterized by infections), a different paradigm for assessing causality was developed. The criteria include strength of association (measured by statistically significant RR or OR), temporally correct association (exposure precedes outcome), dose-response (increased exposure reduces the rate of disease), consistency (same findings are replicated in different populations and geographic areas), and biological plausibility (there is a logical scientifically sound theory that could explain the effect of the exposure on the outcome). The first three criteria can be applied to a specific study, whereas the last two usually are applied to a collection of studies. For example, to assess whether there is support for a causal relationship between physical activity and coronary heart disease mortality, the criteria of causality could be applied in the following way:

- Several studies determined that physically active people had a statistically significant lower mortality rate than physically inactive people (strength of association).
- Physical activity status was assessed before the development of disease (temporally correct).
- Those with higher levels of physical activity had even lower levels of mortality (dose response).
- This relationship was found in different populations and in different geographical areas (consistency).
- A proposed mechanism for the relationship could be explained by either a cellular effect or by animal models (biological plausibility) (Box 2.3).

Measuring Physical Activity

One of the challenges facing physical activity epidemiologists is developing accurate measures of activity. A true measure of the intensity of any physical activity is relative to an individual's capacity. In a laboratory setting, a researcher can measure individual capacity and then determine the relative effort that each subject exerts for a particular activity and assign an appropriate intensity value to that activity. In epidemiology studies, however, the size of the study population usually precludes this type of mea-

BOX 2.3. Criteria for Causality	
Strength of association	Is the measure of association (e.g., relative risk) statistically significant?
Temporally correct	Does the exposure (cause) occur before the outcome (effect)?
Dose-response	Do higher levels of exposure result in increased outcome?
Consistency	Do studies in various populations and settings have similar results?
Biological plausibility	Is there a biological model or logical explanation for the proposed effect?

surement, so researchers must use other methods of assessing physical activity without knowing the subject's maximum capacity.

Objective Measurement

In field studies, physical activity can be measured using objective techniques such as heart rate monitors, accelerometers, and pedometers, with accompanying diaries or logs. Although these motion detectors have the advantage of verifying movement, none of these methods can assess the maximum physical capacity of the individual subject. Although research studies have found good validity and reliability for objective measures such as heart rate monitors and accelerometers (13, 14), there are practical drawbacks to using these measurement methods. The person has to wear a device and accurately record all activities. The burden of remembering to wear the device and to keep a log of activities corresponding to the time the device is being worn precludes widespread use of these devices in large population-based studies. The most common use for motion detectors in large epidemiologic studies is to validate self-report physical activity questionnaires using a subsample of the study population. Key characteristics of these methods and resources for further information can be found in Table 2.2.

Self-report Questionnaires

Questionnaires have been developed to assess participation in various types of sports or recreational activity, as well as everyday activities of living. Because of their flexibility in assessing physical activity from a number of perspectives, questionnaires have gained acceptance for use in a variety of settings, including face-to-face interviews, telephone administration, or self-administration, either on site or by mail. Most large epidemiologic studies rely on question-

TABLE 2.2.   CHARACTERISTICS OF VARIOUS TYPES OF PHYSICAL ACTIVITY ASSESSMENT TOOLS

Assessment tool	Reliability/Validity (reference)	Researcher/ Respondent Burden	Cost	Measurement Features
Heart rate monitors	15	Moderate	Moderate	Provides relative and absolute intensity but cannot assess type of activity; strong correlation with total energy expenditure, but training state and individual differences in heart rate can affect estimates.
Accelerometers	13	High	High	Provides frequency, intensity, duration (i.e., pattern) of activity but cannot assess type of activity; assesses total energy expenditure but can overestimate energy cost of walking and underestimate other activities.
Pedometers	16, 17	Low	Low	Provides only measures of steps, not energy expenditure or type of activity. Modest correlations of step counts with estimated energy expenditure or minutes of activity.
Questionnaires, records, or logs	18–21	Moderate	Low-moderate	Relies on self-report type, frequency, and duration; intensity estimated from type of activity or as reported by self-assessed subject.

naires to assess physical activity. It is true that questionnaire data are subject to self-report issues, but many physical activity questionnaires have been validated and found to provide fairly accurate estimates of physical activity or energy expenditure, especially for the purpose of separating active people from inactive people (20). A detailed collection of questionnaires used to measure physical activity, along with the related reliability and validity for each instrument, can be found in a supplemental issue of Medicine and Science in Sports and Exercise published in 1997 (18).

Because of the complex logistics of conducting studies on large population-based samples, most epidemiology studies of adult populations rely on questionnaires. When dealing with children, however, the reliability of self-report questionnaires is low, and other methods are more useful for assessing physical activity. For very young children, direct observation (i.e., the researcher watches the child and keeps detailed notes of what the child does) has been used, but this technique is very time-intensive, and the results often are not comparable between studies. Objective measurement using heart rate monitors, accelerometers, or pedometers are suggested as effective for measuring total energy expenditure in children and teenagers, and much work is ongoing in the area of physical activity measurement in children (22).

Fitness

Because physical activity is so difficult to measure, some studies use fitness, measured using a standard treadmill protocol, in place of physical activity (23, 24). One of the largest data sets with available treadmill data is from the Cooper Institute for Aerobics Research in Dallas, Texas. Many important studies have been published based on these data, which have been collected since the early 1970s. Fitness status (measured by treadmill time duration) and change in fitness status have been shown to be associated with all-cause mortality and a number of other outcomes, including coronary heart disease (24).

The Literature on Physical Activity on Health

The very earliest medical literature includes recommendations regarding the importance of physical activity or exercise. However, in the early part of the 20th century, the most attention was given to the threat of infectious diseases that quickly killed otherwise healthy individuals and were the leading cause of death. As infectious diseases began to be controlled with the use of antibiotics, attention shifted to the study of chronic diseases, particularly heart disease as it became the leading cause of death.

Occupational Studies

The earliest studies of physical activity and health were conducted by observing workers in occupations that required varying levels and intensity of movement. In 1953, Morris and coworkers published a landmark article that used observational epidemiology methods to identify the differential coronary heart disease experiences of the drivers and ticket takers on London buses (25). The drivers sat all day, whereas the ticket takers climbed up and down the double-decker buses collecting fares, suggesting that physical activity was associated with health. Other studies followed in which occupation was used to classify level of physical activity (26, 27). Although these studies demonstrated an association between physical activity and lower risk of coronary heart disease they were criticized because of what is known as the "healthy worker" effect, which postulates that workers are healthier in general than nonworkers and those who work at jobs requiring heavy labor may be in better health than those who work at less physically demanding jobs.

These occupational studies would be hard to replicate today, because the physical activity required in most jobs do not require high physical demands. Because of these studies, however, and related work in exercise science, it became clear that physical activity was associated with health benefits, particularly cardiorespiratory fitness. Coronary heart disease, the leading cause of death, was increasing, and attention shifted to the study of leisure time physical activity because most jobs did not require sustained physical activity.

Population Studies

Because of the known effects of activity on overall health, particularly cardiorespiratory fitness, several large population studies on heart disease incorporated measures of physical activity or fitness into their data collection schemes. In 1987, a summary of the published studies on physical activity and coronary heart disease concluded that physical inactivity was a risk factor for coronary heart disease (28). (Of the 43 studies reviewed, only five studies analyzed and presented the data on women separately.) A couple of years after this summary, a meta-analysis reinforced the findings that the relative risk of coronary heart disease among less active adults compared to their active peers was 1.9 and that studies with better measures of physical activity found a stronger effect (29). These studies demonstrated that the relative risk of coronary heart disease due to physical inactivity was similar in magnitude to that of hypertension, high serum cholesterol, and smoking. During this time there was very little published consensus on the role of physical activity in children, or among older adults.

Importance of Moderate Intensity Physical Activity

The recognition of physical activity as one of the major risk factors for heart disease by many federal and public organizations led the way for additional research funding to more

fully understand the role of physical activity in preventing coronary heart disease and extending life (8, 30). The research took two main tracks: the exercise science studies continued to identify short-term effects, whereas population-based studies continued to follow cohorts, tracking physical activity patterns throughout the lifespan, to identify long-term heath effects. Some of the initial key studies done during this period began to answer some of the questions regarding intensity issues.

Meanwhile, the scientific community began to look at ways to measure the intensity of an activity. A system was devised to measure metabolic equivalents (**METs**), in which 1 MET is equal to the activity metabolic rate divided by the resting metabolic rate. By the early 1990s it was clear that vigorous physical activity (> 6 METS, or 6 times the resting metabolic rate) was conclusively associated with longevity, particularly because of its effect on the cardiorespiratory system and coronary heart disease. However, in 1995, a joint statement by the Centers for Disease Control and Prevention and the American College of Sports Medicine highlighted the health benefits of physical activity that was at least moderate in intensity (approximately 3–6 METS or equivalent to brisk walking for most people [30]). This recommendation was based on the observation that many epidemiologic studies found increased health benefits as subjects began to increase their physical activity levels from the most sedentary category to the next level. Documented improvements in overall morbidity and mortality as well as coronary heart disease morbidity and mortality occurred at even low levels of exercise intensity or total energy expenditure. A higher volume or intensity of activity produced greater improvements, but the improvements seen at lower intensity levels changed the way scientists began thinking of the relation between physical activity and health.

Although many excellent studies of physical activity and physical fitness and health benefits have been performed, only a few studies on all-cause mortality and stroke among men are highlighted in Table 2.3. These studies found that physical activity was associated with lower all-cause mortality (31–33) and strokes (34–37). However, the amount and intensity issues were still in question. In studies of Harvard alumni, it appeared that total activity was related to reduced mortality, but that vigorous activity was the most important component. However, in the British Regional Heart Study, even regular walking or gardening was associated with lower risk of all-cause mortality among men who had established coronary heart disease. The results were similar for stroke, except that the intensity of the activity was not as important; most studies found an effect from moderate levels of physical activity (34–36). In the Physicians' Health Study, only vigorous activity was measured; it was found to reduce stroke risk (37). A careful review of the measurement definitions used in these studies may explain the differences. For example, the way total energy expenditure is classified and used in the analysis varies between these and

TABLE 2.3.   SELECTED EPIDEMIOLOGIC STUDIES OF PHYSICAL ACTIVITY AND HEALTH IN MEN

Authors	Population	Physical Activity Measure	Outcome	Major Findings
All-cause Mortality				
Lee et al., 1995 (31)	17,321 men (mean age 46) followed to 1988; Harvard Alumni Study	Total energy expenditure from vigorous and from nonvigorous physical activity	All-cause mortality (n = 3728)	Inverse relationship between total physical activity and mortality; vigorous but not nonvigorous activities associated with longevity
Lee and Paffenbarger, 2000 (32)	13,485 men (mean age 57.5) followed to 1992; Harvard Alumni Study	1. Distance walked/ stories climbed 2. Light, moderate, vigorous activities	All-cause mortality (n = 2539)	1. Distance walked and stories climbed independently predicted longevity 2. Moderate or vigorous, but not light, activity predicted longevity
Wannamethee et al., 2000 (33)	772 men with established coronary heart disease; British Regional Heart Study	6 categories based on energy expenditure of activities: inactive; occasional; light; moderate; moderately vigorous; vigorous	All-cause mortality (n = 131)	Light or moderate activity in men with established coronary heart disease was associated with lower risk of all-cause mortality. Regular walking and moderate or heavy gardening were sufficient to achieve this benefit.
Stroke				
Wannamethee and Shaper, 1992 (34)	7735 men aged 40–59 followed for 9.5 years; British Regional Heart Study	6 categories based on energy expenditure of activities: inactive; occasional; light; moderate; moderately vigorous; vigorous	Fatal and nonfatal strokes (n = 128) Heart attacks (n = 612)	Moderate physical activity significantly reduced the risk of stroke and heart attack in men both with and without pre-existing ischemic heart disease. Vigorous activity did not confer any further protection.
Wannamethee et al., 1998 (35)	7142 men aged 40–59 followed for up to 15 years; British Regional Heart Study	6 categories based on energy expenditure of activities: inactive; occasional; light; moderate; moderately vigorous; vigorous	Fatal and nonfatal coronary heart disease, stroke, and diabetes (n = 1766)	Compared to inactive men, those who do any physical activity have a longer disease-free survival
Lee and Paffenbarger, 1998 (36)	11,130 healthy Harvard alumni (mean age 58) followed to 1977-88	Kilocalories/wk of energy expenditure	Incidence of strokes (n = 378)	Physical activity was associated with a decreased risk of stroke; moderate and vigorous intensity, but not light activities, was related to decreased risk of stroke
Lee et al., 1999 (37)	21,823 men aged 40–84 without cancer, stroke, or CHD at baseline; Physicians Health Study	Exercise vigorous enough to work up a sweat (times/wk).	Stroke occurrence (n = 533)	Vigorous physical activity reduces the risk of developing stroke; however, the effect was mediated through beneficial effects on body weight, blood pressure, serum cholesterol, and glucose tolerance.

other studies of physical activity and health. In spite of these differences, there appears to be a strong and consistent relationship between physical activity and all-cause mortality.

Evolving Focus on Special Populations: Women, Children, Elderly

Another major change in the 1990s was the call for research among "special populations," that is, those groups who had not been the focus of research when the major health benefit of physical activity was thought to be coronary heart disease. As it became clear that the rate of heart disease was as high in women as in men, and when the multiple benefits of physical activity became widely known, research studies multiplied and a more diverse population was in-

cluded. This change highlighted some measurement issues that are particularly relevant for women, minority populations, and older populations (38).

There are now many large population studies of women. A few of these, which focus on coronary heart disease, all-cause mortality, and breast cancer, are summarized in Table 2.4. Many of the same associations between physical activity and coronary heart disease and all-cause mortality first found for men have also been found to be true for women. There are notable exceptions with regard to intensity, however. For women, the reduced risk of coronary heart disease and all-cause mortality associated with physical activity was achieved with moderate intensity activities; vigorous intensity activities did not provide additional benefit (39–41). There also is emerging evidence that physical activity may confer protection from breast cancer, at least among older women with stable weight (11, 43).

TABLE 2.3. SELECTED EPIDEMIOLOGIC STUDIES OF PHYSICAL ACTIVITY AND HEALTH IN WOMEN

Authors	Population	Physical Activity Measure	Outcome	Major Findings
Coronary Heart Disease Or All-Cause Mortality				
Manson et al., 1999 (39)	72,488 women aged 30–55 residing in 11 large U.S. states; Nurses' Health Study	MET hours/wk for total physical activity, for walking and for vigorous exercise	Incidence of coronary events, fatal or nonfatal (n = 645)	Sedentary women who became active later in life had a lower risk of coronary events than those who remained sedentary. Brisk walking and vigorous exercise had similar effects.
Lee et al., 2001 (40)	39,372 women, age ≥45 (1992–95) followed to 1999; Women's Health Study	Energy expenditure from all activity, vigorous activity, and walking	Coronary heart disease (n = 244) incident events)	Even light-to-moderate activity was associated with lower CHD rates; at least 1 hour of walking, regardless of pace, was associated with reduced risk of CHD.
Rockhill et al., 2001 (41)	80,348 women (aged 30–55 in 1976), follow-up in 1996; Nurses' Health Study	1. Number of hours/wk of physical activity 2. Number of hours/wk of walking	All-cause mortality and cardiovas-cular (n = 923); cancer (n = 2727); respiratory (n = 181); other (n = 1040)	1. Inverse relationship between hours/wk of physical activity and all-cause deaths and specific causes, except cancer. 2. Inverse relationship between hours/wk walked and all-cause mortality, even the lowest group, 1–2.9 hours/wk.
Kushi et al., 1997 (42)	40,417 Iowan post-menopausal women aged 55–69 in 1986	1. Regular physical activity to keep fit 2. Time spent in moderate or vigorous physical activity	All-cause mortality	1. Inverse relationship between physical activity and all-cause mortality; RR = 0.77 (0.66–0.90) 2. RR = 0.59 (0.51–0.67) for moderate and RR = 0.62 (0.42-0.90) for vigorous
Breast Cancer				
Rockhill et al., 1999 (43)	Women aged 30–55 in 1976 followed for 16 years; Nurses' Health Study	Number of hours/wk in moderate or vigorous activity	Invasive breast cancer (n = 3137)	RR = 0.82 (0.70–0.97) for women who reported moderate or vigorous activity ≥ 7 hours/wk compared to < 1 hour/wk
Carpenter et al., 1999 (11)	Postmenopausal women aged 55–64 in Los Angeles County, 1987–1989	Average MET hours/wk for four time periods to assess lifetime physical activity	Breast cancer (n = 1123) Controls (n = 904) Case-control study	Lifetime consistent exercise, exercise ≥ 4 hours/wk for at least 12 years, or strenuous exercise in past 10 years reduced breast cancer risk among women with stable weight.

Another change in the focus of research studies was the increasing awareness of the role of physical activity in maintaining functional status among older adults (44). With the population in the United States living longer than ever before, it became apparent that strength and flexibility, in addition to moderate intensity activity, were important components of a physically active lifestyle. This realization led to an American College of Sports Medicine (ACSM) position statement in 1998 that stressed the role of aerobic activity but also encouraged the addition of weight or resistance training to increase or maintain muscle mass (45). This recommendation is important for men as well as women, but women have the disadvantage of starting out with less muscle mass than men and also, on average, live several years longer than men.

There are still many unanswered questions regarding the benefits of physical activity for children and adolescents, in spite of a 1994 consensus conference called to assess the amount and type of physical activity required for a healthy lifestyle (46). This conference concluded that due to lack of other information, the recommendations that apply to adults (moderate intensity physical activity for 30 or more minutes most days of the week and vigorous intensity physical activity for 20 or more minutes at least 3 days per week) should be appropriate for adolescents. However, the 2000 Dietary Guidelines published by the U.S. Department of Agriculture and U.S. Department of Health and Human Services propose 60 minutes of physical activity daily for children and adolescents (47). The bottom line is that physical activity is recognized as an important component of health for children as well as adults. Appropriate physical activity actually may be even more important for children, because it may help to offset obesity and related chronic conditions (e.g., diabetes and heart disease) that are starting to appear at younger ages.

What Lies Ahead?

Epidemiology as a science is evolving constantly to answer new questions and to further understand the etiology of disease. The challenges associated with determining the optimal type of activity and the dose required for health benefits will continue to be studied. Advances in computer hardware and software will permit routine use of complex modeling and analyses that will allow interpretation of multiple interacting factors into the physical activity and health relationship. Mapping programs will provide enriched opportunities to view physical activity patterns in the context of neighborhood environment and other social conditions (e.g., crime rate, access to facilities).

Three areas in physical activity epidemiology that will be particularly prominent in the near future: research into identifying how environment structure interacts with personal activity behavior; using new technology to enhance the measurement of physical activity; and understanding the complex connection between physical activity and weight control.

Environmental Structures

Among the emerging research areas are ways to use the methods of epidemiology to study how environmental structure and policies that support active lifestyles influence physical activity. Although the decision to be active is an individual choice, this behavior is influenced by many factors outside of an individual's control. Furthermore, just knowing that physical activity has important health benefits is not enough to change individual behavior. Future studies may assess neighborhood structure as an important element to support a physically active lifestyle. Examples of environmental structures that promote physical activity are activity-friendly and safe green spaces, availability of walking and jogging trails, and bike paths that lead to commercial areas, schools, and recreational facilities. This type of structural change could support increased physical activity for the whole family, and such changes in the environment are likely to have more effect on overall physical activity patterns than those targeted to changing individual behavior.

The physical environment is only one aspect. Most adults spend much of the day away from home. Worksites that provide opportunities for employees to be active during the day (either through on-site facilities or supportive policies) may provide an important strategy for increasing physical activity among adults (48). Within the medical setting, counseling individuals about the importance of physical activity and providing specific guidelines can be extremely important in encouraging sedentary people to at least begin thinking about ways to become more active (49). For children, schools offer an excellent opportunity to become active and to learn skills that last a lifetime. However, most schools are reducing physical education programs in favor of academic subjects. In addition, school facilities often are not available to the community during nonschool hours. Worksites, medical settings, and schools offer important venues for encouraging physical activity, but research on their overall impact is lacking.

Measurement Techniques

Another major field of research that may enrich epidemiologic studies is the emerging area of measurement. With the technological advances that are expected to materialize in the next several years, questionnaire assessment of physical activity in large-scale epidemiologic studies may be replaced or supplemented by innovative strategies (e.g., electronic mechanisms that send data directly to researchers' labs for analysis). Using anticipated technological changes to improve measurement and reduce recall problems, studies will be able to sort out the key elements of physical activity and determine whether it is total energy expenditure or the intensity of the activity that is the most important parameter for specific diseases and conditions. Advances in measurement will enable epidemiologists to conduct large studies of health outcomes with much more accurate measures of energy expenditure than have been possible in the past.

Impact of the Obesity Epidemic

Participation in physical activity is low and has not changed much in the last decade (9), whereas obesity rates (generally defined for adults as BMI $\geq$ 30 kg/m^2) increased substantially in the United States between 1991 and 1998 (50). With the onset of an "obesity epidemic" in the United States, new attention has been given to physical activity as part of an overall weight management strategy. In 2000, for the first time, physical activity was included as a separate entry in the dietary guidelines published by the U.S. Department of Agriculture (47). This added interest has generated a variety of studies designed to sort out the role of energy expenditure in conjunction with maintaining a healthy diet as a strategy to control body weight. These studies are identifying a major lack of understanding of the nature of obesity and may find that the answer is more complicated than a simple relation between energy intake and energy expenditure. Although an individual's metabolic rate is a critical factor in weight control, it may be altered by lifestyle choices (e.g., smoking, physical activity). The answers to curbing this epidemic, therefore, may well lie in applying epidemiologic methods to the problem. For example, prospective studies that can identify characteristics of normal-weight individuals who become overweight or obese in terms of diet, geographic location, occupation, physical activity, or past history of physical activity may lead the way for successful interventions that prevent weight gain as people age.

Summary

This chapter discusses some of the methods used in epidemiology and illustrates how epidemiology has played a major role in documenting the health effects of various types and intensities of physical activity among diverse populations. Although much work remains to be done, there is sufficient information to support the design of programs and infrastructures to assist the most sedentary component of the population to become more active.

REFERENCES

1. MMWR Surveillance Summaries. Youth Risk Behavior Surveillance — United States, 2001. MMWR Morb Mortal Wkly Rep 2002;51(SS04);1–64.
2. Macera CA, Pratt M. Public health surveillance of physical activity. Res Quart Exerc Sport 2000;71:S97–S103.
3. Raffle PAB, Lee WR, McCallum RI, Murray R, eds. Hunter's Diseases of Occupations. London: Edward Arnold, 1991.
4. Shottenfeld D, Fraumeni JF. Cancer Epidemiology and Prevention. Philadelphia: WB Saunders, 1982.
5. Hennekens CH, Buring JF. Epidemiology in Medicine. Boston: Little, Brown and Company, 1987.
6. Timmreck TC. An Introduction to Epidemiology. 3rd Ed. Sudbury, MA: Jones and Bartlett Publishers, 2002.
7. CDC. Physical activity and the prevention of coronary heart disease. MMWR Morb Mortal Wkly Rep 1993;42:669–672.
8. U.S. Department of Health and Human Services. Physical Activity and Health: A Report of the Surgeon General. Atlanta: Centers for Disease Control and Prevention, 1996.
9. CDC. Physical activity trends—United States, 1990–1998. Morb Mortal Wkly Rep 2001;50:166–169.
10. Yeager KK, Anda RF, Macera CA, et al. Sedentary lifestyle and state variation in coronary heart disease mortality. Public Health Reports 1995;110:100–102.
11. Carpenter CL, Ross RK, Paganini-Hill A, Bernstein L. Lifetime exercise activity and breast cancer risk among post-menopausal women. Br J Cancer 1999;80:1852–1858.
12. Dunn AL, Marcus BH, Kampert JB, et al. Comparison of lifestyle and structured interventions to increase physical activity and cardiorespiratory fitness: a randomized trial. JAMA 1999;281:327–334.
13. Bassett DR, Ainsworth BE, Swartz AM, et al. Validity of four motion sensors in measuring moderate intensity physical activity. Med Sci Sports Exerc 2000;32:S471–S480.
14. Ainsworth BE, Bassett DR, Strath SJ, et al. Comparison of three methods for measuring time spent in physical activity. Med Sci Sports Exerc 2000;32:S457–S464.
15. Strath SJ, Swartz AM, Bassett DR, et al. Evaluation of heart rate as a method for assessing moderate intensity physical activity. Med Sci Sports Exerc 2000;32:S465–S470.
16. Bassett DR, Cureton AL, Ainsworth BE. Measurement of daily walking distance: questionnaire versus pedometer. Med Sci Sports Exerc 1999;32:1018–1023.
17. Welk GJ, Differding JA, Thompson RW, et al. The utility of the Digi-Walker step counter to assess daily physical activity patterns. Med Sci Sports Exerc 2000;32:S481–488.
18. Pereira MA, FitzGerald SJ, Gregg EW, et al. A collection of physical activity questionnaires for health-related research. Med Sci Sports Exerc 1997;29:S3–S205.
19. Ainsworth BE, Haskell WH, Whitt MC, et al. Compendium of physical activities: an update of activity codes and MET intensities. Med Sci Sports Exerc 2000;32:S498–S516.
20. Jacobs DR, Ainsworth BE, Hartman TJ, Leon AS. A simultaneous evaluation of ten commonly used physical activity questionnaires. Med Sci Sports Exerc 1993;25:81–91.
21. Brownson RC, Eyler AA, King AC, et al. Reliability of information on physical activity and other chronic disease risk factors among U.S. women aged 40 years or older. Am J Epidemiol 1999;149:379–391.
22. Trost SG. Objective measurement of physical activity in youth: current issues, future directions. Exerc Sports Sci Rev 2001;29:32–36.
23. Sandvik L, Erikssen J, Thaulow E, et al. Physical fitness as a predictor of mortality among healthy, middle-aged Norwegian men. N Engl J Med 1993;328:533–537.
24. Blair SN, Kohl HW, Barlow CE, et al. Changes in physical fitness and all-cause mortality. JAMA 1995;273:1093–1098.
25. Morris JN, Heady JA, Raffle PAB, et al. Coronary heart disease and physical activity of work. Lancet 1953;2:1053–1057, 1111–1120.
26. Paffenbarger RS, Laughlin ME, Gima AS, Black RA. Work activity of longshoremen as related to death from coronary heart disease and stroke. N Engl J Med 1970;282:1109–1114.
27. Paffenbarger RS, Hale WE. Work activity and coronary heart mortality. N Engl J Med 1975;292:545–550.
28. Powell KE, Thompson PD, Caspersen CJ, Kendrick JS. Physical activity and the incidence of coronary heart disease. Annu Rev Public Health 1987;8:253–287.
29. Berlin JA, Colditz GA. A meta-analysis of physical activity in the prevention of coronary heart disease. Am J Epidemiol 1990;132:612–628.
30. Pate RR, Pratt M, Blair SN, et al. Physical activity and public health: a recommendation from the Centers for Disease Control and Prevention and the American College of Sports Medicine. JAMA 1995;273:402–407.
31. Lee I-M, Hsieh C-C, Paffenbarger RS Jr. Exercise intensity and longevity in men: The Harvard Alumni Health Study. JAMA 1995;273:1179–1184.
32. Lee I-M, Paffenbarger RS. Associations of light, moderate, and vigorous intensity physical activity with longevity. Am J Epidemiol 2000;151:293–299.
33. Wannamethee SG, Shaper AG, Walker M. Physical activity and mortality in older men with diagnosed coronary heart disease. Circulation 2000;102:1358–1363.
34. Wannamethee G, Shaper AG. Physical activity and stroke in British middle aged men. Br Med J 1992;304:597–601.
35. Wannamethee SG, Shaper AG, Walker M, Ebrahim S. Lifestyle and 15-year survival free of heart attack, stroke, and diabetes in middle-aged British men. Arch Intern Med 1998;158:2433–2440.
36. Lee I-M, Paffenbarger RS. Physical activity and stroke incidence: The Harvard Alumni Health Study. Stroke 1998;29:2049–2054.
37. Lee I-M, Hennekens CH, Berger K, et al. Exercise and risk of stroke in male physicians. Stroke 1999;30:1–6.
38. Ainsworth BE, Irwin ML, Addy CL, et al. Moderate physical activity patterns of minority women: the Cross-Cultural Activity Participation Study. J Women Health Gender-Based Med 1999;8:805–813.
39. Manson JE, Hu FB, Rich-Edwards JW, et al. A prospective study of walking as compared with vigorous exercise in the prevention of coronary heart disease in women. N Engl J Med 1999;341:650–658.
40. Lee I-M, Rexrode KM, Cook NR, et al. Physical activity and coronary heart disease in women. JAMA 2001;285:1447–1454.
41. Rockhill B, Willett WC, Manson JE, et al. Physical activity and mortality: a prospective study among women. Am J Public Health 2001;91:578–583.
42. Kushi LH, Fee RM, Folsom AR, et al. Physical activity and mortality in postmenopausal women. JAMA 1997;277:1287–1292.
43. Rockhill B, Willett WC, Hunter DJ, Manson JE, Hankinson SE, Colditz GA. A prospective study of recreational physical activity and breast cancer risk. Arch Intern Med 1999;159:2290–2296.
44. Huang Y, Macera CA, Blair SN, Brill PA, Kohl HW, Kronenfeld JJ. Physical fitness, physical activity, and functional limitation in adults aged 40 and older. Med Sci Sports Exerc 1998;30:1430–1435.
45. Pollock ML, Gaesser GA, Butcher JD, et al. The recommended quantity and quality of exercise for developing and maintaining cardiorespiratory and muscular fitness and flexibility in healthy adults. Med Sci Sports Exerc 1998;30:975–991.

46. Sallas JF, Patrick K. Physical activity guidelines for adolescents: consensus statement. Ped Exerc Sci 1994;6:302–314.

47. U.S. Department of Agriculture and U.S. Department of Health and Human Services. Nutrition and Your Health: Dietary Guidelines for Americans. Home and Garden Bulletin No. 232, 5th Ed. Government Printing Office, Washington, D.C., 2000.

48. Cole G, Leonard B, Hammond S, Fridinger F. Using "stages of behavioral change" constructs to measure the short-term effects of a work-site-based intervention to increase moderate physical activity. Psychol Rep 1998;82:615–618.

49. Mullen PD, Evans D, Forster J, et al. Settings as an important dimension in health education/promotion policy, programs, and research. Health Educ Quart 1995;22:329–345.

50. Mokdad AH, Serdula MK, Dietz WH, Bowman BA, Marks JS, Koplan JP. The spread of the obesity epidemic in the United States, 1991–1998. JAMA 1999;282:1519–1522.

SUGGESTED READINGS

Gail MH, Benichou J, eds. Encyclopedia of Epidemiologic Methods. New York: John Wiley & Sons, 2000.

Gordis L. Epidemiology. 2nd Ed. Philadelphia: WB Saunders, 2000.

Kelsey JL, Thompson WD, Evans AS. Methods in Observational Epidemiology. New York: Oxford University Press, 1986.

Last JM. A Dictionary of Epidemiology. 4th Ed. New York: Oxford University Press, 2001, pp 1–196.

Selvin S. Statistical Analysis of Epidemiologic Data. New York: Oxford University Press, 1991.

Szklo N. Epidemiology: Beyond the Basics. 2nd Ed. Aspen, 2000.

CARDIOVASCULAR DISEASES AND DISORDERS

Ischemic Cardiovascular Disease

Carl Foster, John P. Porcari, Kristi Cadwell, Stefanie Hatcher, Arna E. Karlsdottir, Carla Theusch, Pedro Recalde, Stacie Voelker

SEARCHABLE KEY TERMS

Endocardium

Epicardium

Exercise Intensity

Exercise Prescription

Exertional Ischemia

Ischemia

Ischemic Cardiovascular Disease

Myocardial Infarction (MI)

Myocardial Perfusion

Rescue Angioplasty

Silent Ischemia

Thrombolytic Agents

Ventilatory Threshold

Ventricular Function

Overview

Ischemic cardiovascular disease is the most common degenerative disease in the developed world, and the leading cause of death among adults. It has several basic variations of presentation. Most of these are related to narrowing of the coronary arteries secondary to the development of atherosclerotic plaques. This narrowing can lead to exertional ischemia when the available lumen of the affected coronary artery is too small to provide for adequate blood flow to regions of the myocardium during periods of enhanced demand (e.g., exercise, meals, sexual activity, strong emotions). It also may cause resting ischemia when the lumen of the affected artery is too small, either due to severe narrowing of the coronary artery or to transient reductions in the size of the coronary artery lumen secondary to spasm, to unstable angina or myocardial infarction following acute total reductions in regional myocardial blood flow, often attributable to plaque rupture or thrombus formation.

Myocardial Infarction

Myocardial infarction (MI), often called "heart attack," is the death of myocardial muscle cells following a reduction in blood supply that is sustained for more than a few moments. For the most part, MI is attributable to the abrupt closure of one or more of the coronary arteries secondary to the rupture of an atherosclerotic plaque, often with thrombus formation as a consequence of the plaque rupture. The development of irreversible damage to the myocardium takes some time following the acute reduction in blood flow. This time lag forms the logic underlying contemporary treatment options such as thrombolysis and rescue angioplasty. It also forms the logical basis for treatment with simple anticoagulants such as aspirin. The use of acute therapies such as morphine and beta-blockers is based on reducing the metabolic requirements of the myocardium, thus minimizing the metabolic significance of the profound reduction in blood flow that caused the MI. The severity of a MI depends on a number of factors, including the mass of myocardium rendered ischemic, the duration of ischemia, the metabolic requirements of the myocardium during the period of reduced blood flow, and the ability for blood flow to be provided to the affected myocardium via collateral vessels. These factors all act to determine how much myocardial tissue ultimately is lost during the MI. Because of the pattern of the coronary blood flow, the first tissue rendered ischemic during a reduction in blood flow is the **endocardium** (the innermost layer of the myocardium). The **epicardium** (the outer layers of the heart muscle) becomes ischemic as a relatively late feature during acute reductions in blood flow. Typically, the ischemia during a MI is relatively focused in one location, with profound ischemia surrounded by areas of progressively milder ischemia. A mild MI, usually referred to as a subendocardial MI, does not involve the full thickness of the myocardium and usually has a smaller mass of necrotic (or dead) tissue. A more severe MI leads to tissue necrosis throughout the full thickness of the myocardium, often over a wider area. This type usually is referred to as a transmural MI. Electrocardiographically, a subendocardial MI is marked by early ST elevation, which may evolve into either persistent T wave inversion or to an electrocardiogram (ECG) that appears relatively normal. On the other hand, a transmural MI usually has severe ST elevation, which evolves into persistent T wave inversion and Q waves in leads representing the affected area of the myocardium. In both types of MI, there usually is some loss of the R wave in the leads representing the area of the MI.

In the United States and Western Europe, first MIs in men between the ages of 35 and 74 occur at an overall rate of about 4 per 1000 per year. In women the rate is about 2 per 1000 per year. The rate varies substantially within the population, depending on the presence of well-identified risk factors. Among middle-aged and older individuals with multiple risk factors, the rate of first MI can exceed 100 per 1000 persons per year. Data from the Framingham study indicate that in men about one third of all MIs are fatal (15% within the first 2 hours, e.g., sudden death; and 20% who survive the first 2 hours but fail to survive hospitalization). In women, the risk of a fatal first presentation of heart disease is somewhat less, about 10%. The majority of early mortality from MI is related to arrhythmias. Mortality related to pump failure is seen mainly in those patients who survive long enough to reach the hospital, but who develop cardiogenic shock secondary to the loss of a critically large mass of myocardium. Death can also occur secondary to rupture of the myocardium at the site of the MI, leading to cardiac tamponade and acute pump failure. The incidence of cardiogenic shock and myocardial rupture as a cause of fatal myocardial infarction is low compared to deaths attributable to arrhythmia. Late mortality from MI is, likewise, primarily related to the development of arrhythmias, which are attributable to residual ischemia or to conduction abnormalities caused by the scar at the site of the MI.

Nonfatal MIs vary widely in their clinical course, depending on the amount of myocardium lost, the presence or absence of cardiogenic shock, the nature and magnitude of arrhythmias, and the presence or absence of residual ischemia. The rate of subsequent MI is higher than the rate of primary MI, and the clinical course of subsequent MIs is often more difficult than for the primary MI, if for no other reason than the progressive loss of myocardial tissue.

Most patients who survive MI can be discharged from the hospital within a week. Longer hospital stays usually are secondary to the factors listed earlier that determine the clinical course of nonfatal MI. In general, most patients can resume activities of daily living within a few weeks of hospital discharge. There is a general perception among medical personnel that the site of the MI takes about 6 weeks to scar fully, and that activity should be relatively restricted during this period of time. Some data suggest that the tendency of the myocardial scar to extend and to lead to development of a myocardial aneurysm is negatively influenced by too much activity during this time period. More recent data do not support this concept, however, and, in fact, suggest that controlled increases in activity may lead to a reduced likelihood of myocardial remodeling (1).

Therapy for Myocardial Infarction

During hospitalization, the primary medical therapy for MI involves attempts to limit the extent of damage to the heart, by administration of **thrombolytic agents** or **rescue angioplasty**, and by attempts to reduce the myocardial oxygen demands by administration of beta-blockers, nitrates, and narcotic pain relievers. In patients with evidence of pump failure, medical therapy is focused on providing pharmacologic or mechanical inotropic support or pharmacologic afterload reduction. Once the patient has survived the initial MI, early management of the patient revolves around surveillance for residual ischemia, hemodynamic instability that might suggest pump failure, and the development of arrhythmias. In the presence of residual ischemia, the patient usually is considered for cardiac catheterization with the intent of determining whether significant additional myocardium remains at risk. Systematic ambulation of the patient while still in the hospital (Phase I rehabilitation), particularly in conjunction with hemodynamic and electrocardiographic monitoring, is very effective in identifying patients who may be candidates for early invasive evaluation (2, 3). This same role also may be served by either heart rate–limited or symptom-limited graded exercise testing prior to hospital discharge.

During the early posthospitalization period, one of the primary values of rehabilitation programs is surveillance for new or continuing ischemia as the patient's activity level returns to normal. Although telemetric ECG has always been considered to be of low value relative to identifying ischemia, recent evidence suggests that it is better than formerly believed (4). Each rehabilitation session can be viewed as a mini-stress test. When ischemia or other medical problems are identified, the patient can be referred back to his or her physician for early treatment, often avoiding the risk associated with a recurrent infarction. During the course of a 12-week rehabilitation program, it is common to refer 25% to 40% of patients back to their physicians for unscheduled office visits (5, 6). After 20 years of use, telemetric ECG monitoring is still a primary means of surveillance (7).

After the patient has survived the MI and the early posthospitalization phase, the goals of therapy switch somewhat, to the management of residual ischemia or arrhythmias and the treatment of risk factors that might predispose the patient to the development of a subsequent MI. Medical management can be quite complex and tailored to the patient's individual pathophysiology. Virtually every patient is put on aspirin, or some other form of anticoagulation therapy, because the dominant mechanism of subsequent MIs is, like the primary MI, plaque rupture and occlusive thrombus formation. Beta blockade remains a primary treatment of residual ischemia and angina pectoris, because it has the secondary advantage of reducing the patient's likelihood of developing clinically meaningful arrhythmias. Afterload reduction is an option in the patient with some degree of left ventricular dysfunction. If the patient is hyperlipidemic, aggressive treatment with HMG Co-A reductase inhibitors (e.g., statins) is indicated, as is pharmacologic treatment for hypertension and glucose intolerance. Advice to discontinue the use of tobacco products and to exercise systematically round out the therapeutic approach. Although the issue of whether actual regression of atherosclerotic plaques occurs remains controversial, there is ample evidence that very aggressive management of risk factors, either with lifestyle changes or

pharmacologically, can significantly alter the subsequent clinical course of patients after MI (8–10).

Exercise Therapy Following Myocardial Infarction

Evaluation Criteria

Exercise testing should be performed before the patient is discharged, as part of an evaluative work-up designed to determine whether the patient needs invasive evaluation and therapy, or can be discharged and referred for rehabilitation (11, 12). Either symptom-limited, heart rate-limited (generally rest + 30 bpm), or workload-limited (usually 5 METs) exercise tests may be performed with good information yield. As a general rule, the initial loading and rate of progression of the exercise test should be comparatively gentle, allowing the patient's responses to be evaluated before proceeding to the next exercise stage. Limitation of the exercise test at a workload of 5 METs is less popular today than formerly, because this cutoff may represent a maximal test in the most unstable patients and may be unnecessarily limiting in patients with an uncomplicated clinical course. As a general rule, the presence of angina pectoris, changes in the ST segment of the ECG, abnormalities of the blood pressure response, the development of more severe arrhythmias, or the presence of a very low functional capacity indicate that the patient should be referred for cardiac catheterization with the view toward invasive therapy. Recent studies evaluating the interaction of exercise capacity and ischemic markers, the magnitude and shape of the heart rate increases and decreases during the test, and the rate of blood pressure decline after exercise also have been demonstrated to provide valuable prognostic information (13–15). Individuals with an inability to achieve an adequate increase in heart rate with exertion (e.g., chronotropic incompetence) or with delays in the recovery of either heart rate or systolic blood pressure during recovery have been demonstrated to have a poorer prognosis, independently of ECG evidence of exertional ischemia. Individuals with a relatively poor exercise capacity, adjusted for the presence and magnitude of ST segment depression or angina, also have been demonstrated to have a poor prognosis. The prognostic situation guides the overall approach to therapy.

Myocardial Perfusion

Myocardial perfusion scans are performed during exercise or pharmacologic stress testing with the idea of determining whether there is additional myocardium at risk following the resolution of the primary MI. The presence of a stress-related perfusion deficit indicates a risk of residual angina pectoris or subsequent MI. However, stress-related perfusion defects, such as angina pectoris and electrocardiographic ST segment depression, are more indicative of high-grade coronary stenoses, which, in turn, are more associated with exertional angina. These lesions are comparatively less likely to rupture and lead to subsequent MI. Unfortunately, good exercise testing criteria do not exist for identifying the 30% to 50% lesion which is likely to rupture and produce an MI, although a variety of techniques for augmenting the interpretation of the exercise test, particularly for prognosis, are becoming recognized (15–18).

Ventricular Function

Ventricular function studies also may be performed following MI, using either radionuclide ventriculography or echocardiography. The absolute value of markers of left ventricular function, usually ejection fraction, are powerful prognostic tools. With poor left ventricular function (e.g., left ventricular ejection fraction [LVEF] < 30%) or left ventricular function that deteriorates with exertion, survival with medical therapy is not good (19). In the presence of any abnormal exertional ventricular function, invasive therapy should be considered to improve myocardial perfusion or pharmacologic afterload reduction.

Ischemic Disease Without Myocardial Infarction

Many of the same therapeutic principles apply in the patient with ischemic syndromes that do not involve MI. **Ischemia** without MI is related primarily to coronary arteries that have a lumen inadequate to satisfy the needs of the myocardium. This problem usually is related either to the focal narrowing that is a feature of atherosclerotic coronary artery disease, to coronary artery spasm, or to some combination of the two. Ischemia that is provoked by increases in the myocardial oxygen demands (e.g., exercise, meals, sexual activity, strong emotions) is more likely to be related to coronary artery narrowing, whereas ischemia occurring at rest typically is related to coronary artery spasm. The pathophysiologic sequelae of myocardial ischemia are well illustrated by the concept of the ischemic cascade (20). Within this model of the pathophysiologic responses to ischemia, the first abnormality after the development of a perfusion deficit is diastolic dysfunction in the ischemic myocardial tissue. As the magnitude of the perfusion deficit increases (i.e., increasing myocardial demand in the face of an already maximal coronary artery blood flow) regional systolic dysfunction (wall motion abnormalities) follow, then decreases in global ventricular function (ejection fraction), then ST segment changes, then angina pectoris, then myocardial damage leading to necrosis (MI). The realization that the myocardium can be ischemic long before the development of angina pectoris has led to the concept of **silent ischemia**. This disorder apparently is very common and can be just as dangerous as symptomatic ischemia in terms of provoking arrhythmias (21, 22). Until the development of myocardial

necrosis, all of the steps in the ischemic cascade potentially are fully reversible, although there are data suggesting that repeated ischemic insults can lead to fibrotic changes in the myocardium without causing a MI (23).

Treatment options for **exertional ischemia** focus on strategies for increasing myocardial blood flow (e.g., nitrates, angioplasty, bypass surgery), for reducing myocardial oxygen demand (e.g., beta-blockers, nitrates, afterload reducers), or for preventing coronary artery spasm (e.g., calcium blockers). Although there is evidence that ischemia is reduced following warm-up (24, 25), abundant evidence suggests that exercise-related complications are related to exercising with ischemia (26). This has led to the general concept that exercise should be organized to avoid intensities associated with ischemia.

Principles of Exercise Prescription

The basis of **exercise prescription** is to provide enough of a challenge to the patient to provoke changes in his or her physiology, but to avoid most of the potential side effects of exercise, in particular those associated with exertional ischemia. The theory is illustrated by the ancient story of Milo of Crotona, a farm boy who lifted a newly foaled bullock to his shoulders and walked around the barnyard. The next day he lifted the now marginally larger bullock, and the next and the next, until he was able to lift a fully grown bull to his shoulders, becoming the strongest man in the world in the process. The point of the story, of course, is that humans are marvelously adaptable to exercise as long as it is presented in a systematic and progressive manner. The goal of prescription of exercise is similar to that of the prescription of pharmacologic agents (i.e., to secure the desired effects while avoiding the side effects). The parameters of exercise prescription are the *f*requency, the *i*ntensity, the *t*ime (or duration), and the *m*ode (or type) of exercise; they can be remembered using the anagram FITM.

Frequency

The frequency of exercise can vary quite dramatically over the time course of recovery from a MI, and often parallels the intensity and duration of exercise. In the early post-MI period, while the patient is still in the hospital, it is normal for exercise to be performed 2 or even 3 times per day, but at very low intensity and for very brief periods of time. Even in the early posthospital discharge period, it is normal to recommend that the patient ambulate at low intensity and for a short time, several times per day. The primary goals during this period are to prevent bedrest deconditioning by imposing frequent orthostatic stress and to reduce the likelihood of embolic events secondary to prolonged venous stasis. Ambulation during this period also is critical to the patient's state of mind. Following MI, it is quite usual to be depressed. If the patient is able to see that he or she is not going to be a cardiac cripple and can see day-to-day progress, the likelihood of depression may be reduced. As the patient begins formal rehabilitation, ideally during the first or second week posthospital discharge, it is normal to reduce the frequency of exercise somewhat to allow for one, more extensive, training session three to five times per week. However, even during this period, the usual recommendation is to make sure that the patient ambulates several times daily. By several weeks posthospital discharge, the goal is to have the patient pursuing normal activities (which obviates the need for structured ambulation) and to be performing structured exercise training three to five times per week. Thus, over the space of several weeks, the frequency of exercise may be expected to decrease from three to five times per day to three to five times per week. In the patient diagnosed with non–MI-related ischemia, the general recommendation is to exercise three to five times per week, although with tight control of exercise intensity to prevent exertional ischemia.

Intensity

Exercise intensity during hospitalization and during the immediate posthospital phase is relatively less important than exercise frequency. The intensity during this period should be very low (<50% of maximal exercise capacity) and well below the level that causes angina, dyspnea, or undue residual fatigue. If ECG monitoring is available during this period, exercise of sufficient intensity to cause ST segment changes or arrhythmias should be avoided. As a general guideline, a heart rate 20 beats above standing rest should be the upper limit heart rate achieved during ambulation sessions. Likewise, the rating of perceived exertion should probably stay in the easy to moderate range (2–3 or 10–12 on the new and old scales, respectively). The concern with intensity at this stage is that if the plaque that caused the MI is unstable, it may rupture again, causing a second MI. Further, although there has been limited documentation of myocardial rupture during exercise following MI, there is a theoretically valid concern that high intracardiac pressures could lead to myocardial rupture following transmural MI. Lastly, catecholamine release associated with heavy exercise may predispose toward arrhythmias.

After about 6 weeks, during which time the myocardial scar at the site of the MI has time to stabilize, the goal of exercise therapy shifts from preventing deterioration to the recovery of functional capacity and the prevention of further cardiovascular events. During this period, the exercise prescription is highly related to the patient's functional capacity, ideally determined from a symptom-limited graded exercise test. During this period the relative intensity should be in the range of 60% of maximal exercise capacity in METs, or 70% of the $\dot{V}O_2$ reserve. If direct measures of $\dot{V}O_2$ are available, an intensity of about 90% of the ventilatory threshold probably is more appropriate than a predefined percentage

of the $\dot{V}O_2$ reserve. The intensity associated with the ventilatory threshold is linked much more closely to the patient's perception of effort, to the likelihood for elevated catecholamines during exercise, and to the general acceptability of exercise than to any arbitrary percentage of the $\dot{V}O_2$ reserve. Usually the heart rate at these metabolic reference points is used as a monitoring strategy, with 60% to 70% of the maximal heart rate being the default value. These objective markers of exercise intensity should be matched by an appropriate subjective effort, as reflected by a rating of perceived exertion of moderate to somewhat hard (3–4 or 12–14 on the new or old scales, respectively). If the patient experiences angina or shortness of breath, the exercise intensity should be reduced to avoid these symptoms. If ST segment changes are noted, the target heart rate should be set at least 10 beats below the first evidence of ST segment changes, because ST segment changes (and angina) are relatively late manifestations of exertional ischemia (20). A variety of data, from both the rehabilitation literature and that on the triggering of MI support the concept that complications related to exertion are intensity-related, and that exercise with myocardial ischemia should be avoided (27–29). Although there are data supporting the concept that myocardial ischemia generally gets better with warm-up or with continued effort (24, 25), and that left ventricular function may be well-preserved even in the face of mild ischemia (30), the risk of complications precludes intentionally training with ischemia.

Recent data suggest that the **ventilatory threshold** often is reached before the ischemic threshold (31), supporting the idea that an intensity of about 90% of the ventilatory threshold is a reasonable approximation of the optimal intensity for exercise training. We recently have demonstrated that the ability to carry on a conversation (i.e., the "talk test") is closely related to the ventilatory threshold (32–35), suggesting a simple low-tech approach to estimating the ventilatory threshold. The patient is required to recite a simple paragraph of 30 to 100 words, then asked "can you still speak comfortably?" Failure to unequivocally answer "yes" suggests that the ventilatory threshold has been exceeded. As a simple device, we have used recital of the Pledge of Allegiance, with which most people in American culture are familiar, as a simple speaking challenge.

An additional objective technique for exercise prescription relates to the pattern of the heart rate increase with an increase in workload. Most healthy individuals show a negatively accelerated heart rate performance curve at about the intensity associated with the second lactate threshold or second ventilatory threshold. Training at intensities above this point seems to be associated with an inability to continue exercise without a progressive increase in blood lactate. Interesting, many individuals with cardiovascular disease demonstrate a positively accelerated heart rate performance curve at about this same exercise intensity (13, 14). This positive acceleration is consistently associated with deterioration of left ventricular function. The positive acceleration of the heart rate performance curve at this point probably is an attempt to defend cardiac output in the face of a declining stroke volume (36). Given the concerns voiced earlier regarding exercising with an ischemic myocardium, it probably is reasonable to suggest that exercising with deteriorating ventricular function also is unwise, and to suggest that the workload at the breakpoint of the heart rate performance curve (particularly a positively accelerated break point) may represent the upper limit of exercise intensity for patients after any sort of cardiovascular disease.

The intensity of exercise should be progressed cautiously over a period of several weeks. There are several standard strategies for progressing the intensity of exercise. One is to allow the upper limit heart rate to be a higher percentage of the maximal heart rate, so that perceived exertion stays about the same. This is a somewhat empirical approach, effectively equivalent to suggesting that the perceived exertion during exercise should remain in the range of moderate to somewhat hard (e.g., 3–4 or 13–15 on the new and old versions of the Borg scale, respectively). If respiratory gas exchange data are available, the upper intensity of exercise training probably should remain just below that associated with the ventilatory threshold. The percentage of maximal heart rate associated with the deflection of the heart rate performance curve point is variable, suggesting that exercise prescription based on fixed percentages of the maximal heart rate is a fundamentally flawed technique (37).

There is a role for higher-intensity training in the rehabilitation of patients following MI. Such training is associated with profound improvements in clinical status and functional capacity. However, high-intensity training has been accomplished only in very highly selected patients, with a preliminary background of lower-intensity training without exertional ischemia, and usually with the desire to return to recreational level competitive athletics (38–40). Such high levels of training often are associated with very good results relative to the other risk factors, so it probably should not be discouraged if the patient expresses the desire to undertake such extensive efforts. It certainly is superior to regressing back to a sedentary lifestyle or to maintaining untreated risk factors. However, as a practical safety consideration, such high-intensity training probably should only take place once exertional ischemia has been ruled out, and once the patient has established a clear history of lower-intensity training so that the risk of triggering another MI is minimized (27–29).

Duration

The duration of exercise probably is the least important of the three primary markers of the exercise prescription. Certainly, during the early period of high-frequency, low-intensity ambulation while the patient is still in the hospital or in the early posthospital period, the duration of exercise can be quite brief. During this period, the goals of exercising are related primarily to preventing bedrest deconditioning and embolic events, and, in addition, the patient may not yet be very tolerant of sustained exercise. Sometimes only 5 minutes of ambulation or other rehabilitation activity may be entirely appropriate.

As soon as the patient enters formal rehabilitation, the primary early strategy for progressing the exercise load is extending the duration of exercise, while keeping the intensity relatively low. During the first 6 weeks, when the myocardium is healing from the MI, it probably is inadvisable to increase the intensity of exercise very much, but the exercise load can be progressed significantly by increasing the duration from 5 to 10 minutes all the way to 40 to 60 minutes. This has the broad benefits of favorably affecting skeletal muscle, of making exertion-related plaque rupture with subsequent higher-intensity exercise less likely, and of allowing the patient to see relatively significant progress at a time when overcoming the depression that frequently accompanies MI is an important goal of therapy. This same increase in exercise capacity can also often be used to reassure the patient and his or her spouse regarding the safety of resuming sexual relations, a significant but often ignored problem following MI. In patients with ischemia not related to MI, the duration of exercise can begin at about 20 minutes and be progressed to a target of about 40 minutes per session fairly quickly. The main concern with exercise duration is the time available to the patient and the need to avoid orthopaedic injury from too rapid increases in exercise duration.

Mode of Exercise

The primary type of exercise recommended for patients following MI is steady-state aerobic exercise, using either cycle ergometry, treadmill walking, or free-range ambulation. These activities not only are simple, but they provide a comparatively small hemodynamic challenge. Lastly, the intensity of these types of exercise can be regulated fairly easily. The treadmill has the advantage of being able to use either speed or grade to increase the intensity of exercise. For patients who may be unsteady on their feet or uncomfortable with rapid walking, a fairly predictable training workload can be achieved by varying the grade of the treadmill belt. As the patient becomes more stable during the weeks following the MI, other steady-state aerobic activities, including upper extremity exercises, may be added to the exercise program. Recent data have demonstrated that left ventricular function is very stable during conventional resistance exercise, including overhead exercise, in clinically stable patients (41).

Beginning with postsurgical patients, and later extended to patients with congestive heart failure, the last decade has been marked by the use of interval training for patients with cardiovascular disease (42–44). In post-MI patients, once they have passed the 6-week myocardial healing period and if they do not have evidence of ischemia or hemodynamic instability during steady-state aerobic exercise, interval training may be used to good effect. Interval training allows higher-intensity training to be done by the skeletal muscles, without an unreasonable overall metabolic load. The "secret" of using interval training is to keep the duration of the hard segments quite short (<30 seconds). The intensity is best set by a rapidly incremented ramp test on the cycle ergometer, but also may be the highest workload achieved during a normal incremental exercise test. The intensity of the easy segments is very low (~10W on the cycle ergometer). It is even acceptable to rest or to straddle the treadmill belt if the treadmill rather than the cycle ergometer is used for interval training. With nominal durations of 30 seconds hard, 60 seconds easy exercise (30s/60s), most patients find the intensity of exercise very acceptable, and the metabolic responses to such interval training programs are consistent with an average intensity below the ventilatory threshold (43, 44). If 30s/60s proves to be too difficult, then modification of the hard/easy segment duration to 20s/70s or even 10s/80s is very acceptable. Studies in postsurgical patients have demonstrated that the rate of improvement of functional capacity is more rapid in patients using interval training than in patients using only steady-state aerobic training (42). Although these results have not been extended specifically to post-MI patients, it would seem to be reasonable to include this patient group.

Although there has been historical concern regarding the use of resistance training in patients with cardiovascular disease, recent clinical experience suggests that in well-selected patients who are already performing aerobic exercise at a good level, the addition of resistance exercise is well-tolerated and results in an improved clinical status (45). Because of the largely theoretical concerns regarding the risk of myocardial rupture and because of the fairly high blood pressure observed during resistance exercise, it remains prudent to wait until 6 weeks post-MI before beginning more than the most rudimentary of upper extremity range-of-motion exercises. After this time, resistance exercise may add to the patient's self-efficacy (46, 47), regardless of when resistance exercise is added to the program, without substantial risk of inducing left ventricular dysfunction (40).

Complications Related to Exercise Testing and Training

The risks of exercise testing and training have been well reviewed by a number of authors (48–51) and summarized within the last year (52). In general, studies from the 1970s suggested that exercise training had a risk of complications of about 0.4 per 10,000 hours of training, or 50 times less than the well-established risk of exercise testing. Studies published in the mid-1980s suggested that the risk of complications during exercise training was on the order of 0.10 per 10,000 hours, or about 150 times less than the risk of exercise testing. The most recent studies suggest a rate of complications of about 0.16 per 10,000 hours, or about 100 times less than the risk of exercise testing. These latter studies doubtless reflect the effects of better medical management and the addition of revascularized patients to the rehabilitation literature. As a conservative average, the risk of

exercise training in the post-MI patient probably is 0.2 to 0.3 per 10,000 hours, or 50 to 100 times less risky than exercise testing. The bad news is that the presentation of complications in patients with known cardiovascular disease, of whatever variety, usually is in the form of a sudden arrhythmia leading to sudden cardiac death, whereas the presentation of complications in patients without known cardiovascular disease usually is in the form of MI. Thus, although the absolute risk of exercise training is quite low, those involved in exercising this population need to be prepared to deal with relatively severe complications.

For many years, there was concern that exercise training in post-MI patients might lead to an extension of the infarct, or to remodeling of the myocardium in such a way as to promote the risk of aneurysm formation. The most recent data, using nuclear magnetic resonance (NMR) reconstruction technology, effectively lays this concern to rest (1). In contemporary management of acute MI, it is very unlikely that exercise training would be started until the MI has either run its course or been successfully stopped.

Outcomes Related to Exercise Testing and Training

There were several early randomized clinical trials of exercise training following MI. In general, the results of these trials were disappointing, in that although they generally demonstrated improved mortality in patients participating in exercise and risk factor management programs, the results did not achieve statistical significance. In 1988, Oldridge (53) and O'Connor (54) published independent meta-analyses of the data from these trials, which demonstrated that participation in rehabilitation programs improved mortality. The magnitude of reduction in risk, about 20%, was of the same order of magnitude as the effect of stopping smoking or taking beta-blockers, both of which are standard therapies for patients with MI. Interestingly, Oldridge demonstrated a small, statistically insignificant, increase in the incidence of nonfatal reinfarction in the exercising patients. Given our current knowledge of how to prescribe exercise in this patient group, our current understanding of the factors leading to the triggering of MI, and knowledge of the effect of aggressive lipid-lowering therapy on the stability of atherosclerotic plaques, it seems likely that there is now less cause for concern about these findings from Oldridge than when the primary studies were conducted.

Reduction in Symptoms

A variety of early studies in patients with residual angina pectoris following MI demonstrated that systematic exercise training leads to a reduction in symptoms during ordinary activities, primarily by reducing the myocardial oxygen demands of ordinary activities. Given the change in medical therapy of patients with MI since these early studies, this effect of exercise training on symptom management is probably no longer an important consideration. Although exercise is an effective therapy for angina pectoris, other options that have a quicker and more reliable effect are available.

Increase in Exercise Capacity

Together with studies of the reductions in symptoms in patients with angina pectoris following MI, the early literature is replete with studies demonstrating the substantial increase in exercise capacity following training in patients with MI. Current studies are complicated, in that studies of the rate of recovery of functional capacity involve several types of patients. One factor consistent in all studies is the observation of relatively large increases in exercise capacity attributable to exercise training and of relatively faster recovery of exercise capacity (55, 56). However, many studies also have demonstrated a certain degree of spontaneous recovery of functional capacity even without a formal exercise program. Exercise training also has been shown to influence the self-efficacy of physical activity, even in patients long healed from the primary clinical episode. Because self-efficacy more than the objective functional capacity determines the likelihood of a patient engaging in an activity, the role of exercise training in enhancing self-efficacy can hardly be minimized.

Summary

Exercise training is an important therapeutic strategy in the patient who has survived acute MI. In general, the exercise prescription should favor the use of exercise that is comparatively frequent and of longer duration, with careful increases in intensity beginning about 6 weeks following the MI. Although exercise probably is not important as a primary therapy for angina pectoris, post-MI patients who participate in exercise programs may have a better prognosis and may recover normal exercise capacity more rapidly than nonparticipating patients. The risks of exercise training are relatively low, on the order of 100 times less than the risk of exercise testing. The risks of exercise are primarily related to inappropriately intense exercise, which can trigger the rupture of unstable atherosclerotic plaques. The intensity of exercise training probably should be defined in terms of individual physiologic responses such as the ventilatory threshold or heart rate performance curve, or from simple behavioral surrogates of these indices such as the talk test or rating of perceived exertion, rather than arbitrarily defined percentages of the maximal heart rate or maximal working capacity.

CASE STUDY

Mr. Schwartz is a 55-year-old man who suffered a nontransmural MI 3 months ago. He was treated initially with thrombolytic agents at a community hospital, responded well, and refused early cardiac catheterization. His history is remarkable for 30 pack-years of smoking, although he had quit 2 years prior to his MI, and a serum cholesterol at the time of admission of 235 mg/dL with an LDL of 150 mg/dl and HDL of 35 mg/dl. He was discharged on aspirin, Lopid, Tenormin (25 mg b.i.d.) and sublingual nitroglycerin p.r.n. However, he removed himself from the beta-blocker because of erectile difficulties and found the headache associated with nitrate use unacceptable. He was enrolled in a rehabilitation program beginning 3 weeks after hospital discharge, but has not progressed well. Currently, in the rehab program, he is walking 30 minutes at 3.0 mph, 2.5% grade and cycling for 20 minutes at 90 watts. He denies angina, but reports "breathlessness" early in the workout. At home, he walks for 20 minutes at a rather slow pace, and reports feeling apprehensive regarding extending his exercise program. He is an accountant, but has not returned to work because he feels apprehensive about the "stress" of the job.

Mr. Schwartz has been referred for exercise testing to define his exercise capacity and to determine whether there is any residual ischemia. He performed a maximal cycle ergometer exercise test using a modified Jones protocol (3 minutes at 15 watts + 15 watts/min), completing a total of 11 minutes at a power output of 135 watts. He quit because of general fatigue, with breathlessness similar to his presenting symptoms. His heart rate (HR) increased from 60 to 171 beats per minute (104% predicted) (Figure 3.1). His blood pressure increased from 135/88 to 163/90 mm Hg at 8 minutes, with a decrease to 157/90 mm Hg at peak exercise (Figure 3.2). At rest, his ECG revealed normal sinus rhythm at a rate of 60. There was poor R wave progression in V2-V4 consistent with anteroseptal MI. There were no Q waves, and the T waves were normally configured. With exercise, there was ST segment depression evident in V4-V6 beginning at 8 minutes at an

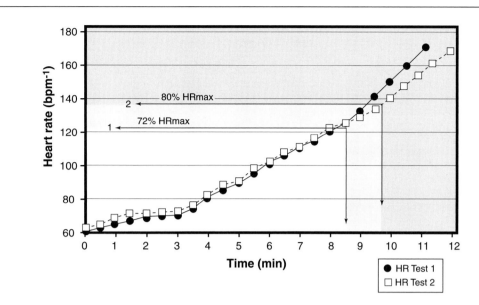

FIGURE 3.1.   Heart rate performance curves for the pre- and post-percutaneous transluminal coronary angioplasty (PTCA) exercise tests. Note that although the peak heart rate does not change significantly, the upward deflection occurs at a higher power output and heart rate and is less marked after PTCA.

HR of 125. At peak exercise, the maximal extent of the ST depression was 1.5 mm (Figure 3.3). The peak $\dot{V}o_2$ was 1.915 L/min, representing 19 ml/m/kg (5.4 METs), which is 71% of predicted for age and gender (Figure 3.4). His HR performance curve demonstrated an upward deflection after HR reached 125 (Figure 3.1). His $V_E/\dot{V}o_2$ demonstrated an upward deflection at 8:30 consistent with a $\dot{V}o_2$ of 1.650 L (4.7 METs) (Figure 3.5). His LV ejection fraction, measured by gated blood pool radionuclide imaging was below normal (>55%) at rest, responded normally until an HR of approximately 125, then decreased significantly to 35% at peak exercise with anterolateral wall motion abnormalities (Figure 3.6). The results are consistent with exertional ischemia beginning at an HR of about 125.

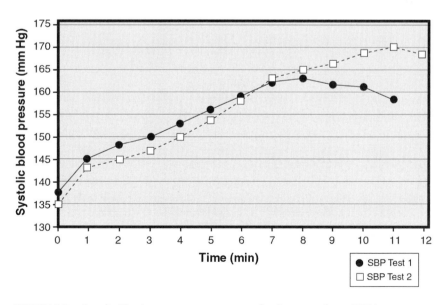

FIGURE 3.2.   Systolic blood pressure response curves for the pre- and post-PTCA exercise tests. Note the significant "rollover" of systolic blood pressure in the original test, consistent with a limitation of cardiac output.

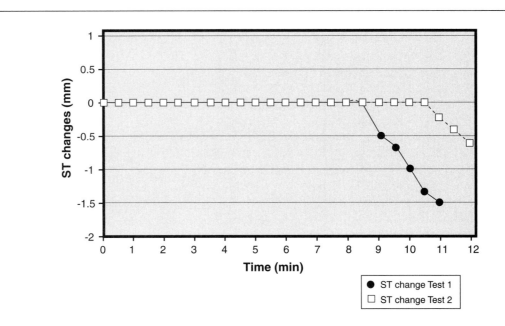

FIGURE 3.3.   Pattern of ST segment changes during the course of the pre- and post-PTCA exercise tests. Note that the ST depression occurs earlier and is of greater magnitude prior to therapy. In test #2, although there was observable ST depression, it did not reach a clinically significant magnitude.

The patient was advised that his results suggested residual ischemia and a fairly unfavorable prognosis on his current therapy. He was offered either cardiac catheterization with potential percutaneous transluminal coronary angioplasty (PTCA) or medical therapy including beta- and calcium blockers and long-acting nitrates. Given his previous problems with pharmacologic therapy, he elected cardiac catheterization. During catheterization, a residual 70% lesion was noted in the circumflex artery distribution, and was reduced to 20% with angioplasty. Repeat exercise testing demonstrated a significant increase in exercise capacity, to 150 watts, and $\dot{V}o_2$ peak to 2.4 L/min (6.9 METs), which is 93% of predicted for age and gender. The peak HR was not changed, but the

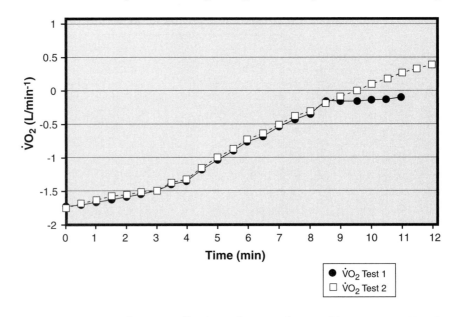

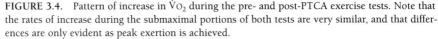

FIGURE 3.4.   Pattern of increase in $\dot{V}o_2$ during the pre- and post-PTCA exercise tests. Note that the rates of increase during the submaximal portions of both tests are very similar, and that differences are only evident as peak exertion is achieved.

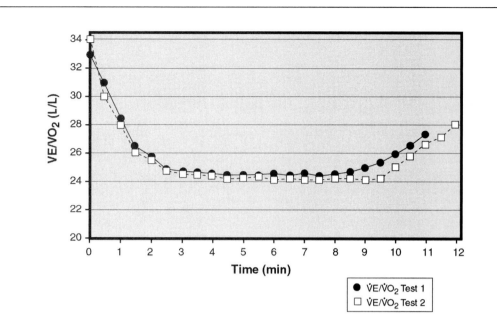

FIGURE 3.5. Pattern of changes in the $V_E/\dot{V}O_2$ during the pre- and post-PTCA exercise tests. Note the rightward shift in the sudden increase in $V_E/\dot{V}O_2$ in the post-PTCA exercise test.

nature of the HR performance curve was changed, with an increase in slope after a rate of 135. This matched the change in the $V_E/\dot{V}O_2$ during exercise. During the repeat exercise test there were nonsignificant ST segment changes or decreases in LV ejection fraction, and the blood pressure response to exercise was more nearly normal.

The patient was returned to the rehabilitation program with an exercise prescription of cycling at 105 watts and an HR of 125 to 135. After 2 weeks in the program he has reported making significant progress, has noted a lessening of symptoms and apprehension regarding exercise, and is planning on returning to work. His serum cholesterol on Lopid is now 170 mg/dl with an LDL fraction of 95 mg/dl and an HDL fraction of 40 mg/dl.

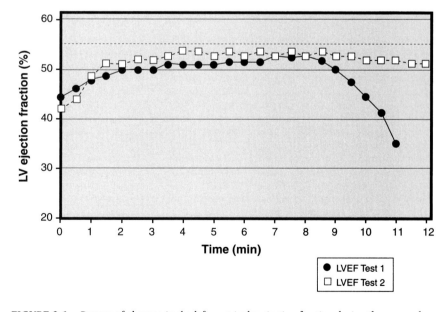
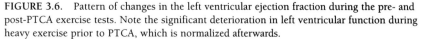

FIGURE 3.6. Pattern of changes in the left ventricular ejection fraction during the pre- and post-PTCA exercise tests. Note the significant deterioration in left ventricular function during heavy exercise prior to PTCA, which is normalized afterwards.

REFERENCES

1. Myers J, Goebbels U, Dzeikan G, et al. Exercise training and myocardial remodeling in patients with reduced ventricular function: one-year follow up with magnetic resonance imaging. Am Heart J 2000;139:252–261.

2. Dion WF, Grevenow P, Pollock ML, et al. Medical problems and physiological responses during supervised inpatient cardiac rehabilitation. Heart Lung 1982;11:248–255.

3. Silvidi GE, Squires RW, Pollock ML, Foster C. Hemodynamic responses and medical problems associated with early exercise and ambulation in coronary artery bypass graft surgery patients. J Cardiopulm Rehabil 1982;2:355–362.

4. Crenshaw B, Porcari JP, Foster C, et al. Comparison of telemetric monitoring to stress electrocardiography [abstract]. J Cardiopulm Rehabil 2000;20:301.

5. Dolatowski RP, Squires RW, Pollock ML, et al. Dysrhythmia detection in myocardial revascularization surgery patients. Med Sci Sports Exerc 1983;15:282–286.

6. Sennett SM, Pollock ML, Pels AE, et al. Medical problems of cardiac patients in an outpatient rehabilitation program. J Cardiopulm Rehabil 1987;458–465.

7. Grall SK, Porcari JP, DeRocco P, et al. The efficacy of continuous ECG monitoring in risk stratified Phase II cardiac rehabilitation patients. Clin Exerc Physiol 2000;2:133–140.

8. Ornish D, Brown SE, Scherwitz LW, et al. Can lifestyle changes reverse coronary heart disease? Lancet 1990;336:129–133.

9. Niebauer J, Hambrecht R, Velich T, et al. Attenuated progression of coronary artery disease after 6 years of multifactorial risk intervention: role of physical exercise. Circulation 1997;96:2534–2541.

10. Haskell WL, Alderman EL, Fair JM, et al. Effects of intensive multiple risk factor reduction on coronary atherosclerosis and clinical cardiac events in men and women with coronary artery disease: The Stanford Coronary Risk Intervention Project (SCRIP). Circulation 1994;89:975–990.

11. DeBusk RF, Davidson DM, Houston N, Fitzgerald J. Serial ambulatory electrocardiography and treadmill exercise testing after uncomplicated myocardial infarction. Am J Cardiol 1980;45:547–554.

12. Starling MR, Crawford MH, Kennedy GT, O'Rourke RA. Treadmill exercise tests predischarge and six weeks post myocardial infarction t detect abnormalities of known prognostic value. Ann Intern Med 1981;94:721–727.

13. Pokan R, Hofmann P, Preidler K, et al. Correlation between deflection of heart rate/performance curve and myocardial function in exhaustive bicycle ergometry. Eur J Appl Physiol 1993;67:385–388.

14. Pokan R, Hofmann P, von Duvillard SP, et al. The heart rate performance curve and left ventricular function during exercise in patients after myocardial infarction. Med Sci Sports Exerc 1998;30:1475–1480.

15. Amon KW, Richards KL, Crawford MH. Usefulness of the postexercise response of systolic blood pressure in the diagnosis of coronary artery disease. Circulation 1984;70:951–956.

16. Mark DB, Shaw L, Harrell FE, et al. Prognostic value of a treadmill exercise score in outpatients with suspected coronary artery disease. N Engl J Med 1991;325:849–853.

17. Cole CR, Blackstone EH, Pashkow FJ, et al. Heart rate recovery immediately after exercise as a predictor of mortality. N Engl J Med 1999;341:1351–1357.

18. Lauer MS, Francis GS, Okin PM, et al. Impaired chronotropic response to exercise stress testing as a predictor of mortality. JAMA 1999;281:524.

19. Jones RH, Floyd RD, Austin EH, Sabiston DC. The role of radionuclide angiocardiography in the preoperative prediction of pain relief and prolonged survival following coronary artery bypass grafting. Ann Surg 1983;197:743–754.

20. Nestor

21. Williams KA, Tailon LA, Carter JE. Asymptomatic and electrically silent myocardial ischemia during upright leg cycle ergometry and treadmill exercise (clandestine myocardial ischemia). Am J Cardiol 1993;72:1114–1120.

22. Gottlieb SO. Association between silent myocardial ischemia and prognosis: Insensitivity of angina pectoris as a marker of coronary artery disease activity. Am J Cardiol 1987;60:33J–38J.

23. Geft IL, Fishbein C, Ninomiya. Intermittent brief periods of ischemia have a cumulative effect and may cause myocardial necrosis. Circulation 1982;66:1150–1153.

24. McAlpine RN, Kattus AA. Adaptation to exercise in angina pectoris. Circulation 1966;33:183–201.

25. Tomai F, Crea F, Danesi A, et al. Mechanisms of the warm-up phenomenon. Eur Heart J 1996;17:1022–1027.

26. Hassock K, Hartwig R. Cardiac arrest associated with supervised cardiac rehabilitation. J Cardiopulm Rehabil 1982;2:402–408.

27. Willich SN, Lewis M, Lowel H, et al. Physical exertion as a trigger of acute myocardial infarction. N Engl J Med 1993;329:1684–1690.

28. Mittleman MA, Maclure M, Tofler GH, et al. Triggering of acute myocardial infarction by heavy physical exertion: protection against triggering by regular exertion. N Engl J Med 1993;329:1677–1683.

29. Albert CM, Mittleman MA, Chae CU, et al. Triggering of sudden death from cardiac causes by vigorous exertion. N Engl J Med 2000;343:1355–1361.

30. Foster C, Gall RA, Murphy P, et al. Left ventricular function during exercise testing and training. Med Sci Sports Exerc 1997;297–305.

31. Meyer K, Samek L, Pinchas A, et al. Relationship between ventilatory threshold and onset of ischemia in ECG during stress testing. Eur Heart J 1995;16:623–630.

32. Dehart-Beverley MM, Foster C, Porcari JP, et al. Relationship between the talk test and ventilatory threshold. Clin Exerc Physiol 2000;2:34–38.

33. Shafer NN, Foster C, Porcari JP, Fater DCW. Comparison of talk test to ventilatory threshold [abstract]. J Cardiopulm Rehabil 2000;20:289.

34. Voelker S, Foster C, Porcari JP, et al. Relationship between the talk test and ventilatory threshold in cardiac patients. Clin Exerc Physiol (in press).

35. Recalde PT, Foster C, Skemp KM, et al. The talk test as a simple marker of ventilatory and lactate threshold. Int J Sports Med (in press).

36. Foster C, Spatz P, Georgakopoulos N. Left ventricular function in relation to the heart rate performance curve. Clin Exerc Physiol 1999;1:29–32.

37. Hofmann P, von Duvillard SP, Seibert FJ, et al: %HRmax target heart rate is dependent on heart rate performance curve deflection. Med Sci Sports Exerc (in press).

38. Kavanagh T, Shephard RJ, Kennedy J. Characteristics of post coronary marathon runners. Ann NY Acad Sci 1977;301:455–465.

39. Ehsani AA, Martin WH, Heath GW, Coyle EF. Cardiac effects of prolonged and intense exercise training in patients with coronary artery disease. Am J Cardiol 1982;50:246–254.

40. Coyle EF, Martin WH, Ehsani AA, et al. Blood lactate threshold in some well trained ischemic heart disease patients. J Appl Physiol 1983;54:18–23.

41. Karlsdottir AE, Foster C, Porcari JP, et al. Left ventricular function during aerobic and resistance exercise. J Cardiopulm Rehabil 2002;22:170–177.

42. Meyer K, Lehmann M, Sunder G, et al. Interval versus continuous exercise training after coronary bypass surgery: a comparison of training induced acute reactions with respect to the effectiveness of the exercise methods. Clin Cardiol 1990;13:851–861.

43. Meyer K, Samek L, Schwaibold M, et al. Physical responses to different modes of interval exercise in patients with chronic heart failure—application to exercise training. Eur Heart J 1996;17:1040–1047.

44. Meyer K, Foster C, Georgakopoulous N, et al. Left ventricular function during interval and steady state exercise in patients with chronic heart failure. Am J Cardiol 1998;82:1382–1387.

45. Pollock ML, Franklin BA, Balady GJ, et al. Resistance exercise in indi-

viduals with and without cardiovascular disease: benefits, rationale, safety and prescription. Circulation 2000;101:828–833.

46. Hatcher S, Theusch C, Porcari JP, et al. Effects of a 10 week resistance training program on functional performance of female cardiac patients [abstract]. J Cardiopulm Rehabil 2000;20:292.

47. Theusch C, Hatcher S, Porcari JP, et al. Effectiveness of a 10 week resistance training program in female cardiac patients [abstract]. J Cardiopulm Rehabil 2000;20:294.

48. Rochemis P, Blackburn H. Exercise tests: a survey of procedures, safety and litigation experiences in approximately 170,000 tests. JAMA 1971;217:1061–1066.

49. Myers J, Voodi L, Ulmann T, Froelicher VF. A survey of exercise testing: methods, utilization, interpretation and safety in the VAHCS. J Cardiopulm Rehabil 2000;251–258.

50. Haskell WL. Cardiovascular complications during exercise training of cardiac patients. Circulation 1978;57:920–925.

51. van Camp SP, Peterson RA. Cardiovascular complications of outpatient cardiac rehabilitation programs. JAMA 1986;256:1160–1163.

52. Foster C, Porcari JP. The risks of exercise training. J Cardiopulm Rehabil 2001;21:347–352.

53. Oldridge NB, Guyatt GH, Fischer ME, Rimm AA. Cardiac rehabilitation after myocardial infarction. JAMA 1988;260:945–950

54. O'Connor GT, Buring JE, Yusuf S, et al. An overview of randomized trials of rehabilitation with exercise after myocardial infarction. Circulation 1989;80:234–244.

55. Foster C, Pollock ML, Anholm JD, et al. Work capacity and left ventricular function during rehabilitation from myocardial revascularization surgery. Circulation 1984;69:748–755.

56. Foster C, Oldridge NB, Dion W, et al. Time course of recovery during cardiac rehabilitation. J Cardiopulm Rehabil 1995;15:209–215.

CHAPTER 4

Chronic Heart Failure

Carl Foster, Arna E. Karlsdottir, John P. Porcari, Katharina Meyer

SEARCHABLE KEY TERMS	
ACE Inhibitors	Ischemic Cardiomyopathy
Aerobic Exercise	Left Ventricular (LV) Ejection Fraction
Afterload	Myocardial Ischemia
Beta Blockers	Preload
Chronic Heart Failure (CHF)	Resistance Training
Diastolic Heart Failure	Respiratory Muscle Strength
Digoxin	Skeletal Muscle
Diuretics	Sodium
Ergoreceptors	Systolic Heart Failure
Idiopathic Dilated Cardiomyopathy	Transplant Criteria
Interval Training	

Overview

Chronic heart failure (CHF) is a serious, life-limiting illness with a progressive functional decline and very high mortality rates. Over 4 million American adults currently have been diagnosed with chronic heart failure (CHF) with more than 400,000 new cases diagnosed annually and approximately 200,000 deaths per year attributed to CHF. The incidence and prevalence of CHF increases with age—CHF is the leading cause of hospital admissions in patients older than 65 years. The annual health care costs attributable to CHF are approximately $10 billion annually in the United States, and are increasing rapidly.

Pathophysiology of Chronic Heart Failure

Chronic heart failure is the inability of the heart to pump sufficient blood to body tissues to meet ordinary metabolic demands. Acutely, it often presents as cardiogenic shock following a severe myocardial infarction (MI), or as a relatively sudden clinical decompensation secondary to other damage to the heart (e.g., viral myocarditis, valve failure). Chronic heart failure often is described as a syndrome in which pathophysiologic and compensatory mechanisms designed to maintain an adequate ejection of blood from the left ventricle become pathogenic, and, instead of acting acutely, function chronically. It is manifested by a volume overload with either exertional or postural dyspnea and decreased exercise tolerance as the primary symptoms. *Chronic* heart failure may be distinguished from *congestive* heart failure by pulmonary congestion, jugular venous distention, and increased pulmonary capillary wedge pressure, which results when blood fails to be pumped forward to such a degree that congestion occurs on the venous side.

Etiology

CHF may develop as a result of either direct myocardial damage or nonishcemic myocardial damage.

Direct Myocardial Damage

Chronic heart failure resulting from direct myocardial damage is called **ischemic cardiomyopathy**. It is characterized by extensive **myocardial ischemia**, with or without myocardial infarction or ventricular aneurysm. This type of CHF usually is a consequence of infarction or severe and prolonged unstable ischemic insult, leading to stunning or hibernation, depending on how long it takes the myocardium to recover following restoration of appropriate myocardial perfusion. The functional consequence is a localized abnormality of ventricular contractility.

Nonischemic Myocardial Damage

Chronic heart failure resulting from nonischemic myocardial damage often is referred to as **idiopathic dilated cardiomyopathy**. The pathophysiology is less clear, but it invariably includes damage to the myocytes in patients with a history of hypertension, diabetes, excessive alcohol intake, or cancer therapy. Nonischemic cardiomyopathies also can result from autoimmune responses to viral infections, and they may occur postpartum, possibly as an immune response in the mother to fetal tissue that somehow enters the maternal circulation. The functional consequences of the nonischemic CHF is a more diffuse and global abnormality of ventricular contractility. Sustained pressure or volume overload resulting in an increased left ventricular pressure with consequent hypertrophy can cause nonischemic cardiomyopathy. Pressure overload can be caused by aortic stenosis, sustained hypertension, or coarctation of aorta. Volume overload can be a result of mitral regurgitation, aortic regurgitation, or ventricular septal defect. Left ventricular filling restrictions resulting in an inability of the ventricles to fill readily with blood ejected from the atria during diastole attributable to mitral stenosis, pericardial restriction or constriction, or severe hypertro-

phy can cause nonischemic cardiomyopathy and lead to CHF.

Regardless of etiology, from a functional standpoint there are two types of heart failure: systolic and diastolic. In **systolic heart failure**, impaired contraction of the ventricles during systole produces an inefficient expulsion of blood, which leads to a backup of blood in the lungs, because venous return can outpace forward cardiac output. This sequence usually is marked by a decrease in the left ventricular ejection fraction or some other marker of contractility. Patients can have abnormally low LV ejection fraction values without having heart failure, however. **Diastolic heart failure** is caused by an inability of the ventricles to readily accept the blood ejected from the atria during diastole. Diastolic dysfunction usually is diagnosed based on abnormalities of the early filling period seen on Doppler echocardiographic examination. A patient may have both types of CHF simultaneously.

The inappropriately low cardiac output stimulates the chain of compensatory mechanisms that form the pathophysiologic picture of CHF. First, the sympathetic nervous system increases peripheral vascular vasoconstriction to improve venous return. This is a baroreceptor-mediated reflex that occurs in an attempt to improve cardiac output. Stimulation of the sympathetic nervous system also results in increased heart rate, likewise intended to increase cardiac output. Both of these reactions, which are normal compensatory physiologic responses to transiently low cardiac output (e.g., the onset of exercise or standing up quickly from a sitting position) act to compound the problem. The result often is a reduction in cardiac output because of an increase in the amount of blood in poorly contracting or already filling ventricles (increased **preload**) and an increase in the amount of work imposed on the heart, both because of increased peripheral vascular vasoconstriction (increased **afterload**) and increased heart rate that makes the heart work harder. Increased ventricular filling pressure can drive blood backward into the lungs, producing pulmonary edema and leading to the dyspnea that is characteristic of CHF, and into other areas, producing jugular venous distention and peripheral edema, which also are characteristic of CHF. Because of decreased cardiac output, the kidneys respond with water and sodium retention, further increasing the problem of volume overload. This response pattern results in a chronic overactive sympathetic stimulation that eventually desensitizes the heart to beta-adrenergic receptor stimulation and decreases the inotropic effect normally associated with sympathetic stimulation. As part of the cycle of poor cardiac output leading to increased catecholamine release, the patient with CHF often winds up with chronically elevated blood catecholamines (i.e., catecholamine poisoning), which may predispose the heart to arrhythmias, often the mechanism of death in CHF. The confounding effects of renal fluid retention, increased neurohumoral activity, deconditioning secondary to the discomfort of exercising, and musculoskeletal abnormalities (which may be primary features of CHF), as well as abnormalities of hematologic, hepatic, pancreatic, and biochemical function, further impair cardiac performance and the exercise tolerance of patients with CHF.

Reasons for Limitation of Exercise Capacity

One of the main features of patients with chronic heart failure is reduced exercise capacity, characterized by shortness of breath and general fatigue or both. The underlying mechanism seems to be very complex in its origins and has been studied extensively.

Central Hemodynamics

Because of ventricular dysfunction, the heart's pumping ability is reduced. Less blood and, therefore, an inadequate amount of oxygen are delivered to the working muscle. This ventricular dysfunction results in an increased ventricular filling pressure due to vascular constriction (1, 2). This vascular constriction results in less aerobic energy supply, phosphagen depletion, early lactate accumulation, shortness of breath, and fatigue (3). Nevertheless, studies have found a weak relation between indices of central hemodynamics and exercise capacity (4–7). Although most patients with CHF have a reduced left ventricular ejection fraction, there is a very poor correlation between left ventricular ejection fraction and maximal oxygen uptake or the presence of CHF.

Pulmonary Function

The ventilatory response to exercise in patients with chronic heart failure has been shown to be abnormal. Minute ventilation (V_E) is higher than in normal subjects at any given level of exercise (2, 5, 7). At any given level of carbon dioxide production, V_E is increased, resulting in a higher than normal $V_E/\dot{V}CO_2$ slope that correlates with exercise capacity in patients with chronic heart failure (8–10). The $V_E/\dot{V}CO_2$ slope has been shown to be prognostically useful (11, 12). A complete explanation of the mechanism underlying this abnormal ventilatory response to exercise is still lacking, although many hypotheses have been proposed. Although a cause–effect relationship has not been established, there usually is an increase in physiologic dead space in patients with CHF. Surprisingly, in view of the tendency to back up blood into the lungs, there is not a diagnostically consistent pattern of elevation of the pulmonary capillary wedge pressure in CHF, or a particularly consistent response to the pulmonary capillary wedge pressure during exercise.

Skeletal Muscle

Studies of **skeletal muscle** in patients with CHF have revealed widespread abnormalities that may contribute to the exercise intolerance of CHF. Early onset of exertional fatigue is commonly reported in CHF. The muscle changes have similarities to those seen in individuals who have been immobilized and have developed disuse atrophy (13). Muscle mass has been shown to be a determinant of exercise capacity in normal subjects (14), and, because muscle atrophy appears to be common in patients with CHF, it seems reasonable to attribute at least part of the exertional intolerance to simple loss of muscle tissue. Studies have found severe muscle atrophy, whether calf, thigh, or total muscle atrophy. These studies have used sensitive procedures such as computed tomography, magnetic resonance imaging, and dual energy X-ray absorptiometry. This muscle atrophy seems to appear in all stages of CHF, regardless of whether the CHF is mild, moderate, or severe (15–18).

Histology

Reduced skeletal muscle oxidative capacity has been observed in patients with CHF. An increase in type II muscle fiber distribution is accompanied by reductions in fiber size. This contributes to reductions in exercise capacity, because Type II fibers tire more easily than Type I (19–21). Drexler et al. (21) also found reduced volume density of mitochondria and surface density of mitochondrial cristae, especially in patients with severe heart failure, likely related to the duration of heart failure. This finding implies a reduced oxidative capacity of skeletal muscles compared to those of healthy individuals. Early lactate accumulation during exercise, which is very common in patients with CHF, has been related to reduced oxidative capacity of the skeletal muscles, to hyperventilation, and to exercise intoleranc e (22–25).

Skeletal Muscle Ergoreflex

Ergoreceptors are afferent nerve endings sensitive to metabolic products of muscular exercise (26). When these receptors are stimulated by metabolites of exercise, there is both a hemodynamic (BP, HR) and ventilatory response. Studies have revealed that these receptors are overactive in patients with CHF during both arm and leg exercise, further explaining the increased ventilatory response during exercise in these patients (27–29).

Respiratory Muscle Strength

Reduced **respiratory muscle strength** has been reported in patients with CHF (30, 31), although the studies have been criticized on methodologic grounds. A recent study by Hughes et al. (32), using investigative methods and protocols that were less difficult for participants, revealed a mild reduction in diaphragm strength, which the investigators related to a possible increase in proportion of slow-twitch (type I) fibers, although the overall strength of the respiratory muscles was well preserved.

Exercise Response

Acute Cardiopulmonary Responses

The exercise capacity of patients with CHF is limited by many factors. They show reduced maximal oxygen uptake for age, and have a high breathing reserve, reduced oxygen uptake/work rate relation, a steep heart rate/oxygen uptake relation, and inefficient ventilation. In addition, they show chronotrophic incompetence, low cardiac output, and an attenuated blood pressure response, but a higher central arteriovenous difference (22, 33–35).

Left Ventricular Function

Studies have revealed that impaired resting left ventricular (**LV**) **ejection fraction** is not necessarily an indicator of further LV deterioration during exercise. Patients with CHF can increase their LV stroke volume through Frank-Starling augmentation from an increased end-diastolic volume. Alternatively, **LV ejection fraction** remains essentially stable throughout exercise (34–37).

Responses During Steady State Exercise

There are limited data on LV function during steady state exercise in patients with CHF. Meyer et al. (38) showed significant increases in heart rate and systolic blood pressure. The patients increased their LV ejection fraction and cardiac output significantly. Lactate levels also have been shown to increase. Importantly, the pattern of changes in LV ejection fraction during steady state exercise in CHF patients is substantially similar to those documented in patients with stable coronary heart disease and in healthy individuals, although at a lower absolute LV ejection fraction (38). The most significant exercise limitation of patients with CHF is an intolerance for sustained exercise. Probably because they are always at an unfavorable part of the length-tension relationship of the sarcomeres in the left ventricle, any further increases in the length of these sarcomeres (such as occurs with increases in the left ventricular end diastolic volume) is likely to be poorly tolerated.

Responses During Resistance Exercise

During isometric exercise, the systemic vascular resistance and mean arterial pressure increase to a great extent. This increase in afterload can potentially result in deleterious effect on the left ventricle (reduced stroke volume and LV ejection fraction). During dynamic resistance exercise for the lower body, systolic blood pressure, diastolic blood pressure, and heart rate have all been shown to increase significantly. Cardiac output has been shown to increase significantly, with the LV ejection fraction remaining stable. The larger increase in afterload during resistance exercise compared to steady-state exercise does not seem to result in left ventricular deterioration (39–42).

Therapeutic Approaches to Chronic Heart Failure

The usual pharmacologic approach in patients with CHF includes ACE inhibitors, beta blockers, digitalis, diuretics, and salt restriction. The goal is to decrease both the preload and the afterload and to reduce the toxic effects of a chronically overactive sympathetic nervous system, prevent recurrent hospitalizations due to worsening heart failure, decrease edema and mortality, and increase the quality of life in these patients.

ACE Inhibitors

Angiotensin II induces vasoconstriction and increases sodium and water retention, resulting in an increased afterload. The angiotensin-converting enzyme (ACE) inhibitors affect hemodynamics favorably by reducing this afterload, and also prevent ventricular remodeling and enlargement (43). Large pharmaceutical trials have demonstrated that **ACE inhibitors** reduce hospitalization and mortality (44–46).

Beta-blockers

Studies have shown that when **beta-blockers** are added to conventional therapy (e.g., ACE inhibitors, diuretics, and digitalis), cardiac function (e.g., LV ejection fraction) improves, and mortality and morbidity are reduced. Patients with heart failure have a chronically overactive sympathetic system; beta-blockers act to antagonize this overactivity and therefore protect the myocytes from catecholamine toxicity. Among other benefits, beta blockers reduce the incidence of arrhythmias in patients with CHF.

Digoxin

Digoxin has a positive ionotropic effect, increasing cardiac output both at rest and during exercise, whether in combination with ACE inhibitors or alone. These effects are sustained during chronic therapy. Digoxin has not been shown to increase survival but has been shown to decrease the incidence of hospitalization due to worsening heart failure (47, 48).

Diuretics

By decreasing preload, **diuretics** improve cardiovascular hemodynamics and relieve symptoms. Long-term use reduces left heart filling pressure during exercise with no alterations in cardiac output (49, 50).

Salt Restriction

The kidneys respond to reduced cardiac ouput by retaining water and **sodium**. Even patients with mild heart failure are unable to secrete salt normally if they consume a high-salt diet (51). The usual advice is to limit sodium diet to 3 g/d, by adding no salt to foods when cooking, and avoiding foods known to have a high sodium content. In the case of severe volume overload, it is necessary to restrict sodium intake to less than 2 g/d. Without these restrictions, the effects of diuretics are reduced, leading to the need to increase the dose of diuretics (52).

Transplant Criteria

Exercise capacity has been shown to be an independent prognostic factor in patients with CHF. A peak exercise $\dot{V}O_2$ value of 14 ml/kg/min has been recognized as the cutpoint for considering transplantation (53), based on data indicating that patients with lower $\dot{V}O_2$ values have a very poor prognosis (1-year survival < 50%). Recent studies have revealed, however, that other cutpoints, ranging between 10 and 17 ml/kg/min, are as effective as a peak $\dot{V}O_2$ of 14 ml/kg/min (54, 55). Other criteria have been recommended, including a $\dot{V}O_{2max}$ of less than 50% of the age- and gender-predicted level. This remains an area of active investigation, because the number of patients who could potentially benefit from transplantation greatly exceeds the number of available organs.

Exercise Therapy

Historical Perspective

Up until the late 1980s, bed rest and restriction of physical activity were commonly prescribed for patients with CHF. Exercise was considered harmful, and the exercise intolerance secondary to heart failure was viewed as a warning symptom. One reason for this belief was a study in patients who had experienced large anterior wall MIs (56). This study showed that exercise training led to myocardial wall thinning, infarct expansion, further asynergy, and reduced ejection fraction. More recently, studies have shown that exercise training does not lead to a further worsening of ventricular function (57, 58) or to myocardial remodeling.

Aerobic Training

Most training studies in patients with CHF have been based on **aerobic exercise**. None of these studies have demonstrated adverse effects that could be related to the exercise, implying that endurance training is safe in patients with CHF, and aerobic training is still the approach most widely used for patients with CHF. Most patients participating in these studies have been of class II-III on the New York Heart Association (NYHA) Heart Failure Classification scale. Patients in NYHA class IV have not been considered candidates for exercise training. Most of the patients studied have been men. Exercise trials usually have lasted from 4 weeks up to 1 year. In most, the exercise intensity has been between 40% and 85% of $\dot{V}O_2$ peak or heart rate reserve, with each session lasting 20 to 60 minutes, and the training occurring on 3 to 5 days per week. The training mode has usually been cycling or walking (59). An increase in $\dot{V}O_{2max}$ usually has been reported following training (58, 60–63). This increase in exercise capacity has been related to several factors, but is due primarily to peripheral adaptations. In these studies few patients have been taking beta-blockers. The increase in cardiac output has been related to increases in maximum heart rate, small increases in maximal stroke volume, and a reduction in systemic vascular resistance. Left ventricular contractility, on the other hand, seems to be unchanged at rest and during exercise (58, 64–66). Widening of the maximal a-v O_2 difference has been observed, implying better oxygen extraction in the metabolically active muscle (58, 65, 66). The ventilatory threshold has been shown to increase, implying more effective metabolism (67, 68). Hambrecht et al. found an increase in total volume density of mitochondrial cristae and an increase in the volume density of cytochrome C oxidase-positive mitochondria after exercise training for 6 months. This result suggests that exercise training improves muscle oxidative capacity. In another study, Hambrecht et al. found that endurance training resulted in a reshift in fiber type ratio (e.g., fiber type I/fiber type II shifted from 48%/52% at baseline to 52%/48% after 6 months of training) (69, 70). Kiilavuori et al., on the other hand, observed no changes in fiber type distribution in patients with CHF after endurance training lasting 6 months (71). Endurance training has been shown to decrease V_E at a fixed submaximal work and decrease the $V_E/\dot{V}CO_2$ slope, thereby improving ventilatory efficiency. This is an important finding, because patients with heart failure often are limited by dyspnea or a sense of breathlessness (65, 66, 72). Endurance training has been shown to correct endothelial dysfunction and decrease peripheral resistance (73, 74). Endurance training also has been shown to have a positive effect on the already overactive sympathetic nervous system, resulting in decreased noradrenalin levels at rest and during submaximal exercise and reductions in resting levels of neurohormones (angiotensin II, vasopressin, atrial natriuretic peptide) (69, 73, 75, 76). This type of training also has resulted in improved quality of life.

Resistance Training

Aerobic training does not reliably result in increased muscle strength. Activities of daily living require both endurance and strength. Therefore, it is logical to think that **resistance training** would be of value for this group of patients as it is for others. Added to the overall muscle atrophy that is related to their decreased functional capacity, patients with CHF show both a decrease in fiber type I distribution and, because CHF usually is a disease of elderly persons, a decrease in fiber type II distribution associated with increasing age. Resistance training should, therefore, be considered a potentially beneficial treatment for patients with CHF. There has been concern that increased afterload during resistance training would be poorly tolerated and harmful for CHF patients. The studies that have been published using either solely resistance training or a combination of aerobic and resistance training have shown promising results, however, with no evidence of adverse events during training sessions or that could be related to the exercise sessions. Forearm muscle training has even been shown to decrease ergoreflex contributions, positively affecting breathing (27).

Because patients with CHF have a low cardiac reserve, several investigators have proposed that whole body training might not be an optimal training method for this group of patients. The use of a single muscle group produces lower demand on the heart than whole body work and better blood flow to the working muscle. Studies that have used single muscle group training have shown good results without side effects. The training periods have lasted 8 to 12 weeks, with exercise sessions 3 to 4 times a week. Some, but not all, of these studies have shown increases in $\dot{V}O_{2max}$. All of the studies have shown increases in strength, improved oxidative capacity in the muscle, and decreased blood lactate concentration during submaximal exercise, and have found no evidence that exercise worsens the underlying heart failure (77–80). As in cardiac patients with normal left ventricular function, circuit weight training in patients with heart failure has resulted in improved strength, delayed anaerobic threshold and lower oxygen consumption at submaximal workloads, even though $\dot{V}O_{2max}$ has not increased (81, 82).

To obtain a positive effect on most of the factors related to the decreased exercise capacity of patients with CHF, a combination of both endurance and strength training would seem to be the best and most effective approach. The studies published have revealed that this combination leads to a significantly greater increase in functional capacity than aerobic training alone, leading to both higher work capacity and peak oxygen uptake, and, in addition, increased strength. None of these studies reported any adverse effects related to training (83–85).

Interval Training

Most activities of daily living are intermittent in nature. It is of interest that in patients who have very low initial exercise capacity at baseline, traditional exercise testing results usually preclude endurance training from being of a higher intensity than what the patients are already accustomed to during their activities of daily living.

Interval training has been shown to be more effective than steady-state training in improving exercise capacity and decreasing lactate at submaximal levels in patients after bypass surgery (86). Because training effects in patients with CHF are primarily peripheral, interval training has been proposed as a method to fully stress the working muscles without causing cardiac overstrain. Meyer et al. (86–88) have shown that, during this type of training, the work rate during training can be much higher than the traditional 75% of peak oxygen uptake, allowing more exercise stimuli on peripheral muscles while still producing minimal cardiac strain. They have developed a special steep ramp test to determine work intensity for work phases in interval training. During that test, patients achieve a work rate 43% to 121% higher than during a traditional ramping exercise test, while cardiac stress remains significantly lower. Different work phases during intervals have been studied, following a protocol using 30-second work /60-second recovery phases. The resistance is set at 50% of the maximal power achieved during the steep ramp test for the work phases and 10 watts during the recovery phases. These studies have shown that the metabolic demands are higher, evidenced by higher lactate accumulation; the hemodynamic and gas exchange responses are no different from those during steady-state training; and the LV function remains stable or unchanged, at least in pattern, compared to that of patients with normal left ventricular function, indicating that this type of training is safe.

CASE STUDY

Mr. S. is a 47-year-old man with precocious coronary heart disease. He had an anterior wall MI at age 42, without invasive follow-up. At age 44 he had an anterolateral wall MI. His hospital course was complicated by what appeared to be inferior extension of this infarct and the development of cardiogenic shock. Cardiac catheterization following this MI revealed a totally occluded left anterior descending artery and a proximal 80% lesion in the circumflex artery. His left ventricular ejection fraction was estimated to be 22%. He was treated with percutaneous transluminal coronary angioplasty of the circumflex lesion with a stent and placed on ACE inhibitors, diuretics, and digitalis. After a difficult hospital course, which involved placement of an intra-aortic balloon pump for 2 days, he stabilized and finally was discharged 12 days after admission. Following 2 weeks of rest at home he was referred for rehabilitation.

Despite regular attendance his early course in rehabilitation has been unsatisfactory. He is still quite weak and develops dyspnea after only 5 minutes of slow walking. He reports that he is sleeping with three pillows and often has edema in his ankles. He would like to return to work as an office manager, but at this time he does not see how or when he might be able to do this. He was referred to the heart failure unit for evaluation and modification of his medical management and exercise program.

Mr. S. presented to the exercise laboratory saying that he was having a "good day." His height was 170 cm, and he weighed 93 kg. He was still taking ACE inhibitors, diuretics, and digitalis. His resting electrocardiogram revealed sinus rhythm with a left bundle branch block pattern. He performed a Stage 1 cycle ergometer test. After 3 minutes of unloaded pedaling, the power output was increased in increments of 17 watts per minute until he stopped pedaling, after 11 minutes, at a power output of 98 watts. His hemodynamic response was notable for a large HR reserve (67% predicted HR achieved) (Figure 4.1). His VO$_2$ response revealed a peak VO$_2$ of 1.35 L/min or 14.7 ml/min/kg and a ventilatory threshold of 1.13 L/min or 12.1 ml/min/kg (Figure 4.2). No arrhythmias occurred during the exercise test. Because of the left bundle branch block pattern, the exercise test

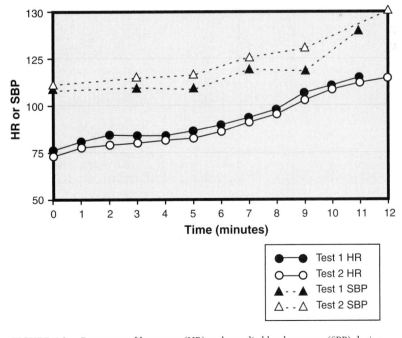

FIGURE 4.1. Responses of heart rate (HR) and systolic blood pressure (SBP) during incremental ergometry demonstrating the overall normality of the response pattern (although with a large HR reserve) and the slight improvement evident from Test 1 to Test 2 (i.e., before and after the exercise program included interval and resistance exercise).

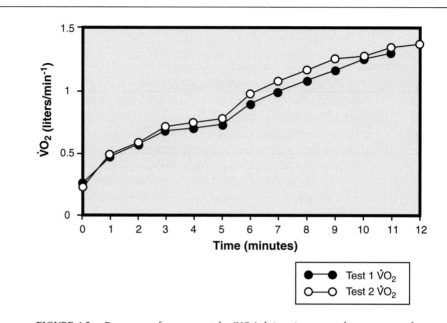

FIGURE 4.2. Responses of oxygen uptake (VO$_2$) duirng incremental ergometry and the improvement from Test 1 to Test 2. The improvement in VO$_2$ (5%) was small, however, compared to the improvement in muscular power evident in the steep ramp test (180 to 270 watts, or 50%).

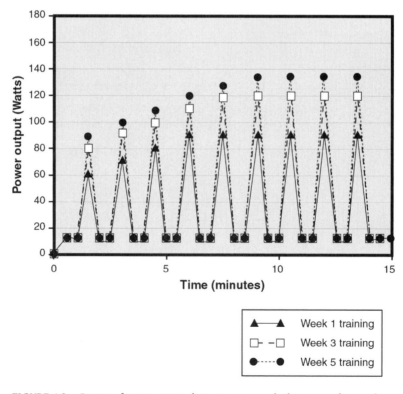

FIGURE 4.3. Pattern of power output during training at the beginnng of interval training, after the adjustment at the end of week 2, and after the adjustment at the end of week 4. Note that the first several repetitions are always easier—to allow for warm-up—and that the 60-second recovery segments remain the same (10 watts) throughout the training program.

was nondiagnostic for ischemia. After resting for 30 minutes, Mr. S. performed a steep ramp cycle test to a power output of 180 watts. On the basis of these findings, the dosage of his diuretics was increased slightly, and he was referred for interval and resistance exercise in the rehabilitation center.

Mr. S. reported to the rehabilitation center for 4 weeks on a daily (Monday through Friday) basis. After a general warm-up involving range-of-motion exercises, he performed interval training on the cycle ergometer. The pattern of power output during the initial training session was 90 watts for 30 seconds followed by 10 watts for 60 seconds, repeated for 15 minutes (Figure 4.3). Additionally, following the interval training, he performed two sets of 10 repetitions at 60% of 1RM of the following exercises: arm press (unilateral); leg press (bilateral); biceps curls (one arm at a time); and modified squats. The rest time between sets was adjusted to minimize dyspnea. After 2 weeks the steep ramp test was repeated (achieving a workload of 240 watts) because the workloads needed to be modified, as they had begun to feel very easy.

After 4 weeks Mr. S. was restudied in the exercise laboratory. At that time he achieved a peak power output of 115 watts with a peak VO_2 of 1.42 L/min or 15.3 ml/min/kg and a ventilatory threshold of 1.22 L/min or 13.1 ml/min/kg. During the steep ramp test, he achieved a power output of 270 watts. He reported much less difficulty walking on his own, and was sleeping on only one pillow. Without consulting his physicians, he had begun to visit his office for an hour or so on his way home from the exercise program.

On the basis of these results, his formal exercise program was reduced to 3 days per week, with advice to walk easily for 15 to 20 minutes on other days of the week. Furthermore, he was advised to continue trying to increase his time at the office.

Summary

Patients with CHF respond to exercise training much like patients with other forms of cardiovascular disease. In general, they are very debilitated at program entry, respond very well to brief bouts of exercise training, and probably are better managed by using perceived exertion than by some arbitrary percentage of the maximal heart rate. Because the periphery is where most training-related adaptations can take place, resistance training and interval training hold great promise. Although these forms of training are alarming conceptually to many physicians, if they are managed in very brief work periods they seem to cause a reliable increase in functional capacity without evidence of left ventricular functional or other clinical deterioration. It must be remembered that patients with CHF are inherently unstable and will periodically "go sour." However, such clinical deterioration seems to be related not to exercise training, but to the natural history of CHF. This underlying instability suggests that careful clinical evaluation of CHF patients before each training session is appropriate to rule out new instability.

REFERENCES

1. Weber KT, Kinasewitz GT, Janicki JS, Fishman AP. Oxygen utilisation and ventilation during exercise in patients with chronic cardiac failure. Circulation 1982;65:1213–1223.
2. Sullivan MJ, Higginbotham MB, Cobb FR. Increased exercise ventilation in patients with chronic heart failure: intact ventilatory control despite haemodynamic and pulmonary abnormalities. Circulation 1988;77:552–559.
3. Myers J. Effect of exercise training on abnormal ventilatory responses to exercise in patients with chronic heart failure. Congest Heart Fail 2000;6:243–249, 255.
4. Franciosa JA, Park M, Levine TB. Lack of correlation between exercise capacity and indices of resting left ventricular performance in heart failure. Am J Cardiol 1981;47:33–39.
5. Franciosa JA, Leddy CL, Wilden M, et al. Relation between hemodynamic and ventilatory responses in determining exercise capacity in severe congestive heart failure. Am J Cardiol 1984;53:127–134.
6. Weber KT, Wilson JR, Janicki J, Likoff MJ. Exercise testing in the evaluation of the patient with chronic cardiac failure. Am Rev Resp Dis 1984;129(suppl):S60–S62.
7. Higginbotham MB, Morris KG, Conn EH, et al. Determinants of variable exercise performance among patients with severe left ventricular dysfunction. Am J Cardiol 1983;51:52–60.
8. Buller NP, Poole-Wilson PA. Mechanism of the increased ventilatory response to exercise in patients with chronic heart failure. Br Heart J 1990;63:281–283.
9. Davies SW, Emery TM, Watling MIL, et al. A critical threshold of exercise capacity in the ventilatory respone to exercise in heart failure. Br Heart J 1991;65:179–183.
10. Harrington D, Coats JS. Mechanisms of exercise intolerance in congestive heart failure. Curr Opin Cardiol 1997;12:224–232.
11. Kleber FX, Vietzke G, Wernecke KD, et al. Impairment of ventilatory efficiency in heart failure. Prognostic impact. Circulation 2000;101:2803–2809.
12. Francis DP, Shamim W, Davies LC, et al. Cardiopulmonary exercise testing for prognosis in chronic heart failure: continuous and independent prognostic value from VE/VCO(2) slope and peak VO(2). Eur Heart J 2000;21:154–161.
13. Harrington D, Coats JS. Skeletal muscle abnormalities and evidence for their role in symptom generation in chronic heart failure. Eur Heart J 1997;18:1865–1872.

14. Shepard R, Bouhlel E, Vandewalle H, Monod H. Muscle mass as a factor limiting physical work. J Appl Physiol 1988;64:1472–1479.

15. Mancini D, Walter G, Reichek N, et al. Contribution of skeletal muscle atrophy to exercise intolerance and altered muscle metabolism in heart failure. Circulation 1992;85:1364–1373.

16. Miyagi K, Asanoi H, Ishizak S, et al. Loss of skeletal muscle mass is a major determinant of exercise tolerance in chronic heart failure. Circulation 1991;84(suppl II): II-74.

17. Minotti JR, Pillay P, Oka R, et al. Skeletal muscle size: relationship to muscle function in heart failure. J Appl Physiol 1993;75:373–381.

18. Magnusson G, Isberg B, Karlberg K, Sylven C. Skeletal muscle strength and endurance in chronic congestive heart failure secondary to idiopathic dilated cardiomyopathy. Am J Cardiol 1994;73:307–309.

19. Yancy CW Jr, Parsons D, Lane L, et al. Capillary density, fiber type and enzyme composition of skeletal muscle in congestive heart failure. J Am Coll Cardiol 1989;13(suppl):38A.

20. Sullivan MJ, Green HJ, Cobb FR. Skeletal muscle biochemistry and histology in ambulatory patients with long-term heart failure. Circulation 1990;81:518–527.

21. Drexler H, Riede U, Munzel T, et al. Alterations of skeletal muscle in chronic heart failure. Circulation 1992;85:1751–1759.

22. Sullivan MJ, Hawthorne M. Exercise intolerance in patients with chronic heart failure. Prog Cardiovasc Dis 1995;38:1–22.

23. Myers J, Froelicher VF. Hemodynamic determinants of exercise capacity in chronic heart failure. Ann Intern Med 1991;115:377–386.

24. Sullivan MJ, Cobb FR. The anaerobic threshold in chronic heart failure: Relation to blood lactate, ventilatory basis, reproducibility and response to exercise training. Circulation 1990;81(suppl II):II47–II58.

25. Sullivan MJ, Green HJ, Cobb FR. Altered skeletal muscle metabolic response to exercise in chronic heart failure. Circulation 1991;84:1597–1607.

26. Piepoli M, Clark AL, Coats AJS. Muscle metaboreceptor in the haemodynamic, autonomic and ventilatory responses to exercise in men. Am J Physiol 1995;38:H1428–1436.

27. Piepoli M, Clark AL, Volteranni M, et al. Contribution of muscle afferents to the hemodynamic, autonomic and ventilatory responses to exercise in patients with chronic heart failure. Effects of physical training. Circulation 1996;93:940–953.

28. Piepoli M, Ponikowski P, Clark AL, et al. A neural link to explain the "muscle hypothesis" of exercise intolerance in chronic heart failure. Am Heart J 1999;137:1050–1056.

29. Grieve DAA, Clark AL, McCann GP, Hillis WS. The ergoreflex in patients with chronic stable heart failure. Int J Cardiol 1999;68:157–164.

30. Ambrosino N, Opasich C, Crotti P, et al. Breathing pattern, ventilatory drive and respiratory muscle strength in patients with chronic heart failure. Eur Respir J 1994;7:17–22.

31. McParland C, Khrishnan B, Wang Y, Gallagher C. Inspiratoy muscle weakness and dyspnea in chronic heart failure. Am Rev Respir Dis 1992;146:467–472.

32. Hughes PD, Polkey MI, Harris ML, et al. Diaphragm strength in chronic heart failure. Am J Respir Crit Care Med 1999;160:529–534.

33. Myers JN. Applications in cardiovascular and pulmonary disease. In: Essentials of Cardiopulmonary Testing. Champaign, IL: Human Kinetics, 1996;109–131.

34. Kitzman DW, Higginbotham MB, Cobb FR, et al. Exercise intolerance in patients with heart failure and preserved left ventricular systolic function: failure of the Frank-Starling mechanism. J Am Coll Cardiol 1991;17:1065–1072.

35. Higginbotham MB, Morris KG, Conn EH, et al. Determinants of variable exercise performance among patients with severe left ventricular dysfunction. Am J Cardiol 1983;51:52–60.

36. Port S, McEwan P, Cobb FR, Jones RH. Influence of resting left ventricular function on the left ventricular response to exercise in patients with coronary artery disease. Circulation 1981;63:856–863.

37. Conn EH, Williams RS, Wallace AG. Exercise responses before and after physical conditioning in patients with severely depressed left ventricular function. Am J Cardiol 1982;49:296–300.

38. Meyer K, Foster C, Georgakopoulos N, et al. Comparison of left ventricular function during interval versus steady-state exercise training in patients with chronic congestive heart failure. Am J Cardiol 1998;82:1382–1387.

39. Reddy HK, Weber KT, Janicki JS, McElroy PA. Hemodynamic, ventilatory and metabolic effects of light isometric exercise in patients with chronic heart failure. J Am Coll Cardiol 1988;12:353–358.

40. Keren G, Katz S, Gage J, et al. Effect of isometric exercise on cardiac performance and mitral regurgitation in patients with severe congestive heart failure. Am Heart J 1989;118:973–979.

41. McKelvie RS, McCartney N, Tomlinson C, et al. Comparison of hemodynamic responses to cycling and resistance exercise in congestive heart failure secondary to ischemic cardiomyopathy. Am J Cardiol 1995;76:977–979.

42. Meyer K, Hajric R, Westbrook S, et al. Hemodynamic responses during leg press exercise in patients with chronic congestive heart failure. Am J Cardiol 1999;83:1537–1543.

43. Cohn JN. Heart failure: future treatment approaches. Am J Hypertens 2000;13:74S–78S.

44. Effect of enalapril on survival in patients with reduced left ventricular ejection fractions and congestive heart failure. The SOLVD Investigators. N Engl J Med 1991;325:293–302.

45. Effect of enalapril on mortality and the development of heart failure in asymptomatic patients with reduced left ventricular ejection fractions. The SOLVD Investigators. N Engl J Med 1992;327:685–691.

46. Effects of enalapril on mortality in severe congestive heart failure. Results of the Cooperative North Scandinavian Enalapril Survival Study (CONSENSUS). The CONSENSUS Trial Study Group. N Engl J Med 1987;316:1429–1435.

47. The Digitalis Investigators Group. The effect of digoxin on mortality and morbidity in patients with heart failure. N Engl J Med 1997;336:525–533.

48. Gheorghiade M. Digoxin therapy in chronic heart failure. Cardiovasc Drugs Ther 1997;11:279–283.

49. Silke B. Haemodynamic impact of diuretic therapy in chronic heart failure. Cardiology 1994;84(suppl 2):115–123.

50. Kramer BK, Schweda F, Riegger GAJ. Diuretic treatment and diuretic resistance in heart failure. Am J Med 1999;106:90–96.

51. Volpe M, Tritto C, DeLuca N, et al. Abnormalities of sodium handling and of cardiovascular adaptations during high salt diet in patients with mild heart failure. Circulation 1993;88:1620–1627.

52. Lenihan DJ, Uretsky BF. Nonpharmacologic treatment of heart failure in the elderly. Clin Geriatric Medicine 2000;16:477–487.

53. Mancini DM, Eisen H, Kussmaul W, et al. Value of peak exercise oxygen consumption for optimal timing of cardiac transplantation in ambulatory patients with heart failure. Circulation 1991;83:778–786.

54. Myers J, Gullestad L, Vagelos R, et al. Clinical, hemodynamic, and cardiopulmonary exercise test determinants of survival in patients referred for evaluation of heart failure. Ann Intern Med 1998;129:286–293.

55. Myers J, Gullestad L, Vagelos R, et al. Cardiopulmonary exercise testing and prognosis in severe heart failure: 14 ml/kg/min revisited. Am Heart J 2000;139:78–84.

56. Judgutt BI, Michorowski BL, Kappagoda CT. Exercise training after anterior Q wave myocardial infarction: Importance of regional left ventricular function and topography. J Am Coll Cardiol 1988;12:362–372.

57. Belardinelli R, Reorgiou D, Cianci G, et al. Effects of exercise training on left ventricular filling at rest and during exercise in patients with ischemic cardiomyopathy and severe left ventricular systolic dysfunction. Am Heart J 1996;132:61–70.

58. Dubach P, Myers J, Dziekan G, et al. Effect of exercise training on myocardial remodeling in patients with reduced left ventricular function after myocardial infarction: Application of magnetic resonance imaging. Circulation 1997;95:2060–2067.

59. Piepoli MF, Flather M, Coats AJS. Overview of studies of exercise training in chronic heart failure: the need for a prospective randomized multicentre European trial. Eur Heart J 1998;19:830–841.

60. Coats AJS, Adamapoulos S, Meyer TE, et al. Effects of physical training in chronic heart failure. Lancet 1990;335:63–66.

61. Belardinelli R, Georgiou D, Scocco V, et al. Low intensity exercise training in patients with chronic heart failure. J Am Coll Cardiol 1995;26:975–982.

62. Keteyian SJ, Levine AB, Brawner CA, et al. Exercise training in patients with heart failure. A randomized, controlled trial. Ann Intern Med 1996;124:1051–1057.

63. Belardinelli R, Georgiou D, Cianci G, Purcaro A. Randomized, controlled trial of long-term moderate exercise training in chronic heart failure. Effects on functional capacity, quality of life and clinical outcome. Circulation 1999;99:1173–1182.

64. Keteyian SJ, Brawner CA, Schairer JR, et al. Effects of exercise training on chronotropic incompetence in patients with heart failure. Am Heart J 1999;138:233–240.

65. Coats AJS, Stamatis A, Radaelli A, et al. Controlled trial of physical training in chronic heart failure— exercise performance, hemodynamics, ventilation and autonomic function. Circulation 1992;85:2119–2131.

66. Sullivan MJ, Higginbotham MB, Cobb FR. Exercise training in patients with severe left ventricular dysfunction: hemodynamic and metabolic effects. Circulation 1988;78:506–515.

67. Sullivan MJ, Higginbotham MB, Cobb FR. Exercise training in patients with heart failure delays ventilatory anaerobic threshold and improves submaximal exercise performance. Circulation 1989;79:324–329.

68. Kiilavuori K, Sovijarvi A, Naveri H, et al. Effect of physical training on exercise capacity and gas exchange in patients with chronic heart failure. Chest 1996;110:985–981.

69. Hambrecht R, Niebauer J, Fiehn E, et al. Physical training in patients with stable chronic heart failure: effects on cardiorespiratory fitness and ultrastructural abnormalities of leg muscles. J Am Coll Cardiol 1995;25:1239–1249.

70. Hambrecht R, Riehn E, Yu J, et al. Effects of endurance training on mitochondrial ultrastructure and fiber type distribution in skeletal muscle of patients with stable chronic heart failure. J Am Coll Cardiol 1997;29:1067–1073.

71. Kiilavuori K, Naveri H, Salmi T, Harkonnen M. The effect of physical training on skeletal muscle in patients with chronic heart failure. Eur J Heart Failure 2000;2:53–63.

72. Davey P, Meyer T, Coats A, et al. Ventilation in chronic heart failure: effects of physical training. Br Heart J 1992;68:473–477.

73. Hambrecht R, Gielen S, Linke A, et al. Effects of exercise training on left ventricular function and peripheral resistance in patients with chronic heart failure. A randomized trial. JAMA 2000;283:3095–3101.

74. Hambrecht R, Fiehn E, Weigl C, et al. Regular physical exercise corrects endothelial dysfunction and improves exercise capacity in patients with chronic heart failure. Circulation 1998;98:2709–2715.

75. Kiilavuori K, Näveri H, Leinonen H, Härkonen M. The effect of physical training on hormonal status and exertional hormonal response in patients with chronic congestive heart failure. Eur Heart J 1999;20:456–464.

76. Braith FW, Welsch MA, Feigenbaum MS, et al. Neuroendocrine activation in heart failure is modified by endurance exercise training. J Am Coll Cardiol 1999;34:1170–1175.

77. Koch M, Doward H, Broustet J-P. The benefit of graded physical exercise in chronic heart failure. Chest 1992;101:231S–235S.

78. Magnusson G, Gordon A, Kaijser L, et al. High intensity knee extensor training, in patients with chronic heart failure. Eur Heart J 1996;17:1048–1055.

79. Gordon A, Tyni-Lenné R, Persson H, et al. Markedly improved skeletal muscle function with local muscle training in patients with chronic heart failure. Clin Cardiol 1996;19:568–574.

80. Tyni-Lenné R, Gordon A, Europe E, et al. Exercise-based rehabilitation improves skeletal muscle capacity, exercise tolerance and quality of life in both women and men with chronic heart failure. J Cardiac Failure 1998;4:9–17.

81. Cider Å, Tygesson H, Hedberg M, et al. Peripheral muscle training in patients with clinical signs of heart failure. Scand J Rehab Med 1997;29:121–127.

82. Hare DL, Ryan TM, Selig SE, et al. Resistance exercise training increases muscle strength, endurance, and blood flow in patients with chronic heart failure. Am J Cardiol 1999;83:1674–1677.

83. Delargadelle C, Feiereisen P, Krecké R, et al. Objective effects of a 6 months´endurance and strength training program in outpatients with congestive heart failure. Med Sci Sports Exerc 1999;31: 1102–1107.

84. Maiorana A, O´Driscoll G, Cheetham C, et al. Combined aerobic and resistance exercise training improves functional capacity and strength in CHF. J Appl Physiol 2000;88:1565–1570.

85. Barnard KL, Adams KJ, Swank AM, et al. Combined high-intensity strength and aerobic training in patients with congestive heart failure. J Strength Conditioning Res 2000;14:383–388.

86. Meyer K, Lehmann M, Sünder G, et al. Interval versus continuous exercise training after coronary bypass surgery: A comparison of training-induced acute reactions with respect to the effectiveness of the exercise methods. Clin Cardiol 1990;13:851–861.

87. Meyer K, Samek L, Schwaibold M, et al. Interval training in patients with severe chronic heart failure: analysis and recommendations for exercise procedures. Med Sci Sports Exerc 1997;29:306–312.

88. Meyer K, Foster C, Georgakopoulos N, et al. Comparsion of left ventricular function during interval versus steady-state exercise training in patients with chronic congestive heart failure. Am J Cardiol 1998;82:1382–1387.

Lipid and Lipoprotein Disorders

Peter Grandjean, Stephen F. Crouse

CHAPTER 5

SEARCHABLE KEY TERMS

Antihyperlipidemic Drugs	Functional Foods
Apolipoproteins	Hepatic Lipase
Atherogenesis	High-Density Lipoproteins (HDL)
Atherosclerosis	HMG-CoA Reductase Inhibitors
Atherosclerotic Lesion	Homocysteine
Bile Acids	Hypercholesterolemia
Bile Acid Binding Resins	Hyperlipidemia
Cardiovascular Diseases (CVD)	Hypertriglyceridemia
Chemotaxic	Intermediate-Density Lipoproteins (IDL)
Cholesterol	Lecithin:Cholesterol Acyltransferase
Cholesterol Esters	(LCAT)
Cholesterol Ester Transfer Protein (CETP)	Lipoproteins
Chylomicrons	Lipoprotein(a) [Lp(a)]
Coronary Heart Disease (CHD)	Lipoprotein Lipase
Coronary Artery Disease (CAD)	Lipoprotein Receptors
CVD risk factors	Low-Density Lipoproteins (LDL)
Dyslipidemias	Macrophages
Dyspepsia	Metabolic Syndrome
Familial Dyslipidemia	Micelles
Fatty Acids	Mitogenic
Flushing	Monounsaturated Fatty Acids
Foam Cell	Morbidity
Forward Cholesterol Transport	Mortality
Free Cholesterol	Myalgia

Myocardial Infarction	Postprandial
Myopathy	Primary Dyslipidemia
Nonpolar Lipid	Pruritus
Oxidation	Reverse Cholesterol Transport
Peptic Ulcers	Saturated Fatty Acid
Phospholipids	Secondary Dyslipidemia
Plant Stanols	Soluble Fiber
Plant Sterols	Statins
Polar Lipid	Triglycerides
Polyunsaturated Fatty Acid	Vascular Thrombi
Population Attributable Risk	Very Low-Density Lipoproteins (VLDL)

Overview

Currently, **coronary heart disease (CHD)** is a tremendous burden in the United States, accounting for approximately 500,000 deaths and over $100 billion in health care costs annually. Over the last several decades much has been done to identify and address risk factors for the development of CHD and other **cardiovascular diseases (CVD)** in an attempt to reduce the number of cases and improve the quality of life. Diet, exercise, and other lifestyle modifications, as well as pharmacological interventions, have been developed to reduce **morbidity** and **mortality** precipitated by high blood pressure, smoking, obesity, physical inactivity, and high plasma cholesterol. Of these CVD risk factors, high cholesterol has the greatest **population attributable risk** (Figure 5.1). Elevated plasma cholesterol, particularly cholesterol from **low-density lipoproteins (LDLC)**, is strongly related to CHD. The positive and exponential relationship between cholesterol concentrations and CVD-related mortality is illustrated in Figure 5.2. The risk for CVD is even greater for those individuals with high plasma cholesterol and other risk factors or metabolic diseases. On the other hand, **high-density lipoproteins (HDL)** protect against CVD, and the cholesterol associated with these lipoproteins (HDLC) is inversely related to the development of CHD—even in the presence of elevated LDLC (Figure 5.3).

Laboratory research and clinical interventions consistently have shown that treating plasma lipid disorders can reduce the incidence and severity of CHD. In this regard, current pharmacologic interventions have proven to be very

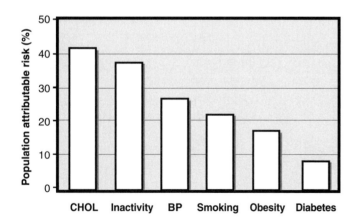

FIGURE 5.1. Cardiovascular disease risk factors and population attributable risk. The population attributable risk is an estimate of the percentage of deaths that would not occur if a risk factor was eliminated. BP, blood pressure; CHOL, blood cholesterol; inactivity, physical inactivity. (Data from Powell [271] and Smith and Pratt [272].)

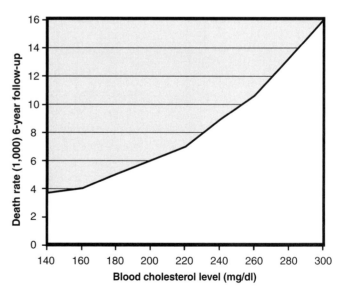

FIGURE 5.2. Relationship between blood cholesterol levels and mortality. (Data from Martin et al. [273].)

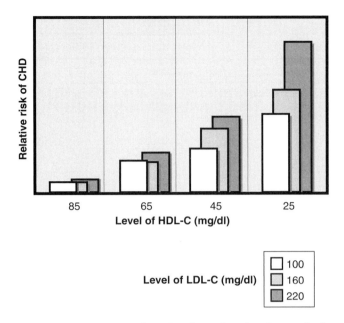

FIGURE 5.3. Interaction of LDLC and HDLC on the relative risk of CHD. This figure illustrates the protective effect of high HDLC levels even with increasing LDLC (see row 1 from left to right). The relative risk of CHD increases with greater LDLC levels as the HDLC levels diminish (rows 2, 3, and 4). (Data from Gordon et al. [45].)

effective. However, other lifestyle changes involving diet and exercise are strongly encouraged as part of an overall therapeutic regimen for managing the most common forms of **dyslipidemias.**

This chapter provides the clinical exercise physiologist with a background in lipid metabolism and transport and an overview of plasma lipid disorders, and describes the current interventions and treatment strategies used in the management of high plasma cholesterol and other dyslipidemias (Box 5.1).

Composition and Function of Lipoproteins

Lipids serve many important biological functions in the human body. **Phospholipids** and **cholesterol** serve as cellular components and precursors of hormones, whereas **triglycerides** provide **fatty acids**, which are a source of energy in metabolically active tissues. Because of their chemical composition, however, lipids are not transported independently in aqueous mediums such as blood, interstitial fluid, and lymph. Thus, the primary function of **lipoproteins** is to transport water-insoluble lipids from their site of absorption or synthesis to target tissues. Plasma lipoproteins are a heterogeneous group of aggregate molecules made up of various lipids and specialized proteins called **apolipoproteins** (1, 2). The outer surface of the lipoprotein is generally comprised of hydrophilic **polar lipids**, such as phospholipids and **free cholesterol**. The lipoprotein core is made up of hydrophobic **nonpolar lipids**, such as triglycerides and **cholesterol esters** (3). The various apolipoproteins help stabilize the lipoprotein in transit, serve as ligands for lipid delivery to various tissues throughout the body, and act as cofactors in enzymatic reactions of lipoprotein metabolism (1, 4, 5).

Plasma lipoproteins are classified according to particle size and density as well as lipid and protein composition (5). The larger, more buoyant lipoproteins are characterized by a higher percentage of nonpolar core lipids and a relatively small protein mass. As particle size diminishes, the density increases, due to greater relative protein mass and lower lipid content. Consequently, lipoproteins most often are classified according to their buoyant density (g/mL) as determined by ultracentrifugation (1, 2). Table 5.1 lists lipoproteins commonly found in human plasma according to their buoyant density and relative protein and lipid mass.

Each of the lipoprotein classes has specialized functions in the transport and delivery of lipids. These functions are mediated, at least in part, by the specific apolipoprotein component of the lipoprotein. Table 5.2 lists the lipoprotein distribution and function of apolipoproteins.

Lipoprotein Transport Pathways

Plasma lipoprotein transport is a complex system that is regulated by apolipoproteins, intravascular enzymes, lipid transfer proteins, and **lipoprotein receptors** that are found in cells throughout the body. Two major pathways often are used to explain the metabolic steps, lipid transfers, and apolipoprotein exchanges that take place in this dynamic process. **Forward cholesterol transport**, first described by Brown and Goldstein (6), is a process in which lipoproteins of intestinal or hepatic origin deliver cholesterol to peripheral tissues (1, 2, 7). **Reverse cholesterol transport** is the process in which cholesterol is removed from peripheral tissues and carried back to the liver (8–11). Although these

TABLE 5.1.   GENERAL CLASSIFICATIONS AND COMPOSITION OF LIPOPROTEINS

Lipoprotein Classification		Surface Lipids and Proteins			Core Lipids	
LIPOPROTEIN	DENSITY (g/mL)	PROTEIN (%)	FC (%)	PL (%)	CE (%)	TG (%)
Chylomicron	< 1.000	3	2	6	4	85
VLDL	< 1.006	10	7	16	12	55
IDL	> 1.006 but < 1.019	18	7	22	22	31
LDL	> 1.019 but < 1.063	25	9	21	41	4
HDL	> 1.063 but < 1.210	52	3	26	17	2
HDL$_2$	> 1.063 but < 1.120	43	5	30	20	2
HDL$_3$	> 1.120 but < 1.210	55	3	25	16	1

Lipoproteins are classified according to their buoyant density and relative protein and lipid masses (% of total lipid and protein content).
CE, cholesterol ester; FC, free cholesterol; HDL, high-density lipoprotein; HDL$_{2\&3}$, subfractions of high-density lipoproteins; IDL, intermediate-density lipoprotein; LDL, low-density lipoprotein; PL, phospholipids; TG, triglyceride; VLDL, very low-density lipoprotein.
Data from Fielding P, Fielding C (1) and Havel R, Kane J (5).

pathways are discussed as distinct routes of lipid transport, the lipids and proteins are in a continuous dynamic flux among lipoprotein fractions and the various organs and tissues. A general understanding of these pathways is funda-

TABLE 5.2.   THE DISTRIBUTION AND FUNCTION OF APOLIPOPROTEIN (APO)

Apolipoprotein	Lipoprotein Distribution	Function
Apo A-I	HDL	Cofactor of LCAT
Apo A-II	HDL	Phospholipid binding; possible inhibitor of LCAT
Apo A-IV	HDL	Unknown
Apo B-100	VLDL, LDL	Lipoprotein–cell receptor binding
Apo B-48	Chylomicrons	Lipoprotein–hepatic cell receptor binding
Apo C-I	VLDL, HDL	Possible cofactor adipose tissue LPL
Apo C-II	Chylomicrons, VLDL, HDL	Cofactor of LPL
Apo C-III	Chylomicrons, VLDL, HDL	Inhibits LPL, activates LCAT
Apo D	HDL	Possible role in CE metabolism
Apo E2	Chylomicrons, VLDL, HDL	Lipoprotein–cell receptor binding
Apo E3	Chylomicrons, VLDL, HDL	Lipoprotein–cell receptor binding
Apo E4	Chylomicrons, VLDL, HDL	Lipoprotein–cell receptor binding

CE, cholesterol ester; HDL, high-density lipoprotein; HDL$_{2\&3}$, high-density lipoprotein subfractions; HTGL, hepatic triglyceride lipase; IDL, intermediate-density lipoprotein; LCAT, lecithin:cholesterol acyltransferase; LDL, low-density lipoprotein; LPL, endothelial-bound lipoprotein lipase; TG, triglyceride; VLDL, very low-density lipoprotein.
Data from Fielding and Fielding (1) and Dufaux et al. (269).

mental to understanding lipoprotein and lipid disorders, because modification of key steps or components in forward and reverse cholesterol transport may lead to an accumulation of cholesterol in the arterial vessel walls and, ultimately, to the development of **atherosclerosis**. Figure 5.4 presents a schematic representation of forward and reverse cholesterol transport.

Forward Cholesterol Transport

Cholesterol is derived either exogenously (from the diet) or endogenously (de novo synthesis). Exogenous cholesterol is absorbed through the intestine and secreted in triglyceride-rich **chylomicrons**. Chylomicrons are secreted with apolipoproteins (apo) apo B-48, apo E, and apo A-I. Once in the plasma, the apo E content increases, apo A-I is lost rapidly, and the apo C proteins equilibrate between HDL and the chylomicrons (1). The addition of apo C-II activates the chylomicron for intravascular lipolysis by acting as a cofactor for the enzyme **lipoprotein lipase**. Triglyceride from the chylomicron is hydrolyzed rapidly by muscle and adipose tissue lipoprotein lipase, and the remaining chylomicron remnants are taken up by the liver through receptor-mediated endocytosis (1, 7, 12–14). Thus, chylomicrons appear in the circulation only a few minutes after a meal and rarely are observed in plasma obtained in a fasted state.

The liver secretes triglyceride-rich **very-low-density lipoproteins** (VLDL), which contain apo B-100, hepatically produced apo A-I, and the apo C proteins. Once VLDLs reach the peripheral circulation, apo A-I is rapidly lost, and the VLDL progressively accumulates apo E and apo C proteins through interactions with HDL (1, 4). Like the chylomicrons, VLDL triglycerides are hydrolyzed in

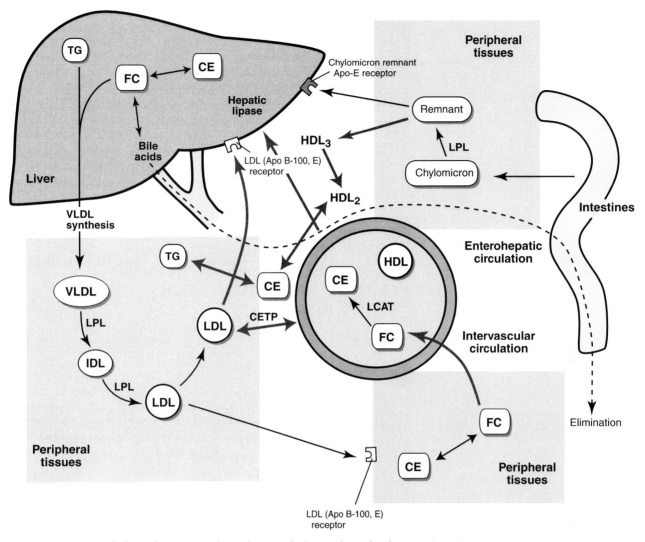

FIGURE 5.4. Major cholesterol transport pathways between the liver and peripheral tissues. Steps in reverse cholesterol transport are distinguished by bold lines; forward cholesterol transport is illustrated by lighter lines. CE, cholesterol ester; CETP, cholesterol ester transfer protein; FC, free cholesterol; HDL, high-density lipoprotein; $HDL_{2\&3}$, high-density lipoprotein subfractions; HL, hepatic lipase; IDL, intermediate-density lipoprotein; LCAT, lecithin:cholesterol acyltransferase; LDL, low-density lipoprotein; LPL, endothelial-bound lipoprotein lipase; TG, triglyceride; VLDL, very-low-density lipoprotein.

the capillary beds of muscle and adipose tissue by lipoprotein lipase, and the free fatty acids are taken up for oxidative metabolism or storage (7, 13). The loss of core and surface lipids reduces the size and increases the density of the VLDL particle, eventually transforming it into an **intermediate-density lipoprotein (IDL)**. Intermediate-density lipoproteins may be hydrolyzed further in the peripheral circulation, giving rise to LDL, or it may be taken up by the liver and extrahepatic cells (2, 7). Thus, LDL is formed in the circulation by the hydrolysis of VLDL and IDL particles (1, 2, 5, 12). Low-density lipoprotein is characterized by a single copy of apo B-100 and a relatively large cholesterol ester mass. It is the major transporter of cholesterol in humans and is absorbed by extrahepatic cells and the liver through apo B receptor endocytosis (1, 6, 7).

Reverse Cholesterol Transport

Because extrahepatic tissues cannot metabolize cholesterol, there must be some means of eliminating this lipid to maintain cholesterol homeostasis. Glomset (8) first proposed the reverse cholesterol transport pathway as a physiologically essential mechanism for the uptake of peripheral cholesterol and its subsequent return to the liver for reutilization or clearance. It has been recognized that reverse cholesterol transport, including the dynamic exchange of cholesterol and other lipids among all lipoproteins, depends on the presence of HDL particles (10, 15, 16). High-density lipoproteins are central to the process of reverse cholesterol transport, because this lipoprotein class can remove cholesterol from peripheral cells and sites of atherosclerotic plaque, compete with LDL in the binding of apo B/E receptors, and transfer cholesterol esters to larger lipoproteins for transport back to the liver. In addition, HDL may help to prevent atheroma formation by serving as an antioxidant (17, 18).

There are several sources of HDL. Nascent HDL containing apo A-I or apo A-II may be secreted by the intestine or the liver. In addition, free apo A-I and apo E can be secreted into the circulation from the intestine or liver. The free apolipoproteins eventually may form HDL particles by taking on lipids through cell-surface interactions with peripheral tissues. Remnant particles from the intravascular hydrolysis of triglyceride-rich lipoproteins also can give rise to HDL particles by associating with the free apolipoproteins or with other nascent HDL (1, 2, 12).

In the circulation, HDL accepts free cholesterol from peripheral tissues, and additional surface and core lipids are obtained from remnant particles that have been produced from the intravascular hydrolysis of VLDL and chylomicrons. Free cholesterol, primarily obtained from the tissues, is esterified by **lecithin:cholesterol acyltransferase (LCAT)**. The newly formed cholesterol esters are either internalized by the HDL or transferred to other lipoproteins by **cholesterol ester transfer protein (CETP)** (8, 19). The internalized cholesterol esters contribute to the conversion of nascent HDL to HDL$_3$, and HDL$_3$ to the more buoyant HDL$_2$ molecule (20–22). The dynamic exchange of nonpolar lipids and apolipoproteins essentially remodels the HDL molecule in the circulation. Mature HDL particles are characterized by a greater cholesterol ester and triglyceride content and the presence of apo A-II and apo E. This remodeling provides several mechanisms for the hepatic uptake of HDL and its lipids. First, apo E allows for HDL uptake via apo B/E receptors (1, 16). Second, the lipolytic action of **hepatic lipase** enables the liver to take up HDL-triglyceride and cholesterol ester (23). Third, a recently identified HDL receptor in the liver allows for the hepatic uptake of triglyceride and cholesterol ester, without removing the HDL particle from the circulation (15, 17).

Most of the cholesterol ester that is produced by LCAT in HDL is transferred to VLDL and LDL in exchange for triglyceride. This exchange of nonpolar lipids among lipoproteins is facilitated by CETP (19, 24). The cholesterol ester that is transferred to VLDL and LDL may undergo either of two fates: cholesterol esters that are transferred to VLDL may remain with the particle as it is remodeled to LDL and redeposited in the peripheral tissue (5, 12, 19, 25); or the LDL cholesterol esters can be returned to the liver via receptor-mediated endocytosis (2). Reverse cholesterol transport is greatly enhanced by this process, because one third of LDL cholesterol is taken up by the liver.

Plasma Lipid Disorders

Modifications in the number or function of apolipoproteins, intravascular enzymes, lipid transfer proteins, and lipoprotein receptors result in a variety of plasma lipid disorders,

---

BOX 5.2. Definitions of Dyslipidemias

Hypercholesterolemia—elevated blood cholesterol concentrations. This term is generally reserved for those individuals with cholesterol concentrations ≥240 mg/dl.

Hypertriglyceridemia—elevated fasting blood triglyceride concentrations. Although different standards exist for what constitutes hypertriglyceridemia versus modestly elevated triglyceride concentrations, this term is generally reserved for those individuals with fasting triglyceride concentrations ≥200 mg/dl.

Hyperlipidemia—elevated cholesterol and triglyceride concentrations.

Dyslipidemia—general term used to identify many abnormal blood lipid disorders.

The following terms are used with hypercholesterolemia, hypertriglyceridemia, hyperlipidemia, and dyslipidemia:

Familial—inherited or of genetic origin

Primary—dyslipidemia arising from a primary cause. Interventions aimed at treating the dyslipidemia are generally appropriate (e.g., genetic, dietary, lipid-lowering drug therapy)*

Secondary—dyslipidemia arising from another condition or problem. Interventions aimed at treating the existing condition or problem will generally resolve the dyslipidemia (e.g., treating diabetes mellitus, hypothyroidism, etc.).*

Exercise helps to modify blood lipids as well as to impart many other health benefits in primary and secondary interventions.

---

termed **dyslipidemias** (Box 5.2). Excessive dietary intake of saturated fatty acids and cholesterol accounts for approximately 80% of **primary dyslipidemias** (26). Inherited genetic disorders constitute another group of primary plasma lipid and lipoprotein abnormalities; these are called **familial dyslipidemias** (Table 5.3). **Secondary dyslipidemias** may arise from metabolic disorders such as diabetes mellitus and hypothyroidism, or systemic and organ diseases such as systemic lupus erythematosus, nephritic syndrome, renal failure, and acute hepatitis. Secondary dyslipidemias also may occur as a result of pharmacologic interventions for other purposes. For example, some forms of beta-blockers, estrogens, progestins, anabolic steroids, and corticosteroids may increase LDLC and triglycerides (TG) or cause a reduction in HDLC (Box 5.3).

As mentioned previously, most cases of primary dyslipidemia are of alimentary origin. There is considerable evidence that populations consuming high amounts of saturated fat have elevated cholesterol, whereas lower plasma cholesterol levels are reported for populations that eat very little saturated fat (27, 28). Of all nutrients, saturated fatty acids seem to have the greatest influence on cholesterol levels, particularly cholesterol found in LDL (29). Recently it has been estimated that plasma cholesterol concentrations are increased approximately 3 mg/dl for each 1% percent of the total caloric intake contributed by saturated fats (30,

TABLE 5.3.   FAMILIAL DYSLIPOPROTEINEMIAS

Type/Classification Changes	Biochemical Mechanism	Blood Lipoprotein and Lipid
I Familial hypertriglyceridemia	Deficiency in LPLa or apo CII resulting in ↓ LPLa	↑ chylomicron, ↓ TG
IIA Familial hypercholesterolemia	Defect in LDL-receptor number or activity resulting in ↓ LDL uptake	↑ LDL, ↑ cholesterol
IIB Familial combined hyperlipidemia	Defect in LDL-receptor number or activity resulting in ↓ LDL uptake, unknown mechanism for elevated TG	↑ VLDL, ↑ TG, ↑ LDL, ↑ cholesterol
III Familial hyperlipoproteinemia	Homozygous for apo E2, interfering with the clearance of chylomicron remnants and VLDL, ↓ HLa	↑ VLDL, ↑ TG, ↑ cholesterol
IV Familial hypertriglyceridemia	↑ synthesis and ↓ clearance of VLDL	↑ VLDL, ↑ TG
V Familial hyperlipidemia	↑ synthesis of VLDL-TG and ↓ clearance of TG-rich lipoproteins	↑ chylomicron, ↑ TG, ↑ VLDL, ↑ cholesterol
Elevated Lp(a)	Macrophage/foam cell uptake of modified LDL particle and ↓ fibrinolytic activity of plasma	↑ Lp(a), ↑ cholesterol
Hyperalphalipoproteinemia	CETP deficiency resulting in an accumulation of cholesterol in HDL	↑ HDL, ↑ cholesterol
Hypoalphalipoproteinemia	Abnormal apo AI, AII, and CIII metabolism, LCAT deficiency	↓ HDL, ↓ cholesterol, ↓ TG
Hyperbetalipoproteinemia	↑ synthesis of VLDL and apo B	↑ VLDL, ↑ TG, ↑ LDL
Hypobetalipoproteinemia	No synthesis of apo B 48 and B100	↓ chylomicron, ↓ TG, ↓ VLDL, ↓ cholesterol, ↓ LDL
Abetalipoproteinemia	No secretion of apo B 48 and B100	↓ chylomicron, ↓ TG, ↓ VLDL cholesterol, ↓ LDL

CETP, cholesterol ester transfer protein; HDL, high-density lipoprotein; HLa, hepatic lipase activity; LCAT, lecithin:cholesterol acyltransferase; LDL, low-density lipoprotein; Lp(a), lipoprotein (a); LPLa, lipoprotein lipase activity; TG, triglyceride, VLDL, very low-density lipoprotein.
Data from Pauciullo P, Mancini M (74) and Nicolosi RJ, Kritchevsky D, Wilson TA (270).

31). By comparison, dietary cholesterol has only a modest influence on plasma cholesterol concentrations. For example, recent findings suggest that plasma cholesterol concentrations increase only 2 to 3 mg/dl for each 100 mg of dietary cholesterol (32). Both dietary saturated fat and

BOX 5.3.   Drugs Prescribed for Other Conditions That Influence Lipids and Lipoproteins

Oral hypoglycemic agents (OHGAs)—diabetes in which there is a relative insulin insufficiency. OHGAs can help increase HDLC and reduce triglyceride concentrations.

Levothyroxine—used in the treatment of hypothyroidism, can reduce TC and LDLC that is secondary to the condition. Levothyroxine may also increase HDLC and reduce triglyceride concentrations.

Anabolic steroids and corticosteroids—may reduce HDLC and elevate triglyceride concentrations. Total cholesterol and LDLC may also increase with use of these drugs.

Estrogens—can elevate both HDLC and triglyceride concentrations

Progestins—reduce HDLC

β-blockers—without sympathomimetic activity can lower HDLC and elevate triglyceride concentrations

Diuretics—may elevate total cholesterol, LDLC, and triglyceride levels with little effect on HDLC

cholesterol seem to elevate plasma cholesterol by reducing LDL-receptor number or interfering with normal LDL-receptor activity (33). However, the exact mechanisms by which dietary saturated fat influences LDL-receptor activity are not completely understood.

No matter what the underlying cause, the practitioner should recognize that virtually all dyslipidemias, particularly elevated cholesterol, increase the risk of cardiovascular disease by accelerating the development of atherosclerosis. Therefore, we include a brief overview of the relationship between lipoproteins, lipids and the atherosclerotic process.

Lipids, Lipoproteins, Atherosclerosis, and Cardiovascular Disease

Evidence Linking Lipids and Lipoproteins to Cardiovascular Disease

Atherosclerosis affecting the coronary vessels, often referred to as **coronary artery disease (CAD)**, is the most prevalent cause of heart disease in Western societies. Strong epidemiologic evidence supports a continuous and graded association between blood cholesterol, LDLC, and **atherogenesis** (34–36). Evidence also exists to show that small, denser LDL particles may be more atherogenic than larger, more buoyant LDL (37), and excess **lipoprotein(a) [Lp(a)]**, the modified form of LDL containing the glycoprotein apo(a), is a strong predictor of premature CAD (38). High triglyceride concentration also may be an independent predictor of CAD, especially when accompanied by low HDLC values (39–42). The presence of elevated **postprandial** triglyceride-rich lipoproteins may indicate a significant risk of CAD (43, 44).

The level of HDLC is inversely related to the incidence of CAD, and is, statistically, a more powerful predictor of CAD than LDLC (35, 45–50). Low HDLC concentrations are predictive of **myocardial infarction** even in subjects with low total cholesterol concentrations (51). It has been estimated that CAD risk increases 3% to 4% with each 1% drop in blood HDLC (52). Expressing either the blood total cholesterol or LDLC as a ratio of HDLC concentration, which relates the anti-atherogenic aspects of HDLC to the atherogenic potential of total and LDL cholesterol, is a stronger predictor of CAD in both men and women than total or HDL cholesterol alone (48, 53). Furthermore, inverse relationships between CAD and the HDL subfractions HDL$_2$C and HDL$_3$C have been reported in prospective studies, and both subfractions are significantly associated with myocardial infarction (48, 54, 55).

There also is evidence to support the measurement of apolipoproteins for determining cardiovascular disease risk. However, these measures generally are limited to research laboratories and are not commonly included in primary clinical lipid screenings. Apolipoprotein A-I, the major peptide found on HDL, is reported to be lower in patients suffering acute myocardial infarction, and a good discriminator of angiographically documented CAD (56, 57). In addition, apo B, the major peptide found in LDL, is elevated in individuals with CAD (58), and the ratio of apo B to apo A-I has been shown to be related to the presence and severity of angiographically defined CAD (59). Apolipoprotein E may protect from CAD through a number of mechanisms, but the extent of the effect is strongly influenced by genetic variation in this peptide (60).

Lipids, Lipoproteins, and the Atherosclerotic Process

The consensus at the current time is that atherosclerosis is an inflammatory disease arising in response to endothelial injury. The related literature is voluminous, and an in-depth review is beyond the scope of this chapter. Fortunately for the interested reader, several excellent reviews have been published (18, 61–65). It is generally agreed that the classic **atherosclerotic lesion** has its origin in the so-called "fatty streak," composed of monocyte-derived **macrophages** and T-lymphocytes. These fatty streaks can develop early, as evidenced by their appearance in arteries of children. With aging, the natural progression of the fatty streak seen in response to repeated endothelial injury is a cycle of mononuclear cell accumulation, smooth muscle cell migration, and proliferation in the lesion, and the formation of fibrous tissue. This progressive change in the lesion results in a gradual increase in size until the lesion develops a fibrous cap covering a core of lipid and necrotic tissue—the advanced, complicated lesion. Not only

does the lesion cause a mechanical narrowing of the arterial lumen with obvious impairment in arterial flow, but fissuring or rupture of the fibrous cap may precipitate **vascular thrombi** formation and sudden death.

But what factors induce these deleterious changes in the arteries? Good evidence exists that endothelial injury and dysfunction can be caused by free radical exposure, hypertension, tobacco use, diabetes mellitus, elevated plasma **homocysteine**, and infections (e.g., herpesvirus). Excessive amounts of circulating cholesterol and triglycerides, as well as the manner in which these lipids are distributed among the lipoprotein carrier molecules, induce and promote endothelial injury, inflammation, and **atherogenesis**.

The weight of the evidence points to the circulating lipoproteins, mainly LDL, as the source of lipid that accumulates in the atherosclerotic lesion. Most cells of the body, including macrophages and arterial smooth muscle cells, which migrate to the site of endothelial injury through a series of steps brought about by **chemotaxic** and **mitogenic** signals, have tightly regulated surface receptors (LDL receptors) to bind LDL, which is then transported by endocytosis into the cell as a receptor-LDL complex. Cellular cholesterol synthesis normally is inhibited when LDL occupies its receptor. Ordinarily, the concentration of circulating LDL is high enough to repress the rate of cellular cholesterol production to very low levels. Therefore, cellular cholesterol synthesis is thought to contribute little to the cholesterol accumulation characteristic of **foam cell** development (6, 66, 67).

Macrophages also possess scavenger receptors capable of binding both acetylated and oxidatively modified LDL. In contrast to the LDL receptor, scavenger receptor activity is not regulated by cell cholesterol content, and may, therefore, lead to massive cholesterol accumulation and foam cell formation, particularly in the presence of excess LDL (6, 68). The macrophage also can bind and ingest lipid through a chylomicron remnant receptor, through a specialized receptor for VLDL, and by the process of phagocytosis following the formation of aggregated LDL particles (69). Additional evidence for the importance of receptor upregulation comes from animal models for atherosclerosis, in which mRNA for scavenger receptors and VLDL receptors were highly induced in atherosclerotic lesions (70). Each of these processes can contribute to macrophage- and smooth muscle cell–derived foam cell formation, and thereby to the development of the mature atherosclerotic lesion.

Several reports from animal experiments, pathological observations, and clinical studies provide metabolic and molecular evidence linking circulating lipids to atherogenesis. **Hypercholesterolemia** contributes to detrimental ultrastructural changes in the endothelium, and LDL, particularly following **oxidation**, exhibits direct cytotoxic effects on endothelial tissue (65, 71, 72). Thus, lipoproteins, especially LDL, increase the growth of mitogen-stimulated arterial smooth muscle cells, in part by providing the cholesterol that is deposited in these tissues. Hence, excess cholesterol deposition from circulating sources and ineffi-

TABLE 5.4. NEW NCEP-ATPIII CLASSIFICATION OF TC, LDLC, HDLC, AND TG CONCENTRATIONS

Total Cholesterol		LDLC		TG*		HDLC
		Optimal *	< 100			Low* < 40
Desirable	< 200	Near optimal	100–129	Normal	< 150	
Borderline High	200–239	Borderline high	130–159	Borderline high	150–199	
High	≥ 240	High 1	160–189	High	200–499	High ≥ 60
		Very high	≥ 190	Very high	≥ 500	

* = Updated lipid classification.
Data from NCEP-ATPIII (76).

cient removal of excess cholesterol are the most frequent contributing factors for the development of atherosclerosis. In contrast to the enabling influence of LDL, there is some evidence that HDL may play a role in restricting arterial smooth muscle cell growth and division (73).

Therapeutic Lifestyle Changes and Pharmacologic Interventions

Systematic approaches to lipid management have been developed in light of the strong scientific evidence that links dyslipidemias to development of CHD, as well as the equally compelling evidence supporting the efficacy of lipid-lowering therapies for reducing the incidence and severity of CHD. Common components of the various recommendations for lipid lowering include dietary interventions, the use of functional foods, increased physical activity and exercise, weight loss, and drug therapy (26, 74). The National Cholesterol Education Program (NCEP) Adult Treatment Panel II (75) and the recently released update from the NCEP Adult Treatment Panel III (NCEP-ATP III) (76) emphasize the use of proper nutrition for the initial treatment of elevated plasma cholesterol and other dyslipidemias in low-risk individuals. The

NCEP guidelines recommend a more aggressive approach, using **antihyperlipidemic drugs**, when treatment goals are not met with dietary intervention alone and in those who are at higher risk for CHD. Physical activity and exercise, as outlined in recent reports from the U.S. Surgeon General (77), and the joint consensus statement from the American College of Sports Medicine and Centers for Disease Control (78) are recognized in the NCEP report as enhancing nutritional and pharmacologic interventions for improving lipid profiles. Unless contraindicated, physical activity and exercise should be incorporated into all lipid-lowering regimens, because many CVD risk factors are addressed concurrently.

The NCEP-ATP III guidelines continue to focus on lowering LDLC, for both primary and secondary prevention of CHD. The most recent report presents a more intensive approach to lowering LDLC in persons with CHD and those with multiple risk factors. The latest report reclassifies LDLC, HDLC, and TG concentrations, updates the goals for LDLC based on known disease and CHD risk, and introduces a nine-step method for determining appropriate lipid-lowering strategies—including special considerations for individuals with metabolic syndrome. Treatment strategies for elevated TG and low HDLC are recommended after LDLC is addressed (Tables 5.4

TABLE 5.5. NEW NCEP-ATPIII CLASSIFICATION OF LDLC GOALS AND CUTPOINTS FOR TLC AND DRUG THERAPY

Risk Category	LDLC Goal	LDLC Level at Which to Initiate TLC	LDLC Level at Which to Consider Drug Therapy
CHD or CHD risk equivalents (10-year risk > 20%)	< 100 mg/dl	≥ 100 mg/dl	≥ 130 mg/dl (100–129 mg/dl: drug optional)*
2 or more risk factors (10-year risk ≤ 20%)	< 130 mg/dl	≥ 130 mg/dl	10-year risk 10–20% ≥ 130 mg/dl; 10-year risk < 10% ≥ 160 mg/dl
0 or 1 risk factor (10-year risk assessment is not necessary because most in this category have < 10% risk)	< 160 mg/dl	≥ 160 mg/dl	≥ 190 mg/dl (160–189 mg/dl: LDL-lowering drug optional)

TLC, therapeutic lifestyle changes; See Table 5.7 for CHD and CHD Risk Equivalents and Risk Factors; See Table 5.8 for 10-year risk based on Framingham Model; * If < 100 mg/dl cannot be achieved by TLC, LDLC-lowering drugs, TG and HDLC modifying drugs, or deferring drug therapy are appropriate based on the clinical situation.
Data from NCEP-ATPIII (76).

TABLE 5.6.   THE 9-STEP LIPID-LOWERING APPROACH FOR CORONARY HEART DISEASE RISK REDUCTION

Step 1.	Determine lipoprotein lipid levels from fasted blood sample.
Step 2.	Identify presence of coronary heart disease (CHD) or CHD risk equivalents (see box in Step 3).
Step 3.	Determine presence of major risk factors other than elevated LDLC:

    1. Cigarette smoking

    2. Hypertension (blood pressure 140/90 mm Hg or on antihypertensive medication)

    3. HDLC < 40 mg/dl (*NOTE: HDLC > 60 mg/dl counts as a negative risk factor; its presence removes one risk factor from the total*)

    4. Family history of premature CHD (CHD in male first-degree relative < 55 years; CHD in female first-degree relative < 65 years)

    5. Age ≥ men 45 years; women ≥ 55 years)

       Note: Peripheral arterial disease, abdominal aortic aneurysm, symptomatic carotid artery disease, diabetes mellitus, and multiple risk factors that confer a 10-year CHD risk of > 20% are regarded as a CHD Risk Equivalent

Step 4.	Determine 10-year CHD risk from Framingham Model if 2 or more risk factors are present without CHD or CHD risk equivalent (see Table 5.8).
Step 5.	Determine "risk category" (see Table 5.6).
Step 6.	Initiate TLC if LDLC is above goal.
Step 7.	Consider adding drug therapy if LDLC exceeds levels shown in Table 5.6.
Step 8.	Identify and treat metabolic syndrome, if present, after 3 months of TLC. Metabolic syndrome is considered to be present with any 3 of the following characteristics:

Risk Factor	Defining Level
Abdominal obesity	Waist Circumference
Men	> 102 cm (40 in)
Women	> 88 cm (35 in)
Triglycerides	≥ 150 m/dl
HDL Cholesterol	
Men	< 40 mg/dl
Women	< 50 mg/dl
Blood pressure	≥ 130/85 mm Hg
Fasting glucose	≥ 110 mg/dl

Step 9.	Treat elevated TG (see Table 5.5).

Condensed version of the recent NCEP-ATPIII recommendations for CHD risk reduction through lipid lowering.
Data from NCEP-ATPIII (76).

through 5.7). The clinical exercise physiologist is encouraged to read the report in its entirety (76). Here we present a more thorough discussion of each therapeutic modality: diet, exercise, and drug therapy.

The Lipid and Lipoprotein Response to Diet

It would seem that reducing the amount of fat in the diet would be a simple solution to the problem of high blood cholesterol and triglycerides. But, as often is the case when dealing with complex systems such as human fat and cholesterol metabolism, the solution is not as simple as it appears. First, it must be recognized that cholesterol and fat are not bad in and of themselves. Cholesterol is essential for health and is found in all cells of the body; cellular synthesis, not the diet, provides the greater part of whole body cholesterol. Many other lipid forms, such as phospholipids and fatty acids, are essential components of all cell membranes and also serve as important fuel for cellular metabolism. The real problem, then, is not whether cholesterol or other lipids are present in the body, but whether or not they are present in excess. Outside of genetic disorders in which

the body mishandles or overproduces cholesterol and lipids, the primary cause of this "excess" problem is an overabundance of calories in the diet, especially fat calories.

NCEP and AHA Diets

As mentioned earlier, the NCEP-ATPIII has established a classification system for identifying persons in need of therapy to modify lipids and lipoprotein-lipids (see Tables 5.4 and 5.5). The NCEP ATP II and ATP III reports support a two-step dietary approach to reduce blood total cholesterol (TC) and LDLC concentrations. Step 1 is recommended for the general population, and especially for individuals with LDLC above 160 mg/dl (4.1 mmol/L). The Step 1 diet limits fat intake to 30% of total caloric intake, saturated fat to less than 10%, and cholesterol to less than 300 mg/d. It is estimated that the average American would need to lower animal fat intake by one third to meet these recommendations. Step 2 is recommended for individuals who are not able to reduce LDLC on the Step 1 diet. The Step 2 diet further limits saturated fat to less than 7% of total calories and cholesterol to less than 200 mg/d. Additional recommendations for both Step 1 and Step 2 diets include: 55% of total calories from carbohydrates, 15% from

TABLE 5.7.   FRAMINGHAM 10-YEAR CHD RISK ESTIMATE WORKSHEET

☐	+	☐	+	☐	+	☐	+	☐	+	☐	=	☐
Age		HDL-C		SBP		TC		Smoking		Total Points		10-Year Risk (%)

Women					Men				
AGE (y)	**POINTS**	**HDLC (mg/dl)**		**POINTS**	**AGE (y)**	**POINTS**	**HDLC (mg/dl)**		**POINTS**
20–34	− 7	. 60		− 1	20–34	− 9	> 60		− 1
35–39	− 3	50–59		0	35–39	− 4	50–59		0
40–44	0	40–49		1	40–44	0	40–49		1
45–49	3	< 40		2	45–49	3	< 40		2
50–54	6	SBP (mm Hg)			50–54	6	SBP (mm Hg)		
55–59	8	**mm Hg**	**Treated**	**Untreated**	55–59	8	**mm Hg**	**Treated**	**Untreated**
60–64	10	< 120	0	0	60–64	10	< 120	0	0
65–69	12	120–129	1	3	65–69	11	120–129	0	1
70–74	14	130–139	2	4	70–74	12	130–139	1	2
75–79	16	140–159	3	5	75–79	13	140–159	1	2
		> 160	4	6			> 160	2	3

Points for Total Cholesterol at Each Age Category (y)

TC (mg/DL)	20–39	40–49	50–59	60–69	70–79	20–39	40–49	50–59	60–69	70–79
< 160	0	0	0	0	0	0	0	0	0	0
160–199	4	3	2	1	1	4	3	2	1	0
200–239	8	6	4	2	1	7	5	3	1	0
240–279	11	8	5	3	2	9	6	4	2	1
>280	13	10	7	4	2	11	8	5	3	1

Points for Smoking Classification at Each Age Category (y)

	20–39	40–49	50–59	60–69	70–79	20–39	40–49	50–59	60–69	70–79
Nonsmoker	0	0	0	0	0	0	0	0	0	0
Smoker	9	7	4	2	1	8	5	3	1	1

Predicted 10-Year CHD Risk from Point Total

Women		Men	
POINT TOTAL	**10-YEAR RISK (%)**	**POINT TOTAL**	**10-YEAR RISK (%)**
< 9	< 1	< 0	< 1
9–12	1	0–4	1
13–14	2	5–6	2
15	3	7	3
16	4	8	4
17	5	9	5
18	6	10	6
19	8	11	8
20	11	12	10
21	14	13	12
22	17	14	16
23	22	15	20
24	27	16	25
≥25	≥ 30	≥ 17	≥ 30

Add points from each category to estimate 10-year CHD risk. Scores for women are obtained on the left side of the tables, for men on the right. HDLC, high-density lipoprotein cholesterol; SBP, systolic blood pressure; TC, total cholesterol.
Adapted from NCEP-ATPIII (76).

protein, 10% from **polyunsaturated fatty acids**, 15% from **monounsaturated fatty acids**, and a total caloric intake at a level required to achieve and maintain a desirable body weight (75). The individual response and effectiveness of this diet is quite variable; indeed, dietary intervention may prove completely ineffective in some individuals. Response variability has been attributed to baseline TC, LDLC concentrations, age, gender, and apo A-IV and apo E heterogeneity (79–84).

Nutrients

Other dietary factors may alter the individual lipid responsiveness to dietary interventions. Simply substituting carbohydrate for fat calories generally leads to an increase in TG and reduction in HDLC concentrations, clearly an undesirable side effect with respect to atherosclerotic risk factors (85, 86). Furthermore, all fats do not affect circulating lipids and lipoprotein-lipids in the same way. A high consumption of **saturated fatty acids** (46%) is associated with an increased concentration of HDLC and larger, cholesterol-enriched LDL, along with a decrease in TG and VLDL (87). When polyunsaturated fats are substituted for saturated fats, LDLC, HDLC, HDL_2C, and apo A-I may be reduced. However, when saturated fats in the diet are replaced with monounsaturated fats, LDLC may be decreased, but HDLC does not change (88, 89). Interestingly, it has been shown that varying the ratio of monounsaturated to saturated fatty acids consumed in a single meal does not acutely affect the resulting postprandial lipid metabolism for at least 9 hours after the test meal (90). This could be interpreted to suggest that changes in lipid metabolism occur only after chronic exposure to dietary interventions. To add to this complicated dietary picture, trans-isomers of monounsaturated fatty acids appear to affect lipoprotein-lipids differently than do cis-isomers. For example, elaidic acid, a trans-isomer, raises LDLC and Lp(a), whereas oleic acid, a cis-isomer, is associated with a reduction in LDLC. Fish oil (especially omega-3 fatty acids), dietary fiber, and plant-derived steroids (e.g., stanol and sterol esters) also may beneficially modify circulating lipids. Dietary intake of antioxidants, such as vitamin E, may reduce the susceptibility of LDL to oxidation, thereby reducing the atherogenicity of this lipoprotein (89). Thus, it should be clear to the reader that many dietary factors have the potential to impact, either for better or worse, blood cholesterol and lipid concentrations associated with the risk for atherosclerosis. As a corresponding benefit, it is important to consider the fact that weight reduction often accompanies a reduction of fat in the diet. Because obesity is itself a CVD risk factor, this would be considered a positive outcome of altering the diet that is coincident with any direct benefit the diet may have on lipid metabolism.

Interaction Between Diet and Exercise

The independent effects of exercise on lipids and lipoprotein-lipids are reviewed elsewhere in this chapter. The question naturally arises, "What, if any, is the combined effect of diet and exercise on these atherosclerotic risk factors?" Exercise increases caloric expenditure, primarily from oxidation of lipids (fatty acids) and carbohydrates. As noted in other parts of this chapter, HDLC concentration is increased and TG decreased in response to exercise training and a single session of exercise. In theory, the increased energy turnover necessitated by physical exercise could alter the transport, storage, and utilization of lipid (and carbohydrate) fuels, thus linking the antiatherogenic lipid profiles of those who exercise regularly with the energy requirements of physical activity.

Currently, the independent and interactive effects of diet and exercise on lipids and lipoprotein-lipids are not well-defined. It has been known for quite some time that dietary practices cannot explain the low-risk lipid profile commonly found in those who exercise. In fact, exercisers typically consume more calories per day than their sedentary counterparts, and a higher proportion of total calories from carbohydrate. Yet, as noted previously, HDLC concentrations typically are higher and TG concentrations lower in those who exercise, in spite of higher daily energy and carbohydrate intake (91). Others have shown that dietary variables do not predict HDLC concentrations in well-trained runners, and that distance run, not dietary variables, is a good predictor of both HDLC and TG concentrations (92, 93). These findings suggest that the impact of diet on lipids in actively training individuals may be blunted. Given this evidence, it has been suggested that exercise may counteract the negative effects of high carbohydrate diets on HDLC and TG (94, 95).

Contrasting findings have been reported, however, from longitudinal diet and exercise studies lasting weeks to months. Published evidence from studies in which diets very low in fat (<10%) and high in complex carbohydrates were combined with daily walking exercise for 3 weeks demonstrated that TC, LDLC, and TG concentrations can be reduced, and LDL particle diameter increased, by such treatment. However, HDLC concentrations concomitantly fall with this diet, and more so in women, an undesirable change with respect to atherogenic risk. This suggests that walking exercise, even though performed daily, may not counteract the generally negative effects of high-carbohydrate diets on HDLC concentrations (96, 97).

Corroboration for these findings with respect to the negative influence of high-carbohydrate diets on lipids and lipoprotein-lipids comes from studies in well-trained individuals on diets of longer duration. Brown et al. (98) reported that high-carbohydrate diets consumed by well-trained cyclists for 3 months resulted in an increase in circulating TG and TC concentrations. High-fat diets had no negative effects on any circulating lipid or lipoprotein-lipid measured in this study. Leddy et al. (99) compared the results of feeding high-fat (42% fat) and low-fat (16% fat) diets to men and women runners who continued to train throughout the 4-week diet periods. Adiposity, weight, blood pressure, TG, TC, LDLC, and apo B did not change in response to the high-fat diet. However, compared to those eating high fat, those consuming low fat had lower HDLC and apo A-I concentrations, and higher ratios of TC to HDLC. Furthermore, runners who increased their fat intake from 16% to 42% raised HDLC without affecting other lipoproteins.

What about the influence of diet on the acute lipid response to a single session of exercise? In one of the few studies to be published in which this question was addressed, Bounds et al. (100) fed moderately trained exercisers high-fat (60% fat) and high-carbohydrate (63% carbohydrate) isoenergetic diets for 2 weeks in a randomized cross-over design. Individuals continued to train while on each diet. At the end of each 2-week diet period, subjects completed an experimental endurance exercise session, and blood was drawn for lipid analysis just before, immediately after, and 24 and 48 hours after the exercise. Diet alone did not affect TC, LDLC, TG, HDLC, HDL_2C, or HDL_3C concentrations. Nor did diet influence the lipid response to exercise: HDLC and HDL_3C rose, and TG and TC fell, 24 to 48 hours after a single session of endurance exercise, regardless of diet. These data corroborate the results published by Leddy et al. (99)—that a high-fat, low-carbohydrate diet did not adversely affect the atherosclerotic lipid risk profiles of individuals engaged in regular endurance exercise. However, Bounds et al. (100) reported that HDLC concentration was not reduced after a high-carbohydrate diet, a finding that conflicts with that reported by Leddy et al. (99). Reasons for these interstudy differences are currently not known.

It would be of interest to the clinical practitioner seeking optimal strategies for the prevention of atherosclerotic disease to know whether or not combining exercise with the NCEP dietary recommendations can be effective. In a large, well-controlled study, men and postmenopausal women with high-risk lipoprotein profiles were assigned at random to one of four groups for a year: NCEP Step 2 diet alone; exercise training alone (10 miles per week walk/jog); NCEP Step 2 diet and exercise combined; or a no-diet, no-exercise control group. At the end of 1 year, neither blood HDLC and TG concentrations, nor the TC to HDLC ratio was different among the treatment groups. Despite the lack of effect on these lipid variables, there were other beneficial effects: LDLC concentration was reduced in the diet and exercise treatment group compared to the control group, with the reduction occurring in both men and women. However, the NCEP Step 2 diet alone did not result in a reduction in LDLC. Thus, the favorable change in LDLC in this population of high-risk men and postmenopausal women occurred only if exercise was combined with the NCEP Step 2 diet (101). These results clearly show the importance of adding exercise to dietary programs targeted at reductions in lipid-related atherosclerotic risk.

In general, dietary interventions account for modest reductions in plasma cholesterol of 3% to 4% (26, 102–104).

Reports from epidemiologic studies suggest a somewhat greater influence of diet on blood lipid profiles and CAD risk reduction than do findings from clinical trials (105–107). Dietary intervention alone usually is less effective at improving lipid profiles than diet combined with pharmacologic therapy (102, 104, 108). In addition to the type of dietary regimen and individual variation in response to diet that were discussed previously, other factors may account for the lack of change in lipid profiles that occur with dietary modification. These factors, such as patient education, the clinician's ability to establish a good relationship with the patient, and the limited means of verifying subject compliance are all related to the fact that dietary interventions are extremely difficult to undertake and maintain (26). With respect to diet and exercise, the increased caloric expenditure that accompanies regular exercise may blunt any influence, either good or bad, of diet on circulating lipids and lipoprotein lipids in trained individuals, although this cannot be stated with absolute certainty. The weight of the literature published to date supports the conclusion that a diet high in fat typically will not result in an adverse change in the lipid profile of those who engage in regular endurance exercise. In contrast, a diet high in carbohydrates and low in fat may reduce HDLC in trained individuals. Acute changes in lipids or lipoprotein-lipids after a single session of exercise are not altered by diet (100). Moreover, when individuals at high lipid risk begin a diet very low in fat, such as the NCEP Step 2 diet, regular exercise may be required to optimize any benefits on the lipid profile that may occur as a result of intervention (76).

The Lipid and Lipoprotein Response to Functional Foods

Functional foods are foods that impart medicinal or health benefits beyond basic nutrition (109, 110). These foods contain biologically active components that appear promising in the prevention and treatment of cardiovascular disease and some forms of cancer. Of particular interest are those functional foods that seem to be effective at reducing the risk of CVD, including sources of **soluble fiber**, **plant stanols**, and **plant sterols**. A considerable amount of research in recent years has shown functional foods to lower CVD risk by lowering total and LDL cholesterol, preventing LDL oxidation, slowing atherosclerotic plaque formation, reducing clot formation by inhibiting platelet aggregation, and improving arterial compliance (109).

Functional foods are attractive to the clinician and patient because they do not seem to have major side effects and, therefore, can be incorporated into the diet safely. In addition, functional foods can impart health benefits when substituted for or added to the current diet without major alterations in eating habits or changes in nutrient intake (110). Moreover, the lipid-lowering effects of drug therapy are augmented when combined with functional foods (111,

112), because the physiologic mechanisms by which functional foods exert their effects are different from the mechanisms of the **antihyperlipidemic drugs** (113, 114).

Soluble Fiber

Soluble fiber is fiber that dissolves readily in aqueous solutions found in the digestive tract. Soluble fiber has been shown to have a direct effect on lowering LDLC by changing the chemical composition of bile acids and increasing **bile acids** in the intestine (see Figure 5.4) (113). The changes in bile acid composition and flux are thought to aid the liver in eliminating cholesterol. Existing research shows that LDLC can be lowered 5% to 10% by ingesting 7 to 10 g/d of soluble fiber from sources such as oats, oat bran, psyllium, various legumes and beans, citrus fruit, strawberries, and apples (115–117).

Plant Stanols and Sterols

Margarine-like spreads containing plant stanols and sterols are a processed form of functional foods derived from pine wood pulp and soybeans. Plant sterols, or phytosterols, were discovered in the 1800s, and their ability to reduce blood cholesterol was realized in the 1950s (110). The lipid-lowering benefits of plant sterols and stanols, which are a fully saturated form of plant sterol, have been substantiated over the last several decades. However, the ability to process and mass produce the plant extracts in a palatable, margarine-like form was developed only recently. These spreads are now commercially available under the trade names Benecol and Take Control. Other food products containing these plant extracts are in the making.

Plant stanols and sterols lower LDLC by incorporating more readily into **micelles** that form in the small intestines during digestion of fats (114). Incorporation of the plant stanols/sterols into these lipid transport molecules displaces cholesterol, thereby inhibiting intestinal absorption of dietary cholesterol and cholesterol that reenters the intestine through the enterohepatic circulation (see Figure 5.4) (114, 118). The current evidence indicates that 1.6 to 2.5 g/d of these margarine-like spreads can reduce total and LDL cholesterol by 10% to 14% (119–122). This daily amount, which may be ingested in one serving or multiple daily servings (122), can exert a noticeable effect on blood lipids in as little as 2 weeks. Particularly appealing features of this functional food are that blood cholesterol levels are lowered regardless of the initial cholesterol concentration (121) and that it is effective with familial forms of **hyperlipidemia** (111).

The Lipid and Lipoprotein Response to Drug Therapy

Lowering blood cholesterol with antihyperlipidemic drugs leads to a decrease in mortality and morbidity from CAD (103, 123, 124). Aggressive cholesterol-lowering therapy has been shown to be effective in reducing the rate of atherosclerotic disease progression in native coronary arteries (125, 126), and in patients with venous coronary artery bypass grafts (127, 128). Lowering total cholesterol and LDLC in patients who already have experienced a coronary event reduces the incidence of death from CAD (129, 130), even in patients with average pretreatment blood LDLC concentrations (131). Furthermore, antihyperlipidemic interventions have been shown to reduce the rate of infarct recurrence in those with elevated TG (132) and decrease CHD risk in patients with low HDLC (133).

Whether or not to initiate drug therapy, the choice of antihyperlipidemic medication(s), and the dosage are decisions left up to the physician and should be based on treatment strategies outlined in the most recent NCEP-ATPIII report. Factors that influence the physician's decision are the patient's current lipid profile; the presence of known cardiovascular, metabolic, liver or kidney disease; the level of CVD risk; the patient's response to dietary and exercise intervention; and other special considerations, such as pregnancy, menopausal status, drug tolerance, and drug interactions (26, 74, 76). Therefore, it is up to the clinical exercise physiologist and other clinicians to communicate with the patient and, as appropriate, with other clinical team members and the physician to ensure that drug therapy is safely and effectively incorporated with lifestyle changes for CVD risk reduction. An overview of the therapeutic effect, side effects, and mechanisms of action of the most common antihyperlipidemic agents is provided to aid the clinical exercise physiologist in this endeavor (Table 5.8).

Statins

Statins are the most effective of the antihyperlipidemic agents at reducing LDLC (134). Their primary effect is to reduce LDLC from 20% to 60% in a dose-dependent fashion at dosages ranging from 20 to 80 mg/d (26, 74). In general, statins have only a modest effect on TG and HDLC levels; the more recent versions, however, show greater promise in favorably modifying these lipids (135, 136). The use of statins in primary and secondary interventions has demonstrated prolonged survival rates in otherwise healthy hyperlipidemics (137) and those with preexisting CHD (129). Statins improved the outcomes in coronary artery bypass patients and slowed or reversed the rate of atherosclerotic development in those with hypercholesterolemia (125, 128).

Statins are **HMG-CoA reductase inhibitors**, which interfere biochemically with cholesterol synthesis in the liver. Other possible mechanisms for reducing CHD that may result from preventing cholesterol synthesis include an up-regulation of LDL-receptors in the liver and peripheral tissues, stabilizing atherosclerotic lesions by reducing in the atherogenic processes of macrophages, reducing platelet ag-

TABLE 5.8. DRUGS USED IN THE TREATMENT OF DYSLIPIDEMIAS

Drug Type	Mechanism of Action	Examples	Trade Names	Common Range of Dosages	Effects on Lipoproteins/Lipids	Advantages/Benefits	Side Effects	Contraindications
HMG-CoA reductase inhibitor	Blocks cholesterol synthesis; increases tissue LDL-receptors	Fluvastatin Pravastatin Lovastatin Simvastatin Cerivastatin Atorvastatin	Lescol Pravachol Mevacor Zocor Baycol Lipitor	20–80 mg 20–40 mg 20–80 mg 20–80 mg 0.4–0.8 g 10–80 mg	↓ TC 15–40% ↓ LDLC 20–60% ↓ TG 7–20% ↑ HDLC 5–15%	Convenient dosage schedule; useful in those with multiple risk factors; low drug interaction potential; low level of system toxicity	Affects liver enzymes; myopathy; myalgia; dyspepsia	Chronic liver disease; pregnancy; in some instances, use with erythromycin, antifungal agents, cyclosporine
Fibric acid derivatives	↓ triglyceride synthesis and VLDL production; ↑ lipoprotein lipase activity	Clofibrate Fenofibrate Gemfibrozil Bezafibrate	Atromid-S Tricor Lopid Bezalip	1000 mg b.i.d. 200 mg 600 mg b.i.d. 200 mg	↓ TC 5–30% ↓ LDLC 10–30% ↓ TG 10–20% ↑ HDLC 10–30%	Used with well-controlled diet to reduce the number of small, dense atherogenic LDL particles; is generally better tolerated than niacin; also affects fibrinogen levels	GI distress; gallstones; myopathy; increases excretion of uric acid	Renal disease; Liver disease
Nicotinic acid	↓ VLDL production; ↓ liver clearance of HDL particles	Niacin	Niaspan Nico-400 Nicotinex Niacinamide	375–2000 mg 500–2000 mg 500–2000 mg 500–2000 mg	↓ TC 15–25% ↓ LDLC 15–25% ↓ TG 30–40% ↑ HDLC 15–25%	Low cost and availability (OTC); favorably improves all atherogenic components of the lipid profile; often used with bile acid binding resins	Flushing; GI distress; hyperglycemia; hyperuricemia	Severe hypotension; Liver disease; diabetes; gout; hyperuricemia; active peptic ulcer
Bile acid sequestrants	Binds bile acids in the intestine	Cholestyramine Colestipol	Questran Colestid	4–16 g 5–20 g	↓ TC 15–25% ↓ LDLC 20–35% TG no Δ or ↑ HDLC no Δ	Low system toxicity; use is permitted in children and pregnancy	GI distress; constipation; interferes with absorption of warfarin, digoxin and thyroxine	Bile duct obstruction; Dybetalipoproteinemia; TG > 200 mg/dl

GI, gastrointestinal; HDLC, high-density lipoprotein cholesterol; LDLC, low-density lipoprotein cholesterol; TC, total cholesterol; VLDL, very low-density lipoproteins; OTC, over the counter; TG, triglycerides; b.i.d., two times per day.
Data from NCEP-ATPIII (76) and PDR Nurse's Drug Book (138).

gregation, and decreasing endothelial dysfunction of blood vessels (26, 74, 134).

The most common side effects reported with statin therapy are elevated liver enzymes, **myalgia**, **myopathy**, and **dyspepsia**. Statins should be avoided or discontinued in patients with liver disease or elevated liver enzymes and during pregnancy (138).

Fibric Acid Derivatives

Fibric acid derivatives, or fibrates, generally are not as effective as other antihyperlipidemic drugs at reducing LDLC; however, their efficacy in reducing TG and elevating HDLC may be underlying reasons for the decrease in CHD mortality and lower rate of nonfatal myocardial infarction (MI) in both primary and secondary prevention trials (139, 140). In secondary prevention trials, fibrates in combination with niacin were more effective than fibrates alone in reducing CHD mortality (132, 140). Bezafibrate, a newer-generation fibrate, may exert an added benefit in CHD risk reduction, since this drug has been shown to increase the exercise-induced vasodilation of coronary arteries (141).

The exact mechanism(s) by which fibric acid derivatives modify abnormal lipid profiles are not fully understood. However, it is thought that this class of drugs reduces fatty acid uptake by the liver and slows hepatic TG synthesis and VLDL production (134, 138). Another mechanism that may account for the lower TG and greater HDLC observed with fibric acid derivatives is a stimulation of lipoprotein lipase (26).

Fibrates often are used in treating type IV hyperlipidemia and dyslipidemic individuals who are unresponsive to diet, exercise, weight loss, and other antihyperlipidemic agents (138). The effects of fibric acid derivatives are similar to those of niacin, but to a lesser extent. Fibric acid derivatives usually are better tolerated than niacin, however, and often are considered as the next drug of choice when niacin treatment results in undesirable side effects (26, 74). Common side effects of fibrates include constipation, myalgia, myopathy, and dyspepsia. This class of drugs is contraindicated for people with hepatic or renal dysfunction (134, 138).

Niacin

The advantages of **niacin** in lipid-lowering therapy are that it is very effective at improving all lipid concentrations in an atherogenic lipid profile, it is available over the counter, and it is relatively inexpensive compared to other antihyperlipidemic agents (26, 134). Among people with documented CAD, niacin therapy is particularly effective at reducing CHD mortality in hypertriglyceridemic patients (132). When used in combination with bile acid sequestrants or fibrates, niacin has been shown to induce regression in atherosclerotic plaque in those with previous CAD (127). Although its efficacy in secondary prevention of

CHD is well documented, the evidence for primary CVD prevention is lacking.

Niacin is thought to reduce TG and LDLC by suppressing hepatic synthesis of VLDL. In addition, recent discovery of a hepatic SRB1-receptor indicates that niacin may increase HDLC by allowing for the return of TG and cholesterol to the liver without eliminating the HDL particle from the circulation (17). The maintenance of HDL in the circulation is thought to enhance reverse cholesterol transport and increase the cholesterol content found in this lipoprotein fraction.

The major drawback of niacin is that it is not well tolerated (26, 74). Niacin therapy often results in **flushing**, skin rashes, gastrointestinal problems, and **pruritus** (138). Niacin is not recommended for individuals with hypotension, liver dysfunction, or peptic ulcers, or those with diabetes mellitus, as it often causes increases in blood glucose concentrations (134, 138).

Bile Acid Sequestrants

Bile acid sequestrants are resins that promote cholesterol elimination through the digestive tract by binding bile acids in the intestine. In primary and secondary trials this class of antihyperlipidemic drugs was demonstrated to be effective at lowering CAD risk by reducing cholesterol and improving lipid profiles (103, 108). However, bile acid sequestrants are most effective when combined with niacin or statins (26, 74).

The use of bile acid sequestrants is limited because they interfere with the absorption of digoxin, thyroid hormones, and Coumadin, among other drugs. In addition, they are least effective of the antihyperlipidemic drugs at changing HDLC, they tend to elevate TG concentrations, and constipation and gastrointestinal disturbances are common (26, 138).

The Lipid and Lipoprotein Response to Exercise

Evidence for the beneficial effects of exercise comes from a number of different types of studies. Early studies often were cross-sectional in design. In the cross-sectional studies, it was common to compare well-trained subjects with those who were untrained. A weakness of this study design is that one cannot completely rule out effects of other factors and personal characteristics in addition to exercise that could alter circulating lipids. For example, physically active individuals often have lower body weights, less body fat, and different diets than those who are inactive, all factors that may influence blood lipids independent of exercise training. In contrast, conclusions are much more definitive when derived from longitudinal studies. One example of this type of study would be one in which untrained individuals are recruited to be subjects, and randomly assigned to either exercise training groups or a control group. Individuals in the control group typically are instructed not to exercise regularly, but they perform all other study activities, such as exercise testing and blood analyses. Thus, at the beginning of the study individuals in both groups are identical with respect to blood lipids as well as factors, such as body weight and aerobic fitness, that could influence blood lipids. It logically follows that any differences in blood lipids and any other variables measured (e.g., body fat, aerobic fitness) among the groups at the end of the study can reasonably be attributed to exercise training. More recently, studies have been designed to explore the effects of a single session of exercise, often called an "acute effect of exercise," on blood lipids. In these studies, blood is first drawn from the subjects at rest for lipid analyses. The subjects then are asked to complete a single exercise session comparable in intensity and duration to a single training session, after which blood is drawn daily for lipid analyses for up to 3 days afterward. No exercise is allowed for the days that blood is sampled. This design was used in several published studies to test the effect of a single session of exercise on blood lipids in both trained and untrained individuals.

Cross-sectional Evidence for an Exercise Effect

In general, blood lipid profiles of physically active groups reflect a reduced risk for the development of cardiovascular disease when compared to their inactive counterparts (78, 142, 143). For example, there is limited evidence to suggest that those who are physically active exhibit lower concentrations of total cholesterol and LDLC than those who are less active (145–150). However, a well-recognized problem with observational studies is that, by design, they do not account for confounding factors, such as group differences in body weight and body fat, caloric intake, nutrient composition of diets, alcohol intake, smoking habits, and other potentially lipid-altering lifestyle characteristics. In fact, the group differences in TC and LDLC diminish and often cease to be significant when these factors are statistically controlled (148, 151, 152). Moreover, a majority of cross-sectional studies indicate smaller, nonsignificant differences in total cholesterol and LDLC levels between exercise-trained and inactive individuals (144, 153). In addition, regression analyses of data from large-scale epidemiologic investigations have failed to demonstrate a consistent relationship between physical activity and TC and LDLC in normo- and hyperlipidemic groups (154, 155).

In contrast to the variable total and LDL cholesterol results, observational data provide stronger evidence for lower triglyceride and greater HDLC concentrations in physically active individuals. Triglyceride levels almost always are lower in endurance athletes, aerobically trained people, and physically active individuals when compared to sedentary controls. Significant triglyceride differences be-

tween these groups range from 18 mg/dl to 77 mg/dl (19–50%) in over half of all related cross-sectional studies. Blood levels of HDLC are 4 mg/dl to 24 mg/dl (9–59%) higher in those having physically demanding jobs and individuals engaged in endurance exercise compared to their less active counterparts (143, 144).

Lipid Changes With Exercise Training— Evidence From Longitudinal Studies

In longitudinal studies, total cholesterol and LDLC rarely change with exercise training in either men or women. When these lipid fractions are altered with exercise training, the reductions are minimal or moderate, averaging 6 mg/dl to 13 mg/dl (4–7%), when compared to nonexercising control subjects (143, 144, 156). A meta-analysis of lipid changes in normo- and hyperlipidemic groups suggests that exercise training may be expected to lower total cholesterol and LDLC by about 4 mg/dl (156).

Based on the frequency of reported changes, HDLC and TG are more responsive to regular exercise than total cholesterol and LDLC. Significantly greater HDLC concentrations are reported after exercise training in over half of the manuscripts reviewed, and reductions in TG levels are found in a third of the related literature (143, 144). When HDLC is significantly elevated after exercise training, the increases are similar in both men and women, ranging from 2 mg/dl to 8 mg/dl (4–22%). Likewise, significant reductions in TG concentrations range from 5 mg/dl to 38 mg/dl (4–37%) after exercise in men. The magnitude of change can be similar in women, but it occurs less frequently. Results from a recent meta-analysis suggest, however, that the effects of exercise training on HDLC and triglyceride favored the more conservative ends of these ranges, with HDLC increases averaging 2 mg/dl and TG decreases averaging 9 mg/dl (156). Although these lipid changes may seem modest, they have been associated with a 2% to 4% reduction in CVD risk (45, 157).

Gender Differences in Lipid Responses to Exercise

Several investigators have demonstrated that exercise can alter HDLC and TG equally in men and women (158–160); however, favorable changes in HDLC and TG are reported less often in women (161). Women also may be more resistant to exercise-induced changes in total and LDL cholesterol than their male counterparts (162, 163). The reasons for less consistent findings in women are not completely clear. Some physiologic and metabolic factors that can influence lipid metabolism, such as smaller muscle and greater fat mass, different fat distribution, menstrual cycle fluctuations, the use of oral contraceptives in premenopausal women, menopausal status, and the use of hormone replacement therapy in postmenopausal women, are thought to contribute to a greater variance in the lipid response to exercise in women (164–166).

The Influence of Baseline HDLC Concentrations on Changes with Exercise

Individuals with initially low HDLC (<35 mg/dl) appear to be resistant to exercise-induced changes in HDLC. Raz et al. (167) reported that aerobic exercise training was ineffective in modifying HDLC in young men with low HDLC. Williams and colleagues (168) found that exercise training increased HDLC to a lesser extent in men with low versus normal baseline HDLC. Others have demonstrated that HDLC responds most favorably to exercise in men with normal initial HDLC values (>38 mg/dl) and is resistant to change in men with baseline HDLC values lower than 37 mg/dl (169–171). Similar studies have not been conducted in women; however, elevations in HDLC have been observed in women with moderate baseline HDLC (172–174) and in those with high preexisting HDLC levels after large increases in exercise training volume (175, 176). Therefore, it appears that exercise training may be most effective at elevating HDLC in those with HDLC levels that are normal or above average prior to beginning an exercise program. There is not currently enough evidence to suggest that baseline total cholesterol, LDLC, or triglyceride concentrations influence lipid responses to exercise training in either gender (156).

The Influence of Body Weight and Body Fat on Lipid Responses to Exercise

Inverse relationships have been established between body mass index (BMI), percent body fat, regional body fat measured at baseline, and the extent to which blood lipids and lipoprotein levels change with exercise training (171, 177, 178). In particular, exercise-induced changes in blood lipids seem to be more modest in individuals with greater BMI, more body fat, or more central fat distribution. These observations have led some to suggest that body weight and body fat reductions must occur during exercise training in order for blood lipid concentrations to be significantly altered (153). Although body weight or body fat loss may augment the lipid changes that occur with exercise (179–183), reductions in body weight or fat do not necessarily have to occur for exercise to improve blood lipid profiles. For example, in several exercise training studies, total cholesterol and LDLC were significantly reduced in the absence of change in body weight or body fat (163, 184–189). In addition, total cholesterol and LDLC often were unchanged after exercise training programs in which body weight and body fat were lowered significantly (169, 173, 175, 177, 190–199). In men, favorable changes in HDLC and TG occur with equal frequency when body weight and body fat are reduced (167, 169, 177, 184, 193,

198–204) or when body weight or body fat does not change with exercise (170, 185, 205–214). In women, TG and HDLC changes also have been demonstrated in the absence of body weight and fat loss (172, 175, 176, 196, 215, 216).

Interestingly, lower total cholesterol and LDLC are observed more often when substantial weight loss occurs through a combination of diet and exercise (181–183, 199, 203, 217–219). It is unclear, however, whether the reductions in TC and LDLC after these interventions are due to greater caloric deficits and weight loss than what is generally reported after exercise alone, or if a decrease in dietary saturated fat and cholesterol intake is more strongly associated with these lipid changes (177, 178, 182, 199). The HDLC level will decrease (181, 182, 217), increase (168, 183, 220), or not change (101, 218) when weight loss is induced by dietary means, alone or in combination with exercise. To make sense of the variable HDLC responses to diet and exercise-induced weight loss, some have suggested that exercise may prevent a decrease in HDLC when combined with dietary means of weight or body fat reduction (182, 217).

Currently, it does not appear that body weight or body fat loss is necessary for exercise to have a beneficial effect on any blood lipid variable. However, reductions in body weight and body fat may augment the exercise-induced lipid changes in those who are overweight or obese (179-183). Furthermore, exercise may enhance the favorable lipid changes that may result from dietary regimens designed to lower body weight and body fat (182, 217).

The Influence of Exercise Intensity and Volume on Lipid Responses

It is difficult to evaluate the effects of exercise intensity on blood lipid changes, because most training studies were conducted with intensities greater than 60% of maximum heart rate or $\dot{V}o_{2max}$. As a result, most of the improvements in blood lipids have been reported with exercise at these training intensities. Despres and colleagues (201), however, observed significant reductions in total and LDL cholesterol with a low-intensity/high-volume training regimen. Others have compared the effects of training intensities, ranging from 40% to 85% of $\dot{V}o_{2max}$ and did not find an intensity effect on any blood lipid variable (158, 191, 216, 221, 222). Stein et al. (209) and Tomiyasu et al. (211) report greater improvements in lipid profiles with high- versus moderate-intensity training; however, a failure to control for the exercise volume in both of these studies makes their findings hard to interpret. When energy expenditure and training volume are controlled, exercise intensity has not been shown to influence lipid changes in men or women (158, 172, 191, 216, 222).

Training volume, specifically as it relates to energy expenditure, seems to be the primary stimulus for blood lipid responses to exercise. Total cholesterol and LDLC are not generally expected to change with exercise training; however, significantly higher HDLC and lower TG levels are observed most often after exercise training programs requiring 1000 to 2000 kcal/week (143, 144). In men, HDLC and TG changes usually do not occur with training volumes less than 1500 kcal/week (186, 202, 209, 223). However, training volumes that elicit 1000 to 1200 kcal/week in energy expenditure also may elevate HDLC in sedentary and moderately fit women (166, 174, 195, 196, 215, 216).

Lipid Changes With Resistance Exercise Training

Blood lipids and lipoproteins usually are not altered after resistance training programs (224–228). Although total cholesterol and LDLC reportedly have decreased after several weeks of resistance training (229–231), the sample sizes in these studies were small and, other than the results of Hurley et al., (231) these findings have been generally limited to women (229, 230). Resistance exercise, in general, may be less effective than endurance activities for modifying blood lipid levels, because relatively fewer calories are expended in resistance versus aerobic activity. The work of Blumenthal et al. (225) and Smutok et al. (224) has shown that lipids and lipoproteins changes should not be expected after low-volume exercise interventions of either resistance or aerobic activities.

Acute Lipid Responses to Exercise

Mobilization from lipid stores and oxidation of lipids provide an important fuel substrate for performance of aerobic exercise. It can reasonably be expected, therefore, that a single session of exercise, and especially aerobic exercise, will affect lipid metabolism and modify blood lipid-lipoprotein levels. In fact, it has been postulated that the characteristic antiatherogenic lipid profile of exercise-trained individuals may be, at least in part, a consequence of a short-term (hours) or delayed (days) response to their last session of exercise independent of chronic exercise training (232). Early support for this "acute response" hypothesis came from studies showing that blood TG concentration was reduced for up to 44 hours after a single session of aerobic exercise, and that this beneficial reduction was evident even in hyperlipidemic men (232–234). Importantly with respect to atherosclerotic risk, early investigators showed that HDLC concentrations were higher and total cholesterol concentrations lower shortly after a single session of exhaustive exercise (235–237).

Results of subsequent studies exploring the acute exercise response vary widely. This is not surprising when one considers that many factors other than exercise may influence lipid metabolism and circulating lipoprotein-lipid concentrations. For example, subject characteristics in published studies differ in age, gender, training status, body weight, body composition, diet, and preexisting lipid concentrations, all of which are factors that have been shown to affect circulating lipids and lipoprotein concentrations (144, 238–241). The time at which blood samples were collected before and after exercise varies among studies from minutes to days. Furthermore, baseline (preexercise) blood samples often are collected without regard for the timing of previous exercise sessions. Studies differ in mode, duration, intensity, and volume (energy expenditure) of the exercise stimulus, and blood concentrations of lipid variables may or may not be corrected for postexercise changes in plasma volume. All of these factors, which have the potential to affect lipid and lipoprotein-lipid concentrations after exercise, should be considered when interpreting results of published studies related to the lipid response to a single session of exercise.

With few exceptions (242) subsequent studies corroborate earlier work showing that a single session of endurance exercise promotes significant reductions in blood TG concentrations (100, 238, 239, 243–247). This exercise effect appears to be robust, and is noted in trained and untrained subjects after moderate and high intensity exercise performed using various aerobic modalities. Some evidence exists to suggest a threshold of about 350 kcal of energy must be expended to promote significant changes in blood TG, but this finding is not universal. Regardless of mode or intensity, the exercise effect is lost after about 48 to 72 hours (245). Existing evidence also suggests a relationship between preexercise TG concentration and the magnitude of the postexercise change—i.e., subjects with elevated preexercise TG values show the greatest postexercise change, whereas those with relatively low preexercise TG concentrations show only modest or no change after exercise (243, 248–250). Despite the paucity of research in women, some gender differences in responsiveness have been reported. There is evidence that when exercise of low and high intensity is performed by young, premenopausal women, a rise in TG concentration is seen immediately after exercise, a finding in contrast to the postexercise fall generally reported in men (241, 251). However, a delayed drop in blood TG concentrations below preexercise values may occur in women as early as 1 hour and up to 48 hours after exercise (252).

The conclusions related to total and LDL cholesterol responses to exercise can be stated with less assurance. Several well-controlled studies show that a reduction in total cholesterol may follow a single session of exercise. When a cholesterol reduction is noted, it is relatively small (3–5%), and short-lived (<24 hours). Postexercise reductions in total cholesterol have been reported for male and female, trained and untrained, hyper- and normocholesterolemic subjects (100, 238, 239, 241, 243, 249). More lasting TC reductions (up to 120 hours postexercise) may accompany exercise when caloric expenditure is very high, particularly in trained women (245, 251). It is important to note, however, that a reasonable number of conflicting reports have been published (242, 244, 246, 247, 252). In fact, increases in blood TC concentrations 24 to 48 hours after exercise have been found in untrained men with normal and elevated blood cholesterol (238, 243, 249). It is likely that some individuals have heritable traits that make them relatively resistant to exercise-induced changes in blood total cholesterol; i.e., they are "nonresponders" to exercise.

In view of the variable response noted for total cholesterol, it is not surprising that the lipoprotein responsible for carrying the bulk of circulating cholesterol, LDLC, exhibits a highly variable response as well. Reductions in LDLC ranging from none to 38% have been reported in trained men immediately and up to 72 hours after completing intense endurance events (100, 244–247). In contrast, LDLC concentration may increase or decrease by 5% to 8% in hypercholesterolemic men after exercise (238, 239, 243), with the conflicting responses possibly due to interstudy differences in the caloric costs (volume) of exercise, and training status of the subjects. It also is possible that some types of hypercholesterolemia are differentially affected by exercise, but this hypothesis currently requires additional research to verify. Although published research in women is sparse, LDLC concentration was reportedly reduced 24 hours after exercise of relatively high intensity and volume (241, 251). However, LDL density, as assessed by ultracentrifugation, was not altered in either normal or hypercholesterolemic women by a single session of aerobic exercise (253). An increase in LDL particle size has been shown to follow completion of a marathon in some men, but not in women, for reasons that currently are unclear (254). In contrast to the research that generally supports a beneficial effect of exercise, data exist that suggest that circulating LDL is more susceptible to harmful oxidation after very intense, long-duration exercise, such as a marathon (255).

A single session of exercise appears to be an effective stimulus for raising HDLC. The benefit of exercise accrues in men and women with normal blood cholesterol concentrations as well as in men with elevated cholesterol. The postexercise increase in HDLC ranges from 4% to 34%, reaching its zenith 24 to 48 hours after exercise, and may be sustained up to 72 hours before returning to preexercise levels (100, 238, 239, 243–247, 249, 251). The volume of exercise per session required to elicit beneficial HDLC changes has been shown to be about 350 kcal to 400 kcal in moderately trained men, and up to 1000 kcal in well-trained men (238, 244, 247). This suggests that an HDLC change threshold exists that varies with the functional capacity of the subjects, a hypothesis yet to be verified experimentally. When HDLC subfractions have been investigated, concentrations of HDL_2-C, HDL_3-C, or both have been shown to be elevated after a single session of exercise (100, 238, 239, 243–247). The HDL density reportedly is reduced for up to 2 days after aerobic exercise in women

with normal or high cholesterol, a finding that provides further evidence that exercise acutely alters intravascular lipid metabolism (253). Which HDLC subfraction is elevated after exercise may depend on the training status of the subjects. In one study, HDL_2-C was elevated in trained men, whereas in untrained men HDL_3-C was higher after exercise (249). Based on the existing literature, it is reasonable to propose that the magnitude of the exercise effect is influenced by the training status of the subjects and volume of exercise performed.

Conclusions regarding the effect of a single session of exercise on apolipoproteins are equivocal at best, because so few studies on this topic have been published to date. Existing evidence shows that in men with elevated total cholesterol concentrations, moderate exercise results in a 4% to 9% increase in apo B concentration (238, 243). In contrast, apo B concentration apparently is unchanged in well-trained men after strenuous exercise (245). Apo A-I and A-II concentrations reportedly were 25% lower immediately after long-duration exercise, but rose 10% to 20% above preexercise values throughout the eight recovery days that followed (245). Others have reported that apo A-I rose slightly (3%) or did not change after moderate amounts of exercise (238, 243, 246). Effects of a single session of exercise on other important lipoproteins have not been carefully studied.

It is well-established that elevated blood Lp(a) is a strong risk factor for CVD (256, 257). Given the similarity of Lp(a) to LDL, it has been hypothesized that exercise might beneficially modify circulating levels of this lipoprotein, and thereby lower cardiovascular disease risk. However, current evidence shows Lp(a) to be resistant to the exercise stimulus (258, 259).

How much exercise is enough, and at what intensity must exercise be performed to effect a beneficial change in lipid levels? With regard to exercise intensity, surprisingly few well-controlled studies have been published to date. Furthermore, interpretation of study results often is confounded by a lack of experimenter control for unequal caloric expenditure (volume of exercise) between intensity groups (260–262). For example, it is not uncommon in published studies to find that exercise duration was identical for subjects exercising at either low or high intensity. Clearly, when this is the case, those exercising at high intensity expend more calories during exercise. In trained runners, greater postexercise increases in HDLC concentrations reportedly follow high-intensity than low-intensity exercise (260, 263). Equally convincing studies suggest this is not the case, however (242, 243). In addition, some evidence exists to show that the pattern and magnitude of lipid changes following a session of exercise may be altered by training (238). Current evidence favors the notion that the effect of exercise intensity depends, to some degree, on training status, but it is difficult to separate this effect from the influence of exercise volume (caloric expenditure).

Published research shows that the acute effect of exercise lasts no more than 3 days, even after the most demanding exercise by trained athletes (245). When exercise is withheld from endurance-trained athletes, blood TG, VLDL cholesterol, and the total cholesterol-to-HDLC ratio are all higher at both 60 hours and 6.5 days after their last training session than at 15 hours postexercise. Postprandial lipemia also is increased in endurance athletes when exercise is withdrawn for several days (264). These data suggest that the beneficial influence of exercise on lipid metabolism is an acute phenomenon that is lost rather quickly after cessation of exercise, even in the most highly trained individuals. The message for the exercise practitioner is that exercise must be repeated at least every 3 days, and probably every other day, to maintain the acute benefit.

Potential Physiological Adaptations and Associated Mechanisms

The biochemical mechanisms underlying the lipid response to exercise remain to be clearly elucidated. Current theory suggests that changes in lipid regulatory enzyme activities (or mass) in response to the metabolic demands of exercise produce the postexercise changes in circulating lipids and lipoprotein-lipids noted in exercise studies. The enzymes and transfer proteins most often studied include lipoprotein lipase (LPL), hepatic lipase (HL), lecithin: cholesterol acyltransferase (LCAT), and cholesterol ester transfer protein (CETP). A link between the decrease in circulating TG concentration, the increase in HDLC (especially HDL_2-C) after exercise, and LPL has been firmly established. Exercise induces the formation of LPL protein in muscle, and LPL activity is acutely increased after a single session of exercise (265). The increase in LPL activity reaches its zenith approximately 24 hours after exercise, a temporal change closely linked with the nadir of the postexercise TG concentration curve. Concurrently, HL activity generally is shown to be reduced or not changed for up to 72 hours after exercise (239, 244, 246, 247, 249). The decrease in HL activity may result in a prolonged survival time for HDL, and a consequent increase in circulating HDL concentration. Again, this would be consistent with the observed data that HDLC is increased after a single session of exercise.

Because CETP plays an important role in intravascular remodeling of circulating lipoproteins by facilitating cholesterol and triglyceride exchange between HDL and triglyceride-rich lipoproteins, it could affect the short-term changes in blood lipoprotein-lipid concentrations after exercise. Few studies have been published in which this possibility was explored, and those that exist do not resolve the issue. Published results demonstrate that CETP activity is unchanged after a single session of exercise. However, there is evidence that CETP mass may be reduced up to 2 days after exercise (239, 245). Such a reduction in mass would, presumably, decrease the cholesterol transfer from HDL to TG-rich lipoproteins, thereby leading to an increase in cholesterol carried in HDL. Although this conclusion is attractive, additional research is required to confirm the current findings.

The response of LCAT activity to exercise is somewhat ambiguous as well. An increase in LCAT activity was reported after an endurance run by trained subjects. In contrast, no change was noted in recreational runners and untrained men after exercise (240, 266–268). From the existing literature, it seems reasonable to conclude that if a single session of exercise has an effect on LCAT at all, it is likely to be one encompassing a large volume of exercise.

Exercise Prescription Options

Caloric expenditure seems to be the general stimulus by which exercise exerts an effect on blood lipids, particularly HDLC and triglyceride concentrations (143, 150–153). Therefore, it seems reasonable to expect that the physical activity and exercise that results in substantial energy expenditure would be most suited for inclusion in an overall strategy for modifying blood lipids. Thus, any mode that includes large muscle groups, is rhythmic and dynamic in nature, and can be sustained for several minutes is preferred, because this type of physical exertion enhances the rate of caloric expenditure. In this regard, weight-bearing modes that augment the rate of caloric expenditure would have an advantage over non–weight-bearing exercise. Exercise intensity does not seem to influence exercise-induced blood lipid changes, so low-to-moderate intensities are just as effective as high-intensity, as long as energy is expended. The mode or intensity is not the primary focus, however. Any exercise that results in significant energy expenditure is likely to produce more favorable blood lipid profiles (Box 5.4).

Resistance training, by itself, usually is not effective at modifying blood lipids, because this form of exercise does not result in substantial energy expenditure. However, resistance exercise can increase muscle mass and, therefore, may enhance the effect of aerobic exercise on HDLC and triglyceride concentrations. A greater muscle mass may influence these lipid concentrations by elevating the rate of caloric expenditure at rest and any given exercise intensity. Resistance exercise also may increase insulin sensitivity and glucose disposal, both of which can have beneficial influences on blood lipid profiles.

The clinical exercise physiologist should keep in mind that the effect of exercise on HDLC and triglyceride is transient, usually lasting up to 48 hours after exertion. Therefore, an exercise regimen of at least every other day is warranted. If other diseases or risk factors are present, such as diabetes, obesity, and hypertension, daily physical activity and exercise may provide additional health benefits.

The choice of exercise progression should relate directly to the goals and needs of the client. Increasing exercise in-

BOX 5.4. Exercise Prescription Options

Mode

Any mode that includes large muscle groups and is dynamic and rhythmic in nature. Weight-bearing exercises are preferred to increase the rate of caloric expenditure.

Weight-bearing exercise (examples): brisk walking, jogging, stair stepping, elliptical trainer, aerobics classes

Nonweight bearing exercise (examples): cycling, rowing, swimming

Frequency

Daily is preferred; however, at least every other day to maintain the transient benefit of exercise on HDLC and triglyceride concentrations.

Daily exercise may be most effective, especially when other risk factors or diseases are present, such as obesity, hypertension, and diabetes mellitus.

Intensity

Moderate-intensity exercise ranging from 50% to 85% of $\dot{V}O_{2max}$, or 40% to 75% of HRR or $\dot{V}O_2R$.

RPE (11 to 14) may be used, particularly when multiple modes are incorporated into the exercise program.

Duration

30 to 60 minutes of moderate-intensity exercise corresponds to an exercise energy expenditure of 350 to 500 kcal (depending on body mass and fitness level). The total exercise time can be accumulated throughout the day.

Progression

The total volume of exercise, as it relates to energy expenditure, is the primary objective of exercise for blood lipid management. Any combination of intensity and time to meet energy expenditure goals is ok.

The choice of increasing intensity or duration should be based on the client's tolerance and preference.

Other Considerations

Educate your client about the role of exercise in lipid management programs so that reasonable goals and expectations are developed.

Determine the type(s) of medications that are being used for lipid lowering.

Be aware of the possible adverse effects of medications prescribed for other conditions on blood lipids.

Encourage your client to drink plenty of fluids, especially if the client is on a weight-reduction program.

Educate your client on the importance of exercise for added health benefits.

tensity usually is not the best choice when injury and adherence are issues. However, exercise of high intensity, rather than low or moderate intensity, can help boost resting energy expenditure for several hours or even days after completing the exercise. For individuals with other special considerations, such as obesity, hypertension, or diabetes (which can often be the case), progressively increasing the total amount of activity, rather than intensity, may be the best option. The total volume of physical activity does not necessarily have to come from added exercise time. Be sure to recommend additional daily physical activity such as stair climbing, walking, gardening, yard work, and any other physical exertion that results in significant caloric expenditure.

What We Know About Exercise and Lipid Disorders

1 The changes in HDLC and triglyceride concentrations that are observed after one exercise session and with regular exercise training seem to occur as a result of elevated lipoprotein lipase activity in skeletal muscle and adipose tissue. Changes in other lipoprotein enzymes and transfer proteins also may occur; however, they are less consistent than the increase in postexercise lipoprotein lipase activity.

2 In most normo- and hyperlipidemic individuals, HDLC can reasonably be expected to increase 5% to 10% after a single exercise session of sufficient volume. The volume of exercise needed to induce HDLC changes seems to be related to the individual's fitness level. Less fit individuals may observe HDLC increases with energy expenditures of 350 kcal, whereas those who are more cardiovascularly fit may need to expend 800 to 1000 kcal. Reasonable triglyceride reductions of 10% to 20% also may be observed after exercise of similar energy expenditure, although triglyceride changes are observed more often in men than in women. Changes in total cholesterol and LDLC are not often reported in research settings and should not be expected to change with one exercise session.

3 A single exercise session of low to moderate intensity can help clear the elevated triglycerides that are observed shortly after a meal.

4 Regular aerobic exercise training alters HDLC and triglyceride concentrations in the same direction and to the same magnitude that has been reported for a single exercise session. Interestingly, these blood lipid changes often are reported in studies that required weekly exercise energy expenditure of 1000 to 2000 kcal. This weekly energy expenditure correlates nicely with single exercise sessions of 350 kcal performed four or five times per week. There is not enough evidence to show that exercise training alone can consistently lower total and LDL cholesterol.

1 How does exercise influence the liver's synthesis and clearance of apolipoproteins, triglycerides, cholesterol, and other lipoproteins?

2 The blood lipid profiles of some individuals respond excellently to exercise training, whereas others are very resistant. Are there physiologic and metabolic factors that we can measure prior to prescribing exercise that will help us to predict "responders" and "non-responders"?

3 Can resistance training combined with aerobic training enhance blood lipid changes reported for aerobic exercise training alone?

4 Is there an optimal mode for exercise designed to alter blood lipid profiles favorably?

5 Some individuals have orthopaedic limitations that prevent them from using large muscle groups during exercise. Can exercise with smaller muscle mass (e.g., dynamic upper body exercise) versus larger muscle mass (e.g., dynamic lower body exercise) of the same caloric expenditure affect blood lipids to the same extent?

6 Can exercise enhance the effect of functional foods and lipid-lowering drugs in hyperlipidemic individuals?

Summary

Dyslipidemias, particularly elevated LDLC concentrations, are associated with increased rates of CHD morbidity and mortality. Other lipid abnormalities, such as increased triglyceride levels and low HDLC, also are strongly related to CHD outcomes. Treatment of dyslipidemias often results in a slowing or reversal of the atherosclerotic process, and, therefore, a reduction in CHD risk. Primary treatment strategies for dyslipidemias include nutritional considerations, such as a reduction in saturated fat and cholesterol intake and incorporating functional foods in the diet. Pharmacologic agents often are used when additional lipid lowering is warranted. Regular exercise and physical activity should be included as part of an overall plan for modifying blood lipid profiles, because increased caloric expenditure through physical exertion often results in elevated HDLC and lower triglyceride concentrations. In addition, exercise may enhance the influence of dietary and pharmacologic interventions for dyslipidemias. However, the best reason for including exercise in blood lipid management programs is the additional health benefits that will be gained from increasing daily physical activity.

DISCUSSION QUESTIONS

1 Assuming the best outcomes, how much would the following intervention strategies reasonably be expected to alter total cholesterol, LDLC, HDLC, and triglyceride concentrations?
a. NCEP Step 1 diet
b. NCEP Step 2 diet
c. Weight loss of 20 lbs by following a nutritionally balanced hypocaloric diet
d. The recommended use of stanol ester spreads
e. The recommended use of soluble fiber
f. The use of low-dose lipid-lowering drugs (statins, niacin, fibrates, bile sequestrants)
g. Daily, moderate-intensity aerobic exercise for 30 to 60 minutes

2 Which combination(s) of the following intervention strategies would be best suited for initiating a primary prevention program aimed at maintaining healthy blood lipid levels?
a. NCEP Step 1 diet
b. NCEP Step 2 diet
c. Weight loss of 20 lbs by following a nutritionally balanced hypocaloric diet
d. The recommended use of stanol ester spreads
e. The recommended use of soluble fiber
f. The use of low-dose lipid-lowering drugs (statins, niacin, fibrates, bile sequestrants)
g. Daily, moderate-intensity aerobic exercise for 30 to 60 minutes

3 Which combination(s) of the intervention strategies listed in question #1 might be reasonable for a lipid-lowering program in clients with:
a. diet-induced hypercholesterolemia?
b. hypertriglyceridemia?
c. elevated cholesterol, triglycerides and low HDLC?

4 How might regular aerobic and resistance exercise enhance blood lipid profiles in postmenopausal women on estrogen/progestin therapy?

5 How might regular aerobic and resistance exercise enhance blood lipid profiles in clients with metabolic syndrome? (See Table 5.6 for characteristics of metabolic syndrome.)

CASE STUDY

Patient Information

Paul is a 36-year-old owner of a computer store. He weighs 245 lbs and is 71 inches tall. Paul recently completed his annual check-up with his primary care physician. His doctor indicated that Paul had a few health issues that needed to be addressed, but otherwise he was healthy. Paul's physician works out in your hospital wellness center and recommended that Paul visit and consult you about an exercise program, and Paul has followed his advice and approached you about starting an exercise program. In his preexercise screening, Paul indicated on his health history questionnaire that his father died of a heart attack at age 54. He also indicated that he had been taking Tenormin for just over a year to control his elevated blood pressure. Paul said that he has tried to exercise on his own in the past, but never really "stuck with it." In the initial tour of your facilities, he mentioned that he knows he should begin a regular exercise program and is looking forward to your help.

Assessments

Results from Paul's preliminary physiological testing and information released from his doctor's office were as follows:

$BP_{resting}$ = 146/92 mm Hg
$HR_{resting}$ = 76 bpm
Skinfold estimate of body fat: 28%
Waist circumference: 46 inches
Cholesterol = 225 mg/dl
LDL-C = 165 mg/dl
HDL-C = 38 mg/dl
TG = 188 mg/dl
Fasting blood glucose = 120 mg/dl

> *Tenormin (atenolol) is a β-blocker that may have adverse effects on HDLC and triglyceride concentrations. Make sure Paul is aware that exercise may not be very effective at increasing HDLC or reducing triglyceride levels while taking the Tenormin. However, make it clear that his physician has determined that the benefits of taking Tenormin (i.e., controlling blood pressure) outweigh the adverse effects. Encourage Paul to discuss his prescription further with his physician.*

> *Your initial exercise prescription should be designed to encourage regular exercise. Changes in blood lipid profiles, reduced blood pressure, body weight reduction, and any other measurable health aspect may not occur immediately. Have Paul focus initially on goals aimed at frequency and exercise session completion. The health benefits will follow.*

Questions

1. Clearly identify (a) Paul's readiness to exercise and (b) his risk stratification (see *ACSM's Guidelines for Exercise Testing & Prescription*, 6th Ed.). Include supporting information for each of your answers.

2. List the primary objective(s) for Paul's INITIAL exercise program. If there is more than one, list the objectives in order of importance. (These objectives will be used to formulate your ExRx for Paul.)

3. List Paul's LONG-TERM OBJECTIVES. If there is more than one, list the objectives in order of importance. (These objectives will also be used to formulate your ExRx for Paul.)

4. List specific INITIAL exercise recommendations for aerobic exercise (i.e., mode[s], intensity, duration, and frequency). For intensity, include heart rate reserve (HRR) and

$\dot{V}o_{2R}$ ranges (if applicable), along with any other measure of intensity you determine appropriate to use. Remember to provide a rationale for each of your initial recommendations.

5. List specific INITIAL resistance training and flexibility recommendations. Again, provide a rationale for your prescription.

6. List the precautions you will take to make Paul's exercise safe.

7. List some strategies you might introduce to promote Paul's enjoyment and adherence to the program you have designed.

8. List any other lifestyle modifications that you would suggest for Paul. Items you list should address Paul's primary ExRx goals and his health and safety.

REFERENCES

1. Fielding P, Fielding C. Dynamics of lipoprotein transport in the circulatory system. In: Vance D, Vance J, eds. Biochemistry of Lipids, Lipoproteins and Membranes. Edmonton, Alberta, Canada: Elsevier Science Publishers, 1991: 427–459.

2. Jackson R, Morrisett J, Gotto A. Lipoprotein structure and metabolism. Physiol Rev 1976;56:259–316.

3. Despopoulos A, Silbernagl S. Nutrition and Digestion. Color Atlas of Physiology. 4th Ed. Stuttgart, Germany: Georg Thieme Verlag, 1991: 196–230.

4. Davis R. Lipoprotein structure and secretion. In: Vance D, Vance J, eds. Biochemistry of Lipids, Lipoproteins and Membranes. Edmonton, Alberta, Canada: Elsevier Science Publishers, 1991: 403–426.

5. Havel R, Kane J. Introduction: Structure and Metabolism of Plasma Lipoproteins. In: Scriver C, Beaudet A, Sly W, Valle D, eds. The Metabolic Bases of Inherited Disease. 7th Ed. New York: McGraw-Hill, 1995: 1841–1851.

6. Brown M, Goldstein J. A receptor-mediated pathway for cholesterol homeostasis. Science 1986;232:34–47.

7. Schneider W. Removal of lipoproteins from the plasma. In: Vance D, Vance J, eds. Biochemistry of Lipids, Lipoproteins and Membranes. Edmonton, Alberta, Canada: Elsevier Science Publishers, 1991: 461–487.

8. Glomset J. The plasma lecithin: cholesterol acyltransferase reaction. J Lipid Res 1968;9:155–167.

9. Bleicher J, Lacko A. Physiologic role and clinical significance of reverse cholesterol transport. J Am Osteopath Assoc 1992;92:625–632.

10. Fielding C, Fielding P. Molecular physiology of reverse cholesterol transport. J Lipid Res 1995;36:211–228.

11. Reichl D, Miller N. Pathophysiology of reverse cholesterol transport. Insights from inherited disorders of lipoprotein metabolism. Arteriosclerosis 1989;9:785–797.

12. Shepherd J. Lipoprotein metabolism: an overview. Ann Acad Med 1992;21:106–113.

13. Nilsson-Ehle P. Lipolysis and lipoprotein metabolism. In: Paoletti R, ed. Drugs Affecting Lipid Metabolism. Heidelberg, Germany: Springer-Verlag, 1987: 83–87.

14. Dixon J, Ginsberg H. Regulation of hepatic secretion of apolipoprotein B-containing lipoproteins: information obtained from cultured liver cells. J Lipid Res 1993;34:167–179.

15. Eisenberg S. High density lipoprotein metabolism. J Lipid Res 1984;25:1017–1058.

16. Gotto A. High-density lipoproteins: biochemical and metabolic factors. Am J Cardiol 1983;52:2B–4B.

17. Kwiterovich P. The antiatherogenic role of high-density lipoprotein cholesterol. Am J Cardiol 1998;82:13Q–21Q.

18. Lusis AJ. Atherosclerosis. Nature 2000;407:233–241.

19. Tall A. Plasma lipid transfer proteins. J Lipid Res 1986;27:361–367.

20. Patsch J, Gotto A, Olivecrona T, Eisenberg S. Formation of high density lipoprotein$_2$-like particles during lipolysis of very low density lipoproteins in vitro. Proc Natl Acad Sci USA 1978;75:4519–4521.

21. Rajaram O, Barter P. Increases in the particle size of high-density lipoproteins induced by purified lecithin:cholesterol acyltransferase: effect of low-density lipoproteins. Biochem Biophys Acta 1986;877:406–414.

22. Cheung M, Wolf A. In vitro transformation of apo A-I-containing lipoprotein subpopulations: role of lecithin: cholesterol acyltransferase and apo B-containing lipoproteins. J Lipid Res 1989;30:499–509.

23. Tikkanen M, Nikkila E. Regulation of hepatic lipase and serum lipoproteins by sex steroids. Am Heart J 1987;13:562–567.

24. Barter P, Hopkins G, Ha Y. The role of lipid transfer proteins in plasma lipoprotein metabolism. Am Heart J 1987;13:538–542.

25. Cook T, Laporte R, Washburn R, et al. Chronic low level physical activity as a determinant of high density lipoprotein cholesterol and subfractions. Med Sci Sports Exerc 1986;18:653–657.

26. Borgia M, Medici F. Perspectives in the treatment of dyslipidemias in the prevention of coronary heart disease. Angiology 1998;49:339–348.

27. Keys A, Menotti A, Aravanis C, et al. The seven countries study: 2,289 deaths in 15 years. Prev Med 1984;13:141–154.

28. People's Republic of China–United States Cardiovascular and Cardiopulmonary Epidemiological Research Group. An epidemiological study of cardiovascular and cardiopulmonary disease risk factors in four populations in the People's Republic of China: baseline report from the PRC-USA [Collaborative Study]. Circulation 1992;85:1083–1096.

29. Grundy S, Vega G. Plasma cholesterol responsiveness to saturated fatty acids. Am J Clin Nutr 1988;47:822–824.

30. Keys A, Anderson J, Frande F. Serum cholesterol response to changes in the diet. Metabolism 1965;14:776–787.

31. Hegsted D, McGandy R, Myers M. Quantitative effects of dietary fat on serum cholesterol in man. Am J Clin Nutr 1965;17:281–295.

32. Howell W, McNamara D, Tosca M. Plasma lipid and lipoprotein responses to dietary fat and cholesterol: a meta-analysis. Am J Clin Nutr 1997;65:1747–1764.

33. Spady D, Dietschy J. Interaction of dietary cholesterol and triglycerides in the regulation of hepatic low density lipoprotein transporter in the hamster. J Clin Invest 1988;81:300–309.

34. Anderson K, Castelli W, Levy D. Cholesterol and mortality: 30 years of follow-up from the Framingham Study. JAMA 1987;257:2176–2180.

35. Pekkanen J, Linn S, Heiss G, et al. Ten-year mortality from cardiovascular disease in relation to cholesterol level among men with and without preexisting cardiovascular disease. N Engl J Med 1990;322:1700–1707.

36. Stamler J, Wentworth D, Neaton J. Is the relationship between serum cholesterol and risk of premature death from coronary artery disease

continuous and graded? Findings in 356,222 primary screens of the Multiple Risk Factor Intervention Trial (MRFIT). JAMA 1986;256:2823–2828.

37. Lamarche B, Tchernof A, Moorjani S, et al. Small, dense low-density lipoprotein particles as a predictor of the risk of ischemic heart disease in men. Circulation 1997;95:69–75.

38. Bostom AG, Cupples LA, Jenner JL, et al. Elevated plasma lipoprotein(a) and coronary heart disease in men aged 55 years and younger. JAMA 1996;276:544–548.

39. Gaziano JM, Hennekens CH, O'Donnell CJ, et al. Fasting triglycerides, high-density lipoprotein and risk of myocardial infarction. Circulation 1997;96:2520–2525.

40. Jeppesen J, Hein HO, Suadicani P, Gyntelberg F. Triglyceride concentration and ischemic heart disease. An eight-year follow-up in the Copenhagen Male Study. Circulation 1998;97:1029–1036.

41. Patsch J. Is hypertriglyceridemia atherogenic? Atheroscler Reviews 1993;25:331–339.

42. Patsch J. Triglyceride-rich lipoproteins and atherosclerosis. Atherosclerosis 1994;110:S23–S26.

43. Cohn JS. Postprandial lipemia: emerging evidence for atherogenicity of remnant lipoproteins. Can J Cardiol 1998;14:18B–27B.

44. Karpe F. Postprandial lipoprotein metabolism and atherosclerosis. J Intern Med 1997;246:341–355.

45. Gordon T, Castelli W, Hjortland M, et al. High density lipoprotein as a protective factor against coronary heart disease. Am J Med 1977;62:707–714.

46. Castelli W, Doyle J, Gordon T, et al. HDL cholesterol and other lipids in coronary heart disease: The Cooperative Lipoprotein Phenotyping Study. Circulation 1977;55:767–772.

47. Castelli W, Garrison R, Wilson P, et al. Incidence of coronary heart disease and lipoprotein cholesterol levels: the Framingham Study. JAMA 1986;256:2835–2838.

48. Stampfer MJ, Sacks F, Salvini S, et al. A prospective study of cholesterol, apolipoproteins, and the risk of myocardial infarction. N Engl J Med 1991;325:373–381.

49. Jacobs D, Mebane IL, Bangdiwala SI, et al. High-density lipoprotein cholesterol as a predictor of cardiovascular disease mortality in men and women: The follow-up study of the Lipid Research Clinics Prevalence Study. Am J Epidemiol 1990;131:32–47.

50. Miller GJ, Miller NE. Plasma high-density lipoprotein concentration and development of ischaemic heart disease. Lancet 1975;1(7897)16–19.

51. Abbott RD, Wilson PW, Kannel WB, Castelli WP. High density lipoprotein cholesterol, total cholesterol screening and myocardial infarction—The Framingham Study. Arteriosclerosis 1988;8:207–211.

52. Wilson PW. High-density lipoprotein, low-density lipoprotein and coronary artery disease. Am J Cardiol 1990;66:7A–10A.

53. Manninen V, Tenkanen L, Koskinen P, et al. Joint effects of serum triglyceride and LDL cholesterol and HDL cholesterol concentrations on coronary heart disease risk in the Helsinki Heart Study. Circulation 1992;85:37–45.

54. Buring JE, O'Connor GT, Goldhaber SZ, et al. Decreased HDL$_2$ and HDL$_3$ cholesterol, Apo A-I and Apo A-II, and increased risk of myocardial infarction. Circulation 1992;85:22–29.

55. Lamarche B, Moorjani S, Cantin B, et al. Associations of HDL$_2$ and HDL$_3$ subfractions with ischemic heart disease in men. Arterioscler Thromb 1997;17:1098–1105.

56. Fager G, Wikund O, Olofsson S, et al. Serum apolipoprotein levels in relation to acute myocardial infarction and its risk factors. Arterioscler 1980;36:67–74.

57. Maciejko JJ, Holmes DR, Kottke BA, et al. Apolipoprotein A-I as a marker of angiographically assessed coronary-artery disease. N Engl J Med 1983;309:385–389.

58. DeBacker G, Rosseneu M, Deslypere JP. Discriminative value of lipids and apoproteins in coronary heart disease. Atheroscler 1982;42:197–203.

59. Noma A, Yokosuka T, Kitamura K. Plasma lipids and apolipoproteins as discriminators for presence and severity of angiographically defined coronary artery disease. Atheroscler 1983;49:1–7.

60. Davignon J, Cohn JS, Mabile L, Bernier L. Apolioprotein E and atherosclerosis: insight from animal and human studies. Clin Chem Acta 1999;286:115–143.

61. Hamilton MT, Etienne J, McClure WC, et al. Role of local contractile activity and muscle fiber type on LPL regulation during exercise. Am J Physiol 1998;275:E1016–E1022.

62. Hazzard W, Ettinger W Jr. Aging and atherosclerosis: changing considerations in cardiovascular disease prevention as the barrier to immortality is approached in old age. Am J Geriat Cardiol 1995;(July/August):16–36.

63. Ross R, Glomset J. The pathogenesis of atherosclerosis. N Engl J Med 1976;295:369–377.

64. Ross R. The pathogenesis of atherosclerosis. Nature 1993;362:801–809.

65. Ross R. Atherosclerosis—An inflammatory disease. N Engl J Med 1999;340:115–126.

66. Slotte JP, Chait A, Bierman E. Cholesterol accumulation in aortic smooth muscle cells exposed to low-density lipoproteins. Arterioscler 1988;8:750–758.

67. Van Lenten B, Fogelman A. Processing of lipoproteins in human monocyte-macrophages. J Lipid Res 1990;31:1455–1466.

68. Goldstein J, Brown M. Regulation of low-density lipoprotein receptors: Implications for pathogenesis and therapy of hypercholesterolemia and atherosclerosis. Circulation 1987;76:504–507.

69. Gianturco SH, Gotto A, Bradley WA. Hypertriglyceridemia: lipoprotein receptors and atherosclerosis. Adv Exper Med Biol 1985;183:47–71.

70. Hiltunen TP, Luoma JS, Nikkari T, Yla-Herttuala S. Expression of LDL receptor, VLDL receptor, LDLreceptor-related protein and scavenger receptor in rabbit atherosclerotic lesions. Circulation 1998;97:1079–1086.

71. Rosenfeld ME. Oxidized LDL affects multiple atherogenic cellular responses. Circulation 1991;83:2137–2140.

72. Rosenfeld ME, Khoo J, Miller E, et al. Macrophage-derived foam cells freshly isolated from rabbit atherosclerotic lesions degrade modified lipoproteins, promote oxidation of low-density lipoproteins, and contain oxidation-specific lipid-protein adducts. J Clin Invest 1991;87:90–99.

73. Tammi M, Ronnemaa T, Vihersaari T, et al. High-density lipoproteinemia due to vigorous physical work inhibits the incorporation of [3H] thymidine and the synthesis of glycosaminoglycans by human aortic arch smooth muscle cells in culture. Atheroscler 1979;32:23–32.

74. Pauciullo P, Mancini M. Treatment challenges in hypercholesterolemia. Cardiovasc Drugs Ther 1998;12:325–337.

75. National Cholesterol Education Program. Second Report of the Expert Panel on Detection, Evaluation, and Treatment of High Blood Cholesterol in Adults (Adult Treatment Panel II). Circulation 1994;89:1331–1445.

76. National Cholesterol Education Program. Third Report of the Expert Panel on Detection, Evaluation, and Treatment of High Blood Cholesterol in Adults (Adult Treatment Panel II). NIH Publication No. 01-3305. Bethesda, MD: U.S. Department of Health & Human Services. National Institutes of Health. NHLBI, 2001.

77. U.S. Department of Health & Human Services. Physical activity and health: a report of the Surgeon General. Atlanta: U.S. Department of Health and Human Services, 1996.

78. Pate R, Pratt M, Blair S. Physical activity and public health. JAMA 1995;273:402–407.

79. Boyd NF, Cousins M, Beaton M, et al. Quantitative changes in dietary fat intake and serum cholesterol in women: Results from a randomized, controlled trial. Am J Clin Nutr 1990;52:470–476.

80. Cobb MM, Teielebaum H, Risch N, et al. Influence of dietary fat, apolipoprotein E phenotype, and sex on plasma lipoprotein levels. Circulation 1992;86:849–857.

81. Dixon LB, Shannon BM, Tershakovec AM, et al. Effects of family history of heart disease, apolipoprotein E phenotype and lipoprotein(a) on the response of children's plasma lipids to change in dietary lipids. Am J Clin Nutr 1997;66:1207–1217.

82. Jenkins D, Hegele R, Jenkins A, et al. The apolipoprotein E gene and the serum low-density lipoprotein cholesterol response to dietary fiber. Metabolism 1993;42:585–593.

83. Minihane A, Khan S, Leigh-Firbank E, et al. Apo E polymorphism and fish oil supplementation in subjects with an atherogenic lipoprotein phenotype. Arterioscler Thromb 2000;20:1990–1997.

84. Krauss R. Understanding the basis for variation in response to cholesterol-lowering diets. Am J Clin Nutr 1997;65:885–886.

85. Jeppesen J, Schaaf P, Jones C, et al. Effects of low-fat, high carbohydrate diets on risk factors for ischemic heart disease in postmenopausal women. Am J Clin Nutr 1997;65:1027–1033.

86. Schlierf G, Arab L, Oster P. Influence of diet on high-density lipoproteins. Am J Cardiol 1983;52:17B–19B.

87. Dreon DM, Fernstrom HA, Campos H, et al. Change in dietary saturated fat intake is correlated with change in mass of large low-density lipoprotein particles in men. Am J Clin Nutr 1998;67:828–836.

88. Ehnholm C, Huttunen JK, Pietinen P, et al. Effect of a diet low in saturated fatty acids on plasma lipids, lipoproteins, and HDL subfractions. Arterioscler 1984;4:265–269.

89. LaRosa JC. The role of diet and exercise in the statin era. Prog Cardiovasc Dis 1998;41:137–150.

90. Roche H, Zampelas A, Jackson K, et al. The effect of test meal monounsaturated fatty acid: saturated fatty acid ratio on postprandial lipid metabolism. Br J Nutr 1998;79:419–424.

91. Thompson P, Lazarus B, Cullinane E, et al. Exercise, diet, or physical characteristics as determinants of HDL-levels in endurance athletes. Atheroscler 1983;46:333–339.

92. Hagan R, Gettman L. Maximal aerobic power, body fat, and serum lipoproteins in male distance runners. J Cardiac Rehab 1983;3:331–337.

93. Sady S, Cullinane E, Herbert P, et al. Training, diet and physical characteristics of distance runners with low or high concentrations of high-density lipoprotein cholesterol. Atheroscler 1984;53:273–281.

94. Hardman A. Interaction of physical activity and diet: Implications for lipoprotein metabolism. Public Health Nutr 1999;2:369–376.

95. Singh RB, Shama V, Gupta K, Singh R. Nutritional modulators of lipoprotein metabolism in patients with risk factors for coronary heart disease: Diet and Moderate Exercise Trial. J Am Coll Nutr 1992;11:391–398.

96. Barnard RJ. Effects of lifestyle modification on serum lipids. Arch Intern Med 1991;151:1389–1394.

97. Beard CM, Barnard J, Robbins DC, et al. Effects of diet and exercise on qualitative and quantitative measures of LDL and its susceptibility to oxidation. Arterioscler Thromb 1996;16:201–207.

98. Brown RC, Cox CM. Effects of high fat versus high carbohydrate diets on plasma lipids and lipoproteins in endurance athletes. Med Sci Sports Exerc 1998;30:1677–1683.

99. Leddy J, Horvath P, Rowland J, Pendergast D. Effect of a high or a low-fat diet on cardiovascular risk factors in male and female runners. Med Sci Sports Exerc 1997;29:17–25.

100. Bounds RG, Martin SE, Grandjean PW, et al. Diet and short-term plasma lipoprotein-lipid changes after exercise in trained men. Int J Sport Nutr Exerc Metab 2000;10:114–127.

101. Stefanick M, Mackey S, Sheehan M, et al. Effects of diet and exercise in men and postmenopausal women with low levels of HDL cholesterol and high levels of LDL cholesterol. N Engl J Med 1998;339:12–20.

102. Goldman L, Cook EF. The decline in ischemic heart disease mortality rates. An analysis of the comparative effects of medical interventions and changes in lifestyle. Ann Intern Med 1984;101:825–836.

103. Lipid Research Clinics Program. The Lipid Research Clinics Coronary Primary Prevention Trial results. I. Reduction in incidence of coronary heart disease. JAMA 1984;251:351–364.

104. Watts JF, Lewis B, Brunt JN. Effects on coronary artery disease of lipid-lowering diet, or diet plus cholestyramine in the St. Thomas Atherosclerosis Regression Trial. Lancet 1992;339:563–569.

105. Miettinen M, Turpeinen O, Karvonen MJ. Effect of cholesterol lowering diet on mortality from coronary artery disease and other causes. A 12-year clinical trial in men and women. Lancet 1972;2:835–838.

106. Renaud S, De Lorgeril M. Dietary lipids and their relation to ischemic heart disease: From epidemiology to prevention. J Intern Med 1989;225:39–46.

107. Hjermann I, Velve Byre K, Holme I. Effects of diet and smoking intervention on the incidence of coronary heart disease: Report from the Oslo Study Group of a randomized trial in healthy men. Lancet 1981;2:1303–1310.

108. Brensike JF, Levy RI, Kelsey SF. Effects of therapy with cholestyramine on progression of coronary arteriosclerosis: results of the NHLBI Type II Coronary Intervention Study. Circulation 1984;69:313–324.

109. Hasler CM, Kundrat S, Wool D. Functional foods and cardiovascular disease. Curr Atheroscler Rep 2000;2:467–475.

110. Cooper KH. Controlling Cholesterol the Natural Way. New York: Bantam Books, 1999.

111. Vuorio AF, Gylling H, Turtola H, et al. Stanol ester margarine alone and with simvastatin lowers serum cholesterol in families with familial hypercholesterolemia caused by the FH-North Karelia mutation. Arterioscler Thromb 2000;20:500–506.

112. Blair S, Capuzzi DM, Gottlieb SO, et al. Incremental reduction of serum total cholesterol and low-density lipoprotein cholesterol with the addition of plant stanol ester-containing spread to statin therapy. Am J Cardiol 2000;86:46–52.

113. Everson GT, Daggy BP, McKinley C, Story JA. Effects of psyllium hydrophilic muciloid on LDL-cholesterol and bile acid synthesis in hypercholesterolemic men. J Lipid Res 1992;33:1183–1192.

114. Heinemann T, Kullak-Ublick GA, Pietruck B, von Bergmann K. Mechanisms of action of plant sterols on inhibition of cholesterol absorption. Comparison of sitosterol and sitostanol. Eur J Clin Pharmacol 1991;40:S59–S63.

115. Brown L, Rosner B, Willett W, Sacks F. Cholesterol-lowering effects of dietary fiber: A meta-analysis. Am J Clin Nutr 1999;69:30–42.

116. Olson BH, Anderson SM, Becker MP, et al. Psyllium-enriched cereals lower blood total cholesterol and LDL cholesterol, but not HDL cholesterol in hypercholesterolemic adults: results from a meta-analysis. J Nutr 1997;127:1973–1980.

117. Jensen CD, Haskell W, Whittam JH. Long-term effects of water-soluble dietary fiber in the management of hypercholesterolemia in healthy men and women. Am J Cardiol 1997;79:34–37.

118. Gylling H, Miettinen TA. Absorption and metabolism of cholesterol in familial hypercholesterolemia. Clin Sci (Colch) 1989;76:297–301.

119. Hallikainen MA, Sarkkinen ES, Gylling H, et al. Comparison of the effects of plant sterol and plant stanol ester-enriched margarines in lowering serum cholesterol concentrations in hypercholesterolemic subjects on a low-fat diet. Eur J Clin Nutr 2000;54:715–725.

120. Hallikainen MA, Sarkkinen ES, Uusitupa MI. Plant stanol esters affect serum cholesterol concentrations of hypercholesterolemic men and women in a dose-dependent manner. J Nutr 2000;130:767–776.

121. Hendricks HF, Westrate JA, van Vliet T, Meijer GW. Spreads enriched with three different levels of vegetable oil sterols and the degree of cholesterol lowering in normocholesterolaemic and mildly hypercholesterolaemic subjects. Eur J Clin Nutr 1999;53:319–327.

122. Plat J, Van Onselen EN, Van Heugten MM, Mensink RP. Effects on serum lipids, lipoproteins and fat soluble antioxidant concentrations of consumption frequency of margarines and shortenings enriched with plant stanol esters. Eur J Clin Nutr 2000;54:671–677.

123. Hunninghake D. Therapeutic efficacy of lipid lowering armamentarium: The clinical benefits of aggressive lipid-lowering therapy. Am J Med 1998;104:9S–13S.

124. Eisenberg DA. Cholesterol lowering in the management of coronary artery disease: the clinical implications of recent trials. Am J Med 1998;104:2S–5S.

125. Blackenhorn DH, Azen SP, Kramsch DM, et al. Coronary angiographic changes with Lovastatin therapy. Ann Intern Med 1993;119:969–976.

126. Waters D, Higginson L, Gladstone P, et al. Effects of monotherapy with an HMG-CoA reductase inhibitor in the progression of coronary

atherosclerosis as assessed by serial quantitative arteriography. Circulation 1994;89:959–968.

127. Blackenhorn DH, Nessin SA, Johnson RL. Beneficial effects of combined colestipol-niacin therapy on coronary atherosclerosis and coronary venous bypass grafts. JAMA 1987;257:3233–3240.

128. Herd A, Cocanougher MK, Dunn K. The effect of aggressive lowering of low-density lipoprotein cholesterol levels and low-dose anticoagulation on obstructive changes in saphenous-vein coronary artery bypass grafts. N Engl J Med 1997;336:153–162.

129. Pedersen TR, Kjekshus J, Berg K, et al. Randomized trial of cholesterol lowering in 4444 patients with coronary heart disease: The Scandinavian Simvastatin Survival Study (4S). Lancet 1994;344:1383–1389.

130. MAAS Investigators. Effects of simvastatin on coronary atheroma: the multicentre Anti-Atheroma Study (MAAS). Lancet 1994;344:633–638.

131. Sacks F, Pfeffer MA, Moye LA, et al. The effect of pravastatin on coronary events after myocardial infarction in patients with average cholesterol levels. N Engl J Med 1996;335:1001–1009.

132. Carlson LA, Rosenhamer G. Reduction of mortality in the Stockholm Ischemic Heart Disease Secondary Prevention Study by combined therapy with clofibrate and nicotinic acid. Acta Med Scand 1988;223:405–418.

133. Downs JR, Clearfield M, Weise S. Primary prevention of acute coronary events with lovastatin in men and women with average cholesterol levels. JAMA 1998;279:1615–1622.

134. Witztum JL. Drugs used in the treatment of hyperlipoproteinemias. In: Hardman JG, Gilman AG, Limbird LE, eds. Goodman and Gilman's The Pharmacological Basis of Therapeutics. 9th Ed. New York: McGraw-Hill, 1996:875–897.

135. Nawrocki JW, Weiss SR, Davidson MH. Reduction of LDL cholesterol by 25 to 60% in patients with primary hypercholesterolemia by atorvastatin, a new HMG-CoA reductase inhibitor. Arterioscler Thromb 1995;15:678–682.

136. Bakker-Arkema RG, Davidson MH, Goldstein RJ. Efficacy and safety of a new HMG-CoA reductase inhibitor, atorvastatin, in patients with hypertriglyceridemia. JAMA 1996;275:128–133.

137. Shepherd J, Cobbe SM, Ford I. Prevention of coronary heart disease with pravastatin in men with hypercholesterolemia. N Engl J Med 1995;333:1301–1307.

138. Spratto GR, Woods AL. PDR Nurse's Drug Handbook. 2001 Edition ed. Montvale, NJ: Delmar Publishers & Medical Economics Co., 2001.

139. Manninen V, Elo MO, Frick M. Lipid alterations and decline in the incidence of coronary heart disease in the Helsinki Heart Study. JAMA 1988;260:641–651.

140. Coronary Drug Project Research Group. Clofibrate and niacin in coronary heart disease. JAMA1975;231:360–381.

141. Seiler C, Suter TM, Hess OM. Exercise-induced vasomotion of angiographically normal and stenotic coronary arteries improves after cholesterol-lowering therapy with bezafibrate. J Am Coll Cardiol 1995;26:1615–1622.

142. Fletcher G, Blair S, Blumenthal C, et al. Benefits and recommendations for physical activity programs for all Americans. A statement for health professionals by the Committee on Exercise and Cardiac Rehabilitation of the Council on Clinical Cardiology, American Heart Association. Circulation 1992;86:340–344.

143. Durstine J, Crouse S, Moffatt R. Lipids in exercise and sports. In: Driskell J, Wolinsky I, eds. Energy-Yielding Macronutrients and Energy Metabolism in Sports Nutrition. Boca Raton, FL: CRC Press, 2000: 87–117.

144. Durstine J, Haskell W. Effects of exercise training on plasma lipids and lipoproteins. In: Holloszy J, ed. Exercise and Sports Science Reviews. Philadelphia: Williams & Wilkins, 1994:477–521.

145. Wood P, Haskell W, Stern M, et al. Plasma lipoprotein distributions in male and female runners. Ann NY Acad Sci 1977;301:748–763.

146. Martin R, Haskell W, Wood P. Blood chemistry and lipid profiles of elite distance runners. Ann NY Acad Sci 1977;301:346–360.

147. Hartung G, Foreyt J, Mitchell R, et al. Relation of diet to high-density-lipoprotein cholesterol in middle-aged marathon runners, joggers, and inactive men. N Engl J Med 1980;302:357–361.

148. Lakka T, Salonen J. Physical activity and serum lipids: a cross-sectional population study in Eastern Finnish men. Am J Epidemiol 1992;136:806–818.

149. Kokkinos P, Holland J, Pittaras A, et al. Cardiorespiratory fitness and coronary heart disease risk factor association in women. J Am Coll Cardiol 1995;26:358–364.

150. Kokkinos P, Holland J, Narayan P, et al. Miles run per week and high-density lipoprotein cholesterol levels in healthy middle-aged men: a dose-response relationship. Arch Intern Med 1995;155:415–420.

151. Leclerc S, Allard C, Talbot J, et al. High-density lipoprotein cholesterol, habitual physical activity and physical fitness. Atherosclerosis 1985;57:43–51.

152. Williams P. Relationships of heart disease risk factors to exercise quantity and intensity. Arch Intern Med 1998;158:237–245.

153. Superko H. Exercise training, serum lipids and lipoprotein particles: Is there a change threshold? Med Sci Sports Exerc 1991;23:677–685.

154. Gordon D, Witztum D, Hunninghake D. Habitual physical activity and high-density lipoprotein cholesterol in men with primary hypercholesterolemia. Circulation 1983;67:512–520.

155. Gordon D, Probstfeld J, Rubenstein C. Coronary risk factors and exercise test performance in asymptomatic hypercholesterolemic men: Application of proportional hazards analysis. Am J Epidemiol 1984;120:210–224.

156. Halbert J, Silagy C, Finucane P, et al. Exercise training and blood lipids in hyperlipidemic and normolipidemic adults: a meta-analysis of randomized controlled trials. Eur J Clin Nutr 1999;53:514–522.

157. Gordon D, Knoke J, Probstfeld J, et al. High-density lipoprotein cholesterol and coronary heart disease in hypercholesterolemic men: the Lipid Research Clinics Coronary Primary Prevention Trial. Circulation 1986;74:1217–1225.

158. King A, Haskell W, Young D, et al. Long-term effects of varying intensities and formats of physical activity on participation rates, fitness, and lipoproteins in men and women aged 50 to 65. Circulation 1995;91:2596–2604.

159. Seip R, Moulin P, Cocke T, et al. Exercise training decreases plasma cholesterol ester transfer protein. Atheroscler Thromb 1993;13:1359–1367.

160. Sunami Y, Motoyama M, Kinoshita F, et al. Effect of low-intensity aerobic training on the high-density lipoprotein cholesterol concentration in healthy elderly subjects. Metabolism 1999;48:984–988.

161. Krummel D, Etherton T, Peterson S, Kris-Etherton P. Effects of exercise on plasma lipids and lipoproteins of women. Proc Soc Ex Biol Med 1993;204:123–137.

162. Ponjee G, Janssen E, Hermans J, van Wersch J. Effect of long-term exercise of moderate intensity on anthropometric values and serum lipids and lipoproteins. Eur J Clin Chem Clin Biochem 1995;33:121–126.

163. Hill J, Theil J, Heller P, et al. Differences in effects of aerobic exercise training on blood lipids in men and women. Am J Cardiol 1989;63:254–256.

164. Taylor P, Ward A. Women, high-density lipoprotein cholesterol, and exercise. Arch Intern Med 1993;153:1178–1184.

165. Grandjean PW, Crouse SF, O'Brien BC, et al. The effects of menopausal status and exercise training on serum lipids and the activities of intravascular enzymes related to lipid transport. Metabolism 1998;47:377–383.

166. Binder E, Birge S, Kohrt W. Effects of endurance exercise and hormone replacement therapy on serum lipids in older women. J Am Geriatric Soc 1996;44:231–236.

167. Raz I, Rosenblit H, Kark J. Effect of moderate exercise on serum lipids in young men with low high density lipoprotein cholesterol. Arteriosclerosis 1988;8:245–251.

168. Williams P, Stefanick M, Vranizan K, Wood P. The effects of weight loss by exercise or by dieting on plasma high density lipoprotein (HDL) levels in men with low, intermediate, and normal-to-high HDL at baseline. Metabolism 1994;43:917–924.
169. Houmard J, Bruno N, Bruner R, et al. Effects of exercise training on the chemical composition of plasma LDL. Atheroscler Thromb 1994;14:325–330.
170. Zmuda J, Yurgalevitch S, Flynn M, et al. Exercise training has little effect on HDL levels and metabolism in men with initially low HDL cholesterol. Atherosclerosis 1998;137:215–221.
171. Nicklas B, Katzel L, Busby-Whitehead J, Goldberg A. Increases in high-density lipoprotein cholesterol with endurance exercise training are blunted in obese compared with lean men. Metabolism 1997;46:556–561.
172. Duncan J, Gordon N, Scott C. Women walking for health and fitness. How much is enough? JAMA 1991;266:3295–3299.
173. Lewis S, Haskell W, Wood P, et al. Effects of physical activity on weight reduction in obese middle-aged women. Am J Clin Nutr 1976;29:151–156.
174. Hardman A, Hudson A, Jones P, Norgan N. Brisk walking and high density lipoprotein cholesterol concentration in previously sedentary women. Br Med J 1989;299:1204–1205.
175. Rotkis T, Boyden T, Stanforth P, et al. Increased high-density lipoprotein cholesterol in women after 10 weeks of training. J Cardiac Rehabil 1984;4:62–66.
176. Goodyear L, Fronsoe M, Van Houten D, et al. Increased HDL-cholesterol following eight weeks of progressive endurance training in female runners. Ann Sports Med 1986;3:33–38.
177. Schwartz R. The independent effects of dietary weight loss and aerobic training on high density lipoproteins and apolipoprotein A-I concentrations in obese men. Metabolism 1987;36:165–171.
178. Coon P, Bleecker E, Crinkwater D, et al. Effects of body composition and exercise capacity on glucose tolerance, insulin, and lipoprotein lipids in healthy older men: A cross-sectional and longitudinal intervention study. Metabolism1989;38:1201–1209.
179. Lamarche B, Despres J, Pouliot M-C, et al. Is body fat loss a determinant factor in the improvement of carbohydrate and lipid metabolism following aerobic exercise training in obese women? Metabolism 1992;41:1249–1256.
180. Buono M, McKenzie T, McKenzie R. Effects of a diet and exercise program on blood lipids, cardiorespiratory function, and body composition in obese women. Clin Kinesiology 1988;42:22–25.
181. Andersen R, Wadden T, Bartlett S, et al. Effects of lifestyle activity vs. structured aerobic exercise in obese women. JAMA 1999;281:335–340.
182. Nieman D, Haig J, Fairchild K, et al. Reducing-diet and exercise-training effects on serum lipids and lipoproteins in mildly obese women. Am J Clin Nutr 1990;52:640–645.
183. Wood P, Stefanick M, Williams P, Haskell W. The effects on plasma lipoproteins of a prudent weight-reducing diet, with or without exercise, in overweight men and women. N Engl J Med 1991;325:461–466.
184. Baker T, Allen D, Lei K, Wilcox K. Alterations in lipid and protein profiles of plasma lipoproteins in middle-aged men consequent to an aerobic exercise program. Metabolism 1986;35:1037–1043.
185. Kiens B, Jorgenson I, Lewis S, et al. Increased plasma HDL-cholesterol and Apo A-I in sedentary middle-aged men after physical conditioning. J Clin Invest 1980;10:203–209.
186. Lopez A, Vial R, Balart L, Arroyave G. Effect of exercise and physical fitness on serum lipids and lipoproteins. Atherosclerosis 1974;20:1–9.
187. Nye E, Carlson K, Kirstein P, Rossner S. Changes in high density lipoprotein subfractions and other lipoproteins induced by exercise. Clin Chim Acta 1981;113:51–57.
188. Peltonen P, Marniemi J, Hietanen E, et al. Changes in serum lipids, lipoproteins, and heparin releasable lipolytic enzymes during moderate physical training in man: a longitudinal study. Metabolism 1981;30:518–526.
189. Moll M, Williams S, Lester R, et al. Cholesterol metabolism in non-obese women. Atherosclerosis 1979;34:159–166.
190. Bassett-Frey M, Doerr B, Laubach L, et al. Exercise does not change high-density lipoprotein cholesterol in women after 10 weeks of training. Metabolism 1996;31:1142–1146.
191. Crouse S, O'Brien B, Grandjean P, et al. Training intensity, blood lipids and apolipoproteins in men with high cholesterol. J Appl Physiol 1996;82:270–277.
192. Franklin B, Buskirk E, Hodgson J, et al. Effects of physical conditioning on cardiorespiratory function, body composition, and serum lipids in relatively normal-weight and obese middle-aged women. Int J Obes 1979;3:97–109.
193. Leon A, Conrad J, Hunninghake D, Serfass R. Effects of a vigorous walking program on body composition, carbohydrate and lipid metabolism of obese young men. Am J Clin Nutr 1979;32:1776–1787.
194. Milesis C, Pollock M, Bah M, et al. Effects of different durations of physical training on cardiorespiratory function, body composition, and serum lipids. Res Q 1976;47:716–725.
195. Whitehurst M, Menendez E. Endurance training in older women. Physician and Sports Medicine 1991;19:95–103.
196. Van der Eems K, Ismail A. Relationships between age and selected serum lipids and lipoproteins in women before and after a physical fitness programme. Br J Sports Med 1985;6:43–45.
197. Wirth A, Diehm C, Hanel W, et al. Training-induced changes in serum lipids, fat tolerance, and adipose tissue metabolism in patients with hypertriglyceridemia. Atherosclerosis 1985;54:263–271.
198. Wood P, Haskell W, Blair S, et al. Increased exercise level and plasma lipoprotein concentrations: a one year randomized, controlled study in sedentary middle-aged men. Metabolism 1983;32:31–39.
199. Wood P, Stefanick M, Dreon D, et al. Changes in plasma lipids and lipoproteins in overweight men during weight loss through dieting as compared with exercise. N Engl J Med 1988;319:1173–1179.
200. Despres J-P, Moorjani S, Tremblay A, et al. Heredity and changes in plasma lipids and lipoproteins after short-term exercise training in men. Arterioscler. 1988;8:402–409.
201. Despres J-P, Moorjani S, Lupien P, et al. Regional distribution of body fat, plasma lipoproteins, and cardiovascular disease. Arterioscler. 1990;10:497–511.
202. Huttunen J, Lansimies E, Voutilainen E, et al. Effect of moderate physical exercise on serum lipoproteins: a controlled clinical trial with special reference to serum high-density lipoproteins. Circulation 1979;60:1220–1229.
203. Schwartz R, Cain K, Shuman W, et al. Effect of intensive endurance training on lipoprotein profiles in young and older men. Metabolism 1992;41:649–654.
204. Wynne T, Bassett-Frey M, Laubach L, Glueck C. Effect of a controlled exercise program on serum lipoprotein levels in women on oral contraceptives. Metabolism 1980;29:1267–1271.
205. Aellen R, Hollmann W, Boutellier U. Effects of aerobic and anaerobic training on plasma lipoproteins. Int J Sports Med 1993;14:396–400.
206. Dressendorfer R, Wade C, Hornick C, Timmis G. High-density lipoprotein cholesterol in marathon runners during a 20-day road race. JAMA 1982;247:1715–1717.
207. Higuchi M, Hashimoto I, Yamakawa K, et al. Effect of exercise training on plasma high-density lipoprotein cholesterol level at constant weight. Clin Physiol 1984;4:125–133.
208. Pollock M, Tiffany J, Gettman L, et al. Effects of frequency of training on serum lipids, cardiovascular function and body composition. In: Franks BD, ed. Exercise & Fitness. New York: Athletic Institution, 1969: 161–177.
209. Stein R, Michielli D, Glantz M, et al. Effects of different exercise training intensities on lipoprotein cholesterol fractions in healthy middle-aged men. Am Heart J 1990;119:277–283.
210. Sutherland W, Nye E, Woodhouse S. Red blood cell cholesterol levels, plasma cholesterol esterification rate and serum lipids and lipoproteins in men with hypercholesterolaemia and normal men during 16 weeks physical training. Atheroscler 1983;47:145–157.

211. Tomiyasu K, Ishikawa T, Ikewaki K, Nakamura H. Effects of exercise on plasma lipases and cholesterol ester transfer protein activities in normolipidemic male subjects. Nutr Metab Cardiovasc Dis 1996;6:13–20.

212. Thompson P, Cullinane E, Sady S, et al. Modest changes in high-density lipoprotein concentrations and metabolism with prolonged exercise training. Circulation 1988;78:25–34.

213. Thompson P, Yurgalevitch S, Flynn M, et al. Effect of prolonged exercise training without weight loss on high-density lipoprotein metabolism in overweight men. Metabolism 1997;46:217–223.

214. Weintraub M, Rosen Y, Otto R, et al. Physical exercise conditioning in the absence of weight loss reduces fasting and postprandial triglyceride-rich lipoprotein levels. Circulation 1989;79:1007–1014.

215. Blumenthal J, Emery C, Madden D. Effects of exercise training on cardiorespiratory function in men and women > 60 years of age. Am J Cardiol 1991;67:633–639.

216. Blumenthal J, Rejeski J, Walsh-Riddle M, et al. Comparison of high- and low-intensity exercise training early after acute myocardial infarction. Am J Cardiol 1988;61:26–30.

217. Weltman A, Matter S, Stamford B. Caloric restriction and / or mild exercise: Effects on serum lipids and body composition. Am J Clin Nutr 1980;33:1002–1009.

218. Vermeulen A. Plasma lipid and lipoprotein levels in obese postmenopausal women: Effects of a short-term low-protein diet and exercise. Maturitas 1990;12:121–126.

219. Warner J, Ullrich I, Albrink M, Yeater R. Combined effects of aerobic exercise and omega-3 fatty acids in hyperlipidemic persons. Med Sci Sports Exerc 1989;21:498–505.

220. Sopko G, Jacobs D, Jeffery R, et al. Effects of blood lipids and body weight in high risk men of a practical exercise program. Atheroscler 1983;49:219–229.

221. Gaesser G, Rich R. Effects of high- and low-intensity exercise training on aerobic capacity and blood lipids. Med Sci Sports Exerc 1984;16:269–274.

222. Savage M, Petratis M, Thompson W, et al. Exercise training effects on serum lipids of prepubescent boys and adult men. Med Sci Sports Exerc 1986;18:197–204.

223. Marti B, Suter E, Riesen W, et al. Effects of long-term, self-monitored exercise on the serum lipoprotein and apolipoprotein profile in middle-aged men. Atheroscler 1990;81:19–31.

224. Smutok A, Reece C, Kokkinos P, et al. Aerobic versus strength training for risk factor intervention in middle-aged men at high risk for coronary heart disease. Metabolism 1993;42:177–184.

225. Blumenthal J, Matthews K, Fredrikson M, et al. Effects of exercise training on cardiovascular function and plasma lipid, lipoprotein, and apolipoprotein concentrations in premenopausal and postmenopausal women. Arterioscler Thromb 1991;11:912–917.

226. Kokkinos P, Hurley B, Smutok A, et al. Strength training does not improve lipoprotein-lipid profiles in men at risk for CHD. Med Sci Sports Exerc 1991;23:1134–1139.

227. Kokkinos P, Hurley B, Vaccaro P, et al. Effects of low- and high-repetition resistive training on lipoprotein-lipid profiles. Med Sci Sports Exerc 1988;20:50–54.

228. Manning J, Dooly-Manning C, White K, et al. Effects of a resistive training program on lipoprotein-lipid levels in obese women. Med Sci Sports Exerc 1991;23:1222–1226.

229. Boyden T, Pamenter R, Going S, et al. Resistance exercise training is associated with decreases in serum low-density lipoprotein cholesterol levels in premenopausal women. Arch Intern Med 1993;153: 97–100.

230. Goldberg L, Elliot D, Schutz R, Kloster F. Changes in lipid and lipoprotein levels after weight training. JAMA 1984;252:504–506.

231. Hurley B, Hagberg J, Goldberg A, Seals D, Ehasani A, Brennan R, et al. Resistive training can reduce coronary risk factors without altering VO2max or percent body fat. Med Sci Sports Exerc 1988;20: 150–154.

232. Oscai L, Patterson J, Bogard D, et al. Normalization of serum triglycerides and lipoprotein electrophoretic patterns by exercise. Am J Cardiol 1972;30:775–780.

233. Holloszy J, Skinner J, Toro G, Cureton T. Effects of a six month program of endurance exercise on lipids in middle aged men. Am J Cardiol 1964;14:753–760.

234. Carlson LA, Mossfeldt F. Acute effects of prolonged, heavy exercise on the concentration of plasma lipids and lipoproteins in man. Acta Physiol Scand 1964;62:51–59.

235. Enger S, Stromme S, Refsum H. High density lipoprotein cholesterol, total cholesterol, triglycerides in serum after a single exposure to prolonged heavy exercise. Acta Med Scand 1981;645:57–64.

236. Kirkeby K, Stromme S, Bjerkedal I, et al. Effects of prolonged, strenuous exercise on lipids and thyroxine in serum. Acta Med Scand 1977;202:463–467.

237. Thompson P, Cullinane E, Henderson O, Herbert P. Acute effects of prolonged exercise on serum lipids. Metabolism 1980;29:662–665.

238. Crouse S, O'Brien B, Grandjean P, et al. Effects of exercise training and a single session of exercise on lipids and apolipoproteins in hypercholesterolemic men. J Appl Physiol 1997;83:2019–2028.

239. Grandjean PW, Crouse SF, Rohack JJ. Influence of cholesterol status on blood lipid and lipoprotein enzyme responses to aerobic exercise. J Appl Physiol 2000;89:472–480.

240. Grandjean PW, Crouse SF, O'Brien BC, et al. Short-term changes in plasma lipids and lipases after aerobic exercise: Impact of obesity [abstract]. Med Sci Sports Exerc 1999;31(Suppl):S135.

241. Pronk N, Crouse S, O'Brien B, Rohack J. Acute effects of walking on serum lipids and lipoproteins in women. J Sports Med Phys Fitness 1995;35:50–58.

242. Davis P, Bartoli W, Durstine J. Effects of acute exercise intensity on plasma lipids and apolipoproteins in trained runners. J Appl Physiol 1992;72:914–919.

243. Crouse S, O'Brien B, Rohack J, et al. Changes in serum lipids and apolipoproteins after exercise in men with high cholesterol: Influence of intensity. J Appl Physiol 1995;79:279–286.

244. Ferguson M, Alderson N, Trost S, et al. Effects of four different single exercise sessions on lipids, lipoproteins, and lipoprotein lipase. J Appl Physiol 1998;85:1169–1174.

245. Foger B, Wohlfarter T, Ritsch A, et al. Kinetics of lipids, apolipoproteins and cholesteryl ester transfer protein in plasma after a bicycle marathon. Metabolism 1994;43:633–639.

246. Sady S, Thompson P, Cullinane E, et al. Prolonged exercise augments plasma triglyceride clearance. JAMA 1986;256:2552–2555.

247. Visich P, Goss F, Gordon P, et al. Effects of exercise with varying energy expenditures on high-density lipoprotein cholesterol. Eur J Appl Physiol Occup Physiol 1996;72:242–248.

248. Cullinane E, Lazarus B, Thompson P, Saritelli A. Acute effects of a single exercise session on serum lipids in untrained men. Clin Chim Acta 1981;109:341–344.

249. Kantor M, Cullinane E, Sady SH, et al. Exercise acutely increases high density lipoprotein-cholesterol and lipoprotein lipase activity in trained and untrained men. Metabolism 1987;36:188–192.

250. Grandjean PW, Crouse SF, Rohack JJ. Lipid responses to a single bout of exercise in type IIa and IIb hypercholesterolemic men [abstract]. Med Sci Sports Exer 2000;32(Suppl):S1877.

251. Goodyear L, Van Houten D, Fronsoe M, et al. Immediate and delayed effects of marathon running on lipids and lipoproteins in women. Med Sci Sports Exerc 1990;22:588–592.

252. Hughes RA, Housh TJ, Hughes RJ, Johnson GO. The effect of exercise duration on serum cholesterol and triglycerides in women. Res Q Exerc Sport 1991;62:98–104.

253. Crouse SF, Cockrill SL, Grandjean PW, et al. LDL and HDL densities after exercise in postmenopausal women with normal and high cholesterol [abstract]. Med Sci Sports Exerc 1999;31(Suppl): S370.

254. Lamon-Fava S, McNamara J, Farber H, et al. Acute changes in lipid, lipoprotein, apolipoprotein, and low-density lipoprotein particle size after an endurance triathlon. Metabolism 1989;38:921–925.

255. Liu M, Bergholm R, Makimattila S, et al. A marathon run increases the susceptibility of LDL to oxidation in vitro and modifies plasma antioxidants. Am J Physiol 1999;276:E1083–E1091.

256. Hoefler G, Harnoncourt F, Paschke E, et al. Lipoprotein(a): A risk factor for myocardial infarction. Arterioscler 1988;8:398–401.
257. Seman LJ, DeLuca C, Jenner JL, et al. Lipoprotein(a)-cholesterol and coronary heart disease in the Framingham Heart Study. Clin Chem 1999;45:1039–1046.
258. Gruden G, Olivetti C, Taliano C, et al. Lipoprotein(a) after acute exercise in healthy subjects. Inter J Clin Lab Res 1996;26:140–141.
259. Hubinger L, Mackinnon LT, Barber L, et al. Acute effects of treadmill running on lipoprotein(a) levels in males and females. Med Sci Sports Exerc 1997;29:436–442.
260. Hicks A, MacDougal J, Muckle T. Acute changes in high-density lipoprotein cholesterol with exercise of different intensities. J Appl Physiol 1987;63:1956–1960.
261. Hughes R, Thorland W, Housh T, Johnson G. The effect of exercise intensity on serum lipoprotein responses. J Sports Med Phys Fitness 1990;30:254–260.
262. Tsetsonis NV, Hardman A. The influence of the intensity of treadmill walking upon changes in lipid and lipoprotein variables in healthy adults. Eur J Phys 1995;70:329–336.
263. Gordon P, Goss F, Visich P, et al. The acute effects of exercise intensity on HDL-C metabolism. Med Sci Sports Exerc 1994;26:671–677.
264. Hardman A, Lawrence J, Herd SL. Postprandial lipemia in endurance-trained people during short interruption to training. J Appl Physiol 1998;84:1895–1901.
265. Greiwe JS, Holloszy J, Semenkovich C. Exercise induces lipoprotein lipase and GLUT-4 protein in muscle independent of adrenergic-receptor signaling. J Appl Physiol 2000;89:176–181.
266. Berger G, Griffiths M. Acute effects of moderate exercise on plasma lipoprotein parameters. Int J Sports Med 1987;8:336–841.
267. Dufaux B, Order U, Muller R, Hollmann W. Delayed effects of prolonged exercise on serum lipoproteins. Metabolism 1986;35:105–109.
268. Frey I, Baumstark M, Berg A, Keul J. Influence of acute maximal exercise on lecithin:cholesterol acyltransferase activity in healthy adults of differing aerobic performance. Eur J Appl Physiol 1991;62:31–35.
269. Dufaux B, Assmann G, Order U, et al. Plasma lipoproteins and physical activity: A review. Int J Sports Med 1982;3:123–136.
270. Nicolosi RJ, Kritchevsky D, Wilson TA. The pathobiology of hypercholesterolemia and atherosclerosis. In: Rippe JM, ed. Lifestyle Medicine. Malden, MA.: Blackwell Science, 1999: 25–39.
271. Powell KE. Population attributable risk of physical inactivity. In: Leon A, ed. Physical Activity and Cardiovascular Health. Champaign, IL: Human Kinetics, 1997: 40–46.
272. Smith CA, Pratt M. Cardiovascular disease. In: Brownson RC, Remington PL, Davis JR, eds. Chronic Disease Epidemiology and Control. Washington, DC: American Public Health Association, 1993: 83–107.
273. Martin MJ, Hulley S, Browner WS. Serum cholesterol, blood pressure, and mortality: Implications from a cohort of 361,662 men. Lancet 1986;2:933–936.

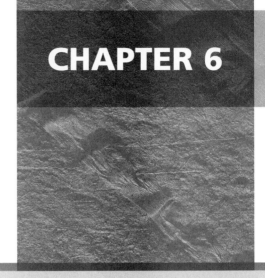

CHAPTER 6

Cardiomyopathies

Antonio Pelliccia

Overview

In 1980, the World Health Organization and the International Cardiology Task Force produced the first definition of cardiomyopathy, describing it as "heart muscle disease of unknown causes." They divided the cardiomyopathies into three broad classifications based on the characteristic anatomic findings of the heart: dilation, hypertrophy, and restriction (Table 6.1). The rationale behind these divisions was that the different cardiomyopathies had distinct pathophysiologic mechanisms, natural histories, and medical treatment. A fourth group, "unclassified cardiomyopathies," included cases that did not easily fit into one of these categories. In 1996, a new categorization was released, in which arrhythmogenic right ventricular cardiomyopathy was added (1).

In athletes or physically active individuals, certain cardiomyopathies have major interest, e.g., hypertrophic car-diomyopathy (HCM), dilated cardiomyopathy (DCM), and arrhythmogenic right ventricular cardiomyopathy (ARVC). These pathologic conditions are responsible for sudden and unexpected death in young individuals, often in association with exercise and sport participation (2–4). Indeed, these cardiomyopathies mimic certain morphologic cardiac features of the "athlete's heart." As a result, questions have emerged regarding the differential diagnosis between a pathologic condition with adverse clinical consequences and a physiologic, benign cardiac adaptation to intensive athletic conditioning (5).

Hypertrophic Cardiomyopathy

Hypertrophic cardiomyopathy (HCM) is a primary cardiac disease with the characteristic morphologic pattern of a hypertrophied and nondilated left ventricle (LV) (6). The

TABLE 6.1.   WORLD HEALTH ORGANIZATION CLASSIFICATION OF CARDIOMYOPATHIES

Hypertrophic
Dilated
   Idiopathic
   Familial/genetic
   Viral/immune
   Alcohol/toxic
Right ventricular
   Arrhythmogenic right ventricular cardiomyopathy
   Uhl disease
Restrictive
   Idiopathic myocardial fibrosis
   Endomyocardial and Loffler endocardial fibrosis
Unclassified
   Fibroelastosis
   Noncompacted myocardium
   Systolic dysfunction with minimal dilatation
   Mitochondrial myopathies
Specific
   Ischemic
   Valvular
   Hypertensive
   Inflammatory
   Tachycardia-induced
   Metabolic
   Peripartal

prevalence of this disease in the general population is estimated to be 0.2%. This prevalence is greater than previously thought, because in recent years noninvasive testing (especially echocardiography) and the techniques of molecular diagnosis have recognized a wider spectrum of morphologic and clinical alterations associated with this disease.

Genetic Defects

Hypertrophic cardiomyopathy can be caused by several **mutations** in any one of different genes that encode proteins of the **cardiac sarcomere** (7–10). The abnormalities related to the thick filament include beta-myosin heavy chain on chromosome 14. Those related to the thin filament include cardiac troponin T on chromosome 1, troponin I on chromosome 19, and alfa-tropomyosin on chromosome 15. Other genetic abnormalities include those related to the skeleton of the sarcomere, which comprise myosin-binding protein C on chromosome 11, cardiac actin on chromosome 15, and titin on chromosome 2. Available data suggest that mutations in the beta-myosin heavy chain are the most common alterations and may account for about 35% to 50% of all familial HCMs. Mutations in cardiac myosin-binding protein C and troponin T account for an additional 15% to 20% each; mutations in the other genes are less common and account for 10% in total.

All of the known mutations in HCM involve genes that encode proteins of the sarcomere. This finding represents a unifying principle that allows scientists to regard these diverse genetic alterations as a single disease entity. Genetic defects appear to eventually cause impaired myocardial contractility, which triggers the cascade of events that results in the compensatory hypertrophy of myocytes and the proliferation of fibroblasts. Environmental factors also can affect the HCM phenotypes and explain why the hypertrophy is mostly restricted to the LV, despite the equal abundance of mutant proteins in the right ventricle, as well as the reduction in wall thickness and cardiac mass in patients in whom the LV outflow gradient had been eliminated by septal alcohol injection (6, 9, 10).

Morphologic Alterations

Left ventricular hypertrophy traditionally has been regarded as the gross anatomic marker and the determinant of many clinical features and consequences in patients with HCM (6, 11).

Left Ventricular Wall Thickness

The maximum left ventricular wall thickness ranges from mildly increased (>13 mm) to massively increased (>35 mm), including the most substantial hypertrophy observed in any cardiac disease (60 mm), but in most patients the thickness averages 20 to 22 mm (11). However, a substantial minority of persons (particularly family members identified in the course of pedigree mapping) show only mild LV wall thickening (13 to 15 mm), which may create diagnostic ambiguity, particularly in young subjects involved in athletic activities (12). The distribution of hypertrophy usually is asymmetrical, and virtually all possible patterns of LV wall thickening may occur.

Left ventricular wall thickening usually becomes evident during adolescence, with spontaneous increases in the magnitude and extent of wall thickening in association with accelerated body growth and maturation. Consequently, most children with HCM do not show LV hypertrophy (as assessed by two-dimensional echocardiography) until adolescence (6). Although in most HCM patients LV remodeling is complete by about 18 years of age, a few genetically affected individuals (particularly those with mutations in the gene for cardiac myosin-binding protein C) show little or no hypertrophy (in them, the maximum LV wall thickness is ≤13 mm) during adulthood and present with a late onset of the hypertrophic process in midlife or beyond (7, 9, 10). On the contrary, a late *decrease* in LV wall thickness in adult HCM patients identifies a subset of individuals with decreasing LV systolic function and worsening of the clinical course (the "end-stage" disease [13]).

Left Ventricular Cavity

The LV cavity usually is reduced in size and shows an abnormal and sometimes bizarre shape as a consequence of asymmetric thickening of the LV walls. Indeed, increased LV chamber stiffness and abnormal **LV filling** (as evaluated by Doppler echocardiography) are present in most patients with HCM (6). Typically, the early peak of transmitral flow-velocity (E) is decreased, the deceleration time of the early peak is prolonged, the late (atrial, A) peak is increased, and the E/A ratio is inverted. In HCM, diastolic dysfunction is not strictly related to the severity and distribution of LV hypertrophy, and may be present in cases with only mild hypertrophy and no symptoms. Other morphologic alterations include malformation of the mitral valve apparatus, with enlargement and elongation of the leaflets in various patterns, anomalous papillary muscles inserted directly into the anterior mitral leaflet, or abnormal intramural coronary arteries with thickened walls and a narrowed lumen (6).

Differential Diagnosis Between Hypertrophic Cardiomyopathy and "Athlete's Heart"

In athletes, LV remodeling is the consequence of hemodynamic overload associated with chronic exercise training. The intense exercise training causes an increase in LV dimensions, including wall thickness above the upper normal limits predicted by age and body size (14, 15). Specifically, absolute LV wall thickness may be 13 mm or more, falling in a range compatible with the diagnosis of HCM, in a small, but important, subset of elite athletes (16). Differentiation between HCM and "athlete's heart" may convey ethical, economic, and legal implications. For example, the diagnosis of HCM is the basis for disqualification of an athlete from competition in an effort to minimize the risk of sudden cardiac death (17). On the other hand, the identification of physiologic LV hypertrophy associated with "athlete's heart" may avoid an unnecessary withdrawal of the athlete from competition, and the unjustified loss of the varied (including economic) benefits derived from sport.

Several criteria have been devised that may offer a measure of clarification for this clinical dilemma (5) (Figure 6.1).

Maximum Left Ventricular Wall Thickness

The maximum LV wall thickness found in highly trained athletes may reach 15 or 16 mm, which probably represents the upper limit of physiologic LV wall thickening (16). In patients with HCM, LV wall thickness usually is greater and averages 20 to 22 mm (11); however, an important minority of patients may show only mild hypertrophy, with wall thickness in a "gray zone" of 13 to 15 mm (11, 12). This overlaps the LV dimensions found in elite athletes.

In athletes, the distribution of LV hypertrophy is substantially symmetric and regular, and differences among various segments of LV walls are small (≤2 mm) (16). In

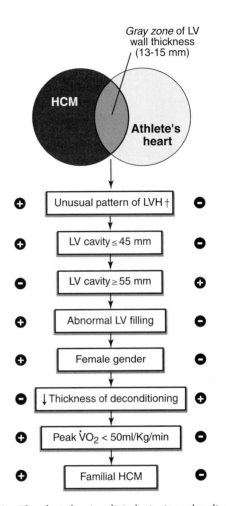

FIGURE 6.1. Flowchart showing clinical criteria used to distinguish HCM from "athlete's heart" when left ventricular (LV) wall thickness is in the "grayzone" of overlap consistent with both diagnoses.
† Unusual pattern of hypertrophy includes heterogeneous distribution of LV hypertrophy, in which asymmetry is prominent and adjacent regions may be of greatly different thicknesses, with sharp transition evident between segments; also, patterns in which the anterior ventricular septum is spared from the hypertrophic process and the predominant thickening may be in the posterior portion of the septum, or anterolateral or posterior free wall, or the apex. LA, left atrium; LV, left ventricle; ↓, decreased.

HCM patients, the distribution of hypertrophy is characteristically asymmetric and heterogeneous, and contiguous portions of LV walls may show different thicknesses, with an abrupt transition between adjacent segments.

Left Ventricular Cavity

The LV cavity in the "athlete's heart" usually is enlarged (i.e., end-diastolic diameter ≥55 mm) (15) and maintains the physiologic ellipsoid shape (18), with the mitral valve normally positioned, and there is no evidence of LV outflow obstruction. In patients with HCM, the LV cavity dimension is within normal limits or even small (the end-diastolic diameter often is <45 mm), with the cavity shape often greatly distorted and the mitral valve displaced interiorly (11).

Left Ventricular Filling

Trained athletes with physiologic LV hypertrophy consistently show normal LV filling, as evaluated by Doppler echocardiography (19). In contrast, abnormalities in LV filling have been described in as many as 80% of HCM patients (20). Therefore, in an athlete with borderline LV wall thickening, the presence of an abnormal Doppler diastolic waveform strongly suggests the diagnosis of HCM. A normal diastolic LV filling is not useful for differential diagnosis, because it may be compatible with either "athlete's heart" or HCM.

Dynamic Changes in Left Ventricular Hypertrophy

Serial echocardiographic studies in athletes demonstrate dynamic changes in LV dimensions related to changes in the training load and, specifically, a reduction of LV wall thickness after deconditioning. In fact, elite and highly trained rowers examined at peak conditioning (when maximum LV wall thickness averaged 13–15 mm) and later after an average 3-month complete deconditioning period showed a significant reduction in wall thickness (2–5 mm, mean 3 mm) (21). The potential for normalization of physiologic LV wall thickening was confirmed by a recent study in which investigators prospectively assessed LV remodeling by echocardiography in athletes over a 6-year period after the cessation of their athletic careers. A complete normalization of LV hypertrophy with wall thickness returning to normal values (i.e., ≤12 mm) in each athlete was reported (22).

In HCM patients, however, no substantial changes in LV wall thickness are expected to occur in response to changes in their habitual physical activity. Consequently, a brief period of complete deconditioning combined with serial echocardiographic studies may be useful in distinguishing physiologic from pathologic LV hypertrophy. This approach, however, requires high-quality echocardiographic images and the athlete's compliance with a temporary interruption of the training program.

Type of Sport and Peak Oxygen Consumption

Physiologic LV hypertrophy is virtually restricted to highly trained athletes engaged in endurance disciplines (primarily rowing, canoeing, and cycling) (16). Elite athletes engaged in these disciplines have superior exercise performance and often attain a high peak oxygen consumption (e.g., a $\dot{V}o_{2max}$ > 50 ml/kg/min, and often > 70 ml/kg/min). On the other hand, asymptomatic patients with HCM and only mild LV hypertrophy (in a range of 13 to 16 mm) show a reduced aerobic power (i.e., $\dot{V}o_{2max}$ < 50 ml/kg/min) (23).

Gender

Gender itself may be a diagnostic criterion. In a large cohort of 600 highly trained women athletes engaged in a variety of different sport disciplines, borderline LV wall thickening (13 to 15 mm) was virtually absent (24); therefore, this finding in female athletes is unlikely to represent the physiologic consequence of physical training and is more likely to be an expression of pathologic hypertrophy.

Genetic Testing

Recent advances in molecular biology have raised the possibility of DNA diagnosis in individuals suspected of having HCM (7–10). Currently, a variety of mutations in 10 genes have been described in familial HCM, and more than 200 individual disease-causing mutations have been reported for these genes. The identification of genetic alterations responsible for HCM has increased the expectation for widespread DNA testing as the definitive method to resolve the uncertainty of clinical diagnosis; however, due to the substantial genetic heterogeneity of the disease and the complex, time-consuming, and expensive techniques needed for genetic screening, DNA analysis currently is restricted to research-oriented genotyping of selected pedigrees and is not yet routinely available for clinical practice.

Clinical Presentation and Natural History

Hypertrophic cardiomyopathy shows a broad spectrum of clinical expressions due to different pathophysiologic mechanisms, including LV diastolic dysfunction of the hypertrophic and noncompliant left ventricle, which results in impaired LV filling; asymmetric thickening of the ventricular septum and dynamic obstruction of the LV outflow; thickened and narrowed intramural coronary arteries with impaired coronary vasodilator reserve and myocardial ischemia; and supraventricular and ventricular arrhythmias (particularly atrial fibrillation and ventricular tachycardia). The contribution of these different determinants to the presence and severity of cardiac symptoms may be different among patients (6).

The clinical course of an individual patient with HCM generally follows one of the following pathways: (1) congestive symptoms of heart failure and progressive functional limitation as a consequence of diastolic dysfunction in the presence of preserved systolic function; (2) remodeling of the hypertrophied LV with progressive cavity dilatation and depressed systolic function (the "end-stage" phase); (3) consequences of atrial fibrillation (syncope and embolic events); and (4) sudden cardiac death. In a population of young (and adult) HCM patients, impaired consciousness with syncope or presyncope, along with palpitations, which usually are the consequence of rapid atrial or ventricular tachyarrhythmias, are clinical events of major interest and require immediate attention. Sudden and unexpected death (not associated with heart failure) occurs in the natural history of this disease without premonitory symptoms or progressive deterioration of the clinical course, and may represent the first clinical manifestation of the disease (6). Sudden death usually occurs in HCM patients between age of 12 and 35 years, but rarely in the first decade of life.

Risk Stratification for Sudden Death

A substantial proportion of the patients who die suddenly collapse during or just after vigorous physical activity. This observation is consistent with the finding that HCM is the most common cause of sudden death in young competitive athletes in the United States (2, 3). Therefore, because intense physical activity during training and competition seems to be a trigger for this event, the American Heart Association recommends that athletes with HCM should be excluded from competitive sports (17).

The greatest risk for sudden cardiac death in HCM patients seems to be associated with one of the following factors: a previous episode of cardiac arrest; a family history of multiple sudden deaths; multiple or repetitive bursts of **nonsustained ventricular tachycardia**, or **sustained ventricular tachycardia** on ambulatory Holter ECG; massive LV hypertrophy (i.e., maximum wall thickness > 35 mm); impaired blood pressure response at exercise; or certain malignant genotypes (e.g., Arg403Gln of beta-myosin heavy-chain) (25, 26).

When the risk assessed by these criteria is judged to be sufficiently high for therapeutic intervention, current treatment options are limited to long-term pharmacological therapy with amiodarone or an **implantable cardioverter-defibrillator** (ICD). The ICD represents the most definitive option, based on recent studies that have proved its efficiency in preventing the incidence or recurrence of cardiac arrest in patients at risk (27).

Dilated Cardiomyopathy

Dilated cardiomyopathy (DCM) is a myocardial disorder characterized by LV dilatation and impaired systolic function. Dilated cardiomyopathy includes disorders that are familial or genetic in origin, or secondary to infection or inflammation, exposure to toxic substances, metabolic disorders, or, finally, may be idiopathic (Table 1). The prevalence of this disease is estimated to be 4 cases per 10,000 people (28).

Genetic Defects

About 30% to 50% of the cases of DCM are inherited, presenting with either an autosomal dominant, autosomal recessive, X-linked, or mitochondrial transmission (9). Genes for the autosomal dominant DCM have been mapped to six different loci localized in 1q32, 2p31, 9q13, 10q21-q23, 1p1-1q1 and 3p22-3p25. Two genes for X-linked cardiomy-

opathy have been identified: the dystrophin gene (dystrophin is a large protein part of the sarcolemma), which also is responsible for Duchenne and Becker muscular dystrophy, and G4.5 in Barth syndrome. To date, the genes for X-linked and autosomal dominant DCM have been mapped, demonstrating genetic heterogeneity. Recently, mutations in cardiac actin located in chromosome 15q14 have been identified. In these cases, DCM may result from a defective transmission of force in cardiac myocytes.

Morphologic Alterations

DCM is characterized by LV chamber dilatation and a diminution in systolic function (29). The total mass of the heart is increased as a result of a disproportionately increased cavity size with respect to the ventricular walls, which are normal or mildly thickened. Dilatation of the LV cavity chamber, when substantial, is associated with an abnormal, spherical shape. In addition, the mitral annulus enlarges with resultant valvular regurgitation. Myocardial LV remodeling is associated with diminished systolic function (with an ejection fraction far less than 50%), a reduced stroke volume, and an increased end-diastolic chamber pressure. These changes trigger the neurohormonal aberrations typical of the heart failure milieu.

Histologic changes usually are nonspecific, but certain features are commonly found, e.g., hypertrophied myocytes associated with areas of necrosis, large interstitial fibrosis and, occasionally, small cluster of lymphocytes in the interstitial or perivascular areas.

Differential Diagnosis

The differential diagnosis between "athlete's heart" and DCM occasionally must be reviewed when the patient under consideration is a trained athlete, based on the echocardiographic recognition of a markedly enlarged LV cavity size (i.e., end-diastolic diameter ≥ 60 mm) (30). The enlarged LV cavity is compatible with physiologic LV enlargement due to intensive athletic conditioning, but it may instinctively suggest a diagnosis of DCM. The protocol shown in Figure 6.2 encompasses the morphologic and clinical criteria that may offer a measure of clarification for this differential diagnosis.

Left Ventricular Morphology

In patients with DCM, the LV cavity is disproportionately enlarged compared to the wall thickness and the right ventricular cavity, and the LV chamber modifies to a more spherical shape (29). In trained athletes, LV cavity enlargement may be in the same range of absolute values as in DCM patients, but LV cavity dilation is associated with mild wall thickening and an enlargement of the right ventricle.

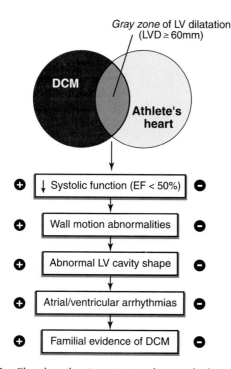

FIGURE 6.2.   Flowchart showing criteria to distinguish idiopathic dilated cardiomyopathy (DCM) from "athlete's heart" when LV cavity dimension is enlarged and in the "gray zone" of overlap consistent with both diagnoses. EF, ejection fraction; LV, left ventricle.

Indeed, the physiologically dilated LV cavity maintains the normal ellipsoid shape, with the mitral valve normally positioned and without mitral regurgitation (18, 30).

Left Ventricular Function

The most definitive evidence for DCM is the presence of global systolic dysfunction (i.e., ejection fraction < 50%), or evidence of segmental wall motion abnormalities. Instead, athletes with physiologic LV cavity enlargement do not show global systolic dysfunction, segmental wall motion abnormalities, or an abnormal diastolic filling pattern (30).

Knowledge of the athlete's type of sport and training profile may be relevant to the diagnosis. Left ventricular cavity enlargement (with end-diastolic diameter ≥ 60 mm) is common in athletes training in largely aerobic disciplines, such as cycling, cross-country skiing, rowing, or long-distance running, and is associated with normal or superior physical performance (30). Patients with DCM, on the other hand, usually present reduced exercise tolerance.

Clinical Presentation and Natural History

In young DCM patients, arrhythmias are common and may occur at any level of disability, even before LV dysfunction is clinically evident. Life-threatening ventricular and supraventricular tachyarrhythmias typically represent the clinical presentation of this disorder (31, 32). Chest pain

also is common and affects up to one third of DCM patients with normal coronaries; this angina may be, in part, a consequence of the reduced coronary vascular reserve. Eventually, sudden death may occur in patients with DCM, including young individuals engaged in physical exercise and sport activities (31, 32).

Most adult DCM patients present clinically with signs and symptoms of fluid congestion and low cardiac output, including reduced exercise tolerance and dyspnea. Occasionally, patients may present with right-sided heart failure symptoms and mesenteric congestion, which can be mistaken for a gastrointestinal disorder. Finally, pulmonary and systemic thromboembolism occurs at a variable rate of 1% to 6% per year in adult patients without anticoagulation.

It is difficult to predict the natural history of DCM, but the average 5-year survival rate is approximately 50%. The predictors of poor outcome in DCM include markedly reduced ejection fraction (i.e., <30%); recurrent syncopal episodes, or sustained ventricular tachycardia; reduced cardiac index (<2.5 L/min) and maximum oxygen uptake ($\dot{V}O_{2max}$ <12 ml/kg), with increased pulmonary wedge pressure (>20 mm Hg); and increased plasma levels of norepinephrine or atrial natriuretic factor. Management options include digoxin, angiotensin-converting enzyme (ACE) inhibitors, diuretics, angiotensin II receptor blockers, beta-blockers and antiarrhythmics, and anticoagulants.

Arrhythmogenic Right Ventricular Cardiomyopathy

Arrhythmogenic right ventricular cardiomyopathy (ARVC) is a heart muscle disorder characterized pathologically by fibrofatty replacement primarily affecting the right ventricle, and clinically by life-threatening ventricular arrhythmias in young people (33). The prevalence of ARVC in the general population is unknown, but is estimated to be approximately 1 in 5000.

Genetic Alterations

A positive family history is present in about one third of patients with ARVC. The most common pattern of inheritance is autosomal dominant, although the recessive pattern has also been reported. To date, linkage analyses have identified genetic abnormalities on chromosome 1q42-q43, 2q32-q32.2, 3p23, 10p12-p14, 14q23-q24, and q12-q22 in the dominant pattern, and 17 in the recessive variant. However, some families are not linked to these genetic loci, which suggests further genetic heterogeneity. The cardiac ryanodine receptor gene (RyR2), which is responsible for catecholamine-induced ventricular tachycardia, also has been implicated recently in ARVC and offers potential insight into the association of ventricular tachyarrhythmias with this disease (9).

Morphologic Alterations

The morphologic abnormalities usually are confined to the right ventricle, although in adult patients the LV also may be involved (34). Macroscopically, the right ventricular cavity is dilated, and segmental thinning of the free wall is present, mostly at the inflow tract, apex, or infundibular region. When the LV is involved, the gross morphology resembles that of DCM. Morphologic alterations of ARVC usually begin in the subepicardium or mediomural layer and move to the endocardium with a progressive, noninflammatory loss of myocytes. The myocytes are replaced with collagen and adipose tissue, which leaves strands of myocytes inside areas of fibrosis or fat. In a subset of patients, patchy infiltrates with dead myocytes and inflammatory cells (mostly lymphocytes) also have been described (33, 34). Recently, apoptosis (a highly regulated process that leads to programmed cell death) has been postulated to trigger the cascade of events that results in these degenerative changes.

Diagnosis of Arrhythmogenic Right Ventricular Cardiomyopathy and Differentiation From "Athlete's Heart"

Clinical diagnosis of ARVC may be difficult, and an expert consensus panel has proposed major and minor criteria (Table 6.2) (35).

Diagnosis of ARVC currently is based on the recognition of two major criteria, or one major plus two minor criteria, or four minor criteria. These criteria encompass morphologic, histologic, electrocardiographic, and genetic findings. Although these guidelines represent a valuable contribution to a difficult clinical diagnosis, assessment of the sensitivity and specificity of these criteria still requires prospective clinical evaluation.

The differential diagnosis between ARVC and "athlete's heart" often emerges in athletes showing an enlarged right ventricular cavity or an abnormal ECG pattern, with inverted T waves in the anterior precordial leads (V_1 to V_3) (36, 37). In these instances, clinical differentiation of ARVC from "athlete's heart" may be difficult, but critical assessment of the ECG pattern and right ventricular morphology (as assessed by imaging techniques) provides some clues that can be helpful in this differentiation.

Plain and Signal-Averaged Electrocardiogram

The electrocardiogram is abnormal in more than 50% of patients with ARVC. The most common abnormalities include the presence of inverted T waves in the right precordial leads (V_1 to V_3) in individuals over the age of 12 years, an association with increased QRS duration (>110 msec), and an incomplete right bundle branch block pattern (34, 36). However, these changes are not specific, and trained athletes occasionally may show inverted T waves in the ante-

TABLE 6.2. CRITERIA FOR DIAGNOSIS OF ARRHYTHMOGENIC RIGHT VENTRICULAR CARDIOMYOPATHY

I. Global or regional dysfunction and structural alterations*
Major
Severe dilatation and reduction of RV ejection fraction with no (or only mild) LV impairment.
Localized RV aneurysms (akinetic or dyskinetic areas with diastolic bulging)
Severe segmental dilatation of the RV
Minor
Mild global RV dilatation or ejection fraction reduction with normal left ventricle
Mild segmental dilatation of the RV
Regional RV hypokinesia

II. Tissue characterization of walls
Major
Fibrofatty replacement of myocardium on endomyocardial biopsy

III. Repolarization abnormalities
Minor
Inverted T waves in right precordial leads (V_2 and V_3), in people older than 12 yr and in the absence of right bundle branch block

IV. Depolarization and conduction abnormalities
Major
Epsilon waves or localized prolongation (>110 ms) of the QRS complex in right precordial leads (V_1 and V_3)
Minor
Late potentials (signal-averaged ECG)

V. Arrhythmia
Minor
Left bundle branch block type ventricular tachycardia (sustained and nonsustained) (ECG, Holter, exercise testing)
Frequent ventricular extrasystoles (>1000/24 h) (Holter)

VI. Family history
Major
Familial disease confirmed at necropsy or surgery
Minor
Familial history of premature sudden death (<35 years of age) due to suspected ARVC.
Familial history (clinical diagnosis based on present criteria)

---

*Detected by echocardiography, angiography, magnetic resonance imaging, or radionuclide scintigraphy.

ARVC, arrhythmogenic right ventricular cardiomyopathy; ECG, electrocardiogram; LV, left ventricular; RV, right ventricular

Data from McKenna WJ, Thiene G, Nava A, et al. (35).

rior precordial leads and right ventricular conduction delays in the absence of this disease (37). Indeed, in patients with ARVC, the QRS duration is longer in right precordial leads (V_1 to V_3) compared to the left leads (V_5 to V_6), with a difference (i.e., QT dispersion) of greater than 50 msec. Finally, in a subset of ARVC patients (5–10%) a small discrete potential (called an epsilon wave) is evident just after the QRS complex in the right precordial leads. This is thought to be the consequence of delayed activation within the abnormal right ventricle (36). Late potentials on the **signal-averaged ECG** represent the counterpart of the epsilon waves on the 12-lead ECG. The presence of late potentials is more common in ARVC patients with severe histologic changes and a reduced right ventricular ejection fraction, and this finding commonly is associated with ventricular tachyarrhythmias (36, 38). Late potentials are absent in trained athletes with a physiologically enlarged right ventricle.

Imaging Techniques

Cine-MRI is considered the method of choice for the diagnosis of ARVC, because it may identify tissue areas of altered signal intensity and segmental wall motion abnormalities consistent with fibrofatty replacement. However, this technique does have methodologic and economic limitations: the MRI may have insufficient spectral resolution to quantify right ventricular thickness adequately, and the normal presence of epicardial and pericardial fat may cause difficulty in identifying intramyocardial fat. Finally, the cost of testing is substantial, which restricts this technique to selected cases.

In patients with ARVC, echocardiography may show an even mildly enlarged right ventricular cavity, segmental abnormalities (such as thinning, bulging and aneurysm formations in the free wall), and wall motion abnormalities (36). Athletes engaged in endurance disciplines, on the other hand, show an enlarged right ventricular cavity (which is associated with an enlarged left ventricular cavity), normal free wall thickness, and no wall motion abnormalities.

Clinical Presentation and Natural History

Arrhythmogenic right ventricular cardiomyopathy presents clinically in almost 80% of patients before the age of 40; the most common symptoms are palpitations, presyncope or syncope, and sudden death. Most of the arrhythmic symptoms are explained by ventricular tachycardia (VT) originating from the right ventricle with a left bundle branch block configuration (38). Occasionally, multiple VT morphologies may be found, because the disease may be widespread in the right ventricle and may produce multiple arrhythmogenic foci. Sudden unexpected death may occur in young ARVC patients without premonitory symptoms (4, 34). The mechanism of sudden death is related to acceleration of VT, usually in association with exercise and sport participation. Right heart failure may occur in adult ARVC patients, usually in the 4th and 5th decades of life, and develops as a consequence of right ventricular dilatation, wall thinning, and progressive loss of contractile function. When extensive myocardial damage also affects the LV, biventricular heart failure that closely resembles idiopathic dilated cardiomyopathy occurs (38).

Management is designed to control the clinical manifestations of the disease. Ventricular arrhythmias can be treated with antiarrhythmic agents such as amiodarone or sotalol. Patients considered at high risk for sudden death should receive an implantable automatic cardioverter defibrillator. These patients include those who have been resuscitated from cardiac arrest, have a history of recurrent syncope, or present with threatening VTs not controlled by pharmacologic therapy.

What We Know
About Cardiomyopathies

1 Cardiomyopathies represent a broad spectrum of primary cardiac diseases, often with a genetic basis. They are characterized by muscle cell alterations, including hypertrophy, degeneration, and necrosis.

2 Functionally, cardiomyopathies are associated with muscle cell dysfunction and a variable degree of impairment in cardiac function (e.g., LV diastolic dysfunction, left or right ventricular systolic dysfunction, and wall motion abnormalities).

3 Clinically, a varied spectrum of symptoms may be present, including palpitations, syncope, dyspnea, fatigability, and angina.

4 These diseases have great clinical relevance in the young and adult population because they represent the most common cause of sudden and unexpected cardiac death.

5 The diagnosis of cardiomyopathies is based on the accurate evaluation of the distinctive morphologic cardiac abnormalities and differentiation from physiologic cardiac changes associated with chronic athletic conditioning (i.e., "athlete's heart").

What We Would Like to Know
About Cardiomyopathies

1 Is the incidence of arrhythmogenic right ventricular cardiomyopathy as high as that of hypertrophic cardiomyopathy? Is this a unique cardiomyopathy, or does it represent a spectrum of cardiac diseases with similar morphologic abnormalities?

2 Will genetic testing for DNA abnormalities be implemented in clinical practice for the diagnosis of familial cardiomyopathies?

3 What is the clinical significance of a genetic abnormality in a young individual who does not present evidence of morphologic cardiac abnormalities?

4 Do we have reliable criteria for assessing the risk for sudden death in asymptomatic or mildly symptomatic patients with cardiomyopathies?

5 Is exclusion from regular physical training and sport participation an effective method to reduce the incidence of sudden death and to prolong the life of young patients with cardiomyopathies?

Summary

Cardiomyopathies represent a spectrum of primary myocardial diseases, usually with a genetic basis, that are characterized by cardiac hypertrophy, dilatation, or right ventricular abnormalities. The prevalence of cardiomyopathies is greater than previously expected; statistics reveal an incidence of about 0.2% for HCM. The clinical relevance of cardiomyopathies is based on the recognition that they represent the most common cause of sudden and unexpected cardiac death in young, competitive athletes. The diagnosis of cardiomyopathies is based on an accurate evaluation of the distinctive morphologic abnormalities and the differentiation from physiologic cardiac changes associated with chronic athletic conditioning (i.e., "athlete's heart").

A varied spectrum of symptoms may be present in patients with cardiomyopathies, including syncope, dyspnea, fatigability, and angina. However, a substantial subset of patients present only mild (or no) symptoms. The treatment of cardiomyopathies is directed toward the reduction of sudden cardiac death risk by controlling the incidence of arrhythmias and includes the exclusion of patient from regular and highly intense athletic activities.

CASE STUDY

Patient Information

Linda is a 20-year-old volleyball player. She was athletically active during childhood and young adulthood, participating in school and college sport activities (volleyball, aerobic dance classes, and swimming). She recently decided to play competitive volleyball and was required to pass a preparticipation medical evaluation before entering a regular training program and competition.

Assessments

Linda did not report any symptoms or impairment in physical performance. Family history was negative for cardiac diseases or premature sudden death. At physical examination, a murmur was heard in the left ventricular outflow area that was variable with postural changes. The 1st and 2nd sounds were normal, and her blood pressure was 120/80 mm Hg. The remaining physical examination was unremarkable. In consideration of the cardiac murmur, the physician prudently requested a 12-lead ECG. The 12-lead ECG was markedly abnormal (Figures 6.3 and 6.4), showing increased R and S wave voltages in the anterior precordial leads (V_1 to V_3), and an abnormal repolarization pattern with flat T wave in the lateral precordial leads (V_5 and V_6) and in peripheral leads L_1 and aVL.

The abnormal 12-lead ECG is suggestive for the presence of structural cardiac disease. Specifically, a combination of increased R and S wave voltages and an abnormal repolarization pattern suggests the presence of LV hypertrophy. Although trained athletes may show abnormal ECG patterns compatible with the presence of physiologic LV hypertrophy, this finding is inconsistent with Linda's type and intensity of physical training.

Questions

1. How would you evaluate Linda's cardiac murmur and abnormal 12-lead ECG? What possible diagnosis might you take into consideration?

2. What tests must be considered to confirm any clinical suspicions?

3. What recommendations might you offer regarding Linda's participation in intense physical activities?

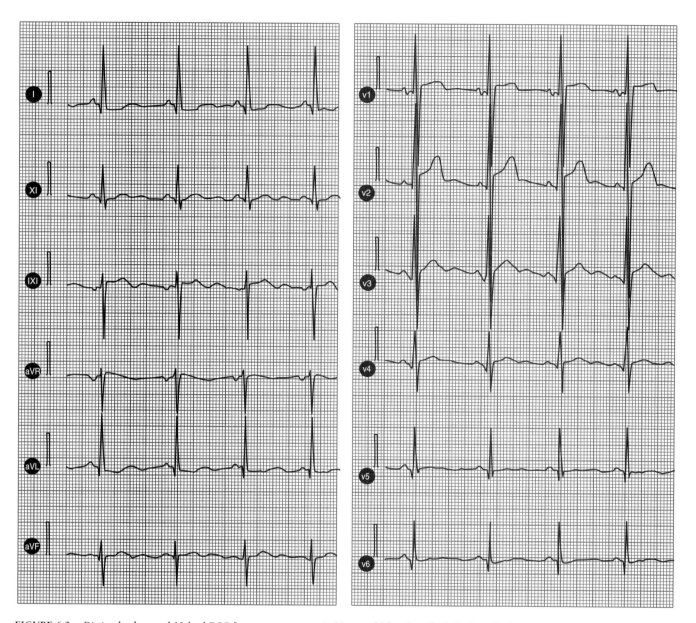

FIGURE 6.3. Distinctly abnormal 12-lead ECG from an asymptomatic 20-year-old female volleyball player highly suggestive for cardiac disease (such as HCM). The 12-lead ECG shows increased R and S wave voltages in anterior precordial leads (V_1 to V_3), abnormal repolarization pattern with flat T wave in lateral precordial leads (V_5 and V_6), and peripheral leads L_1 and aVL.

DISCUSSION QUESTIONS

1 What morphologic cardiac abnormalities are characteristic of the different cardiomyopathies (i.e., hypertrophic, dilated, and right ventricular)?

2 What is the clinical course of the different cardiomyopathies?

3 What are the mechanisms leading to sudden death in hypertrophic/right ventricular cardiomyopathy?

4 Does exercise play a role in the clinical course of cardiomyopathies? If so, how?

5 What are the most reliable criteria for the differential diagnosis of HCM and physiologic LV hypertrophy associated with "athlete's heart"?

6 What are the clinical criteria for assessing the risk of sudden death in young asymptomatic patients with HCM?

7 What is the recommended treatment for young HCM patients with recurrent syncope?

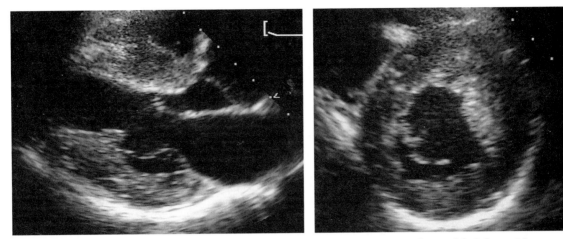

a. Long-axis parasternal view of the left ventricle   b. Short-axis parasternal view of the left ventricle

FIGURE 6.4   The parasternal long- and short-axis (a, b) views in the same athlete as in Figure 6.3. A diffuse myocardial hypertrophy is evident, which includes several segments of the left ventricle; the maximum wall thickening (24 mm) is present at level of anterior ventricular septum (AVS) and anterolateral free wall (ALFW). The left ventricular cavity is reduced in size (end-diastolic diameter 34 mm) and greatly distorted, due to the abnormal thickening of anterior and lateral free wall. The overall morphologic pattern is consistent with diagnosis of hypertrophic cardiomyopathy. ALFW, anterolateral free wall; AVS, anterior ventricular septum; LV, left ventricle; PFW, posterior free wall; VS, ventricular septum.

REFERENCES

1. Report of the 1995 World Health Organization/International Society and Federation of Cardiology Task Force on the definition and classification of cardiomyopathies. Circulation 1996;93:841–842.
2. Maron BJ, Shirani J, Poliac LC. Sudden death in young competitive athletes. Clinical, demographic, and pathological profiles. JAMA 1996;276:199–204.
3. Burke AP, Farb V, Virmani R, et al. Sports-related and non-sports-related sudden cardiac death in young adults. Am Heart J 1991;121:568–575.
4. Corrado D, Thiene G, Nava A, et al. Sudden death in young competitive athletes: clinicopathologic correlations in 22 cases. Am J Med 1990;89:588–596.
5. Maron BJ, Pelliccia A, Spirito P. Cardiac disease in young trained athletes: insights into methods for distinguishing athlete's heart from structural heart disease, with particular emphasis on hypertrophic cardiomyopathy. Circulation 1995;91;1596–1601.
6. Maron BJ. Hypertrophic cardiomyopathy. The Lancet 1997;50:127–133.
7. Marian AJ, Roberts R. Recent advances in the molecular genetics of hypertrophic cardiomyopathy. Circulation 1995;92:1336–1347.
8. Maron BJ, Moller JH, Seidman CE, et al. Impact of laboratory molecular diagnosis on contemporary diagnostic criteria for genetically transmitted cardiovascular diseases: hypertrophic cardiomyopathy, long-QT syndrome, and Marfan syndrome. Circulation 1998;98:1460–1471.
9. Priori SG, Barhanin J, Hauer RNW, et al. Genetic and molecular basis of cardiac arrhythmias. Impact on clinical management. Eur Heart J 1999;20:174–195.
10. Roberts R, Sigwart U. New concepts in hypertrophic cardiomyopathies, part I. Circulation 2001;104:2113–2116.
11. Klues HG, Schiffers A, Maron BJ. Phenotypic spectrum and patterns of left ventricular hypertrophy in hypertrophic cardiomyopathy: morphologic observations and significance as assessed by two-dimensional echocardiography in 600 patients. J Am Coll Cardiol 1995;26:1699–1708.
12. Maron BJ, Kragel AH, Roberts WC. Sudden death due to hypertrophic cardiomyopathy in the absence of increased left ventricular mass. Br Heart J 1990;63:308–310.
13. Spirito P, Maron BJ, Bonow RO, et al. Occurrence and significance of progressive left ventricular wall thinning and relative cavity dilatation in patients with hypertrophic cardiomyopathy. Am J Cardiol 1987;60:123–129.
14. Henry WL, Gardin JM, Ware JH. Echocardiographic measurements in normal subjects from infancy to old age. Circulation 1980;62:1054–1061.
15. Gardin JM, Savage DD, Ware JH, et al. Effect of age, sex, body surface area on echocardiographic left ventricular wall mass in normal subjects. Hypertension 1987;9(suppl II):II36–II39.
16. Pelliccia A, Maron BJ, Spataro A, et al. The upper limit of physiologic cardiac hypertrophy in highly trained elite athletes. N Engl J Med 1991;324:295–301.
17. Maron BJ, Mitchell JH. 26th Bethesda Conference: recommendations for determining eligibility for competition in athletes with cardiovascular abnormalities. J Am Coll Cardiol 1994;24:845–899.
18. Pelliccia A, Avelar E, De Castro S, Pandian N. Global left ventricular shape is not altered as a consequence of physiologic remodeling in highly trained athletes. Am J Cardiol 2000;86:700–702.
19. Lewis JF, Spirito P, Pelliccia A, et al. Usefulness of Doppler echocardiographic assessment of diastolic filling in distinguishing "athlete's heart" from hypertrophic cardiomyopathy. Am J Cardiol 1992;68:296–300.
20. Maron BJ, Spirito P, Green KJ, et al. Noninvasive assessment of left ventricular diastolic function by pulsed Doppler echocardiography in patients with hypertrophic cardiomyopathy. J Am Coll Cardiol 1987;10:733–742.
21. Maron BJ, Pelliccia A, Spataro A, et al. Reduction in left ventricular wall thickness after deconditioning in highly trained Olympic athletes. Br Heart J 1993;69:125–128.
22. Pelliccia A, Maron BJ, De Luca R, et al. Remodeling of left ventricular hypertrophy in elite athletes after long-term deconditioning. Circulation 2002;105:944–949.
23. Sharma S, Elliott PM, Whyte G, et al. Utility of metabolic exercise testing in distinguishing hypertrophic cardiomyopathy from physiologic left ventricular hypertrophy in athletes. J Am Coll Cardiol 2000;36:864–870.
24. Pelliccia A, Maron BJ, Culasso F, et al. The athlete's heart in women: echocardiographic characterization of 600 highly trained and elite female athletes. JAMA 1996;276:211–215.

25. Spirito P, Seidman CE, McKenna WJ, Maron BJ. The management of hypertrophic cardiomyopathy. N Engl J Med 1997;336:775–785.

26. Elliott PN, Poloniecki J, Dickie S, et al. Sudden death in hypertrophic cardiomyopathy: Identification of high risk patients. J Am Coll Cardiol 2000;36:2212–2218.

27. Maron BJ, Shen W-K, Link MS, et al. Efficacy of implantable cardioverter-defibrillators for the prevention of sudden death in patients with hypertrophic cardiomyopathy. N Engl J Med 2000;342:365–373.

28. Manolio TA, Baughman KL, Rodeheffer R, et al. Prevalence and etiology of idiopathic dilated cardiomyopathy. Am J Cardiol 1992;69:1458–1466.

29. Gavazzi A, De Maria R, Renosto G, et al. The spectrum of left ventricular size in dilated cardiomyopathy: Clinical correlates and prognostic implications. Am Heart J 1993;125:410–422.

30. Pelliccia A, Culasso F, Di Paolo FM, Maron BJ. Physiologic left ventricular cavity dilatation in elite athletes. Ann Intern Med 1999;130:23–31.

31. Lauer MS, Evans CE, Levy D. Prognostic implications of subclinical left ventricular dilatation and systolic dysfunction in men free of overt cardiovascular disease (the Framingham Heart Study). Am J Cardiol 1992;70:1180–1184.

32. Redfield MM, Gersh BJ, Bailey KR, Rodeheffer RJ. Natural history of incidentally discovered, asymptomatic idiopathic dilated cardiomyopathy. Am J Cardiol 1994;74:737–739.

33. Thiene G, Nava A, Corrado D, et al. Right ventricular cardiomyopathy and sudden death in young people. N Engl J Med 1988;318:129–133.

34. Corrado D, Basso C, Thiene G, et al. Spectrum of clinicopathologic manifestations of arrhythmogenic right ventricular cardiomyopathy/dysplasia: a multicenter study. J Am Coll Cardiol 1997;30:1512–1520.

35. McKenna WJ, Thiene G, Nava A, et al. Diagnosis of arrhythmogenic right ventricular dysplasia/cardiomyopathy. Br Heart J 1994;71:215–218.

36. Marcus FI. Right ventricular dysplasia: evaluation and management in relation to sports activities. In: Estes NAM, Salem DN, Wang PJ, eds. Sudden Cardiac Death in the Athlete. New York: Futura Publishing, 1998:277–284.

37. Pelliccia A, Maron BJ, Culasso F, et al. Clinical significance of abnormal electrocardiographic patterns in trained athletes. Circulation 2000;102:278–284

38. Nava A, Bauce B, Basso C, et al. Clinical profile and long-term follow-up of 37 families with arrhythmogenic right ventricular cardiomyopathy. J Am Coll Cardiol 2000;36:2226–2233.

SUGGESTED READINGS

Thompson PD. Exercise and Sports Cardiology. New York: McGraw-Hill, 2001.

Estes NAM III, Salem DN, Wang PJ. Sudden Cardiac Death in the Athlete. New York: Futura Publishing, 1998.

Topol EJ. Textbook of Cardiovascular Medicine. Philadelphia: Lippincott-Raven, 1998.

CHAPTER 7

Cardiac Valvular Disease

Bernard A. Clark

Overview

The human heart is a muscular pump—actually two interdependent pumps that operate in series. During maximal exercise, a normal heart has the capacity to increase cardiac output to at least four to five times the resting level to meet metabolic demand. The cardiac valves play a key role in the efficient function of the pump, promoting forward blood flow and preventing retrograde or regurgitant flow.

The atrioventricular (AV) valves lie between the atrial and ventricular chambers, with the bileaflet **mitral valve** on the left and the trileaflet **tricuspid valve** on the right. The free edges of the valve leaflets are tethered by strong **chordae tendineae** to the papillary muscles, pyramidal projections from the walls of the ventricles. During ventricular systole, the thin leaflets of the AV valves coapt tightly and prevent blood in the ventricular chambers from regurgitating into the low pressure atrial chambers. The chordae are tightened by the contracting papillary muscles, facilitating leaflet coaptation. During diastole, the thin valve leaflets open widely, allowing the free flow of blood from the thin-walled atria to the muscular ventricles, nearly creating a single diastolic chamber. The large area of the supporting fibrous annulus offers little resistance to flow during diastolic filling.

The **semilunar valves** separate the ventricular chambers from the great arteries that exit the heart—the **aortic valve** on the left and the **pulmonic valve** on the right. The three cuplike leaflets, or cusps, of the semilunar valves are supported by the fibrous annulus and the proximal wall of the artery. During systole, the leaflets open widely against the artery wall and provide a large, slightly triangular opening through which blood is forcefully ejected from the ventricle. In diastole, the higher arterial pressure causes the leaflets to coapt tightly, preventing the regurgitation of blood back into the relaxed ventricular chambers. The openings of the left and right coronary arteries are in the aortic root, directly above two of the aortic valve cusps.

There are two forms of cardiac valvular dysfunction, regurgitation (or "insufficiency") and stenosis. Causes of valve abnormalities can be broadly classified as either **congenital valvular disease** or **acquired valvular disease**. A congenital disorder results from abnormal fetal development. Such disorders may be clinically apparent immediately after birth if severe, or may manifest decades later after degenerative changes accrue. Acquired abnormalities result from injury to valve tissue secondary to infection, inflammation, or degeneration. Significant dysfunction may occur acutely, as can happen with infection of a valve by a virulent bacterial organism such as *Staphylococcus aureus*. However, the progression of the functional abnormality may be gradual, as may happen after valve involvement during acute rheumatic fever or with degenerative calcification of the leaflets with atherosclerosis. The etiology and clinical course of specific lesions are discussed later in this chapter.

Valvular regurgitation occurs when the leaflets fail to coapt properly or prolapse. The resulting backward flow of blood may cause a number of hemodynamic problems of varying severity, depending on the degree of regurgitation and acuity of the lesion. Insufficiency of the atrioventricular or semilunar valve results in volume overload of the ventricular chamber. This leads to enlargement of the chamber (to accommodate the normal incoming venous flow and the volume of blood that has leaked through the diseased valve). Severe or longstanding volume overload ultimately weakens systolic function, possibly irreversibly, and may result in heart failure. Efficiency of the ventricular pump also is compromised with limitation of peak cardiac output.

Stenosis occurs when the valve leaflets fail to open adequately, reducing the area of the valve orifice. The areas of the **atrioventricular valves** are large compared with those of the semilunar valves. Diastolic inflow to the ventricles from the atria is driven by a relatively low atrioventricular pressure gradient. A large valve orifice and longer diastolic time interval facilitate adequate ventricular filling. The aortic and pulmonic valve areas are smaller because ejection of blood is driven by a much larger pressure gradient generated by ventricular systole. Stenotic valvular lesions create a higher resistance to flow across the orifice and lead to el-

evation of pressure in the chamber proximal to the affected valve. Ventricular **pressure overload** due to stenosis of a semilunar valve causes hypertrophy of the ventricular walls and ultimately may lead to weakening of systolic function and heart failure. Stenosis of an atrioventricular valve increases resistance to atrial emptying and an elevation of pressure in the atrial chamber. This, in turn, elevates the pressure in the veins leading to the atrium and may cause signs and symptoms of venous congestion. The ability to increase cardiac output appropriately may be compromised and, as dysfunction becomes more severe, may be reduced even at rest.

The clinical presentation of cardiac valve disorders varies depending on the particular valve involved, the type and severity of the dysfunction, the demands placed on the circulatory system, and the presence or absence of other cardiac or noncardiac conditions. It is not unusual to have combined regurgitant and stenotic lesions or multivalvular involvement that creates a more complicated circulatory derangement.

Specific Valvular Abnormalities

The various valvular disorders are considered separately in the following sections. More attention is given to the left-sided abnormalities because mitral and aortic valve disease are responsible for most of the morbidity and mortality and a major cause of clinical concern for those evaluating the risks of exercise.

Detailed discussions of valvular disease, including etiology, natural history, and management, can be found in standard internal medicine and cardiology textbooks. Interested readers also may find a wealth of information concerning these topics in practice guidelines from a combined American College of Cardiology and American Heart Association Task Force published in the journal *Circulation* in November 1998 (1). In January 1994, recommendations concerning eligibility for competition in athletes with cardiovascular abnormalities were developed by the American College of Cardiology (ACC) and the American College of Sports Medicine (ACSM) at the 26th Bethesda Conference. These recommendations were published in a series of articles in the October 1994 issue of the *Journal of the American College of Cardiology* (2). Table 7.1 classifies individual sports according to their dynamic and static exercise intensity (low, moderate, and high) (3). There are limitations to this classification system, as have been pointed out by its authors. One cannot readily account for contribution of emotional stress on the cardiovascular system or the athlete's level of training. In team sports, the level of static or dynamic stress may vary depending on the position played (3). As specific valve disorders are discussed, recommendations concerning participation in sports activities will be made based on the severity of the physiologic derangement, using Table 7.1 as a reference.

TABLE 7.1. CLASSIFICATION OF SPORTS BASED ON PEAK DYNAMIC AND STATIC COMPONENTS DURING COMPETITION

Low Dynamic	Moderate Dynamic	High Dynamic
Low Static		
Billiards	Baseball	Badminton
Bowling	Softball	Cross-country skiing
Cricket	Table tennis	(classic technique)
Curling	Tennis (doubles)	Field hockey
Golf	Volleyball	Orienteering
Riflery		Race walking
		Racquetball
		Running (long
		distance)
		Soccer
		Squash
		Tennis (singles)
Moderate Static		
Archery	Fencing	Basketball
Auto racing	Field events (jumping)	Ice hockey
Diving	Figure skating	Cross-country skiing
Equestrian	Football (American)	(skating technique)
Motorcycling	Rodeoing	Football (Australian
	Rugby	rules)
	Running (sprint)	Lacrosse
	Surfing	Running (middle
	Synchronized	distance)
	swimming	Swimming
		Team handball
High Static		
Bobsledding	Body building	Boxing
Field events (throwing)	Downhill skiing	Canoeing/kayaking
Gymnastics	Wrestling	Cycling
Karate/judo		Decathlon
Luge		Rowing
Sailing		Speed skating
Rock climbing		
Waterskiing		
Weight lifting		
Windsurfing		

Adapted from Mitchell JH, Haskell WL, Raven PB (3).

Aortic Stenosis

Aortic stenosis (AS) is an important cause of death in young athletes during physical exertion. Sudden cardiac death as an initial presentation of AS is rare, and a number of studies have found that when it occurred, there had been antecedent symptoms (1). It is more likely to occur in the setting of severe congenital stenosis that has not been detected prior to the event. Aortic stenosis in adults is due to rheumatic disease or to the calcification of a normal trileaflet valve or congenitally bicuspid valve (4).

The normal adult aortic valve has an opening area of about 3 to 4 cm^2 (Figures 7.1 and 7.2). Significant effects on circulation usually do not occur until the valve area has been reduced to about one fourth of normal size (1). The crucial point varies among individuals depending upon

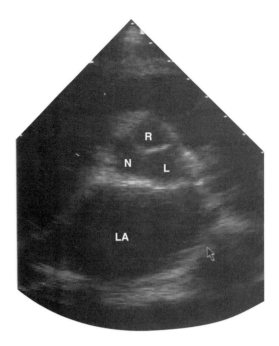

FIGURE 7.1. Two-dimensional echocardiographic view of a normal valve in the closed position during diastole. L, left coronary leaflet; LA, left atrium; N, noncoronary leaflet; R, right coronary leaflet.

their body size. For purposes of grading the severity of stenosis in adults, an area larger than 1.5 cm^2 is considered mild stenosis, an area greater than 1.0 cm^2 to 1.5 cm^2 is moderate stenosis, and an area of 1.0 cm^2 or less is severe stenosis (1). Transvalvular systolic pressure gradients also are used to classify the degree of stenosis. In congenital AS,

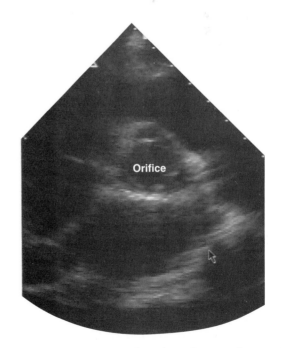

FIGURE 7.2. Two-dimensional echocardiographic view of a normal aortic valve in the open position during diastole. A roughly triangular shaped opening (orifice) is seen.

the peak instantaneous gradient (Figure 7.3) is used to classify severity, with a gradient of 50 mm Hg or more indicative of severe stenosis (5). Peak gradients of 20 mm Hg or less indicate mild stenosis, and gradients from 21 to 49 mm Hg are classified as moderate stenosis. In acquired (degenerative or rheumatic) disease, a mean gradient of 40 mm Hg or more (see Figure 7.3) indicates severe stenosis. These criteria apply in the setting of a normal cardiac output—reduced transvalvular flow (as occurs as the left ventricle fails) will produce a lower gradient and, as a result, lead to underestimation of the severity of AS.

The cardinal clinical presentations of aortic stenosis are syncope, angina (chest discomfort), and congestive heart failure. Aortic stenosis usually progresses over a long asymptomatic period, and the appearance of these symptoms warns of a grave prognosis if the AS is not treated surgically, with death usually occurring in 2 to 5 years (6). In the presence of severe AS, the peripheral vasodilation induced by physical exertion may lead to hypotension and cerebral hypoperfusion, causing lightheadedness or syncope. In addition, reduced aortic root pressure (coronary perfusion pressure) in combination with high left ventricular pressure (LV) and increased oxygen demand may result in myocardial ischemia, provoking angina or serious cardiac dysrhythmias.

The diagnosis of AS is established by findings on physical examination and specialized testing. Severe aortic stenosis delays and reduces the amplitude of the arterial pulses. A palpable thrill, or vibration, may be appreciated in the carotid pulse or over the upper chest adjacent to the sternum. A harsh mid- to late-peaking systolic murmur with a single second heart sound is characteristic of AS. The electrocardiogram (ECG) typically demonstrates findings consistent with left ventricular hypertrophy. Two-dimensional (2D) and Doppler echocardiography are valuable and diagnostic, demonstrating valvular thickening and calcification with leaflet immobility (Figures 7.4, 7.5, and 7.6). The transvalvular systolic pressure gradient and calculated valve area can be determined using Doppler and 2D echocardiographic findings (7, 8). Cardiac catheterization, if necessary, can be used to measure the systolic pressure gradient and determine valve area. The calcified and immobile valve leaflets may be seen on fluoroscopy. The role of exercise testing in subjects with AS has been somewhat controver-

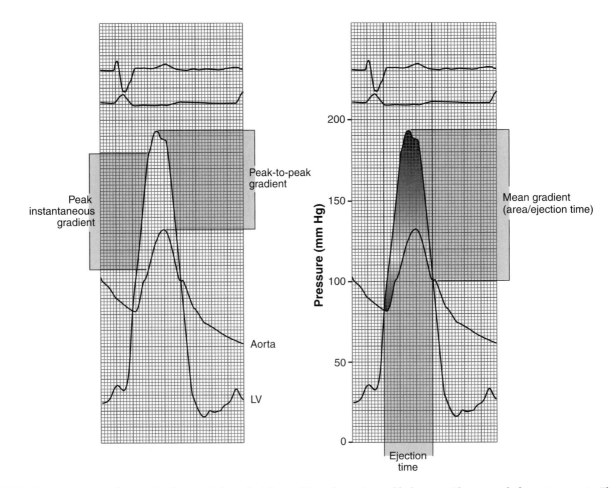

FIGURE 7.3.   Pressure tracing obtained simultaneously from the left ventricle and aorta in an elderly man with severe calcific aortic stenosis. The measurements used to determine peak instantaneous gradient, peak-to-peak gradient, and mean gradient across the aortic valve are illustrated.

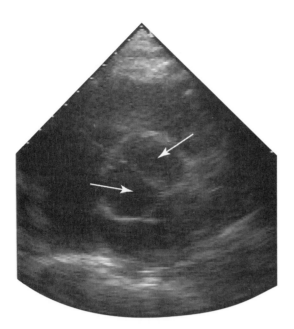

FIGURE 7.4. Two-dimensional echocardiographic view of a congenital bicuspid aortic valve in the closed position during diastole. Two leaflets are visualized (*arrows*) with a central closure line.

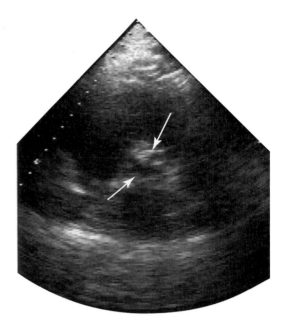

FIGURE 7.6. Two-dimensional echocardiographic view of a severely calcified and stenotic aortic valve. The degenerative acquired disorder is due to atherosclerotic change in a tri-leaflet aortic valve, resulting in thickening and calcification of the leaflets (*arrows*).

sial because of concerns about safety and the predictive value of ECG changes (9–12).

Recommendations for Competition in the Presence of Congenital Aortic Stenosis

In the absence of ECG abnormalities, exercise-related chest pain, syncope, or symptomatic dysrhythmias, the athlete

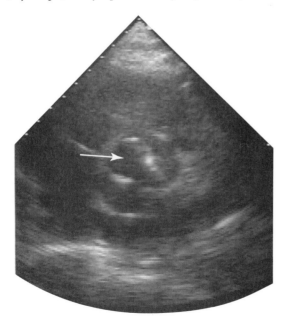

FIGURE 7.5. Two-dimensional echocardiographic view of a congenital bicuspid aortic valve in the open position during diastole. The opening is irregular and reduced in size (*arrow*), and the leaflets are thickened.

with congenital aortic stenosis, including discrete **subaortic stenosis** and **supravalvular stenosis**, may participate in all **competitive sports** as long as he or she has normal exercise tolerance and mild aortic stenosis. If moderate AS is present, the athlete may participate in low static, low and moderate dynamic, or moderate static, low dynamic competitive sports only if there is, at most, mild left ventricular hypertrophy without a strain pattern on ECG, a normal exercise test (i.e., no exercise-induced arrhythmias or ischemic changes, normal exercise duration and blood pressure response), and absence of symptoms. Athletes with severe congenital AS should not participate in competitive sports (5).

Recommendations for Competition in the Presence of Acquired Valvular Aortic Stenosis

Athletes with asymptomatic mild AS may participate in all competitive sports. If moderate stenosis is present, the athlete may participate in all low static, low dynamic competitive sports (see Table 7.1). These athletes may participate in low and moderate static, low and moderate dynamic sports if an exercise tolerance test to at least the expected level of exertion does not provoke symptoms, dysrhythmias, significant ST segment changes on ECG, or hypotension. All competitive sports should be avoided in the presence of severe AS or symptomatic moderate AS. If there is a history of syncope (even with mild AS), a careful evaluation by a cardiologist is necessary to evaluate for serious dysrhythmias that could result in sudden death. If the athlete has supraventricular tachycardia or complex ventricular dysrhythmia, he or she should be limited to low static, low dynamic sports (13).

Aortic Regurgitation

Diseases affecting the aortic valve leaflet, annular ring, or the ascending aorta can lead to **aortic regurgitation (AR)**. Among the common etiologies of leaflet dysfunction are congenitally bicuspid aortic valve, rheumatic heart disease, and infective endocarditis. Aortic root and annular causes include ascending aortic aneurysm or dissection, Marfan syndrome, systemic hypertension, and rheumatoid spondylitis (13). Aortic regurgitation increases left ventricular diastolic volume and stroke volume, the latter ejected during systole against systemic resistance. Compensatory LV hypertrophy and chamber dilatation results, and the AR may be well tolerated over a long period, particularly if it is not severe. Congestive heart failure due to the chronic volume overload develops over time as systolic LV function deteriorates. The onset of LV failure often is insidious, and full recovery of systolic performance may not occur after valve replacement. As diastolic filling time decreases during exercise, the volume of regurgitation may decrease. The reduction in systemic resistance also tends to improve forward flow. However, with severe chronic AR, the demand for coronary flow may exceed the capacity of the coronary circulation, resulting in myocardial ischemia. Angina pectoris and serious ventricular dysrhythmias may occur, with possible syncope or sudden death (13). High-intensity static exercise will increase the volume of regurgitation due to elevation of aortic pressure. Acute AR is caused by leaflet or annular damage (e.g., infection, trauma, aortic root dissection) and presents as congestive heart failure or circulatory shock.

The diagnosis and hemodynamic severity of AR can be established by physical examination and noninvasive cardiac testing. A high-pitched decrescendo murmur along the left sternal border, which begins with the second heart sound and may last through the duration of diastole, is typical of AR. When the regurgitation is more severe (or with left ventricular failure), the murmur may end earlier in diastole. A systolic flow murmur also is present in most cases due to the increased stroke volume caused by the AR. The peripheral pulses may be bounding in character due to an increase in pulse pressure (increased systolic and decreased diastolic blood pressure) and vigorous left ventricular contraction. Electrocardiographic features of LV hypertrophy are the rule with chronic significant AR, with increased voltage and repolarization abnormalities. The chest x-ray and echocardiogram demonstrate enlargement of the left ventricular chamber and the ascending aorta. Doppler echocardiography is very helpful in the diagnosis and management of AR (Figure 7.7). An accurate assessment of left ventricular size and function and gradation of the severity of regurgitation are provided, and the exami-

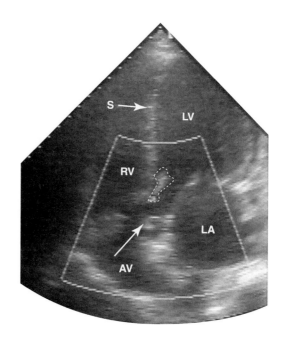

FIGURE 7.7.   Two-dimensional and Doppler echocardiographic view of a small jet of aortic insufficiency during diastole. The jet is outlined. AV, aortic valve; LA, left atrium; LV, left ventricle; RV, right ventricle; S, ventricular septum.

nation can easily be repeated for serial evaluations over time (14).

Recommendations for Competition in the Presence of Chronic Aortic Regurgitation

For athletes with chronic aortic regurgitation, an exercise test to at least the expected level of exertion during competition is recommended to assess functional capacity and screen for symptoms. The athlete must report any symptoms that may indicate the development of ventricular dysfunction (e.g., fatigue, shortness of breath) or dysrhythmias (e.g., palpitations, lightheadedness, syncope). In addition to symptom evaluations, serial echocardiographic studies (initially at 6 months and yearly thereafter) should be performed to determine the stability of LV dimensions and function. If the athlete with mild or moderate AR has left ventricular dimensions that are normal or only mildly increased, he or she may participate in all competitive sports. In the presence of moderate left ventricular enlargement (with stable dimensions on serial studies), asymptomatic athletes with adequate exercise capacity may participate in low and moderate static and low, moderate, and high dynamic competitive sports (see Table 7.1). If there is evidence of progressive LV chamber enlargement on serial echo studies, he or she should not engage in competitive sports. Likewise, athletes with severe AR, those with mild to moderate AR with symptoms, or those with marked dilation of the proximal ascending aorta should not engage in competitive sports. If ventricular arrhythmias are present at rest or with exertion, the athlete with mild or moderate AR should be restricted to low static, low dynamic sports only. Athletes with Marfan syndrome and AR should be restricted according to the criteria outlined above with additional considerations (e.g., avoidance of sports with risk of bodily collision) due to the possibility of aortic rupture (13, 15).

Mitral Stenosis

Mitral stenosis (MS) in adults is almost exclusively due to rheumatic heart disease, with scarring and fusion of the mitral leaflets and subvalvular chordae tendineae. A significant reduction in valve area leads to elevation in left atrial (LA) and pulmonary venous pressure. Progressive elevation of pulmonary arterial pressure occurs because of chronic pulmonary venous hypertension and may result in right heart failure. Atrial fibrillation occurs commonly with chronic MS and may be responsible for further hemodynamic derangement and the formation of clot within the LA chamber and LA appendage. The increased forward blood flow and decreased diastolic filling times that result from exertion may cause a marked elevation of LA and pulmonary capillary pressures, leading to interstitial (or frank alveolar) edema and dyspnea. Severe mitral stenosis usually produces significant exertional dyspnea, discouraging competitive athletic endeavors. However, persons with mild to moderate MS may be asymptomatic, even during strenuous activity, or may be motivated to the point of denying symptoms (13). Graded exercise testing is a valuable means of accurately assessing functional capacity and evaluating for exertional symptoms. Doppler echocardiography, combined with exercise, provides a noninvasive appraisal of mitral valve anatomy and function and a method to measure transvalvular gradients, calculate a valve area, and estimate pulmonary artery pressures (Figure 7.8).

The diagnosis of mitral stenosis may be difficult to establish on physical examination because the auscultatory findings are often subtle and easily missed. These findings include a loud first heart sound, an opening snap following the second heart sound, and a low-pitched apical diastolic murmur ("rumble").

The chest x-ray and ECG may demonstrate evidence of left atrial enlargement or, in later stages of the disease, enlargement of the right-sided chambers. Mitral stenosis is classified as mild, moderate, or severe based on calculation or measurement of valve area and the level of systolic pulmonary artery (PA) pressure or exercise pulmonary artery wedge pressure (an estimate of left atrial pressure). The normal mitral valve area approaches 5 cm^2; symptoms usually result when that area is less than 2.5 cm^2. Mild MS is defined as a valve area larger than 1.5 cm^2 or an exercise PA wedge pressure of 20 mm Hg or less or rest PA systolic pressure below 35 mm Hg. With moderate MS the valve area is between 1.1 cm^2 and 1.4 cm^2, or the exercise PA wedge pres-

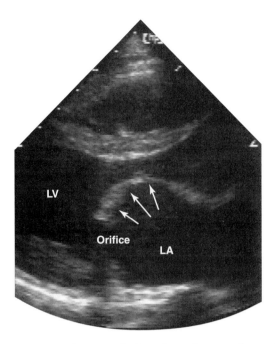

FIGURE 7.8. Two-dimensional echocardiographic view of a mitral valve deformed by rheumatic valvitis. During diastole, the valve has a "domed" appearance (*arrows*) due to scarring and fusion of the leaflets.

sure is 25 mm Hg or less, or the rest PA systolic pressure is 50 mm Hg or less. Severe MS is present if the valve area is smaller than 1.1 cm^2, the exercise PA wedge pressure is greater than 25 mm Hg, or the rest PA systolic pressure is greater than 50 mm Hg. The presence of a PA systolic pressure higher than 80 mm Hg indicates a severe hemodynamic derangement secondary to the MS and an increased risk of serious effects on right ventricular function (13). Mitral valve area and PA systolic pressure usually can be determined by Doppler echocardiography. If necessary, cardiac catheterization may be used to obtain the data.

Recommendations for Competition in the Presence of Mitral Stenosis

If the degree of mitral stenosis is mild and the athlete is in sinus rhythm, he or she may participate in all competitive sports. Under the following conditions, the athlete may participate in low and moderate static, low and moderate dynamic competitive sports (see Table 7.1): presence of atrial fibrillation with mild MS; sinus rhythm or atrial fibrillation with moderate MS; and peak PA pressure at rest or during exercise less than 50 mm Hg. If the peak PA systolic pressure is between 50 and 80 mm Hg, the athlete should be restricted to low and moderate static, low dynamic sports. If severe MS is present or if the PA systolic pressure exceeds 80 mm Hg, the athlete should not participate in competitive sports. Those on anticoagulant therapy should avoid sports that risk bodily collision (13).

Mitral Regurgitation (MR)

Regurgitation of the mitral valve can be caused by a number of disorders affecting the valve leaflets, the chordae tendineae, or the valve annulus. **Mitral valve prolapse** (MVP), the most common cause of clinically important MR, is due to thickening and redundancy of the mitral leaflets and elongation of the supporting chordae (Figure 7.9). Mitral valve prolapse has been overdiagnosed in the past due to the use of rather liberal echocardiographic criteria, with a reported prevalence in the range of 2% to 6% (1). However, a recent reference from the Framingham Heart Study, performed to eliminate selection bias, found "classic" MVP in only 1.3% of their population (16). Mitral valve prolapse usually is a benign disorder, with serious mechanical complications (e.g., acute chordal rupture, bacterial endocarditis) confined largely to those patients with the most severe valvular pathology, particularly in men over the age of 45 with left ventricular and left atrial enlargement (1, 17). Sudden cardiac death in MVP is uncommon, occurring in less than 2% of known cases over long-term follow-up. However, it is not a trivial concern because of the relatively high prevalence of the condition in the general population (18). Rheumatic heart disease, Marfan syndrome and other connective tissue disorders, infective endocarditis, coronary artery disease, and dilated cardiomyopathy are additional important causes of MR (13).

The major problems caused by MR are due to volume overload of the left ventricle with enlargement of the LV and left atrium. A portion of the left ventricular stroke volume (referred to as the "regurgitant fraction") is ejected retrograde into the LA during systole, decreasing forward flow and increasing left atrial volume. This impairs the heart's ability to increase forward cardiac output and elevates left atrial and pulmonary capillary pressure, leading to pulmonary congestion and edema. The excessive LV volume overload due to chronic MR ultimately may decrease contractility and cause left heart failure. The elevations in pulmonary pressure also may produce right heart failure. Because the left atrial pressure is considerably lower than the end-diastolic aortic pressure, the LV can eject blood into the LA against little resistance. Consequently, the LV ejection fraction, a commonly used measure of systolic function, may remain in the "normal" range even as contractile dysfunction develops. When the ejection fraction decreases below the normal range, the degree of functional deterioration may be significant and irreversible (1). Increases in LA size and pressure will increase the risk of developing atrial fibrillation.

A harsh or blowing apical holosystolic murmur radiating to the left axillary region is typical of MR. The physical examination with mitral valve prolapse may reveal single or multiple mid-systolic "clicks," with or without a late systolic murmur. The left ventricle may be enlarged on chest x-ray. Doppler echocardiography has a high level of sensitivity in detecting MR and is generally helpful in grading severity (Figure 7.10). Eccentric jets of MR directed toward the smooth endocardial surface of the LA may not disperse as widely, leading to an underestimation of the MR severity. Sophisticated Doppler techniques can be used to determine the volume of regurgitation and assess LV systolic function and may provide an estimate of pulmonary artery systolic pressure (19). The echocardiogram (transthoracic or transesophageal) also provides important anatomic data about mitral valve structure and function as well as left ventricular and left atrial chamber size and LV contractility. Studies should be repeated at intervals (in the athlete and nonathlete) to assess for changes in LV dimensions and systolic function. Radionuclide ventriculography can also be used to assess LV function.

Dyspnea may occur during exercise because of elevated pulmonary venous and capillary pressure. During static exercise, the elevation in systemic vascular resistance may increase the volume of regurgitation, thereby raising pulmonary pressure. The effect of dynamic exercise on MR is complex as the increase in LV contractility (the force driving the regurgitation) may be balanced in part by a reduction in systemic resistance (which would favor more forward flow). However, the increase in heart rate (more systolic periods of regurgitation) and reduced diastolic filling time (less time for the left atrium to empty) would tend to elevate LA and pulmonary venous pressure. There is concern that the increases in volume load induced by repetitive bouts of exercise could accelerate the progression of LV dysfunction. Exercise testing is useful to assess the functional

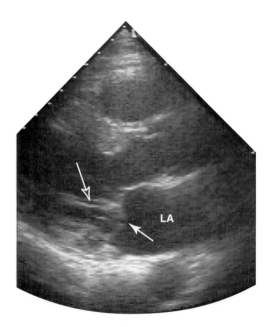

FIGURE 7.9.   Two-dimensional echocardiographic view of mitral valve prolapse during systole. The valve closure line puckers into the left atrium (LA), and leaflet separation can be seen (*arrow*). The mitral leaflets are thickened, and the chordae (*open arrow*) is stretched and elongated.

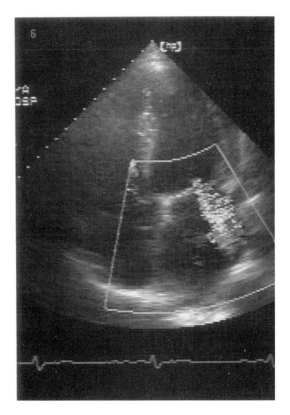

FIGURE 7.10. Two-dimensional and Doppler echocardiographic view of mitral regurgitation during systole. A moderately large jet of MR is seen on Doppler examination (*arrow*). LA, left atrium; LV, left ventricle; MV, mitral valve.

capacity and evaluate for symptoms during exertion. Color and spectral Doppler echocardiography during exercise can detect the presence or worsening of MR with exertion by providing a semiquantitative evaluation of severity and assess LV systolic performance. However, the use of these techniques in the management of MR remains investigational (19).

Recommendations for Competition in the Presence of Mitral Regurgitation

For athletes with mitral regurgitation, a noninvasive assessment of LV and LA size and LV systolic function is necessary prior to beginning a vigorous program of exercise or participating in competitive sports. If the athlete is in sinus rhythm and has normal LV dimensions and systolic function (LVEF >60%), he or she can participate in all competitive sports (see Table 7.1). Individuals with mild LV enlargement and normal systolic function at rest can participate in low and moderate static, low and moderate dynamic exercise (whether in sinus rhythm or atrial fibrillation). Selected athletes from this group (with appropriate functional capacity on exercise testing) may also participate in high dynamic exercise. The exercise test is useful in ath-

letes with atrial fibrillation to ensure that the heart rate response during exertion will not be excessive. If there is more than a mild degree of LV enlargement or evidence of LV systolic dysfunction at rest, the athlete should not participate in competitive sports. Sports carrying a risk of bodily contact should be avoided in those on anticoagulants (e.g., in atrial fibrillation) (13). Because of the variety of causes of MR, there may exist concerns that require additional consideration. For example, persons with MR secondary to LV dilation because of ischemic heart disease will have limitations due to the presence of coronary artery disease as well as the valvular regurgitation. If the MR is a result of bacterial endocarditis, the valve leaflets may be fragile and prone to further injury. Rupture of thinned, attenuated chordae may occur in patients with significant valvular prolapse.

Recommendations for Competition in the Presence of Mitral Valve Prolapse

In addition to restrictions based on the presence of the mitral regurgitation, recommendations for athletes with mitral valve prolapse from a separate ACC/ACSM task force were developed by the participants of the 26th Bethesda Conference (15). Athletes with MVP and a structurally abnormal valve (leaflet thickening and elongation) can engage in all competitive sports as long as none of the following factors are present: a history of syncope due to documented cardiac dysrhythmia; a family history of sudden cardiac death associated with MVP; repetitive episodes of sustained or nonsustained supraventricular tachyarrhythmias (particularly if exaggerated by exercise); moderate to severe MR; and prior embolic event. In the presence of any of the above, the athlete should be restricted to low static, low dynamic competitive sports. These additional recommendations arise from additional risks involved in those with MVP.

Pulmonic Stenosis

Unlike left-sided valvular lesions, abnormalities of the pulmonary valve are due largely to congenital malformation. In congenital **pulmonic stenosis** (PS), the valve leaflets are fused, giving the valve a domed or cone-shaped appearance during systole. In some cases, the leaflets are thickened and poorly mobile. Children and adolescents with PS (even severe) are usually asymptomatic. Dyspnea and fatigue may be present in adults with longstanding disease because of a limited ability to increase cardiac output with exercise (1). Syncope and light-headedness with exertion may occur, but sudden cardiac death is rare. Right ventricular (RV) failure and tricuspid insufficiency may occur as a consequence of chronic PS.

In mild PS a systolic ejection murmur and ejection click may be present on auscultation. The ECG may be normal or demonstrate some evidence of right ventricular hypertrophy. The severity of PS is classified by the peak instantaneous gradient (see Figure 7.1), which can be obtained by cardiac catheterization or Doppler echocardiography. Mild stenosis is indicated by a peak gradient less than 40 mm Hg. Gradients between 40 and 70 mm Hg are seen with moderate PS, and severe stenosis is indicated by a gradient above 70 mm Hg. Balloon **valvotomy** or surgical **valvuloplasty** usually is performed if the gradient is at least 50 mm Hg (5).

Recommendations for Competition in the Presence of Pulmonic Stenosis

Asymptomatic athletes with pulmonic stenosis can participate in all competitive sports as long as the peak systolic gradient is less than 50 mm Hg and RV function is normal. These athletes should be reevaluated annually to assess for symptoms and an increasing systolic gradient. In the presence of a peak gradient greater than 50 mm Hg, the athlete can participate in low static, low dynamic sports. Athletes who undergo surgical valvotomy or balloon valvuloplasty, have adequate relief of obstruction, and have normal RV function can participate in all competitive sports after a period of recovery (about 1 month for balloon valvuloplasty and 3 months for surgical valvotomy). If severe stenosis persists (peak gradient >50 mm Hg), the athlete should only participate in low intensity competitive sports (5).

Pulmonic Regurgitation

Pulmonic regurgitation (PS), or regurgitation of the pulmonic valve, can occur as a consequence of valvotomy or valvuloplasty for PS, but it also may be due to primary or idiopathic dilation of the pulmonary artery (a congenital abnormality). Unlike aortic regurgitation, PR usually is well tolerated because pulmonary vascular resistance and pulmonary artery pressures are normally low. Rarely, RV volume overload may occur, leading to a need for pulmonary valve replacement. There have been instances of heart failure, complex ventricular dysrhythmias, and late sudden death among persons with long-standing PR after successful surgical repair of tetralogy of Fallot, a complex congenital malformation that includes PS or pulmonary outflow obstruction (1).

A diastolic decrescendo murmur may be audible along the upper left sternal border but may be difficult to appreciate due to the low diastolic gradient across the valve. Mild PR is commonly seen even in persons without valvular disease and is easily detected by Doppler echocardiography.

Recommendations for Competition in the Presence of Pulmonic Regurgitation

Athletes with pulmonic regurgitation may participate in all competitive sports as long as they have no symptoms at-

tributable to PR (e.g., RV overload and failure). If severe PR develops after repair of tetralogy of Fallot, participation should be limited to low static, low dynamic competitive sports (5).

Tricuspid Stenosis

Tricuspid stenosis (TS), or stenosis of the tricuspid valve, in adults is most likely due to rheumatic fever and is associated with rheumatic MS (a more common consequence of rheumatic valvular disease). A diastolic rumble may be present on physical examination but may not be distinguishable from the murmur of the coexisting MS. The Doppler echocardiogram will demonstrate the anatomic and flow abnormalities typical of TS, with leaflet thickening, fusion, and reduced mobility.

Recommendations for Competition in the Presence of Tricuspid Stenosis

Any restrictions for participating in competitive sports in athletes with rheumatic TS should be based on the severity and symptoms related to the associated MS (13).

Tricuspid Regurgitation

Acquired **tricuspid regurgitation** (TR) is unusual in adolescents and young adults and usually is the result of trauma, infective endocarditis secondary to intravenous drug abuse, or a small ventricular septal defect. In an older population, TR may occur as a consequence of chronic pressure overload and dilation of the right ventricle as a result of PS or pulmonary hypertension. The latter may be an idiopathic disorder or secondary to chronic left-sided valve disease, such as mitral stenosis. Tricuspid regurgitation also may occur as a consequence of rheumatic fever. Most cases of significant TR in the younger population are congenital and are due to **Ebstein's anomaly** (a malformation of the tricuspid valve) with variable deformity of the tricuspid valve. In the presence of severe TR with marked elevation in right atrial pressure, there is right-to-left shunting of blood across the atrial septum, leading to systemic arterial oxygen desaturation and cyanosis. Right ventricular volume overload and congestive heart failure may ensue, with low cardiac output and premature death. At the other end of the spectrum of severity are those with a mild deformity of the valve, less TR, and a favorable prognosis. In addition to the valve abnormalities, persons with Ebstein's anomaly also may have atrioventricular bypass tracts that can cause cardiac dysrhythmias.

A blowing holosystolic murmur may be appreciated along the left sternal border, varying with respiration. In addition, prominent systolic neck vein pulsations ("cannon V waves") may be seen in the jugular venous pattern. The Doppler echocardiogram demonstrates the systolic regurgitant jet and is useful in quantifying the severity of TR (Figure 7.11). An acquired (e.g., from endocarditis or rheumatic disease) or congenital (e.g., Ebstein's anomaly) etiology can be established as well. Valve repair or replacement is possible and may be necessary if there is significant RV overload or congestive failure. In the absence of marked elevation of right atrial and systemic venous pressure, TR may be well tolerated.

Recommendations for Competition in the Presence of Tricuspid Regurgitation

In the absence of congestive signs and symptoms or evidence of markedly elevated right atrial pressures, the athlete with TR can participate in all competitive sports (13). Specific recommendations for athletes with Ebstein's anomaly were established by the 26th Bethesda Conference (5). Those with a "mild" expression of the anomaly who do not have cyanosis or evidence of dysrhythmia and have a nearly normal heart size can participate in all competitive sports. If the TR is of moderate severity and there are no dysrhythmias detected by ambulatory ECG monitoring, the athlete can participate in low static, low dynamic competitive sports. If the anomaly is severe, the athlete should not participate in competitive sports. After surgical repair, the athlete may participate in low static, low dynamic sports if residual TR is at most mild, heart size is not significantly increased, and rhythm abnormalities are not present on ambulatory monitoring and exercise testing.

Multivalve Disease

Several conditions may be associated with dysfunction of more than one heart valve. Multiple valves may be affected as a sequel to acute rheumatic fever, with combined lesions of the mitral and aortic valves being most common. Tricuspid involvement may lead to TR, or the insufficiency may result from dilation of the RV secondary to pulmonary hypertension late in the course of mitral stenosis. In addition, myxomatous valvular changes and infective endocarditis may affect multiple valves. Combined valve abnormalities create derangements in circulatory function that may be complex, requiring more extensive testing (e.g., cardiac catheterization, 2D and Doppler echocardiography) for evaluation.

Recommendations for Competition in the Presence of Multivalve Disease

As a general rule, athletes with multivalve dysfunction should not participate in competitive sports. In selected cases, some athletes may be able to compete after a thorough evaluation by a cardiologist, preferably one with expertise in sports medicine. The restrictions for participation usually will be based on the athlete's most serious valve disorder. However, moderate dysfunction of multiple valves may create serious hemodynamic derangement, more severe than that of a single valve lesion (13).

Athletes With Mechanical or Bioprosthetic Heart Valves

Valve replacement may be done with **mechanical heart valves** or **bioprosthetic heart valves**. Following successful valve replacement surgery, most patients experience an improvement in circulatory function. However, a pressure gradient usually persists across the prosthetic valves because the effective valve opening is smaller than that of a normal native valve. During exercise, the transvalvular pressure gradients may increase significantly, and the rise in cardiac output may be blunted, limiting functional capacity. Various prosthetic valves differ in terms of valve areas and pressure gradients developed at higher rates of blood flow (20). Exercise stress testing to the level of exertion anticipated during competition is valuable to ensure that circulatory function will be adequate and to screen for effort-related symptoms (21). Uncertainty exists concerning the effects of repeated bouts of exercise on prosthetic valve longevity and ventricular function (22), a fact that needs to be considered by the potential competitive athlete.

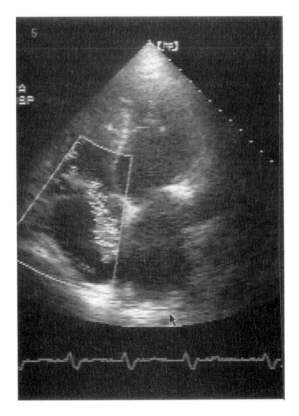

FIGURE 7.11. Two-dimensional and Doppler echocardiographic view of tricuspid regurgitation during systole. An eccentric jet of TR is seen on Doppler examination (*arrow*). RA, right atrium; RV, right ventricle; TV, tricuspid valve.

Recommendations for Competition in the Presence of Prosthetic Heart Valves

An athlete with a mechanical or bioprosthetic mitral valve who has normal valve function, is not taking an anticoagulant medication, and has at least near-normal ventricular function can participate in low and moderate static, low and moderate dynamic competitive sports (see Table 7.1). Athletes with prosthetic valves who require anticoagulant therapy should not participate in sports that have a risk of bodily collision. If the athlete has a bioprosthetic or mechanical aortic valve, is not taking an anticoagulant, and has normal valve function and at least near-normal ventricular function, he or she can participate in low static and low dynamic sports. Some selected athletes, after careful evaluation, may be able to participate in low and moderate static, low and moderate dynamic competitive sports (13). As a practical consideration, most athletes with a mechanical prosthetic valve do require anticoagulation therapy to prevent valve thrombosis.

Mitral Valvuloplasty for Mitral Valve Prolapse or Mitral Regurgitation

Advances in surgical technique and intraoperative evaluation by transesophageal echocardiography have enabled cardiothoracic surgeons to repair, rather than replace, the mitral valve in selected cases of mitral regurgitation. Valve competence can be restored by removing redundant, prolapsing valve tissue and implanting a prosthetic "ring" to reduce the size of the annulus. After surgery, there is no requirement for long-term anticoagulation. However, because of the abnormal, myxomatous character of the valve tissue, there is a concern that the trauma associated with contact sports could injure the repaired valve and cause serious dysfunction.

Recommendations for Competition After Mitral Valve Repair (Valvuloplasty)

Because of the risk of valve tissue injury, athletes who have had MV repair should not engage in sports with a risk of bodily collision. In general, the athlete can participate in low static, low dynamic sports, and selected athletes can participate in low and moderate static, low and moderate dynamic competitive sports (see Table 7.1) (13).

What We Know
About Exercise and Valvular Heart Disease

1 Normal function of the heart valves plays a major role in the effectiveness of the heart as a pump.

2 Abnormal valvular function (regurgitation or stenosis) limits forward cardiac output during exercise and reduces functional capacity.

3 Significant dysfunction of the left sided heart valves (mitral or aortic) causes shortness of breath (dyspnea) with physical exertion because of elevation of pulmonary venous and capillary pressure.

4 Certain valvular abnormalities (aortic stenosis and aortic insufficiency) may increase the risk of sudden death during physical exertion.

5 Multiple tests may be necessary to accurately assess the severity of valvular dysfunction, including 2D and Doppler echocardiography, cardiac catheterization, and graded exercise testing.

6 Guidelines have been established to assist in determining the appropriate level of competition for athletes with valvular heart disease.

What We Would Like to Know
About Exercise and Valvular Heart Disease

1 Will repeated bouts of exertion associated with competitive sports accelerate the deterioration of left ventricular function in athletes with valvular conditions that cause left ventricular volume overload (e.g., aortic insufficiency and mitral insufficiency)?

2 Can the increased pressure load caused by vigorous physical activity acutely damage valve tissue weakened by a congenital or acquired abnormality?

3 Can pharmacotherapy reduce the risk of adverse events in selected athletes with more severe valvular abnormalities and allow them to compete safely in competitive sports?

Summary

Diseases of the heart valves may have a significant impact on the hemodynamic function of the cardiac pump and place the athlete at risk of sudden death or other serious adverse events. Symptoms may develop late in the course of disease because many disorders worsen gradually and may escape detection on a cursory examination. Motivated athletes may ignore or deny symptoms that develop insidiously. Fortunately, most serious valve abnormalities are associated with physical findings that can prompt the careful examiner to the need for a more thorough evaluation. Two-dimensional and Doppler echocardiographic techniques are valuable tools that aid immensely in the diagnosis and gradation of severity of valve lesions.

Graded exercise testing also is very useful to assess the severity of the hemodynamic derangement and the functional capacity of the athlete. Cardiac catheterization may be necessary when the results of noninvasive testing are inconclusive or equivocal. Consensus recommendations adopted by the American College of Cardiology and the American College of Sports Medicine at the 26th Bethesda Conference provide a basis for decision-making concerning participation in competitive sports (2). However, these guidelines cannot account for all variables, such as the emotional stresses of competition, differences in skill levels, efficiency, and the intensity of training and practice. Collaboration among professionals (including coach, trainers, sports medicine physician, and cardiologist) along with the athlete are necessary to ensure the safety of competition.

CASE STUDY

Patient Information

George, a 16-year-old high school student, is trying out for the varsity track team along with several of his friends. He has not had any serious illnesses. His medical clearance form was completed by a general practitioner who has seen him in the past only for routine visits and immunizations. George has participated on the golf team and jogs regularly at a low intensity but does not engage in strenuous exercise. On the first day of practice, he noted a sensation of tightness in the mid-chest and became breathless while sprinting on the track. The symptoms passed quickly and he did not report them to his coach. The following day, he became very lightheaded at the end of the 50-yard dash and blacked out for a few seconds, falling to the ground. He appeared very pale, was short of breath, and was transiently disoriented after the incident. The local ambulance squad was called, but George felt well by the time of arrival and declined to go to the hospital. His coach insisted that he see a physician before returning to the team. He decided to see Dr. Roberts, the school's team physician.

Assessments

Dr. Roberts obtained a detailed history from George and discovered that he had tended to avoid heavy physical activities in the past because of breathlessness. He admitted that he would occasionally feel lightheaded and breathless after running up a flight of stairs. On physical examination, his carotid pulses were somewhat delayed and reduced in amplitude. An early systolic ejection click was heard over the upper left border of the sternum, followed by a harsh and loud late-peaking systolic murmur. A soft diastolic, decrescendo murmur also was heard along the left sternal border when George held his breath after exhaling. The second heart sound had two components, but the aortic closure sound was soft. An ECG was obtained and had features consistent with left ventricular hypertrophy. Dr. Roberts ordered a 2D and Doppler echocardiogram. This study confirmed the presence of left ventricular hypertrophy and demonstrated normal ventricular function. The aortic valve leaflets were thickened, and the valve had a dome shape during systole, with limited excursion of the cusps. Doppler interrogation of the left ventricular outflow tract and aortic valve yielded a peak instantaneous gradient across the valve of 45 mm Hg. The color Doppler study also revealed the presence of mild aortic regurgitation.

Questions

1. What valvular disorder does George have? Is it a congenital or acquired problem?
2. How would you classify the severity and symptomatic status of George's valve disease? What were the likely causes of his symptoms during and after running?
3. Should George be allowed to compete in track events? Can he participate in any other competitive sports?
4. Would it be possible for George to participate in competitive sports in the future?

REFERENCES

1. Bonow RO, Carabello B, de Leon AC Jr, et al. ACC/AHA guidelines for the management of patients with valvular heart disease: executive summary. A report of the American College of Cardiology/American Heart Association Task Force on Practice Guidelines (Committee on Management of Patients with Valvular Heart Disease). Circulation 1998;98:1949–1984.

2. Maron BJ, Mitchell JH. 26th Bethesda Conference: Recommendations for determining eligibility for competition in athletes with cardiovascular abnormalities. J Am Coll Cardiol 1994;24:845–899.

3. Mitchell JH, Haskell WL, Raven PB. 26th Bethesda Conference: Recommendations for determining eligibility for competition in athletes with cardiovascular abnormalities. Classification of sports. J Am Coll Cardiol 1994;24:864–866.

4. Otto CM. Aortic stenosis. Clinical evaluation and optimal timing of surgery. Cardiol Clin 1998;16:353–366.

5. Graham TP, Bricker JT, James FW, Strong WB. 26th Bethesda Conference: Recommendations for determining eligibility for competition in athletes with cardiovascular abnormalities. Task Force 1: Congenital heart disease. J Am Coll Cardiol 1994;24:867–873.

6. Frank S, Johnson A, Ross J Jr. Natural history of valvular aortic stenosis. Br Heart J 1973;35:41–46.

7. Zoghbi WA, Farmer KL, Soto JG, et al: Accurate noninvasive quantification of stenotic aortic valve area by Doppler echocardiography. Circulation 1986;73:452–459.

8. Oh JK, Taliercio CP, Holmes DRJ, et al. Prediction of the severity of aortic stenosis by Doppler aortic valve area determination: prospective Doppler-catheterization correlation in 100 patients. J Am Coll Cardiol 1988;11:1227–1234.

9. Otto CM, Burwash IG, Legget ME, et al. Prospective study of asymptomatic valvular aortic stenosis: Clinical, echocardiographic, and exercise predictors of outcome. Circulation 1997;95:2262–2270.

10. Barlow JB, Jankelow D. Prospective study of asymptomatic aortic stenosis. Circulation 1998;97:1651–1652.

11. Carabello BA. Prospective study of asymptomatic aortic stenosis: response. Circulation 1998;97:1652–1653.

12. Otto CM. Prospective study of asymptomatic aortic stenosis: Response. Circulation 1998;97:1653.

13. Cheitlin MD, Douglas PS, Parmley WW. 26th Bethesda Conference: Recommendations for determining eligibility for competition in athletes with cardiovascular abnormalities. Task Force 2: Acquired valvular heart disease. J Am Coll Cardiol 1994;24:874–880.

14. Bonow RO. Chronic aortic regurgitation. Role of medical therapy and optimal timing for surgery. Cardiol Clin 1998;16:449–461.

15. Maron BJ, Isner JM, McKenna WJ. 26th Bethesda Conference: Recommendations for determining eligibility for competition in athletes with cardiovascular abnormalities. Task Force 3: Hypertrophic cardiomyopathy, myocarditis and other myopericardial diseases and mitral valve prolapse. J Am Coll Cardiol 1994;24:880–885.

16. Freed LA, Levy D, Levine RA, et al. Prevalence and clinical outcome of mitral-valve prolapse. N Engl J Med 1999;34:1–7.

17. Jeresaty RM, Edwards JE, Chawla SK. Mitral valve prolapse and ruptured chordae tendineae. Am J Cardiol 1985;55:138–142.

18. Jeresaty RM. Mitral-valve prolapse. N Engl J Med 1999;341:1471–1472.

19. Quiñones MA. Management of mitral regurgitation. Optimal timing for surgery. Cardiol Clin 1998;16:421–435.

20. Silberman S, Shaheen J, Fink D, et al. Comparison of exercise hemodynamics among nonstented aortic bioprostheses, mechanical valves, and normal native aortic valves. J Card Surg 1998;13:412–416.

21. Lehmann G, Kölling K. Reproducibility of cardiopulmonary exercise parameters in patients with valvular heart disease. Chest 1996;110:685–692.

22. Landry F, Habel C, Desaulniers D, et al. Vigorous physical training after aortic valve replacement: analysis of 10 patients. Am J Cardiol 1984;53:562–566.

Pacemakers

Romualdo Belardinelli

Overview

The first pacemaker was implanted in 1958. Since that time, there have been important advances in cardiac pacemaker technology, and the spectrum of clinical applications has broadened significantly. Currently, about 1 million patients in the United States have a cardiac pacemaker, and almost 500,000 pacemakers are implanted worldwide each year (1).

As cardiac pacemaker technology has evolved, increasing attention has been paid to the improvement of hemodynamic function. The first pacemakers were programmed at a fixed **heart rate**, not synchronized to the atrial activity (asynchronous ventricular pacing), because their aim was to prevent bradyarrhythmias. The ventricular pacing mode,

however, did not allow **cardiac output** to improve in response to an increased metabolic demand, as, for instance, during exercise (Figure 8.1). The ability to increase heart rate during exercise is of crucial importance for increase in cardiac output. This response not only indicates the efficiency of the cardiovascular system, but also reflects the level of functional capacity. Cardiac output increases linearly with **oxygen uptake**, with a slope of approximately 6 L/min (6 L cardiac output per 1 L oxygen uptake per minute). At peak exercise, cardiac output for a normal sedentary adult increases by a factor of 5, from 5 L/min to 25 L/min. In elite athletes, the increase may be as much as 8 to 10 times the resting rate. Because cardiac output is the product of heart rate and **stroke volume**, both variables play a role in its increase. In normal untrained individuals,

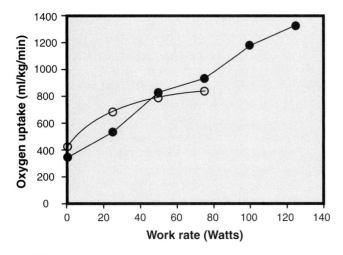

FIGURE 8.1. Oxygen uptake during a symptom-limited exercise test on a cycle ergometer in a middle-aged cardiac patient with normal left ventricular systolic function during asynchronous fixed-rate ventricular pacing (VOO, open circles) and during atrial synchronized ventricular pacing (VAT, closed circles). During VOO pacing, heart rate remained at 72 beats/minute throughout the exercise test. During VAT pacing, heart rate increased from 72 to 148 beats/minute. Note the marked difference in oxygen uptake increase during exercise between the 2 pacing modes.

stroke volume accounts for the early increase in cardiac output during isotonic incremental exercise, reaching a plateau at about 40% of peak oxygen uptake. Any further increase in cardiac output above this level until peak exercise is reached depends entirely on heart rate. In cardiac patients, stroke volume may be significantly lower at rest, and it fails to rise appropriately with work rate increase. In this setting, heart rate becomes even more crucial as a determinant of cardiac output increase to meet a higher metabolic demand. From an analysis of functional capacity related to

different cardiac pacing modes, it appears that ventricular rate response is the single most important factor in increasing exercise capacity in patients with permanent cardiac pacemakers, and that the way in which rate responsiveness is achieved is relatively unimportant (2).

This chapter presents a brief description of cardiac pacemakers, their clinical applications, and cardiac hemodynamics during different pacing modes. It also presents the physiologic and pathophysiological response of cardiac permanently-paced patients to acute and chronic exercise.

Permanent Pacemakers

A pacemaker is a system composed of a pulse generator (battery) that delivers electric stimuli over leads with electrodes in contact with the heart (Figure 8.2). The pulse generator is crucial, because it produces electric stimuli. This generator is simply a battery, most commonly a lithium iodine battery. A battery causes a potential difference, which produces a current flow through a conductor. Lithium iodine batteries have a capacity of 0.8 to 3.0 ampere hours, and last for 4 to 15 years, depending on resistances and voltage output. In one study (3), the longest duration was nuclear plutonium– or promethium-powered pacemakers, with 72% still functioning by 217 months after implantation. The briefest was mercury-zinc (no longer in use), with a 50% survival 36 months after implantation. The lithium iodine–powered pacemakers have a longer duration when output impedance is maintained at 510 ohms, when paced mode is 50% of time functioning, output programming is between 5 μJ and 200 μJ, and battery drain is low. Pulse duration also is important. At 2.5 V and 0.25 ms pulse duration, the estimated longevity of a common lithium iodine cardiac pacemaker is 28 years for a 510-ohm

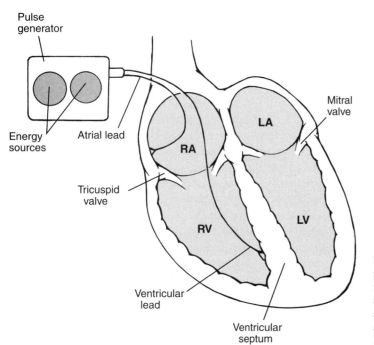

FIGURE 8.2. Schematic representation of a dual-chamber cardiac pacemaker. The pulse generator usually is implanted in the subcutaneous tissue in a pocket developed in the prepectoralis fascia. Atrial and ventricular leads are advanced through the subclavian vein and are positioned in the right atrial appendage and right ventricular apex, respectively. LA, left atrium; LV, left ventricle; RA, right atrium; RV, right ventricle.

TABLE 8.1. THE NORTH AMERICAN SOCIETY OF PACING AND ELECTROPHYSIOLOGY (NASPE) AND BRITISH PACING AND ELECTROPHYSIOLOGY GROUP (BPEG) CARDIAC PACEMAKERS CODE

Position	1	2	3	4	5
Function	Chamber paced	Chamber sensed	Response to sensing	Rate response, programmability	Antitachyarrhythmic function(s)
Specific aims	0 (none) A (atrium) V (ventricle) D (dual—atrium and ventricle)	0 (none) A (atrium) V (ventricle) D (dual—atrium and ventricle)	0 (none) T (triggered) I (inhibited) D (dual—triggered and inhibited)	0 (none) P (programmable) M (multiprogrammable) C (communicating) R (rate modulation)	0 (none) P (programmable) M (multiprogrammable) C (communicating) R (rate modulation)

0, none; A, atrium; C, communicating; D, dual; I, inhibited; M, multiprogrammable; P, programmable; R, rate modulation; T, triggered; V, ventricle

load. At 10 V and 1.0 ms output, however, the calculated longevity of the same pacemaker model drops to 2.3 years.

Cardiac pacemakers are programmed to stimulate the heart at a selected frequency, called the pacing rate. The pacing rate is chosen by the physician, depending on the type of cardiac disease, and usually is between 50 and 80 beats per minute. The most physiologic cardiac pacing is the one that mimics the normal conduction system as much as possible, and provides **atrioventricular synchrony**. It is important to maintain an **atrioventricular interval** in pacemakers with two leads, one in the right atrium and the other in the apex of the right ventricle (i.e., dual chamber pacing) to achieve a normal hemodynamic response to exercise.

Cardiac Pacing Code

The **cardiac pacing code** uses specific abbreviations to code cardiac pacemakers. These abbreviations indicate the cardiac chamber(s) paced, the chamber(s) sensed, the response to sensing, programmability, and antiarrhythmic function(s) (Table 8.1) (4). According to the North American Society of Pacing and Electrophysiology/British Pacing and Electrophysiology Group (NASPE/BPEG) classification, the first letter refers to the chamber or chambers being paced, and the second letter refers to the chamber or chambers being sensed. The letter A indicates atrial pacing or sensing, the letter V refers to ventricular pacing or sensing, and the letter D stands for dual-chamber (i.e., atrial and ventricular) pacing or sensing. The third letter refers to the response to a sensed event—the pacemaker can either inhibit (I) pacing output from one or both leads, or trigger (T) pacing at a programmable interval after the sensed event. The fourth letter represents either the type of programmability or rate-responsive pacing. Finally, the fifth letter indicates the capability to interrupt atrial or ventricular tachyarrhythmias (4). A pacemaker coded as AAI, for example, stimulates the atrium (A), senses the atrium (A) (and not the ventricle), and inhibits (I) pacing output from the atrial lead. A VVI pacing indicates that the right ventricle is the paced chamber (first V) as well as the sensed

chamber (second V), and it inhibits pacing output from the ventricular lead. A pacemaker coded DDD has dual pacing (atrial and ventricular) (first D), with dual sensing (atrial and ventricular)(second D), and it can trigger or inhibit from both leads (third D).

Clinical Indications

Pacing systems can also be classified as single-lead (atrial, AAI, or ventricular, VVI) and dual-chamber (DDD). Modern pulse generators can be programmed to a variety of **single-chamber pacing** as well as dual-chamber modes. This multi programmability greatly improves the accuracy and flexibility of cardiac pacing. The selection of pacing mode is mandatory to obtain the best clinical results. When pacing is appropriate, it is cost-effective in terms of relief of symptoms, prolongation of life, and improvement of the quality of life (5). Table 8.2 shows optimal pacing, aside alterna-

TABLE 8.2. RECOMMENDATIONS FOR OPTIMAL PACEMAKER MODE

Diagnosis	Optimal	Alternative	Inappropriate
SND	AAIR*	AAI	VVI VDD
AVB	DDD	VDD	AAI DDI
SND and AVB	DDDR DDIR	DDD DDI	AAI VVI AAI
Chronic AF with AVB	VVIR	VVI	DDD VDD
CSS	DDI	DDD VVI	AAI VDD AAI
MVVS	DDI	DDD	VVI VDD

*From the British Cardiac Pacing and Electrophysiology Group. AF, atrial fibrillation, AVB, atrioventricular block; CSS, carotid sinus syndrome; MVVS, malignant vasovagal syndrome; SND, sinoatrial node disease.
*See Table 8.1 for pacemaker codes.

tive, and inappropriate pacing modes. In addition to the classical indications for permanent pacing, which include atrioventricular block, sinus node dysfunction, bifascicular and trifascicular block, hypersensitive carotid sinus, and neurocardiac syndromes, cardiac pacing now is used more frequently in hypertrophic cardiomyopathies, in chronic heart failure with dilated cardiomyopathy, and to prevent atrial fibrillation (6–12).

Hemodynamic Function

The new generation of cardiac pacemakers is programmed not only for the traditional aim, prevention of an excessive reduction in heart rate, but also to maintain cardiocirculatory hemodynamics within physiologic limits in either normal or pathological conditions. Many variables can affect cardiac hemodynamic function and functional capacity in patients with a cardiac pacemaker; of these, some are related to the pacemaker system, whereas others are related to characteristics of the individual patient (Table 8.3). PPM-related factors include atrioventricular synchrony, atrioventricular interval, rate-responsiveness, and **site of pacing**.

Atrioventricular Synchrony

The most physiologic cardiac pacing is the one that mimics the normal conduction system as much as possible, and provides atrioventricular synchrony. At rest, atrioventricular synchrony contributes 20% to 25% of the cardiac output, depending on several factors, such as heart rate, left ventricular systolic and diastolic function, left ventricular filling pressure, left atrial size, contractility, retrograde ventriculoatrial conduction, and the timing between atrial and

TABLE 8.3. VARIABLES THAT AFFECT HEMODYNAMIC FUNCTION

Pacemaker-related
Atrioventricular synchrony
Atrioventricular interval
Rate responsiveness
Pacing site

Patient-related
Physiologic
  Age
  Sex
  Body weight
  Fitness level
Pathologic
  Cardiac disease
  Respiratory disease
  Oxygen transport
  Peripheral
  Medications

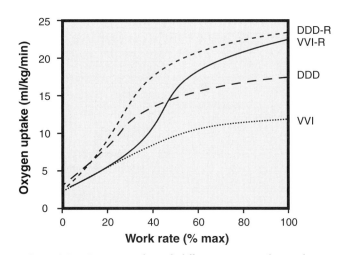

FIGURE 8.3. Oxygen uptake with different pacing modes at relative submaximal and maximal work rate increase during incremental (ramp) cycle-ergometry stress testing in 141 cardiac patients (mean age 61 ± 15 years). The hemodynamic response is improved with DDD-R and VVI-R pacing modes as compared with DDD. Fixed-rate pacing (VVI) determines the smallest increase in oxygen uptake. Although oxygen uptake is similar with DDD-R and VVI-R pacing modes at peak exercise, it is higher at submaximal work rate intensities in DDD-R mode, due to AV synchrony.

ventricular contractions (13). Peak exercise oxygen uptake is significantly higher when the atrium is paced maintaining synchrony (Figure 8.3). The cardiac index also improves resampling oxygen uptake increase (14). However, atrioventricular synchrony gradually becomes less important as cardiac output increases at higher exercise intensities, primarily due to the increased contribution of heart rate. No significant difference has been demonstrated between DDD and rate-matched VVI pacing with regard to central hemodynamics, cardiac sympathetic activity, and myocardial oxygen consumption at rest and during acute submaximal exercise (15). During chronic submaximal exercise (daily activities), patients with high-degree atrioventricular (AV) block have similar mean exercise time and respiratory rate with DDD and VVI-R pacing modes (16).

The hemodynamic advantage of sequential atrioventricular pacing over single-chamber (VVI) pacing is more clearly evident in patients with sick sinus syndrome than in those patients with complete atrioventricular block. In the former condition, retrograde ventriculoatrial conduction is common, because atrioventricular conduction is intact. Atrial-based pacing seems to be associated with a lower incidence of adverse cardiac events, including atrial fibrillation, congestive heart failure, and stroke. Quality of life also is improved, and cardiac mortality is lower in these patients (17).

The Pacemaker Syndrome

The maintenance of atrioventricular synchrony is fundamental for avoidance of the **pacemaker syndrome** (18).

This syndrome is characterized by a combination of several signs and symptoms that develop as a consequence of atrioventricular synchrony loss, and the presence of ventriculoatrial conduction. Atrial systole against closed atrioventricular valves causes a rapid rise in pulmonary venous pressure, atrial distention with atrial fibrillation, and reflex vasodepressor effects. Many patients may adapt to the pacemaker syndrome when mild symptoms are present. Exercise capacity also is depressed because of the rapid rise in pulmonary wedge pressure and dyspnea. In some cases, the symptoms are attenuated or disappear after the cardiac pacemaker is reprogrammed in dual-chamber mode (DDD instead of VVI) (19). This change is associated with important improvement in oxygen uptake, heart rate, and **ventilation** at peak exercise.

Atrioventricular Interval

The optimal atrioventricular interval for normal PR intervals is 150 ±15 ms (20). To achieve a normal hemodynamic response to exercise, the sensed AV interval should be programmed 40 to 50 ms shorter than the paced AV interval, because the P wave is delayed relative to the start of the AV interval due to the conduction time between sinus node and atrial electrode. Because PR interval shortens as the heart rate increases during exercise (5 ms every 10 beats) (20), modern pacemakers automatically shorten the AV delay, depending on the chronotropic response. This allows cardiac output to increase during exercise and exercise capacity to be greater compared with the constant AV interval pacing mode (21, 22). In patients with enlarged hearts and left ventricular systolic dysfunction (dilated cardiomyopathy), cardiac output response to isotonic exercise does not change over a wide range of AV intervals (50–200 ms) (23). In contrast, patients with diastolic dysfunction (hypertension) may take advantage of an optimized AV interval (24) based on daily physical activities.

Rate Responsiveness

Rate responsiveness (coded as R in Table 8.1) is the ability of a pacemaker to increase the lower heart rate in response to physiologic stimuli so it can provide a more physiologic hemodynamic response to face an increased metabolic demand, as, for instance, during physical exertion (25). The increase in heart rate during exercise is a crucial determinant of cardiac hemodynamic response (see Figure 8.3). In patients with normal left ventricle function, single-chamber ventricular pacing with neither rate-responsiveness nor AV synchrony (VVI mode) is less efficient in increasing cardiac output or oxygen uptake during incremental cycle-ergometer exercise as compared with VVI-R pacing mode, which provides rate-responsiveness without AV synchrony (26). Both cardiac output

and peak oxygen uptake are increased significantly during VVI-R pacing (16% and 18%, respectively, $P < 0.05$ for both). These results have been confirmed in another study, in which cardiac output was monitored at rest and during incremental exercise in patients with multiprogrammable DDD units implanted for complete AV block (25). Three pacing modes were selected: VVI pacing at 70 beats per minute; atrial-triggered pacing (VDD); and VVI pacing at a rate matched to the rate achieved at each stage of work rate increase during VDD pacing. At rest and submaximal work rate corresponding to 25% of the total workload, cardiac output was similar in the three pacing modes. At higher submaximal work rates and at peak exercise, cardiac output was identical with VDD and VVI-rate matched pacing, and was significantly greater than that achieved with VVI pacing (11.2 L/min vs 13.8 L/min). The increases in heart rate obtained with both VDD and VVI-rate matched pacing modes were similar, which can explain the higher cardiac output during submaximal and maximal exercise intensities as compared to VVI pacing. Rate-responsiveness was the main determinant of cardiac output increase. In fact, the addition to AV synchrony (VDD) did not determine any significantly greater cardiac output response than VVI rate-matched pacing. In another study, the improvement in exercise capacity obtained with a rate-matched AV synchronous pacing unit (VAT) was no different from that obtained with a rate-matched unit (VVIR), indicating that rate responsiveness is more important than AV synchrony for increasing work rate (2, 27, 28).

Rate-response pacing units have sensors that inform the pacemaker of an increased metabolic demand requiring a higher heart rate. There are several sensors, each of which is very sensitive to detect a peculiar parameter, including physical activity or catecholamines, QT interval, respiratory rate or minute ventilation, blood pH or temperature, oxygen content of mixed venous blood, stroke volume, and right atrial pressure (29–39). All of these sensors have limitations, and a time delay in the range of 30 to 60 seconds after the onset of exercise. Some systems can calculate the optimal rate-response program on the basis of a light physical activity (brief walk) and the level of activities of daily living. Newer pacemakers include dual sensors, combining an activity sensor with short response delay, and a physiologic sensor (e.g., Q-T interval, ventilation) with a longer delay. However, they are more accurate at higher heart rates. These new sensors use automatic algorithms to control rate responsiveness and are more rapid to increase heart rate with exercise.

In summary, **dual-chamber pacing** improves functional capacity compared with fixed-rate ventricular pacing, but not compared with rate-adaptive ventricular pacing (40, 41). The explanation may be that the cardiocirculatory response to exercise is due to mostly heart rate increase. For instance, in patients with complete atrioventricular block, ventricular rate does not increase adequately with exercise.

Site of Pacing

High right ventricular septal pacing determines a greater cardiac output increase during isotonic exercise than low septal pacing. Septal pacing may allow ventricular depolarization via the His-Purkinje system and determine a more efficient contractile function than right ventricular apical pacing (42). In patients with chronic heart failure with dilated cardiomyopathy, both ventricular activation and mechanical efficiency are abnormal. The electrical activation of myocardial cells is delayed as a consequence of inhomogeneous ventricular conduction across fibrotic tissue. Both intraventricular and interventricular dyssynchrony develop, which can worsen left ventricular systolic function (43, 44). There is evidence that **atrial synchronized biventricular pacing** (i.e., multisite pacing at the level of the right atrium, right ventricular apex, and left ventricle) in patients with dilated cardiomyopathy and left bundle branch block can correct interventricular dyssynchrony and improve left ventricular performance (45). The magnitude of improvement in interventricular synchrony is correlated with improvement in ejection fraction (46). The simultaneous activation of the right and left ventricles may improve interventricular septum coordination, resulting in an increased ejection fraction as well as exercise capacity. The site of pacing in the left ventricle seems particularly important to guarantee an enhanced contractility (47, 48). In fact, left ventricular free-wall pacing improves contractility, whereas pacing at the anterior wall does not seem to be efficient. Recent evidence suggests that both peak $\dot{V}O_2$ and the anaerobic threshold during cycle ergometer exercise stress testing are increased with biventricular pacing, whereas the traditional dual chamber pacing (DDD-R) determines significantly less improvement in functional capacity (unpublished data).

Patient-Related Factors

Physiologic and pathologic variables can influence the cardiocirculatory response to exercise in patients with a cardiac pacemaker (see Table 8.3).

Age

In most people, exercise capacity improves from childhood to the third decade of life, after which it starts to decline steadily, depending on the amount of physical activity performed and the patient's lifestyle characteristics. It is assumed that peak oxygen uptake declines by 10% each decade after the third. The decline in functional capacity is due to age-related decrements in both central and peripheral physiologic factors that are involved in oxygen transport and utilization. However, subjects who regularly perform exercise have a measured peak oxygen uptake approximately 25% higher in each age category as compared to sedentary subjects of the same age, gender, and body size (49, 50).

Gender

Exercise capacity in women is 15% to 30% less than that of men. The difference in aerobic capacity between women and men matched for age and body mass is 25% in sedentary and 22% in trained individuals (51). This difference can be explained by body composition and hemoglobin concentration. In women, fat-free body mass and hemoglobin concentration are 37% and 10% to 14% lower, respectively, than that in men. Over two decades, peak oxygen uptake declines 22% in trained women and 20% in trained men (51). The difference in aerobic capacity between men and women is largely a function of muscle mass.

Body Weight

Exercise capacity is reduced in overweight–obese individuals. On average, it has been estimated that oxygen uptake during unloaded pedaling on a cycle ergometer increases by about 6 ml/min/kg of extra body weight. At peak exercise, absolute peak oxygen uptake is 20% to 30% lower than that in normal-weight subjects of the same age and gender. Heart rate response to exercise is steeper, and the heart rate/oxygen uptake slope exceeds normal values, whereas stroke volume increase is within normal limits. In a group of 204 healthy subjects between 20 and 70 years of age, prediction of peak oxygen uptake is not improved by the addition of weight as an independent variable to age, gender, and height (52).

Fitness Level

Trained subjects have higher functional capacity than sedentary individuals matched for age, gender, and body size. For any decade of age, peak oxygen uptake is two to three times greater and heart rate response to exercise is flatter at any relative work rate in a trained subject. These responses are achieved independent of age and gender, and are related to cardiovascular and peripheral adaptations induced by physical activity (53).

Left Ventricular Function

Although there is no relation between ejection fraction and peak oxygen uptake, cardiac diseases usually reduce peak oxygen uptake as well as cardiac output at peak exercise. We performed 550 consecutive exercise tests with gas exchange analysis in our laboratory in a heterogeneous group of individuals with various cardiac diseases. Patients with coronary artery disease and normal left ventricular function had a peak oxygen uptake 18% lower than that of normal subjects matched for age, gender, and body weight (22 ± 6 ml/kg/min vs 18 ± 5 ml/kg/min; $P < 0.05$). Patients with left ventricular dysfunction had an even more marked reduction in peak oxygen uptake (16 ± 4.5

ml/kg/min). When patients with left ventricular systolic dysfunction are compared with patients with normal ejection fraction and left ventricular diastolic dysfunction, peak oxygen uptake is found to be 50% higher in the latter group. Other factors related to oxygen transport can influence exercise capacity.

Respiratory Diseases

Patients with pulmonary diseases have a reduced exercise capacity because of their respiratory limitation. Both peak oxygen uptake and anaerobic threshold are reduced, as well as peak work rate. Patients with restrictive physiology have a depressed $\dot{V}O_2$/**work rate slope** (<10 ml/min/watt), an increased respiratory frequency, and a low breathing reserve (54). Patients with obstructive lung disease have a high physiologic dead space (VD/VT), a positive arterial-end-tidal CO_2 difference during exercise (normally it is negative), and high ventilatory equivalents at the anaerobic threshold point and at peak exercise (55). In both cases, pao_2 decreases during exercise, and peak exercise workload is depressed (56).

Oxygen Transport

The transport of oxygen from blood to mitochondria is crucial to maintain an adequate diffusion gradient of oxygen between the capillary bed and skeletal muscle. Cardiac output is not the only factor that plays a key role in the oxygen supply to the cells—other factors also are important, such as blood flow distribution to working muscles, partial pressure of oxygen in the capillary blood, hemoglobin concentration in the blood, and hemoglobin's affinity for oxygen (57). In cardiac patients with a pacemaker, it is common for the concomitant presence of one or more pathological conditions to affect the oxygen transport pathway. Optimization of pacemaker programming, **exercise training**, and medications all contribute to improve exercise capacity (58).

Peripheral Factors

In normal subjects, during exercise peripheral blood flow is diverted to the active skeletal muscles, and the fraction perfusing organs such as the kidney, liver, and gastrointestinal tract is decreased (59). A shift of the oxyhemoglobin dissociation curve to the right (Bohr effect) due to metabolic acidosis favors oxygen diffusion from the capillaries into the mitochondria, where adenosine triphosphate (ATP) is synthesized aerobically. In a patient with a cardiac pacemaker with no rate-responsiveness option, oxygen supply to the periphery can be insufficient for working muscles, a situation that is compensated for by preferential blood flow distribution and higher oxygen extraction. In patients with

heart failure, both functional and structural alterations of skeletal muscles that reduce the capability to produce external work can develop (60–63).

Medications

Many drugs can affect cardiovascular response to exercise. Beta-blockers and calcium antagonists can reduce cardiac output and exercise capacity. In contrast, vasodilators improve cardiovascular hemodynamics during exercise.

In summary, the hemodynamic response to exercise of cardiac patients with a permanent pacemaker depends on several factors, so that it is impossible to identify an unequivocal response. Modern pacemakers have automatic functions, such as a rapid resetting of AV interval and rate responsiveness, that allow optimal hemodynamic response during exercise stress testing as well as physical activities of daily living.

Functional Capacity and Quality of Life

The results of the most important controlled studies comparing the effects of physiologic and ventricular pacing during acute bicycle or treadmill exercise in patients with advanced atrioventricular block and sinoatrial disease with atrioventricular node dysfunction are summarized in Table 8.4. Exercise capacity is greater during dual-chamber pacing than during fixed-rate ventricular pacing (VVI) (64). However, as previously mentioned, dual-chamber pacing

TABLE 8.4. FUNCTIONAL CAPACITY IN DUAL-CHAMBER VS VENTRICULAR PACING

Authors	No. Patients	Exercise Type	Exercise Tolerance
DDDS *vs* VVI			
Rediker[64]	19	T	+
Perrins[65]	13	C	+
Yee[66]	8	T	−
Kristensson[40]	44	C	+
Pehrsson[67]	14	C	+
Total[67]	98		
DDD vs VVI-R			
Fenanapazir	14	T	−
Linde-Edelstam[28]	17	C	−
Oldroyd[15]	10	T	−
Menozzi[16]	14	C	−
Sulke[70]	22	T	−
Jutzy[71]	14	T	−
Total	91		

C, cycle ergometer; DDD, dual-chamber pacing; T, treadmill; VVI, ventricular pacing; VVI-R, ventricular pacing with rate-adaptive response; +, improvement; −, no improvement.

does not significantly improve functional capacity as compared with rate-adaptive ventricular pacing (VVI-R) (65). In patients with chronotropic incompetence, dual-chamber pacing is more effective than asynchronous fixed-rate pacing in improving functional capacity, because only the former allows heart rate to increase during exercise (66). However, heart rate increase is crucial to improve cardiac output—more than any other programmable parameter—as suggested by the similar absolute workload at peak exercise with dual-chamber pacing and rate-adaptive ventricular pacing in patients with the same cardiac disease (67).

Exercise capacity usually is correlated with quality of life in cardiac patients (68). In patients with a cardiac pacemaker, quality of life, assessed with questionnaires, usually improves in parallel to functional capacity improvement. Dual-chamber pacing seems more effective than ventricular pacing, whether or not the rate-adaptive function is programmed (69–73). This finding is not in complete agreement with the results of studies on exercise tolerance reported in Table 8.4. Some biases can explain this different result, such as, for instance, small sample size and objective difficulty in keeping patients blinded. In patients with heart failure, resynchronization therapy by biventricular pacing has been demonstrated to improve New York Heart Association (NYHA) functional class as well as quality of life scores (Minnesota). In a study performed in our laboratory, quality of life improved by 59% and peak $\dot{V}O_2$ by 23% (unpublished data).

Cardiopulmonary Exercise Testing

Exercise is a physiologic stimulus that stresses the cardiovascular system to meet an increased metabolic demand. In normal subjects and patients with intact left ventricular function, cardiac output increases fourfold from resting values, and external work is produced according to previously described factors. To meet the increased demand, the cardiovascular system must increase cardiac output as well as oxygen extraction by working skeletal muscles.

Cardiac output is the product of heart rate and stroke volume. Heart rate increases at the beginning of exercise by vagal withdrawal, accounting for a rapid increase in cardiac output until approximately 40% of peak exercise capacity has been reached. Above that level, the response takes much longer. After a few minutes, heart rate increase depends on augmented sympathetic nervous activity. Stroke volume increases quite early, from about 70 ml/beat at rest to a maximum of 110 to 120 ml/beat, and reaches a plateau at approximately 40% of peak exercise. After this point, heart rate accounts entirely for any increase in cardiac output, until peak exercise is reached. Cardiac output increases relatively linearly with oxygen uptake ($\dot{V}O_2$). According to Fick's principle, $\dot{V}O_2$ = cardiac output $\times$ **arteriovenous oxygen difference**. In normal, fit individuals, heart rate increases almost linearly with $\dot{V}O_2$ by a slope of 3.5 to 4 beats

per ml/kg/min of oxygen. The slope indicates stroke volume between 40% and 80% of $\dot{V}O_2$ increase during isotonic exercise. In Figure 8.4, the four determinants of $\dot{V}O_{2max}$ are cardiac output, heart rate, stroke volume, and A-$\dot{V}O_2$ difference. In cardiac failure, cardiac output increase only doubles from rest, heart rate increases steeply, stroke volume does not increase or increases less than 50% than normal, and A-$\dot{V}O_2$ difference at peak exercise is not different from that in normal individuals. By contrast, in athletes, cardiac output increases 8 to 10 times from rest, because of an increase in stroke volume, while heart rate response is flatter. Arteriovenous oxygen difference at peak exercise does not differ from that of normal subjects.

Noninvasive, continuous monitoring of metabolic, ventilatory, and hemodynamic variables during exercise in cardiac patients with a permanent pacemaker provides more accurate information in these patients than traditional ECG stress testing, and also allows a more complete definition of the cardiocirculatory response to exercise, as well as functional capacity limitation. Modern cardiac pacemakers are multiprogrammable and can change atrioventricular delay automatically through a sensor-mediated mechanism when metabolic demand increases. Measuring ventilation as well as gas exchange during exercise can quantify the individual metabolic response, evaluate the appropriateness of pacemaker programming, and also prescribe exercise training programs.

Functional capacity can be expressed as oxygen uptake at peak exercise or maximal oxygen uptake ($\dot{V}O_{2max}$) as well as exercise duration or maximal workload achieved at peak exercise. In addition, $\dot{V}O_{2max}$ represents a measure of cardiovascular performance, because it is the product of heart rate by stroke volume (cardiac output) by A-$\dot{V}O_2$ difference. Peak $\dot{V}O_2$ is increased when rate-variable pacing is compared with fixed-rate pacing (see Figure 8.1). It has been calculated that a 42% rise in heart rate from resting values during incremental isotonic exercise is associated with a 22% increase in $\dot{V}O_{2max}$ and a 13% increase in the anaerobic threshold (29). The improvement in $\dot{V}O_{2max}$ reflects not only the chronotropic response to exercise, but also peripheral adjustments. With rate-responsive pacing, lactate production is decreased in working muscles as compared to fixed-rate pacing, as a consequence of oxygen supply improvement. The improved hemodynamic response to exercise in patients with rate-responsive pacing also can be documented by another index of cardiovascular performance. Oxygen uptake increases during exercise in relation to work rate by a slope of approximately 10 ml/min/watt in normal subjects. In patients with a cardiac pacemaker, the $\dot{V}O_2$/W slope changes with the pacing mode. During incremental exercise in fixed-rate pacing mode, the slope is approximately 30% lower than during rate-variable pacing. Ventilation also improves with rate-responsive pacing. This improvement is reflected by higher minute ventilation at peak exercise and by a less steep ventilatory equivalent for carbon dioxide above the anaerobic threshold. Heart rate increase during isotonic incremental exercise is related

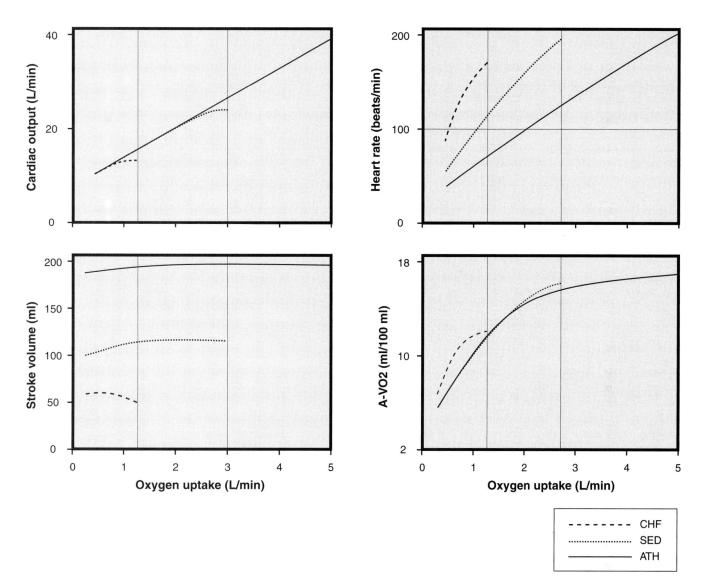

FIGURE 8.4. The four determinants of maximal oxygen uptake ($\dot{V}_{O_{2max}}$) during symptom-limited exercise in chronic heart failure patients (dotted line, CHF), normal sedentary (thin continuous line, SED) and athletes (thick continuous line, ATH). For details, see text.

to $\dot{V}_{O_2}$ increase. The slope HR/$\dot{V}_{O_2}$ is 3.5 to 4 beats/mL/kg/min in normal subjects. In patients with chronotropic incompetence (HR/$\dot{V}_{O_2}$ <2) with DDD pacing, the HR/$\dot{V}_{O_2}$ slope during exercise is steeper when the pacing mode is shifted toward rate-responsive function as compared with patients with a normal slope. Peak $\dot{V}_{O_2}$ is significantly higher in patients with a HR/$\dot{V}_{O_2}$ slope >2 in DDD mode. However, despite similar heart rate at peak exercise, peak $\dot{V}_{O_2}$ is not different when DDDR pacing is compared below and above the two HR/$\dot{V}_{O_2}$ slopes. **Heart rate/$\dot{V}_{O_2}$ slope** can be used to optimize rate-variable pacing systems. In 66 patients with VVI-R pacing who underwent a symptom-limited cardiopulmonary exercise test (CPX) in our laboratory, heart rate/$\dot{V}_{O_2}$ slope was 5.5 ± 1.9 beats/mL/kg, significantly steeper than that measured in normal controls (3.8 ± 1.6 beats/mL/kg). This discrepancy may lead to overestimation

of the pacing rate needed to perform physical activities in cardiac patients with chronic rate-responsive pacing. These results indicate that gas exchange analysis can give additional information to standard ECG stress testing, and also identify patients who can benefit most from rate-variable pacing.

Exercise Training

In cardiac rehabilitation centers, it is quite common to find patients with coronary artery disease or chronic heart failure who also have a cardiac pacemaker. Before starting an exercise training protocol, it is important to know the type of **pacemaker** and its programming. If the device is old and without rate modulation, the hemodynamic response to exercise is depressed, and so is functional capacity, as discussed earlier in this chapter. In these cases, either a symptom-limited exercise testing protocol with small increments in work rates or a submaximal constant work rate protocol can be chosen, to avoid early onset of fatigue and underestimation of functional capacity. If the device is of new generation (multiprogrammability and rate modulation), it is important to know the type of sensor(s). Activity sensors have a piezoelectric crystal that converts detected motions into an electrical signal processed by an automatic algorithm. Physical activity causes vibrations that indicate the need to modulate heart rate. A delayed response may be present when small muscle groups are activated at low work rates (e.g., early stage cycle ergometer) (34). For motion sensors, treadmill protocols with increments in both grade and speed should be preferred, because they do not respond to changes in grade only (35). For cardiac patients without chronic pacing, exercise protocols with a smooth increase in work rate (ramp) are preferable to those with large step increases in workload (e.g., Astrand, Bruce). In fact, they can underestimate exercise capacity when patients are overweight or unfit, and fatigue rapidly develops. The upper rate of cardiac pacemakers also should be taken into account. The pacemaker should be programmed so that it allows a sufficient amount of external work. If the heart rate response is steep and exceeds the upper-rate limit, a Wenckebach pattern may develop to maintain a higher heart rate. A 2:1 rhythm can determine a rapid decrease in heart rate, and early fatigue.

Theoretically, all patients with a cardiac pacemaker can benefit from cardiac rehabilitation, but benefits depend on three groups of variables related not only to the type of cardiac pacemaker, but also to the patient's clinical characteristics and protocol design (74, 75).

Inclusion and Exclusion Criteria

Exercise programs should be started 10 to 15 days after pacemaker implantation in those patients who do not have local or general complications. Clinical stability in the preceding 4 weeks is a requisite for obtaining advantages from training. All new pacemakers are multiprogrammable and can be tailored to patient needs. For instance, a young patient with rate-adaptive dual pacing and normal left ventricular function should have a higher upper-rate limit than a sedentary patient with inducible myocardial ischemia. Exclusion criteria are unstable angina, uncontrolled hypertension or diabetes, recent acute heart failure, tachyarrhythmias or complex ventricular arrhythmias, neuromuscular or orthopaedic limitations that do not allow regular exercising.

Intensity

Exercise intensity is chosen on the basis of the clinical picture and the desired goal. The objective of exercise training programs is to improve the patient's functional capacity and quality of life, and also to help patients to accept living with a cardiac pacemaker through educational and psychological supports. In middle-aged, pacemaker-dependent patients with normal cardiac function, exercise intensity can be calculated at 60% to 70% of peak $\dot{V}O_2$ measured on a preliminary CPX. An alternative method is to calculate the heart rate reserve (heart rate at peak exercise − heart rate at rest) × (intensity [i.e., 50–80% of peak heart rate) + heart rate at rest. However, because patients with VVI pacemakers may have little or no chronotropic reserve, it is preferable to use systolic blood pressure as the reference (74). In patients with left ventricular dysfunction and an enlarged ventricle, the intensity should be lower, especially during the initial 2 to 3 weeks. After this period, work intensity can be increased on the basis of individual progress and stabilized at 50% to 60% of peak $\dot{V}O_2$. The precise calculation and correct choice of exercise training intensity for the patient are important to avoid high heart rate levels and to prevent a Wenckebach pattern from developing. Patients with coronary artery disease who develop myocardial ischemia during exercise can take advantage of interval training, with intermittent exercise bouts at the ischemic threshold (5-minute on-off protocol, with an initial 5-minute loadless warm-up). For instance, if the ischemic threshold is stable at 100 watts, requiring the heart rate to increase to 120 beats/min, exercise intensity can be calculated as 5-minute sessions of cycling at 90 watts, followed by 5 minutes of subthreshold exercise at 50% of the threshold intensity (in this specific case, 50 watts). In total, three 5-minute exercise bouts, each followed by a 5-minute subthreshold exercise, can be performed per session.

Exercise Type

Warm-up calisthenics should be performed before the patient starts cycling or treadmill exercise. The warm-up is important to improve muscular tone, avoid dyspnea, and delay muscle acidosis. Moreover, in patients with inducible myocardial ischemia, warm-up exercise usually increases the ischemic threshold and may allow greater external work. After 15 to 20 minutes of warm-up, isotonic exercise can be started on a cycle ergometer or treadmill and done for 40 minutes, considering an initial loadless exercise (5 minutes) and a final loadless cool-down (5 minutes). For patients with a nonphysiologic sensor, treadmill exercise at the selected intensity is preferable to cycling, because of the more rapid increase in heart rate due to movement. Stationary cycling may not provide a sufficient stimulus for sensors to increase heart rate. Treadmill exercise intensity should be arranged by changing speed more than grade.

Methodology

It is preferable for patients just beginning an exercise program to perform supervised exercise at the hospital facilities. In all patients, at the beginning and at the end, we perform blood chemistry, an ECG, and cardiopulmonary exercise testing. The initial and final evaluations are crucial to monitor changes induced by the training program, to determine the individual exercise intensity, and to measure the amount of benefit each patient can achieve (Figure 8.5). Educational support and dietary counseling are provided by skilled operators. During exercise sessions, room temperature should be maintained at 22°C with humidity constant at 50%. Heart rate and blood pressure are taken at rest before starting the program, during aerobic exercise, and during recovery. Excessive increases in blood pressure during exercise should be avoided. For instance, if blood pressure rises during stationary cycling above 180/90 mm Hg

from rest, the workload should be reduced to stabilize it around 160/90 mm Hg. Heart rate during exercise should be monitored for the same reason, to avoid exercise intensities above the target level and possible adverse events, especially arrhythmias and myocardial ischemia. Heart rate monitoring (telemetry) is recommended for all patients at the beginning of training protocol, and must be maintained throughout the entire training period in those patients who have arrhythmias or inducible ischemia. Adequate rehydration with isotonic beverages at the end of each session also should be recommended. In our laboratory, adverse events are rare—the most common are postexercise hypotension (5%) and benign arrhythmias (18%). Compliance with exercise sessions varies between 60% and 90% in our hospital. The duration of training is 8 weeks, sometimes less. In our program, we perform three sessions per week, because we believe that requiring more sessions is likely to increase the dropout rate.

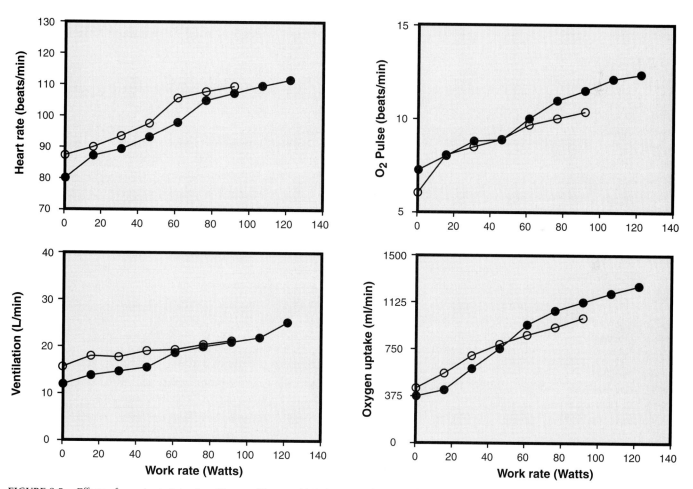

FIGURE 8.5. Effects of exercise training in a 54-year-old man with ischemic cardiomyopathy and chronic heart failure who has had a biventricular pacing system implanted. After an 8-week supervised exercise training program at 60% of peak oxygen uptake, an improvement of functional capacity, expressed by a 25% improvement in peak oxygen uptake and a 33% increase in work tolerance, was noted. These improvements were not accompanied by any change in heart rate and ventilatory responses, but O_2 pulse was improved significantly. Because O_2 pulse is a good approximation of stroke volume, this change indicates that the improvement in peak oxygen uptake in this patient was due entirely to a training-induced improvement in left ventricular systolic function. *Open circles,* initial study; *closed circles,* results after exercise training.

Results

Patients with heart failure, advanced age, restrictive diastolic filling, extensive peripheral obstructive arterial disease, and obesity with multiple risk factors gain less benefit from these exercise programs than those without these characteristics. The results are not significantly different from patients with the same underlying cardiac disease without permanent pacing. Peak $\dot{V}O_2$ increases by 15% to 25%, exercise time by 18% to 26%, and the anaerobic threshold by 12% to 20%. Total cholesterol is not significantly changed, but HDL cholesterol is increased by 9% to 15%, and triglycerides are reduced by 14% to 28%. Patients with the highest improvement in functional capacity are younger than 40 years of age, are male, and have depressed left ventricular systolic function and low peak $\dot{V}O_2$ at initial CPX.

What We Know
About Pacemakers

1 The introduction of cardiac pacemakers into clinical practice provided important new therapeutic strategies in the treatment of bradyarrhythmias.

2 Modern cardiac pacemakers are noninvasively multiprogrammable, rate-responsive, and atrial synchronous. The "plasticity" of permanent pacemakers allows appropriate pacing for individual needs and better hemodynamic function.

3 Pacemaker technology has improved in the last decade, and the rate of complications is lower.

4 New applications of cardiac pacing are heart failure and atrial fibrillation. In heart failure, the insertion of a dual-chamber pacemaker with a third electrode stimulating the coronary sinus (biventricular pacing) generally improves cardiac hemodynamics through a more efficient contractility. Functional capacity also is improved as a result of the reduced cardiac insufficiency. Paroxysmal atrial fibrillation is alleviated when patients are paced in AAI or DDD mode, which "stabilizes" the atrial rhythm. Another potential clinical indication is hypertrophic cardiomyopathy. A reduction in left ventricular outflow gradient and symptoms has been described with dual-chamber pacing in patients with this condition. The septum, abnormally hypertrophic, is depolarized later than it would be during intrinsic conduction, with reduced septal motion and lower gradient. This pathophysiologic "correction" translates into reduced pulmonary congestion and symptoms.

What We Would Like To Know
About Pacemakers

In the evolution of pacemaker therapy, increasing attention has been paid to improvement of hemodynamic function in different clinical situations. Providing atrioventricular synchrony appears to be an advantage, contributing to 20% to 30% higher cardiac output. Atrial-based pacing (AAI or DDD) determines higher cardiac output during exercise than VVI pacing. Patients with pacemakers can improve their exercise tolerance by regular exercising. Both peak oxygen uptake and anaerobic threshold are increased after endurance exercise training programs of moderate intensity. Rate responsiveness is crucial in these patients to allow heart rate increase at the target intensity. It is important to know that modern pacemakers offer the feature of automatically mode switching from DDD mode to either VVI or DDI mode during episodes of supraventricular tachyarrhythmias. With resumption of sinus rhythm, the pacer mode automatically switches back to DDD. Thus, DDDR pacing with mode switching allows higher exercise capacity than VVIR pacing on exercise testing, and it is subjectively preferred by patients.

Pacemaker complications can occur at the time of implantation or later. The most common early complications are pneumothorax, local hematoma, venous thrombosis, infection, and diaphragmatic stimulation. Late complications are lead failure, high thresholds, pacemaker failure, diaphragmatic stimulation, battery depletion, and "pacemaker syndrome." It is very important to check the pacemaker status periodically to prevent late complications.

Electromagnetic interference is a potential source of pacemaker malfunctioning. Cellular phones and electronic equipment can alter pacing rate and cause presyncope, syncope, chest pain, and palpitations. Therapeutic radiation can damage internal circuits at doses greater than 5000 rads. Pacemaker malfunctioning can result in loss of capture, abnormal pacing rate, undersensing, or oversensing. It is important to inspect ECG strips, interrogate the pacemaker, and check pacing and sensing thresholds, lead impedance, battery voltage and magnet rate, and chest radiographs.

A growing number of patients have implantable cardioverter defibrillators (ICD) with antibradycardia pacing, as well as antitachycardia pacing and extensive programmability. These patients may be involved in exercise training programs. In our experience, there is no particular risk of evoking arrhythmias during exercise in ICD holders, if exercise type and intensity are correctly chosen. Functional capacity is improved after exercising three times a week for 4 to 6 weeks on a cycle ergometer at 60% of peak oxygen uptake for 40 minutes. Continuous aerobic exercise does not trigger ICD discharge due to heart rate elevation from resting values, because heart rate increase with this kind of exercise is progressive, not brisk, and the highest heart rate during a session is far below the standard value that will trigger ICD discharge (usually 190 beats/min). However, a patient involved in physical activities requiring short bursts of intense exercise, as when playing tennis or squash, can experience rapid increases in heart rate or induce tachyarrhythmias that can trigger the ICD's discharge. Careful follow-up is required to make sure the devices perform in the manner for which they are intended.

Summary

1. Patients with a cardiac pacemaker often have an underlying cardiac disease that contributes to functional deterioration.
2. Exercise training programs should be tailored to each patient's clinical characteristics and pacemaker type. The main objectives of exercise training are improvements in functional capacity and quality of life.

3. Adverse events during training are relatively rare and generally do not hamper program completion.
4. Educational and psychological support is important.
5. Dietary counseling must be considered.
6. Benefits are more evident with programs combining exercise training with educational, psychological, and dietary support.
7. Limitations are the lack of randomized controlled studies with correct statistical design.

DISCUSSION QUESTIONS

1. How are cardiac pacemakers classified?

2. What is the best cardiac pacemaker mode for patients referred to cardiac rehabilitation?

3. What is the intensity of exercise training in patients with myocardial infarction and permanent DDD-R pacing?

4. What are inclusion and exclusion criteria for cardiac patients with permanent pacing?

5. What benefits do you expect after exercise training in patients with permanent cardiac pacing?

CASE STUDY

Patient Information

Mr. Capri is a 50-year-old man who has been admitted to the emergency unit because of chest pain and asthenia. His body mass index is 23.5. His heart rate was 32/min, blood pressure 160/100 mm Hg. He was mildly hypercholesterolemic (total cholesterol: 225 mg/dl). His ECG showed a third-degree atrioventricular block with ST elevation in D2, D3, and AV_F. The diagnosis was inferior acute myocardial infarction complicated by third-degree AV block. A temporary pacemaker was inserted into the right ventricle via the right femoral vein and programmed at 80 beats/min. Shortly afterward he was conducted to the catheterization laboratory for coronary angiography, which demonstrated an occlusion of the second portion of the right coronary artery and a significant stenosis of the first tract of the left anterior descending artery. A coronary angioplasty was performed, with application of one stent on the right coronary artery and a second stent in the left anterior descending artery. He soon felt better. After 1 week, however, it was necessary to implant a permanent, dual-chamber DDD-R pacemaker because the AV block was persistent.

Assessment

In summary, this is a case of a patient with coronary artery disease with an acute myocardial infarction complicated by a third-degree AV block, treated with coronary angioplasty and permanent dual-chamber pacing. After 15 days, the patient was referred to cardiac rehabilitation.

Questions

1. What factors must you take into consideration before you develop an exercise program for Mr. Capri?

2. Develop a program of exercise training for Mr. Capri. Describe the intensity, frequency, duration, and mode of exercise that would be safe and appropriate. How long should the program last?

3. What other health care professionals might be engaged in assisting Mr. Capri during the time he follows the exercise program?

4. How would you evaluate Mr. Capri's progress at the conclusion of your program? Is it necessary for him to continue a maintenance program at home? How often?

The American Heart Association recommends a program of prevention in patients with acute myocardial infarction (MI) with hypercholesterolemia, like Mr. Capri. In fact, post-MI patients who undergo cardiac rehabilitation have a better life expectancy (25% less mortality over 3 years) than patients who do not. Coronary stenting is not a contraindication for exercise training. As recently reported, 6 months of moderate exercise training does not increase the restenosis rate after coronary angioplasty and does improve functional capacity and quality of life 6 months after training begins. The combination of medications with exercise training and diet counseling seems to reduce the progression of coronary atherosclerosis and also to improve personal wellness. Permanent pacing does not adversely affect functional capacity improvement.

Loss of Capture—A loss of capture is diagnosed on ECG when there is a visible pacing stimulus and no atrial or ventricular depolarization. It depends on leads or the lead–tissue interface. Dislodgment of a lead from its position is the most common cause of loss of capture. Another cause may be an increase in the pacing threshold above the pacing output, as a result of drug therapy, myocardial infarction, or ischemia. Less commonly, a fracture of the lead, insulation breaks or loose set screws, and battery depletion can cause failure of capture. It may require a reprogramming of pacing output, or lead or battery replacement.

Upper-rate limit—In patients with bradyarrhythmias, the pacing rate is set at a level below which the ventricular rate cannot fall. Equally, a pacemaker that stimulates and senses the atrium requires an upper rate limit (URL), defined as the shortest interval between ventricular stimuli or from a spontaneous QRS to the next ventricular stimulus. The URL is a programmable value that generally is set at a rate lower than that corresponding to the total atrial refractory period (the sum of the atrioventricular interval and the postventricular atrial refractory period). When a patient has a sinus tachycardia, the pacemaker tracks the P waves in a 1:1 fashion up to the upper programmed pacing rate or to the pacemaker 2:1 rate. In the latter case, the ventricular response would drop by nearly half, with hemodynamic consequences. For this reason, the total atrial refractory period is programmed to a sufficiently short interval or the URL of the pacemaker is programmed to a rate above the 2:1 atrioventricular conduction rate. Thus, a cardiac pacemaker should be programmed to allow a sufficient amount of external work. If the heart rate response is steep and exceeds the upper-rate limit, a Wenckebach pattern may develop to maintain a higher heart rate. A 2:1 rhythm can determine a rapid decrease in heart rate, drop in blood pressure, and early fatigue.

Pacemaker-induced tachycardia—It is not impossible that, instead of preventing bradyarrhythmias, a pacemaker may induce a tachyarrhythmia. This event is rare but can occur in some situations. An electric stimulus can fall into the vulnerable period of the cardiac cycle and induce tachyarrhythmias such as supraventricular tachycardia, atrial fibrillation or flutter, ventricular tachycardia, or fibrillation. Myocardial sensitivity to stimulation is increased during myocardial ischemia, metabolic imbalance, drug therapy, or intoxication or electrolyte imbalance.

REFERENCES

1. Parsonnet V, Bernstein AD. The 1989 World Survey of Cardiac Pacing. Pacing Clin Electrophysiol 1991;14:2073–2076.
2. Nordlander R, Headman A, Pehrsson SK. Rate responsive pacing and exercise capacity—a comment. Pacing Clin Electrophysiol 1989;12:749–751.
3. Furman S, Garvey J, Hurzeler P. Pulse duration variation and electrode size as factors in pacemaker longevity. J Thorac Cardiovasc Surg 1975;69:382–389.
4. Bernstein AD, Camm AJ, Fletcher R, et al. The NASPE/BPEG generic pacemaker code for antibradyarrhythmia and adaptive rate pacing and antitachyarrhythmia devices. Pacing Clin Electrophysiol 1987;10:794–799.
5. Gregoratos G, Cheitlin MD, Conill A, et al. ACC/AHA guidelines for implantation of cardiac pacemakers and antiarrhythmia devices: a report of the American College of Cardiology/American Heart Association Task Force on Practice Guidelines (Committee on Pacemaker Implantation). J Am Coll Cardiol 1998;31:1175–1209.
6. Barold SS. Indications for permanent cardiac pacing in first degree AV block: class I, II or III. Pacing Clin Electrophysiol 1996;19:747–751.
7. McAnulty JH, Rahimtoola SH, Murphy E, et al. Natural history of "high risk" bundle branch block: final report of a prospective study. N Engl J Med 1982;307:137–143.
8. Kay R, Estiolo M, Wiener I. Primary sick sinus syndrome as an indication for chronic pacemaker therapy in young adults: incidence, clinical features and long term evaluation. Am Heart J 1982;103:338–342.
9. Maloney JD, Jaeger FJ, Rizo-Patron C, Zhu DW. The role of pacing for the management of neurally mediated syncope: carotid sinus syndrome and vasovagal syncope. Am Heart J 1994;127:1030–1037.
10. Jeanrenaud X, Goy JJ, Kappenberger L. Effects of dual-chamber pacing in hypertrophic obstructive cardiomyopathy. Lancet 1992;339:1318–1323.
11. Auricchio A, Sommariva L, Salo RW, et al. Improvement of cardiac function in patients with severe congestive heart failure and coronary artery disease by dual chamber pacing with shortened AV delay. Pacing Clin Electrophysiol 1993;16:2034–2043.
12. Saksena S, Praiash A, Hill M, et al. Prevention of recurrent atrial fibrillation with chronic dual-site right atrial pacing. J Am Coll Cardiol 1996;28:687–694.
13. Karlof I. Hemodynamic effect of atrial triggered versus fixed rate pacing at rest and during exercise in complete heart block. Acta Med Scand 1975;197:195–206.
14. Fananapazir L, Bennett DH, Monks PH. Atrial synchronized pacing: contribution of the chronotropic response to improved exercise performance. Pacing Clin Electrophysiol 1983;6:601–608.
15. Oldroyd KG, Rae AP, Carter AP, et al. Double-blind crossover comparison of the effects of dual chamber pacing (DDD) and ventricular rate adaptive (VVIR) pacing on neuroendocrine variables, exercise performance, and symptoms in complete heart block. Br Heart J 1991;65:188–193.
16. Menozzi C, Brignole M, Moracchini PV, et al. Intrapatient comparison between chronic VVIR and DDD pacing in patients affected by high degree AV block without heart failure. Pacing Clin Electrophysiol 1990;13:1816–1822.
17. Alpert MA, Curtis JJ, Sanfelippo JF, et al. Comparative survival after permanent ventricular and dual chamber pacing for patients with chronic high degree atrioventricular block with and without preexistent congestive heart failure. J Am Coll Cardiol 1986;7:925–932.
18. Furman SS. Pacemaker syndrome. Pacing Clin Electrophysiol 1994;17:1–5.
19. Heldman D, Mulvhill D, Nguyen H, et al. True incidence of pacemaker syndrome. Pacing Clin Electrophysiol 1990;13:1742–1750.
20. Rees M, Haennel RG, Black WR, et al. Effect of rate-adapting AV delay on stroke volume and cardiac output during atrial synchronous pacing. Can J Cardiol 1990;6:445–452.
21. Haskell RJ, French WJ. Optimum AV interval in dual-chamber pacemakers. Pacing Clin Electrophysiol 1986;9:670–675.
22. Ovsyshcher I. Toward physiological pacing: optimization of cardiac hemodynamics by AV delay adjustment. Pacing Clin Electrophysiol 1997;20:861–865.
23. Shinbane JS, Chu E, DeMarco T, et al. Evaluation of acute dual-chamber pacing with a range of atrioventricular delays on cardiac performance in refractory heart failure. J Am Coll Cardiol 1997;30:1295–1300.
24. Modena MG, Rossi P, Carcagni A, et al. The importance of different atrioventricular delay for left ventricular filling in sequential pacing: clinical implications. Pacing Clin Electrophysiol 1996;19:1595–1604.
25. Wirtzfeld A, Schmidt G, Himmler FC, Stangl K. Physiological pacing: present status and future development. Pacing Clin Electrophysiol 1987;10:41–56.
26. Leung SK, Lau CP, Ting MO. Cardiac output is a sensitive indicator of difference in exercise performance between single and dual sensor pacemakers. Pacing Clin Electrophysiol 1998;21:35–41.
27. Linde-Edelstam C, Nordlander R, Pehrsson SK, Ryden L. A double-blind study of submaximal exercise tolerance and variation in paced rate in atrial synchronous compared to activity sensor modulated ventricular pacing. Pacing Clin Electrophysiol 1992;15:905–915.
28. Linde-Edelstam C, Hjemdahl P, Pehrsson SK, et al. Is DDD pacing superior to VVIR? A study on cardiac sympathetic nerve activity and myocardial oxygen consumption at rest and during exercise. Pacing Clin Electrophysiol 1992;15:425–434.
29. Kay GN, Bubien RS, Epstein AE, Plumb VJ. Rate-modulated cardiac pacing based on transthoracic impedance measurements of minute ventilation: correlates with exercise gas exchange. J Am Coll Cardiol 1989;14:1283–1289.
30. Rossi P, Plicchi G, Canducci G, et al. Respiratory rate as a determinant of optimal pacing rate. Pacing Clin Electrophysiol 1983;6:502–507.
31. Lau CP, Tai YT, Fong PC, et al. Clinical experience with an activity sensing DDDR pacemaker using an accelerometer sensor. Pacing Clin Electrophysiol 1992;15:334–342.
32. Stangl K, Wirtzfeld A, Heinze R, et al. A new multisensor pacing system using stroke volume, respiratory rate, mixed venous oxygen saturation, and temperature, right atrial pressure and right ventricular pressure and dP/dt. Pacing Clin Electrophysiol 1988;11:712–724.
33. Katritsis D, Camm AJ. Adaptive rate pacemakers: comparison of sensors and clinical experience. Cardiol Clin 1992;10:671–690.
34. Mehta D, Lau CP, Ward DE, et al. Comparative evaluation of chronotropic responses of QT sensing and activity sensing rate responsive pacemakers. Pacing Clin Electrophysiol 1988;11:1405–1412.
35. Haennel RG, Logan T, Dunne C, et al. Effects of sensor selection on exercise stroke volume in pacemaker dependent patients. Pacing Clin Electrophysiol 1998;21:1700–1708.
36. Bacharach DW, Hilden RS, Millerhages JO, et al. Activity-based pacing: Comparison of a device using an accelerometer versus a piezoelectric crystal. Pacing Clin Electrophysiol 1992;15:188–196.
37. Lau CP. The range of sensors and algorithms used in rate adaptive cardiac pacing. Pacing Clin Electrophysiol 1992;15:1177–1211.
38. Alt E, Matula M, Theres H, et al. The basis for activity controlled rate variable cardiac pacemakers: An analysis of mechanical forces on the human body induced by exercise and the environment. Pacing Clin Electrophysiol 1989;12:1667–1680.
39. Lau CP, Butrous GS, Ward DE, Camm AJ. Comparison of exercise performance of six rate-adaptive right ventricular cardiac pacemakers. Am J Cardiol 1989;63:833–838.
40. Kristensson BE, Arnman K, Smedgard P, Ryden L. Physiological versus single-rate ventricular pacing: a double-blind cross over study. Pacing Clin Eletrophysiol 1985;8:73–84.
41. Leclercq C, Gras D, Le Helloco A, et al. Hemodynamic importance of activation sequence compared to atrioventricular synchrony in left ventricular function. Am Heart J 1995;129:1133–1141.
42. Buckingham T. Right ventricular outflow tract pacing. Pacing Clin Electrophysiol 1997;20:1237–1242.
43. Cazeau S, Ritter P, Pakdach S, et al. Four chamber pacing in dilated cardiomyopathy. Pacing Clin Electrophysiol 1994;17:1974–1979.

44. Blanc JJ, Etienne Y, Gilard M, et al. Evaluation of different pacing sites in patients with severe heart failure: results of an acute hemodynamic study. J Am Coll Cardiol 1997;10:3273–3277.

45. Grines CL, Bashore TM, Boudoulas H, et al. Functional abnormalities in isolated left bundle branch block. The effect of interventricular asynchrony. Circulation 1989;79:845–853.

46. Kass DA, Chen CH, Curry C, et al. Improved left ventricular mechanics from acute VDD pacing in patients with dilated cardiomyopathy and ventricular conduction delay. Circulation 1999;99:1567–1573.

47. Auricchio A, Stellbrink C, Block M, et al. Effect of pacing chamber and atrioventricular delay on acute systolic function of paced patients with congestive heart failure. Circulation 1999;99:2993–3001.

48. Kerwin WF, Botvinick EH, O'Connell WO, et al. Ventricular contraction abnormalities in dilated cardiomyopathy: Effect of biventricular pacing to correct interventricular dyssynchrony. J Am Coll Cardiol 2000;35:1221–1227.

49. Inbar O, Oren A, Scheinowitz M, et al. Normal cardiopulmonary responses during incremental exercise in 20 to 70-yr old men. Med Sci Sports Exerc 1994;26:538–543.

50. Astrand I, Astrand PO, Hallback I, Kilborn A. Reduction in maximal oxygen uptake with age. J Appl Physiol 1073;35:649–654.

51. Astrand PO. Human physical fitness with special reference to sex and age. Physiol Rev 1956;36:307–335.

52. Wasserman K, Whipp BJ. Exercise physiology in health and disease (state of the art). Am Rev Respir Dis 1975;112:219–249.

53. Dehl MM, Bruce RA. Longitudinal variations in maximal oxygen intake with age and activity. J Appl Physiol 1972;33:805–807.

54. Hansen JE, Wasserman K. Pathophysiology of activity limitation in patients with interstitial lung disease. Chest 1996;109:1566–1576.

55. Wasserman K, Brown HV. Exercise performance in chronic obstructive pulmonary disease. Med Clin North Am 1981;65:525–547.

56. Bye PTP, Farkas GA, Roussos CH. Respiratory factors limiting exercise. Am Rev Physiol 1983;45:439–451.

57. Wagner PD. Determinants of maximal oxygen transport and utilization. Ann Rev Physiol 1996;58:21–50.

58. Hammond MD, Gale GE, Kapitan KS, Ries A, Wagner PD. Pulmonary gas exchange in humans during exercise at sea level. J Appl Physiol 1986;60:1590–1598.

59. Grimby G, Nilsson NJ, Saltin B. Cardiac output during submaximal and maximal exercise in active middle-aged athletes. J Appl Physiol 1966;21:1150–1156.

60. Massie BM, Conway M, Yonge R, et al. Skeletal muscle metabolism in patients with congestive heart failure: relation to clinical severity and blood flow. Circulation 1987;76:1009–1019.

61. Harrington D, Coats AJS. Skeletal muscle abnormalities and evidence for their role in symptom generation in chronic heart failure. Eur Heart J 1997;18:1865–1872.

62. Drexler H, Riede U, Munzel T, et al. Alterations in skeletal muscle in chronic heart failure. Circulation 1992;85:1751–1759.

63. Wilson JR, Fink L, Maris J et al. Evaluation of energy metabolism in skeletal muscle of patients with heart failure with gated phosphorus-31 nuclear magnetic resonance. Circulation 1985;71:57–62.

64. Rediker DE, Eagle KA, Homma S, et al. Clinical and hemodynamic comparison of VVI versus DDD pacing in patients with DDD pacemakers. Am J Cardiol 1988;61:323–329.

65. Perrins EJ, Morley CA, Chan SL, Sutton R. Randomized controlled trial of physiological and ventricular pacing. Br Heart J 1983;50:112–117.

66. Yee R, Benditt DG, Kostuk WJ, et al. Comparative functional effects of chronic ventricular demand and atrial synchronous ventricular inhibited pacing. Pacing Clin Electrophysiol 1984;7:23–28.

67. Pehrsson SK. Influence of heart rate and atrioventricular synchronization on maximal work tolerance in patients treated with artificial pacemakers. Acta Med Scand 1983;214:311–315.

68. Belardinelli R, Georgiou D, Cianci G, Purcaro A. Randomized, controlled trial of long-term moderate exercise training in chronic heart failure. Effects on functional capacity, quality of life, and clinical outcome. Circulation 1999;99:1173–1182.

69. Lamas GA, Orav EJ, Stambler BS, et al. Quality of life and clinical outcomes in elderly patients treated with ventricular pacing as compared with dual chamber pacing. N Engl J Med 1998;338:1097–1104.

70. Sulke N, Chambers J, Dritsas A, Sowton E. A randomized double-blind crossover comparison of four-rate responsive pacing modes. J Am Coll Cardiol 1991;17:696–706.

71. Jutzy RV, Florio J, Isaeff DM, et al. Comparative evaluation of rate modulated dual chamber and VVIR pacing. Pacing Clin Electrophysiol 1990;13:1838–1846.

72. Lau CP, Tay YT, Lee PWH, et al. Quality of life in DDR pacing: atrioventricular synchrony or rate adaptation? Pacing Clin Electrophysiol 1994;17:1838–1843.

73. Lukl J, Doupal V, Heinc P. Quality of life during DDD and dual sensor VVIR pacing. Pacing Clin Electrophysiol 1994;17:1844–1848.

74. Superko HR. Effects of cardiac rehabilitation in permanently paced patients with third-degree heart block. J Cardiopulm Rehabil 1983;3:561–568.

75. Estes NA III, Brockington G, Manolis AS, Salem D. Pacemakers and exercise: Current status, future directions and practical implications of physiological pacemakers. Sports Med 1989;8:1–8.

Heart Transplantation

Ray W. Squires

Overview

The first successful human heart transplant was performed by Christian Barnard in 1967 in Cape Town, South Africa (1). The resulting publicity and enthusiasm spurred a number of surgical centers to perform the operation, but long-term survival was poor and the procedure was not widely performed during the 1960s and 1970s. The development, at Stanford University, of the transvenous **endomyocardial biopsy** technique for early detection of acute rejection together with the introduction of the powerful immunosup-

pressant cyclosporine resulted in a marked improvement in survival. These important milestones, and eventual insurance funding of the operation and aftercare in the United States, made the operation an attractive treatment for patients with terminal heart failure.

By the end of 1999, approximately 56,000 heart transplants worldwide had been reported to the Registry of the International Society for Heart and Lung Transplantation (2). Fewer than 200 procedures were reported in 1982, with a rapid increase to approximately 4500 operations during 1993. The total number of transplants has decreased in recent years, with approximately 3500 operations reported for 1999. Worldwide, approximately 220 centers perform heart transplants (of these, 9 centers are in Canada, and 146 centers are in the U.S.). Transplant recipients range from newborn to the eighth decade of life. Approximately 400 operations were performed in the pediatric population (≤17 years of age), most for treatment of congenital heart disease or idiopathic cardiomyopathy. Most recipients, however, are between 35 and 64 years of age. The average age of the donor is approximately 30 years. The median waiting time for an organ depends on the patient's blood type and the degree of medical urgency, with typical wait times varying between 75 and 335 days (3). Unfortunately, the number of potential candidates for heart transplantation far exceeds the available supply of donor organs.

Orthotopic heart transplantation (Figure 9.1) is the usual surgical technique, in which the recipient's diseased heart is removed and the donor heart is anastomosed to the great vessels and atria of the recipient (4). In the extremely rare circumstances of excessively elevated pulmonary vascular resistance with severe pulmonary hypertension, or a significant donor-recipient body weight mismatch, the heterotopic or "piggyback" transplant may be used (Figure 9.2). In the **heterotopic heart transplant**, the recipient's dis-

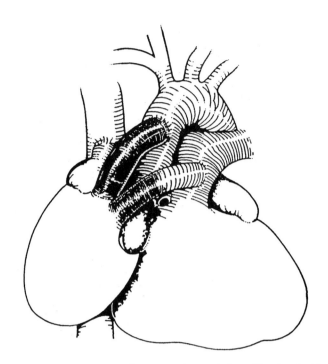

FIGURE 9.2. Heterotopic heart transplant technique. (Reprinted with permission from Squires RW. Exercise training after cardiac transplantation. Med Sci Sports Exerc 1991;23:686–694.)

eased heart is left in place and the donor heart is implanted in parallel to the existing heart. This procedure results in the unique electrocardiographic appearance of two separate "QRS" complexes on the electrocardiogram (ECG). Survival after heterotopic transplantation is much poorer than with the orthotopic technique.

For patients with **end-stage heart failure**, cardiac transplantation is the accepted form of definitive treatment, with 1-year and 5-year survivals of 81% and 68%, respectively (2). The annual mortality through 14 years of follow-up is 4% per year. Early mortality most commonly is due to primary graft failure. Late mortality is due primarily to graft vessel disease and malignancy. The goals of heart transplantation are improved survival, reduced symptoms, and an increased exercise capacity. Approximately 90% of patients who require transplantation suffer from chronic heart failure resulting from either coronary artery disease (**ischemic left ventricular dysfunction**) or **idiopathic dilated cardiomyopathy**. Other conditions that may result in terminal heart failure include hypertension, valvular heart disease, **myocarditis**, alcohol abuse, chemotherapy, acquired immunodeficiency syndrome, complex congenital heart disease, infiltrative diseases of the myocardium (e.g., **cardiac amyloid**, **hemachromatoses**), and peripartum (4).

After recovery from transplantation surgery, most patients report a reasonably favorable quality of life. Many patients return to work, school, or their usual avocational activities, although exercise capacity remains below average (as discussed later in this chapter). In one series of patients

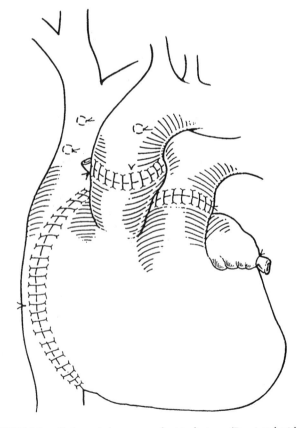

FIGURE 9.1. Orthotopic heart transplant technique. (Reprinted with permission from Squires RW. Exercise training after cardiac transplantation. Med Sci Sports Exerc 1991;23:686–694.)

under 60 years of age, the rate of return to work at 1 and 5 years (for survivors) was nearly 70% (6). However, because of immunosuppressant drugs and other transplant-related factors, patients are prone to develop serious medical problems. Table 9.1 lists the more common problems observed in transplant recipients.

Medication Side Effects and Possible Complications

Immunosuppressants

Immunosuppressants are given to prevent acute rejection of the donor heart (4). Cyclosporine, azathioprine, and prednisone are the medications typically used. Tacrolimus may be substituted for cyclosporine (7), and mycophenolate mofetil may be used in place of azathioprine. These powerful drugs enable the patient to tolerate the donor heart but are associated with several common side effects. For example, cyclosporine may result in renal dysfunction and has general vasopressor effects, resulting in hypertension requiring drug treatment in approximately 67% of patients (8). Prednisone, in the dose range used in transplantation, is particularly bothersome. It alters body fat distribution, with resultant truncal obesity and a "moonfaced" appearance for many patients. Prednisone also may cause mood swings as well as skeletal muscle atrophy and weakness, osteoporosis, and an adverse blood lipid profile. If at all possible, prednisone is tapered and stopped during the first 1 to 2 years after transplantation. Skeletal muscle cramping is another common patient complaint. Table 9.2 lists the immunosuppressants and their common side effects.

Acute Rejection

Acute rejection is characterized by infiltration of the myocardium with **T-lymphocytes** and may result in myocyte injury and necrosis, if not detected early in its course and adequately treated with additional immunosuppressant drugs. Routine, periodic transvenous endomyocardial biopsies are

TABLE 9.2. COMMON IMMUNOSUPPRESSANT DRUGS AND ASSOCIATED SIDE EFFECTS

Drug (Trade name)	Potential Side Effects
Cyclosporine (Gengraf, Neoral, Sandimmune)	Renal dysfunction, tremor, hypertension, hirsutism, gum hyperplasia, muscle cramps, acne
Azathioprine (Imuran)	Nausea/vomiting, leukopenia, thrombocytopenia, anemia
Prednisone	Muscle atrophy/weakness, hypertension, fluid retention, osteoporosis, aseptic necrosis of bone, "moonface" appearance, truncal obesity, increased insulin resistance, cataracts, glaucoma, mood swings, personality change, insomnia, peptic ulcer disease
Tacrolimus (ProGraf)	Tremor, headache, diarrhea, hypertension, nausea, renal dysfunction
Mycophenolate mofetil (CellCept)	Diarrhea, leukopenia, sepsis, vomiting, infection, edema

performed to detect acute rejection early in its course. Based on tissue sample analysis, rejection is graded from mild to severe (Table 9.3). Acute rejection is treated with additional immunosuppressants and may require hospitalization. Severe acute rejection, resulting in substantial **myocyte necrosis** and fibrosis, may produce left ventricular dysfunction and heart failure (4).

Infection and Malignancy Risk

Immunosuppressed transplant patients are at higher risk of opportunistic infections and malignancy than other patients with cardiovascular diseases. During the first several weeks after surgery, pulmonary bacterial infections are common. Late after transplantation, viral, bacterial, and

TABLE 9.1. COMMON MEDICAL PROBLEMS OBSERVED IN HEART TRANSPLANT RECIPIENTS

Condition	Prevalence at 5 Years Posttransplant
Hypertension	67%
Hyperlipidemia	40%
Graft vessel disease	22%
Diabetes mellitus	16%
Renal dysfunction	13%
Malignancy	10%

Data from Hosenpud JD, Bennett LE, Keck BM, et al. (2).

TABLE 9.3. STANDARDIZED CARDIAC BIOPSY ACUTE REJECTION GRADING SCALE

Grade	Findings
0	No rejection
1	Mild rejection
1A	Focal infiltrate without necrosis
1B	Diffuse, sparse infiltrate, no necrosis
2	Moderate rejection, one focus with aggressive infiltration and/or myocyte damage
3	Moderate rejection
3A	Multifocal aggressive infiltrates and/or myocyte damage
3B	Diffuse inflammatory process with necrosis
4	Severe rejection, diffuse aggressive polymorphous infiltrates with necrosis

Modified from Squires RW (4).

fungal infections pose a threat. Special precautions must be taken to minimize the chances of exposure to infectious agents and to individuals with active infections. Patients are encouraged to wear a surgical mask and gloves in public places, particularly during the first 3 months after surgery, as a barrier to infectious organisms. Recurrent hospitalizations for treatment of acute rejection and infection are common during the first year after transplantation. Acute rejection and infection are the most common causes of early mortality in transplant patients.

Malignancy risk is substantial for transplant patients. At 5 years after surgery, approximately 10% of recipients have experienced a malignancy (2).

Accelerated Graft Coronary Disease

Accelerated graft coronary disease, also called cardiac allograft vasculopathy or **graft vessel disease**, is the major limiting factor in long-term survival after transplantation and is the leading cause of death in these patients 1 year or more after surgery. Approximately 25% of patients have angiographic evidence of clinically important disease 5 years after surgery. It is an unusually accelerated form of coronary disease affecting epicardial and intramyocardial coronary arteries and veins (9). The pathophysiology is believed to begin with repetitive endothelial injury from the immune system's response to the graft, ischemia-perfusion injury, viral infection, immunosuppressant medications, and traditional coronary risk factors such as dyslipidemia, insulin resistance, and hypertension. Following injury, the inflammation-repair response of the vessel wall results in intimal thickening, which may become obstructive. The lesions may diffusely involve the entire vessel or may result in more focal obstruction. The process occurs in both pediatric and adult recipients with equal regularity.

Annual coronary angiography is routinely performed in most patients to detect the disease. Revascularization with catheter-based techniques or coronary bypass graft surgery may be effective in patients with discrete, focal lesions. However, because the lesions often are more diffuse in nature, retransplantation is the most common treatment, although survival is not as favorable as with a first transplant.

Statins and Fibric Acid Derivatives

Statin medications (e.g., pravastatin and simvastatin) and **fibric acid derivatives** (e.g., gemfibrozil) may slow progression of accelerated graft coronary disease and improve survival (9–11). In addition, statins have been shown to reduce the incidence of acute rejection and to improve left ventricular function (12–14). These benefits appear to be independent of these drugs' effect in improving the blood lipid profile.

Psychological Factors

The psychological response to the transplant process is understandably intense for most patients (15). During the waiting time for the operation after being accepted as a transplant candidate, emotions range from relief and happiness to anxiety (indefinite waiting time and lack of absolute assurance that the transplant will occur) and thoughts of death. Patients who require continuous hospitalization while waiting for an organ may find the environment supportive or merely tedious and boring. Immediately after transplantation, patients usually are joyous at the prospects for a longer, better quality life.

As the period of postoperative convalescence continues, patients must adjust to the tedium of appointments and procedures. As discussed previously, the immunosuppressant medication prednisone may cause mood swings and personality change. The first episode of acute rejection may result in heightened feelings of anxiety and transient depression. As the recovery from surgery progresses and the degree of medical surveillance decreases, patients generally shift their attention from transplant-related activities to becoming more independent and resuming family roles, as well as occupational and avocational pursuits. The readjustment to life after transplantation requires months, and the 1-year anniversary of the surgery is an important milestone in this process. Most patients are able to return to employment or other productive pursuits.

Responses to Exercise

The responses of heart transplant patients to acute exercise is unique and is related, in part, to the following factors (4, 16):

- At the time of organ harvesting, the transplanted (donor) heart is surgically denervated and receives no direct efferent activity from the autonomic nervous system and provides no direct afferent input to the central nervous system. Months after transplantation, some patients exhibit signs of partial cardiac reinnervation, and this will be discussed later in this chapter.
- The donor heart has undergone ischemic time and reperfusion (during organ harvesting and after transplantation).
- There is no intact pericardium.
- The donor heart may have suffered various amounts of myocyte necrosis resulting from bouts of acute rejection.
- **Diastolic dysfunction** may be present.
- Abnormal skeletal muscle histology and energy metabolism, developed during the course of chronic heart failure, may be present.
- Peripheral and coronary vasodilatory capacity may be impaired.

Heart Rate and Exercise

As a result of the loss of parasympathetic innervation with transplantation, the heart rate at rest is elevated to approximately 95 to 115 beats/min and represents the inherent rate of depolarization of the sinoatrial node (17). With graded exercise, the heart rate typically does not increase during the first several minutes, followed by a gradual rise with peak heart rates slightly lower than normal (approximately 150 beats/min) due to sympathetic nervous system denervation. Many patients achieve their highest exercise heart rates during the first few minutes of recovery from exercise, rather than at the time of the greatest exercise intensity. Heart rate may remain near peak values for several minutes during recovery before gradually returning to resting levels. Regulation of heart rate during exercise occurs via the circulating catecholamines. Figure 9.3 shows the heart rate response of the same patient to graded exercise 1 year before and 3 months after orthotopic transplantation. Note the delayed increase in heart rate during the first few minutes of exercise. During recovery from exercise, the heart rate remains elevated and slowly returns to pre-exercise levels as the concentration of circulating catecholamines returns to baseline. The **chronotropic reserve** (the difference between rest and maximal exercise heart rate) is less than normal.

With orthotopic transplantation, it is possible that the sinoatrial (SA) node of the recipient's heart may be left intact. The depolarization wave from the SA node generally does not pass through the suture line in the right atrium, but the ECG may show two distinct "p" waves (one from the recipient and one from the donor sinoatrial nodes).

Blood Pressure and Vascular Pressures

Blood pressure at rest usually is mildly elevated in post–heart transplant patients, even though most patients receive antihypertensive medications. During exercise, their blood pressure generally increases appropriately, although peak exercise blood pressures usually are slightly lower than expected for normal individuals (18). Vascular resistance is elevated, and intracardiac and pulmonary vascular pressures (particularly right-sided pressures) generally are elevated in transplant patients (19).

Left Ventricular Function

In most heart transplant patients, **left ventricular systolic function**, as measured by ejection fraction, falls in the normal range at rest and during exercise (19). However, **left ventricular diastolic function** is impaired, as evidenced by elevated filling pressure for a given end-diastolic volume. This impairment results in a below normal increase in stroke volume during exercise. The impaired rise in stroke volume, coupled with the below normal heart rate reserve, results in an impaired exercise cardiac output.

Exercise Cardiac Output

When exercise is begun, cardiac output in transplant recipients with complete **cardiac denervation** initially is increased by augmentation of stroke volume via the Frank-Starling mechanism and subsequently by an increase in heart rate (20). Figure 9.4 shows the greater increase relative to controls in left ventricular end-diastolic volume index during exercise in transplant patients that results in the enhanced Frank-Starling effect. However, at rest and during exercise the cardiac index is lower for transplant patients than for normal persons (Figure 9.5).

Skeletal Muscle Structure and Biochemistry

Several skeletal muscle structural and biochemical abnormalities develop during the clinical course of chronic heart failure, including reduced aerobic metabolic enzyme activity, lower capillary density, impaired vasodilation during exercise due to endothelial dysfunction, and conversion of some slow-twitch motor units to fast-twitch motor units with a greater reliance on anaerobic rather than aerobic energy production. These abnormalities generally persist after transplantation, with partial improvement after several months for some patients (21–23).

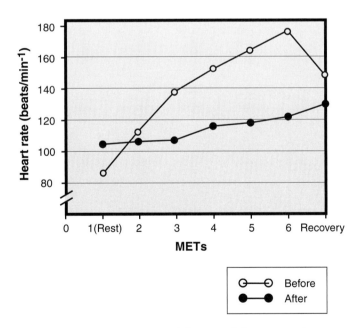

FIGURE 9.3. Heart rates measured during graded exercise in the same patient 1 year before and 3 months after orthotopic heart transplantation. Note the elevated resting heart rate and the delayed increase in heart rate after transplantation consistent with complete denervation. METs, metabolic equivalents. (Reprinted with permission from Squires RW. Cardiac rehabilitation issues for heart transplantation patients. J Cardiopulmonary Rehabil 1990;10:159–168.)

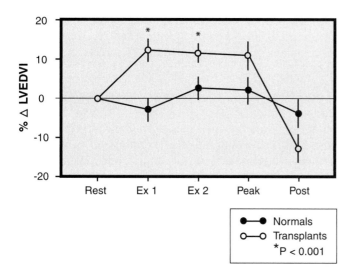

FIGURE 9.4. The change in left ventricular end-diastolic volume index (LVEDVI) during graded supine exercise in heart transplant recipients compared with healthy persons. (Reprinted with permission from Pflugfelder PW, Purves PD, McKenzie FN, et al. Cardiac dynamics during exercise in cyclosporine treated orthotopic heart transplant recipients: assessment by radionuclide angiography. J Am Coll Cardiol 1987;10:336–341.)

Pulmonary Function and Arterial Oxygenation

The efficiency of pulmonary ventilation is below normal during the first several months after transplantation (4), illustrated by an elevation in the ratio of minute ventilation to carbon dioxide production (the ventilatory equivalent for CO_2, VE/VCO_2). This excess ventilation results in a height-ened sense of shortness of breath during exercise. The increase in tidal volume during exercise is blunted, probably due to respiratory muscle weakness, deconditioning, and the effects of corticosteroid medications (24). Diffusion impairment is present in approximately 40% of patients. However, arterial saturation with oxygen at rest and during exercise is normal for the majority of patients (25). A minority of patients with pretransplant diffusion abnormalities experience mild arterial desaturation (to approximately 90%) with exercise (26). Azathioprine may cause anemia in some patients, which may reduce arterial oxygen content (4).

Oxygen Extraction by Exercising Skeletal Muscle

Extraction of oxygen from the arterial blood by metabolically active body tissues, as indicated by the arterial-mixed venous oxygen difference, is normal at rest. However, during exercise the arterial-mixed venous oxygen difference does not increase in a normal manner and reflects abnormalities with both the delivery of capillary blood to exercising skeletal muscle and impairment in the oxidative capacity of the muscle (19).

Oxygen Uptake Kinetics/Peak $\dot{V}O_2$

The rate of increase in $\dot{V}O_2$ (oxygen uptake kinetics) is slower than normal, as a result of an impaired rise in both cardiac output and arterial-mixed venous oxygen difference (27). Peak exercise oxygen uptake is generally below average for age and gender (4, 18). Figure 9.6 shows oxygen up-

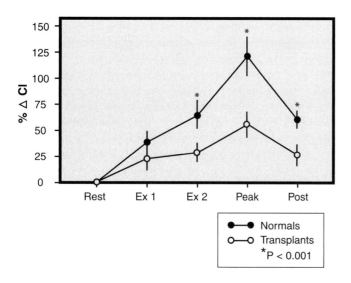

FIGURE 9.5. The change in cardiac index (CI) during graded supine exercise in heart transplant recipients compared with healthy persons. (Reprinted with permission from Pflugfelder PW, Purves PD, McKenzie FN, et al. Cardiac dynamics during exercise in cyclosporine treated orthotopic heart transplant recipients: assessment by radionuclide angiography. J Am Coll Cardiol 1987;10:336–341.)

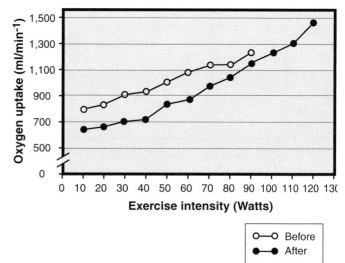

FIGURE 9.6. Oxygen uptake versus cycle ergometer power output for the same patient measured 1 year before and 3 months after orthotopic heart transplantation. (Reprinted with permission from Squires RW. Cardiac rehabilitation issues for heart transplantation patients. J Cardiopulmonary Rehabil 1990;10:159–168.)

take versus cycle ergometer power output during graded exercise for the same patient, measured 1 year before and 3 months after orthotopic transplantation. For any given submaximal power output, oxygen uptake was consistently lower after transplantation, indicating slower $\dot{V}O_2$ kinetics. After transplantation, peak $\dot{V}O_2$ was 18% higher for this patient, however.

Because of the dual abnormalities of an impaired exercise cardiac output and arterial-mixed venous oxygen difference described above, peak oxygen uptake is usually below normal for transplant patients. In a series of 95 patients who performed a cardiopulmonary exercise test in my laboratory at one year after transplantation, the mean age- and gender-predicted peak $\dot{V}O_2$ was approximately 62% (range, 39% to 110% ; 11 to 38 ml/kg/min). Considerable diversity in peak $\dot{V}O_2$ is seen, with some individuals exhibiting above average cardiorespiratory fitness and others with severely impaired capacities (17). Patients with a greater chronotropic reserve generally have a higher peak $\dot{V}O_2$ (28). Athletic performance posttransplant is possible, as evidenced by the return of a 20-year-old elite soccer player to competition after transplantation. Peak $\dot{V}O_2$ for this individual was 12.9 METs (29). Table 9.4 lists common abnormal exercise physiology findings in transplant patients.

Partial Cardiac Reinnervation

Occasionally, a heart transplant patient with graft vessel disease and myocardial ischemia will report typical anginal symptoms, suggesting at least partial afferent **cardiac reinnervation** (30). It also appears that partial cardiac sympathetic efferent reinnervation occurs in many pa-

tients over the first several months to years after surgery. The evidence for this statement is based on neurochemical evaluation of autonomic nervous activity in the heart as well as the observation of improved responsiveness of heart rate during exercise (31, 32). The heart rate reserve (also called the chronotropic response), defined as the difference between the heart rate at rest and at the highest point with exercise, increases during the first 6 weeks after surgery in many patients. In a subset of patients, the heart rate reserve increases further over the next 6 to 12 months. In addition, a more rapid return of heart rate to baseline after exercise is observed in some patients at 1 to 2 years postsurgery.

In my own laboratory, we recently reported data for 95 patients who underwent graded exercise testing approximately 1 year after transplantation (33). Partial normalization of the heart rate response to exercise was defined as an increase in heart rate for each minute of exercise, heart rate max occurring at peak exercise, and a decrease in heart rate during each minute of recovery. Using this definition, 32 subjects (33.7%) exhibited a partial normalization in heart rate response. Maximal heart rate was higher (147 versus 134 beats/min, $P < 0.008$) and exercise test duration was longer (8.2 versus 7.2 minutes, $P < 0.05$) although peak $\dot{V}O_2$ was similar (20.9 versus 19.4 ml/kg/min, P = NS). Figure 9.7 shows the heart rate responses to graded exercise of the same patient at 3 months and 24 months after transplantation. Note the typical denervated response at 3 months and the relatively normalized response at 24 months (partial reinnervation).

TABLE 9.4. ABNORMAL EXERCISE PHYSIOLOGY FINDINGS IN HEART TRANSPLANT PATIENTS

Increased resting heart rate
Delayed heart rate increase at onset of exercise
Blunted maximal heart rate
Delayed return of heart rate to resting level after cessation of exercise
Reduced heart rate reserve
Increased exercise left ventricular end-diastolic pressure (diastolic dysfunction)
Increased exercise pulmonary artery pressure, pulmonary capillary wedge pressure, right atrial pressure
Increased left ventricular end-systolic and end-diastolic volume indices
Impaired stroke volume increase during exercise
Reduced exercise cardiac output
Decreased exercise arterial-mixed venous oxygen difference
Slower oxygen uptake kinetics during exercise
Decreased maximal oxygen uptake
Reduced maximal power output during exercise testing
Decreased ventilatory anaerobic threshold
Increased ventilatory equivalents for oxygen and carbon dioxide

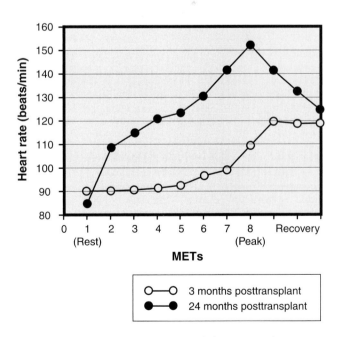

FIGURE 9.7. Heart rate responses to graded exercise in the same patient at 3 months and 24 months after transplantation demonstrating both denervation (at 3 months) and partial reinnervation (at 24 months). METs, metabolic equivalents.

Graded Exercise Testing

Exercise testing after cardiac transplantation is useful in determining the exercise capacity, prescribing exercise training, and in counseling patients regarding the timing of return to work or school or resumption of avocational activities. Due to the recovery and healing processes after surgery and the usual deconditioned state prior to surgery, it is best to wait 4 to 8 weeks after surgery before performing graded exercise testing to maximal effort. In patients with complicated postoperative courses, a longer period of recovery is recommended before performance of an exercise test.

Treadmill or cycle ergometer protocols, with continuous exercise (2- to 3-minute stages), or ramp tests may be used. Arm cranking protocols may also be employed, after adequate sternal healing, for a specific upper extremity fitness evaluation or an arm cranking exercise prescription (18). The initial exercise stage should begin at an intensity of approximately 2 METs, with 1 to 2 MET increments in intensity per stage (18, 30). Continuous multilead ECG monitoring with blood pressure measurement and Borg perceived exertion ratings for each stage is recommended. For precise determination of aerobic capacity and the ventilatory anaerobic threshold, direct measurement of $\dot{V}O_2$ and associated variables is highly desirable. The endpoints of graded exercise tests should be maximal effort (symptom-limited maximum) or traditional signs of exertional intolerance.

In my laboratory we prefer to use a treadmill, beginning at a speed of 2.0 mph with zero percent grade. We employ 2-minute stages and use an active recovery period of three minutes duration (Table 9.5). In a group of 17 patients who underwent orthotopic heart transplantation, participated in a supervised, 3-session per week exercise program that lasted 6 to 8 weeks, and underwent graded exercise testing at the end of the program (less than 3 months after surgery), the following data (means ± SD) were recorded (34):

- Resting heart rate: 101 ± 12 beats/min
- Resting systolic/diastolic blood pressure: 126 ± 8/86 ± 8 mm Hg

TABLE 9.5. MAYO CLINIC CARDIOPULMONARY TREADMILL EXERCISE TEST PROTOCOL

Stage	Duration (min)	Speed (mph)	Grade (%)
1	2.0	2.0	0
2	2.0	2.0	7.0
3	2.0	2.0	14.0
4	2.0	3.0	12.5
5	2.0	3.0	17.5
6	2.0	3.4	18.0
7	2.0	3.8	20.0
8	2.0	5.0	18.0
9	2.0	5.5	20.0
10	2.0	6.0	22.0
Cool down	3.0	1.7	0

From Kaye DM, Esler M, Kingwell B, et al. (31).

- Exercise test duration: 7.5 ± 1.1 minutes
- Peak exercise heart rate: 132 ± 24 beats/min
- Peak blood pressure: 162 ± 12/82 ± 9 mm Hg
- Peak $\dot{V}O_2$: 19 ± 4 ml/kg/min

The ECG of transplant recipients commonly demonstrates right bundle branch block and nonspecific ST-T wave changes (35). The sensitivity of the exercise ECG in these patients is poor, and most transplant cardiologists prefer coronary angiography to determine the presence and severity of graft vessel disease.

Responses to Exercise Training

Heart transplant recipients are excellent candidates for the benefits of exercise training given their pretransplant syndrome of chronic heart failure with its attendant poor exercise tolerance and usual deconditioning and post transplant treatment with corticosteroids resulting in potential skeletal muscle atrophy and weakness. Transplant patients present a clinical problem of physical rehabilitation after open-heart surgery similar to that of patients with coronary or valvular surgery.

Aerobic Exercise Training

The literature includes at least six studies demonstrating the benefit of aerobic exercise training for patients after orthotopic heart transplantation and at least two publications dealing with heterotopic transplantation and exercise training (36–43). In general, transplant recipients respond to training similarly to other cardiac patients. Peak $\dot{V}O_2$ usually improves by approximately 25% after 2 to 6 months of training. Exercise training improves mitochondrial oxidative function in transplant patients but apparently does not increase skeletal muscle capillary density as it does in healthy subjects (44). Potential additional benefits of regular exercise include the following:

- Improved submaximal exercise endurance
- Increased peak cycle power output or peak treadmill exercise workload
- Increased maximal heart rate
- Decreased exercise heart rate at the same absolute submaximal workload
- Increased ventilatory (anaerobic) threshold
- Decreased submaximal exercise minute ventilation
- Reduced exercise ventilatory equivalent for CO_2
- Lessened symptoms of fatigue and dyspnea
- Reduced rest and submaximal exercise systolic and diastolic blood pressure
- Decreased peak exercise diastolic blood pressure
- Reduced submaximal exercise ratings of perceived exertion
- Improved psychosocial function

- Increased lean body mass
- Reduced body fat stores
- Increased bone mineral content

The first study of exercise and heart transplant patients was published in 1983 and involved only two subjects in a case presentation format (36). After a 6-week period of exercise training, ratings of perceived exertion and systolic blood pressure were consistently lower for all submaximal exercise intensities during pre- and post-training graded exercise tests. The majority of early investigations were small and included fewer than 20 subjects. The first large study was by Niset and colleagues in 1988 (38), who studied 62 patients after orthotopic transplantation at approximately 1 month after surgery and again at the 1-year anniversary. Patients were instructed in exercise principles and started in a supervised program. No control group was included in the design of the study. A precise description of the exercise prescriptions and patient adherence to the program was not available. Directly measured peak $\dot{V}O_2$ did increase by 33% ($P < 0.01$).

Kavanagh and associates, in 1988, reported the results of a 16-month exercise training program in 36 transplant recipients (no control group) (42). Exercise training started approximately 7 months after surgery and was carefully supervised. Patients demonstrated many benefits after training, including a 27% increase in peak $\dot{V}O_2$.

Some of the limitations of these early investigations were overcome in a study by Kobashigawa and colleagues reported in 1999 (43). Twenty-seven transplant patients were randomized to an exercise or control group early after surgery. The exercise group underwent supervised exercise training, whereas the control group performed an unstructured home walking program for a period of 6 months. Supervised exercise included both aerobic and muscle strengthening components. Peak $\dot{V}O_2$ improved to a greater extent in the supervised group (+ 4.4 versus + 1.9 ml/kg/min, $P < 0.01$). There were no differences between the groups for the number of episodes of acute rejection or infection. Therefore, supervised exercise programs appear to improve fitness to a greater extent than less structured approaches to training.

One investigation compared aerobic exercise capacity in transplant and coronary bypass patients at the end of phase II cardiac rehabilitation (approximately 3 months after surgery) and at 1 year (34). At the 3-month mark, both groups were similar in aerobic capacity. However, the coronary bypass surgery patients continued to improve in fitness over the course of the first year after surgery and were substantially more fit than the transplant recipients (+ 6 ml/kg/min in peak $\dot{V}O_2$). Thus, even after a supervised exercise program, most transplant patients are less fit than other types of patients who have undergone cardiothoracic surgery. They also apparently do not respond to traditional long-term exercise training as well as patients do after coronary bypass surgery. Novel approaches to training,

such as interval high-intensity training, need further evaluation in these unique patients.

Resistance Exercise

Most heart transplant patients require prednisone for immunosuppression. Unfortunately, potential side effects of this drug are skeletal muscle atrophy and weakness. Resistance exercise partially reverses corticosteroid-related myopathy and improves skeletal muscle strength. Horber and associates found definite evidence of skeletal muscle weakness and atrophy in the lower extremities of renal transplant patients who received prednisone compared with controls (45). Fifty days of isokinetic strength training increased muscle mass and strength substantially. In addition, strength training has been shown to improve bone density and to reduce the potential development of osteoporosis in heart transplant recipients, also caused by prednisone (46).

Effect of Exercise Training on Immune Function and Longevity

An extremely important question concerning exercise training in immunosuppressed heart transplant recipients is the effect of training on immune function. Traditional, moderate exercise training does not increase or decrease the number or severity of episodes of acute rejection (43, 47). In addition, training does not require changes in immunosuppressant treatment. Infection risk is not altered by regular exercise. There are no data to suggest that training either improves or worsens survival after transplantation.

Exercise Programming Suggestions

Pretransplant Graded Exercise Testing and Training

As part of the evaluation process for transplantation, ambulatory patients undergo cardiopulmonary exercise testing. Peak $\dot{V}O_2$ is a powerful prognostic indicator: patients with an aerobic capacity of 14 ml/kg/min (4 METs) or below experience a markedly reduced 1-year survival, independent of left ventricular ejection fraction.

Based on the results of the exercise test, an exercise prescription may be developed for the patient with the goal of maintaining or improving cardiovascular fitness while waiting for a donor organ. Ideally, the exercise program should be carried out under medical supervision, although many patients have performed home-based exercise successfully. The exercise prescription follows the same guidelines used for other patients with chronic heart failure, as described in Chapter 4.

Early Mobilization and Inpatient Exercise Training

After surgery, patients are extubated expeditiously, usually within 24 hours. Passive range of motion for both the upper and lower extremities, sitting up in a chair, and slow ambulation may begin and progress gradually after extubation (48). Walking or cycle ergometry may be gradually increased in duration from 20 to 30 minutes. Exercise intensity is guided using the Borg perceived exertion scale ratings of 11 to 13 ("fairly light" to "somewhat hard" [Table 9.6]), keeping the respiratory rate below 30 breaths/min and arterial oxygen saturation above 90%. Exercise frequency should be two or three sessions per day (4). Patients whose postoperative courses are uncomplicated remain hospitalized for 7 to 10 days.

During inpatient rehabilitation, as well as in the outpatient period, episodes of acute rejection of moderate or greater severity may require alteration of the exercise plan. If the rejection episode is graded as moderate, activity may be continued at the current level but should not progress until after the rejection has resolved with treatment. Severe acute rejection necessitates suspension of all physical activity with the exception of passive range-of-motion exercises.

Outpatient Exercise Training

Heart transplant patients may enter an outpatient cardiac rehabilitation program as soon as they are dismissed from the hospital (4). Patients usually are required by the transplant team to remain near the transplant center for close follow-up for approximately 3 months. Ideally they should exercise in both a supervised environment (up to three sessions/week) and independently (at least three sessions/week).

Continuous monitoring of the ECG during the first few supervised exercise sessions is standard practice. It is not necessary to perform graded exercise testing before beginning the outpatient exercise program. However, graded exercise testing should be performed at approximately 8 weeks after surgery, for patients with relatively uncomplicated recoveries, when the patient has recovered suffi-

ciently from surgery to assess the cardiopulmonary response to exercise and to refine the exercise prescription.

Exercise prescription for heart transplant patients is similar to methods used with other patients who have undergone cardiothoracic surgery. The one exception is that a target heart rate is not used, unless the patient has a partially "normalized" heart rate response, as discussed previously. The typical denervated heart increases its rate slowly during submaximal exercise, and the heart rate may either drift gradually higher during steady-state exercise or plateau after several minutes (17). Ratings of perceived exertion (Borg scale) of 12 to 14 ("somewhat hard") may be used to prescribe exercise intensity (4). The exercise prescription should include standard warm-up and cool-down activities, a gradual increase in aerobic exercise duration to 30 to 60 minutes, with a frequency of four to six sessions per week. Typical modes of aerobic exercise used during the early outpatient recovery period include walking outdoors or in enclosed shopping centers or schools, treadmill walking, cycle ergometry, and stair climbing.

Because of the sternal incision, special emphasis on upper extremity active range-of-motion exercises is required. Approximately 6 weeks after the date of surgery, when sternal healing is nearly completed, rowing, arm cranking, combination arm-leg ergometry, outdoor cycling, hiking, jogging, and swimming are additional exercise options depending on the patient's fitness level. Sports such as tennis and golf may be performed as early as 6 weeks after surgery if patient fitness is adequate (directly measured peak $\dot{V}O_2$ of 5 METs or greater) and sternal healing is nearly completed.

Skeletal muscle weakness in transplant recipients is very common and is related to the following factors:

- Skeletal muscle atrophy, which is a hallmark of advanced heart failure
- Pretransplant deconditioning
- Corticosteroid use posttransplant as part of the immunosuppressant regimen

Muscle strengthening exercises should be incorporated into the exercise program to counteract these factors. For the first 6 weeks after surgery, bilateral arm lifting is restricted to less than 10 pounds to avoid sternal nonunion. At this early stage of rehabilitation, light hand weights are an excellent method of starting resistance exercise. After at least 6 weeks of recovery, patients may be started on weight machines, emphasizing moderate resistance, 10 to 20 slow repetitions per set, one to three sets of exercises for the major muscle groups, with a frequency of two to three sessions per week (4, 18). I recommend using Borg scale ratings of 12 to 14 to set the intensity of lifting. Strength gains of 25% to 50% or greater often result from 8 weeks of strength training in these patients. Performance of strength training immediately following the aerobic portion of the program is recommended. Because transplant recipients are likely to require antihypertensive medications, periodic blood pressure measurement during strength training is recommended.

TABLE 9.6. THE BORG PERCEIVED EXERTION SCALE

6		14	
7	Very, very light	15	Hard
8		16	
9	Very light	17	Very hard
10		18	
11	Fairly light	19	Very, very hard
12		20	
13	Somewhat hard		

Reprinted with permission from Borg G. Physical Performance and Perceived Exertion. Lund, Sweden: Gleerup, 1962.

CASE STUDY

This patient, Michael, was born with complex congenital heart disease, which included transposition of the great arteries, a ventricular septal defect, and pulmonary artery stenosis. He underwent three corrective cardiac surgical procedures, at the ages of 3 months, 5 years, and 12 years. He was small in stature—168 cm in height, 49.9 kg in weight as an adult—but otherwise developed normally. Michael was not as physically active as his peer group and did not participate in physically vigorous sports.

In his late teens and early 20s he became progressively more dyspneic and fatigued. By the age of 29 he was unable to work because of severe symptoms even with minimal exertion. He underwent evaluation for heart transplantation at that time and was too debilitated to perform a graded exercise test. His maximal walking distance was approximately 50 yards.

Michael underwent orthotopic heart transplantation in May of the same year, at the age of 30 years. His posttransplant hospital stay was remarkable for one bout of moderate acute rejection (grade 2), which responded to therapy. While in the hospital (12 days) he began a progressive walking and stationary cycling program, in addition to range-of-motion exercises.

Michael entered the outpatient cardiac rehabilitation program within 1 week of hospital dismissal. He continued in the program for approximately 3 months while he remained in town for close follow-up. He gradually progressed his exercise routine in the program to treadmill walking for 40 minutes at 3.0 mph 2% grade, plus warm-up and cool-down periods of 5 minutes, three times per week. Borg perceived exertion scale ratings of 11 to 14 were used to gauge proper exercise intensity. He also performed general range-of-motion exercises and mild resistance exercise for the arms, beginning with 2-kg handweights and progressing to weight machines at 8 weeks after surgery.

During the 3-month outpatient period after transplantation, Michael underwent several endomyocardial biopsies, echocardiograms, and blood tests that did not indicate clinically significant acute rejection or infection. The graft was functioning well and he was progressing in rehabilitation in a normal fashion. His weight was 61.7 kg. Medications included the following:

- Cyclosporine, 100 mg twice daily
- Azathioprine, 125 mg daily
- Prednisone, 5 mg daily
- Furosemide, 40 mg twice daily
- Lisinopril, 5 mg daily
- Diltiazem ER, 120 mg daily
- Pravastatin, 10 mg daily
- Alendronate, 70 mg weekly

A treadmill cardiopulmonary graded exercise test was performed. Michael exercised 8.6 minutes to a workload of 3.0 mph 17.5% grade. Limiting symptoms were fatigue and moderate dyspnea. Heart rate at rest was 108 beats/min. With exercise, heart rate did not change for the first 4 minutes and then increased gradually to 132 beats/min at peak exercise. During recovery after peak exercise, the heart rate increased to 140 beats/min at 5 minutes post–peak exercise and then gradually decreased thereafter. Blood pressure was 110/90 at rest and 122/84 at peak exercise. The ECG demonstrated right bundle branch block at rest and during exercise with occasional single premature ventricular and supraventricular ectopic beats. Peak $\dot{V}O_2$ was 1.46 L/min or 23.7 ml/kg/min (6.7 METs), which was 53% of normal for a healthy man of his age. Arterial oxygen saturation measured by oximetry was normal.

He was allowed to return to his hometown and was given an exercise prescription for performance of unsupervised exercise. The recommended modes of aerobic exercise included walking (outside or treadmill) and cycle ergometry. He was told to spend at least 5 minutes in warm-up and cool-down and to exercise for 30 to 60 minutes at least four times each week. Intensity of aerobic exercise was prescribed using a Borg perceived exertion scale range of 12 to 14. Michael was also encouraged to perform resistance exercise, one or two sets of 10 to 15 repetitions for the major muscle groups two or three times each week.

Michael returned to the medical center for his 1-year evaluation. He was working full-time at a desk job and was walking at a brisk pace two to four times a week for a duration of approximately 45 minutes. Body weight was 61.4 kg. His coronary angiogram did not reveal any graft vessel disease. The right ventricular biopsy was consistent with mild acute rejection (grade 1A), which was seen routinely in Michael's case. The echocardiogram demonstrated a normal left ventricle with an ejection fraction of 70%. However, the right ventricle was mildly dilated and there was a partial flail of a tricuspid valve leaflet with moderate to severe tricuspid regurgitation (probably due to trauma from the endomyo-cardial biopsy catheter). Moderate pulmonary hypertension was present (52/24 mm Hg compared with normal values of <25 mm Hg systolic and <10 mm Hg diastolic).

His cardiopulmonary graded exercise test was favorable, with a duration of 10 minutes (3.0 mph 17.5% peak workload) with a limiting symptom of fatigue. Heart rate at rest was 87 beats/min and increased normally during exercise to 145 beats/min at the peak workload. During recovery the heart rate decreased normally. Blood pressure was 114/84 at rest and increased to 130/70 at peak exercise. The ECG was unchanged from the previous exercise test. Peak $\dot{V}O_2$ was 1.61 L/min, 26.7 ml/kg/min or 7.6 METs (60% of normal for age and gender). There was no arterial oxygen desaturation during exercise. Based on the favorable exercise test responses, no further treatment was deemed necessary for his tricuspid regurgitation and pulmonary hypertension.

His exercise program was reviewed in detail. Because his heart rate response to graded exercise had normalized, he was given a target heart rate range of 126 ± 6 beats/min (70% using the heart rate reserve technique) to guide intensity in addition to the perceived exertion scale. He was encouraged to perform mild to moderate resistance exercise.

Comment

This case illustrates the interesting clinical course of a patient after successful heart transplantation for the treatment of very severe chronic heart failure. Michael's improvement in exercise capacity after surgery was excellent, although even with regular, mild exercise training he did not attain a normal exercise capacity by 1 year posttransplant. His graded exercise test early after transplantation demonstrated complete cardiac denervation, and a target heart rate was not used in the exercise prescription. However, by the time of his 1-year anniversary graded exercise test, his heart rate response had become more normal (evidence for partial cardiac reinnervation). Therefore, he was given a target heart rate range at that time. Due to the risk of osteoporosis and muscle weakness associated with long-term prednisone use, resistance exercise was strongly encouraged. He will undergo exercise testing and a review of his exercise habits when he returns for his next annual evaluation.

REFERENCES

1. Barnard CN. The operation: a human cardiac transplant: an interim report of a successful operation performed at Groote Schuur Hospital, Cape Town. S Afr Med J 1967;41:1271–1274.
2. Hosenpud JD, Bennett LE, Keck BM, et al. The registry of the International Society for Heart and Lung Transplantation: Seventeenth official report 2000. J Heart Lung Transplant 2000;19:909–931.
3. Kauffman HM, McBride MA, Shield CF, et al. Determinants of waiting time for heart transplants in the United States. J Heart Lung Transplant 1999;18:414–419.
4. Squires RW. Cardiac rehabilitation issues for heart transplantation patients. J Cardiopulmonary Rehabil 1990;10:159–168.
5. Tagusari O, Kormos RL, Kawai A, et al. Native heart complications after heterotopic heart transplantation: Insight into the potential risk of left ventricular assist device. J Heart Lung Transplant 1999;18:1111–1119.
6. Kavanagh T, Yacoub MH, Kennedy J, Austin PC. Return to work after heart transplantation: 12-year follow-up. J Heart Lung Transplant 1999;18:846–851.
7. Penson MG, Winter WE, Fricker FJ, et al. Tacrolimus-based triple-drug immunosuppression minimizes serum lipid elevations in pediatric cardiac transplant recipients. J Heart Lung Transplant 1999;18:707–713.
8. Scott JP, Higenbottam TW, Large S, Wallwork J. Cyclosporine in heart transplant recipients: An exercise study of vasopressor effects. Eur Heart J 1992;13:531–534.
9. Weis M, von Scheidt W. Cardiac allograft vasculopathy: A review. Circulation 1997;96:2069–2077.
10. Wenke K, Meiser B, Thiery J, et al. Simvastatin reduces graft vessel disease and mortality after heart transplantation: A four-year randomized trial. Circulation 1997;96:1398–1402.
11. Stapleton DD, Mehra MR, Dumas D, et al. Lipid-lowering therapy and long-term survival in heart transplantation. Am J Cardiol 1997;80:802–804.
12. Gao SZ, Hunt SA, Schroeder JS, et al. Early development of accelerated graft coronary artery disease: Risk factors and course. J Am Coll Cardiol 1996;28:673–679.
13. Kobashigawa JA, Katznelson S, Laks H, et al. Effect of pravastatin on

outcomes after cardiac transplantation. N Engl J Med 1995;333:621–627.

14. Jenkins GH, Grieve LA, Yacoub MH, Singer DRJ. Effect of simvastatin on ejection fraction in cardiac transplant recipients. Am J Cardiol 1996;78:1453–1456.

15. Kuhn WF, Davis MH, Lippmann SB. Emotional adjustment to cardiac transplantation. Gen Hosp Psychiatry 1988;10:108–113.

16. Niset G, Preumont N. Determinants of peak aerobic capacity after heart transplantation. Eur Heart J 1997;18:1692–1693.

17. Squires RW. Transplant. In: Pashkow FJ, Dafoe WA (eds). Clinical Cardiac Rehabilitation: A Cardiologist's Guide. 2nd Ed. Baltimore: Williams & Wilkins, 1999:175–191.

18. Keteyian SJ, Brawner C. Cardiac transplant. In: American College of Sports Medicine. ACSM's Exercise Management for Persons with Chronic Diseases and Disabilities. Champaign, IL: Human Kinetics, 1997:54–58.

19. Kao AC, Van Trigt P, Shaeffer-McCall GS, et al. Central and peripheral limitations to upright exercise in untrained cardiac transplant recipients. Circulation 1994;89:2605–2615.

20. Pope SE, Stinson EB, Daughters GT, et al. Exercise response of the denervated heart in long-term cardiac transplant recipients. Am J Cardiol 1980;46:213–218.

21. Stratton JR, Kemp GJ, Daly RC, et al. Effects of cardiac transplantation on bioenergetic abnormalities of skeletal muscle in congestive heart failure. Circulation 1994;89:1624–1631.

22. Lampert E, Mettauer B, Hoppeler H, et al. Structure of skeletal muscle in heart transplant recipients. J Am Coll Cardiol 1996;28:980–984.

23. Hanson P, Slane PR, Lillis DL, et al. Limited oxygen uptake post heart transplant is associated with impairment of calf vasodilatory capacity. Med Sci Sports Exerc 1995;27:S49.

24. Brubaker PH, Brozena SC, Morley DL, et al. Exercise-induced ventilatory abnormalities in orthotopic heart transplant patients. J Heart Lung Transplant 1997;16:1011–1017.

25. Squires RW, Hoffman CJ, James GA, et al. Arterial oxygen saturation during graded exercise testing after cardiac transplantation. J Cardiopulmonary Rehabil 1998;18:348.

26. Braith RW, Limacher MC, Mills RM, et al. Exercise-induced hypoxemia in heart transplant recipients. J Am Coll Cardiol 1993;22:768–776.

27. Mettauer B, Zhao QM, Epailly E, et al. $\dot{V}_{O_2}$ kinetics reveal a central limitation at the outset of subthreshold exercise in heart transplant recipients. J Appl Physiol 2000;88:1228–1238.

28. Douard H, Parrens E, Billes MA, et al. Predictive factors of maximal aerobic capacity after cardiac transplantation. Eur Heart J 1997;18:1823–1828.

29. Golding LA, Mangus BC. Competing in varsity athletics after cardiac transplantation. J Cardiopulmonary Rehabil 1989;9:486–491.

30. Kavanagh T. Physical training in heart transplant recipients. J Cardiovasc Risk 1996;3:154–159.

31. Kaye DM, Esler M, Kingwell B, et al. Functional and neurochemical evidence for partial cardiac sympathetic reinnervation after cardiac transplantation in humans. Circulation 1993;88:1110–1118.

32. Scott CD, Dark JH, McComb JM. Evolution of the chronotropic response to exercise after cardiac transplantation. Am J Cardiol 1995;76:1292–1296.

33. Squires RW, Leung TC, Cyr NS, et al. Partial normalization of the heart rate response to exercise after cardiac transplantation: frequency and relationship to exercise capacity. Mayo Clin Proc 2002;77:1295–1300.

34. Daida H, Squires RW, Allison TG, et al. Sequential assessment of exercise tolerance in heart transplantation compared with coronary artery bypass surgery after phase II cardiac rehabilitation. Am J Cardiol 1996;77:696–700.

35. Ehrman JK, Keteyian SJ, Levine AB, et al. Exercise stress tests after cardiac transplantation. Am J Cardiol 1993;71:1372–1373.

36. Squires RW, Arthur PA, Gau GT, et al. Exercise after cardiac transplantation: a report of two cases. J Cardiopulmonary Rehabil 1983;3:570–574.

37. Degre S, Niset GL, Desmet JM, et al. Effects de lentrainment physique sur le coeur humain denerve apres transplantation cardiaques orthotopique. Ann Cardiol Angeol (Paris) 1986;35:147–149.

38. Niset G, Cousty-Degre C, Degre S. Psychological and physical rehabilitation after heart transplantation: 1 year follow-up. Cardiology 1988;75:311–317.

39. Sieurat P, Roquebrune JP, Grinneiser D, et al. Surveillance et readaptation des transplantes cardiaques heterotopiques a la periode de convalescence. Arch Mal Couer 1986;79:210–216.

40. Kavanagh T, Yacoub MH, Mertens DJ, et al. Exercise rehabilitation after heterotopic cardiac transplantation. J Cardiopulmonary Rehabil 1989;9:303–310.

41. Keteyian S, Shepard R, Ehrman J, et al. Cardiovascular responses of heart transplant patients to exercise training. J Appl Physiol 1991;70:2627–2631.

42. Kavanagh T, Yacoub MH, Mertens DJ, et al. Cardiorespiratory responses to exercise training after orthotopic cardiac transplantation. Circulation 1988;77:162–171.

43. Kobashigawa JA, Leaf DA, Lee N, et al. A controlled trial of exercise rehabilitation after heart transplantation. N Engl J Med 1999;340:272–277.

44. Lampert E, Mettauer B, Hoppeler H, et al. Skeletal muscle response to short endurance training in heart transplant recipients. J Am Coll Cardiol 1998;32:420–426.

45. Horber FF, Scheidegger JR, Grunig BF, et al. Evidence that prednisone-induced myopathy is reversed by physical training. J Clin Endocrinol Metab 1985;61:83–88.

46. Braith RW, Mills RM, Welsch MA, et al. Resistance exercise training restores bone mineral density in heart transplant recipients. J Am Coll Cardiol 1996;28:1471–1477.

47. Zhao QM, Mettauer B, Epailly E, et al. Effect of exercise training on leukocyte subpopulations and clinical course in cardiac transplant patients. Transplant Proc 1998;30:172–175.

48. McGregor CGA. Cardiac transplantation: surgical considerations and early postoperative management. Mayo Clin Proc 1992;67:577–585.

CHAPTER 10

Pediatric Cardiac Problems

Thomas W. Rowland

Overview

Regular exercise is important for the health and well-being of children with heart abnormalities. In most of these children, disease is not severe enough to interfere with normal exercise capacity. However, those with more severe defects experience exercise intolerance, and in others there is a specific risk for sudden death with intense activities. It is important that children at risk be identified and guided into appropriate exercise activities. This chapter examines the means in which the different forms of heart disease in children can influence exercise capacity as well as the risks and benefits of physical activities in these children.

Introduction

The **heart** and **circulation** play an integral role in supporting the muscular activity of **exercise**, providing not only energy substrate and oxygen supply but also temperature control, removal of metabolic wastes, and hormonal influences. It is not unexpected, then, that individuals with abnormalities in cardiac anatomy or function might suffer from limitations of exercise capacity. Exercise places a strain on **cardiac function** to perform these functions, an effect which may place the heart at risk. And, seemingly paradoxically, regular **physical activity** may play a role in prevention of **heart disease** as well as ameliorate the severity of pre-existing heart illness.

This complex interplay of salutary and adverse effects between heart disease and exercise exists in **children** as well as in adults. The forms of heart disease seen in the two age groups differ, however. Whereas adults suffer principally from coronary atherosclerotic disease and hypertension, most cardiac illness in the pediatric age group is in the form of **congenital heart disease**, defined as structural malformations that are present at birth and that result from errors in cardiac development early in gestation These are misadventures in embryogenesis, mistakes in the complex and poorly understood mechanisms by which the normal heart is formed by the end of the second month of pregnancy.

This chapter reviews the impact of the various forms of congenital heart disease on exercise capacity, as well as the risks and benefits of exercise for children with heart disease. Information regarding heart–exercise issues in children is limited compared with what is known about adult heart disease. The philosophy of care, however, remains the same—optimizing the health benefits of regular physical activity, even if that activity must be limited, while acting to protect individuals with heart disease from undue risk during exercise.

Congenital Heart Disease: A Primer

The influences, risks, and salutary effects of exercise in children with congenital heart disease are best discussed in re-lation to the different pathophysiologies created by the various forms of heart defects. It is appropriate, then, to begin with a brief overview of the nature of and the physiologic insults created by congenital heart abnormalities.

The incidence of congenital heart disease at birth is approximately 8 per 1000 children, or slightly less than 1%. Little is known regarding the etiology of these structural abnormalities, which presumably reflect some environmental insult on a genetically predisposed fetus. Maternal viral infections (particularly rubella), medications (e.g., thalidomide), maternal diabetes mellitus, and high altitude have been identified as environmental influences associated with congenital heart disease. And virtually all of the chromosomal abnormalities (e.g., Down syndrome, Turner syndrome) have a high associated incidence of congenital heart abnormalities. In a **pediatric cardiology** clinic, however, these explanations account for only a small percentage of patients; the rest have no discernible cause for their defects.

Congenital heart disease is detected clinically by either symptoms (e.g., **cyanosis**, signs of **congestive heart failure**) or findings on physical examination (e.g., **heart murmur**, abnormal pulses). The clinical significance of these anomalies varies, from insignificant and trivial to life-threatening. Many children with minor abnormalities never need therapeutic intervention, some require immediate surgical help as an emergency life-saving measure, and still others have indications for elective surgery to prevent future complications.

Dramatic progress in surgical techniques has provided at least some help for virtually all children with serious heart disease. As a result, babies who in the past would have succumbed early from their complex anomalies now are surviving into childhood, adolescence, and young adulthood. Although the long-term outlook for these patients remains questionable, they are presenting important and difficult new issues of health care—including recommendations for physical activity and sports play—that have not previously been encountered.

Surgery for significant congenital heart disease typically is performed in early infancy; consequently, issues regarding participation in sports often surround postoperative cardiac status rather than the hemodynamics of the original malformation. For example, **tetralogy of Fallot**, an abnormality that might have caused exercise limitation from **hypoxemia** in a 5 year old, now is typically repaired within the first two years of life. Questions regarding the appropriateness of sports play surround potential postoperative concerns in these patients such as ventricular **dysrhythmias** or right ventricular dysfunction rather than oxygen desaturation.

There are many forms of congenital heart disease, but the physiologic insults created by these anomalies generally fall into one or more of three categories: left-to-right shunts, right-to-left shunts, and obstructions. Each has its own particular impact on exercise capacity, and the risks of **sports** play in some cases also may be physiology-specific.

Left-to-Right Shunts

In a patient with a left-to-right shunt, systemic venous blood normally returns to the right atrium and ventricle and is pumped to the lungs. There it is oxygenated and returned to the left side of the heart, where some is pumped out the aorta. Some blood, however, finds a way to return back to the right heart and is pumped to the lungs again. Such a shunt occurs when there is an embryologic error that creates a communication between the two pumps, and the blood passes from left to right because the pressures are greater on the left. Such a defect can occur at the atrial (atrial septal defect), ventricular (ventricular septal defect), or great vessel level (patent ductus arteriosus).

The magnitude of blood being shunted in these conditions is largely a factor of the size of the communication. The two principal pathophysiologic effects of a large left-to-right shunt are (1) pulmonary vascular overload with **pulmonary hypertension** and increased lung weight, creating increased ventilatory work, and (2) a volume overload on one or both cardiac ventricles. In an atrial septal defect with shunting of blood from the left atrium to the right, for example, the right ventricle must pump not only the systemic venous blood returning in the vena cavae but also the blood crossing the defect. In a large defect, this may amount to three to four times the normal volume entering the ventricle.

This pathophysiology of a large left-to-right shunt is manifested clinically by signs described as congestive heart failure. These signs include tachypnea, tachycardia, cardiomegaly, hepatomegaly, and failure to thrive. Large defects causing these findings require cardiac surgery to close the defect, usually in early infancy. In some situations shunts can be closed nonsurgically by devices placed by catheters (i.e., coil closure of patent ductus arteriosus). Defects of moderate size may cause no symptoms but often are closed on an elective basis at some time during early childhood to prevent the long-term effects of chronic volume overload. Small left-to-right shunts usually require no intervention and are compatible with a normal life.

Right-to-Left Shunts

In defects causing a right-to-left shunt, blood gets from the right side of the heart out to the systemic circulation, bypassing the lungs. The resulting cardinal feature of these defects, as a result, is hypoxemia and cyanosis. Most of these forms of congenital heart disease are serious and require surgical intervention within the first days or weeks of life.

There are several different forms of right-to-left shunting. Some involve obstructions to blood flow on the right side of the heart in association with a communication between the two sides of the heart. An example is tetralogy of Fallot, in which a large ventricular septal defect (opening in the wall between the ventricles) occurs with significant narrowing of outflow of the right ventricle (**pulmonary stenosis**). Low-saturated blood entering the right ventricle from the right atrium "prefers" to pass from right to left through the ventricular septal defect and out the aorta rather than facing the more restricted route out the pulmonary artery. The result is systemic hypoxemia.

In **transposition of the great arteries**, cyanosis occurs because of the failure of the systemic and pulmonary circulations to mix. The aorta arises off the right ventricle, and the left ventricle gives rise to the pulmonary artery. This creates two independent circulations, a situation that, unless some surgical provision is made for mixing, is incompatible with life. Infants with this anomaly therefore require emergency procedures performed shortly after birth.

A third form of cyanotic congenital heart disease involves those defects that cause both a right-to-left and left-to-right shunt. For instance, patients who are born with a single ventricle have mixing of systemic and pulmonary venous blood as both right and left atria dump blood into the single chamber. This blood with low oxygen saturation is then pumped preferentially to the pulmonary circulation because of the lower resistance compared with that of the systemic circulation. Clinically these abnormalities are expressed by signs of congestive heart failure and mild cyanosis.

Obstructions

Many forms of abnormal heart development in utero result in a blockage of blood flow within the heart or great vessels. Most commonly this involves the aortic or pulmonary valves, when fusion of raphe create a limited excursion of the valve leaflets and left and right ventricular outflow obstruction (or stenosis), respectively.

Such obstructions create augmented heart work. In **aortic valve stenosis**, for example, it is obligatory that all blood pass by the obstructed outflow site. To accomplish this, the ventricle must increase the pressure generated and becomes thickened (hypertrophied). During the pediatric years, the ventricular myocardium is very capable of doing this, but if significant obstructions are left untreated, heart muscle failure will eventually occur, often in the adult years. If the obstruction is significant, intervention may be nonsurgical, involving dilation of the valve with a balloon catheter inserted at the time of cardiac catheterization. Most patients with obstructions such as aortic and pulmonary valve stenosis have no symptoms; these defects are detected by the associated obvious findings (e.g., a loud heart murmur) on physical examination.

Effect of Congenital Heart Defects on Exercise Performance

The great majority of children with congenital heart disease tolerate exercise normally. They are able—and should be encouraged—to participate fully in the usual activities of childhood as well as on sports teams. Nonetheless, in some cases the disturbed hemodynamics created by heart defects interfere with expected exercise capabilities.

Sustained exercise performance demands an adequate supply of oxygenated blood to contracting muscle. Any impairment in circulatory pump function, volume of blood flow, or level of systemic arterial oxygenation can be expected, therefore, to result in impaired exercise fitness. It follows that all of the different pathophysiologic groups of congenital heart disease, if sufficiently severe, can manifest clinically as exercise intolerance. The mechanism for inability to perform sustained exercise is different for each type of disease, however (Figure 10.1).

This section presents the effect of the different forms of congenital heart disease on exercise capacity, using a specific type of defect as an example. It should be recognized that limitations of physical capacity in children with congenital heart defects depends not only on the severity of the defect but also on the type of exercise being performed. Most habitual activity by children is characteristically short-burst and limited in duration. Because such anaerobic-type activities usually are not limited by cardiovascular function or systemic oxygenation, even children with severe forms of heart abnormalities may show little difficulty with normal lifestyle activities. Once they attempt more sustained, aerobic activities, however (e.g., the 1-mile run in gym class, participation on a competitive soccer team), serious limitation in exercise capacity will become evident.

It should also be appreciated that lack of **physical fitness** in children with heart disease is not necessarily related en-

tirely to their cardiac abnormality per se. Young people with heart disease may shun exercise activities, from either fear or disinterest, leading to low levels of fitness, increasing hypoactivity, and progressively declining exercise capacity.

Atrial Septal Defects

Most large left-to-right shunts (e.g., ventricular septal defect, patent ductus arteriosus) cause congestive heart failure and pulmonary hypertension in the first few months of life. Patients with these defects undergo early surgical repair, and typically these repaired hearts have no impact on physical activities in later childhood and adolescence. Similarly, when these defects are minor (i.e., a small ventricular septum) the degree of excessive pulmonary blood flow and ventricular volume overwork is insufficient to affect cardiovascular responses to exercise adversely (1).

The natural course of patients with a large communication in the septum between the atria (**atrial septal defect**) often is different. For reasons that are not altogether clear, these children tolerate large interatrial shunts and increased pulmonary blood flow without pulmonary hypertension or congestive heart failure, although these complications often appear later, in young adulthood (2). And, because they sometimes produce abnormalities that are subtle on physical examination, the diagnosis of an atrial septal defect may be missed initially.

Sustained exercise involves a volume overload on both the heart and lungs to meet the circulatory needs of exercising muscle. A left-to-right shunt from an atrial septal defect, in effect, creates the same physiologic stressors—a volume overload on the heart (in this case, the right ventricle) and excessive pulmonary blood flow. It would be expected, then, that the ability of the heart and lungs in a patient with an atrial septal defect to respond to the augmented cardiac and ventilatory work of exercise would be limited. That is, the restricted cardiopulmonary reserve available for exercise response in a child or adolescent with a substantial left-to-right shunt is diminished, and, as a consequence, exercise tolerance may be reduced.

Most children and adolescents with atrial septal defects are asymptomatic and will not report any problems with exercise (3). The aforementioned hemodynamic effects of a large interatrial communication may, however, negatively influence capabilities in highly competitive endurance sports. Consequently, a cardiac assessment is an appropriate part of the medical evaluation of a young athlete who is inappropriately fatigued with training in distance events.

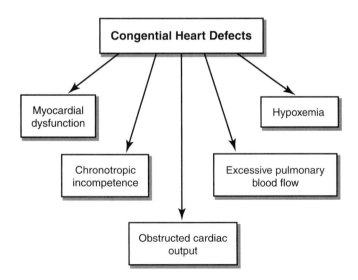

FIGURE 10.1. Congenital heart disease can affect exercise performance negatively by several mechanisms.

Tetralogy of Fallot

Patients with tetralogy of Fallot demonstrate right-to-left shunting with systemic hypoxemia. Early surgery typically is successful in correcting this abnormality, usually leaving the child with a mild degree of pulmonary stenosis and valvular insufficiency.

Not unexpectedly, arterial oxygen desaturation dramatically depresses exercise tolerance by limiting aerobic metabolism. If a child with unoperated tetralogy exercises, the problem of low oxygen delivery to the muscles is compounded. Systemic venous return from the exercising limbs is markedly low in oxygen content, and this desaturated blood is preferentially shunted right-to-left through the ventricular septal defect (because of the pulmonary stenosis) and out the aorta. Consequently, systemic arterial saturation falls drastically with increasing exercise intensity. If the older child with tetralogy of Fallot is for some reason inoperable, exercise intolerance will be a major concern. Sports play will be impossible, and even participation in normal daily activities will be limited.

Fortunately, most patients with tetralogy of Fallot receive early surgical repair, with the result that hypoxemia and its negative influence on exercise performance are not an issue during childhood. However, other postoperative aspects of this disease may affect the ability in some children to tolerate exercise. Right ventricular dysfunction has been observed in some patients. However, this may reflect previous timing of surgery, at 5 years of age or older, which is now avoided by improved surgical techniques that permit repair in early infancy. **Chronotropic incompetence**, or a limited ability to raise heart rate with exercise, is not uncommon following tetralogy repair (4). This can limit **cardiac output** responses and lower $\dot{V}O_{2max}$. For most patients with early, successful repair, however, these influences are mild and cause no important limitations in exercise capacity or ability to participate in sports (5).

Ventricular ectopy has been observed in as many as 5% to 10% of children following repair of tetralogy of Fallot, usually in those with an inadequate hemodynamic surgical result. Although this dysrhythmia does not, in itself, impair exercise performance, risks involved with provocation of ventricular tachyarrhythmias during exercise may make it necessary to restrict these children from sports play. (This restriction is discussed later in respect to risks imposed by congenital heart disease by sports participation.)

Transposition of the Great Arteries

Fifty years ago, transposition of the great arteries was a universally fatal abnormality, with newborns succumbing in the first days of life to progressive hypoxemia and metabolic acidosis. The introduction of the Mustard operation in the 1960s, however, dramatically changed this picture. In this procedure, a baffle is placed within the atria to direct systemic venous return (flow in the inferior and superior vena cavae) through the mitral valve and into the left ventricle. This leaves the highly oxygenated pulmonary venous return to flow across the tricuspid valve into the right ventricle and out the aorta. The result is, in effect, an "atrial switch," which results in normal systemic arterial oxygen saturation.

With a survival rate well over 90%, individuals with transposition did well following the Mustard procedure and typically described normal exercise tolerance in their daily lives. In long-term followup, however, several problems have became apparent, which, in some cases, limit tolerance with more intense or sustained exercise (6). In this operation, the right ventricle continues to serve as the systemic ventricle, and the tricuspid valve acts as the atrioventricular valve on the systemic side. This workload is not always tolerated, as indicated by evidence of right ventricular dysfunction and tricuspid regurgitation, findings used to explain the limited cardiovascular fitness observed in some young people following Mustard repair. Depressed sinus node function, sometimes necessitating implantation of an artificial pacemaker, and problems with recurrent atrial dysrhythmias (particularly atrial flutter) also have been problematic in long-term care of these patients.

These complications following Mustard repair for transposition stimulated the development of a new operative approach, the "arterial switch" operation, in the 1980s. This intuitively more appropriate surgical repair involves exchanging the aorta and main pulmonary at the cardiac base and then transplanting the coronary arteries to the root of the "neo-aorta" on the left side. This procedure, then, essentially reconstructed the anatomy back to a normal arrangement (that is, the pulmonary artery arises off the right ventricle and the aorta off the left) (Figure 10.2).

Long-term followup of patients who have undergone the "arterial switch" operation is not yet available, but early studies indicate normal exercise tolerance (7). Systemic oxygenation is normal, myocardial function is appropriate, coronary insufficiency typically has not been observed, and no significant problems with exercise-induced dysrhythmias have been seen.

Single Ventricle

In a number of forms of congenital heart disease, the malformation effectively results in a single functioning ventricle. This can occur when the tricuspid or pulmonary valve is atretic, resulting in severe underdevelopment of the right ventricle and limited pulmonary blood flow and systemic hypoxemia. Alternatively, the entire left side of the heart can be extremely hypoplastic, with a tiny left atrium and mitral valve, minuscule left ventricle, and aortic valve atresia. This set of anomalies, known as the "hypoplastic left heart syndrome," manifests as severe hypotension and cardiogenic shock in the first days of life as the ductus arteriosus closes, leaving no means of egress of blood from the heart to the body. Children also can be born with a large, single ventricle with mixing of systemic and pulmonary venous blood through normal tricuspid and mitral valves.

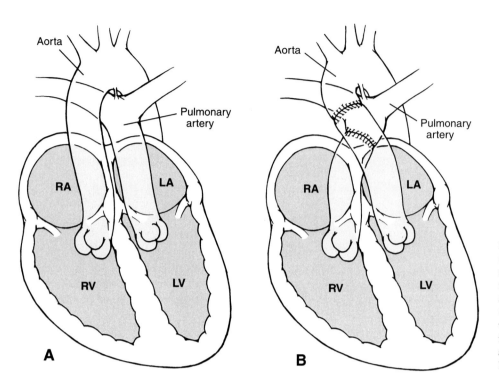

FIGURE 10.2. In patients with transposition of the great arteries (A), the aorta arises off the right ventricle and the pulmonary artery off the left. Following the arterial switch procedure (B), normal ventricle-to-great vessel continuity is restored, with transplantation of the coronary arteries to the base of the "neo-aorta." LA, left atrium; LV, left ventricle; RA, right atrium; RV, right ventricle.

In the past, palliative surgery often permitted a limited life expectancy for patients with such defects, but systemic hypoxemia or poor myocardial function invariably precluded normal exercise activities. The current surgical approach to patients with a single functioning ventricle, the **Fontan procedure**, has altered the survival of these children, but problems with exercise tolerance persist.

In the Fontan procedure, which often is performed in two stages, the superior and inferior venae cavae are connected directly to the pulmonary artery. This directs systemic venous return to the lungs for oxygenation without an intervening pump, leaving the patient's single ventricle to serve only as a systemic pump. Although this results in elevation in central venous pressure, the combined effects of mechanisms such as the skeletal muscle pump and the "suction" effect of ventricular relaxation sustain systemic venous return and cardiac output.

Given this significant rearrangement, it is not surprising that patients demonstrate significant limitations of exercise capacity following the Fontan procedure. This is reflected by a decreased duration of exercise (about 60% predicted) and a maximal oxygen uptake that is 50% of that expected for age. Ability to generate cardiac output with exercise is depressed because heart rate is low, and **stroke volume** declines during a progressive exercise test.

These problems presumably are related to limitations of generating cardiac flow during exercise because oxygenation is now approximately normal. A number of possible mechanisms for exercise limitation in these patients have been presented, but the explanation remains uncertain. The lack of an "auxiliary" pulmonary ventricle would be expected to be an important contributor, but factors such as depressed contractility of the single ventricle, chronotropic incompetence, and abnormalities in skeletal muscle pump function also may play a role.

Aortic Valve Stenosis

Obstructive abnormalities of the heart can limit exercise capabilities by restricting the volume of systemic blood flow. With narrowing of the aortic valve (i.e., aortic valve stenosis) this issue may be confounded by the need to increase coronary blood flow to meet the augmented energy needs of the myocardium during exercise because the orifices of the coronary arteries are immediately downstream from the site of obstruction.

Patients with mild to moderately severe aortic valve stenosis typically have no problems with exercise. Those with more severe obstruction (e.g., a pressure difference, or gradient, between the left ventricle and aorta of >50–60 mm Hg) may demonstrate a blunted stroke volume response to exercise as well as a reduced rise in blood pressure (8). The rise in left ventricular pressure with exercise is exaggerated, and the left ventricle–aorta pressure gradient is more pronounced. Moderate exercise in patients with significant aortic valve stenosis increases the left ventricular outflow tract gradient in direct proportion to the rise in cardiac output. This pattern indicates the influence of a fixed outlet obstruction on the cardiac output responses to exercise.

When a child with significant aortic stenosis exercises, a serious strain may be placed on the balance between the demand for myocardial perfusion and the supply of coronary blood flow (9). The exaggerated increase in left ventricular pressure and the hypertrophied mass of ventricular myocardial tissue combine to escalate myocardial metabolic oxygen demand, which also is increased by the tachycardia and augmented myocardial contractility that occur with increasing exercise intensity. At high levels of exercise, diastolic filling time, when most coronary perfusion occurs, is reduced to about 25% of that at rest. The resulting risk of a mismatch between perfusion supply and myocardial demand predispose the patient to ischemia and ventricular dysrhythmias.

The Risks of Exercise in Patients With Congenital Heart Disease

The increased exercise risks for adults with coronary artery disease, particularly as it relates to **sudden death**, has prompted concern over similar dangers in children and adolescents with congenital heart disease. The concern is raised especially in the context of their participation in intensive organized sports, which strain the limits of cardiac function and trigger high levels of sympathetic stimulation and increases in serum catecholamines. In fact, the risk of sudden death in youngsters with congenital heart disease is low, and most can participate in athletics without concern. It is important, however, to identify those individuals in whom the risks associated with sports play *do* exist and either modify their participation or exclude them from particular sports.

Other potential risks, such as the possible long-term adverse effect of sports training on volume- or pressure-overloaded myocardium, are intuitive but not documented. Similarly, resistance activities that increase systemic blood pressure (e.g., weightlifting, water skiing) seem ill-advised in patients with hypertension or with aortic valve insufficiency, but the level of such risk has not been identified. As noted previously, some children with heart disease are at risk for *not* participating in physical activities out of inappropriate concern regarding the dangers involved (10).

The risk of sudden death from heart disease with physical activity is, in general, confined to limited types of anomalies. In order of risk these include **hypertrophic cardiomyopathy**, congenital anomalies of the **coronary arteries**, **Marfan syndrome**, and valvular aortic stenosis. Specific exercise guidelines for patients with these and other forms of heart disease have been outlined in the report on the 26th Bethesda Conference listed in the Suggested Readings.

The mechanism for sudden death during physical activity in most of these conditions has been presumed to be arrhythmogenic, particularly in ventricular tachycardia or fibrillation. Although exercise increases the chance of sudden death in individuals with these conditions, restriction from physical activity does not, unfortunately, serve to eliminate the risks of such tragedies. In the following sections, the most common causes of sudden cardiac death in young athletes during sports participation are reviewed, with particular attention paid to potential mechanisms.

Hypertrophic Cardiomyopathy

Hypertrophic cardiomyopathy is not, strictly speaking, a form of congenital heart disease because it is characterized by an overgrowth of heart muscle rather than an error in normal cardiac morphogenesis. This abnormality cannot be classified as acquired, either—it is an autosomally dominant inherited condition. The cardiac hypertrophy, which principally involves the ventricular septum, sometimes can be immense, with a thickness exceeding three to four times normal (Figure 10.3).

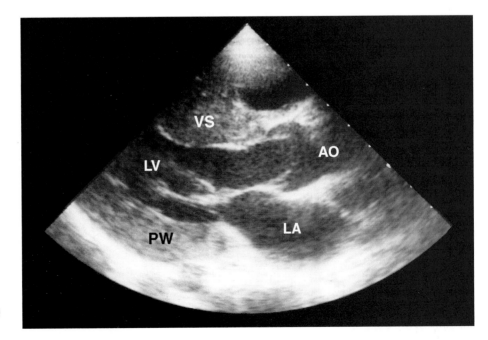

FIGURE 10.3. Two-dimensional echocardiogram of a heart with hypertrophic cardiomyopathy. The ventricular septum (VS) is markedly thickened, as is the posterior wall (PW), while the size of the left ventricle (LV) is compromised. AO, aorta; LA, left atrium.

The cause of sudden death in individuals with hypertrophic cardiomyopathy is not clear. The incidence of sudden death is not related to left ventricular outflow obstruction, which tends to be minimal in young individuals. It is most likely that subendocardial coronary perfusion through the markedly hypertrophied heart becomes limited, particularly in the face of the diastolic time constraints and augmented myocardial demands of physical activity. Relatively ischemic myocardium that is being adrenergically stimulated is at risk for life-threatening ventricular tachyarrhythmias.

In some clinical reports, the statistical risk of sudden death from hypertrophic cardiomyopathy is high, amounting to 2% to 4% per year. Studies in adults indicate that sudden death occurs equally during vigorous physical activity, mild activity, and rest or sleep. Thus, although most patients who die suddenly with this condition do not succumb during intense sports play, a disproportionate number do (11). This finding has led to the recommendation that patients with hypertrophic cardiomyopathy be restricted from organized athletics or exhaustive exercise.

As a first step, individuals with hypertrophic cardiomyopathy must be recognized clinically. Hypertrophic cardiomyopathy is rare in children and adolescents; the reason it ranks as the most common cause of unexpected sudden cardiac death in young athletes is that lack of specific clinical findings renders it difficult to detect on routine physical examination. Physical findings typically are deceptively benign. Accompanying murmurs may sound functional, and pulses usually are normal. A family history of cardiomyopathy or sudden death is an important clue, as is a report of previous symptoms of chest pain or **syncope** with exercise.

Congenital Coronary Artery Anomalies

Young athletes do not suffer from atherosclerotic coronary artery disease, but congenitally misplaced or hypoplastic coronary vessels may create the same risk of ischemic sudden death. Fortunately, such anomalies are rare. Unfortunately, the first clinical sign that such an anomaly is present often is the athlete's sudden collapse and death on the playing field. In some cases, however, athletes have given a history of previous chest pain, dizziness, or syncope during sports participation (12).

The most common anomaly creating such risk is take-off of the left coronary artery from the right aortic sinus. This vessel then courses between the aortic and pulmonary artery roots to provide blood supply to its normal distribution on the left side of the heart. Lack of adequate coronary perfusion with exercise may occur either from compression of the left coronary artery between the enlarged great vessels or as a result of relative stenosis from its acutely angled take off from the aorta.

There are numerous variations of such coronary anomalies, including origin of the left coronary artery from the pulmonary artery. Coronary arteries can be hypoplastic or can become obstructed by fibromuscular hyperplasia. In all these cases, the mechanism of sudden death appears to be an imbalance between supply and demand, with myocardial ischemia and life-threatening ventricular dysrhythmias.

Marfan Syndrome

Marfan syndrome is an hereditary disorder of connective tissue with associated cardiovascular disorders, which, strictly speaking, cannot be considered forms of congenital heart disease. Individuals with Marfan syndrome are identified by a classic constellation of clinical findings that includes tall stature, long arms and fingers (arachnodactyly), hyperflexible joints, musculoskeletal disorders (e.g., pectus excavatum, kyphoscoliosis), dislocated ocular lens, and typical cardiovascular disorders. The latter include mitral valve prolapse, progressive aortic root dilatation and aneurysm formation, and aortic valve insufficiency. The most serious risk to such individuals is rupture of their **aortic root aneurysm** with cardiac tamponade and sudden death.

Participation in sports activities has been considered to increase the risk of these cardiac complications. Consequently, recommendations call for patients with Marfan syndrome to refrain from sports that could involve acutely increased intra-aortic pressure by a blow to the chest (e.g., boxing, football), repetitive sustained cardiac output (e.g., swimming, cross-country running), or sudden surges of systemic blood pressure (e.g., weightlifting, wrestling) (13). The specific level of danger accompanying these activities is unknown, however, making it difficult to prescribe specific limitations in individual patients. The problem of sports restriction in these individuals is compounded further by the fact that many are talented athletes, particularly in sports in which tall stature offers a competitive advantage (e.g., basketball, volleyball).

There is no specific test to identify individuals with Marfan syndrome. The diagnosis is, of course, highly likely in tall individuals who have a family history of other members with this syndrome. Tall athletes with long arms and fingers who possess other characteristics consistent with Marfan syndrome should have a cardiac and genetics evaluation to allow appropriate guidelines for sports play.

Aortic Valve Stenosis

The incidence of sudden death in children with aortic valve stenosis is estimated to be approximately 1%. It generally is limited to patients who have a left ventricular outflow gradient more than 40 to 50 mm Hg, an abnormal electrocardiogram, or symptoms related to aortic valve stenosis (e.g., angina, dizziness, exercise fatigue). As with hypertrophic cardiomyopathy, a disproportionate number of these occurrences are associated with vigorous physical activity, although most happen either with patients at rest or during mild exertion.

Because many of the characteristics of severe aortic stenosis are similar to those of adults with coronary artery disease (e.g., **angina**, ischemic ECG changes), it has been assumed that the most likely mechanism for sudden death in these patients is relative coronary insufficiency with **myocardial ischemia** and terminal ventricular tachyarrhythmia. Certainly the coronary supply and demand imbalance that occurs with exercise in severe aortic stenosis should be expected to predispose to this pathogenesis. The demand for myocardial perfusion is exaggerated in this situation, both by exercise and the expanded mass of hypertrophied muscle, and coronary flow may be limited by the significant degree of aortic outflow obstruction. This obstruction is, of course, fixed and does not adjust to increased needs for cardiac output during exercise.

An alternative explanation for sudden death in patients with aortic stenosis involves the triggering of prominent vagal reflexes by augmented left ventricular pressures with exercise. Left ventricular baroreceptors are sensitive to increases in chamber pressures, particularly in conditions of low blood volume (as occurs with dehydration in sports play). These receptors stimulate a vagal reflex that causes hypotension and, in most cases, syncope. It is conceivable, however, that in situations of particularly high ventricular pressure, as occurs in patients with significant left ventricular outflow obstruction, that this reflex might effect sufficient hypotension and bradycardia to cause sudden death.

Patients with at least moderately severe aortic stenosis traditionally have been restricted from intense sports participation because of the risk for sudden death. The rarity of these events and lack of accurate predictive clinical markers, however, has led to a good deal of subjectivity in making these recommendations. Additionally, it is recognized that most episodes of sudden death in patients with aortic stenosis do not occur during sports play, and there is no evidence that restriction from athletics is truly effective in preventing these events. Any possible protective value of exercise restriction needs to be weighed against the potential physical, psychological, and social benefits that might be gained from sports participation.

Dysrhythmias

Abnormal heart rhythms in children often are associated with structural heart disease, and the risk of life-threatening dysrhythmias is identified by the type of heart abnormality (e.g., ventricular tachycardia or fibrillation presumably is the terminal mechanism of sudden death in conditions such as hypertrophic cardiomyopathy, coronary disease, and aortic stenosis). In other situations, the appearance of a rhythm disturbance itself raises the question of safety of participation in sports and vigorous physical activities.

In general, few cardiac dysrhythmias pose serious risk and need for restriction from sports play. These typically involve those that pose a risk for ventricular tachycardia and fibrillation.

Beneficial Effects of Exercise in Congenital Heart Disease

Regular exercise, including participation in organized sports, provides important health benefits. For young individuals, participation in physical activities may pay long-term dividends of decreasing risk of atherosclerotic vascular disease, obesity, hypertension, type 2 diabetes, and osteoporosis. Regular exercise is important for emotional health as well, optimizing enjoyment of life and enhancing self-esteem. Involvement in sports can provide an opportunity for social growth and development of self-discipline and psychological resilience.

Preventive Cardiology With Congenital Heart Disease

Children with congenital heart disease can benefit from these salutary effects of a physically active lifestyle in the same way as those with normal hearts. In fact, certain considerations indicate a particular importance of such exercise for such youngsters. Those with decreased levels of physical fitness due to cardiac limitations can maximize their ability to perform exercise by being regularly active. As life expectancy improves in those with repaired complex forms of heart disease (such as with the Fontan procedure), such patients will be encountering the added risks of adult coronary artery disease. The effects of superimposed atherosclerotic ischemic disease on pre-existing myocardial dysfunction from congenital heart abnormalities may prove especially disadvantageous. Therefore, efforts to prevent coronary artery disease in these patients through regular exercise, proper diet, and avoidance of obesity and smoking are particularly pertinent.

Children and adolescents with congenital heart abnormalities may experience emotional reactions to their illness, which can include anxiety, depression, and lack of self-confidence. Regular exercise carries the potential for improving such emotional disorders and enhancing social development, making promotion of exercise especially important for these patients.

Cardiac Rehabilitation Programs

Exercise rehabilitation programs (**cardiac rehabilitation**) for adults who have suffered a myocardial infarction have proven successful in improving physical capacity as well as increasing quality of life based on enhanced mood, self-concept, and social confidence. Whether these programs accomplish this through a direct action on myocardial function or amelioration of the atherosclerotic process remains controversial.

Although the pathophysiology of serious congenital heart defects in children and adolescents differs from that of adult patients post-MI, certain features such as myocardial dysfunction, impaired exercise tolerance, and psychosocial disorders often are shared. This observation has stimulated interest in utilizing similar exercise rehabilitation programs for youth with congenital heart disease.

Reports from the centers conducting such programs are largely anecdotal and suffer from small patient numbers, lack of "untreated" controls, and inclusion of varying types of heart defects. Nonetheless, they suggest that a careful organized exercise program for pediatric patients can improve the child's functional capacity to perform and enjoy physical activities, develop self-esteem and social confidence, and provide the child and family with realistic information regarding the child's limits for physical activity (14).

Organized programs may be particularly effective in providing the psychosocial benefits of participation in regular exercise that occur in a group setting. They also provide an assurance of safety to parents who may be concerned about the risks of exercise in their children.

What We Know About Exercise for Children With Heart Disease

1 Most children with heart disease tolerate exercise normally, and they should be encouraged to maintain regular habits of physical activity as part of a healthy lifestyle.

2 A growing number of youth who have survived surgery for complex heart defects will be limited in their exercise capacity. Although participation in sports activities may not be possible, these patients should be offered guidance as to which activities they will be able to tolerate.

3 A small number of heart defects create a risk for sudden death with sports play. Individuals with these abnormalities need to be identified and restricted from athletic participation.

4 Limited experience with exercise rehabilitation programs for children with serious heart disease indicates their potential for improving physical fitness and combating emotional disorders in these patients.

What We Would Like to Know About Exercise for Children With Heart Disease

1 It would be helpful in understanding risks and benefits of heart disease in children to possess a better insight into the mechanisms by which heart abnormalities affect normal exercise performance.

2 The efficacy of exercise rehabilitation programs needs to be documented by adequate research studies. Information regarding the appropriate types and levels of exercise intensity in such programs is also needed.

3 An effective means of identifying youth at risk for sudden unexpected cardiac death during sports participation needs to be developed.

Summary

The great majority of children with heart disease do not experience exercise intolerance and can participate in intense exercise and sports without undue risk. Among the different forms of heart defects, various pathophysiologies can, however, negatively influence exercise performance when these abnormalities are severe. This is particularly true following surgery for complex forms of cyanotic congenital heart disease. These patients need to understand that they will be limited in their ability to participate in some forms of physical activities, but they should be encouraged and guided into those types of exercise that they can tolerate. In a very few cases, heart disease poses a significant risk for sudden death during exercise. Youth at risk need to be identified and restricted from sports play.

DISCUSSION QUESTIONS

1 What arguments should be offered to the child with minor heart disease who appears to be refraining from physical activity because of fear of a "heart attack"?

2 What methods can be used to clinically detect heart disease that would place a would-be athlete at risk during preparticipation screening?

3 What forms of heart disease would be expected to benefit the most from an exercise rehabilitation program?

CASE STUDY

Patient Information

A 10-year-old boy was born with tricuspid atresia (completely blocked tricuspid valve at the exit of the right atrium) with a markedly underdeveloped right ventricle. He has undergone the Fontan operation to connect his superior and inferior vena cavae directly to the right pulmonary artery, leaving the left ventricle as the systemic pump. He has problems running the mile in gym class testing, but otherwise his parents describe his daily physical activities as normal. In fact, he participated on a community soccer team (with a short field) last summer without difficulties. He now wants to join a higher level competitive soccer team, but his parents are concerned about possible risks.

Assessments

Physical examination reveals a healthy-appearing boy, well-nourished and without cyanosis or tachypnea. Vital signs are normal, and pulse oximetry indicates an oxygen saturation of 92%. His cardiac examination is normal except for a single second heart sound. The electrocardiogram shows a sinus rhythm with left ventricular hypertrophy. An echocardiogram confirms his abnormal heart anatomy. Left ventricular function is low normal, and there is a mild degree of mitral insufficiency. There is no dilatation of the superior or inferior vena cava. On a treadmill exercise test he demonstrates a low endurance time with a $\dot{V}O_{2max}$ of 26 ml/kg/min. No ectopy nor ischemic changes are seen on the electrocardiogram during exercise.

This is a boy who has the expected low level of endurance or aerobic fitness typically seen in patients following the Fontan operation. He has been able to tolerate exercise reasonably well in his daily life, however, because such activities generally are short-term and do not rely heavily on aerobic fitness. Now he wants to participate in an endurance activity that is unlikely to be tolerated. An honest discussion is needed to give him and his parents a realistic view of the role that physical activities will play in his life, both positive and negative.

Questions

1. What would you tell his parents about the risks of participating on the soccer team?
2. How would you counsel him regarding physical activities?
3. Are there means of improving his exercise fitness?

REFERENCES

1. Mertens L, Reybrouck T, Dumoulin M, et al. Cardiopulmonary exercise testing after surgical closure of a large ventricular septal defect [abstract]. Pediatr Exerc Science 1996;8:89.
2. Oelberg DA, Marcotte F, Kreisman H, et al. Evaluation of right ventricular systolic pressure during incremental exercise by Doppler echocardiography in adults with atrial septal defect. Chest 1998;113:1459–1465.
3. Matthys D. Pre- and postoperative exercise testing of the child with atrial septal defect. Pediatr Cardiol 1999;20:22–25.
4. Perrault H, Davignon A, Grief G, et al. Disturbance of heart rate during exercise following intracardiac repair: contribution of cardiopulmonary bypass. Pediatr Exerc Science 1992;4:270–280.
5. Wessel HU, Paul MH. Exercise studies in tetralogy of Fallot: a review. Pediatr Cardiol 1999;20:39–47.
6. Paul MH, Wessel HU. Exercise studies in patients with transposition of the great arteries after atrial repair operations (Mustard/Senning): a review. Pediatr Cardiol 1999;20:49–55.
7. Weindling SN, Wernovsky G, Colan SD, et al. Myocardial perfusion, function, and exercise tolerance after the arterial switch operation. J Am Coll Cardiol 1994;23:424–433.
8. Doyle EF, Arumugham P, Lara E, et al. Sudden death in young patients with congenital aortic stenosis. Pediatrics 1974;53:481–489.
9. Cueto L, Moller JH. Haemodynamics of exercise in children with isolated aortic valvular disease. Br Heart J 1973;35:93–98.
10. Bergman AB, Stamm SJ. The morbidity of cardiac nondisease in schoolchildren. N Engl J Med 1967;276:1008–1013.
11. Maron BJ, Roberts WC, Epstein SE. Sudden death in hypertrophic cardiomyopathy: a profile of 78 patients. Circulation 1982;65:1388-1394.
12. Basso C, Maron BJ, Corrado D, Thiene G. Clinical profile of congenital coronary artery anomalies with origin from the wrong aortic sinus leading to sudden death in young competitive athletes. J Am Coll Cardiol 2000;35:1493–1501.
13. Braverman AC. Exercise and the Marfan syndrome. Med Sci Sports Exerc 1998;30 (Suppl):S387–S395.
14. Barber G. Training and the pediatric patient: a cardiologist's perspective. In: Blimkie JR, Bar-Or O, eds. New Horizons in Pediatric Exercise Science. Champaign, IL: Human Kinetics Publishers, 1995: 137–146.

SUGGESTED READINGS

26th Bethesda Conference: recommendations for determining eligibility for competition in athletes with cardiovascular abnormalities. January 6-7, 1994. Med Sci Sports Exerc 1994;26(10 Suppl):S223–S283.

Conwell JA, Bricker JT. Exercise in children after surgery for congenital heart disease. In: Thompson PD (ed). Exercise and Sports Cardiology. New York: McGraw-Hill, 2000:264-297.

Estes NAM, Link MS, Homoud M, Wang PJ. Electrocardiographic variants and cardiac rhythm and conduction disturbances in the athlete. In: Thompson PD, ed. Exercise and sports cardiology. New York: McGraw-Hill, 2000:211–232.

Reybrouck T, Gewillig M. Exercise testing and daily physical activity in children with congenital heart disease. In: Armstrong N, van Mechelen W, eds. Paediatric exercise science and medicine. Oxford: Oxford University Press, 2000:313–322.

Rowland TW. Sudden unexpected death in sports. Pediatr Ann 1992;21:189–195.

Rowland TW. Congenital obstructive and valvular heart disease. In: Goldberg B (ed). Sports and exercise for children with chronic health conditions. Champaign, IL: Human Kinetics Publishers, 1995:225–236.

Rowland TW. Exercise and children's health. Champaign, IL: Human Kinetics Publishers, 1990:181–192.

Washington RL. Dysrhythmic heart disease. In: Goldberg B, ed. Sports and exercise for children with chronic health conditions. Champaign, IL: Human Kinetics Publishers, 1995:237–246.

PULMONARY DISEASES AND DISORDERS

Chronic Obstructive Pulmonary Disease

Frank W. Cerny, Su Zhan

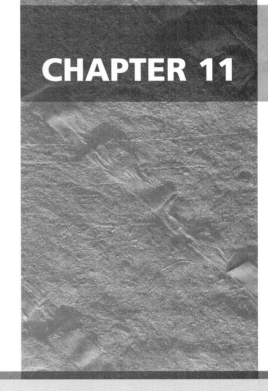

Overview

Chronic obstructive pulmonary disease (COPD), which includes diseases such as **chronic bronchitis** and **emphysema**, affects over 16 million people in the United States. The 110,000 annual deaths attributed to COPD make it the 4th leading cause of mortality in the United States, after heart disease, lung cancer, and cerebrovascular disease (1). Approximately $10 billion is spent annually for care of people with COPD, and more than that is lost due to decreased productivity of people with COPD (2). Between 80% and 90% of COPD cases are caused by cigarette smoking. Chronic bronchitis is characterized by excessive mucus secretion, generally caused by chronic irritation of the airways that leads to persistent cough. In addition to the mucus-related narrowing of the airways, chronic bronchitis may be associated with narrowing due to swelling of the airway wall and active contraction of the smooth muscle surrounding the airway. Chronic bronchitis accounts for about 12 million of the total cases of COPD in the United States.

Pathophysiology of Chronic Obstructive Pulmonary Disease

Chronic bronchitis, a long-lasting **inflammation** of the bronchi, is caused by prolonged irritation of the bronchial mucosa. Diagnosis is based on the presence of cough and sputum production for more than 3 months out of 2 consecutive years. The diagnosis is strengthened with **pulmonary function tests** showing the presence of airflow obstruction (3). This obstruction is reflected in a reduction in measures of maximal airflow (FEV_1, $FEF_{25-75\%}$) and increases in **airway resistance** (Raw) and decreases in specific conductance (sGaw) (Table 11.1). Enlarged mucus-secreting glands and an increase in the number of mucus-secret-

ing cells, the **goblet cells** lining the walls of the trachea and larger bronchi, characterize this disease. The disease is associated with **chronic cough** and increasing **mucus expectoration** as the disease progresses.

Emphysema is characterized by permanent destruction of parts of the gas-conducting system, the airways, and the gas exchange units of the lung, the alveoli. The damage is permanent because of the irreversible destruction of the lung protein **elastin**. Elastin is involved in maintaining the structure of the alveolar walls, and when this protein is absent the smallest part of the airways, the **bronchioles**, collapse, making it difficult to move air into and out of the alveoli. The consequent narrowing of the airways combined with increased obstruction due to mucus accumulation increases the forces necessary to move air through the airways—that is, the flow-resistive work of breathing increases. To minimize this flow-resistive work, breathing is controlled to reduce breathing frequency and increase tidal volume to attain any given level of ventilation. Unfortunately, other changes in the lung, discussed later in this section, also increase the work of breathing associated with increasing tidal volume so that these patients run out of options for effectively increasing ventilation, particularly during exercise.

In addition to the changes in the airways, the convoluted structure of the alveoli also is destroyed, leaving the gas exchange units extremely compliant and dramatically decreasing the area available to exchange O_2 and CO_2. The destruction of alveolar spaces increases the area that is ventilated, but into a space where no gas exchange takes place, the **dead space** (Vd). As the lung disease progresses, the Vd increases, necessitating increases in ventilation to move enough air to overcome the "wasted ventilation" of the Vd and still maintain ventilation to the gas exchange units, the alveoli.

The lung destruction and increase in **lung compliance** contribute to a condition of **hyperinflation**, in which these patients breathe at high lung volumes. By breathing at high

TABLE 11.1. COMMON PULMONARY FUNCTION TESTS AND THEIR USE IN THE ASSESSMENT OF CHRONIC OBSTRUCTIVE PULMONARY DISEASE

Test	What it Measures	Use in COPD
Forced vital capacity (FVC)	Total amount of air that can be moved into and out of the lung	1) Assess loss of lung volume 2) Used to calculate other volumes (see below)
Forced expiratory flow in 1 second (FEV_1)	The rate of airflow through the larger (>2 mm) airways	Determine the degree of airway obstruction
Forced expiratory flow between 25% and 75% of FVC ($FEF_{25-75\%}$)	The rate of airflow through the smaller (<2 mm) airways	Determine the degree of airway obstruction
Functional residual capacity (FRC)	The amount of air left in the lungs at the end of a normal exhalation	Assess the degree of hyperinflation
Residual volume (RV)	The air left in the lung at the end of a maximal exhalation	Assess the degree of hyperinflation
Total lung capacity	Lung capacity for holding air	Assess loss of lung volume
Airway resistance (Raw)	The resistance to airflow in the airways	Determine the degree of airway obstruction
Specific conductance of the airways (sGaw = 1/Raw/FRC)	The resistance to airflow in the airways	Determine the degree of airway obstruction

lung volumes, increased forces are required to move the elastic structures (the lung and chest wall) of the pulmonary system—that is, the elastic work of breathing increase. To minimize this elastic work, breathing is controlled to reduce tidal volume and increase breathing frequency to attain any given level of ventilation. This breathing strategy increases the flow-resistive work of breathing, however, which already is high in these patients. The high flow-resistive work and high elastic work contribute to the sense of breathlessness or shortness of breath associated with COPD.

Hyperinflation is reflected in pulmonary function measures of lung volume as decreases in the volume of air that can be breathed in and out (FVC) and increases in the amount of air in the lungs at the end of a tidal (FRC) and maximal exhalation (RV) (see Table 11.1). This hyperinflation increases the energy cost of breathing and limits the ability to increase **tidal volume** (Vt). An agonizing paradox is established, whereby the poor gas exchange and increased Vd require increases in ventilation, but because of the **airway obstruction** and hyperinflation the lung is unable to respond. The inability to increase ventilation leads to further decreases in gas exchange, promoting a downward cycle in function.

Both chronic bronchitis and emphysema generally are progressive, particularly if the source of irritation—smoking—continues. The airway irritation in chronic bronchitis leads to a chronic inflammatory process that can progress to emphysema. As emphysema progresses, an increasing amount of the lung is destroyed, to the point that the patient may have to be placed on supplemental oxygen during exercise and eventually even at rest. The progression of the disease can be slowed if the patient stops smoking, but recovery of the destroyed lung is impossible. Besides smoking cessation, treatment of COPD includes the use of inhaled β-agonists, anticholinergics, corticosteroids, and antibiotics for treatment of acute exacerbations (Table 11.2).

Healthy young adults, even at maximal exercise, use only about 80% of the gas exchange capacity of the lung. The remaining 20% reserve capacity is important in understanding the insidious progression and functional consequences of the disease. The young smoker may destroy parts of the lung and not notice any consequences until this reserve is lost. Even at that, most smokers do not exercise sufficiently to feel the effects of a loss of 20% or more of the lung. It is not until the destruction progresses to such a point that shortness of breath is noticed during activities of daily living that the patient may even notice the disease. By then, a considerable capacity of the lung may have been destroyed without the patient's knowledge. This finding emphasizes the importance of an exercise test in the evaluation of these patients.

Exercise Testing

Exercise testing in COPD is used to assist in the evaluation of disease severity, to identify specific functional deficits, and to evaluate the effectiveness of therapy (4, 5). Tests commonly used include the standard **graded, progressive incremental test** (**GXT**), similar to that associated with stress testing for cardiac patients, single stage tests, and several field tests.

The GXT is useful for identification of functional limitations in patients with COPD (6). The incremental tests are used primarily for determining the level of exercise at which a patient may not respond appropriately, providing some indication of the degree of disease-related dysfunction. Standardized GXTs are available for treadmill or cycle ergometer testing. The graded, incremental nature of these tests allows observation of the patient's response at each exercise level so that the exercise intensity, and the heart rate at that intensity, at which an abnormal response occurs is noted. In addition, these tests allow determination of the patient's peak exercise capacity and possible factors that may limit that capacity. The selection of work rate increment can influence both the response to each work increment and the peak work rate achieved (7). A test performed with very small increments, prolonging the time to reach peak capacity, can result in increased levels of **minute** ventilation (V_E), heart rate (HR), **dyspnea**, and leg fatigue at lower work intensities and a lower peak work capacity than a test with larger increments. A test with increments that are too large may lead to termination of the test before sufficient measurements can be made to characterize the patient's ventilatory response to exercise. Facilities without a testing laboratory can perform an incremental shuttle test in a hallway. This test requires a patient to walk between two marked points in a specified time, with the rate progressively increasing, providing work increments as in a laboratory test.

To avoid the risks of cardiac arrhythmia, heart attack, or large decreases in **arterial** O_2 levels that may be associated with a peak work capacity test, it is sometimes desirable to use a test that will predict peak work capacity from exercise performed at several submaximal exercise levels (8). These tests generally require that the patient exercise at two or more low levels of exercise intensity. On the basis of the heart rate response to these loads, the peak workload that could be achieved at a predicted peak heart rate is estimated. Submaximal tests to predict maximum capacity are used infrequently in the pulmonary setting because it is likely that the lung disease would limit exercise capacity well before the level predicted by these tests would be reached. Submaximal tests are used, however, to assess the effects of therapy. To evaluate the effects of therapy, it is not necessary to perform a peak exercise test. Positive training effects can be identified for a patient who has decreased arterial oxygen levels at a specific exercise load prior to therapy by performing an exercise assessment after therapy at that same load and at a level somewhat above that load. This is just one example of how changes in symptoms and function over time can be assessed reliably by making measurements at several submaximal exercise levels (4).

The distance covered in a specific time can also be used to document the peak work capacity of a patient. The most

TABLE 11.2.   MEDICATIONS USED IN THE TREATMENT OF CHRONIC OBSTRUCTIVE PULMONARY DISEASE

Drug	Comments	Side Effects
β-agonists		
Epinephrine (Primatene Mist)	Short-acting; serves as an emergency medication	Peripheral vasodilation, increased heart rate, increased skeletal muscle tremor, increased insulin, free fatty acid and glucose, decreased Pao_2 (worsened $\dot{V}/\dot{Q}$ matching), myocardial necrosis
Albuterol, terbutaline, pirbuterol, metaproterenol	Intermediate-acting	Same as epinephrine
Salmeterol	Long-acting	Same as epinephrine
Theophylline		
	Long-acting—sustained bronchodilation over a 24-hour period	Headache, seizures, cerebral vasoconstriction, gastrointestinal irritations, increased myocardial irritability
Anticholinergics		
Atropine methonitrate, atropine sulfate, ipratropium bromide (Atrovent), oxitropium bromide, glycopyrrolate bromide (Robinul)	Response is not as immediate as to a β-agonist. Using β-agonist and anticholinergics together can produce an additive and a more sustained effect than using large doses of either class alone.	Uncommon at therapeutic dose; dryness of mouth
Anti-inflammatory		
Corticosteroids	Effect on COPD is still controversial	Hypothalamic-pituitary-adrenal axis suppression, altered body shape (centripetal obesity), muscle atrophy, osteoporosis, hypertension
Beclomethasone dipropionate (BDP), triamcinolone (TAA), budesonide (BUD), flunisolide (FLU)		
Cromolyn		
Cromolyn sodium, nedocromil	Inhibits IgE-dependent histamine release from mast cells, blocks neuronal reflexes in the lung, and decreases airway reactivity; not a bronchodilator	Gastrointestinal irritations, increased cough, headache, dermatitis
Antibiotics		
Ampicillin	Used for acute exacerbations of bronchitis in COPD patients	Anaphylactic shock, urticaria, rash, pseudomembranous enterocolitis
Trimethoprim-sulfamethoxazole (Bactrim)	Used for acute exacerbations of bronchitis in COPD patients	Gastrointestinal irritations, skin rashes
Mucolytic-expectorant-mucoregulating drugs		
Acetylcysteine (Mucomyst)	A mucolytic drug that breaks down the polymeric structure of mucus	Severe bronchospasm if not accompanied by a β-agonist
Iodides	Expectorants increasing the flow of mucus	Iodide sensitivity—acneiform rash and hypothyroidism
Saturated solution of potassium iodide (SSKI), iodopropylene glycerol (Organidin)		
Guaifenesin	Same	
S-carboxymethylcysteine	A mucoregulating drug that favorably alters the constituents of mucus	

commonly used test is a 6-minute test that can be performed in the hallway of most facilities. Although it is more difficult under these circumstances than during a laboratory test, heart rate can be monitored during these tests using a heart rate monitor, and arterial **oxygen saturation** (Sao_2) can be measured by oximetry. These tests have the advantage that they are more functional and may give the clinician a better idea than a laboratory test as to how a patient will respond to activities of daily living.

It is important to monitor changes in arterial blood gases (arterial oxygen and carbon dioxide pressures—Pao_2 and $Paco_2$, respectively) during exercise in patients with pulmonary diseases. This can be done relatively cheaply and noninvasively using modern technology. Changes in arterial oxygen levels can be estimated using a **pulse oximeter**. This instrument passes light of specific wavelength through the patient's finger, ear, or other easily accessible surface of the skin to determine the level of arterial oxygen saturation

(SaO_2) of the hemoglobin (Hb). Because of the well-known relationship between PO_2 and SO_2 the PaO_2 can be estimated from measurements made during the systolic pulse. Knowing whether a pulmonary patient desaturates is the equivalent of knowing whether a cardiac patient shows ECG arrhythmias during exercise. The $PaCO_2$ is monitored using breath-by-breath measurements of **end-tidal** CO_2 ($P_{ET}CO_2$), where air is sampled at the mouth during exhalation so that the CO_2 measured at the end of a tidal breath reflects alveolar CO_2. In patients with COPD, $P_{ET}CO_2$ is not as precise an estimate of $PaCO_2$ as in healthy individuals, but it can provide information regarding the degree of **hyperventilation** or **hypoventilation** (CO_2 retention) during the exercise test. It is easier to monitor these physiologic variables during exercise in pa-

tients riding on a cycle ergometer, but the treadmill is a more natural movement for most patients and the results are better applied to daily living. Criteria for termination of the test include the inability of the patient to continue, a decrease in saturation below 75%, and cardiovascular abnormalities such as a decrease in pulse pressure or an ECG arrhythmia.

Exercise Response

The progressive nature of COPD is not reflected directly in changes in exercise capacity (Figure 11.1). Exercise capacity remains near normal until the **lung dysfunction** becomes severe. This lack of a linear relationship between ex-

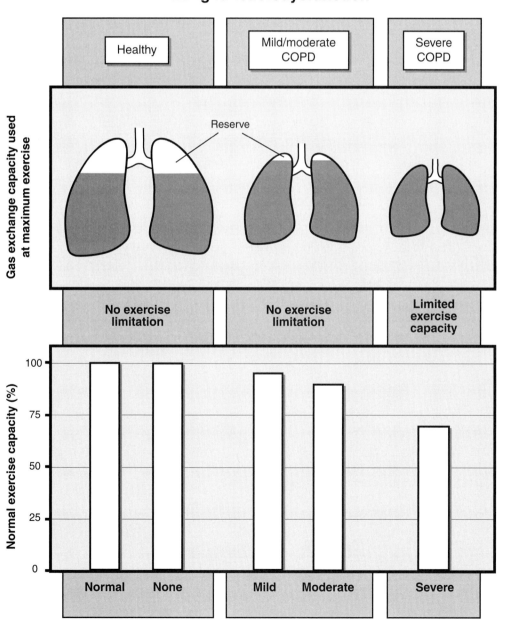

FIGURE 11.1. The concept and the effect of disease severity on **pulmonary reserve** is shown. The difference between the maximal available gas exchange capacity and the maximum used (i.e., reserve) is shown at the top in relation to the degree of lung dysfunction. Disease reduces and eventually eliminates this reserve until so little of the lung is left that exercise capacity is dramatically reduced in patients with severe lung dysfunction (*bottom*). COPD, chronic obstructive pulmonary disease.

ercise capacity and lung dysfunction probably is due to the lung function reserve discussed earlier. At maximal exercise in healthy individuals, approximately 20% of the lung's capacity to exchange gases is not used, but as the lung disease of COPD progresses this reserve is diminished and eventually disappears. It is only well after a considerable amount of the lung capacity has been lost that exercise capacity will be significantly reduced.

The response to exercise in COPD patients is characterized by a higher than normal minute ventilation ($\dot{V}_E$), an attenuated Vt response, and, in many patients, a decrease in arterial oxygen pressure (PaO_2) and an increase in carbon dioxide pressure ($PaCO_2$) (Figure 11.2). The basis for these changes is the destruction of the lung and consequent increases in Vd. These altered responses become progressively worse as the disease progresses and Vd increases.

Figure 11.3 describes the disease-related mechanical and gas exchange alterations that effect decreases in exercise capacity in COPD. The COPD-related obstruction results in airflow limitation and a decreased capacity to increase ventilation to meet the demands of exercise. The COPD-related lung destruction results in a loss of lung recoil (increased lung compliance), leading to pulmonary hyperinflation, which limits the mechanical effectiveness of the inspiratory muscles. This limitation results because the diaphragm is constantly in a shortened position. In some cases, the hyperinflation and loss of muscle effectiveness may lead to an increased susceptibility to diaphragm fatigue (9). The increased respiratory muscle energy required to breathe at the high lung volumes associated with hyperinflation is minimized by an increase in breathing frequency, which means that less of each breath reaches the alveoli, increasing dead space ventilation in the conducting airways such that the volume of each breath that simply moves in and out of the airways in

each breath (Vd/Vt) increases. The lung destruction also causes large increases in physiological Vd. Consequently, these patients increase $\dot{V}_E$ (see Figure 11.2A) in an attempt to maintain alveolar ventilation ($\dot{V}_A$) in the face of this increased Vd. The limited Vt response to exercise (see Figure 11.2B) reflects an inability to increase lung volume in the face of existing hyperinflation. The hyperinflation, in combination with expiratory airflow limitation, further limits the ability to increase ventilation. In addition to the mechanical disadvantage of the respiratory muscles, there is an independent effect of the disease on both respiratory and nonrespiratory muscles that may be related to malnutrition (10). The typical COPD patient with severe disease shows considerable muscle atrophy due, in part, to malnutrition.

The exercise-related decreases in PaO_2 and increases in $PaCO_2$ (see Figure 11.2C) are a result of the destructive process in the gas exchange units. The lung destruction leads to inhomogeneous distribution of both $\dot{V}_A$ and **lung perfusion** ($\dot{Q}$) in the lung and poor matching of $\dot{V}_A$ and $\dot{Q}$ ($\dot{V}_A/\dot{Q}$) (11–14). This creates areas of the lung with high levels of $\dot{V}_A$, but little or no $\dot{Q}$ (looking like Vd) and other areas with little or no $\dot{V}_A$, but considerable $\dot{Q}$ (looking like shunt), both contributing to decreased PaO_2. In this environment of poor $\dot{V}_A/\dot{Q}$ matching, a lower $P\bar{v}O_2$, such as occurs during exercise, will promote further reductions in PaO_2. Ultimately the situation evolves to a system that is unable to respond to the increased demands placed on it, thereby limiting exercise capacity.

In addition to these ventilatory-related exercise limitations, there is increasing evidence that alterations in peripheral blood flow and or limitations in O_2 extraction may affect exercise capacity in some patients with severe COPD (15). A plateau in leg $\dot{V}O_2$ during incremental cycle exercise, in spite of increasing total body $\dot{V}O_2$, indicates that a

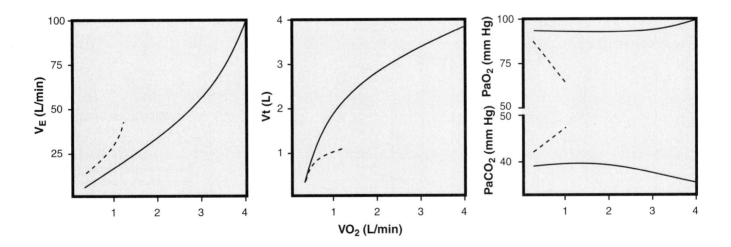

FIGURE 11.2. The ventilatory response to exercise, shown on the abscissa as oxygen consumption, in a healthy person (*solid line*) and in a person with severe COPD (*dashed line*). (**A**) minute ventilation; (**B**) tidal volume; (**C**) arterial oxygen and carbon dioxide levels.

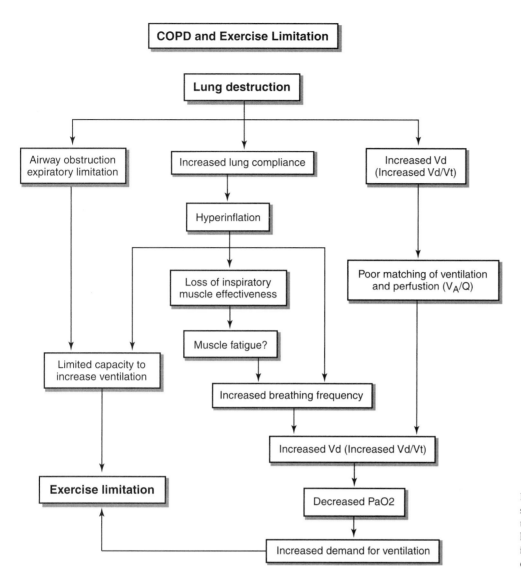

FIGURE 11.3. The dynamic relationships between the effects of COPD on the lung (i.e., airway obstruction and lung destruction) and the alterations in physiology that ultimately result in exercise limitation in these patients.

greater energy demand elsewhere may be compromising the ability of the body to increase perfusion to the working muscles. It has been hypothesized that the increased work of breathing in some patients with severe COPD may demand elevated blood flow, thereby depriving the working muscles of needed flow. Alternatively, a reduced tissue diffusion (16) of O_2 to the working muscles may account for the limitation in leg Vo_2 in selected patients. In either case, alterations in peripheral factors cannot be eliminated as possible exercise limiting factors in certain patients with COPD.

The ventilatory demand during exercise can be altered by diet and exercise mode. A high-carbohydrate diet, by elevating the **respiratory exchange ratio** (RER = $\dot{V}co_2/\dot{V}o_2$), increases the ventilatory requirement to expel CO_2. The ventilatory demand also is greater with walking than with cycling for patients with COPD (17). This exercise modality–dependent ventilatory response must be kept in mind when prescribing exercise for these patients.

Exercise Prescription

It would be tempting to assume that principles of exercise prescription appropriate for cardiac rehabilitation would also be appropriate for patients with COPD. Unfortunately, this is not true for all patients with COPD. Dyspnea (shortness of breath) and arterial desaturation make estimates of work capacity difficult, so that prescribing exercise at a standard percentage of peak is not possible (18). Likewise, the inability to define a lactate threshold in many of these patients makes this variable a less useful tool for establishing training exercise intensity (19). Finally, comorbid conditions (e.g., unstable heart disease, cor pulmonale) may preclude some patients from participation in rehabilitation.

Patients with mild disease, who do not desaturate or show no signs of CO_2 retention during exercise, show variable degrees of exercise limitation (see Figure 11.1). Patients with mild to moderate lung dysfunction are able to follow the standard recommendations for exercise in cardiac patients. These patients start exercise at an exercise intensity of 60% to 65% of peak work capacity and progress to an intensity of 75% to 80% of peak capacity as their conditioning levels increase.

When a patient with cardiac disease exercises, it is important to monitor the ECG for possible arrhythmias and the blood pressure for hypertension. The equivalent measure for patients with COPD, without heart disease, is the level of oxygen in the arterial blood. The need to insert an arterial sampling line has been eliminated through the use of noninvasive oxygen saturation monitors. Because there is a direct relationship between SaO_2 and PO_2, this provides an estimate of the level of oxygenation in the arterial blood. Chronically low SaO_2 can result in pulmonary hypertension and heart failure. To avoid this, many patients are required to use portable oxygen delivered through nasal cannula to avoid decreases in SaO_2 below 85% to 90%.

Patients with severe lung dysfunction who desaturate during exercise are exercised with more caution and with a more individualized prescription but seem to benefit considerably from participation in a comprehensive rehabilitation program (20). It is necessary to decide whether supplemental oxygen is required to maintain SaO_2 levels. In general, O_2 supplementation is required when SaO_2 decreases below 90% during exercise and sufficient O_2 is administered through nasal cannula to maintain SaO_2 at or above 90%. In some patients with extreme dysfunction, it becomes impossible to supply sufficient O_2 to prevent exercise-related desaturation, and exercise must be curtailed.

Rehabilitation

There is no cure for COPD. Goals are to improve function, reduce symptoms, and improve the patient's quality of life. The complexity of pulmonary rehabilitation requires a team approach. The team must include individuals with expertise in not only the medical treatment of these patients but also their psychological and social well-being (21). The team should include a pulmonary physician; respiratory, physical, and occupational therapists; dietitians; and psychologists (22, 23). The first step in rehabilitation is to promote smoking cessation, which reduces the decline in lung function (3). Patients, spouses, and others involved in the care of a patient should receive information regarding the disease, including its progression and treatment. If an exercise program is being considered, these individuals also should receive information from the GXT (if performed) and the implications of the disease in terms of quality of life. Admission to rehabilitation programs may require a physician's referral, and this has been shown to unnecessarily eliminate many patients from participation due to conservative attitudes among primary care physicians. This can be overcome through self-referral (24).

Hyperinflation is one of the primary factors causing exercise limitation (see Figure 11.3). Some clinicians advocate measures to reduce hyperinflation as the first step in rehabilitation. **Bronchodilators** can decrease hyperinflation by reducing airway resistance, improving airflow, and promoting lung emptying. Reducing the need to buffer **hypoxia**-induced lactic acid also may delay exercise-related hyperinflation. Supplemental oxygen decreases reliance on nonoxidative metabolism and minimizes the production of lactic acid. Of course, improvement of aerobic capacity through exercise training also can reduce this metabolic load.

Aerobic training for as little as 6 weeks improves exercise capacity and quality of life in patients with COPD who can tolerate high-intensity (25) as well as lower-intensity (26) exercise. High-intensity aerobic training also results in improvements in measures of peripheral muscle strength (25). Adding strength training to a standard aerobic training program appears to add little benefit in terms of exercise capacity or quality of life (26). According to one report, the benefits of 6 months of respiratory muscle and exercise training include a decrease in shortness of breath, an improvement in 6-minute walk time, and an improvement in quality of life that persisted for 2 years (27). The benefits of exercise training are intensity-related, such that unsupervised programs, which are associated with lower-intensity exercise, result in less—but still significant—change than supervised programs in which exercise intensity can be monitored and enforced (28).

Exercise training improves respiratory muscle performance, and respiratory muscle training improves exercise performance. Because dyspnea is a factor that limits exercise in most patients with COPD, it is important that rehabilitation attempt to reduce these symptoms. Regular camp exercise (29) and regular supervised exercise training result in increased respiratory muscle strength and endurance (30). Conversely, inspiratory muscle training in patients with COPD improves exercise capacity (31–33), although it is unclear whether this improvement is due to the training or other factors, such as desensitization to the fear of dyspnea, improved coordination, or group interaction, that are involved in rehabilitation programs (33). In any case, it appears that either general training that might emphasize training the respiratory muscles or specific training of the respiratory muscles should be part of rehabilitation in COPD patients. Pulmonary rehabilitation programs that include exercise may show little or no improvement in pulmonary function but consistently show improvements in dyspnea, exercise capacity, sleep, and appetite (34–37). One recent study (38) has reported that in some patients with COPD, exercise training may result in a limitation in the ability to neutralize exercise-produced oxygen-free radicals. Further research is needed to determine the implications of this research.

Depression, anxiety, and other psychiatric symptoms common to COPD can be improved with a comprehensive pulmonary rehabilitation program (39). The high incidence of these disorders suggests that a psychosocial component should be part of the pulmonary rehabilitation program (40). Short-term stress management and relaxation therapy (41–44) have not demonstrated long-term benefits, with one exception (45). These data suggest that, although these therapies alone have little or no effect on psychological profiles, when viewed in conjunction with other therapy and education programs they may contribute to a long-term positive impact on the quality of living in patients with COPD (46).

Pulmonary rehabilitation programs usually are structured in the same way as those that have been developed for cardiac rehabilitation (Table 11.3). For patients who are extremely ill and hospitalized for an acute exacerbation of their disease, the program should begin during this period of hospitalization (Phase I). Hospitalizations can be as short as several days but may last as long as several weeks. The activity that can be tolerated at this stage may be extremely limited, even with supplemental oxygen. Activity should include normal activities of daily living and should progress as quickly as possible to walking in the hallway. During this phase, physical therapy should progress as quickly as possible from passive to active range of motion and even active resistance exercises. Patients should be monitored for Sao_2 and heart rate if possible.

Phase II includes patients who have been discharged from inpatient care but who still show considerable disability. These patients should be exercised in a clinical setting where monitoring is still possible. Exercise prescription should be made with an exercise test with a GXT, if possible. Patients who are recovering from an acute exacerbation of their disease may progress rapidly in a Phase II program.

Other patients with severe lung dysfunction and dependency on supplemental O_2 may require phase II monitoring indefinitely. Patients with moderate lung dysfunction, or those who show good lung function after progressing through a Phase II program, may continue in a Phase III program. The objective of Phase III is to wean the patient from monitoring, if possible. Some patients in Phase III may continue in their need for oxygen supplementation, but the flow rate required to maintain Sao_2 at or above 90% should be determined with an exercise test. Finally, patients who have little lung dysfunction and normal exercise capacity and who require no monitoring should be encouraged to participate in activity in the community (Phase IV). Outpatient rehabilitation programs are effective in improving the patient's self-efficacy and perception of dyspnea as well as physical working capacity (47).

Cost Effectiveness

Pulmonary rehabilitation is cost-effective, with financial benefits to Medicare and other third-party payers and, most importantly, to COPD patients themselves (48). COPD is caused primarily by cigarette smoking. It causes over 100,000 deaths and costs over $20 billion dollars for direct care and for lost productivity annually. A rehabilitation program that results in smoking cessation can decrease both the human and financial costs. Pulmonary rehabilitation programs have been shown to reduce the number of hospital days, emergency department visits, doctor's office visits, and reliance on other health care services. Pulmonary rehabilitation programs also may help

TABLE 11.3. STRUCTURE AND CRITICAL ELEMENTS OF A REHABILITATION PROGRAM FOR PATIENTS WITH CHRONIC OBSTRUCTIVE PULMONARY DISEASE

Phase	Activity	Education	Psychosocial
I Inpatient	Bedside or in-room activity Active range of motion Progress to resistance to movement Monitor Sao_2 Supplement oxygen as necessary	Smoking cessation Self-reliance skills Teach awareness of dyspnea and methods to relieve	Treat depression and anxiety as needed
II Ambulation allowed; program under supervision	Progress to independence for self-care Progress to regular exercise of moderate (55–70% peak) intensity Monitor Sao_2 Supplement oxygen as necessary	Reinforce smoking cessation Diet and cooking Lung disease and work Employment issues Present community resources	Treat depression and anxiety as needed Assist in developing social skills necessary to integrate into community Employment issues
III Move from supervised to unsupervised program	Progress to increased involvement in activities of personal choice in the home and community Monitor Sao_2 at start, but wean as indicated Supplement oxygen as necessary	Reinforce smoking cessation Employment issues Reinforce previous concepts	Treat depression and anxiety as needed.
IV Community-based	Participate in normal activities in home and community Supplement oxygen as necessary		Treat depression and anxiety as needed

patients with COPD return to work and delay disability or early retirement. Individuals seeking pulmonary rehabilitation usually are older workers and generally are not good candidates for vocational rehabilitation training. Despite the limitation of age, after receiving pulmonary rehabilitation either as inpatients or outpatients, 25% of patients with COPD in one study were able to return to full-time employment, while only 3% of COPD patients could work full time without receiving pulmonary rehabilitation. Moreover, 19% of these patients with COPD who completed a pulmonary rehabilitation program were independent in self-care, compared with only 5% of patients without pulmonary rehabilitation (49). These statistics indicate that pulmonary rehabilitation programs have the potential to make a significant contribution to the well-being of patients and reduce the financial costs associated with this disease.

What We Know
About COPD and Exercise

1 It is clear that exercise capacity decreases as the lung dysfunction of COPD worsens. The decrement in exercise capacity, however, is not linear, with a relatively normal capacity in patients with mild to moderate dysfunction.

2 Once the disease reduces the normal reserve in gas exchange capacity, exercise capacity is reduced more dramatically.

3 Virtually all patients can benefit from exercise rehabilitation. Although the lung destruction associated with the disease will not be reversed, increases in muscle capacity, including the respiratory muscles, can effect improvements in the patient's ability to perform tasks of everyday living.

What We Would Like to Know
About COPD and Exercise

1 Chronic obstructive pulmonary disease is not a homogenous disease. We still do not know whether patients who are affected by the disease in one way will respond differently to rehabilitation than those who have a somewhat different disease process.

2 It is uncertain whether specific rehabilitation protocols may be more beneficial to some patients than oth-

ers. This knowledge would help us optimize rehabilitation for specific patients.

3 Finally, more research is needed to identify specific deficiencies in patients with COPD—for example, upper body tasks—and how rehabilitation can be tailored to address these weaknesses.

Summary

Chronic obstructive pulmonary disease is a debilitating disease that results in destruction of the lung. Exercise testing should be used along with pulmonary function testing to assess the status, the effects of therapy, and the progression of the disease in patients with COPD. Noninvasive monitoring of arterial oxygen levels using pulse oximetry is important during exercise testing and activity in patients with COPD. Knowing the level at which O_2 levels decrease during exercise is important in establishing safe activity intensity levels and in determining whether supplemental O_2 is necessary to maintain or increase arterial O_2 during periods of activity.

Exercise prescription should be made on the basis of exercise and pulmonary function status and should include a variety of aerobic activities of progressively increasing intensity. The progression should be determined on the basis of the response to exercise, using arterial O_2 levels as a guide. The rehabilitation program for patients with COPD should include education, rhythmic aerobic exercise, and, if desired, resistive exercise. The goal is to improve exercise tolerance and, if appropriate, return to work. Multidisciplinary programs have been shown to be effective in maintaining work capacity and reducing the health care costs of the disease.

DISCUSSION QUESTIONS

1. The total cost of COPD is estimated to be over $20 billion per year. What is included in this cost estimate?

2. What is the primary cause of COPD, and what are the mechanisms leading to a reduction in exercise capacity?

3. What are the critical variables to monitor during an exercise test, and what are some of the uses of an exercise test in patients with COPD?

4. What are the critical elements of a rehabilitation program during the different phases of pulmonary rehabilitation?

CASE STUDY

Patient Information

Mr. Stanley is a 75-year-old, 168-cm, 65-kg ex-carpenter with a diagnosis of emphysema. He has been a pack-a-day smoker for the past 50 years. He has a 35-year history of coughing and mucus production, with frequent upper respiratory infections. He has not worked for the past 10 years because he was unable to perform the demands of the job. More recently, he has been short of breath when performing low-level activities such as walking. His most recent pulmonary function tests show severe lung dysfunction.

Assessments

Test	Absolute Value	% Predicted
FVC	3.03 L	82%
FEV_1	1.1 L	38%
$FEF_{25-75\%}$	0.66 L/sec	24%
FRC	6.56 L	198%
Sao_2	88%	

His physician has requested a progressive exercise test with full monitoring of ventilatory variables, including minute ventilation ($\dot{V}_E$), tidal volume (Vt), frequency (Fb) and arterial oxygen saturation (Sao_2), and ECG. You select a modified Balke protocol with treadmill speed at 2.0 mph and 2% grade increments every 2 minutes.

Mr. Stanley reached a grade of 4% (3 METS) at a heart rate of 121 bpm. The test was terminated at that time because his Sao_2 had decreased to 72%.

Problem

Mr. Stanley's ventilatory results indicated **severe** COPD. His $\dot{V}_E$ is 110% of that expected at rest and remains higher than expected throughout the test, reaching 135% of expected at his peak load. His higher $\dot{V}_E$ was accomplished primarily through an increase in breathing frequency, with almost no increase in Vt from rest to exercise. His resting Vd/Vt ratio, an indication of dead space ventilation, was 46%, compared with a normal of 30%, and instead of decreasing to less than 10% at peak exercise, as in a healthy person, his Vd/Vt increased to over 50%. His increased $\dot{V}_E$ was not unexpected and probably was caused by the increase in Vd. However, on the basis of his airway obstruction you would have predicted a much greater increase in Vt than Fb. Your rationale was that the best strategy to minimize the increased resistance to airflow would have been to minimize increases in flow by increasing Vt.

Questions

1. How would you explain the unexpected breathing pattern?
2. At what phase in the rehabilitation program would you place Mr. Stanley, and what would your exercise prescription include?

REFERENCES

1. Hurd S. The impact of COPD on lung health worldwide: epidemiology and incidence. Chest 2000;117(2 Suppl):1S–4S.
2. Sullivan SD, Ramsey SD, Lee TA. The economic burden of COPD. Chest 2000;117 (2 Suppl):5S–9S.
3. Anthonisen NR, Connett JE, Kiley JP, et al. The Lung Health Study Research Group: effects of smoking intervention and the use of an inhaled anticholinergic bronchodilator on the rate of decline of FEV_1. JAMA 1994;272:1497–1505.
4. Covey MK, Larson JL, Wirtz S. Reliability of submaximal exercise tests in patients with COPD. Med Sci Sports Exerc 1999;31: 1257–1264.
5. Oga T, Nishimura K, Tsukino M, et al. The effects of oxitropium bromide on exercise performance in patients with stable chronic obstructive pulmonary disease. Am J Respir Crit Care Med 2000;161: 1897–1901.
6. Gallagher CG. Exercise limitation and clinical exercise testing in chronic obstructive pulmonary disease. Clin Chest Med 1994;15: 305–326.
7. Debigare R, Maltais F, Mallet M, et al. Influence of work rate incremental rate on the exercise responses in patients with COPD. Med Sci Sports Exerc 2000;32:1365–1368.
8. ACSM's Guidelines for Exercise Testing and Prescription. 6th Ed. Philadelphia: Lippincott Williams & Wilkins, 2000.

9. Mador MJ, Kufel TJ, Pineda LA, Sharma GK. Diaphragmatic fatigue and high-intensity exercise in patients with chronic obstructive pulmonary disease. Am J Respir Crit Care Med 2000;161:118–123.

10. Gosselink R, Troosters T, Decramer M. Distribution of muscle weakness in patients with stable chronic obstructive pulmonary disease. J Cardiopulmonary Rehabil 2000;20:353–360.

11. Mithoefer JC, Ramirez C, Cook W. The effect of mixed venous oxygenation on arterial blood in chronic obstructive pulmonary disease: the basis for a classification. Am Rev Respir Dis 1978;117:259–264.

12. Minh V-D, Lee HM, Dolan GF, et al. Hypoxemia during exercise in patients with chronic obstructive pulmonary disease. Am Rev Respir Dis 1979;120:787–794.

13. Raffestin B, Escourrou P, Legrand A, et al. Circulatory transport of oxygen in patients with chronic airflow obstruction exercising maximally. Am Rev Respir Dis 1982;125:426–431.

14. Wagner PD, Rodriguez-Roisin R. Clinical advances in pulmonary gas exchange. Am Rev Respir Dis 1991;143:883–888.

15. Simon M, LeBlanc P, Jobin J, et al. Limitation of lower limb VO_2 during cycling exercise in COPD patients. J Appl Physiol 2001;90:1013–1019.

16. Roca J, Hogan MC, Story D, et al. Evidence for tissue diffusion limitation of VO_{2max} in normal humans. J Appl Physiol 1989;67:291–299.

17. Palange P, Forte S, Onorati P, et al. Ventilatory and metabolic adaptations to walking and cycling in patients with COPD. J Appl Physiol 2000;88:1715–1720.

18. Simmons DN, Berry MJ, Hayes SI, Walschlager SA. The relationship between % HR_{peak} and % VO_{2peak} in patients with chronic obstructive pulmonary disease. Med Sci Sports Exerc 2000;32:881–886.

19. Zacarias EC, Neder JA, Cendom S, et al. Heart rate at the estimated lactate threshold in patients with chronic obstructive pulmonary disease: effects on the target intensity for dynamic exercise training. J Cardiopulmonary Rehabil 2000;20:369–376.

20. Niderman MS, Clemente PH, Fein AM, et al. Benefits of a multidisciplinary pulmonary rehabilitation program. Improvements are independent of lung function. Chest 1991;99:798–804.

21. Lyth JR. Model of the team approach. In: Banja JD, Jann BB, Wolf L, eds. Rehabilitation Medicine: Contemporary Clinical Perspectives. Philadelphia: Lea & Febiger, 1992.

22. Pulmonary rehabilitation: joint ACCP/AACVPR evidence-based guidelines. ACCP/AACVPR. Pulmonary Rehabilitation Guidelines Panel. American College of Chest Physicians. American Association of Cardiovascular and Pulmonary Rehabilitation Chest 1997;112:1363–1396.

23. Resnikoff PM, Ries AL. Pulmonary rehabilitation for chronic lung disease. J Heart Lung Transplantation 1998;17:643–650.

24. Bickford LS. National pulmonary rehabilitation survey. Respiratory Care 1988;33:1030–1042.

25. Gimenez M, Servera P, Vergara P, et al. Endurance training in patients with chronic obstructive pulmonary disease: a comparison of high versus moderate intensity. Arch Phys Med Rehabil 2000;81:102–109.

26. Bernard S, Whittom F, Leblanc P, et al. Aerobic and strength training in patients with chronic obstructive pulmonary disease. Am J Respir Crit Care Med 1999;159:896–901.

27. Guell R, Casan P, Belda J, et al. Long-term effect of outpatient rehabilitation of COPD: a randomized trial. Chest 2000;117:976–983.

28. Puente-Maestu L, Sanz ML, Sanz P, et al. Comparison of effects of supervised versus self-monitored training programmes in patients with chronic obstructive pulmonary disease. Eur Respir J 2000;15:517–525.

29. Keens TG, Krastins IR, Wannamaker EM, et al. Ventilatory muscle endurance training in normal subjects and patients with cystic fibrosis. Am Rev Respir Dis 1977;116:853–860.

30. Orenstein DM, Franklin BA, Doershuk CF, et al. Exercise conditioning and cardiopulmonary fitness in cystic fibrosis: the effects of a three-month supervised running program. Chest 1981;80:392–398.

31. Belman MJ, Mittman C. Ventilatory muscle training improves exercise capacity in chronic obstructive pulmonary disease patients. Am Rev Respir Dis 1980;121:273–280.

32. Pardy RL, Rivington RN, Despas PJ, Macklem PT. Inspiratory muscle training compared with physiotherapy in patients with chronic airflow limitation. Am Rev Respir Dis 1981;123:421–425.

33. Levine S, Weiser P, Gillen J. Evaluation of a ventilatory muscle endurance training program in the rehabilitation of patients with chronic obstructive pulmonary disease. Am Rev Respir Dis 1986;133:400–406.

34. Hodgkin J. Benefits and the future of pulmonary rehabilitation. In: Hodgkin JE, Connors GL, Bell CW, eds. Pulmonary Rehabilitation: Guidelines to Success. Philadelphia: JB Lippincott, 1993.

35. Carter R, Nicotra B, Clark L, et al. Exercise conditioning in the rehabilitation of patients with chronic obstructive pulmonary disease. Arch Phys Med Rehabil 1988;69:118–122 .

36. Cockroft AE, Saunders MJ, Berry G. Randomised controlled trial of rehabilitation in chronic respiratory disability. Thorax 1981;36:200–203.

37. Casaburi R. Exercise training in chronic obstructive lung disease. In: Casaburi R, Petty TL (eds). Principles and Practice of Pulmonary Rehabilitation. Philadelphia: WB Saunders, 1993:204–224.

38. Rabinovich RA, Ardite E, Troosters T, et al. Reduced muscle redox capacity after endurance training in patients with chronic obstructive pulmonary disease. Am J Respir Crit Care Med 2001;164:1114–1118.

39. Gift AG, McCrone SH. Depression in patients with COPD. Heart Lung 1993;22:289–297.

40. Emery CF, Leatherman NE, Burker EJ, MacIntyre NR. Psychological outcomes of a pulmonary rehabilitation program. Chest 1991;100:613–617.

41. Blake RL Jr, Vandiver TA, Braun S, et al. A randomized controlled evaluation of psychosocial intervention in adults with chronic lung disease. Family Medicine 1990;22:365–370.

42. Sassi-Dambron DE, Eakin EG, Ries AL, Kaplan RM. Treatment of dyspnea in COPD. A controlled clinical trial of dyspnea management strategies. Chest 1995;107:724–729.

43. Renfroe KL. Effect of progressive relaxation on dyspnea and state anxiety in patients with chronic obstructive pulmonary disease. Heart Lung 1988;17:408–413.

44. Gift AG, Moore T, Soeken K. Relaxation to reduce dyspnea and anxiety in COPD patients. Nursing Research 1992;41:242–246.

45. Tandon MK. Adjunct treatment with yoga in chronic severe airway obstruction Thorax 1978;33:514–517.

46. Emery CF, Schein RL, Hauck ER, MacIntyre NR. Psychological and cognitive outcomes of a randomized trial of exercise among patients with chronic obstructive pulmonary disease. Health Psychology 1998;17:232–240.

47. Scherer YK, Schmieder LE. The effect of a pulmonary rehabilitation program on self-efficacy, perception of dyspnea, and physical endurance. Heart Lung 1997;26:15–22.

48. Radovich JL, Hodgkin JE, Burton GG, Yee AR. Cost-effectiveness of pulmonary rehabilitation program. In: Hodgkin J (ed). Pulmonary Rehabilitation: Guidelines to Success. Philadelphia: JB Lippincott, 1993:548–561.

49. Hass A, Cardon H. Rehabilitation in chronic obstructive pulmonary disease. Med Clin North Am 1969;53;593–606.

CHAPTER 12

Cystic Fibrosis

Matthias Huetler, Ralph Beneke

Overview

Cystic fibrosis (CF) is the most common life-limiting genetic disorder in Caucasians (Box 12.1). This autosomal recessive disease is found in about 1 in 2000 to 4000 in live births. The central feature of this chronic progredient disease is the presence of an abnormal, highly adherent, viscous mucus in epithelium-lined organs. The organs most often affected are the lungs, pancreas, intestines, and sweat glands. Clinical hallmarks are **chronic pulmonary disease**, **exocrine pancreatic insufficiency**, and high sodium and chloride content in the sweat (1). Most of the morbidity and mortality of CF can be attributed to the effects of the disease in the lungs. Currently, the life expectancy of persons with CF is between 30 and 40 years (2).

Cystic fibrosis is caused by mutations in a single gene encoding for the CF transmembrane conductance regulator (CFTR) on chromosome 7 (3). This protein, which primar-

Cystic fibrosis is a progressive multiorgan disease. The primary affected organs are the lungs, pancreas, intestines, and sweat glands. Impaired lung function and malnutrition are the deciding factors for the clinical aspect of the disease, hospitalization, and survival rate.

ily acts as a chloride channel, is expressed in epithelial cells and is central in determining transepithelial salt transport, fluid flow, and ion concentrations (1). The most common CFTR mutation, found in two thirds of cases (2), leads to a disruption of CFTR biosynthesis, which is associated with the classic severe CF phenotype.

The disease is marked by a great variability in the frequency and severity of clinical manifestations and complications (4). Diagnosis is suggested by clinical manifestations of exocrine pancreatic insufficiency or chronic pulmonary disease and then confirmed by a positive result on sweat or genetic testing (5). The genotype not only determines severity and progress of the disease but also seems to be an independent factor of exercise tolerance (6). Approximately 80% to 90% of patients have an exocrine pancreatic insufficiency. The resulting gastrointestinal complications usually are the first signs of CF to be noted and lead to the diagnosis before the age of 1 year in 70% of cases (4). Malnutrition and poor weight gain and growth are subsequent complications. Almost all patients have chronic sinopulmonary disease. The pulmonary aspect of CF is characterized by excessive mucus production, airway obstruction, chronic endobronchial infection, and airway inflammation leading to progressive lung destruction (7), fibrosis, and, finally, **respiratory failure** (4). Typical symptoms are **dyspnea**, cough, wheezing, and recurrent infections. The pulmonary disease is the primary cause of death for most patients with CF (4) and is responsible for 75% of all hospital admissions (8).

Care and Therapy

Careful monitoring of pulmonary, nutritional, and metabolic parameters coupled with a complex standardized therapy in specialized care centers (Box 12.2) can lead to

BOX 12.2. **Care and Therapy for Cystic Fibrosis**

Treatment aims for patients with CF are to prevent or to slow down the decline of lung function, to improve nutritional status, and to optimize quality of life. In end-stage disease, transplantation of the primarily affected organ is the only therapeutic option for intermediate-term survival.

increased life expectancy for the patient with CF. There is a correlation between nutritional state, pulmonary state, and survival figures (9). Treatment aims are to prevent or slow the decline of lung function and improve nutritional status but also to optimize quality of life.

Regular tests of pulmonary function are used to monitor the progression of airway disease and response to treatment. One generally recognized measure of loss of pulmonary function is a decline of the forced expiratory volume in 1 second, usually expressed as a percentage of the predicted volume (FEV_1). A reduced FEV_1 with signs of obstruction as well as overinflation with an increased total lung capacity and **residual volume** is typical in CF (10). The FEV_1 is used to describe severity of lung disease in CF and is one of the most important outcome criteria in the clinical evaluation of patients with CF. Simple anthropometric measures such as body weight, body mass index, or growth in children are used to monitor nutritional status.

Conventional Therapy

The effects of cystic fibrosis on the lungs are the most threatening. **Antibiotics**, **mucolytics**, and standard chest physiotherapy are used to keep the airways clear of excessive secretions and to treat intercurrent infections effectively (11). Anti-inflammatory medication and **bronchodilators** are used to treat inflammation and reversible lung obstruction. Oxygen supplementation is necessary intermittently in advanced disease and continuously in end-stage disease.

Adequate attention to nutrition is essential in the patient with CF. Standard management of the characteristic exocrine pancreatic insufficiency includes supplementation of pancreatic enzyme, fat-soluble vitamin supplementation, and a high-calorie diet. If caloric intake fails to meet the requirement, more aggressive approaches include nocturnal enteral feeding (e.g., by gastrostomy) or parenteral nutrition. Medication with positive effects on nitrogen balance is discussed for special cases. In about 10% of patients the exocrine pancreatic insufficiency is associated with endocrine insufficiency (**diabetes mellitus**), requiring diabetic control and therapy. Diabetes tends to develop late in the course of the disease.

Transplantation

In end-stage disease, transplantation of the primarily affected organ remains the only therapeutic option for intermediate-term survival. Because it is the lung aspect of the disease that causes most of the mortality, CF is a major indication for lung transplantation, with a 5-year survival rate of about 50% (8).

The Exercise Response

Exercise response is extremely variable in patients with CF because it is related to the severity of the disease, which significantly modulates exercise capacity (Box 12.3).

In the mildly affected patient exercise capacity and the ability to perform tasks of daily life often are normal. Patients, most of whom are young, can participate in sports activities and social life. As the disease progresses, exercise capacity and the ability to perform the physical work of daily living decrease (12). Normally the ventilatory system becomes the major exercise-limiting factor. The patient's lifestyle becomes more sedentary, leading to deconditioning. This loss of conditioning combined with the **malnutrition** that often gets worse with disease progression contributes to further limitation of exercise (13). In end-stage disease, exercise capacity is nearly lost.

The observed range of exercise capacity in terms of peak oxygen uptake or peak work load is wide. Peak data range from more or less normal values in mildly affected patients to extremely low in severely affected patients (14). The exercise response in mild-moderate lung disease is nearly comparable to that of healthy controls. In moderate-severe disease the decline in lung function and the patient's nutritional status become the performance-limiting factors (13). The influence of malnutrition may be mediated by loss of muscle mass and decreased muscle function (14, 15). Decreased muscle strength (16), muscle force (17), and abnormalities in oxygen (18) or energy metabolism (19) have been reported in patients with CF. Ventilatory muscle strength and endurance normally are preserved or even increased in most patients (20, 21).

As the lung disease progresses, the structural and functional changes lead to an increase in deadspace ventilation. To maintain the effective alveolar ventilation at any given level of exercise, the total ventilatory demand increases depending on the severity of the disease. The peak minute ventilation often approaches or exceeds the resting maximal voluntary ventilation, indicating no further ventilatory reserve.

BOX 12.3. The Exercise Response in Cystic Fibrosis

The exercise response in patients with CF is extremely variable. It is related to the severity of the disease, mainly lung function and nutritional status. In the mildly affected patient, exercise capacity and the ability to perform activities of daily living often are normal. With disease progression, exercise capacity and the ability to perform the physical work of daily living decrease. The subsequent more sedentary lifestyle amplifies all aspects of deconditioning. In end-stage disease, the exercise capacity is nearly lost. Successful clinical therapy improves exercise capacity, but it may impair acute response and adaptation to exercise training.

Ventilation becomes the limiting factor for oxygen transport and exercise (22). The **restrictive** lung changes cause relative low tidal volume and high respiratory rate at a given exercise level. In severe disease, tidal volume often is near maximal at rest, and the increase in ventilation is achievable only by increasing respiratory rate (23). An exercise-induced bronchoconstriction is observed only rarely (24).

In most patients the increase in **cardiac output** with exercise is adequate (25). With advanced disease, the **stroke volume** response may become compromised (26) Maximal heart rate can be lower than predicted, indicating that the cardiovascular system is not exercise limiting (22). The heart rate response to increasing workload in patients with CF has been found to be similar to that of healthy subjects (27).

Patients with moderate to severely impaired lung function indicated by an $FEV_{1\%}$ of less than about 60% (28) regularly experience **exercise-induced hypoxemia (EIH)**. The extent of EIH cannot be predicted and a possible related effect on cardiac function is not clear. An interrelationship between hypoxemia and fall in stroke volume cannot be excluded (29). However, it has been suggested that brief exercise periods of EIH are not harmful (23, 30). In severely affected patients not only EIH but also **exercise-induced hypercapnia** is frequently observed (31). Resting hypercapnia is acutely worsened by exercise.

Impact of Therapy

Successful clinical therapy clearly improves exercise capacity (32, 33). Based on the clear relationship among lung function, nutritional status, and exercise capacity, therapeutic options that have the potential to improve lung function may also increase peak exercise capacity and decrease the physiologic and psychophysical strain of any given submaximal exercise.

Conventional Therapy

The chronic use of significant amounts of highly potent medication probably has other effects on exercise response, both direct and indirect. However, few data are available on this topic. Chronic application of **corticosteroids** is known to induce **myopathy**, which is characterized by loss of leg muscle, muscle weakness, and decreased muscle strength and endurance.

The main caloric energy source used in dietary supplementation also may influence the metabolic response to exercise by favoring either the lipid or carbohydrate metabolism. Fat-dominated caloric supplementation reduces the ratio between metabolic glycogen and fat utilization. This slightly increases oxygen demand, requiring higher ventilation at given workloads. Improvement of nutritional status—for example, via a gastrostomy—may increase performance capacity. However, irritations of the skin, peristomal leaking, or the location of the gastrostomy itself may cause discomfort, reducing exercise compliance and performance.

If severe EIH occurs during exercise, oxygen supplementation has been reported to reduce the magnitude of desaturation and decrease minute ventilation and heart rate during submaximal work. In severely affected patients peak exercise capacity can be increased by supplemental oxygen (34).

Transplantation

Transplantation for end-stage disease with nearly lost exercise capacity completely changes performance-limiting factors. After successful organ transplantation, the organ that previously was most severely impaired no longer plays a primarily limiting role for exercise. Medication becomes increasingly important and may influence the exercise response. Immunosuppressive therapy contributes to the markedly reduced muscle function in lung transplant recipients (35). **Arterial hypertension** may occur in the posttransplant period, and the enormous influence of **antihypertensive medication** on exercise response must be considered.

Is Maximal Exercise Testing Recommended?

On principle, every exercise program should be safe, and the exercise prescription should be based on appropriate and objective testing results (Box 12.4). In pulmonary disease the evaluation of exercise tolerance, physical limitations, and especially the requirement for supplemental oxygen is recommended before the patient begins any exercise training program (36, 37). Commonly used tests are incremental, submaximal, or maximal exercise tests or ramp test protocols, submaximal steady-state constant workload tests, and timed distance walk tests. Absolute and relative contraindications are comparable with those in cardiac patients (38).

BOX 12.4.   Is Maximal Exercise Testing Recommended?

Exercise testing to maximum levels can be safely conducted even in severely affected patients with CF. Submaximal testing may be impossible due to minimized exercise capacity. In severely impaired patients any increase of the metabolic rate above rest may provoke physical strain.

Safe testing procedure:

- knowledge of the patient's medical history, current status, and medication
- a test program considering the severity of the patient's disease and current therapy
- adequate monitoring.

Incremental exercise testing, the method most commonly used to determine a baseline performance capacity, makes it possible to evaluate the functional impact of any interventional process. Generally accepted submaximal measures of performance such as anaerobic ventilatory or lactate threshold may be affected by the individual pattern of the patient's CF or specific impacts of therapy on exercise-induced acute reactions. This may impair interpretability and validity of such submaximal parameters (39). Severely impaired patients may not show any submaximal measure of performance capacity. Any type of testing may provoke maximal physical strain due to these patients' minimized exercise capacity. Independently of such limitations, the identification of limiting factors and the real level of individual performance reserve require symptom-limited (i.e., disease-specific) maximal exercise testing. Both identification of limiting factors and knowledge of the performance reserve are prerequisites for prescribing safe and effective exercise programs on an individual basis, and for valid documentation of any program outcome.

Exercise testing to maximum levels can be conducted safely even in severely affected patients. Maximal exercise tests typically are performed on treadmill or electronically braked bicycle ergometer. The initial workload—and, more importantly, workload increments—should be selected according to the patient's age, anthropometric measures, and disease severity as expressed by FEV_1 (40) to ensure meaningful testing results. Workload usually is increased in increments of 1 to 2 minutes. Relevant measures are workload capacity and spirometric measures such as oxygen uptake, tidal volume, breathing frequency, expired ventilation, end-tidal carbon dioxide partial pressure ($petCO_2$), oxygen saturation, and heart rate, measured via electrocardiogram (ECG). Transcutaneous pulse oximetry can be used to monitor oxygen saturation noninvasively if limitations are considered (41).

Constant load tests at submaximal workloads to measure maximal performance time and timed distance walk tests to determine maximal walking distance per a given period of time are alternate tools for performance testing. They do not enable direct determination of maximum workloads or walking velocities, but they are useful supplementary tools to evaluate the external validity of previous exercise prescriptions. The latter may be of special relevance because the individual pattern of multifactorial diseases such as CF and consecutive therapeutic consequences may significantly affect the time-related response to given workload intensities.

Exercise Programming Options

General Recommendations

Regular exercise is generally recommended in patients with CF of all ages and all disease stages (Box 12.5). The capacity to benefit from regular exercise is assumed to be normal in

BOX 12.5. **Exercise Programming Options**

Regular exercise usually is recommended for patients with CF of all ages and all disease stages. Every exercise program should be safe. Training programs should be progressively designed. Exercise prescriptions should follow general recommendations with respect to volume, frequency, and intensity and need to be based on objective testing results. Endurance, resistance, and circuit training have been proved to be successful methods of training. New exercise prescriptions require evaluation during subsequent training sessions.

Special recommendations and potential adverse effects of exercise apply to different disease aspects, as follows:
- Lung: hypoxia, hypercapnia, bronchoconstriction, pneumothorax, hemoptysis
- Diabetes mellitus: hypo- or hyperglycemia
- Malnutrition: inadequate caloric intake, negative nitrogen balance
- Osteoporosis, osteopenia: fractures
- Liver/spleen: bleeding, hematoma
- Sweat glands: dehydration, electrolyte loss

mild to moderate disease (42). In severe disease, the benefit may be even more pronounced, because the degree of improvement is inversely related to initial fitness (23). The exercise program should be designed to increase or maintain the patient's overall fitness but also to influence specific disease-related problems positively. In general, the exercise program should be designed progressively, which can be best realized in supervised programs. The progression may relate to exercise frequency, exercise duration, and intensity (38). In patients with CF, all studies using a progression have reported positive effects of the training program (42–44).

Aerobic endurance training and resistance training are the two major elements of exercise programs for patients with CF. The traditional outcome measures in studies on the effect of regular exercise are exercise tolerance, lung function, ventilatory muscle function, **sputum** expectoration, and breathlessness. In the recent past, psychological well-being and peripheral muscle function have gained increasing interest and are now included in the list of outcome measures. Peripheral muscle function is a useful measure because appropriate muscle training can be used to influence a muscular detraining state associated with increasing sedentary lifestyle, medication-induced myopathia, and osteoporosis or osteoporosis-associated phenomena. **Osteoporosis** and **osteopenia** are common findings in adults with CF (45)

Using all the available clinical data and paying special attention to previous exercise testing, the exercise program should be prescribed individually for each patient, taking into consideration that person's disease severity, initial fitness level, and exercise response as important determinants. An initial program should have a minimum duration

of 8 to 12 weeks to ensure that substantial training gains can be achieved. Appropriate supervision helps to optimize the success of an exercise program. The latter is a particularly important problem in home exercise programs.

Special recommendations pertain to EIH and salt loss during exercise. The general recommendation is to maintain the oxygen saturation level in arterial blood above 90% (40). In patients with more severe impairment, however, lower levels of arterial oxygen saturation cannot always be avoided even when oxygen supplementation is used. Such short episodes, which also can be observed in daily life, have not yet been proved to be harmful. Furthermore, due to the underlying pathophysiology of CF, special care should be taken to maintain adequate fluid and salt intake, particularly during exercise in hot climates and during endurance events.

Endurance Exercise Program

The traditional way to increase cardiovascular fitness is performance of aerobic exercise involving large muscle masses (Boxes 12.6 and 12.7). Studies have demonstrated increased fitness from any kind of training using swimming, walking and jogging (42, 46–48), ergometer training (44, 49), nonspecific sports, or trampoline exercise (48, 50). Running is suitable only for mildly to moderately impaired patients, because minimum exercise capacity (i.e., an oxygen uptake of more than 20–25 ml/kg/ min) is necessary for running (51). Ideally, each training session consists of three phases: warm-up (5–10 minutes); an endurance phase (20–60 minutes); and cool-down (5–10 minutes). A recreational phase is optional.

The minimum total exercise time needed to maintain physical fitness is 60 to 90 minutes per week. The duration and frequency may vary from 5 to 10 minutes once or twice a day in severely ill patients to 30 to 40 minutes 2 to 3 times a week in mildly affected patients. Ideally, 20 to 60 minutes 3 to 5 times a week are recommended to increase physical fitness in healthy subjects (38). In patients with CF, successful exercise programs were described as using 5 to 60 minutes two or three times a week (42, 43, 46–48; see Boxes 12.6 and 12.7), 10 to 20 minutes 5 times a week (44, 52), 15 minutes daily (53), and "regular" (49, 54). Realization of these goals depends, however, on disease severity, total program duration, **supervision** mode, patient motivation, and daily time already spent for therapy. As the number of hours spent on therapy per day is negatively correlated with quality of life (55), additional time constraints may adversely affect patient **compliance** and **adherence**.

The exercise intensity of prolonged endurance training should be submaximal, and the results of the initial exercise test should be used to prescribe intensity individually using standard recommendations (38). In CF the heart rate is the measure most often used to prescribe exercise intensity (42, 43, 47, 48, 52). Exercise duration may vary, from 10 to 30

BOX 12.6. Results of a 3-Month Training Program

Study design: nonrandomized, controlled
Number of subjects: n = 21 (control, n = 10)
Age of subjects: 10–30 years
Disease severity: FEV_1: 32–81% of vital capacity
Program duration and type: 3 months, institution
Exercise mode: main component walking, jogging
Exercise duration: 60 minutes, including 5–10 minutes for
   warm-up, 10–30 minutes aerobic activity, 5 minutes for
   cool-down
Exercise frequency: 3 times a week
Exercise intensity: 70–85% of HR_{peak}
Progression: yes
Supervision: each session
Main training effect: (1) improved exercise tolerance;
   (2) lower HR at given workload

Data from Orenstein et al. (42)

minutes, at exercise intensities between 50% and 80% of maximum heart rate, or 45% and 75% of heart rate reserve, or peak oxygen uptake. In severely affected patients the lower limits of standard recommendations should be used for prescription. Prediction based on estimated rather than measured values should be avoided (40). The prescription should be reviewed after the first sessions and adapted if necessary, particularly in patients with severe disease. Maximal workload also has been used as a basis for intensity prescription (44, 52).

Interval training can be used as an alternative in cardiovascular training. In severely impaired patients it may be the only possible mode of endurance training. The change between more intense exercise and low or no exercise enables the patient to recover in between the more intense elements. This form of training often is the most practical form of training in severely affected patients with low exercise capacity. One possible prescription for cycle ergometer training is 2-minute intervals 6 to 8 times per session at an intensity of 50% of maximum workload, with 1-minute intervals of 25% or no exercise in between the higher-intensity intervals. No studies about the effect of longer-term interval training in patients with CF are available.

Resistance Training

In addition to training for muscle strength and endurance, resistance training related to the lung aspect of the disease is to be considered in patients with CF.

The general training program consists of exercises that train the major muscle groups of the body. The lung disease–related program consists of training focused on the upper body (38), and specific ventilatory muscle training. The effect of nonspecific training on ventilatory muscle

function is similar to that of the specific training. Consequently, specific training is reserved for special cases, particularly patients with markedly decreased muscle strength (38). Voluntary normocapnic hyperpnea and breathing through a high inspiratory resistance are methods of the specific ventilatory muscle training (20, 56–58). The exercise prescription for nonspecific resistance training is essentially the same as that recommended for healthy subjects (38). Exercise frequency should be 2 or 3 times a week. The resistance training program should allow for three sets of 10 to 15 repetitions per muscle group. Every contraction should be coordinated with expiration to minimize the possibly increased risk of a **pneumothorax**. Children should not be excluded from supervised resistance training programs (59).

Circuit Training

Circuit training combines elements of endurance and weight training and has corresponding benefits. Because it is a highly physically demanding and effective training method, it should be done no more than once a week. The exercises usually are easy with respect to coordinative tasks. This training method can be used in any age group as long as exercises are selected appropriately. The workload should be individually adjusted based on the individual patient's performance capacity. Four to eight exercises using different muscle groups can be combined. Each exercise normally lasts 30 seconds, with a subsequent break of 60 to 120 seconds, depending on disease severity.

BOX 12.7. A Home Exercise Program

Study design: randomized, controlled
Number of subjects: n = 30 (control, n = 35)
Age: 13.4 ± 3.9 yrs (range, 7–19)
Disease severity: mild-moderate, FEV_1 > 40% pred
mean 89 ± 20% pred
Program duration and type: 3 years, home exercise
Exercise mode: free choice, with jogging, swimming, cycling,
   football recommended
Exercise duration: 5 minutes for warm-up, at least 20 minutes
   aerobic activity, 5 minutes for cool-down
Exercise frequency: at least 3 times a week
Exercise intensity: 70–80% of HR_{max} corresponding to about
   150 bpm
Progression: no
Supervision: (1) telephone contact every 4-6 weeks; (2) self-
   recorded physical activity in a daily diary; (3) other sup-
   portive activities
Main training effect: (1) slower lung function decline; (2) no
   effect on exercise tolerance

Data from Schneiderman-Walker et al. (48)

Potential Physiological Adaptations and Associated Mechanisms

Regular exercise training of at least 6 weeks, regardless of training mode, intensity, and duration, has been shown to improve cardiorespiratory fitness and muscle performance and to provide psychological benefits. The influence on lung function is small but still exists (Box 12.8).

Cardiorespiratory Fitness

Exercise conditioning has been reported to improve peak work capacity (42–44, 47, 53), peak oxygen uptake (42, 44, 53), peak heart rate, peak oxygen pulse (53), and peak ventilation (44). These effects have been observed for a wide range of disease severity and age, in short- and long-term studies, and using various exercise modes and prescriptions. However, only a few studies were controlled and supervised (42, 43, 47). With respect to the progression of chronic diseases in long-term studies, a training effect may be reflected not only by an increased but also by an unchanged exercise tolerance (48, 49, 60). Further indicators of successful conditioning are decreased heart rate (42) and diminished sensations of breathlessness (61) at given submaximal levels of workload indicating a reduced physiological strain.

Lung Function

The effects of exercise conditioning on lung function are small. However, it has been suggested that exercise may contribute to stabilization of lung function (42, 48, 60). One causal factor of this stabilizing effect may be a positive effect on airway clearance (44, 62, 63). Another one may be an exercise-induced increase in water content of the mucus in the lung (64). The **residual volume** has been found to be decreased after nonspecific, whole-body exercises (60, 61, 65) or resistance training (66). Possible mechanisms are an improved lung ventilation pattern (60) or increased chest wall mobility (66). The decrease of **residual volume** could improve ventilatory muscle function and sensation of breathing.

> **BOX 12.8. Potential Physiologic Adaptations and Associated Mechanisms**
>
> General beneficial effects on the cardiorespiratory system and peripheral muscles can be detected from specific aspects of the disease, such as improved sputum expectoration and airway clearance, altered ventilatory patterns, chest wall mobility, stabilized lung function, and also psychological well-being.

Ventilatory Muscle Function

Respiratory muscle strength or endurance can be increased by specific muscle training (20, 56–58), upper body exercise (20), or an aerobic exercise program (20, 42, 46, 65). The effect does not depend on the specificity of the training stimulus, indicating that even the ventilatory demand of nonspecific exercise appears to be beneficial for the respiratory muscles (20, 42). Independent of beneficial results the effect of specific respiratory muscle training on measures of lung function and exercise performance remains unclear (20, 40, 56–58), but may depend on program duration (57).

Peripheral Muscle Function

Muscle strength has been shown to be improved after 6 months of resistance training 3 times per week (66) but also improves after 6 months of nonspecific cycling training done for 20 minutes 5 times per week (52). The effect of the cycling program was confined to the muscle groups mainly involved in cycling. Increased muscle mass (66), remodeling of muscle, and improved neuromuscular coordination have been thought to contribute to the improvement (52). In general, approximately 20 units of resistance training appear to be the minimum needed to gain an effect on muscle mass (67). Although not measured, the improved muscle performance may help to reduce the physiological and psychological strain of a given level of submaximal exercise (68).

Well-Being

Physical fitness is related to the feeling of well-being in patients with CF (69). Positive influences of exercise conditioning on factors contributing to this sense of well-being have been reported in children and adults of varying disease status (44, 48, 52, 53, 60).

Limitations

The results of studies on the effect of exercise conditioning in patients with CF are not consistent. One widely accepted suggestion is that the effects of exercise are small but do exist. Multiple factors including study design, studied populations, investigated measures, and lung function may have impaired the clarity of results (Box 12.9).

Study Design

Only few studies have been done utilizing a **controlled** study design, sufficient sample size, adequate exercise programming, and a mode of supervision (42, 48). Exercise conditioning in a clinical setting differs from home exercise

BOX 12.9. **Exercise Limitations in CF**

Current literature on the effect of exercise conditioning in patients with CF does not report consistent results. One reason may be a variety of limitations in the design of previous studies. In part these limitations result from the fact that CF is associated with a multifactorial impairment of health and performance is strongly affected by the therapeutic situation.
Training adaptations also may be diminished by progression of the disease.

training programs in many ways, and comparisons between them are difficult. Supportive therapy, exercise prescription, duration of the program, mode of supervision, and compliance are important aspects to be taken into consideration.

Study Population

Although CF is the most common genetic disorder in Caucasians, it often is difficult to investigate a sufficient number of patients to allow for general conclusions. The significant drop-out rates reported (up to about 35% [44]) add to this difficulty. Minimizing this rate is a special challenge and is particularly important in long-term home exercise programs. The typical CF population involves patients from childhood to young adult (42). When evaluating the effect of training, the possible influence of development and maturation must be considered (52). The wide variability of disease in CF makes it difficult to clearly identify effects of a given training program on specific aspects of the disease and physical fitness. Additionally, the large variability makes it difficult to perform a controlled study design by using **matching pairs**. Using patients as their own controls, carryover effects as well as acute changes or progression in disease aspects are potential **confounders**.

Measures of Training Effects

Most studies have focused on improvement of peak exercise values and lung function. Few data are available on the effect of exercise conditioning on submaximal exercise. Everyday activities, however, are mostly submaximal. Accordingly, a reduction of the physiological and psychological strain of a given level of submaximal exercise is probably the more important aspect for daily life. The influence of an exercise program on factors contributing to the patient's well-being is another important aspect in the individual's life and should be included in future studies as a relevant outcome measure. In long-term studies an unchanged outcome measure may be discussed as a positive effect of the training program because it maintains the patient's physical capabilities. This, however, requires a well-controlled, **randomized** study with a sufficient number of subjects (48).

Influence of Lung Function on Exercise

The clear relationship between lung function and exercise tolerance is important in the evaluation of exercise effects. If the effect of exercise conditioning on lung function is only stabilizing, acute disease- or therapy-related changes in lung function must always be considered in interpreting results of exercise conditioning programs. Acute changes make it difficult to identify the true effects of regular exercise.

What We Know
About Cystic Fibrosis and Exercise

1 Cystic fibrosis is a genetically polymorphic, progressive multiorgan disease primarily affecting the lungs, pancreas, intestines, and sweat glands and leading to an early death. Physical fitness is positively associated with prognosis in CF. In end-stage disease transplantation of the primarily affected organ remains the only therapeutic option for intermediate-term survival.

2 Exercise capacity and the ability to perform the physical work of daily living decrease as CF progresses. In severely impaired patients, any increase of the metabolic rate above rest may provoke intense physical strain.

3 Regular exercise usually is recommended for patients with CF of all ages and all disease stages. The type of exercise prescribed should be based on objective testing results. Safe testing requires knowledge of the patient's medical history, current status, and medication; a program designed specifically for the patient, considering the severity of his or her disease and current therapy; and adequate monitoring. New exercise prescriptions must be evaluated after the patient's first few training sessions.

4 Exercise produces positive results that include beneficial effects on the cardiorespiratory system and peripheral muscles, sputum expectoration, airway clearance, ventilatory patterns, and chest wall mobility, as well as psychological well-being.

What We Would Like to Know
About Cystic Fibrosis

1 The patient's genotype influences the severity and progression of the disease and seems to be a factor independent of exercise tolerance, but neither the effects of genetics nor those of exercise can be predicted.

2 The perfect exercise program has not been developed yet. The results of studies on the effect of exercise conditioning reported in the recent literature are not consistent. Exercise may help to stabilize lung function.

3 The extent of exercise-induced hypoxemia (EIH), cannot be predicted and a possible effect of EIH on cardiac function is not clear. Whether or not the short episodes of EIH that often can be observed in daily life in patients with CF are harmful is not known.

4 The potential effects of the chronic use of large amounts of highly potent medications on exercise response have not been sufficiently investigated.

Summary

Patients with CF can benefit from regular exercise. Favorable effects on various aspects of physical fitness as well as psychological well-being have been reported. Moreover, regular exercise seems to stabilize lung function and delay the progress of lung disease, the most threatening aspect of the disease. This finding is underlined by the positive association between physical fitness and prognosis in patients with CF (70, 71). Based on the results of training and epidemiologic studies it is recommended that exercise be integrated into the patient's daily life. Home exercise programs may play an essential role in the realization of this recommendation but have not been well investigated (72).

CASE STUDY

Patient Information

Paul is a 27-year-old man who has been known to have CF since birth. Disease progression is characterized by a slight but constant decline in FEV_1 and body weight. His FEV_1 is now 30% predicted, and his body weight is 51 kg with a body mass index (BMI) of 18. The lung aspect is the dominant feature of his disease. On average he has one or two acute pulmonary infections per year. Paul is monitored in a specialized CF care center and gets complex standardized therapy. A gastrostomy was inserted 2 years ago to improve his nutritional status. He has no need for oxygen supplementation in daily life. Paul is married, has no children, and is on early disability. He has not been engaged in regular exercise since leaving school. Up to the age of 25 years he focused more or less exclusively on education and work. Paul enjoys exercising. For two brief periods, he went to a fitness studio two or three times a week, but he lost motivation without an adequate training group. He has heard that exercise may have beneficial effects on his health status and wants to start again with regular exercise in a newly opened fitness studio near his home. He now wants to know what kind of exercise is recommended for him, how he should proceed, and if there are any restrictions.

Before Planning the Exercise Program
General Considerations

Paul has exercise experience, a positive attitude toward exercise, and good motivation. His main reason for quitting the fitness studio trials, loss of motivation by training alone, must be recognized. He probably needs more specific supervision. Good motivation and supervision are crucial aspects of a successful exercise program. Paul's disease status can be described as severe but relatively stable. Therapy is probably optimized. In patients with severe disease an exercise test should always be performed before planning an exercise program. This provides the essential information to identify reasons for exercise limitations, the facts required to prescribe a safe exercise program, and a framework for evaluating progress or negative side effects. The main constraints for the design of his exercise program are Paul's pulmonary (FEV_1) and muscular (BMI) limitations.

Athletic Activities

Patients with mild disease can perform almost all kinds of sports with very few exceptions. (Exceptions would include activities that are potentially harmful in combination with disease aspects such as scuba diving in a patient in whom the lungs are primarily affected or contact sports in those who are most severely affected in the liver or spleen.) In more severe disease (such as Paul's) exercise is limited to individual sports. Participation in classic team sports is unrealistic because of the patient's diminished performance capacity, which requires frequent breaks and the possible need for oxygen supplementation. Some team sports allow for modifications to adapt to the specific needs of severely impaired patients, but such approaches usually are not feasible because they require not only extremely skilled supervisors but also a sufficient number of patients with common interests and comparable impairments of performance. Every individual sports program should include a warm-up period, a main exercise portion, and a cool-down period. Warm-up and cool-down are more important as preparation than for energy metabolism. The training program should address mainly endurance and strength but also flexibility and coordination. Integration in a training group that consists not of other patients but rather of casual members of a normal gym offers Paul a positive psychological effect, potentially increasing his motivation and compliance.

Exercise Prescription

Exercise prescriptions require measurement of performance because predicted values often are misleading in severe, multifactorial chronic diseases. For aerobic exercise, standard recommendations can be applied. As with a severely impaired patient, Paul's prescribed program should begin at the lower limits of exercise intensity. It may be that even these limits are misleading and too high for the specific combination of limitations of his pulmonary and muscular conditions. Resistance training can be prescribed following standard recommendations.

Expected Benefits

Potential benefits are improved or at least diminished loss of performance capacity and the modification of specific aspects of the disease. The effect of adequate training on cardiorespiratory fitness and muscular strength is balanced by the progression of the chronic disease. Therefore, improvements such as those reported in some relevant literature cannot be always expected. For Paul improved cardiorespiratory and muscular fitness combined with a positive effect on psychological well-being would be an optimal outcome. The exercise program should improve sputum expectoration, airway clearance, and chest wall mobility. An unchanged or only slightly decreased performance capacity is considered a successful outcome of the training program if the decrease occurs with increased severity of disease.

Planning the Exercise Program
Location and Equipment

Paul discovered a well-equipped fitness studio. He decided to do his resistance training with training machines rather than with dumbbells, because he felt that the dumbbells that he was able to use look inadequate compared with those handled by other men at the gym. His resistance training follows usual recommendations, with series of 8 to 15 repetitions and adequate weights. He perceives jogging as inadequate, so he decided to do his endurance exercises with an electronically braked cycle ergometer. The ergometer training is prescribed based on clinical exercise testing.

Exercise Testing and Prescription

Testing protocol: initial load of 0.3 W/kg, stage duration of 2 minutes, increments of 0.3 W/kg

Measures: workload (W), heart rate (HR), **rate of perceived exertion (RPE)**, oxygen saturation (SO_2), VO_2, and minute ventilation (VE).

Rationale: An exercise protocol with small increments permits evaluation of the acute response to different exercise intensities, even though performance capacity is rather low.

All measures help to describe exercise limitations and thus to prescribe exercise. Additionally, HR, RPE, and SO_2 can be used under training conditions and may serve to monitor the training. This makes it possible to compare testing results and exercise prescriptions with the real training procedure. The combination of objective (HR, SO_2) with subjective (RPE) responses assists in review of test results and recommendations and for potential modifications of exercise prescriptions, which may be of special importance for patients like Paul in a more severe stage of the disease.

Pre-testing values: HR, 93 beats per minute (bpm); VO_2, 5.8 ml/kg/min); VE, 14 L/min; SO_2, 95%.

Peak exercise values: workload, 1.87 W/kg; HR, 167 bpm (87% predicted); VO_2, 28.9 ml/kg/min; VE, 47 L/min (110% of maximal voluntary ventilation); SO_2, 80%.

Interpretation: Resting HR, VE and metabolic rate are slightly increased compared to healthy subjects comparably accustomed to the exercise testing procedure. Performance and cardiorespiratory response are impaired mainly by pulmonary function.

Prescription: Prolonged endurance training up to 15 minutes should be restricted to light to moderate exercise intensity to prevent a long-lasting drop of SO_2 during the training session. Such training should correspond to 50% to 60% of HR (130–140 bpm) or VO_2 reserve (about 17–20 ml/kg/min). This should be perceived as an RPE value between 11 and 12. Paul was advised to perform prolonged cycling at 50 W equivalent to approximately 53% of his peak workload.

Training Experience

After his first (unsupervised) training session Paul complained that the prescription for endurance exercise was wrong. He insisted that the exercise intensity was too high. He reported that his heart was banging, that he had severe breathing problems, and that he would describe the training as having an RPE value of 19, not 12. In addition, he developed muscle soreness the following day.

Paul is known as a patient who normally does not dramatize discomfort, who is able to apply prescriptions correctly, and who has no problems using technical equipment. Consequently his report that the prescribed exercise intensity was too high was taken seriously.

Control Training Session

A 15-minute endurance training at a constant workload of 50 W was conducted in the exercise testing laboratory. After 15 minutes, HR (150 bpm), RPE (14), and VO_2 (22 ml/kg/min) were higher than the predicted range. This was combined with a relevant decrease of SO_2 (82%). The results indicate an underestimation of Paul's acute response to prolonged workload and an inadequate oxygen transport capacity for a prolonged oxygen demand even in the setting of light to moderate exercise intensity.

Revised Exercise Prescription

A general recommendation for the feasibility of prolonged exercise training is that the SO_2 should be kept over 90%. This can be achieved by reducing the relative exercise intensity but also by increased availability of oxygen. Paul considered these alternatives and rejected the proposal of reducing the workload by 10%. He felt that the initially prescribed workload had been a challenge due to breathlessness but no real problem with respect to leg power. Paul decided to stay with the initial exercise prescription but to combine this training with oxygen supplementation and SO_2 and HR monitoring in the fitness studio.

Control Training Session in the Fitness Studio

A 15-minute endurance training session was conducted at a constant workload of 50 W combined with supplementation of oxygen and documentation of SO_2, HR, and RPE. After

15 minutes, HR (143 bpm) and RPE (12) were slightly higher than predicted. Paul's SO_2 was 90% or above throughout the training session, and the flow rate of oxygen was between 2 and 3 L/min. The results of this training control indicate that the training prescription has been sufficiently adjusted. Later SO_2 measurement during selected subsequent training sessions permits adjustment of a progressive training program.

REFERENCES

1. Sheppard DN, Welsh MJ. Structure and function of the CFTR chloride channel. Physiol Rev 1999;79(S1):S23–S45.
2. Quinton PM. Physiological basis of cystic fibrosis: a historical approach. Physiol Rev 1999;79(S1): S3–S22.
3. Ma J, Davis PB. What we know and what we do not know about cystic fibrosis transmembrane conductance regulator. Clin Chest Med 1998;19:459–471.
4. Mickle JE, Cutting R. Clinical implications of cystic fibrosis transmembrane conductance regulator mutations. Clin Chest Med 1998;19:443–458.
5. Rosenstein BJ. What is a cystic fibrosis diagnosis? Clin Chest Med 1998;19:423–443.
6. Selvadurai HC, McKay KO, Blimkie CJ, et al. The relationship between genotype and exercise tolerance in children with cystic fibrosis. Am J Respir Crit Care Med 2002;165:762–765.
7. Konstan MW. Therapies aimed at airway inflammation in cystic fibrosis. Clin Chest Med 1998;19:505–513.
8. Dark J, Corris P. Transplantation. In: Shale D (ed). Cystic Fibrosis. London: BMJ Publishing Group, 1996:120–133.
9. Corey M, McLaughlin FJ, Williams M, Levison H. A comparison of survival, growth, and pulmonary function in patients with cystic fibrosis in Boston and Toronto. J Clin Epidemiol 1988;41:583–591.
10. Shale D. Management in adults. In: Shale D (ed). Cystic Fibrosis. London: BMJ Publishing Group, 1996:14–31.
11. Hiller EJ. Management in children. In: Shale D (ed). Cystic Fibrosis. London: BMJ Publishing Group, 1996:1–13.
12. Lands LC, Coates AL. Cardiorespiratory and skeletal muscle function and their effects on exercise limitation. In: Yankaskas JR, Knowles MR (eds). Cystic Fibrosis in Adults. Philadelphia: Lippincott-Raven, 1999:365–382.
13. Coates AL, Boyce P, Muller D, et al. The role of nutritional status, airway obstruction, hypoxia, and abnormalities in serum lipid composition in limiting exercise tolerance in children with cystic fibrosis. Acta Paediatr Scand 1980;69:353–358.
14. Cropp GJ, Pullano TP, Cerny FJ, Nathanson IT. Exercise tolerance and cardiorespiratory adjustments at peak work capacity in cystic fibrosis. Am Rev Respir Dis 1982;126:211–216.
15. De Meer K, Jeneson JA, Gulmans VA, et al. Efficiency of oxidative work performance of skeletal muscle in patients with cystic fibrosis. Thorax 1995;50:980–983.
16. Boas SR, Joswiak ML, Nixon PA, et al. Factors limiting anaerobic performance in adolescent males with cystic fibrosis. Med Sci Sports Exerc 1996;28:291–298.
17. De Meer K, Gulmans VA, van der Laag J. Peripheral muscle weakness and exercise capacity in children with cystic fibrosis. Am J Respir Crit Care Med 1999;159:748–754.
18. Moser C, Tirakitsoontorn P, Nussbaum E, Newcomb R, Cooper DM. Muscle size and cardiorespiratory response to exercise in cystic fibrosis. Am J Respir Crit Care Med. 162(5):1823–1827, 2000.
19. Boas SR, Danduran MJ, McColley SA. Energy metabolism during anaerobic exercise in children with cystic fibrosis and asthma. Med Sci Sports Exerc 31(9):1242–1249, 1999.
20. Keens TG, Krastins IR, Wannamaker EM, Levison H, Crozier DN, Bryan AC. Ventilatory muscle endurance training in normal subjects and patients with cystic fibrosis. Am Rev Respir Dis 116:853–860, 1977.

21. Lands LC, Heigenhauser GJF, Jones NL, Heigenhauser GJ. Respiratory and peripheral muscle function in cystic fibrosis. Am Rev Respir Dis 147:865–869, 1993.
22. Godfrey S, Mearns M. Pulmonary function and response to exercise in cystic fibrosis. Arch Dis Child 1971;46:144–151.
23. Webb AK, Dodd ME. Exercise and training in adults with cystic fibrosis. In: Hodson ME, Geddes DM (eds). Cystic Fibrosis. London: Chapman & Hall, 1995:397–409.
24. MacFarlane PI, Heaf D. Changes in airflow obstruction and oxygen saturation in response to exercise and bronchodilators in cystic fibrosis. Pediatr Pulmonol 1990;8:4–11.
25. Lands LC, Geigenhauser GJF, Jones NL. Cardiac output determination during progressive exercise in cystic fibrosis. Chest 1992;102: 1118–1123.
26. Perrault H, Coughlan M, Marcotte JE, et al. Comparison of cardiac output determinants in response to upright and supine exercise in patients with cystic fibrosis. Chest 1992 ;101:42–51.
27. Cerny FJ, Pullano TP, Cropp GJA. Cardiorespiratory adaptations to exercise in cystic fibrosis. Am Rev Respir Dis 1982;126:217–220.
28. Freeman W, Stableforth DE, Cayton RM, Morgan MD. Endurance exercise capacity in adults with cystic fibrosis. Respir Med 1993;87:541–549.
29. Siassi B, Moss AJ, Dooley RR. Clinical recognition of cor pulmonale in cystic fibrosis. J Pediatr 1971;78:794–805
30. Coates AL. Oxygen therapy, exercise and cystic fibrosis. Chest 1992; 101:2–4.
31. Coates AL, Canny G, Zinman R, et al. The effects of chronic airflow limitation, increased dead space, and the pattern of ventilation on gas exchange during maximal exercise in advanced cystic fibrosis. Am Rev Respir Dis 1988;138:1524–1531.
32. Cerny FJ, Cropp GJA, Bye MR. Hospital therapy improves exercise tolerance and lung function in cystic fibrosis. Am J Dis Child 1984;138:261–265.
33. Pike SE, Prasad SA, Balfour-Lynn IM. Effects of intravenous antibiotics on exercise tolerance (3-min step test) in cystic fibrosis. Pediatr Pulmonol 2001;32:38–43.
34. Marcus CL, Bader D, Stabile MW, et al. Supplemental oxygen and exercise performance in patients with cystic fibrosis with severe pulmonary disease. Chest 1992;101:52–57.
35. Landis et al., 1998.
36. American Association of Cardiovascular and Pulmonary Rehabilitation. Guidelines for pulmonary rehabilitation programs. 2nd Ed. Champaign, IL: Human Kinetics, 1998.
37. Orenstein DM. Exercise testing in cystic fibrosis. Pediatr Pulmonol 1998;25:223–225.
38. American College of Sports Medicine. ACSM's Guidelines for Exercise Testing and Prescription. 6th Ed. Philadelphia: Lippincott Williams & Wilkins, 2000.
39. Nikolaizik WH, Knöpfli B, Leister E, et al. The anaerobic threshold in cystic fibrosis. Pediatr Pulmonol 1998;25:147–153.
40. Cerny FJ, Orenstein D. Cystic fibrosis. In: Skinner JS (ed). Exercise Testing and Exercise Prescription for Special Cases. 2nd Ed. Philadelphia: Lea & Febiger, 1993:241–250.
41. Orenstein DM, Curtis SE, Nixon PA, Hartigan ER. Accuracy of three pulse oximeters during exercise and hypoxemia in patients with cystic fibrosis. Chest 1993;104:1187–1190.

42. Orenstein DM, Franklin BA, Doerchuk CF, et al. Exercise conditioning and cardiopulmonary fitness in cystic fibrosis. The effects of a three-month supervised running program. Chest 1981;80:392–398.

43. Edlund LD, French RW, Herbst JJ, et al. Effect of a swimming program on children with cystic fibrosis. Am J Dis Child 1986;140:80–83.

44. Salh W, Bilton D, Dodd M, Webb AK. Effect of exercise and physiotherapy in aiding sputum expectoration in adults with cystic fibrosis. Thorax 1989;44:1006–1008.

45. Conway SP, Morton AM, Oldroyd B, et al. Osteoporosis and osteopenia in adults and adolescents with cystic fibrosis: prevalence and associated factors. Thorax 2000;55:798–804.

46. Zach MS, Purrer B, Oberwaldner B. Effect of swimming on forced expiration and sputum clearance in cystic fibrosis. Lancet 1981;2: 1201–1203.

47. Braggion C, Cornacchia M, Miano A, et al. Exercise tolerance and effects of training in young patients with cystic fibrosis and mild airway obstruction. Pediatr Pulmonol 1989;7:145–152.

48. Schneiderman-Walker J, Pollock SL, Corey M, et al. A randomized controlled trial of a 3-year home exercise program in cystic fibrosis. J Pediatr 2000;136:304–310.

49. Heijerman HG, Bakker W, Sterk PJ, Dijkman JH. Long-term effects of exercise training and hyperalimentation in adult cystic fibrosis patients with severe pulmonary dysfunction. Int J Rehab Res 1992;15:252–257.

50. Stanghelle JK, Hjeltnes N, Bangstad HJ, Michaelsen H. Effect of daily short bouts of trampoline exercise during 8 weeks on the pulmonary function and the maximal oxygen uptake of children with cystic fibrosis. Int J Sports Med 1988;9(Suppl):32–36.

51. Di Prampero PE. The energy cost of human locomotion on land and in water. Int J Sports Med 1986;7:55–72.

52. Gulmans VA, de Meer K, Brackel HJ, et al. Outpatient exercise training in children with cystic fibrosis: physiological effects, perceived competence, and acceptability. Pediatr Pulmonol 1999;28:39–45.

53. De Jong W, Grevink RG, Roorda RJ, et al. Effect of a home exercise training program in patients with cystic fibrosis. Chest 1994;105:463–468.

54. Stanghelle JK, Michaelsen H, Skyberg D. Five-year follow-up of pulmonary function and peak oxygen uptake in 16-year-old boys with cystic fibrosis, with special regard to the influence of regular physical exercise. Int J Sports Med 1988;9(Suppl.):19–24.

55. Staab D, Wenninger K, Gebert N, et al. Quality of life in patients with cystic fibrosis and their parents: what is important besides disease severity? Thorax 1998;53:727–731.

56. Asher MI, Pardy RL, Coates AL, et al. The effects of inspiratory muscle training in patients with cystic fibrosis. Am Rev Respir Dis 1982;126:855–859.

57. Sawyer EH, Clanton TL. Improved pulmonary function and exercise tolerance with inspiratory muscle conditioning in children with cystic fibrosis. Chest 1993;104:1490–1497.

58. De Jong W, van Aalderen WM, Kraan J, et al. Inspiratory muscle training in patients with cystic fibrosis. Respir Med 2001;95:31–36.

59. Rowland TW. Muscle strength and endurance. In: Rowland TW (ed). Exercise and Children's Health. Champaign, IL: Human Kinetics, 1990:85–95.

60. Andreasson B, Jonson B, Kornfalt R, et al. Long-term effects of physical exercise on working capacity and pulmonary function in cystic fibrosis. Acta Paediatr Scand 1987;76:70–75.

61. O'Neill PA, Dodd M, Phillips B, et al. Regular exercise and reduction of breathlessness in patients with cystic fibrosis. Br J Dis Chest 1987;81:62–69.

62. Baldwin DR, Hill AL, Peckham DG, Knox AJ. Effect of addition of exercise to chest physiotherapy on sputum expectoration and lung function in adults with cystic fibrosis. Respir Med 1994;88:49–53.

63. Cerny FJ. Relative effects of chest physiotherapy and exercise for in-hospital care of cystic fibrosis. Phys Ther 1989;69:633–639.

64. Hebestreit A, Kersting U, Basler B, et al. Exercise inhibits epithelial sodium channels in patients with cystic fibrosis. Am J Respir Crit Care Med 2001;164:443–446.

65. Zach MS, Oberwaldner B, Hausler F. Cystic fibrosis: physical exercise versus chest physiotherapy. Arch Dis Child 1982;57:587–589.

66. Strauss GD, Osher A, Wang CI, et al. Variable weight training in cystic fibrosis. Chest 1987;92:273–276.

67. Beneke R. Krafttraining—ausgewählte Methoden und ihre Wirkung. Forschende Komplementärmedizin. Res Complement Med 1998;5:5–11.

68. Simpson K, Killian K, McCartney N, et al. Randomised controlled trial of weightlifting exercise in patients with chronic airflow limitation. Thorax 1992;47:70–75.

69. Orenstein DM, Nixon PA, Ross EA, Kaplan RM. The quality of well being in cystic fibrosis. Chest 1989;95:344–347.

70. Nixon PA, Orenstein DM, Kelsey SF, Doershuk CF. The prognostic value of exercise testing in patients with cystic fibrosis. N Engl J Med 1992;327:1785–1788.

71. Moorcraft AJ, Dodd ME, Webb AK. Exercise testing and prognosis in adult cystic fibrosis. Thorax 1997;52:291–293.

72. Bar-Or O. Home-based exercise programs in cystic fibrosis: Are they worth it? J Pediatr 2000;136:279–280.

SUGGESTED READINGS

Boas SR. Exercise recommendations for individuals with cystic fibrosis. Sports Med 1997;24:17–37.

Canny GJ, Levison H. Exercise response and rehabilitation in cystic fibrosis. Sports Med 1987;4:143–152.

Cooper DM. Exercise and cystic fibrosis. The search for a therapeutic optimum. Pediatr Pulmonol 1998;25:143–144.

Hodson ME, Geddes DM (eds). Cystic Fibrosis. London: Chapman & Hall, 1995.

Orenstein DM. Cystic fibrosis. In: Goldberg B (ed). Sports and Exercise for Children With Chronic Health Conditions. Champaign, IL: Human Kinetics, 1995.

Webb AK, Dodd ME. Exercise and sport in cystic fibrosis: benefits and risks. Br J Sports Med 1999;3:77–78.

Yankaskas JR, Knowles MR (eds). Cystic Fibrosis in Adults. Philadelphia: Lippincott-Raven, 1999:365–382.

Asthma and Exercise-Induced Asthma

Kenneth W. Rundell, Daniel A. Judelson

Airway Dysfunction
Airway Hyperreactivity
Asthma
Athlete
Atopy
Exercise
Exercise-Induced Asthma

Exercise-Induced Hypoxemia
Eucapnic Voluntary Hyperventilation
Hypoxia
Obesity
Skiers Asthma
Tachyphylaxis
Wheeze

Overview

Asthma is a chronic lung disease that affects an estimated 17 million people in the United States, costs over $11 billion per year, results in the loss of more than 16 million school and work days per year, and kills 14 Americans each day. Asthma is characterized as an inflammatory disorder of the airways in which many cells and cellular elements play a role (Figure 13.1). In particular, **mast cells, eosinophils, T-lymphocytes, macrophages, neutrophils,** and **epithelial cells** may be actively involved in airway **inflammation**.

Asthma can cause spontaneous recurrent episodes of wheezing, breathlessness, chest tightness, and coughing, especially during the morning or at night. Symptoms also present following allergen exposure or exercise. These episodes often are associated with widespread variable airflow obstruction, which often is reversible, either spontaneously or with treatment (1). However, persistent chronic inflammation and airway remodeling often are associated with asthma and exercise-induced asthma (EIA) and can be identified by below-normal **spirometry** or body **plethysmography** resting measurements.

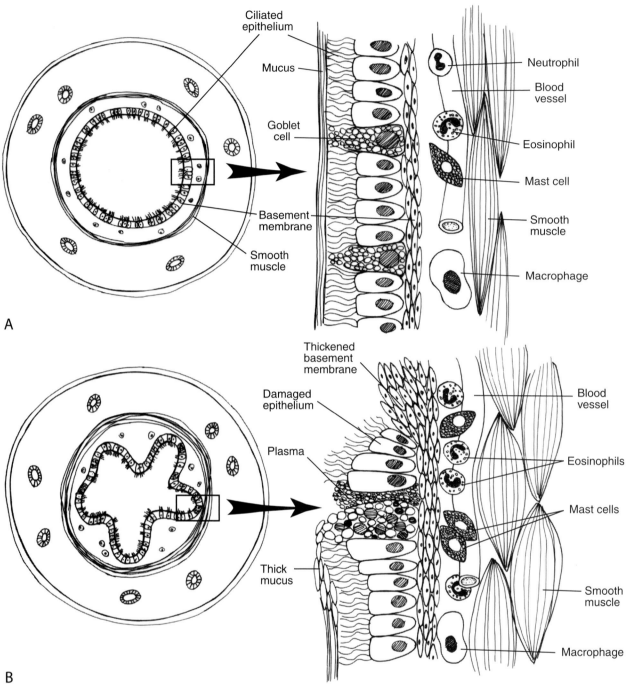

FIGURE 13.1. Schematic of normal airway (**A**) and a constricted airway (**B**) of an asthmatic. Note the smooth muscle constriction, thickened mucosal layer, thickened basement membrane, denuded epithelium, and increased inflammatory cells of the asthmatic airway.

Epidemiology

Although the incidence of asthma is increasing worldwide, epidemiologic studies of asthmatics typically are thought to have limited value. Because there is no universally accepted measure for airway dysfunction, this lack of consistency in asthma diagnosis results in a wide range of reported prevalence estimates. Additionally, the validity of asthma evalua-tion measures can be questionable. For example, positive predictive values (i.e., the likelihood of a patient with a positive test having asthma) for asthma diagnosed by an exercise challenge or an inhaled methacholine (or **histamine**) challenge have been found to be only 40% to 50% (2–4). Likewise, self-reported symptoms have not proven to be sensitive for identifying EIA in athletes (5). Prospects for a universally accepted diagnostic tool for the identification of asthmatics remain bleak until the complete disease pathogenesis is known and understood (6). Despite limitations in measurement, most of the research analyzing asthma in the general population points to a rising severity and incidence (7).

Hygiene Hypothesis

The prevalence of asthma in Western societies has doubled in the last 20 years. Although air pollution is a product of modernization that may aggravate existing asthma, it is unlikely that it is responsible for the asthma epidemic. However, there is strong evidence implicating modern health care in the rise in asthma. This theory has been termed the "hygiene hypothesis." Changes in the view of bacterial and viral infections, altered microflora, and changes in dietary habits (increased consumption of omega-6 fatty acids) seem to be the most likely causes of the increased prevalence of allergic diseases (8). Reduction in infection and generalized contact with the microbial environment during early life appears to affect the functional maturation of the Th-1 (normal) arm of the immune response (9). The diminished microbial exposure during the first years of life that is found in societies with a high standard of living may be disadvantageous in terms of mucosal sensitization to allergy (10).

Predisposition for asthma appears to be determined in early life, with events occurring in utero and in infancy that influence future development of atopy (11). According to the hygiene hypothesis, asthma results directly from the repeated local expression in airway tissues of Th2-polarized T cell immunity to inhaled allergens. These responses are primed in utero and reshaped during postnatal allergen exposure, leading to the emergence of stable allergen-specific T-cell memory, which is polarized toward Th1 (normal) or Th2 (atopic) phenotype. The Th1/Th2 switching process is influenced by a number of host and environmental factors that are not fully understood (12). The development of resistance or sensitivity to environmental antigens depends to a large extent on the nature of immunologic memory that is generated during early antigen encounters in infancy and early childhood (13). The immunologic milieu at the maternofetal interface is naturally skewed toward the Th2 phenotype and appears to be preserved for varying periods into infancy, accounting for a high risk window for allergic sensitization (12). For example, immune system development is influenced by infections in the airway mucosa, which may activate local tissue macrophages and secrete Th-2-inhibitory cytokines, or, conversely, microbial stimulation via gastrointestinal tract commensals and pathogens may trigger postnatal maturation of immune competence. It appears that the speed with which the immune system in human infants attains adult-equivalent competence postnatally is inversely related to risk for primary allergic sensitization to environmental antigens.

Risk Factors

Several risk factors have been identified that help explain recent increases in asthma incidence. Typically, risk factors act synergistically. For example, research suggests that age and gender are intimately related, with a higher prevalence for males at a young age but a higher prevalence for females at an older age. Long-term cohort studies have shown that the majority of childhood asthma begins in infancy, with most children reporting their first wheezing attack before the age of 3 years. In fact, asthma is the most common childhood disease, affecting approximately five million children. Boys seem to be more affected at an early age, with 5.3 per 1000 boys compared with only 2.9 per 1000 girls diagnosed as asthmatic at age 1 (14). Skobeloff et al. (15) reported twice as many hospital admissions for boys less than 10 years old than similarly aged girls. Later in life, however, the prevalence of asthma is greater among females than among males. In the study by Skobeloff et al. (15), women 20 to 50 years of age were admitted to a hospital for asthma three times more often than their male counterparts. Women over 50 years of age were admitted 2.5 times more often than men and were hospitalized for a longer period of time.

Socioeconomic status (SES) and related environmental conditions also have been defined as risk factors for asthma. Low SES often is associated with unfavorable living conditions high in allergens such as pollution, dust mites, cigarette smoke, and cockroaches. Notably, asthma and other allergic conditions are most prevalent in the United Kingdom, Australia, New Zealand, Chile, and southern regions of Europe, all areas where environmental triggers may be high. Asthma severity and premature mortality are twice as common in individuals with low SES and are thought to be related to increased environmental exposure to allergens. Interestingly, asthma prevalence has been found to be greater in the high-SES population (16). This unexpected finding may simply be a side effect of the fact that this population receives better health care and, consequently, more frequent asthma diagnosis.

Race appears to be another important risk factor for asthma. Recent studies (17, 18) have found a higher prevalence of asthma in African-Americans than in any other racial group. High serum IgE levels, a marker of asthma, are characteristic of African-Americans; however, the high IgE level may be related to SES and environmental exposure to allergens rather than race. The reduced lung volume characteristic of the African-American population and a heightened reactivity to methacholine (a drug used to elicit an asthmatic response) also may influence the reported prevalence. African-Americans also suffer from a much higher asthma mortality rate than Caucasians (3.34 vs. 0.65 per 1000). Furthermore, persons of African-American and Hispanic background are at greater risk than Caucasians for both adult and childhood onset of asthma and asthmatic symptoms, even after factors of SES are included (19).

The prevalence of asthma and obesity is increasing in industrialized countries. Several studies have demonstrated an association between the two disorders, which suggests that asthma is a risk factor for obesity (20–22). Airway obstruction and peak flow variability, two important pulmonary variables have shown increases in obese populations. Reductions in fat mass and body mass index, however, elicit improvements in airway responsiveness and function. This relationship between obesity and airway function requires further investigation.

Pathophysiology of Asthma and Exercise-Induced Asthma

Asthma is an airway disorder characterized by chronic inflammation of the airways. The inflammatory response contributes to airway hyperreactivity to stimuli, air flow limitation, a variety of symptoms, and airway remodeling (Figure 13.2). This response can be classified as acute, subacute, or chronic. The acute response can be characterized by a transient recruitment of inflammatory cells to the airway, whereas the subacute response is defined by resident inflammatory cells in the airway causing more persistent inflammation and accompanying symptoms. Chronic inflammation, characteristic of more severe asthma, is defined by resident inflammatory cells, airway remodeling, and persistent respiratory symptoms.

The inflammatory process of asthma is multicellular, involving mast cells, eosinophils, T lymphocytes, macrophages, neutrophils, and epithelial cells. T-helper 2 cells have been identified as being important in the development of allergic airway inflammation. IgE-mediated atopy is highly associated with asthma (23); however, non-IgE-mediated inflammation also may predominate. The airway smooth muscle may be hypertrophied, and the epithelial basement membrane often is thickened by interstitial collagen deposits in the lamina reticularis (24). In asthmatic individuals, episodic wheezing, breathlessness, chest tightness, and coughing are characteristic. Spontaneous episodes typically occur at night or early morning and are characterized by reversible airflow obstruction. This complex, redundant process of inflammation often causes an increase in bronchial hyperreactivity that is triggered by a variety of stimuli. One such stimulus is the drying of the airways from the ventilatory process during exercise. This section explores the specific pathogenesis of airway hyperreactivity triggered by exercise.

Airway inflammation and bronchial hyperreactivity characteristic of exercise-induced asthma most likely are initiated by loss of the airway surface liquid (ASL) as a consequence of humidifying large volumes of inspired air during exercise (25–27). Subsequently, this can result in water loss and **osmolarity** change in airway cells. The influx of water to restore osmolarity, when exercise intensity (ventilation) is reduced, is thought to stimulate the release of inflammatory mediators. These mediators then cause bronchial smooth muscle constriction or edema. A less likely explanation of the mechanism for EIA suggests that thermal events initiate airway narrowing (28–31). The thermal hypothesis states that at the cessation of exercise, rapid rewarming of the airways results in reactive **hyperemia** that narrows the airways. Although it is certain that **ambient** temperature has a role in EIA, the primary effect probably is to recruit smaller airways (beyond generation 10) in warming and humidifying inspired air (26). Nonetheless, it is clear that the severity of EIA is determined by ventilation rate, ambient air water content, and ambient temperature *during exercise*, and the majority of EIA cases probably involve an inflammatory response.

In nonasthmatic individuals, water loss from the airway surface liquid during air humidification is constantly replenished. The most likely and immediate source is the epithelial cell, which has been described as an "osmometer" that enhances the movement of water to the ASL (32). For this process to be effective, epithelial cell water replenishment must keep pace with ASL water loss; the airway submucosa is the most likely source of water for this. Remodeling of the subepithelial basement membrane, identified in cross-country skiers and mild asthmatic subjects (33, 34), may be responsible for a diminished capacity to respond to evaporative water loss of the ASL. Subsequent to this, smaller airways are recruited into the humidification process and may enhance airway hyperreactivity (32). The resulting cellular water loss increases intracellular ion concentrations (e.g., calcium) that are necessary for the release of inflammatory mediators.

The most important cells in mediator release appear to be mast cells. Elevated T-lymphocyte, macrophage, neutrophil, and eosinophil counts obtained from bronchoalve-

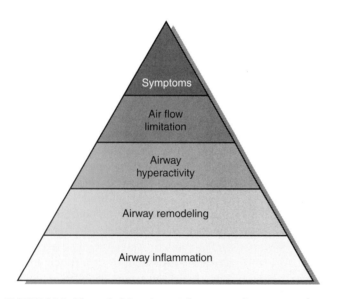

FIGURE 13.2. The underlying airway inflammation characteristic of asthma leads to airway remodeling and airway hyperreactivity. Symptoms and air flow limitation of asthma and EIA are functions of inflammation, remodeling, and hyperreactivity.

olar **lavage** have been reported for frank asthma and "cross-country ski asthma" (33, 35); however, these cells may merely be indicative of chronic airway inflammation and have no relationship to the acute response associated with EIA. The conflicting results concerning differential cell counts obtained from bronchoalveolar lavage (BAL) support this concept. Some EIA studies have identified high mast cell counts with normal neutrophil and eosinophil counts (36), whereas others have reported elevated neutrophil and eosinophil counts with normal mast cell counts (33). It is likely that mast cells are important in the pathogenesis of EIA in both asthmatic and nonasthmatic persons. Mast cell mediator release has been demonstrated to occur by IgE allergen-induced activation as well as by non-IgE–dependent stimuli such as cold dry air (37–39). This is important if mast cells are involved in airway hyperreactivity in the nonatopic subject. However, much evidence exists supporting a role of eosinophils in the pathogenesis of EIA in the chronic asthmatic. Pohunek et al. (40) have demonstrated that elevated serum eosinophilic cationic protein (s-ECP) is related to acute episodic bronchial asthma. Moreover, Fujitaka et al. (41) demonstrated that the ratio of s-ECP to peripheral blood eosinophil counts (the ECP/Eo ratio) was strongly correlated to the severity of asthma. Eosinophils are most likely involved in the development of chronic inflammation in asthma. Because eosinic inflammatory expression occurs several hours after a stimulus, however, it probably does not contribute directly to acute EIA.

Even though all cells of the airway demonstrate potential to be affected by osmolarity change and release inflammatory mediators, there is much evidence supporting mast cell release of the bronchoconstrictor mediators histamine, cysteinyl **leukotrienes**, and **prostaglandins**. These inflammatory agents appear to be the principal cause of EIA, although direct evidence for inflammatory mediator release by detection of the mediators in body fluids (e.g., sputum, blood, urine) following an exercise challenge have been equivocal and not without flaw. More recently, urinalysis has demonstrated potential as a successful method for detecting airway mediator release. Increased urine concentrations of mast cell markers 9α-11β-prostaglandin (PG) F_2, Ntau-methylhistamine, and leukotriene (LT) E_4 (metabolites of PGD_2, histamine, LTC_4, and LTD_4) have been shown to accompany EIA (42–48).

Early studies implicated histamine as a biomarker of mast cell activation and subsequent bronchoconstriction. Elevated postexercise histamine concentrations in blood were identified and assumed to originate from airway mast cells. However, subsequent studies have shown that this elevated postexercise histamine level in asthmatics was due to the circulating basophil degranulation that accompanies exercise. Later, attempts to measure histamine concentrations in the airway BAL fluid or by sputum analysis were made with limited success; these techniques were unable to demonstrate airway histamine release definitively after ex-

ercise. The difficulty in identifying histamine in body fluids could be due to the half-life of histamine (which is a matter of minutes) or the rapid removal of histamine at the airway surface; thus postexercise blood, BAL, or sputum analysis may not fit the time course of histamine release and removal.

Indirect pharmacologic probes provide the most convincing evidence supporting histamine-mediated EIA. Several studies (49–55) using histamine H_1-receptor antagonists have demonstrated varying degrees of protection (30–60%). Interestingly, studies found less protection during exercise than during exercise surrogates using the potent H_1-receptor antagonist terfenadine (53, 54, 56). Terfenadine decreased airway hyperreactivity by 24%, 44%, and 56%, in exercise, hyperventilation, and **hypertonic** saline challenges, respectively (Figure 13.3). This finding strongly implies that other mediators are involved in the EIA response and that these surrogate challenges of EIA are more histamine-dependent than the EIA response from exercise.

The accumulated indirect pharmacologic evidence and the time course of histamine-initiated bronchoconstriction suggest that multiple mediators are involved in EIA. Products of the arachidonic acid pathway have been implicated as key mediators in the expression of EIA. These include the 5-lipoxygenase–generated leukotrienes and the cyclooxygenation derived prostanoids.

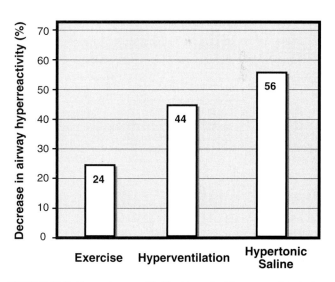

FIGURE 13.3. Protection provided by histamine H_1-receptor blockade (Terfenadine) on airway hyperreactivity for exercise, hyperventilation, and hypertonic saline challenges. The lower protection provided by Terfenadine during exercise suggests that factors other than histamine play a large role in the hyperreactive response to exercise. (Data from Finnerty JP, Wilmot C, Holgate ST. Inhibition of hypertonic saline-induced bronchoconstriction by terfenadine and flurbiprofen. Evidence for the predominant role of histamine. Am Rev Respir Dis 1989;140:593–597, and Finnerty JP, Holgate ST. Evidence of the role of histamine and prostaglandins as mediators in exercise-induced asthma: the inhibitory effect of terfenadine and flurbiprofen alone and in combination. Eur Respir J 1990;3:540–557.)

The final products generated by 5-lipoxygenase are the leukotrienes LTB_4, LTC_4, LTD_4, and LTE_4 (Figure 13.4). One of these, LTB_4, functions in **chemotaxis** transduction and has not been identified as having a role in the expression of EIA. Within eosinophils, mast cells, and alveolar macrophages, LTA_4 is rapidly converted to LTC_4 and then exported to the extracellular space, where it is then cleaved to form LTD_4 and LTE_4. The leukotrienes LTC_4, LTD_4, and LTE_4 are active in bronchoconstriction and mucus secretion, with LTD_4 being the most and LTE_4 the least potent (57–61). Studies using inhaled mediators demonstrate leukotrienes to be 100 to 1000 times more potent than histamine. Data implicating the cysteinyl leukotrienes in the pathogenesis of EIA include postexercise increases of urinary LTE_4 and reduced postexercise **bronchospasm** with antileukotriene treatment (42, 43, 45, 46, 62). The LTD_4-receptor antagonists and 5-lipoxygenase inhibitors were found to be 0 to 90% effective in inhibiting the postexercise bronchoconstriction characteristic of EIA (Figure13.5; 63–65). This supports the concept of multiple mediator involvement in EIA. Roquet et al. (66) defined the major mediators involved in allergen-induced airway obstruction as histamine and leukotrienes. A combination therapy of leukotriene receptor antagonist and antihistamine pro-

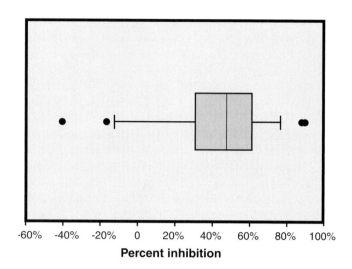

Percent inhibition

FIGURE 13.5. The 5-lipoxygenase inhibitor Zileuton demonstrates a wide range of protection against EIA; this provides strong evidence for a complex, dynamic, and diverse pathology of multiple mediators.

vided significantly more effective treatment than either drug alone, although post-bronchoprovocation obstruction was not completely reversed, indicating still other mediator involvement.

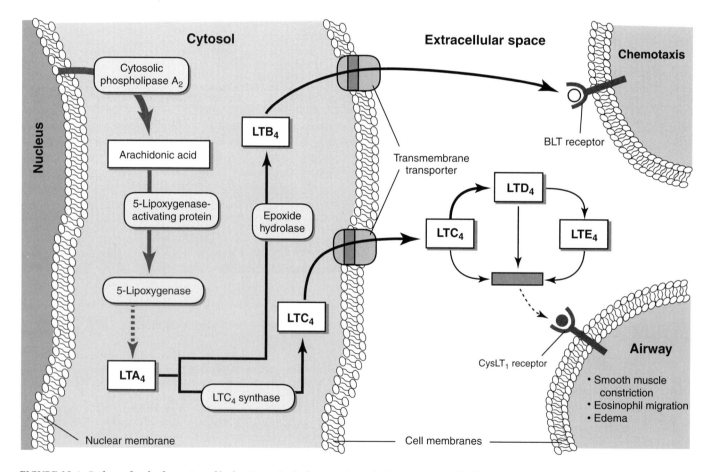

FIGURE 13.4. Pathway for the formation of leukotrienes. In the human airway, leukotriene C_4 and leukotriene D_4 are 10 times more potent than leukotriene E_4. BLT receptor, LTA_4, LTC_4, LTB_4, LTD_4, LTE_4, leukotrienes. (Redrawn from Drazen JM, Israel E, O'Byrne PM. Treatment of asthma with drugs modifying the leukotriene pathway. N Engl J Med 1999;340:197–206.)

PGD$_2$ and thromboxane (Tx)A$_2$ are the primary products of arachidonic acid cyclooxygenation in mast cells. Both are potent bronchoconstrictors but are difficult to identify in plasma or airway fluids because of their short half-lives. However, increased urinary metabolites of PGD$_2$ and TxA$_2$, 9α-11β-PGF$_2$, and TxB$_2$ have been found in relation to acute episodic asthma and EIA (44, 45, 67). Further evidence that prostanoids contribute to EIA is provided by studies using **cyclooxygenase** inhibitors. The inhibitor flurbiprofen has been shown to provide 31% protection against EIA (54), and a TxA$_2$ synthetase inhibitor attenuated EIA for 7 of 11 patients (68). Studies using other cyclooxygenase inhibitors were not successful in demonstrating inhibition of EIA (56, 69), providing more evidence for a complex pathogenesis of multiple mediators in EIA.

The pathogenesis of acute asthma and EIA have many similarities. Questions remain, but it is certain that the release of inflammatory mediators characteristic of allergen-induced asthma occurs in EIA. The mechanism in which inflammatory cells are activated involves ASL dehydration, followed by an osmotic response initiating the release of inflammatory compounds. Remodeling of the subepithelial basement membrane is characteristic of asthmatic as well as nonasthmatic EIA athletes. It is thought that the remodeled basement membrane diminishes the capacity to respond to evaporative water loss of the ASL. It is likely that mast cell degranulation plays a role in airway hyperreactivity. Mast cell mediator release can occur by IgE allergen-induced activation as well as by non–IgE-dependent stimuli such as cold, dry air. Although evidence supports mast cell involvement, elevated T-lymphocyte, macrophage, neutrophil, and eosinophil counts obtained from BAL are found in both the asthmatic and the cold weather athlete. However, whether or not the elevated cell counts are simply indicative of chronic airway inflammation and are not responsible for the acute response associated with EIA cannot be determined. Current scientific evidence supports multiple mediator involvement in the pathogenesis of EIA. The inability of any single mediator therapy to totally inhibit EIA, coupled with the variability in individual response to single drug treatment, supports this concept. The most likely mediators include histamine, leukotrienes, and prostanoids.

Asthma and Exercise

Although most asthmatics are susceptible to airway hyperreactivity initiated by exercise, with appropriate medical intervention the ability to perform routine exercise usually is not limited. However, in many patients in whom resting lung function may be impaired because of chronic inflammation or airway remodeling, exercise performance may be compromised, especially among elite athletes. It is reasonable to assume that asthmatic patients will benefit from routine exercise.

Asthma During Exercise

A primary characteristic defining asthma is a reduction in airway function, which can potentially limit the type and amount of exercise the asthmatic is capable of performing. However, with appropriate medical intervention and knowledge of asthma triggers, most asthmatics are able to exercise symptom-free. In fact, exercise will improve the quality of life for the asthmatic and allow the individual to perform daily activities that otherwise would not be possible. Whether exercise actually improves the asthmatic condition is debatable, but the improvements in exercise tolerance and decreased ventilation rate for a given workload are well documented and will result in an increase in the quality of life for the asthmatic.

Although the hyperreactive airway response to exercise in EIA is thought to occur typically after the cessation of exercise, EIA can and often does occur during exercise and may limit athletic performance. Several factors determine whether asthma is limiting during exercise: the degree of chronic inflammation, the degree of airway reactivity, the mode of exercise (constant workload or interval type), the intensity and duration of exercise, and the environmental conditions in which the exercise is performed. It is known that asthmatics suffer measurable falls in FEV$_1$ and mid-expiratory flows during exercise (70, 71). What is not clear is whether the mild exercise-induced asthmatic is flow-limited during exercise.

The typical EIA response involves exercise bronchodilation during exercise with postexercise falls in expiratory flow rates (72, 73). The initial improvement in lung function at the beginning has been attributed to a withdrawal of vagal tone, followed by a mechanical bronchodilator influence. It is thought that increased tidal volume results in a mechanical coupling between lung tissue and the small airways. The larger tidal volumes cause the airways to be stretched open; thus, the high tidal volumes during exercise provide protection against bronchoconstriction.

Usually it is only after tidal volume decreases that the bronchoconstrictive influences dominate airway function. Beck et al. (70) have shown that during 36 minutes of steady-state exercise, asthmatic subjects exhibit an initial bronchodilation within the first 6 minutes of exercise, followed by a steady decline in airway function during the remaining 30 minutes of exercise (Figure 13.6A). Because the duration of most exercise challenges for EIA diagnosis is 6 to 8 minutes, this observed decline in exercise airway function has effectively gone unnoticed. Of particular interest, and germane to exercise in the real world, is the dynamic airway function by asthmatic subjects during interval-type exercise. Beck et al. (70) performed spirometry on asthmatic subjects during 36 minutes of interval-type exercise consisting of 6-minute sessions alternating moderate and light intensity. The FEV$_1$ and mid-expiratory flows demonstrated an overall gradual fall during the 36 minutes of exercise, with improvement in airway function during the

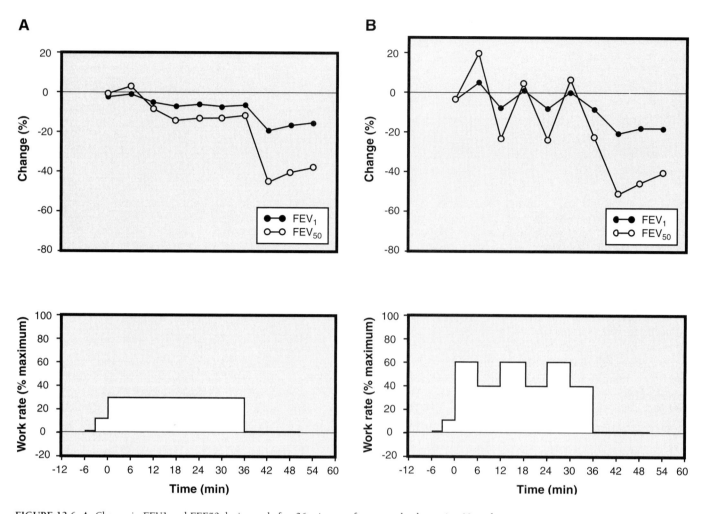

FIGURE 13.6. A. Change in FEV1 and FEF50 during and after 36 minutes of constant load exercise. Note the slight improvement after 6 minutes of exercise, followed by a significant decline in pulmonary function during the remaining 30 minutes of exercise with a further decline after exercise was stopped. **B.** Change in FEV1 and FEF50 during and after 36 minutes of interval type exercise, alternating 6-minute periods of moderate and light intensity exercise. Note the dynamic nature of pulmonary function between exercise intensities, but the overall decline over 36 minutes. (Redrawn from Beck et al. Am J Respir Crit Care Med 1994;149:352–357.)

moderate-intensity period and deterioration during the light-intensity period (Figure 13.6B). This dynamic flux in airway function implicates a bronchodilatory mechanism that is most likely mechanically mediated. However, PGE_2 and NO (produced by the epithelial cells) have known bronchodilatory effects and may provide protection from bronchoconstriction.

Exercise-Induced Asthma

Exercise is the most common trigger of an acute asthma attack among clinically diagnosed asthmatics. It has been estimated that 50% to 90% of all asthmatics are hyperresponsive to exercise. In fact, in mild asthmatics, EIA may be the only apparent expression of the disease. EIA is characterized by transient narrowing of the airways during or—most often—following exercise. Symptoms of cough, wheeze, chest tightness, **dyspnea**, and excess mucus production

may accompany the airway narrowing associated with exercise. Table 13.1 provides a complete list of symptoms.

Other terms often used to describe EIA are *exercise asthma, exercise airway hyperreactivity, exercise-induced bronchospasm or bronchoconstriction (EIB), skier asthma, skier cough, hockey cough,* and *cold-induced asthma*; all of these terms describe essentially the same condition. It has been suggested that the term EIB be used to describe post-exercise airway narrowing in the nonasthmatic population and the term EIA be used in specific reference to the asthmatic population (74). For the purpose of simplicity, in this chapter we will use the term EIA to represent all individuals who suffer from airway hyperreactivity associated with exercise; although it has been suggested that all individuals who have quantitatively defined EIA (measured by post-exercise reductions in pulmonary function) are asthmatic to some degree (75), Nordic skiers demonstrate airway remodeling different from that identified in the frank asthmatic (33, 35).

TABLE 13.1. SYMPTOMS OF ASTHMA AND EXER-CISE-INDUCED ASTHMA[a]

Observable clinical symptoms

Coughing Dyspnea

Wheezing Shortness of breath

Chest tightness Excess mucus

Exercise performance–related symptoms

Climate- or seasonal-related fluctuations in asthma or asthma-like symptoms that may be related to the water content or pollen content in the air

Poor performance for level of conditioning

Feeling of being "out of shape" or of having "heavy legs"

[a] Symptoms may occur more frequently at night or early morning in the asthmatic, or after exercise in both the asthmatic and the exercise-induced asthmatic.

Exercise-induced asthma has been documented since the second century. A high percentage of athletes and most asthmatics (during some stage in their disease) are affected by EIA. The prevalence of EIA has been estimated to be 4% to 20% in the general population (2, 74, 76–82). In specific athlete populations, estimates of 11% to 55% have been reported (83–91). The highest prevalence of EIA within the athlete population is found in winter sports (5, 83–86, 90–92); summer sports report a prevalence similar to that estimated for the general population (88, 90).

The large difference in EIA prevalence between summer and winter athletes supports the concept that specific environmental demands on airways influence the pathophysiology of airway dysfunction (33, 35, 36, 93–96). The airways of outdoor winter athletes are chronically exposed to the insult of cold, dry air at high ventilation rates. Likewise, the ice arena athlete may be exposed to high concentrations of rink air pollutants emitted from gas- or propane-powered ice resurfacing machines (97–104).

Diagnosis of Asthma and Exercise-Induced Asthma

Asthma Diagnosis

The diagnosis of asthma is not accomplished merely by the observation of asthma-like symptoms. True diagnosis is based on the definition of asthma and its components: in addition to basic symptomatology, a patient must demonstrate a medical history consistent with asthma, a variable or partially reversible airflow obstruction, and airway inflammation. Other potential diagnoses (e.g., bronchitis or emphysema) also must be eliminated (105–107).

Symptoms and outward indicators of asthma are diverse and varied. Some patients complain of basic respiratory difficulties, including coughing, wheezing (high-pitched whistling during exhalation), chest tightness, or shortness of breath. Other signs include prolonged difficulty in eliminating upper respiratory infections, difficulty sleeping due to night symptoms, and worsening problems in the presence of certain triggers—exercise, animal dander, house dust mites, mold, smoke, pollen, changes in weather, or airborne chemicals (106–108). Although the presence of these symptoms and a basic physical examination are marginally effective in diagnosing asthma, objective measures of lung function must be obtained for an accurate and reliable diagnosis (105, 108, 109).

It is preferable to obtain these objective measures through the use of standard spirometry, the most effective means to determine the presence or reversibility of airflow obstruction and restriction (105, 106, 110). Bye et al. (111) demonstrated a statistically significant underdiagnosis of airflow obstruction when spirometry was not performed; the importance of this truly objective measure cannot be overstated. The typical procedure calls for a baseline pulmonary function test (PFT), the inhalation of a bronchodilator agent (isoproterenol or a short-acting β_2-agonist), and a final PFT 15 minutes after the bronchodilator is used. Final results are compared with baseline values and percent changes are noted (107). The most useful variables obtained from spirometry are forced expiratory volume in the first second (FEV_1), forced vital capacity (FVC), and the ratio between these values (FEV_1/FVC) (106). A 12% to 15% improvement in FEV_1 strongly suggests reversible airflow (105, 107, 112); moreover, a FEV_1/FVC lower than predicted values indicates airflow obstruction, and a reduced FVC coupled with a normal FEV_1/FVC points to airflow restriction (106). The short-acting bronchodilators used in this test can be replaced by oral corticosteroids, with a 20% improvement in FEV_1 after 10 to 14 days considered indicative of asthma (105).

When full spirometry is not available, the patient's peak expiratory flow (PEF) can be easily, quickly, and inexpensively determined. This measure is more variable and less diagnostic than FEV_1 or FVC, but the PEF can be useful (108). Asthma status based on PEF can be obtained by examining percent improvement after the inhalation of a bronchodilator (>20% improvement = asthmatic) (105) or by analyzing serial measurements over the course of a week to determine PEF variability (see Table 13.2).

Occasionally, because asthma is an episodic disease, individuals with mild symptoms may appear normal during physical examinations and objective spirometry (108). In these cases, other laboratory or hospital tests may be required for diagnosis. Bronchoprovocation tests are used most commonly in such cases (105, 108, 110). These tests involve successive inhalations of a bronchially irritating substance (e.g., methacholine, histamine, nonisotonic aerosols) in increasing dosages. Each inhalation is followed by a PFT. The test ends when the subject reaches a predetermined level of reactivity, in which case the patient is considered asthmatic, or the maximum dose is administered without significant response, in which case the patient is

TABLE 13.2. CLASSIFICATION OF ASTHMA SEVERITY

	CLINICAL FEATURES BEFORE TREATMENT[a]	
Symptoms[b]	**Nighttime Symptoms**	**Lung Function**
Step 4 Severe persistent • Continual symptoms • Limited physical activity • Frequent exacerbations	Frequent	• FEV_1 or PEF ≤60% predicted • PEF variability >30%
Step 3 Moderate persistent • Daily symptoms • Daily use of inhaled short-acting beta₂-agonist • Exacerbations affect activity • Exacerbations ≥2 times a week; may last days	>1 time a week	• FEV_1 or PEF >60–<80% predicted PEF variability >30%
Step 2 Mild persistent • Symptoms >2 times a week but <1 time a day • Exacerbations may affect activity	>2 times a month	• FEV_1 or PEF ≥80% predicted PEF variability 20-30%
Step 1 Mild intermittent • Symptoms ≤2 times a week • Asymptomatic and normal PEF between exacerbations • Exacerbations brief (from a few hours to a few days); intensity may vary	≤2 times a month	• FEV_1 or PEF ≥80% predicted • PEF variability <20%

[a] The presence of one of the features of severity is sufficient to place in that category. An individual should be assigned to the most severe grade in which any feature occurs. The characteristics noted in this figure are general and may overlap because asthma is highly variable. Furthermore, an individual's classification may change over time.

[b] Patients at any level of severity can have mild, moderate, or severe exacerbations. Some patients with intermittent asthma experience severe and life-threatening exacerbations separated by long periods of normal lung function and no symptoms.

From Expert Panel Report 2. Guidelines for the Diagnosis and Management of Asthma, United States Department of Health and Human Services, National Institute of Health, Publication No. 97-4051, July 1997 (106).

considered nonasthmatic. It is important to remember that bronchoprovocation tests, although providing potentially important information, are not purely diagnostic for asthma. Rather, they describe the presence or absence of bronchial hyperresponsiveness to a particular substance (107). Other parameters that may provide information include auscultation of the chest, eosinophilia blood count, chest x-rays, examination of other PFT variables, tests of diffusion capacity, allergy testing, presence of nasal polyps or sinus disease, and the presence of gastroesophageal reflux (106, 108).

Classification of Asthma Severity

A variety of criteria and many different systems have been proposed to classify the severity of asthma. Although experts argue the merits of including frequency and duration of symptoms, persistence or degree of airflow limitation, or indices of morbidity in the "severity algorithm," nearly all agree that a key indicator of asthma severity is the minimum pharmacologic therapy required (105, 108). The most current classification system, approved and endorsed by the

National Institutes of Health (NIH), the National Heart, Lung, and Blood Institute (NHLBI), and the National Asthma Education and Prevention Program (NAEPP) (106), is presented in Table 13.2.

Exercise-Induced Asthma Diagnosis

The large variability in reported EIA prevalence may be explained, in part, by the methodology employed in formulating the diagnosis. The appropriate method for obtaining an accurate and reliable diagnosis of EIA is a debated topic. Typically, the procedure involves a baseline pulmonary function test (PFT), an EIA-provoking challenge, and a series of PFTs following the challenge. Patients are evaluated by comparing postchallenge test results to the prechallenge test results and calculating a percent change from baseline. This basic procedure is fraught with questions, however. Is testing even necessary—that is, is the presence of obvious postexercise symptoms an accurate means of diagnosis? When and at what increments should postchallenge PFTs be completed? What variables and what cutoff criteria should be used to determine the presence of EIA? What form should the EIA-provoking challenge take: pharmacologic, hyperventilation, or exercise? If exercise is used, what should the mode, intensity, and duration be? The answers to these questions present nearly limitless variations in procedure and protocol for the diagnosis of EIA.

Before any details regarding challenge protocol are addressed, the very necessity of the challenge itself should be questioned. With EIA symptoms that are overtly obvious and easily described by the patient, is mere observation of the postexercise signs or symptoms a sufficiently powerful diagnostic tool? Although a few studies (5, 85, 87, 113, 114) have examined whether symptoms are always coexistent with EIA, self-reported symptoms often are the only basis for diagnosis (5, 115, 116). Rundell et al. (5) demonstrated that among elite athletes, a diagnosis based on self-reported symptoms is no more accurate than a coin toss. In that study, 61% of EIA-positive athletes reported having symptoms; 45% of non-EIA athletes, however, also reported having symptoms of EIA. The proportion of EIA-positive and non-EIA athletes reporting two or more symptoms was essentially the same (39% vs. 41%; Table 13.3). A sensitivity/specificity analysis demonstrated that self-reported symptoms were not effective for identifying EIA-positive or excluding EIA-negative athletes (Table 13.4). Moreover, in some cases, respiratory disorders other than EIA result in exercise-related symptoms. One commonly misdiagnosed disorder is vocal cord dysfunction (VCD), in which inspiratory stridor is mistaken for the characteristic wheeze of EIA but is, in fact, a paradoxical closure of the vocal cords. Vocal cord dysfunction occurs during exercise, typically is abrupt in onset, and resolves spontaneously within 2 minutes of exercise cessation.

Because full pre- and postspirometric measurements are required for an accurate and reliable diagnosis of EIA, the appropriate time points of measurement and the cut-off criteria become important. Studies show that the greatest drop

TABLE 13.4. THE EFFECTIVENESS OF SELF-REPORTED SYMPTOMS

Symptom	Proportion of True Diagnosis[a]	Sensitivity[b]	Specificity[c]
Self-reported symptoms			
Cough	0.66	0.61	0.69
Wheeze	0.61	0.17	0.82
Chest tightness	0.63	0.20	0.83
Excess mucus	0.65	0.22	0.85
No. self-reported symptoms			
1 or more	0.57	0.61	0.55
2 or more	0.67	0.44	0.78

[a] Proportion of true diagnoses (those whose reported symptoms match PFT diagnosis)
[b] Sensitivity (the proportion of symptom-positives who tested positive)
[c] Specificity (the proportion of symptom-negatives who tested negative)
Data from Rundell KW, Im J, Mayers LB, et al. (5).

in pulmonary function occurs 5 to 10 minutes postexercise (76, 117). To include these time points, as well as ensure a complete analysis, spirometry can be done immediately, and then 5, 10, and 15 minutes after the cessation of exercise. Frequently, however, the immediate postexercise PFT is not used because of its limited diagnostic potential and the inability of the subject to perform the maneuver with an acceptable effort.

Although PFTs provide a number of variables, only some of these have been used for the determination of EIA. As with asthma testing, FEV_1 has been the variable most studied. Cut-off criteria of a 10% to 15% fall from baseline measures are among the most popular (76, 117), although there is no statistical basis for these numbers. When full spirometry is not available, PEF often is used, with decrements similar to those for FEV_1 being considered diagnostic. Again, the lack of statistical justification is a concern. Finally, mean midexpiratory flow ($FEF_{25-75\%}$) recently has gained acceptance, with drops of 15% to 25% (112, 118) being considered positive for EIA (EIA+). As with the other standards, these numbers are not based on statistical evidence. However, Rundell et al. (5) have presented statistically justified values for the elite athlete population (> 2 standard deviations from the normal, healthy population of elite athletes): drops in FEV_1, $FEF_{25-75\%}$, and PEF of 7%, 12.5%, and 18%, respectively.

Once the measurement schedule and cut-off criteria have been determined, the actual EIA-provoking challenge must be considered. A variety of protocols, modes, and methods have been used, but the challenges fall into four primary categories: pharmacologic, osmotic, hyperventilation, and exercise.

Pharmacologic challenges are identical to the bronchoprovocation tests often used to determine the presence of frank asthma. Two of the most popular pharmacologic challenges use histamine and methacholine to provoke bronchoconstriction. Histamine causes airway obstruction

TABLE 13.3. CUMULATIVE SELF-REPORTED SYMPTOMS FOR PFT-POSITIVE, PFT BORDERLINE, AND PFT NORMAL ATHLETES

	NUMBER (%) OF REPORTED SYMPTOMS			
	1 (%)	**> 2 (%)**	**> 3 (%)**	**> 4 (%)**
PFT+	25 (31)[a]	18 (39)[a]	5 (24)	1 (20)
PFT-B	17 (21)	9 (20)	5 (24)	2 (40)
PFT-N	39 (48)[a,b]	19 (41)[a]	11 (52)	2 (40)
Total	**81**	**46**	**21**	**5**

[a] Indicates significantly different than PFT-B, P <0.05.
[b] Indicates significantly different than PFT+, P<0.05..
PFT+, >10% post exercise fall in FEV_1; PFT-B, PFT borderline (>7% but <10% or >12% post exercise fall in FEV_1 and/or $FEF_{25-75\%}$); PFT-N, PFT normal.
Data from Rundell KW, Im J, Mayers LB, et al. (5).

via the activation of bronchial smooth muscle and secretory receptors; methacholine functions by inducing bronchoconstriction, increased airway inflation pressure, and contraction of the trachealis muscle (119).

Two osmotic challenges that demonstrate promise for evaluation of the hyperreactive airways characteristic of asthma and EIA are the dry powdered mannitol inhalation challenge (120, 121) and the nebulized hypertonic saline challenge (122–125). The mannitol challenge uses the same general protocol as a methacholine or histamine challenge, whereby increasing doses of the stimulating substance are administered, each followed by pulmonary function tests, until an upper-limit dose is reached or PFT cut-off criteria for asthma are met. Mannitol inhalation acts by altering the osmolarity of the ASL, followed by mast cell granulation and inflammatory mediator release (120). Another osmotic challenge designed to identify hyperreactive airways involves the inhalation of nebulized hypertonic saline. This provocation, like the mannitol challenge, alters the tonicity and osmolarity of the airway surface liquid, causing mast cells to release inflammatory mediators (53). Osmotic challenges are popular because they use substances that are economical, stable, and easily obtained (126).

Another category of challenges designed to screen for asthma or EIA that are based on the premise that exercise per se does not cause EIA are the hyperventilation challenges—any activity that increases ventilation rate enough to dry or cool airways will cause bronchoconstriction in susceptible individuals. The hyperventilation protocol involves voluntary breathing at a predetermined rate, typically 60% to 85% of maximal ventilatory rate (MVV). The respiration rate for the challenge is estimated by assuming MVV to be $35 \times FEV_1$. The challenge is administered between pre- and post-PFTs and most often uses a dry air mixture containing 4.5% CO_2 (120, 127). The purpose of the hypercapnic air is to ensure eucapnic voluntary hyperventilation (EVH). This will protect against a hyperventilation-induced hypocapnia, which has been shown to cause bronchoconstriction in both

EIA-positive and EIA-negative subjects (128). A variation on the EVH challenge involves chilling the inspired air, thus potentially causing a greater change in airway osmolarity or vascular response (28).

The final provocation challenge for asthma or, most often, EIA that we will discuss is exercise itself. Although other forms of provocation may be useful (especially for the subject unable to complete an exercise challenge), intuitively it makes sense that the best test for exercise-induced asthma would be exercise (129).

Choosing exercise as the method of bronchial provocation for EIA evaluation does not, however, simplify the diagnosis. Exercise intensity, duration, mode, and environmental conditions are all factors that must be considered. Although exercise intensity originally had been prescribed at approximately 85% of maximum heart rate (76), recent studies suggest that a significantly higher exercise intensity should be used (up to 95% to100% of maximum effort), especially in the athlete population (83, 86, 87, 91). The duration of exercise, originally prescribed at 6 to 8 minutes (111), is consistent with a mathematical model of airway drying devised by Anderson and Daviskas (27) (Figure 13.7). However, successful diagnoses have been obtained using short-duration, high-intensity exercise as the provoking challenge (5, 83, 86, 87, 130). Anderson and Daviskas' airway-drying model provides evidence that high-intensity, high-ventilation exercise can dry the airways sufficiently within 2 minutes and thus provoke a response in susceptible individuals (32).

The mode of exercise also has been shown to be important to the severity of EIA response, although it may be the environment associated with a particular activity that is the primary determinant of the response (87). For example, because swimming occurs in a pool, where ambient conditions often are warm and extremely humid, the prevalence and intensity of EIA should be lessened. However, high airway hyperresponsiveness has been noted in the indoor pool environment; high chlorine levels are thought to be the cause. Another indoor athletic environment, the ice arena, has conditions of cold temperatures and low hu-

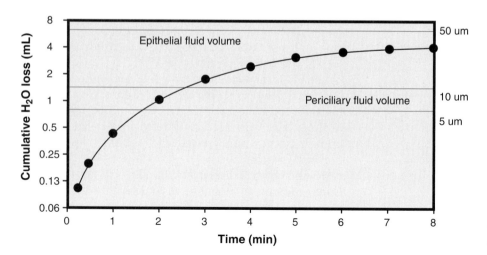

FIGURE 13.7. Mathematical model (Reference 32) estimating water loss from the trachea to the 12th generation of airways. The model assumes either a 5- or 10-μm depth of airway surface liquid (ASL), a ventilation rate of 60 L·min-1 of inspired air at 26°C, 8.8 mg H_2O·L^{-1}. Under these conditions, a calculated net water loss of 7.4 μL H_2O would dehydrate the periciliary fluid within 2 to 3 min.

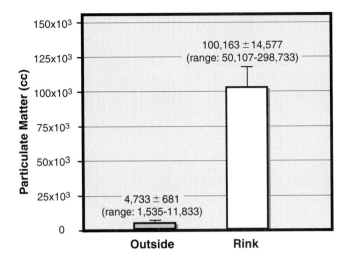

FIGURE 13.8. Particulate matter (PM <1.0 μm diameter) measured in outside air and at ice level in seven ice rinks during prime usage hours (29 measurements). Note that PM concentration in the ice arena air is greater than 20 times that of the ambient air outside of the ice arena. (Reprinted with permission from Williams SD, Judelson DA, Rundell KW. High levels of airborne particulate matter in indoor ice arenas. Med Sci Sports Exerc 2001;33[suppl 5]:S12.)

midity combined with high levels of potentially harmful pollutants released by the ice resurfacing machines (Figure 13.8), conditions that will exacerbate the asthmatic response (5, 104).

Any exercise test of sufficient intensity and duration, under dry-air ambient conditions, can be used to elicit a bronchoconstricting response for EIA screening, but it is best to employ an exercise challenge that matches the subject's actual athletic event (83, 84, 87, 91). Taking this "sport-specific" theory one step farther, actual competitions have been used as the stimulating challenge (87, 91). These studies demonstrated that a subject can experience EIA symptoms during his or her particular sporting event yet be symptom-free during a laboratory exercise challenge (Figure 13.9). Conversely, those who react to a nonexercise laboratory test (e.g., methacholine or EVH challenge) may be asymptomatic during their actual event. To ensure a patient is most appropriately treated to improve his or her condition during athletic performance, a sport-specific challenge may be employed. The efficacy of such challenges (which may vary in intensity, duration, and mode) in comparison with a standardized (6 to 8 min-

FIGURE 13.9. Postexercise pulmonary function values for an actual or simulated race (field-based challenge: FBC) and a 6-8 minute treadmill run at 95% peak HR (laboratory-based exercise challenge: LBC). 78% of the athletes (18/23) who were EIA positive by FBC were EIA normal by LBC.

* Indicates significant difference between FBC and LBC at specific sample time (P <0.05). † Indicates significantly different than 5-minute sample time within exercise challenge mode (P <0.05). ‡ Significantly different than 10-minute sample time within exercise challenge mode (P <0.05). (Reprinted with permission from Rundell KW, Wilber RL, Szmedra L, et al. Exercise-induced asthma screening of elite athletes: field versus laboratory exercise challenge. Med Sci Sports Exerc 2000;32:309–316.)

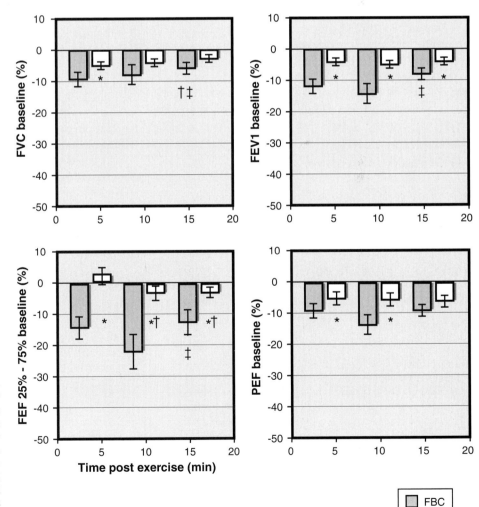

utes of high-intensity exercise in constant environmental conditions) laboratory challenge is still questionable, however.

Therapy of Asthma and Exercise-Induced Asthma

Goals of Therapy

The ultimate goal of any treatment or therapy is the cure or complete removal of the disease; unfortunately, this is not possible with asthma or EIA. However, a number of reasonable goals can be achieved that will allow the asthmatic to lead a normal, physically active life.

The primary purpose of asthma therapy is to control the patient's chronic respiratory symptoms, for example, cough, wheeze, and dyspnea. Closely coupled to this is the desire to limit asthma exacerbations, minimize the use of rescue bronchodilators, and decrease the number of hospitalizations. These goals are best achieved by maintaining baseline pulmonary function at normal or near normal levels. As a result of attaining these goals, normal activity levels (including exercise) can be achieved. The Canadian Asthma Consensus Report published in 1999 reported indicators of controlled asthma to serve as a reasonable goal for most asthmatics (105) (Table 13.5).

It is important to remember that achieving all of these goals may not be possible for all patients. As with diagnosis and pharmacologic prescription, the goals of therapy need to be designed and suited to each individual patient (105).

Medications for Asthma

The pharmacologic approach to the treatment of asthma and EIA can be divided into two primary categories based on the physiology of the disease. Because asthma is considered a disease of chronic airway inflammation, medications in one group, known as controllers, aim to provide long-term control by reducing inflammation. Drugs in this category are taken on a daily basis and provide the foundation for all asthma management (83). The other type of medication, known as relievers, is designed to relieve acute obstruction or bronchoconstriction. Drugs in this category are taken on an as-needed basis and supplement the controllers (105, 106).

Inhaled Corticosteroids

The NIH, NHBLI, and NAEPP define anti-inflammatory medications as "those that cause a reduction in inflammatory markers in airways tissue or secretions...and thus decrease the intensity of airways hyperresponsiveness" (106). Inhaled corticosteroids are the most effective, potent, and often used of the anti-inflammatory medications in the treatment of asthma (83, 108, 110). The inhaled corticosteroids present significantly fewer adverse effects than their orally consumed counterparts and are well tolerated by most people. The small potential risk is far outweighed by the benefits and efficacy of inhaled corticosteroids (106). With long-term use, inhaled corticosteroids will improve pulmonary function in asthmatic individuals. Improvements in resting FEV_1 (131) and PEF (132–134) are observed after prolonged (>3 weeks) treatment with inhaled steroids. Likewise, the frequency of asthma exacerbations (134, 135), beta-2 agonist use (132), and bronchial hyperreactivity (106, 136) diminishes. Corticosteroids inhibit multiple segments of the asthmatic cascade, suppressing the generation of cytokines, reducing the population of airway eosinophils, and preventing inflammatory mediator release (106).

Cromolyn Sodium and Nedocromil Sodium

Cromolyn sodium and nedocromil sodium have been used extensively as long-term controllers and as pretreatment prophylaxis for EIA. They are believed to block chloride ion flux into mast cells, epithelial cells, and neurons (137); inhibit the release of histamines, leukotrienes, and prostaglandins (110, 138); and prevent mast cell degranulation (136). These medications have been shown to improve PEF, reduce nocturnal use of reliever medications (e.g., beta-2 agonists), and also act in prophylactic blockade of the bronchoconstriction following exercise in EIA-positive individuals (108, 139, 140).

Leukotriene Modifiers

Leukotriene modifiers, such as montelukast, zafirlukast, and zileuton, have demonstrated clinically significant attenuation of asthma-related bronchoconstriction (64, 141), relief of asthma symptoms (106), protection against EIA (64), and reduction in the dose of inhaled corticosteroids

TABLE 13.5. INDICATIONS OF ASTHMA CONTROL

Parameter	Frequency or value
Daytime symptoms	< 4 days/week
Nighttime symptoms	< 1 night/week
Physical activity	Normal
Exacerbations	Mild, infrequent
Absence from work or school	None
Need for short-acting β_2-agonist	< 4 doses/week[a]
FEV_1 or PEF	> 85% of personal best, ideally 90%
PEF diurnal variation[b]	< 15% of diurnal variation

[a] May use 1 dose/day for prevention of exercise-induced symptoms.
[b] Diurnal variation is calculated by subtracting the lowest PEF from the highest and dividing by the highest PEF multiplied by 100.
FEV_1, forced expiratory volume in 1 second; PEF, peak expiratory flow obtained with a portable peak flow meter
Data from Canadian Asthma Consensus Report, 1999 (105).

(142). Leukotrienes are clearly implicated in the pathogenesis of asthma and EIA, even though the beneficial effects of leukotriene modifiers have not been 100% in all patients (see Figure 13.5). This finding implies that leukotrienes are not *the* single mediator involved in airway inflammation. Nonetheless, the leukotriene modifiers have been proven clinically to be important in the treatment of asthma. However, these drugs are relatively new, and their efficacy is still under investigation (136).

Beta$_2$-Adrenergic Agonists

Beta$_2$-adrenergic agonists have a potent bronchodilatory effect and are used in treatment of acute asthma exacerbation and for EIA prophylaxis. In fact, β_2-agonists are considered to be the most effective preventative therapy for EIA and have been reported to improve pulmonary function in 90% of subjects suffering from EIA (143). The β_2-agonists typically are administered by metered-dose inhalers or, in the case of salmeterol (a long acting β_2-agonist), by a metered-dose inhaler or a dry powder inhalation device.

The most popular class of quick-relief medication is the short-acting β_2-agonists. Functionally similar to long-acting β_2-agonists (i.e., they increase cAMP activity), short-acting β_2-agonists relax smooth muscle, increase air flow, decrease vascular permeability, and act to moderately inhibit mediator release (106, 108). The use of short-acting β_2-agonists is not without drawbacks, however. These agents have a relatively short duration of action—4 to 6 hours—with the peak bronchodilatory effect occurring within 60 minutes. This pattern, coupled with frequent use, has been shown to worsen the asthmatic condition (106, 108). The NIH, NHLBI, and NAEPP recommend one canister per month as the maximal dosage; anything higher implies the need for better basic asthma control (e.g., inhaled corticosteroids) (106). Other recommendations (112) suggest that if short-acting β_2-agonists are used more than two times per week for rescue or prophylaxis, then a treatment program using corticosteroids should be implemented to address the chronic inflammation of asthma. The efficacy of short-acting β_2-agonists in treating EIA in elite athletes has recently been questioned (144); it was shown that over a 2-year period, short-acting β_2-agonists were ineffective in controlling EIA in elite speed skaters (Figure 13.10). In this study, maximum postexercise falls in 1998 for elite speed skaters taking no medication were no different from postexercise falls in FEV$_1$ in 2000 while using a short-acting β_2-agonist. This study suggests that short-acting β_2-agonists may not provide the best protection in a population of elite athletes who require prophylaxis on a daily basis. Controller medication addressing chronic inflammation may be required to treat this population appropriately.

Long-acting β_2-agonists function similarly to short-acting β_2-agonists by preventing bronchoconstriction (106), improving the expiratory flow rate (145), and lessening the frequency and intensity of asthma or EIA exacer-

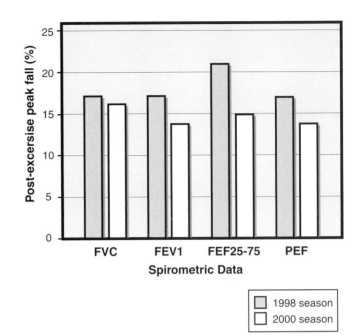

FIGURE 13.10. Postexercise falls in pulmonary function prior to and following short-acting β_2-agonist treatment (N = 8 EIA-positive elite short track speed skaters). Values are for the greatest fall measured at 5, 10, or 15 minutes postexercise. No significant improvements from β_2-agonist intervention were noted for any pulmonary function measured. Initial testing was done during the 1998 season and follow-up testing was done during the 2000 season. (Reprinted with permission from Wilber RL, Rundell KW, Judelson DA. Efficacy of asthma medication regimen in elite athletes with exercise-induced asthma. Med Sci Sports Exerc 2001;33[suppl 5]:S12.)

bation (145, 146). Unlike the short-acting β_2-agonists, long-acting β_2-agonists may be effective for up to 12 hours (145, 147) and are especially useful as supplements to inhaled corticosteroids for patients with intensified nocturnal symptoms (136). The long-acting β_2-agonists salmeterol and formoterol have bronchodilator effects similar to those of albuterol (the commonly used short-acting β_2-agonist) in magnitude and can be used as prophylaxis against EIA for up to 8 hours, superseding multiple daily doses of albuterol. This can be especially important for schoolchildren, who typically have days filled with multiple, often random, unscheduled bouts of exercise. It is important to note that tachyphylaxis in response to salmeterol has been noted after 1 month of daily use (63). However, this study demonstrated that in the short term, within 1 hour of drug inhalation, salmeterol was still effective (63). A summary of anti-inflammatory controllers and their chemical families can be found in Table 13.6.

Other Medications

Other treatments for acute attacks of asthma include oral corticosteroids and ipratropium bromide. Oral corticosteroids are useful in such cases when short-acting β_2-agonists are not providing an adequate response; often, a

TABLE 13.6. ANTI-INFLAMMATORY CONTROLLER MEDICATIONS

Drug	Chemical Family
Beclomethasone dipropionate	Corticosteroid
Budesonide	Corticosteroid
Flunisolide	Corticosteroid
Fluticasone propionate	Corticosteroid
Triamcinolone acetonide	Corticosteroid
Cromolyn sodium	
Nedocromil sodium	
Montelukast	Leukotriene modifier
Zafirlukast	Leukotriene modifier
Zileuton	Leukotriene modifier
Salmeterol	Long acting β_2-agonist
Theophylline	Methylxanthine

short course of oral corticosteroids also is prescribed after an exacerbation requiring hospitalization (136). The use of oral corticosteroids, however, is kept to a minimum because they have potentially severe side effects. Ipratropium bromide may also be suggested in the case of severe exacerbations; it functions by affecting the cholinergic innervation to the airway smooth muscle and reducing bronchial hyperreactivity to inhaled irritants (106, 108). Table 13.7 presents a summary of short-acting relievers and their chemical families.

Most asthma medications are available in both inhaled and systemic forms. The inhaled version is universally preferred because of the increased concentration of medication delivered to appropriate areas, fewer side effects, and a shorter time until onset of action (105, 106).

The Use of Medication According to the Severity of Asthma

Just as a variety of classification schemes to describe the intensity of asthma have been created, so have differing diagnoses based on these systems. The system of drug use currently endorsed by the NIH, NHLBI, and NAEPP (see Table 13.2) is reviewed here (106).

TABLE 13.7. SHORT-ACTING RELIEVER MEDICATIONS

Drug	Chemical Family
Albuterol	Short-acting β_2-agonists
Bitolterol	Short-acting β_2-agonists
Metaproterenol	Short-acting β_2-agonists
Pirbuterol	Short-acting β_2-agonists
Terbutaline	Short-acting β_2-agonists
Methylprednisolone	Oral corticosteroid
Prednisolone	Oral corticosteroid
Prednisone	Oral corticosteroid
Ipratropium bromide	Anticholinergic

Prescribed medication for acute exacerbations of asthma are the same for all categories of asthma severity: short-acting β_2-agonists commensurate with the intensity of symptoms. Only in the long-term control of asthma are there differences between asthmatic severity intensities. Step 4 (Severe Persistent) asthmatics obviously require the most medication of the four groups. Recommended daily medications include high doses of inhaled corticosteroids, a long-acting bronchodilator (e.g., a long-acting β_2-agonist or theophylline), and some form of oral corticosteroids. The prescription for Step 3 (Moderate Persistent) asthmatics is slightly more variable. Depending on individual reaction and preference, medium doses of inhaled corticosteroids may be replaced by the combination of a low-medium dose of inhaled corticosteroids coupled with a long-acting bronchodilator, especially for nighttime use. If necessary, the use of either group of medications may be intensified. The recommendation for Step 2 (Mild Persistent) asthmatics is the use of one of the following: low doses of inhaled corticosteroids, cromolyn or nedocromil sodium, sustained-release theophylline, or a leukotriene modifier. Inhaled corticosteroids are the suggested medication. Step 1 (Mild Intermittent) asthmatics do not require daily medication; the use of a short-acting β_2-agonist for asthma attacks typically is all that is required (106).

For financial and health reasons, minimum pharmacologic intervention is most desirable (105, 108, 136). In addition, preliminary diagnoses and medical prescriptions may not achieve desired results immediately, or the severity of asthma may change over time, requiring changes in the medical intervention. To achieve the best possible treatment, the NIH, NHLBI, and NAEPP provide recommendations on changing medications according to alterations in disease state or patient need: the step-care approach to asthma therapy. Gaining control of the disease is most important and can be achieved in two ways. Patients may be classified (and medicated) at the step most appropriate to their symptoms and intensity, or they may be diagnosed *one step higher* than would be apparent, ideally ensuring control will be attained (106).

If the patient's asthma is in check, treatment should be reviewed every 1 to 6 months and, if possible, medication should be reduced or altered. This is known as the "step-down" method. If there is no change in asthma intensity, eventually a baseline level of medication will be reached below which further reductions in dosage include loss of disease control. If this point is reached, or the original prescription does not sufficiently meet the goals of therapy, medication should be intensified (the "step-up" method). Before the dosage is increased, however, patient medication technique, adherence, and avoidance of potential triggers should be examined. If these considerations are being attended to properly, an increase in medication (dose or the addition of another medication) may be in order (106).

Nonpharmacologic aspects of asthma therapy also require attention. As with any disease, patient education is of the utmost importance. Basic asthma facts, appropriate inhaler or medication technique, and the roles and actions of medications should all be known and understood by the patient. Additionally, self-management plans, action plans for acute exacerbations, and trigger avoidance are necessary, and these are possible only through appropriate education (106).

What We Know
About Asthma and Exercise-Induced Asthma

1 Asthma is a chronic lung disease characterized by inflammation, resident inflammatory cells, airway hyperreactivity to stimuli, reversible air flow obstruction, and a variety of symptoms such as cough, wheeze, excess mucus, dyspnea, and chest tightness.

2 An estimated 17 million people in the United States have asthma, resulting in annual medical costs exceeding $11 billion and 14 deaths each day.

3 Asthma is the most common childhood disease, affecting approximately 5 million children; males seem to be affected more at an early age, whereas the prevalence among females is greater later in life.

4 The inflammatory process of asthma is multicellular, involving mast cells, eosinophils, T lymphocytes, macrophages, neutrophils, and epithelial cells; IgE-mediated atopy is highly associated with, but not exclusive to, asthma and EIA.

5 Airway inflammation and bronchial hyperreactivity characteristic of EIA are most likely initiated by water loss of the airway surface liquid and subsequent osmolarity change in airway cells, ultimately resulting in inflammatory mediator release.

6 The pathogenesis of asthma and EIA supports multiple mediator involvement, with the most likely mediators including histamine, leukotrienes, and prostanoids.

7 Although the typical EIA response is bronchodilation during exercise with postexercise falls in pulmonary function, EIA can occur during exercise and limit athletic performance.

8 The prevalence of EIA among elite winter athletes is more than twice that identified for the general population, ranging from 20% to 50%, depending on the sport surveyed.

9 The diagnosis of asthma and EIA should be based on symptoms, medical history, variable or partially reversible airflow obstruction, or the presence of airway inflammation.

10 Treatment of asthma or EIA should be based on a complete medical evaluation and focused on controlling airway inflammation.

What We Would Like to Know
About Asthma and Exercise-Induced Asthma

1 Is the incidence of asthma really increasing or are we observing a phenomenon related to better asthma awareness, better medical care, and better diagnosis?

2 Is the exercise-induced airway narrowing observed in otherwise asymptomatic healthy individuals the same pathophysiology as the EIA in subjects with clinical asthma?

3 Are the repetitive high ventilation rates of the training elite athlete an underlying cause of EIA, or are inhaled allergens, irritant gases, or airborne particulate matter critical to the development of EIA?

4 Is the performance of the mild exercise-induced asthmatic limited by his or her asthma?

5 How reversible is the airway remodeling observed in asthmatics and in exercise-induced asthmatics?

6 What role do the inflammatory cytokines play in the pathogenesis of EIA and asthma?

7 What are the mechanisms of non-IgE mediated asthma?

Summary

The prevalence of asthma has increased over the last 25 years, to the point of being the most common and most costly illness in the United States. It is the leading cause of chronic illness in children, affecting more than one child in twenty. An equally high percentage of the population suffers from EIA; this is extremely prevalent among elite winter athletes, with 50% of athletes in some sports EIA-positive. Asthma is a chronic inflammatory disease of the airways that is characterized by episodes of coughing, wheezing, dyspnea, chest tightness, and excess mucus formation. These symptoms are associated with bronchial hyperreactivity and chronic or acute airflow obstruction that can reverse spontaneously or with medical intervention. Mast cells, eosinophils, T lymphocytes, macrophages, neutrophils, and epithelial cells are involved in the inflammatory process. Additionally, airway remodeling of the basement membrane that contributes to persistent abnormalities of the lung has been noted both in asthma and in EIA. The pathology of asthma and exercise-induced asthma is complex, involving multiple inflammatory mediators and stimulated by a variety of triggers. However, with appropriate treatment, the asthmatic should be able to control this disease and live a normal, active life.

DISCUSSION QUESTIONS

1 Why are environmental conditions (e.g., temperature, humidity, and airborne pollutants) important determinants of the asthmatic response?

2 Asthma and EIA are similar, but they may not be identical. What are the differences?

3 What is the step-care approach to asthma therapy and why do the NIH, NHLBI, and NAEPP support it?

4 Briefly describe the role airway surface liquid plays in the development and severity of asthma.

5 What questions must be answered in choosing a provoking challenge for the diagnosis of EIA?

6 Does exercise play a role in the treatment of asthma? If so, how?

CASE STUDY

Patient Information

Mike is an 18-year-old ice hockey player. As a freshman at a major college, he has recently begun his preseason conditioning with the ice hockey team. Despite training hard in the off-season to maintain his "game shape" and working hard during practices, the coaches are concerned with Mike's fitness. He seems to have a difficult time recovering between exercise bouts and frequently coughs during and after training. Additionally, Mike feels pressure in his chest during and after exercise, which he describes as "feeling like someone is standing on my chest when I try and breathe." His symptoms are apparent during most training sessions, but those inside the ice arena seem to cause the most trouble for Mike. Discussion of his problems with the team's athletic trainer led to an appointment with the team physician.

Assessments

Despite Mike's strenuous training regime, his actual and perceived fitness levels were not equivalent. This, along with the other respiratory symptoms he was having, caused the team physician to evaluate Mike for exercise-induced asthma. His pre-exercise pulmonary function test revealed a baseline value of FEV_1 that was only 70% of the predicted value for a male of his age and height. Mid-expiratory flow rates were even lower, at 45% of predicted values. After exercise, these already low values were further reduced by 25% (FEV_1) and 20% (FEF50). Additionally, the completion of a maximal exercise test showed only an average $\dot{V}O_{2max}$ value for an 18-year-old male and an arterial saturation of 87% at maximal exercise.

Reduced baseline pulmonary function (<85% predicted) and significant postexercise falls in pulmonary function suggest airway dysfunction. The reduced baseline is more indicative of chronic inflammation (frank asthma), while the post-exercise falls in pulmonary function imply exercise is a potent trigger for bronchoconstriction. The possibly low $\dot{V}O_{2max}$ and below-normal arterial saturation suggest pulmonary limitation to maximal exercise, which may be due to bronchoconstriction or airway inflammation.

Questions

1. What factors must you take into consideration when evaluating Mike's fitness level?
2. What factors must you take into consideration when making recommendations about Mike's training program?

3. What medications would you prescribe so that Mike would be able to live both his athletic and nonathletic lives to the fullest?
4. How would you evaluate the efficacy of the medication/exercise program that you prescribe?

ACKNOWLEDGMENTS

The authors thank Sara Chelland and Barry Spiering for their assistance in the preparation of this chapter.

REFERENCES

1. National Heart Lung and Blood Institute. Global Initiative for Asthma. Bethesda, MD: NIH Publications, 1995. National Institutes of Health Pub No 95-3659.
2. Backer V, Ulrik CS. Bronchial responsiveness to exercise in a random sample of 494 children and adolescents from Copenhagen. Clin Exp Allergy 1992;22:741–747.
3. Backer B, Groth S, Dirksen A, et al. Sensitivity and specificity of the histamine challenge test for the diagnosis of asthma in an unselected sample of children and adolescents. Eur Respir J 1991;4:1093–1100.
4. Pattimore PD, Asher MI, Harrison AC, et al. The interrelationship among bronchial hyperresponsiveness, the diagnosis of asthma, and asthma symptoms. Am Rev Respir Dis 1990;142:549–554.
5. Rundell KW, Im J, Mayers LB, et al. Self-reported symptom and exercise-induced asthma in the elite athlete. Med Sci Sports Exerc 2001;33:208–213.
6. Hartert TV, Peebles RS. Epidemiology of asthma: the year in review. Curr Opin Pulm Med 2000;6:4–9.
7. Lundback B. Epidemiology of rhinitis and asthma. Clin Exp Allergy 1998;Suppl 3:3–10.
8. Strannegard O, Strannegard IL. Why is the prevalence of allergy increasing? Changed microbial load is probably the cause. Lakartidningen 1999;96:4306–4312.
9. Holt PG, Sly PD, Bjorksten B. Atopic versus infectious diseases in childhood: a question of balance? Pediatr Allergy Immunol 1997;8:53–58.
10. Berstad AE, Brandtzaeg P. Does reduced microbial exposure contribute to increased prevalence of allergy? Tidsskr Nor Laegeforen 2000;120:915–919.
11. Howarth PH. Is allergy increasing? —early life influences. Clin Exp Allergy 1998;28(Suppl 6):2–7.
12. Holt PG, Yabuhara A, Prescott S, et al. Allergen recognition in the origin of asthma. Ciba Found Symp 1997;206:35–49 .
13. Holt PG. Infections and the development of allergy. Toxic Lett 1996;86:205–210.
14. Harju T, Keistinen T, Tuuponen T, Kivelda SL. Hospital admissions of asthmatics by age and sex. Allergy 1996;51:693–696.
15. Skobeloff EM, Spivey WH, St Clair SS, Schoffstall JM. The influence of age and sex on asthma admissions. JAMA 1992;268:3437–3440.
16. Volmer T. The socio-economics of asthma. Pulm Pharmacol Ther 2001;14:55-60.
17. Fagan JK, Scheff PA, Hryhorczuk D, et al. Prevalence of asthma and other allergic diseases in an adolescent population: association with gender and race. Ann Allergy Asthma Immunol 2001;86:177–184.
18. Joseph CL, Ownby DR, Peterson EL, Johnson CC. Racial differences in physiologic parameters related to asthma among middle-class children. Chest 2000;117:1336–1344.
19. Litonjua AA, Carey VJ, Weiss ST, Gold DR. Race, socioeconomic factors, and area of residence are associated with asthma prevalence. Pediatr Pulmonol 1999;28:394–401.
20. Von Kries R, Hermann M, Grunert VP, Von Mutius E. Is obesity a risk factor for childhood asthma? Allergy 2001;56:318–322.
21. Camargo CA Jr, Weiss ST, Zhang S, et al. Prospective study of body mass index, weight change, and risk of adult-onset asthma in women. Arch Intern Med 1999;159:2582–2588.
22. Castro-Rodriguez JA, Holberg CJ, Morgan WJ, et al. Increased incidence of asthmalike symptoms in girls who become overweight or obese during the school years. Am J Respir Crit Care Med 2001;163:1344–1349.
23. Sporik R, Holgate ST, Platts-Mills TA, Cogswell JJ. Exposure to house-dust mite allergen (Der p I) and the development of asthma in childhood. N Engl J Med 1990;323:502–507.
24. Roche WR. Fibroblasts and asthma. Clin Exp Allergy 1991;21:545–548.
25. Anderson SD, Schoeffel RE, Follet R, et al. Sensitivity to heat and water loss at rest and during exercise in asthmatic patients. Eur J Resp Dis 1982:63:459–471.
26. Anderson SD, Daviskas E. The mechanism of exercise-induced asthma is. J Allergy Clin Immunol 2000;106:453–459.
27. Anderson SD, Daviskas E. Pathophysiology of exercise-induced asthma: The role of respiratory water loss. In: Weiler JM, ed. Allergic and Respiratory Disease in Sports Medicine. New York: Marcel Dekker, Inc. 1997.
28. Chen WY, Horton DJ. Heat and water loss from the airways and exercise-induced asthma. Respiration 1977;34:305–313.
29. Deal EC, McFadden ER Jr, Ingram RH, et al. Role of respiratory heat exchange in production of exercise-induced asthma. J Appl Physiol 1979;46:467–475.
30. Deal EC, McFadden ER Jr, Ingram RH, Jaeger JJ. Hyperpnea and heat flux: initial reaction sequence in exercise-induced asthma. J Appl Physiol 1979;46:476–483.
31. McFadden ER Jr, Lenner KAM, Strohl KP. Postexertional airway rewarming and thermally induced asthma. New insights into pathophysiology and possible pathogenesis. J Clin Invest 1986;78:18–25.
32. Anderson SD. Airway drying and exercise-induced asthma. In: McFadden ER Jr, ed. Exercise-Induced Asthma. New York: Marcel Dekker, Inc, 1999.
33. Karjalainen EM, Laitinen A, Sue-Chu M, et al. Evidence of airway inflammation and remodeling in ski athlete with and without bronchial hyperresponsiveness to methacholine. Am J Respir Crit Care Med 2000;161:2086–2091.
34. Laitinen LA, Laitinen A, Haatela T. Airway mucosal inflammation even in patients with newly diagnosed asthma. Am Rev Respir Dis 1993;147:697–704.
35. Sue-Chu M, Larsson L, Moen T, et al. Bronchoscopy and bronchoalveolar lavage findings in cross-country skiers with and without "ski-asthma." Eur Respir J 1999;13:626–632.
36. Sue-Chu M, Karjalainen EM, Laitinen A, et al. Placebo-controlled study of inhaled budesonide on indices of airway inflammation in bronchoalveolar lavage fluid and bronchial biopsies in cross-country skiers. Respiration 2000;67:417–425.
37. Peters SP. Mechanism of mast-cell activation. In: Busse WW, Holgate ST, eds. Asthma and Rhinitis. Boston: Blackwell Scientific Publications, 1995.
38. Togias AG, Naclerio RM, Proud D, et al. Nasal challenge with cold dry air results in release of inflammatory mediators. J Clin Invest 1985;76:1375–1381.

39. Togias AG, Proud D, Lichtenstein LM, et al. The osmolality of nasal secretions increases when inflammatory mediators are released in response to inhalation of cold, dry air. Am Rev Respir Dis 1988;157:625–629.

40. Pohunek P, Kucera P, Sukova B, et al. Serum ECP taken in the acute episode of bronchial obstruction can predict the development of bronchial asthma in young children. Allergy Asthma Proc 2001;22:75–79.

41. Fujitaka M, Kawaguchi H, Kato Y, et al. Significance of the eosinophil cationic protein/eosinophil count ratio in asthmatic patients: its relationship to disease severity. Ann Allergy Asthma Immunol 2001;86:323–329.

42. O'Sullivan S, Roquet A, Dahlen B, et al. Evidence for mast cell activation during exercise-induced bronchoconstriction. Eur Respir J 1998;12:345–350.

43. O'Sullivan S. On the role of PGD2 metabolites as markers of mast cell activation in asthma. Acta Physiol Scand Suppl 1999;644:1–74.

44. Nagakura T, Obata T, Schihijo K, et al. GC/MS analysis of urinary excretion of 9alpha,11beta-PGF2 in acute and exercise-induced asthma in children. Clin Exp Allergy 1998;28:181–186.

45. Beasley CR, Robinson C, Featherstone RL, et al. 9 alpha, 11 beta-prostaglandin F2, a novel metabolite of prostaglandin D2 is a potent contractile agonist of human and guinea pig airways. J Clin Invest 1987;79:978–983.

46. Kumlin M, Dahlen B, Bjorck T, et al. Urinary excretion of leukotriene E4 and 11-dehydro-thromboxane in response to bronchial provocations with allergen, aspirin, leukotriene D4 and histamine in asthmatics. Am Rev Respir Dis 1992;146:96–103.

47. Kumlin M, Stensvad F, Larsson L, et al. Validation and application of a new simple strategy for measurements of urinary leukotriene E$_4$ in humans. Clin Exp Allergy 1995;25:467–479

48. Westcott JY. The measurement of leukotrienes in human fluids. Clin Rev Allergy Immunol 1999;17:153–177.

49. Eiser NM. Histamine antagonists and asthma. Pharmacol Ther 1982;17:239–250.

50. Hartley JPR, Norgrady SG. Effect of inhaled antihistamine on exercise-induced asthma. Thorax 1980;35:675–679.

51. Patel KR. Terfenadine in exercise-induced asthma. Br Med J 1987;288:1496–1497.

52. McFarlane PI, Heaf DP. Selective histamine blockade in childhood asthma: the effect of terfenadine on resting bronchial tone and exercise-induced bronchoconstriction. Thorax 1991;46:190–192.

53. Finnerty JP, Wilmot C, Holgate ST. Inhibition of hypertonic saline-induced bronchoconstriction by terfenadine and flurbiprofen. Evidence for the predominant role of histamine. Am Rev Respir Dis 1989;140:593–597.

54. Finnerty JP, Holgate ST. Evidence of the role of histamine and prostaglandins as mediators in exercise-induced asthma: the inhibitory effect of terfenadine and flurbiprofen alone and in combination. Eur Respir J 1990;3:540–557.

55. Ghosh SK, DeVos C, McIlory I, Patel KR. Effect of cetirizine on exercise-induced asthma. Thorax 1991;46:242–244.

56. Finnerty JP, Twentyman OP, Harris A, et al. Effect of GR 32191, a potent thromboxane receptor antagonist, on exercise induced bronchoconstriction in asthma. Thorax 1991;46:190–192.

57. Drazen JM, Austen KF. Leukotrienes and airway responses. Am Rev Respir Dis 1987;136:985–988.

58. Weiss JW, Drazen JM, Coles N, et al. Bronchoconstrictor effects of leukotriene C in humans. Science 1982;216:196–198.

59. Griffen M, Weiss JW, Leitch AG, et al. Effects of leukotriene D on the airways in asthma. N Engl J Med 1983;308:436–439.

60. Smith LJ, Greenberger PA, Patterson R, et al. The effect of inhaled leukotriene D$_4$ in humans. Am Rev Respir Dis 1985;131:368–372.

61. Alderoth E, Morris MM, Hargreave FE, O'Byrne PM. Airway responsiveness to leukotrienes C$_4$ and D$_4$ and to methacholine in patients with asthma and normal controls. N Engl J Med 1986;315:480–484.

62. Finnerty JP, Wood-Baker R, Thomson H, Holgate ST. Role of leukotrienes in exercise-induced asthma. Inhibitory effect of ICI 204219, a potent leukotriene D4 receptor antagonist. Am Rev Respir Dis 1992;145:746–749.

63. Coreno A, Skowronski M, Kotaru C, McFadden ER Jr. Comparative effects of long-acting β$_2$-agonists, leukotriene receptor antagonists, and 5-lipoxygenase inhibitor on exercise-induced asthma. J Allergy Clin Immunol 2000;106:500–506.

64. Drazen JM, Israel E, O'Byrne PM. Treatment of asthma with drugs modifying the leukotriene pathway. N Engl J Med 1999;340:197–206.

65. Meltzer EO, Weiler JM, Widlitz MD. Comparative outdoor study of the efficacy, onset and duration of action, and safety of cetirizine, loratadine, and placebo for seasonal allergic rhinitis. J Allergy Clin Immunol 1996;65:46–50.

66. Roquet A, Dahlen B, Kumlin M, et al. Combined antagonism of leukotrienes and histamine produces predominant inhibition of allergen-induced early and late phase airway obstruction in asthmatics. Am J Respir Crit Care Med 1997;155:1856–1863.

67. Morris JF. Spirometry in the evaluation of pulmonary function. West J Med 1976;125:110–118.

68. Hoshino M, Fukushima Y. Effect of OKY-046 (thromboxane A$_2$ synthetase inhibitor) on exercise-induced asthma. J Asthma 1991;28:19–29.

69. O'Byrne P, Jones G. The effect of indomethacin in exercise-induced bronchoconstriction and refractoriness after exercise. Am Rev Respir Dis 1986;134:69–72.

70. Beck KC, Offord KP, Scanlon PD. Bronchoconstriction occurring during exercise in asthmatic subjects. Am J Respir Crit Care Med 1994;149:352–357.

71. Suman OE, Babcock MA, Pegelow DF, et al. Airway obstruction during exercise in asthma. Am J Respir Crit Care Med 1995;152:24–31.

72. Godfrey S. Exercise-induced asthma. In: Bierman CW, Pearlman DS, eds. Allergic Diseases From Infancy to Adulthood. Philadelphia: WB Saunders, 1988.

73. Stirling DR, Cotton DJ, Graham BL, et al. Characteristics of airway tone during exercise in patients with asthma. J Appl Physiol 1983;54:934–942.

74. Anderson SD, Holzer K. Exercise-induced asthma: is it the right diagnosis in elite athletes? J Allergy Clin Immunol 2000;106:419–428.

75. Godfrey S. Clinical and physiological features. In: McFadden ER, ed. Exercise-Induced Asthma. New York: Marcel Davis, 1999.

76. Anderson SD, Connolly NM, Godfrey S. Comparison of bronchoconstriction induced by cycling and running. Thorax 1971;26:396–401.

77. Haby MM, Anderson SD, Peat JK, et al. An exercise challenge protocol for epidemiological studies of asthma in children: comparison with histamine challenge. Eur Respir J 1994;7:43–49.

78. Haby MM, Peat JK, Mellis CM, et al. An exercise challenge for epidemiological studies of childhood asthma: validity and repeatability. Eur Respir J 1995;8:729–736.

79. O'Donnell, AE, Fling J. Exercise-induced airflow obstruction in a healthy military population. Chest 1993;103:742–744.

80. Rice SG, Bierman CW, Shapiro GG, et al. Identification of exercise-induced asthma among intercollegiate athletes. Ann Allergy 1985;55:790–793.

81. Rupp NT, Guill MF, Brudno DS. Unrecognized exercise-induced bronchospasm in adolescent athletes. Am J Dis Child 1992;146:941–944.

82. Tan RA, Spector SL. Exercise-induced asthma. Sports Med 1998;25:1–6.

83. Mannix ET, Farber MO, Palange P, et al. Exercise-induced asthma in figure skaters. Chest 1996;109:312–315.

84. Mannix ET, Manfredi F, Farber MO. A comparison of two challenge tests for identifying exercise-induced bronchospasm in figure skaters. Chest 1999;155:649–653.

85. Larsson L, Hemmingsson P, Boethius G. Self-reported obstructive airway symptoms are common in young cross-country skiers. Scand J Med Sci Sports 1994;4:124–127.

86. Provost-Craig MA, Arbour KS, Sestilli DC, et al. The incidence of exercise-induced bronchospasm in competitive figure skaters. J Asthma 1996;33:67–71.

87. Rundell KW, Wilber RL, Szmedra L, et al. Exercise-induced asthma screening of elite athletes: field versus laboratory exercise challenge. Med Sci Sports Exerc 2000;32:309–316.

88. Voy RO. The U.S. Olympic Committee experience with exercise-induced bronchospasm, 1984. Med Sci Sports Exerc 1984;18:328–330.

89. Weiler JM, Layton T, Hunt M. Asthma in United States Olympic athletes who participated in the 1996 summer games. J Allergy Clin Immunol 1998;102:722–726.

90. Weiler JM, Ryan EJ III. Asthma in United States Olympic athletes who participated in the 1998 Olympic Winter Games. J Allergy Clin Immunol 2000;106:267–271.

91. Wilber RL, Rundell KW, Szmedra L, et al. Incidence of exercise-induced bronchospasm in Olympic winter sport athletes. Med Sci Sports Exerc 2000;32:732–737.

92. Judelson DA, Williams SD, Rundell KW. Gender differences in pulmonary function of elite ice hockey players. Med Sci Sports Exerc 2001;33(suppl 5):S12.

93. Berk JL, Lenner KA, McFadden ER Jr. Cold-induced bronchoconstriction: role of cutaneous reflexes vs. direct airway effects. J Appl Physiol 1987;63:659–664.

94. Deal EC, McFadden ER Jr, Ingram RH, et al. Airway responsiveness to cold air and hyperpnea in normal subjects and in those with hay fever and asthma. Am Rev Resp Dis 1980;121:621–628.

95. Fitch KD, Godfrey S. Asthma and athletic performance. JAMA 1976;234:152–157.

96. Giesbrecht GG, Younges M. Exercise- and cold-induced asthma. Can J Appl Physiol 1995;20:300–314.

97. Brauer M, Lee K, Spengler JD, et al. Nitrogen dioxide in indoor ice skating facilities: an international survey. J Air Waste Management Assoc 1997;47:1095–1102.

98. Bylin G, Lindvall AT, Rehn T, Sundin B. Effects of short-term exposure to ambient nitrogen dioxide concentrations on human bronchial reactivity and lung function. Eur J Respir Dis 1985;66:205–217.

99. Costa DL, Dreher KL. Bioavailable transition metals in particulate matter mediate cardiopulmonary injury in healthy and compromised animal models. Environ Health Perspect 1997;105(suppl 5):1053–1060.

100. Folinsbee LJ, Bedi JF, Horvath SM. Combined effects of ozone and nitrogen dioxide on respiratory function in man. Am Ind Hyg Assoc J 1981;42:534–541.

101. Folinsbee LJ. Does NO2 exposure increase airways responsiveness? Toxicol Indust Health 1992;8:273–283.

102. Koenig JQ. Air pollution and asthma. J Allergy Clin Immunol 1999;104:717–722.

103. Levy JI, Lee K, Yanagisawa Y, et al. Determinants of nitrogen dioxide concentrations in indoor ice skating rinks. Am J Public Health 1998;88:1781–1786.

104. Williams SD, Judelson DA, Rundell KW. High levels of airborne particulate matter in indoor ice arenas. Med Sci Sports Exerc 2001;33(suppl 5):S12.

105. Boulet LP, Becker A, Bérubé A, et al. Canadian asthma consensus report, 1999. CMAJ 1999;161(suppl 11):S1–S62.

106. National Heart, Lung, and Blood Institute. Expert panel report 2: guidelines for the diagnosis and management of asthma. Bethesda, MD: NIH Publications, 1997.

107. Ortega-Carr D, Bush RK. Asthma in adults and adolescents. In: Rakel RE, ed. Conn's Current Therapy. Philadelphia: WB Saunders, 1995.

108. Williams PV, Shapiro GG. Asthma in children. In: Rakel RE, ed. Conn's Current Therapy. Philadelphia: WB Saunders, 1995.

109. Li JT, O'Connell EJ. Clinical evaluation of asthma. Ann Allergy Asthma Immunol 1996;76:1–15.

110. United States Olympic Committee, Division of Sports Medicine. Asthma. Colorado Springs: 1999.

111. Bye MR, Kerstein D, Barsh E. The importance of spirometry in the assessment of childhood asthma. Am J Dis Child 1992;146:977–978.

112. American Thoracic Society. Lung function testing: selection of reference values and interpretative strategies. Am Rev Respir Dis 1991;144:1202–1218.

113. Heir T, Oseid S. Self-reported asthma and exercise-induced asthma symptoms in high-level competitive cross-country skiers. Scand J Med Sci Sports 1994;4:128–133.

114. Nystad W, Harris J, Borgen JS. Asthma and wheezing among Norwegian elite athletes. Med Sci Sports Exerc 2000;32:266–270.

115. Charpin D, Vercloet D, Charpin J. Epidemiology of asthma in Western Europe. Allergy 1988;43:481–492.

116. Sears MR. Epidemiological trends in bronchial asthma. In: Kaliner MA, Barnes PJ, Persson CGA, eds. Asthma, Its Pathology and Treatment. New York: Marcel Dekker, 1991.

117. Eggleston PA, Rosenthal RR, Anderson SA, et al. Guidelines for the methodology of exercise challenge testing of asthmatics. J Allergy Clin Immunol 1979;64:642–645.

118. Rundell KW, Im J, Wilber RL, et al. Mid expiratory flow rates of cold weather athletes with exercise-induced asthma. Med Sci Sports Exerc 2001;33(suppl 5):S12.

119. Wagner EM, Jacoby DB. Methacholine causes reflex bronchoconstriction. J Appl Physiol 1999;86:294–297.

120. Anderson SD, Brannan J, Spring J, et al. A new method for bronchial-provocation testing in asthmatic subjects using a dry powder of mannitol. Am J Respir Crit Care Med 1997;156:758–765.

121. Brannan JD, Koskela H, Anderson SD, Chew N. Responsiveness to mannitol in asthmatic subjects with exercise- and hyperventilation-induced asthma. Am J Respir Crit Care Med 1998;158:1120–1126.

122. Anderson SD, Smith CM, Rodwell LT, et al. The use of non-isotonic aerosols for evaluating bronchial hyperresponsiveness. In: Spector S, ed. Provocation Challenge Procedures. New York: Marcel Dekker, 1995.

123. Belcher NG, Lee TH, Rees PJ. Airway responses to hypertonic saline, exercise and histamine challenges in bronchial asthma. Eur Respir J 1989;2:44–48.

124. Riedler J, Reade T, Dalton M, et al. Hypertonic saline challenge in an epidemiologic survey of asthma in children. Am J Respir Crit Care Med 1994;150:1632–1639.

125. Smith CM, Anderson SD. Inhalation provocation tests using non-isotonic aerosols. J Allergy Clin Immunol 1989;84:781–790.

126. Rabone SJ, Phoon WO, Anderson SD, et al. Hypertonic saline challenge in an adult epidemiological survey. Occup Med 1996;46:177–185.

127. Crapo RO. Pulmonary-function testing. N Engl J Med 1994;331:25–30.

128. Sterling GM. The mechanism of bronchoconstriction due to hypocapnia in man. Clin Sci 1968;34:277–285

129. Mahler DA. Exercise-induced asthma. Med Sci Sports Exerc 1993;25:554–561.

130. Rundell KW, Judelson DA, Williams SD. Diagnosis of exercise-induced asthma in the athlete. In: Rundell KW, Wilber RL, Lemanske R eds. Asthma and Exercise. Champaign, IL: Human Kinetics, 2002.

131. van Essen-Zandvliet EE, Hughes MD, Waalkens HJ, et al. Effects of a 22 months of treatment with inhaled corticosteroids and/or beta-2-agonists on lung function, airway responsiveness, and symptoms in children with asthma. The Dutch Chronic Non-specific Lung Disease Study Group. Am Rev Respir Dis 1992;146:547–554.

132. Haahtela T, Jarvinen M, Kava T, et al. Comparisons of a beta 2-agonist, terbutaline, with an inhaled corticosteroid, budesonide, in newly detected asthma. N Engl J Med 1991;325:388–392.

133. Barnes NC, Marone G, Di Maria GU, et al. A comparison of fluticasone propionate, 1 mg daily, with beclomethasone dipropionate, 2 mg daily, in the treatment of severe asthma. International Study Group. Eur Respir J 1993;6:877–885.

134. Fabbri L, Burge PS, Croonenborgh L, et al. Comparison of fluticasone propionate with beclomethasone dipropionate in moderate to severe asthma treated for one year. International Study Group. Thorax 1993;48:817–823.

135. Dahl R, Lundback B, Malo JL, et al. A dose-ranging study of fluticasone propionate in adult patients with moderate asthma. International Study Group. Chest 1993;104:1352–1358.

136. The Medical Letter. Drugs for asthma. Med Lett Drugs Ther 2000;42:19–24.
137. Alton EW, Norris AA. Chloride transport and the actions of nedocromil sodium and cromolyn sodium in asthma. J Allergy Clin Immunol 1996;98:S102–S106.
138. Eady RP. The pharmacology of nedocromil sodium. Eur J Respir Dis Suppl 1986;147:112–119.
139. Lal S, Dorow PD, Venho KK, Chatterjee SS. Nedocromil sodium is more effective than cromolyn sodium for the treatment of chronic reversible obstructive airway disease. Chest 1993;104:438–447.
140. Schwartz HJ, Blumenthal M, Brady R, et al. A comparative study of the clinical efficacy of nedocromil sodium and placebo. How does cromolyn sodium compare as an active control treatment? Chest 1996;109:945–952.
141. Gaddy JN, Margolskee DJ, Bush RK, et al. Bronchodilation with a potent and selective leukotriene D4 (LTD4) receptor antagonist (MK-571) in patients with asthma. Am Rev Respir Dis 1992;146:358–363.
142. Israel E, Cohn J, Dube L, Drazen JM. Effect of treatment with zileuton, a 5-lipoxygenase inhibitor, in patients with asthma. A randomized controlled trial. Zileuton Clinical Trial Group. JAMA 1996;275:931–936.
143. Anderson SD, Seale JP, Ferris L, et al. An evaluation of pharmacotherapy for exercise-induced asthma. J Allergy Clin Immunol 1979;64:612–624.
144. Wilber RL, Rundell KW, Judelson DA. Efficacy of asthma medication regimen in elite athletes with exercise-induced asthma. Med Sci Sports Exerc 2001;33(suppl 5):S12.
145. D'Alonzo GE, Nathan RA, Henochowicz S, et al. Salmeterol xinafoate as maintenance therapy compared with albuterol in patients with asthma. JAMA 1994;271:1412–1416.
146. Greening AP, Ind PW, Northfield M, Shaw G. Added salmeterol versus higher-dose corticosteroid in asthma patients with symptoms on existing inhaled corticosteroid. Allen & Hanburys Limited UK Study Group. Lancet 1994;344:219–224.
147. Becker AB, Simons FE. Formoterol, a new long-acting selective beta-2-agonist, decreases airway responsiveness in children with asthma. Lung 1990;168 (suppl):99–102.

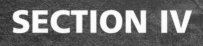

NEUROMUSCULAR DISEASES AND DISORDERS

CHAPTER 14

Stroke

Timothy R. McConnell

Overview

Stroke refers to a potentially fatal reduction or cutoff of the blood supply to part of the brain resulting in brain cell damage and varying severities of impaired neurologic function (1, 2). **Ischemic strokes** are the most common (82% of all strokes) and, similar to that of ischemic heart disease, are the result of a blockage in an artery that supplies blood to the brain. In contrast, **hemorrhagic strokes**, less common but more deadly, occur when an artery carrying blood to the brain bursts (1–3).

Although the survival rate for stroke is quite good, exceeding 70%, a large percentage of stroke patients suffer from **neurologic impairments** that require acute and long-term rehabilitation programs. The associated physical trauma of stroke is variable and may include impairment in language and perception as well as motor, emotional, sensory, and cognitive function (4). Stroke impairments result from upper motor neuron damage causing **paresis, paralysis, spasticity,** and **sensoriperceptual dysfunction** as well as debilitating secondary effects that include **contracture**, impaired voluntary movement, and eventual **disuse muscle atrophy** (5, 6). Moreover, these associated disabilities compromise the individual's ability to maintain **activities of daily living**, let alone return to work and enjoyable recreational physical activities. If not addressed, the long-term residual negatively impacts the patient's cardiorespiratory ability to exercise and diminishes muscular strength below that necessary for maintenance of independent care (5).

To combat the physical deceleration of the poststroke patient, acute and long-term exercise programs are needed to enhance recovery, improve functional status, and optimize **quality of life** for the remainder of the patient's life. Termination of formal rehabilitation after the immediate poststroke phase condemns many patients to the resumption of their previous sedentary lifestyle and prolonged, gradual deterioration in physical function. To avoid the progressing negative impacts of stroke, a greater emphasis must be placed on long-term rehabilitative efforts that promote compliance and improve and maintain physical function. Such long-term initiatives are the focus of this chapter.

Stroke and Loss of Exercise Capacity

A stroke and the resulting hemiparesis produce physiologic changes in muscle fibers and metabolism during exercise that are similar to those that occur with prolonged disuse (5, 7). For example, paretic muscles show a reduced muscle blood flow when compared with nonparalyzed extremities at the same level of physical activity, greater **lactate** production, higher utilization of muscle glycogen, and a diminished capacity to oxidize free fatty acids (8). In addition, paretic muscles activate glycolytic **Type II fibers** to initiate contraction, whereas nonparetic muscles primarily recruit **Type I fibers**. Eventually, this change in recruitment patterns leads to a reduced proportion of Type I fibers, diminished capacity for **oxidative metabolism**, and diminished **exercise endurance**. Other compounding musculoskeletal factors associated with stroke also complicate exercise training, such as muscle strain, spasticity, and joint pain. In addition, hemiparetic disturbances affect gait, imposing excessive energy expenditures (1.5- to 2-fold normal) during routine ambulation (9). Consequently, the amount of oxygen consumed per submaximal workload in **hemiparetic** patients is greater than observed in normal subjects—that is, they are less efficient.

In addition, the physical inactivity associated with hemiparesis results in disuse of nonaffected skeletal muscle groups, further limiting **aerobic capacity**. The diminished use of nonaffected muscle enhances the increased energy cost of movement in these muscles as well. In general, the overall reduced muscular endurance of the affected and nonaffected muscle groups contributes to overall decreased exercise efficiency and greater difficulty performing routine activities of daily living, greater level of fatigue, and decreased willingness to pursue occupational or recreational tasks that require cardiorespiratory endurance and muscular strength (5). In summary, the prolonged muscular disuse following a stroke results in a number of maladaptations:

- Reduced muscle fiber size
- Decreased myofibril firing rate
- Atrophy of Type 2 muscle fibers
- Increased fatigue
- Decreased motor unit numbers
- Altered motor unit recruitment

The response to exercise to training also is affected by the type of **cerebrovascular lesion**, the extent of the disability, and concomitant medications. In addition, there are many confounding comorbidities common to stroke survivors, including obesity, high blood pressure, type 2 diabetes, hyperlipidemia, stress, depression, and social isolation, that negatively impact the patient's willingness and capabilities to comply with efforts to maintain physical function (10). Maintaining functional capacity following a stroke is of particular concern in elderly patients, in whom advancing age and residual neurologic deficits already promote a sedentary lifestyle leading to declining cardiovascular fitness, disuse atrophy, and weakness. The overall goal of long-term exercise training, regardless of confounding influences, is regaining and maintaining independence in basic activities of daily living and quality of life.

Along with the declining endurance capacity subsequent to prolonged inactivity, the stroke patient also succumbs to a loss of **muscular strength**. Ultimately, the loss of strength significantly impairs the person's ability to perform routine daily tasks and ambulatory skills. The relation observed between muscle strength and fat-free mass and improvement in functional status suggests that preservation of fat-free mass is an important determinant of physical function (11). Strength training for the stroke patient is effective for increasing muscle mass and restoring strength of selected muscle groups (12).

Exercise Training After Stroke

Epidemiology

Daily caloric expenditure is strongly associated with a progressively lower risk of stroke, particularly ischemic stroke. As with heart disease, **physical inactivity** consistently emerges as an independent risk factor for initial and recurrent stroke. Individuals who are not physically fit are three times more likely to have a stroke when compared with fit individuals (13). The protective effect of physical activity for stroke is evident for both women and men, young and old, and in all racial and ethnic groups (14).

Although there appears to be a dose-response relationship between physical activity level and incidence of ischemic stroke, establishing a threshold for exercise or activity is difficult. Intense or vigorous activity does not result in any greater benefit in overall mortality from cardiovascular causes than frequent light or moderate activity (14–16). Walking more than 20 km per week, maintaining an energy expenditure of 4,200 kJ per week, and even past participation in college sports appear protective (17–19). Also, becoming active in middle and later adulthood reduces stroke risk (20). Therefore, it appears that being more active, regardless of type or intensity of activity, has a protective effect against stroke (21, 22).

How, exactly, increased activity works to reduce the incidence and complications of stroke is debated and is currently under investigation. Both **passive** and **active exercise** and increased activity in general result in a significant increase in cerebral oxygen saturation, cytochrome enzyme levels, and enhanced cerebral activation and initiation of autoregulatory mechanisms (23). In addition, people who are more active or become more active tend to be more compliant with eliminating other risk factors associated with higher stroke rates (20, 24). Apparently, there is a strong interaction among activity, the physiologic adaptations to physical activity, and many of the primary and secondary risk factors for stroke (Box 14.1) (16, 25, 26).

Forty percent of asymptomatic stroke patients have advanced or severe coronary artery disease, and 46% have

---

BOX 14.1. **Stroke Risk Factor Classification**

Modifiable Risk Factors
Smoking
Hypertension
Dyslipidemia
Physical inactivity/sedentary lifestyle
Hyperhomocysteine abnormality
Sleep apnea
Elevated cholesterol/lipids
Cigarette smoking
Alcohol consumption
Oral contraceptives
Obesity
Abnormal glucose tolerance
Left ventricular hypertrophy by electrocardiographic analysis

Partially Modifiable Risk Factors
Diabetes mellitus
Coronary heart disease, myocardial infarction
Previous stroke
Left ventricular hypertrophy
Hypercoagulable states
Tissue plasminogen activator
Asymptomatic carotid bruit
Cardiac comorbidity
Transient ischemic attacks
Elevated hematocrit
Sickle cell disease

Nonmodifiable Risk Factors
Age
Gender
Race
Positive family history

Nonatherogenic Risk Factors
Sleep apnea
Elevated homocysteine levels
Foramen ovale

---

mild to moderate coronary artery disease (27). Therefore, in addition to exercise therapy, the stroke rehabilitation professional must consider the high incidence of stroke recurrence and the risk of cardiovascular events and be actively involved in patient education and management of cardiovascular risk factors. Involvement of patients with documented coronary artery disease in comprehensive cardiac rehabilitation programs has been shown to reduce the risk of stroke in addition to the risk of other initial or recurrent cardiovascular events (13, 28–31). Therefore, long-term participation in regular structured programs of exercise and education is essential for improvement and maintenance of endurance capacity and muscular strength and for minimizing the risks, symptoms, and problems associated with comorbid cardiovascular disease (32). Subsequently, stroke rehabilitation must be committed not only to the short-term goal of maximizing function and minimizing disability but also to the long-term goal of reducing the risk of stroke recurrence and cardiovascular morbidity and mortality (16).

Endurance

In spite of this potentially irreversible trend for deconditioning, the endurance of stroke patients can improve with long-term, regularly scheduled exercise programs prescribed according to professional guidelines (33). By reversing the decreased metabolic activity, **oxygen uptake**, and increased lactic acid production, endurance exercise training not only improves endurance in both paralyzed and nonparalyzed extremities but also increases overall **maximal oxygen consumption**. In addition, endurance exercise training has the documented health-related benefits of reducing risk for stroke and cardiovascular disease in general (8).

Although most spontaneous recovery occurs in the first 30 days after stroke, recovery overall continues for a much longer period (32). Professional standards for exercise prescription are effective for improving exercise capacity in both acute and chronic phases of stroke recovery. Long-term fitness programs of combined muscular strength and aerobic endurance are appropriate and effective for improving motion efficiency and overall functional capacity for stroke patients (2). As a result, these patients are able to complete their routine activities of daily living at a lower percentage of their peak exercise capacity, require less frequent rest periods, and are less fatigued at the end of the day.

Strength

Stroke-associated motor impairments, coupled with the continuing loss of muscle mass and strength due to disuse atrophy, accelerate the progression of disability, inability to perform activities of daily living, loss of confidence in performing physical tasks, and decreased quality of life. Ultimately, there is loss of self-care ability, as well as loss of the ability to perform tasks requiring mobility such as walking, rising from a chair, and ascending stairs, all of which have been associated with a two-fold greater risk for institutionalization and death (11).

Progressive resistance training improves strength not only in paretic muscle groups but also in nonaffected muscle groups. Performance during strength training also serves as an indicator of functional ability—the number and intensity of repetitions performed is predictive of such functional outcomes as walking as well as overall functional performance (34). Aside from the documented strength increases in specific muscle groups, the resultant improvements in functional capabilities increase the patient's capacity to perform routine activities of daily living.

Moreover, the importance of maintaining or improving gait speed cannot be underestimated. Habitual gait speed is a function of endurance capacity, joint mobility, balance, and lower extremity muscle strength and has been recognized as an indicator of gait performance, self-perceived physical function, independence, social activity, and functional health (35, 36). In addition, patients may feel stronger than they have for many years because before the stroke they had gradually slipped into long-term inactivity.

Traditionally, recovery of motor function has been thought to be nearly complete in the first 3 to 6 months after stroke. Strength training, though, can profoundly improve strength and result in improvements in physical function late in the course of stroke recovery. The positive changes associated with strength training are not maintained without continued training, however (36). Following formalized training, if the patient returns to his or her former sedentary lifestyle, there is a significant loss of strength within only 4 weeks (12). Therefore, to attain optimal function, the stroke patient's convalescence must include a comprehensive program of combined endurance and strength training that the patient will find amenable for long-term compliance.

Emotional and Psychological Aspects of Stroke

In addition to the physiologic benefits, exercise helps with the emotional and psychological aspects of stroke. By 4 years after a stroke, 80% of patients have lost interest in recreational activities, 65% have excessive tiredness, 50% have irritability, and 40% suffer from depression (1). A high valuation of self can result in high aspirations and goal setting and an increased likelihood that the patient will modify behavior to remain more physically and cognitively active (7). Similarly, a low self-efficacy (i.e., confidence to

perform physical tasks) results in a decreased likelihood and willingness to attempt new physical skills (37–39). Self-concept and self-efficacy improve across gender and age as a result of participating in exercise programs, for both healthy individuals and those with cardiovascular disease (7, 40).

Aerobic exercise and an improved functional capacity may alleviate depressive symptoms. Increasing physical activity has been found to be a useful treatment or prevention intervention for depression in individuals with varying disabilities (41, 42). Due to the high prevalence of depressive symptoms in the stroke population, exercise may have the potential to serve as a cost-effective means of addressing physiologic as well as psychological disabilities in adults following a stroke.

In short, for stroke patients to maintain optimal physical, cognitive, and emotional function and ultimately an enhanced quality of life, exercise and physical activity are essential.

Safety

Another patient deterrent to participating in physical tasks is safety. Strength and improved functional capacity, however, are inversely related to the risk of falling during such routine activities as ambulation and transfer (43). General exercise safety guidelines for stroke patients include the following (1):

- Have a thorough medical evaluation before you start your exercise program and at regular intervals thereafter.
- Initially, exercise in a program that offers direct supervision.
- Know the warning signs of a stroke, and seek medical care.
- Know the warning signs of an impending cardiac complication.
- Follow a proper exercise protocol.
- Avoid physical activities that will cause an excessive rise in blood pressure.
- Don't overestimate your abilities and undertake potentially risky exercises—especially without adequate assistance.
- Be aware of other comorbidities and possible effects of medications on the exercise response.
- Monitor progress and notify a physician if unexplained decreases or changes in physical capabilities occur.

In addition, the clinical exercise physiologist must be watchful for abnormal gait patterns, signs of vision deficits, or other considerations that may suggest possible safety hazards. Furthermore, a thorough consultation with the patient's physiatrist concerning patient readiness is strongly recommended.

Exercise Training and Testing Options

Endurance and Aerobic Exercise Training

Endurance training is increasingly recognized as an important component within a comprehensive stroke rehabilitation program, particularly the long-term or maintenance phase (Box 14.2) (2, 25). Therapeutically, many available exercise modalities or assistive devices allow or may be adapted for those with significant neurologic or other orthopaedic deficits (Box 14.3) (2, 5, 9). Proper supportive devices such as adjustable chest braces, handlebars, and seats, and proper foot alignment using toe clips that accommodate braces and large-based shoes may allow effective exercise. The use of equipment with reciprocal bilateral movement of both upper and lower extremities also assists movement of the paretic limb through a range of motion while performing aerobic conditioning. The equipment selected should be safe, provide comfortable support during use, and allow the patient easy mounting and dismounting (Figure 14.1).

Resistance and Strength Training

Ideally, strengthening exercises should resemble the movements or components of the task being trained (Table 14.1)

BOX 14.2. Recommendations for Endurance Training for Stroke Patients

1. Determine comorbidities and their effect on the patient's functional capacity.
2. Determine the patient's ability to walk, in distance and minutes, and his or her ability to use modified equipment.
3. Frequency and duration of aerobic exercise
   a. Start with 2- to 3-minute sessions using two or three modalities, with the goal of increasing each session to 45 minutes.
   b. Three times per week, if patients can walk, for 15 to 20 minutes with or without periods of rest.
   c. Five times per week, twice per day, if a patient cannot tolerate 15 minutes of walking or stationary cycling.
4. Intensity
   a. The target heart rate should be 50% to 70% of the maximum heart rate obtained for 220 − age, or using the heart rate reserve formula [(MHR − RHR) × 0.5 – 0.7] + RHR.
   b. General rule: 15 to 30 beats above the resting heart rate.
   c. Rating of perceived exertion (RPE) of "somewhat hard" (12 to 13 on the 6 to 20 scale; 4 to 5 on the 0 to 10 scale).
5. Always start with warm-up and finish with cool-down exercises for the improvement of range of motion and flexibility. Each should be at least 5 minutes.

BOX 14.3. Improvements as a Result of Endurance Exercise Training

Physical Improvements

Increased gait speed

Increased self-selected walking velocity and activities of transfer

Reduction in the energy requirements to perform standardized walking task

Improved stair-climbing ability

Improved lower extremity muscle tone

Improved measures of impairment and disability

Enhanced independent function

Greater maximal exercise capacity

Greater physical work capacity

Increase in HDL cholesterol and decreased triglycerides

Decreased platelet aggregation and increased fibrinolysis

Weight loss

Decreased resting and submaximal heart rate and blood pressure

Delay in the onset of angina with exercise

Enhanced motor unit recruitment limiting the development of disuse atrophy

Ability to perform daily activities at a lower percentage of maximum exercise capacity

Reduction of cardiovascular risk, including better blood pressure control

Improvements in Perception

Increased activity level at which patients feels comfortable performing routinely or for an extended period of time

Enhanced quality of life

Improved self-confidence and perceived functional abilities

Greater confidence for engaging in physical activities and an increased willingness to attempt physical tasks

(2, 10, 12). For example, programs of muscle strengthening may help to optimize gains in gait speed and functional mobility by combining specific tasks, such as stepping, with strengthening of the muscle groups involved in walking. A training program can be as sophisticated as using weights or resistance machines for designated muscle groups or as simple as doing repetitions of the impaired task, such as activities of transfer (e.g., repeated standing from a chair). A variety of training protocols have been used and found successful (Box 14.4) (2, 34, 44). The key is understanding the patient's needs and triggers for compliance and then developing clear and specific objectives concerning functional improvement. In addition, correct movement patterns must be emphasized. If the patient is unable to perform specific exercises properly, these may be deferred until the patient is better able to accomplish them or until after consultation with the patient's physiatrist.

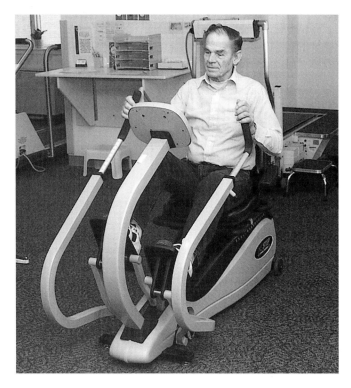

FIGURE 14.1. Equipment that provides comfortable support, easy mounting and dismounting, and reciprocal bilateral movement of both upper and lower extremities. Courtesy of Nu Step, Inc., Ann Arbor, Michigan.

Task-Related Training

Approximately two thirds of stroke survivors have chronic neurologic impairments that affect their mobility and their ability to perform routine tasks of daily living (44). The inability to perform routine tasks can be physically inconvenient and emotionally very frustrating. To promote long-term improvement and maintenance of specific task-oriented function, activities that incorporate specific task improvement must be part of the patient's daily routine. Ideally, the

TABLE 14.1. STRENGTH TRAINING PROGRAMS

Exercises or equipment	Body weight, sandbag, hand weights, Velcro wrist weights and ankle weights, machines, and elastic bands
Intensity	Initial settings of 50% 1 RM or 70% of 10-RM for 2 weeks
	Gradually increase to 80% 1 RM for 8 weeks
Repetition	3 sets of 8 to 10 repetitions
	Increase weight by 10% when able to complete 15 repetitions
Duration	30 minutes per session
	8 to 12 weeks for improvement
	Ongoing for maintenance
Frequency	2 to 3 times each week
	Daily for low-functional patients

Data from Teixeira-Salmela LF et al. (2), Rimmer JH, Hedman G (10), and Fiatarone MA et al. (12).

BOX 14.4.   Improvements as a Result of Strength Training

Improvements in Physical Performance

Faster gait speed

Faster repeated chair-to-stand time

Faster stair climb time

Greater strength of affected lower extremity

No adverse effects of spasticity

Increased total strength

Improvements in Perceptions

Increased activity level at which subject feels comfortable

Improved quality of life

Improved measures of overall impairment and disability

Improved self-confidence

Improved perceived functional abilities

Improved perception of independence

strengthening and endurance exercises used should closely resemble the tasks or components of the task being trained for (i.e., specificity of training) (44).

Muscle- or muscle group–specific strengthening exercises are a critical component of any task-related training program. For instance, to improve walking, task-related training involves strategies to increase strength, coordination, weight-bearing capacity of the affected lower limb, and flexibility and other strategies to provide the opportunity for intensive and repetitive practice, such as walking on a treadmill (44–46). As a result of appropriately designed task-related programs, walking speed and endurance, force production, sit-to-stand, and balance while standing and stepping all improve, and, in addition, patients report that they feel better and are more confident (47). Task-related programs can be performed during a formal rehabilitation program as well as independently at home and may include such activities as these (44, 48):

- Reaching for objects beyond arm's length in sitting position
- Sit-to-stand from various chair heights
- Stepping up and down, forward, and sideways on the flat and onto blocks of various heights
- Performing heel lifts in standing position
- Reaching for objects in standing position, including down to the floor with the base of support constrained
- Doing reciprocal leg flexion and extension in standing position
- Standing up from a chair, walking a short distance, and returning to the chair
- Walking on a treadmill
- Walking over various surfaces and obstacles
- Walking over slopes and stairs

> **BOX 14.5. Treadmill Walking Program**
>
> 1. Partial body support or handrail support.
> 2. Functional ambulatory category improved in all patients.
> 3. Treadmill speed adjusted to comfortable cadence and increased accordingly (at a RPE of no more than 12)
>   a. 15 minutes per session increased to 30 minutes, 5 days per week
>   b. or, as exercise duration increases, 40 minutes per day, 3 times per week

Treadmill Gait Training

Approximately 70% of acutely hospitalized stroke patients are not able to walk independently after stroke (49). Many of those who recover the ability to ambulate without physical assistance are still disabled by their slow walking speed and can only walk short distances with frequent breaks. Over the long term, poor walking skills result in a reduction in community activity involvement, loss of independence, and isolationism. Treadmill training after stroke is beneficial for improving gait mechanics. For those patients who are unable to walk alone due to marked muscle weakness and poor coordination, assistance or partial weight support using an overhead harness may allow the patient many repetitions of a complete gait cycle (Box 14.5) (44, 54–56). As the patient progresses, the degree of support can be decreased gradually, increasing weight bearing (50). Similarly, handrail-supported treadmill walking is a safe and effective modality for long-term aerobic exercise training in patients with mild to moderate hemiparetic gait disturbances (9). Compared with walking overground, the repetitiveness of treadmill training allows hemiparetic stroke patients to achieve more normalized gait symmetry, promotes appropriate timing and a consistent walking speed, and improves gross motor efficiency (Box 14.6) (9, 44, 49, 51, 56). This improved walking efficiency is important because the energy expenditure required to perform routine ambulation is elevated by approximately 1.5- to 2.0-fold in hemiparetic stroke patients (52, 53). By improving walking efficiency, patients better tolerate routine activities of daily living, experience less overall fatigue, and improve their perception of quality of life.

> **BOX 14.6. Advantages of Treadmill Training**
>
> 1. Increased gait velocity, cadence, and stride length
> 2. Improved gait capability
> 3. Task-oriented exercise
> 4. Provides numerous repetitions of a supervised gait pattern
> 5. Forces and improves symmetry between right and left leg step length

Another effective training strategy is placement of obstacles in the walking path or having the patient walk on variable terrain. These strategies encourage further hip and knee extension and flexion and maintenance of balance by forcing longer steps and higher leg-lifting.

Home Exercise Programs

For stroke patients to be able to maintain the gains in physical function accrued during the acute and long-term rehabilitation process, they must receive education and instructions for continued home exercise and activity enhancement. In addition to maintaining the level of physical function they've gained, patients will continue to improve if enhanced activity levels and skills training are adhered to after discharge from formal rehabilitation programs (57). Without specific home exercise guidelines, however, most patients are relegated to a sedentary lifestyle that not only results in a relapse of neuromuscular symptoms but also exacerbates the risk for further cardiovascular events. For continued improvement and maintenance of strength, balance, and endurance, the home exercise program should be structured to encourage more frequent use of the affected extremities (32). The previously described strength and endurance exercises can easily be integrated into a comprehensive home rehabilitation program that may include the following:

- Strength training: hand weights, elastic bands, barbell weights, homemade weights, food cans, water-filled bottles, books
- Endurance: (1) walking, walking, and more walking; (2) home exercise equipment: cycles, rowing machines, steppers or house steps
- Task-related activities: walking, transition from sitting to standing, weight-bearing activities, workstations (multiple physical tasks performed in intervals), walking on variable terrains

Exercise Testing

Cardiovascular comorbidity is prevalent in the stroke population, and cardiac death remains the leading cause for mortality in long-term stroke survivors (58). In spite of the potential cardiovascular risk of exercise, the presence of significant neurologic deficits affecting gait and balance has discouraged systematic exercise testing prior to exercise participation in the paretic stroke patient (58). The question arises whether the information obtained from an exercise test is worth the risks of performing the test, particularly if the patient is unable to give an adequate cardiovascular effort for test results to be valid.

The need for an exercise test should be determined based on the degree of neuromuscular impairment resulting from the stroke, symptoms suggestive of significant coronary heart disease, and the level of intensity at which the patient will be exercising relative to his or her peak exercise capacity (59). During the acute rehabilitative phase, when efforts are focused on specific muscle groups or small task training, the cardiovascular demands of rehabilitation may be minimal. During the later rehabilitative phase, however, when the patient is ambulating freely and the cardiovascular demands of rehabilitation become more intense, an exercise test may be warranted.

Successful exercise testing procedures have been documented for stroke patients. Although debate exists concerning using treadmill walking versus cycle ergometry, the choice is patient-specific. When selecting the type of exercise and protocol to be used, the primary concerns are ensuring patient comfort and safety while at the same time obtaining a level of cardiovascular stress that provides valid diagnostic information concerning the presence of significant cardiovascular disease, functional capacity, and any other limitations to exercise (59). For treadmill use, ambulatory impairments resulting from the stroke may require modifications of standard exercise testing procedures. For some patients, treadmill exercise may be inappropriate. Many stroke patients with altered gait patterns may have difficulty with treadmill walking because the treadmill forces a constant walking speed. Allowing handrail support, however, may provide enough assistance for patients to obtain an adequate level of exercise to provide valid test results. During an easily administered pretest assessment, all patients with self-selected floor walking velocities of 0.5 mph or greater had adequate neurologic function to perform a graded treadmill test with continuous handrail support and no other assistance (58). Aside from the information obtained concerning the patient's cardiovascular risk status, treadmill testing also provides information about the patient's ability to tolerate the stresses of walking throughout their daily routine. In addition to the sample protocol presented in Table 14.2 (58), there are a number of commonly used lower-level testing protocols (33).

For those patients who are unable to perform treadmill walking, other types of exercise may be used or modified (59). Current models of recumbent ergometry are comfortable and stable, and the reciprocal movements of arm and leg levers promote the use of a large muscle mass, include the paretic limbs, and discourage localized fatigue (see Fig-

TABLE 14.2. TREADMILL PROTOCOL—LOW LEVEL

Special Procedures	Handrail support (ad libitum)
Initial workload	0.5 mph/0% grade for 1 minute
Increments	0.1 mph each minute
Monitoring	ECG and blood pressure
	Observe patient's subjective tolerance and gait stability
Endpoint	Volitional fatigue or signs of cardiopulmonary distress
	Exercise duration 6–12 minutes

Data from Macko RF et al. (58).

TABLE 14.3. CYCLE OR COMBINED ARM AND LEG ERGOMETER PROTOCOL

Staging	1 or 2 minutes with 1-minute rest intervals
Initial workloads	0.5 to 1.0 MET (12.5–25 watts)
Increments	0.5 to 1.0 MET (12.5–25 watts)
Monitoring	ECG and blood pressure
	Observe patient's subjective tolerance and symptoms
Endpoint	Volitional fatigue or signs of cardiopulmonary distress
	Exercise duration 6–12 minutes

ure 14.1). Initial workloads and stage increments should be selected that produce the greatest rate-pressure product possible during exercise before the onset of extreme localized fatigue. Using shorter-duration workloads of 1 or 2 minutes with 1-minute rest intervals may delay the onset of localized fatigue and allow greater total work to be performed. After each rest interval, workloads can be increased in increments of 0.5 to 1.0 multiples of resting energy equivalent (METs). In general, regardless of protocol, the best results are obtained when protocols are selected that result in a total exercise time of 6 to 12 minutes (60). Exceeding 12 minutes may result in the onset of localized musculoskeletal fatigue before the maximal level of cardiovascular stress is achieved (Table 14.3).

Ergometer use for exercise testing has the following advantages:

- It is easier to quantify the external workload.
- There is less variation in exercise efficiency.
- A more accurate work-to-$\dot{V}O_2$ ratio can be obtained.
- There is less torso and arm movement, making it easier to record electrocardiogram results and blood pressure.
- It is more comfortable and reassuring for the patient.

The primary disadvantage of cycle ergometry is reduced $\dot{V}O_{2max}$ by 10% to 15% due to localized muscle fatigue.

What We Know
About Stroke and Exercise

1 For hemiplegic individuals to perform functional activities more effectively, they need a higher than normal capacity for energy supply, including a more efficient cardiovascular system and a higher muscular capacity to use oxygen.

2 Combined endurance and strength exercise training is effective for maintaining adequate functional capacity to perform routine activities of daily living, independence, and quality of life.

3 Daily caloric expenditure is strongly associated with a lower risk of stroke and other cardiovascular impairments.

4 Standard professional guidelines for exercise prescription are effective for stroke patients.

5 Training approaches that emphasize task-oriented strengthening and coordination exercises improve not only overall functional capacity but also the ability to perform specific tasks.

6 A low-velocity treadmill test or low-level protocols using alternative exercise modalities can be used effectively for exercise testing many paretic patients.

7 Recumbent ergometers that are safe, comfortable, easy to mount, stable, and have reciprocal limb motion are effective for testing and training stroke patients.

8 For patients to comply with long-term objectives, exercise programs must be inexpensive, easily accessible, or able to be performed at home.

We Would Like to Know
About Stroke and Exercise

---

1 Does systematic long-term exercise training improve and maintain cardiovascular health outcomes and functional mobility in the chronic stroke population?

2 Does treadmill training improve functional mobility and the cardiovascular health profile in the chronic stroke population?

3 Are home-based stroke rehabilitation and exercise programs both cost-effective and functionally effective?

4 Are stroke patients at a high risk of cardiovascular complications during high-intensity exercise programs?

5 Do stroke patients improve muscular strength at a similar rate in paretic versus nonaffected limbs?

Summary

The number of stroke survivors with neuromuscular impairments is increasing, requiring cost-effective means for long-term rehabilitation. The enhancement of functional capabilities improves exercise efficiency, the ability to perform routine activities of daily living, emotional difficulties, and overall quality of life. Without available rehabilitation opportunities, loss of function due to inactivity is accompanied by a greater risk for falls, loss of independence, and higher overall mortality rates. Effective long-term programs must be convenient and easily accessible and promote the improvement and maintenance of endurance and strength with task-specific training modalities.

DISCUSSION QUESTIONS

1 How does task-specific training apply to the stroke patient?

2 What are the components of a comprehensive rehabilitation approach for stroke patients?

3 Many of the muscular changes associated with stroke are similar to those associated with prolonged disuse. What are they, and how does exercise combat or reverse these maladaptations?

4 Should stroke patients have an exercise test before starting an exercise program?

CASE STUDY

Patient Information

Jack is a 65-year-old man with a complex cardiovascular medical history. He has been referred to cardiac rehabilitation and is scheduled to begin exercise classes approximately 6 weeks following coronary artery bypass revascularization surgery and mitral valve replacement. His postsurgical recovery course has been uneventful in terms of the surgical procedure but is complicated by his previous cardiovascular history, which includes a right-sided hemiparesis from a stroke approximately 10 years earlier. During the acute poststroke rehabilitation phase, Jack was found to have a moderate expressive and receptive aphasia, and his right upper and lower extremities showed only trace movement with decreased sensation. The right lower extremity had good strength and the left side had normal strength. The acute poststroke therapy went well, with the patient eventually ambulating independently with some motor return to the right upper extremity complicated by a flexion synergy with some elbow and finger extension. The patient's speech improved, and he showed 100% accuracy in following conversational speech. Jack's progress has continued stable since that time. Other factors that must be taken into consideration are that the patient is an insulin-requiring diabetic and has had multiple previous cardiac-related events, including congestive heart failure, myocardial infarctions, and, in addition, chronic obstructive pulmonary artery disease.

Assessments

The initial program assessment revealed a pleasant gentleman who appeared motivated to comply with our exercise recommendations. He walks with obvious gait impairment and still has limited use of his right arm, and he states that both of these conditions have worsened since the surgery. Since his surgery, Jack has had no apparent angina, and his shortness of breath appears to have improved. The patient's main concern is muscular weakness and associated instability. Current medications include Humulin insulin, 70 units in the morning and 30 units in the evening; Zoloft, 100 mg in the evening; Vasotec, 5 mg once a day; Colace, 100 mg twice a day; aspirin, 81 mg daily; Tenormin, 12.5 mg once a day; and Ativan 0.5 mg as needed. The patient's body weight is 102 kg (224 pounds), with a waist circumference of 116 cm and a waist-to-hip circumference ratio of 1.04. A self-efficacy scale indicates a low self-confidence for performing tasks requiring physical exertion, but his perception of quality of life is within normal ranges.

Jack lives alone. He presents a reasonable knowledge of low-fat food preparation but is not willing to put a lot of time into food preparation. Therefore, a dietary consult will be obtained to discuss efficient food preparation for one. Even though Jack previously drank beer on a daily basis, he now drinks alcohol only on a limited basis (two beers once per week) and has not used tobacco for over 15 years. Throughout his prolonged illnesses, Jack has experienced mild periodic depression for which he has received counseling. Being a very "plain" and withdrawn kind of gentleman, Jack is not very socially active and spends a lot of time alone.

Based on his program entry assessment, Jack's program objectives include improved muscular strength and endurance in the paretic and nonaffected extremities, weight loss, and risk factor lifestyle modifications, particularly emphasizing food selection and preparation and increased physical activity.

An abdominal circumference exceeding 100 cm and a waist-to-hip ratio exceeding 1.0 indicates that Jack is obese and a central fat depositor (android obesity, which predisposes him to future cardiovascular complications). In addition, the obesity may further limit his ambulatory capabilities.

The American College of Sports Medicine recommends that the exercise prescription for those undergoing cardiovascular revascularization and heart valve surgery be based on risk stratification concerning the patient's progress while in the hospital and on his or her acute postrecovery period at home. If the postsurgical course is uneventful, exercise prescription guidelines follow the usual recommendation for the asymptomatic cardiac patient, balancing intensity with duration and frequency. Initially, intensity is 40% to 50% of the maximum oxygen uptake reserve. During the low-intensity phases, the intent of the program will be to increase duration gradually. Initial durations and frequencies can be short-duration exercise bouts (≤5 minutes) performed multiple times each day. As duration is increased to 20 minutes, the intensity will be gradually increased in increments of less than 1 MET (the metabolic equivalent of quiet rest). In the event of medication changes or no preparticipation exercise test, signs and symptoms of possible overexertion should be monitored, with ratings of perceived exertion between "fairly light" and "somewhat hard" (RPE = 11 to 13 on the 6–20 scale).

Questions

1. What factors must be considered when developing Jack's exercise prescription?
2. What educational factors must be emphasized for Jack while he is in the program?
3. What are some concerns for Jack's long-term compliance?

REFERENCES

1. Gordon NF. Stroke, Your Complete Exercise Guide. The Cooper Clinic and Research Institute Fitness Series. Champaign, IL: Human Kinetics, 1993.
2. Teixeira-Salmela LF, Olney SJ, Nadeau S, Brouwer B. Muscle strengthening and physical conditioning to reduce impairment and disability in chronic stroke survivors. Arch Phys Med Rehabil 1999;80:1211–1218.
3. Wood-Dauphinee S. The epidemiology of stroke: relevance for physical therapists. Physiother Can 1985;37:377–386.
4. O'Sullivan S. Stroke. In: O'Sullivan S, Schmitz TJ, eds. Physical Rehabilitation Assessment and Treatment. 3rd Ed. Philadelphia: FA Davis, 1994.
5. Potempa K, Braun LT, Tinkell T, Popovich J. Benefits of aerobic exercise after stroke. Sports Med 1996;21:337–346.
6. Rosenfalk A, Andreassen S. Impaired regulation of force and firing pattern of single motor units in patients with spasticity. J Neurol Neurosurg Psychiatry 1980;43:907–916.
7. Brinkmann JR, Hoskins TA. Physical conditioning and altered self-concept in rehabilitated hemiplegic patients. Physical Therapy 1979;59:859–865.
8. Landin S, Hagenfeldt L, Saltin B, et al. Muscle metabolism during exercise in hemiparetic patients. Clin Sci Mol Med 1977;53:257–269.
9. Macko RF, DeSouza CA, Tretter LD, et al. Treadmill aerobic exercise training reduces the energy expenditure and cardiovascular demands of hemiparetic gait in chronic stroke patients. A preliminary report. Stroke 1997;28:326–330.
10. Rimmer JH, Hedman G. A health promotion program for stroke survivors. Top Stroke Rehabil 1998;5:30–44.
11. Weiss A, Suzuki T, Bean J, Fielding RA. High intensity strength training improves strength and functional performance after stroke. Am J Phys Med Rehabil 2000;79:369–376.
12. Fiatarone MA, Marks EC, Ryan ND, et al. High-intensity strength training in nonagenarians. JAMA 1990;263:3029–3034.
13. Blair SN, Kohl HW, Barlow CE. Low cardiorespiratory fitness and incidence of non-fatal stroke [abstract]. Med Sci Sports Exerc 1989;21:S49.
14. Sacco RL, Gan R, Boden-Albala B, et al. Leisure time physical activity and ischemic stroke risk: The Northern Manhattan Stroke Study. Stroke 1998;29:380–387.
15. Slattery ML, Jacobs DR, Nichaman MZ. Leisure time physical activity and coronary heart disease death: the US Railroad study. Circulation 1989;79:304–311.
16. Goldberg G, Berger GG. Secondary prevention in stroke: a primary rehabilitation concern. Arch Phys Med Rehabil 1988;69:32–40.
17. Lee IM, Paffanbarger RS. Physical activity and stroke incidence: The Harvard Alumni Health Study. Stroke 1998;29:2049–2054.
18. Wannamathee SG, Shaper AG. Physical activity and the prevention of stroke. J Cardiovasc Risk 1999;6:213–216.
19. Paffenbarger RS, Wing AL. Characteristics in youth predisposing to fatal stroke in later years. Lancet 1967;i:753–754.
20. Hu FB, Stampfer MJ, Colditz GA, et al. Physical activity and risk of stroke in women. JAMA 2000;283:2961–2967.
21. Ellekjaer H, Holmen J, Ellekjaer E, Vatten L. Physical activity and stroke mortality in women: ten-year follow-up of the Nord-Trondelag Health Survey, 1984–1986. Stroke 2000;31:14–18.
22. Kiely DK, Wolf PA, Cupples LA, et al. Physical activity and stroke risk: The Framingham Study. Am J Epidemiol 1994;140:608–620.

23. Doering TJ, Resch KL, Steuernagel BB, et al. Passive and active exercises increase cerebral bloodflow velocity in young healthy individuals. Am J Phys Med Rehabil 1998;77:490–493.
24. Paffenbarger RS, Brand RJ, Shultz R, Jung D. Energy expenditure, cigarette smoking and blood pressure level as related to death from specific diseases. Am J Epidemiol 1978;108:12–18.
25. Halar EM. Management of stroke risk factors during the process of rehabilitation. Phys Med Rehabil Clin North Am 1999;10:839–856.
26. Dyken ML, Wolf PA, Barnett HJM, et al. Risk factors in stroke: statement for physicians by Subcommittee on Risk Factors and Stroke. Stroke 1984;15:1105–1111.
27. Hertzer NR, Young JR, Beven EG, et al. Coronary angiography in 506 patients with extracranial cerebrovascular disease. Arch Intern Med 1985;145:849–852.
28. O'Connor G, Buring Y, Yusuf S, et al. An overview of randomized trials of rehabilitation with exercise after myocardial infarction. Circulation 1989;79:234–244.
29. Oldridge NB, Guyatt G, Fischer M, et al. Cardiac rehabilitation after myocardial infarction: Combined experience of randomized clinical trials. JAMA 1988;260:945–950.
30. Abbott RD, Rodriguez BL, Burchfiel CM, et al. Physical activity in older middle-aged men and reduced risk of stroke: The Honolulu Heart Program. Am J Epidemiol 1994;139:881–893.
31. Kujala UM, Kaprio J, Sarn S et al. Relationship of leisure-time physical activity and mortality. JAMA 1998:279:440–444.
32. Duncan P, Richards L, Wallace D, et al. A randomized, controlled pilot study of a home-based exercise program for individuals with mild and moderate stroke. Stroke 1998;29:2055–2060.
33. American College of Sports Medicine. ACSM's Guidelines for Exercise Testing and Prescription. 6th Ed. Philadelphia: Lippincott Williams & Wilkins, 2000.
34. Nugent JA, Schurr KA, Adams RA. A dose-response relationship between the amount of weight bearing exercise and walking outcome following cerebrovascular accident. Arch Phys Med Rehabil 1994;75:399–402.
35. Bozcko M, Mumenthaler M. Modified pendulousness test to assess tonus of high muscles in spasticity. Neurology 1958;8:846–851.
36. Bohannon R, Walsh S. Nature, reliability, and predictive value of muscle performance measures in patients with hemiparesis following stroke. Arch Phys Med Rehabil 1992;73:721–725.
37. Ewart GK, Taylor CB, Reese LB, DeBusk RF. Effects of early post-myocardial infarction exercise testing on self-perception and subsequent physical activity. Am J Cardiol 1983;51:1076–1080.
38. Foster C, Oldridge NB, Dion W, et al. Time course of recovery during cardiac rehabilitation. J Cardiopulmonary Rehabil 1995;15:209–215.
39. Oldridge NB, Rogowski BL. Self-efficacy and in-patient cardiac rehabilitation. Am J Cardiol 1990;66:362–365.
40. McConnell TR, Laubach CA, Szmedra L. Age and gender related trends in body composition, lipids, and exercise capacity during cardiac rehabilitation. Am J Geriatric Cardiol 1997;6:37–45.
41. Coyle CP, Santiago MC. Aerobic exercise training and depressive symptomatology in adults with physical disabilities. Arch Phys Med Rehabil 1995;76:647–652.
42. MacDonald MR, Nielson WR, Cameron MG. Depression and activity patterns of spinal cord injured persons living in a community. Arch Phys Med Rehabil 1987;68:339–343.
43. Luukinen H, Koski K, Laippala P, Kivela SL. Risk factors for recurrent falls in the elderly in long-term institutional care. Public Health 1995;109:57–65.

44. Richards CL, Malouin F, Wood-Dauphinee S, et al. Task specific physical therapy for optimization of gait recovery in acute stroke patients. Arch Phys Med Rehabil 1993;74:612–620.

45. Smith GV, Silver KHC, Goldberg AP, Macko RF. "Task-oriented" exercises improves hamstring strength and spastic reflexes in chronic stroke patients. Stroke 1999;30:2112–2118.

46. Greshem GE, Fitzpatrick TE, Wolf PA, et al. Residual disability in survivors of stroke: The Framingham study. N Engl J Med 1976;293:954–956.

47. Kwakkel G, Wagenaar RC, Twisk JWR, et al. Intensity of leg and arm training after primary middle-cerebral artery stroke: a randomized trial. Lancet 1999;354:191–196.

48. Deam CM, Richards CL, Malouin F. Task-related circuit training improves performance of locomotor tasks in chronic stroke: A randomized, controlled pilot trial. Arch Phys Med Rehabil 2000;81:409–417.

49. Hassid E, Rose D, Commisarow J, et al. Improved gait symmetry in hemiparetic stroke patients induced during body weight-supported treadmill stepping. J Neurol Rehabil 1997;11:21–26.

50. Visintin M, Barbeau H, Korner-Bitensky N, et al. A new approach to retrain gait in stroke patients through body weight support and treadmill stimulation. Stroke 1998;29:1122–1128.

51. Hesse S, Bertelt C, Jahnke MT, et al. Treadmill training with partial body weight support compared with physiotherapy in non-ambulatory hemiparetic patients. Stroke 1995;26:976–981.

52. Corcoran PJ, Jebson RH, Brengelman GL, Simons BC. Effects of plastic and metal leg braces on speed and energy cost of hemiparetic ambulation. Arch Phys Med Rehabil 1970;51:69–77.

53. Gersten J, Orr W. External work of walking in hemiparetic patients. Scand J Rehabil Med 1971;3:85–88.

54. Hesse S, Bertelt C, Schaffrin A, et al. Restoration of gait in nonambulatory hemiparetic patients by treadmill training with partial body-weight support. Arch Phys Med Rehabil 1994;75:1087–1093.

55. Smith GV, Macko RF, Silver KHC, Goldberg AP. Treadmill aerobic exercise improves quadriceps strength in patients with chronic hemiparesis following stroke: a preliminary report. J Neuro Rehab 1998;112:111–117.

56. Waagfjord J, Levangie PK, Certo CME. Effects of treadmill training on gait in a hemiparetic patient. Phys Ther 1990;70:549–560.

57. Fujitani J, Ishikawa T, Akai M, Kakurai S. Influence of daily activity on changes in physical fitness for people with post-stroke hemiplegia. Am J Phys Med Rehabil 1999;78:540–544.

58. Macko RF, Katzel LI, Yataco A, et al. Low-velocity graded treadmill stress testing in hemiparetic patients. Stroke 1997;28:988–992.

59. Moldover JR, Daum MC. Cardiac stress testing of hemiparetic patients with a supine bicycle ergometer: Preliminary study. Arch Phys Med Rehabil 1984;65:470–473.

60. Buchfuhrer M, Hansen J, Robinson T, et al. Optimizing the exercise protocol for cardiopulmonary assessment. J Appl Physiol 1983;55:1558–1564.

SUGGESTED READINGS

Gordon NF. Stroke: Your Complete Exercise Guide. Champaign, IL: Human Kinetics, 1993.

Palmer-McLean K, Wilberger JE. Stroke and Head Injury. In: Durstine JL, ed. ACSM's Exercise management for Persons with Chronic Diseases and Disabilities. Champaign, IL: Human Kinetics, 1997:169–174.

Whaley MH, Kaminsky LA. Epidemiology of physical activity, physical fitness, and selected chronic diseases. In: Roitman JL, ed. ACSM's Resource Manual for Guidelines for Exercise Testing and Prescription, 3rd Ed. Baltimore: Williams & Wilkins, 1998:13-26.

CHAPTER 15

Exercise and Lower Limb Amputation

Kenneth H. Pitetti, Robert C. Manske

SEARCHABLE KEY TERMS

Atherosclerosis	Neuropathies
Category RPE Scale	Osteogenic Sarcoma
Category-Ratio RPE Scale	Percent Heart Rate Reserve
Ischemia	Teratogenic Agent
Maximal Capacity	Valsalva Maneuver

Overview

There are about 311,000 individuals in the United States with lower limb (LL) amputation (1, 2). Lower limb amputations result from any of the following factors: vascular and circulatory disease caused by either type 2 (adult onset) diabetes or peripheral vascular disease (70%); trauma (23%); tumor (4%); and congenital deformity (3%). Table 15.1 lists the classification and description of LL amputations (3).

Pathophysiology

Most persons requiring lower limb amputation are older than 55 years of age (4). In fact, a 10-year (1989–1999)

study (5) of LL amputations by the Veterans Health Administration reported that 87% of LL amputees in that study were above the age of 55 years. These LL amputees, who were patients in Veterans Health Administration hospitals, accounted for 10% of all amputations in U.S. males during this 10-year period. The major causes for LL amputation among these patients were **neuropathies** and peripheral vascular disease secondary to either type 2 diabetes or atherosclerosis (2, 5). It must be remembered that the disease process is not arrested by the amputation. For instance, Kald and colleagues (5) reported a 50% mortality rate only 2 years postoperation, and Bodily and colleagues (6) reported a 20% to 50% risk of losing the contralateral leg due to vascular disease within 5 years after the initial surgical amputation. Therefore, because most amputations in the United States are performed on individuals over the age of 55 years

TABLE 15.1. CLASSIFICATIONS OF LOWER LIMB AMPUTATIONS

Classification	Description
Symes	Amputation of the forefoot or midfoot, usually leaving the heel bones (calcaneus and talus) intact, allowing full weight-bearing onto the heel of the foot
Transtibial	Below the knee (BK)
Transfemoral	Above the knee (AK)
Hip disarticulation	Removal of the leg at the femoral-hip joint
Unilateral amputation	Involves only one leg (e.g., unilateral below-knee; unilateral above-knee)
Bilateral amputation	Involves both legs (e.g., bilateral above-knee; bilateral above-and below-knee; bilateral below-knee)

Data from Pittetti KH (3).

and result from direct complications of type 2 diabetes and atherosclerosis, postsurgical morbidity and mortality become paramount concerns. Accordingly, the goal of exercise regimens for this population, referred to throughout this chapter as *dysvascular LL amputees,* is to preclude or abate the pathogenesis of diabetes or atherosclerosis.

Lower limb amputations not only become necessary by the process of type 2 diabetes and peripheral vascular disease secondary to atherosclerosis, but also can result from trauma, tumors, or congenital deformities. Individuals with amputations from these latter causes are referred to in this chapter as *nonvascular LL amputees.* Traumatic injuries that require LL amputation most often occur to individuals under the age of 50. Trauma itself can cause the acute removal of the lower limb, as, for instance, when a soldier steps on a land mine, but traumatic amputation also can follow acute injury such as a massively crushed limb, massive fractures causing **ischemia** and unreconstructable vasculature, or thermal, chemical, and electrical burns, and frostbite. Curative treatment of tumors, such as a malignant **osteogenic sarcoma** that has not yet metastasized, can require LL amputation. Congenital deformities can occur during the fetal stage of growth due to genetic anomalies or **teratogenic agents** (e.g., thalidomide, alcohol) and require the amputation of a deformed foot or lower leg. A prosthetic limb can then replace the amputated deformed limb and allow for better ambulation.

Because most nonvascular LL amputees are younger than 50 years of age, exercise regimens for them are similar to those for nondisabled persons of this age group. That is, the exercise program focuses on risk reduction for developing secondary disabilities such as cardiovascular disease, type 2 diabetes, high blood pressure, and obesity and, therefore, issues that affect morbidity and mortality. It is important to note that nonvascular LL amputees have a higher risk for developing these secondary cardiovascular-related

disabilities than the nondisabled population due to their predisposition to living a sedentary lifestyle (7, 8).

Upper extremity amputations are not covered in this chapter because upper extremity amputations have little effect on the individual's ambulatory capacity and, therefore, less effect on activity level. In addition, upper extremity amputees have no greater risk of developing peripheral and cardiovascular disease, hypertension, obesity, or type 2 diabetes than able-bodied individuals (7, 8). For information on upper extremity amputation and exercise, Pitetti and Manske's chapter (9) in *ACSM's Resource Manual for Guidelines for Exercise Testing and Prescription* should be consulted.

Behavioral Modifications

Diet and exercise are the most critical behavioral modifications for LL amputees. These become crucial in the months and years following the amputation because: (1) most amputations are due to vascular and circulatory disease, which are conditions caused by the pathogenesis of either type 2 diabetes or peripheral vascular disease; and (2) nonvascular LL amputees have a higher risk of developing type 2 diabetes or peripheral and coronary vascular disease because of a sedentary lifestyle that follows the amputation. Diet and exercise programs for dysvascular amputees are secondary preventative treatments against the ongoing process of diabetes or peripheral vascular disease. For nonvascular amputees, diet and exercise are primary preventative treatments to reduce the risk of developing diabetes, cardiovascular disease, hypertension, and peripheral vascular disease.

Behavioral Modification and Type 2 Diabetes

Type 2 diabetes is a major cause of dysvascular LL amputations, and nonvascular LL amputees are at high risk to develop type 2 diabetes. Type 2 diabetes causes cells throughout the body, especially skeletal muscle, fat, and liver cells, to become less sensitive to insulin. Insulin continues to be made and released into the bloodstream by the pancreas, but becomes progressively less effective at moving glucose from the blood into the cells of the body. This loss of insulin sensitivity is strongly related to both inactivity and obesity. (For more information on type 2 diabetes, see Chapter 21.)

Some simple nutritional guidelines to control weight and reduce the risk of obesity that could lead to or exacerbate type 2 diabetes are found in Box 15.1.

Behavioral Modifications and Vascular Disease

Vascular disease is another common problem for LL amputees, and it is important to address diet and behavioral modifications specific for vascular disease as it pertains to these patients. It has been reported that the prevalence of concomitant coronary vascular disease with lower extremity amputation due to vascular dysfunction caused by atherosclerosis may be as high as 75% (10). Some of the risk factors for vascular disease differ from those for type 2 diabetes. Risk factors for vascular disease include diabetes mellitus, smoking, high blood pressure, and high serum cholesterol, plus the major risk factors of inactivity and obesity.

One obvious way to substantially decrease or prevent vascular problems for many LL amputees with ongoing vascular disease is to quit smoking. However, due to the addictive nature of nicotine, achieving complete abstinence from smoking can be a long, frustrating battle. It may be more prudent and feasible for the LL amputee who is a smoker first to reduce the number of cigarettes smoked per day, with the long-term goal of complete abstinence. High blood pressure can be controlled by a combination of antihypertensive medications, a diet that pays close attention to limiting salt intake, and regular physical exercise. Serum cholesterol can be reduced (decrease in total cholesterol, especially in the serum lipoprotein known as low-density lipoproteins or LDL) or improved (increase in the antiatherosclerotic lipoprotein, called high-density lipoproteins or HDL) by anticholesterol medication, proper diet that encourages an increase in the intake of foods high in soluble fiber and low in saturated fat (e.g., fresh fruits and vegetables), plus exercise. It is important to note that dietary changes and exercise are involved in reducing four of the risk factors for vascular disease—high blood pressure, high serum cholesterol, inactivity, and obesity.

The behavioral modification of exercise also plays a major role for treatment and prevention of diabetes, hypertension, and cardiovascular disease. The primary purpose of prescribing exercise for the prevention and treatment of type 2 diabetes is to burn kilocalories (kcal—for the lay person, most food packages list kcal as "calories"). Because excessive weight or obesity is the key risk factor for type 2 diabetes, exercising combats type 2 diabetes in two ways:

the exercise improves sensitivity to insulin, and exercise, along with a proper diet, reduces body fat.

The Behavioral Modification of Walking for Exercise: Is It Applicable for Lower Limb Amputees?

According to the Centers for Disease Control and Prevention, the normal lifestyle for most nondisabled Americans is sedentary (11). More than 60% of nondisabled American adults do not exercise at a level adequate to promote normal and healthy functioning body systems (e.g., cardiovascular, pulmonary and musculoskeletal systems), and 25% do not exercise at all. As we begin a new millennium, the majority of nondisabled Americans are sedentary, physically unfit, and overweight (12). Associated with an increase in the number of sedentary nondisabled Americans is an increased prevalence of chronic diseases due to heart disease (up 2.8-fold since 1900), a sixfold increase in type 2 diabetes between 1958 and 1993; and a doubling in the number of obese persons in the past 2 decades (12).

The exercise and sports science research community and related professions have new policy documents relating to the maintenance of regular patterns of physical activity that focus on types of physical activity to be sustained and easily integrated into the contexts of people's everyday lives (13). In an attempt to reduce the prevalence of sedentary lifestyles in America, the primary emphasis—increasing population-wide energy expenditure—is related directly to activities that can affect the overall energy expenditure of large populations. Recreational and transport-related walking are being emphasized, because these are activities available to the entire nondisabled American population. However, recreational walking is not a viable or feasible physical activity pattern for most LL amputees.

The energy expenditure of walking is higher for LL amputees than for nondisabled peers or upper limb amputees. This increase in energy expenditure is related directly to the level of amputation. Huang and colleagues (14) reported that when LL amputees choose their own comfortable walking speed, the mean energy cost is 9% higher in unilateral below-knee, 49% higher for unilateral above-knee, and 280% higher for bilateral above-knee amputees when compared with able-bodied peers. Other researchers also have shown that the energy cost of walking is greater for LL amputees than for nondisabled individuals and upper extremity amputees (15–19). In addition, LL amputees chronically suffer from skin breakdowns and hair follicle infections, and these complications can occur more often with the added stress of long periods of walking in their prosthesis. The combination of additional energy expenditure (i.e., physical effort) and the potential painful consequences of skin breakdowns or infections precludes walking as a physical activity pattern that can be maintained and easily integrated into the everyday activities of most LL amputees, especially vascular LL amputees.

Physical Fitness and Functional Evaluations

Guidelines presented in this section and the next section, Exercise Guidelines and Programming, follow the general principles established for both disabled and nondisabled populations in *ACSM's Guidelines for Exercise Testing and Prescription* (20). More specific guidelines regarding management for LL amputees with type 2 diabetes, cardiovascular diseases, or respiratory diseases can be found in *ACSM's Exercise Management for Persons with Chronic Diseases and Disabilities* (21). Pitetti and Manske also have established guidelines for both upper and lower limb amputees specific to the circumstances created by amputation (9).

All dysvascular and nonvascular amputees who are being treated for any cardiopulmonary complication should obtain their physician's consent before beginning an exercise program.

Cardiovascular Evaluations

Mode of Testing

The recommended mode of testing to determine the cardiovascular fitness of LL amputees is an exercise machine that engages the largest amount of muscle mass possible. For unilateral above- or below-knee amputees, bilateral below-knee amputees, and bilateral amputees with one below-knee and one above-knee amputation, the exercise machine of choice would involve both upper and lower body musculature (e.g., arm-leg ergometer, such as Schwinn Air-Dyne [Figure 15.1]).

Lower limb amputees who are unable to involve their lower extremities on an arm-leg ergometer (e.g., bilateral above-knee amputees) should be tested using either an arm crank ergometer (e.g., Monark Arm Ergometer, Model 881), upper body exerciser, or the arm mechanism of an arm-leg ergometer (e.g., Schwinn Air-Dyne). These methods have been shown to elicit similar physiological responses (22).

Testing Protocols

Arm-Leg Ergometer

A maximal test should begin with a 2-minute warm-up at 25 watts (W), followed by incremental increases of 25 W every 2 minutes until volitional exhaustion. Heart rate should be monitored and recorded every minute, blood pressure should be taken after the first minute of each work level (while exercising), and rating of perceived exertion (RPE) should be recorded at the end of the 2nd minute of each work level. If it becomes difficult to measure the patient's blood pressure, exercise should be stopped every 2 minutes, blood pressure measured, and exercise then continued.

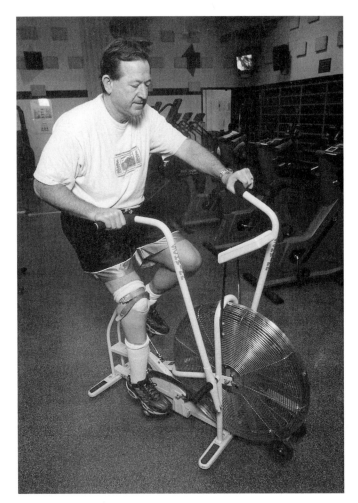

FIGURE 15.1.   Schwinn Air-Dyne Ergometer.

A **submaximal** test should begin with a 2-minute warm-up at an intensity level of 12.5 W followed by incremental increases of 12.5 W every 2 minutes and terminated when the heart rate reaches 65% to 70% of heart rate reserve or 85% of age-adjusted maximal heart rate. (For calculating heart rate reserve or age-adjusted maximal heart rates, consult Huang et al. [22]). If the patient is taking medication that blunts the heart rate response (e.g., beta blockers), the test should be terminated at a Borg scale of 15 when using the **Category RPE Scale** (range of 6–20) or 6 when using the **Category-Ratio RPE Scale** (range of 1–10). Heart rate, blood pressure, and RPE monitoring and recording should follow the same procedure for LL amputees who are classified as low-risk.

Arm Ergometry

Lower limb amputees who perform a maximal exercise test using arm-leg ergometry usually reach maximal or peak heart rates within a 10-beat range (±10 beats) of maximal age-predicted heart rate (220 − age = maximal age predicted heart rate). However, those LL amputees who are tested using arm ergometry may reach only 60% to 70% of age-predicted maximal heart rate, because the metabolic capacity of the smaller contracting muscle mass (i.e., arms, shoulders, and chest) limits exercise performance relative to that seen for those LL amputees using arm-leg ergometry.

A maximal arm ergometry test should begin with a 2-minute warm-up at an intensity level of 0 W at a constant cadence of 50 rpm, with incremental increases of 5 W every 2 minutes until volitional fatigue is reached. In addition, an intermittent exercise protocol should be followed, with 1-minute rest periods between each incremental increase of 5 W. An intermittent protocol is used for three reasons: (1) to allow for clear ECG tracings if electrocardiographic responses are being followed; (2) to allow time for accurate blood pressure measurement; and (3) to avoid early fatigue and allow the LL amputee to reach a greater total volume of high-intensity exercise. The heart rate should be monitored and recorded every minute, blood pressure taken during the 1-minute rest periods, and RPE recorded at the end of the 2nd minute of each work level.

A submaximal arm ergometry protocol would follow the same procedure as the maximal protocol, but would be terminated at a Borg scale of 15 when using the Category RPE Scale or 6 when using the Category-Ratio RPE Scale.

It is extremely important for the heart rate and RPE to be carefully monitored and recorded throughout all tests, because these parameters play a major role in prescribing exercise intensity.

Functional Evaluation: Walking Test

It has been shown that exercise programs improve the walking efficiency of LL amputees (23, 24). An easy way to monitor improved walking ability is to have the LL amputee walk a distance, ranging from 100 to 600 yards, and record the number of steps taken and the time (in seconds) it took to walk the distance. The distance of the walk test depends on the level of amputation. Physically fit unilateral LL amputees (below- and above-knee) should handle a walk of 500 or 600 yards easily. A distance of 100 to 200 yards is appropriate for deconditioned amputees, bilateral amputees, or amputees with a hip disarticulation. The walking test should be performed on a gymnasium floor, tennis court, hallway, or any other location that provides adequate distance and has a smooth, level surface.

Body Composition

Skinfold and Circumference Measurements

Various regression equations have been developed to predict percent body fat from skinfold and circumference measurements. However, these regression equations are derived from and applied to the specific population of able-bodied males and females and, therefore, are not applicable to LL amputees. It is important to note, however, that a decrease in the sum of skinfold thickness or circumference measurements will occur with reduction in body fat for both able-bodied or disabled populations. The sum of seven skinfolds (bicep, tricep, subscapula, chest, axial, hip, and abdomen) should be monitored throughout the exercise program of LL amputees, with decreases in these measurements reflecting a decrease in body fat.

Another simple measure that is associated with increased risk for vascular and metabolic diseases is the waist/hip ratio (i.e., circumference of the waist divided by the circumference of the hips). Target waist/hip ratios are below 0.95 for men and 0.85 for women, for LL amputees as well as able-bodied individuals. Waist girth alone also can be used.

Body Mass Index

Body mass index (BMI) is used to assess weight relative to height and is calculated by dividing body weight in kilograms by height in meters squared (wt/ht^2). The standards established for BMI that identify individuals who are overweight or obese, like the regression formulas to estimate percent body fat by using the sum of skin folds or circumference measures, were established for the nondisabled population. Therefore, BMI should be used like the sum of skinfolds, in that a reduction in BMI indicates an improvement in health status.

Muscle Fitness

Muscle fitness describes the combined status of three variables: muscle strength, muscle endurance, and flexibility. These variables are extremely important for LL amputees, because development of muscular fitness can help maintain and improve posture, prevent or reduce muscle pain in the lower back, and improve the capacity to perform essential daily tasks and live independently.

Muscle Strength

Muscle strength refers to the maximal force (expressed either in pounds or kilograms) that can be generated by a group of muscles. Muscle strength testing can be performed using free weights or weight machines (e.g., Nautilus) that are available in most health clubs. Because most LL amputees are over 55 years of age, free weights present a safety issue, however, and should be used with caution.

Muscle strength can be measured using various one-repetition maximum (1RM) weight-lifting tests. For safety purposes, before starting 1RM tests, LL amputees should have an initial warm-up period (e.g., 5 minutes on an arm-leg ergometer or arm ergometer [Figure 15.2] at low intensities followed by stretching) and sufficient practice time (i.e., performing the weight lifting movement at low to moderate loads) before the actual 1MR or weight is se-

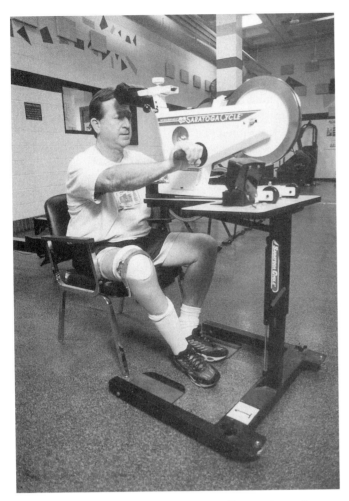

FIGURE 15.2. Saratoga Cycle arm ergometer (Saratoga Access & Fitness, Inc).

lected. Because of the advanced age or poor health and physical condition of many LL amputees, rest periods of 5 to 10 minutes between 1RM tests may be appropriate. The battery of 1RM tests may need to be spread over 2 to 3 days to prevent muscle discomfort or muscle soreness from discouraging the LL amputee from continuing. Proper breathing technique also should be practiced to prevent a Valsalva-type maneuver during lifting that could lead to lightheadedness or syncope.

Suggested lower body 1RM tests that are good for both the noninvolved limb (if unilateral) and the muscles of the amputated leg (for example, knee extension or flexion would not be appropriate for an above-knee amputee or a below-knee amputee with an extremely short stump) are as follows: knee flexion and extension, sitting leg press (if unilateral below-knee, perform with both limbs), and hip flexion and extension.

If the appropriate equipment is available, stomach curl (or sit-ups) and back extension are good trunk 1RM tests. Suggested upper body 1RM tests include sitting military press, bench press, sitting incline press, bicep curl, seated row, sitting latissimus pull down, and tricep extension. Ad-

ditional or substituted upper, trunk, and lower body 1RM tests can be given depending on the available equipment.

Muscle Endurance

Muscle endurance is the ability of a muscle group to perform repeated contractions (i.e., repetitions) during a short time period (30–60 seconds), with termination due to muscle fatigue. These tests involve repeating all the 1RM tests, but using a standard submaximal load such as one's own body weight for push-ups (if applicable) or 60% of the 1RM for weightlifting movements. The same safety precautions used during 1RM testing (e.g., sufficient rest periods between tests) should be followed for endurance testing.

Flexibility

Flexibility is the ability of a joint to move through a range of motion. Consult Corbin (25) for flexibility assessment.

Exercise Guidelines and Programming

Excellent resources for exercise professionals involved in exercise programs for LL amputees are available (26–28). The guidelines presented in this section follow those established in *ACSM's Guidelines for Exercise Testing and Prescription* (20). For LL amputees with type 2 diabetes, cardiovascular or respiratory diseases, the reader is referred to *ACSM's Exercise Management for Persons with Chronic Diseases and Disabilities* (21).

Because most LL amputees who begin to exercise are entering a multicomponent program (e.g., diet, exercise, smoking cessation, reduction of alcohol consumption) of behavioral change, health professionals are strongly urged to review the chapters in *ACSM's Guidelines for Exercise Testing and Prescription* (20) and the *Resouce Manual for Guidelines for Exercise Testing and Pescription* (29) that cover the scientifically validated approaches to health behavior change.

The FITT&P Principles of Exercise

The exercises prescribed for LL amputees focus on the FITT&P principle: Frequency of exercise, or number of days of exercise per week; Intensity of exercise, or the work level (e.g., **percent heart rate reserve**, rating of perceived exertion or RPE, or number of watts used while using a bicycle or rowing ergometer); Time (in minutes), or duration of each exercise session; Type or mode of exercise (e.g., arm-leg ergometer, bicycle ergometer [Figures 15.3–15.5], rowing ergometer, swimming); and Progression or gradual increase in frequency or duration over time (i.e., weeks to months).

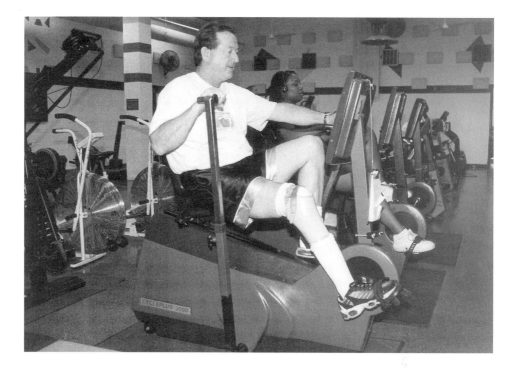

FIGURE 15.3. Cycleplus 3000 (Bioform Engineering).

Cardiovascular Programming: Type or Mode

Modes of exercise chosen for the LL amputee should incorporate the necessary amount of muscle mass to produce improvements in cardiovascular fitness or burn kcal; should be similar in the amount of effort needed (i.e., kcal expended) to similar exercise in able-bodied individuals; and should not cause overuse injuries, pain, or discomfort to nonamputated or amputated limbs.

Table 15.2 presents the recommended types or modes of exercise for improvement in cardiovascular fitness (30).

It is necessary to remember that all amputees who use swimming or upper body ergometry as their mode of exercise initially will elicit only small magnitudes of cardiovascular improvement due to the smaller muscle mass in the upper body. The same is true of unilateral above-knee or hip disarticulation amputees and bilateral above- and below-knee amputees who perform one-leg cycle ergometry. In time, however, strength and endurance of the exercising muscles will gradually increase and, therefore, will develop enough mass to elicit larger magnitudes of cardiovascular improvements. In addition, one of the main purposes of prescribing exercise for the prevention and treatment of type 2 diabetes and obesity for LL amputees is burning kcals. During the initial stages of a category "Z" type of exercise (see Table 15.2), the LL amputee will also be improving the sensitivity of the cells of his or her body to insulin and, when that is combined with a proper diet, reducing body fat.

Box 15.2 presents recommendations for exercise prescription for cardiovascular training in LL amputees.

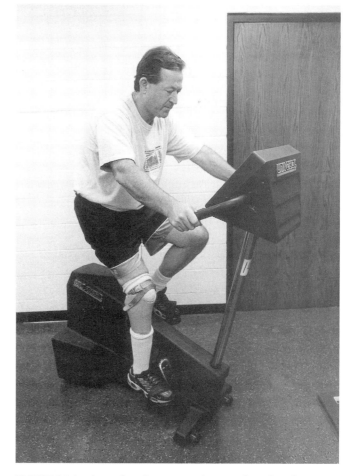

FIGURE 15.4. Sitting bicycle ergometer (Universal Aerobicycle, Universal Products).

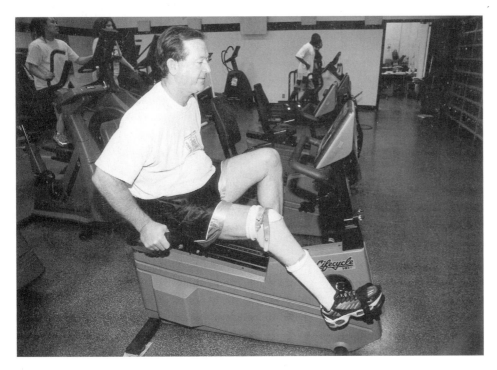

FIGURE 15.5.   Reclining bicycle ergometer (Row Lifecycle, Lifefitness).

Muscular Fitness Programming: Types or Modes

Most health club facilities provide an array of weight machines that can strengthen all the major muscle groups of the body. Table 15.3 lists the body area (e.g., upper body, trunk, and lower body) and the muscle groups that each classification of LL amputee can and should train.

Upper body weight training becomes especially important for amputees using arm crank ergometry or swimming for their cardiovascular training. Initially, these modes may not elicit large magnitudes of cardiovascular improvements due to the small upper body muscle mass. Weight training, in conjunction with swimming or arm crank ergometery, should hasten the increase in upper body muscle mass.

TABLE 15.2.   TYPES OR MODES OF AEROBIC EXERCISE FOR IMPROVING CARDIOVASCULAR FITNESS FOR LL AMPUTEES

	UNILATERAL AMPUTEES			BILATERAL AMPUTEES		
Mode	**Below-Knee, Symes**	**Above-Knee**	**Hip Disarticulation**	**Both Below-Knee, Both Symes**	**One Below-, One Above-Knee**	**Both Above-Knee**
Sitting arm–leg ergometry (Schwinn Air-Dyne)	X	X	X	X	X	O
Standing arm–leg ergometry (Reebok Body Trec)	X	Y	O	Y	O	O
Bicycle ergometry reclined or sitting-up (LifeCycle)	X	Z	Z	X	Z	O
Rowing ergometry (Concept II) (Figure 15.6)	X	X	X	X	Y	Y
Arm ergometry (Monark 881)	Z	Z	Z	Z	Z	Z
Swimming	Z	Z	Z	Z	Z	Z

O, Will most likely be unable to perform
X, Should incorporate sufficient muscle mass to improve cardiovascular fitness
Y, If amputee is capable of performing, should incorporate sufficient muscle mass to improve cardiovascular fitness
Z, Will elicit improvements in cardiovascular fitness, but because it incorporates a smaller muscle mass. The improvements will be of a smaller magnitude than that obtained with categories X and Y.
Data from Franklin BA (29).

- Frequency: 3 to 5 days per week; can be increased gradually to 7 days for those needing weight loss
- Intensity: begin at low intensity—i.e., 540% to 50% of maximal work level reached during cardiovascular evaluation, 40% to 50% heart rate reserve at level 12 or at level 11 ("fairly light") on the RPE category scale
- Time: 10 to 20 minutes per exercise session to start, with a goal of 30 to 60 minutes
- Type: see Table 15.2.
- Progression: Increase frequency and duration gradually on a weekly basis until a level is reached that meets either the individual's goal or time availability. At this point, the individual should consider increasing intensity as tolerated, to as high as 85% of maximal work and/or heart rate reserve, or 17 ("very hard") on the RPE scale. Once a desired level of fitness is reached, exercise frequency can be reduced, and recreational/sports activities (e.g., canoeing) can be substituted.
- It should be noted that an individual with a high fitness level can burn as many calories at a high intensity in a much shorter time than can an individual with a low fitness level who performs at lower intensities.

Recommendations for muscle training can be found in Box 15.3. Recommended "Dos" and "Don'ts" for muscle training are found in Box 15.4.

Stretching

Stretching exercises for upper body, trunk, and lower body should be performed at every exercise session (26). De-

pending on the level of amputation, stretching should involve musculature of the neck, shoulder, trunk and back, and hip, as well as the muscles of the nonamputated limb and residual muscle of the amputated limb.

Putting It All Together: The Personalized Exercise Program for LL Amputees

The co-author of this chapter (KHP) has been an amputee for over 31 years, and has worked with many different disability populations in developing exercise programs to improve their fitness. This section presents the exercise program that he performs, which is easily adjusted to all classifications of LL amputees and their physical fitness levels. It is divided into four parts: muscle/cardiovascular warm-up; stretching and weight training; cardiovascular exercise; short recovery phase; and low-intensity aerobic kcal burn.

The Program

Part 1: Muscle/Cardiovascular Warm-Up

Select the mode or type of exercise that will involve the largest amount of the LL amputee's muscle mass (see Table 15.2). For the first 3 minutes, exercise at a low intensity (30–40 % maximal capacity, 30–40% heart rate reserve, or a Category RPE scale of 7; very, very light). After 3 minutes increase the intensity to 50% maximal capacity, 50% heart rate reserve, or a Category RPE scale of 11; very light. Initially, the duration should be 5 minutes (i.e., 3 minutes RPE scale of 7 followed by 2 minutes of RPE scale of 11), increasing 1 minute every 2 weeks, with a target duration of 10 to 15 minutes. As the weeks progress, the amputee can

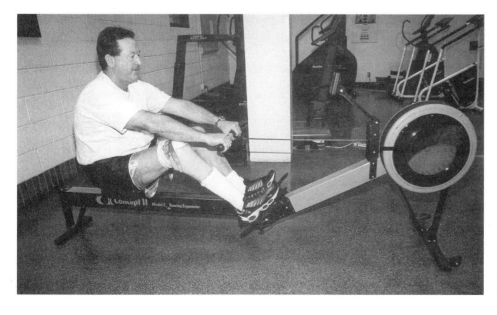

FIGURE 15.6. Concept II rowing ergometer (Concept II Inc).

TABLE 15.3.   MUSCLE GROUPS THAT SHOULD BE EXERCISED USING FREE WEIGHTS OR WEIGHT MACHINES AT LEAST ONCE A WEEK

	UNILATERAL AMPUTEES			BILATERAL AMPUTEES		
Mode	**Below-Knee, Symes**	**Above-Knee**	**Hip Disarticulation**	**Both Below-Knee, Both Symes**	**One Below-, One Above-Knee**	**Both Above-Knee**
Upper Body						
Biceps (curls)	X	X	X	X	X	X
Triceps (dips, arm extension)	X	X	X	X	X	X
Shoulder girdle (sitting and incline military press, bench press, seated row, lat pull, shoulder abduction and adduction)	X	X	X	X	X	X
Trunk						
Abdomen (curls or sit-ups)	X	X	X	X	X*	X*
Back (machine that works lower back)	X	X	X	X	X*	X*
Lower Body						
Quadriceps (leg extension)	Y	Y*	Y*	Z	Z*	O
Hamstring (leg flexor)	Y	Y*	Y*	Z	Z*	O
Hip girdle (adduction, abduction, flexion, extension)	X	X	X	X	X*	X*

O, Will most likely be unable to perform
X, Should be able to perform
X*, Should be able to perform with either adjustments to the machine or assistance from staff personnel
Y, Exercise each leg separately
Y*, Exercise the nonamputated leg
Z, If sufficient stump, exercise each leg separately
Z*, If sufficient stump, exercise the below-knee amputated leg

increase exercise intensity in the following manner: 3 minutes at 30% to 40% of maximal capacity, 30% to 40% heart rate reserve, or RPE of 7; 5 minutes at 50% of **maximal capacity** or RPE of 11; and increasing after 8 minutes to 60% of maximal capacity, 60% heart rate reserve, or RPE of 13, somewhat hard, until the end of the exercise session.

As an example, if the amputee's cardiovascular evaluation determined a maximal capacity of 100 W, then the work levels for this part of the exercise session would be 30 to 40 W for 3 minutes, 50 W for 5 minutes, and 60 W for the remainder of the session.

The purpose of this part of the exercise session is to gradually prepare the muscle for more intensive exercise by increasing blood flow to the working muscles; burn kcals; and, as exercise time is increased, promote cardiovascular fitness.

Part 2: Stretching and Weight Training

Stretching should involve the muscles that will be used during weight training and cardiovascular conditioning. Following stretching, select two weight lifting modes that will work the upper body, one that will work the trunk musculature, and two that will work the lower body (see Table

15.3). On the days that do not include lifting weights, use this time solely for stretching.

Part 3: Cardiovascular Conditioning

Select the same mode used for exercise in Part 1, or, another mode of exercise that also involves a large muscle mass. For instance, a unilateral below-knee amputee may use the Schwinn Air-Dyne for Part 1, but select Body Trec (Reebok) (Figure 15.7) for cardiovascular conditioning. The first 2 minutes of exercise are at 50% of maximal work level; the remainder of Part 3 exercise is at an intensity of 60% to 70% maximal capacity, or 60% to 70% of heart rate reserve, or RPE in Category 13 to 16. Initially, exercise should be a duration of 12 minutes (which includes the first 2 minutes at 50% max), increasing 1 minute every 2 weeks, with a target duration of 20 to 30 minutes.

Part 4: Short Recovery Phase

Part 3 is the "guts" of the workout, and after completion, the LL amputee will be relatively fatigued. Allow a 5- to 10-minute "active" rest period (i.e., not sitting, but walking slowly) before starting Part 5. This is also the time to

- Frequency: 2 to 3 days per week
- Intensity: 60% to 80% 1 RM, or a weight that allows 8 repetitions to be performed. This weight should be used until 12 repetitions can be performed; then the weight should be increased by 5 to 10 pounds, and the patient should return to 8 repetitions.
- Time: At least five separate exercises are to be performed: two upper body (one pushing and one pulling, or antagonistic pairs), one trunk, and two lower body (one flexion and one extension, or antagonistic pairs). Weight training should be performed within 20 minutes.
- Type: See Table 15.3.
- Progression: At first, one should perform one set of 8 repetitions, increasing 1 repetition every 1 to 2 weeks until 12 repetitions can be performed with the same weight. Once 12 repetitions can be performed, increase by 5 to 10 lbs, to a weight at which only eight repetitions can be performed. Depending on the individual's fitness goal or time constraints, he or she can progress to two sets per workout.

guard against dehydration by drinking liberal amounts of water.

Part 5: Low-Intensity Aerobic Caloric Burn

Select the mode of exercise used in Part 1 or Part 3 and exercise at an intensity of 30% to 40% maximal work level, 30% to 40% heart rate reserve, or RPE of 7. Begin at a duration of 5 minutes, adding 1 minute every 2 weeks, with a target duration of 15 to 20 minutes. The purpose of Part 5 is to burn additional kcals.

Time Consideration

Once the amputee reaches target durations, then each part of this protocol can be adjusted depending on the time constraints of each day. For instance, on a day with limited time for exercising, time durations could be limited to 10, 15, and 10 minutes for Parts 1, 3, and 5, respectively, with Part 2 involving only stretching. On a day with few time constraints (e.g., weekend, holiday), time durations should be extended to 15 to 20, 20 to 30, and 15 to 20 minutes for Parts 1, 3, and 5, respectively, with Part 2 including weight training as well as stretching.

Exercise Kilocalorie Counting

Because one of the major purposes of an exercise program for LL amputees is burning kcals, it is important to keep a

log of daily and weekly calories (i.e., kilocalories) burned. For reduction or control of weight the ACSM recommends an expenditure of at least 2000 kcal per week (20). For deconditioned LL amputees, this goal should be approached gradually over a 3- to 6-month period. Initially, the LL amputee may be able to exercise only for 5, 12, and 5 minutes for Parts 1, 3, and 5, respectively. This may only add up to 100 calories a workout, but when done 3 to 5 times per week, the initial weekly caloric expenditure would be 300 to 500 calories. It is important for the LL amputee to be patient but consistent (i.e., stay on task). No matter the initial physical fitness of LL amputees, within 3 to 6 months the target caloric expenditure of 2000 calories per week should be attained, and, for most, probably will be exceeded.

How to Count Calories

Most aerobic exercise machines found in community health clubs have digital readouts of such parameters as work level (usually in watts), exercise time, distance covered (in miles), and kcal (usually described as "calories" on digital readouts) burned for the duration of the time spent exercising. These readouts are not always accurate (they can be off by as much as 10–20%), but they are relatively reliable (i.e., given a specific work level and duration, the exercise machine will show similar kcal readout). For example, in Part 1 of the exercise regimen, a LL amputee can exercise on a machine for 5 minutes at a given work intensity and on

For efficient use of time, weight training should be performed on the same day as cardiovascular training.

At least five separate exercises should be performed per workout: two upper body, one trunk, and two lower body.

For instructional purposes, consider LL amputee training 3 days a week; Monday, Wednesday, and Friday:

Monday: bicep curls, sitting military press (i.e., two upper body exercises), and sit-ups (1 trunk exercise), and hip abduction and adduction (2 lower body exercises)
Wednesday: triceps extensions, and shoulder abduction, a low-back exercise, and hip flexion and extension
Friday: incline military press and lat pulls, abdominal curls, and leg flexion and extension

In this way, all major muscle groups would be exercised within each week.

Weight training should not be performed 2 days in a row, or more than three times per week, to guard against muscle fatigue. For example, if the plan is to exercise 4 days per week, Monday, Wednesday, Friday, and Saturday, weight training should not be performed on both Friday and Saturday. However, cardiovascular/calorie burning training and stretching should be performed on all 4 days.

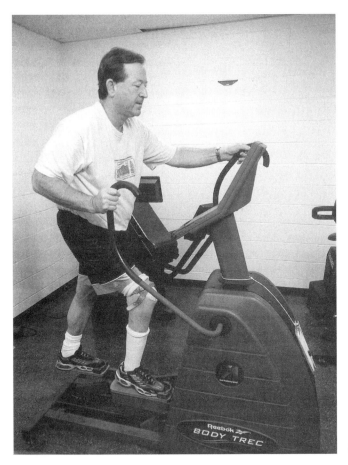

FIGURE 15.7.   Body Trec (Reebok).

completion, the exercise machine shows a kcal readout of 30 calories. The amputee will find that for the next 2 weeks, if the mode, duration, and work level are kept the same, the machine will consistently record a readout at or near 30 kcals (i.e., ±1–2 calories). As the LL amputee continues to exercise on the same machine and at the same work level, but over time extends the duration to 10 minutes, the machine should show a readout at or near 60 kcal, doubling the amount of calories burned. At first, for the initial 5-minute duration, the actual amount of kcals may be only 25 instead of 30 calories, but by the time the duration of the exercise has doubled (from 5 to 10 minutes), the actual amount of kcals burned also has doubled, and the patient's motivation increases.

The LL amputee should maintain a small notepad to record the number of kcals burned after using each machine for each day of the week. Realistic goals of increasing caloric expenditure each week (e.g., 10–50 kcal) should be set, with a weekly caloric goal of 2000 calories or more.

Calories In—Calories Out

Keeping a log that records kcals burned per machine, per day, and per week also helps the LL amputee understand the "cost" of food eaten each day. Most snacks (e.g., candy, peanuts, soda) list the kcal content on the package (note: "calories" on the package actually means kilocalories,). Read it before eating it. A 200-calorie candy bar can equate to 20 to 30 minutes on an exercise machine. Knowing the "cost" of calories in versus calories out can help guide the LL amputee in food selection.

Research Notes

In 1973, James (24) reported that for healthy, male, unilateral above-knee amputees, one-legged (noninvolved leg) bicycle ergometry training improved cardiovascular fitness and walking efficiency, and the asymmetry of the prosthetic gait decreased. In 1987, Pitetti and colleagues (23) reported that when a combination of unilateral below- and above-knee, and bilateral below-and above-knee amputees trained on a Schwinn Air-Dyne ergometer, they improved their cardiovascular fitness and walking efficiency. These findings substantiate that individuals with LL amputations can reduce the energy expenditure of walking and improve their cardiovascular fitness using the methodologies outlined in this chapter.

The red flags specific for type 2 diabetes and peripheral vascular disease are covered in Chapter 21 and in Section II, respectively. However, LL amputees are at higher risk for developing vascular disease caused by atherosclerosis, type 2 diabetes, and high blood pressure than their nondisabled peers due to their predisposition for living a sedentary lifestyle. Therefore, a quick review of preliminary symptoms of these diseases is in order.

Vascular Disease: Atherosclerosis

Arteriosclerosis is a chronic disease of the arterial system characterized by abnormal thickening and hardening of the blood vessel walls. **Atherosclerosis** is a form of arteriosclerosis in which the thickening and hardening of the vessel walls are caused by soft deposits of intraarterial fat and fibrin that harden over time. Atherosclerosis presents with symptoms that result from inadequate blood perfusion of tissues, which is due to obstruction of the blood vessels that supply them. Early in the course of the disease, partial vessel obstruction may lead to momentary ischemic events (e.g., chest pain, shortness of breath), often associated with intense physical activity such as quickly walking or running up flights of stairs, or emotional stress. As the lesion caused by atherosclerosis becomes larger, obstruction increases and may result in tissue infarction—complete blockage of the blood vessel—resulting in a heart attack and stroke.

Atherosclerotic obstruction of the vessels supplying the brain is the major cause of stroke. Early signs of an impending stroke due to transient ischemic attacks that may last for 2 to 30 minutes are loss of or abnormal sensations in an arm or leg on one side of the body; weakness or paralysis of an arm or leg on one side of the body; partial loss of vision or hearing; double vision; dizziness; slurred speech; inability to recognize parts of the body; imbalance and falling; and fainting.

Type 2 Diabetes

The first symptoms of diabetes are related to the direct effects of high blood sugar levels. When blood sugar levels get too high (above 160–180 mg/dl), glucose passes into the urine. When this happens, the kidneys excrete additional water to dilute the large amounts of glucose lost in the urine. Because the kidneys produce excessive urine, a person with diabetes urinates often and at high volume, a condition called *polyuria*. This excessive urination creates abnormal thirst, a condition known as *polydipsia*. In addition, people whose diabetes is poorly controlled are more susceptible to infections.

Hypertension

Hypertension, or high blood pressure, is a "silent killer" because in most people it does not cause any symptoms. There are coincidental occurrences of certain symptoms that are widely—but erroneously—believed to be associated with high blood pressure, such as headaches, nosebleeds, dizziness, flushed face, and tiredness. Although people with high blood pressure may have these symptoms, they occur just as frequently in persons with normal blood pressure.

Untreated high blood pressure increases a person's risk of developing heart disease, kidney failure, blindness, and stroke at an early age. The best way to identify high blood pressure early is to make sure to have blood pressure measured once or twice a year by a trained health professional.

Medications

For vascular amputees, their amputation was a direct result of peripheral vascular disease and type 2 diabetes. The medications specific for these conditions and their effect on exercise response are covered in Chapter 21.

Many amputees experience the phenomenon called "phantom pain." Phantom pain can range from an annoyance to agonizing pain. When the pain is severe, relief is sometimes obtained from medications meant to treat epilepsy or depression, which have little or no effect on the exercise response. Some amputees who suffer excruciating phantom pain may find antidepressants or narcotics (e.g., methadone) necessary to relieve phantom pain. Antidepressants can cause drowsiness, and if amputees use narcotics

for their phantom pain they should consult their physician before continuing an exercise program.

Other Issues

Psychological Considerations

Disbelief is a common first psychological reaction to amputation, especially if the amputation was from trauma. Depression also is seen pre- or postamputation. Much like losing a friend or loved one, amputees go through a formal grieving process. This grieving process should be allowed to run its course, from denial to acceptance. Some amputees may have social fears concerning their future (e.g., employment and financial concerns), continued commitment and response to the amputation from spouse or loved ones, and concerns about body image. The amputee will need reassurance and understanding from family, friends, and all who are associated with their acute rehabilitation at the hospital. More importantly, the amputee will need his family and friends to understand and appreciate the need for lifestyle changes and the monetary and time commitment that accompanies these lifestyle changes (i.e., time and monthly fees of attending a health club).

Lower limb amputees who have made adjustments in their lives and have made lifestyle changes that have enabled them to function successfully in the community and in their professional endeavors are good role models for recent amputees. Social support groups also are available and can be beneficial.

Phantom Limb and Phantom Pain

Both phantom limb sensation and pain associated with the amputated limb are common postsurgery (31, 32). Phantom limb is a sensation in which the amputee feels as though the surgically removed limb is still there. The distal part of the extremity (e.g., the foot for a below-knee amputee) is the area most often felt, with sensations described as numbness, tingling, or pressure.

Phantom pain, on the other hand, is actual pain that feels as if it comes from the amputated limb. This must not be confused with postoperation surgical pain at the distal portion of the stump. Localized pain at the distal end of the stump can be caused by excessive pressure and friction from a nonconforming prosthesis, skin breakdown, or scar tissue. A thorough physical examination should be performed on the residual limb to ensure that the pain emanating from the limb is truly phantom in nature rather than from other local conditions.

Another way in which phantom pain differs from the pain emanating from the distal portion of the stump is that phantom pain appears to originate from the portion of the limb that was amputated. Burning, squeezing, and shooting pain sensations are the most common forms of phantom limb pain. Lower limb amputees are more likely to suffer phantom pain, or feel intensified phantom pain, on days when they have used the prosthesis for long periods of time (e.g., standing, walking, yard work). Aerobic exercises using non–weight-bearing exercise modes (e.g., Schwinn Air-Dyne, arm crank ergometry, swimming, rowing ergometry) should not cause or intensify phantom pain. If weight-bearing modes of exercise such as the StairMaster (Figure 15.8) or Body Trec (Figure 15.7) increase the incidence or intensity of phantom pain, substitution of non–weight-bearing modes of exercise is recommended.

Hygiene

The residual limb should be washed daily, especially following exercise, to prevent hair follicle infections. Thorough hygiene also involves keeping the inside lining of the prosthetic limb clean. Stump socks should be changed daily. Using the right size and number of stump socks also is important for the prevention of skin irritations and blisters. Stump socks should be changed whenever damp or wet.

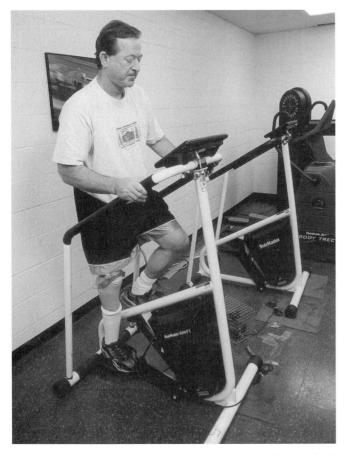

FIGURE 15.8. Stairmaster 4000 PT (Stairmaster Sports Medical Product)

What We Know
About Lower Limb Amputations

1 The main causes for LL amputation—type 2 diabetes and vascular disease—can be prevented by a healthy lifestyle that includes a wholesome diet, no cigarette smoking, and regular exercise.

2 Using the methods outlined in this chapter, a LL amputee can receive the same health benefits from exercise as a nonamputee.

What We Would Like to Know
About Lower Limb Amputations

1 What are the exact causes of phantom pain?

2 What are the best approaches to treatment of phantom pain?

Summary

Exercise training is designed to be rehabilitative for both dysvascular and nonvascular amputees. Exercise regimens are meant to improve muscle strength, endurance, and cardiovascular fitness to allow the amputee to perform a greater range of activities of daily living, to improve the possibility of gaining meaningful employment, or allow the LL amputee to return to his or her previous job.

In addition, exercise for vascular amputees is a secondary preventative treatment against the ongoing process of type 2 diabetes and peripheral vascular disease. For nonvascular amputees, exercise is a primary preventative treatment to reduce the risk of developing diabetes, cardiovascular disease, hypertension, and peripheral vascular disease.

DISCUSSION QUESTION

1 Distinguish between the pathophysiology of dysvascular and nonvascular LL amputees and, therefore, the different roles exercise plays in their lives.

2 Describe the two major lifestyle modifications that LL amputees must make and the effect these changes in lifestyles would have on a dysvascular and nonvascular LL amputee.

3 Why isn't walking recommended as a mode of exercise for LL amputees?

4 A 40-year-old nonvascular unilateral above-knee amputee who lost his leg in a motorcycle accident at the age of 20 wants to begin an exercise program. He has not exercised since his accident, he is 40 pounds overweight, and he does not smoke. What physical fitness and functional evaluations would you perform (cardiovascular, functional, and muscu-

lar), and how would you develop a program of exercise (cardiovascular and muscular) for him?

5 Describe the differences between phantom limb and phantom pain.

CASE STUDY

Patient Information
Preamputation

Herman is a 54-year-old man who lost his leg due to a traumatic amputation of his right foot and lower leg (i.e., unilateral below-knee) while on combat operations in Vietnam in November of 1970. At the time of the amputation, Herman was 24 years old. Throughout his childhood and early adolescence, Herman had played football, baseball, and basketball. He played 4 years of high school football and 3 years of college football. While in high school and college, he had engaged in a rigorous off-season physical training regimen consisting of 3 days of weight training (2 hours of power lifting per workout) and 3 days of running (2-mile run followed by sprint-type conditioning drills per workout) per week. Before going to Vietnam he spent 16 months of arduous infantry training at several military installations in the United States and the Panama Canal Zone. He served as a platoon leader in Vietnam, and his unit had been engaged in constant search-and-destroy missions for 4 months before his injury. Before entering active duty, he had not used tobacco in any manner. He began smoking cigarettes while on active duty and was smoking 1 to 2 packs of cigarettes a day at the time of his injury.

Postamputation

Herman spent 6 months of rehabilitation at an Army hospital in the United States, was fitted with a prosthesis, and returned to civilian life in the spring of 1971. From 1971 to 1982 he taught high school biology, science, and math courses and coached football and basketball. During this time he earned a Master's degree in biology. In 1982 he entered a doctoral program, and he received a Ph.D. in human physiology in 1986. From 1987 to the present time he has been a university professor. Following his return from Vietnam, between 1970 and 1975 he smoked an average of 2 packs a day; in 1975, he stopped smoking and has not smoked since.

From 1971 to 1980, Herman lifted weights two to three times per week (1.5 hours per session), and played half-court and full-court basketball twice weekly when not coaching. He was unable to perform these exercise activities while coaching, however, because of lower limb muscle fatigue and stump soreness and pain. His coaching duties involved 2 to 3 hours per coaching session or game, 4 to 5 times per week, for 5 months of the year.

In 1980, a swimming facility became available in his community, and he substituted swimming for all other noncoaching exercise activities at a frequency of 4 to 6 times per week, for 30 to 60 minutes per session. He was able to continue his swimming routine while coaching because it did not involve his lower extremities.

In 1982 he entered a doctoral program in a location where distance to a swimming facility and time constraints made swimming prohibitive. However, the university where he matriculated had a weight room and stationary bicycle ergometers available on campus. He performed bicycle ergometry 3 to 5 times per week, 30 to 40 minutes per session, and lifted weights (all upper body, see Table 15.3) 3 to 5 times per week, for 25 minutes per session. In 1983 the university purchased a Schwinn Air-Dyne ergometer, and he substituted Schwinn Air-Dyne ergometry for bicycle ergometry. From 1983 to 1992, he coached youth football, soccer, basketball, and baseball.

Medical History

Herman has a family history of heart disease. His maternal grandmother and paternal grandfather died of heart attacks at the age of 54 and 56, respectively. His father survived a heart attack at the age of 54 and suffered a stroke at the age of 64. His mother was diagnosed with congestive cardiomyopathy at the age of 57.

Herman was diagnosed with hypertension (resting blood pressure: 160/110 mm Hg) and hypercholesterolemia (total cholesterol, 270 mg/dl; high-density lipoprotein [HDL], 73 mg/dl; low-density lipoprotein [LDL], 190 mg/dl; triglycerides, 120 mg/dl) at the age of 44. The combination of hypertensive medication and an increase in exercise volume (he currently averages a frequency of 4×2 to 6×2 hours of aerobic exercise per week) has controlled his hypertension: currently, his resting blood pressure is 130/85 mm Hg. He did not choose to take medication for his hypercholesterolemia, and felt he could control it with exercise and diet. His current blood cholesterol is as follows: total cholesterol, 250 mg/dl; HDL, 75 mg/dl; LDL, 170 mg/dl; triglycerides, 110 mg/dl).

Questions

1. Would Herman's few years of smoking have a lasting effect on his risks for cardiovascular diseases, lung cancer, emphysema, and bronchitis or bronchiolitis?

2. Given his history of a high level of physical activity and healthy diet throughout his life, why would he suffer from hypertension and hypercholesterolemia?

3. Why did he opt *not* to take medication to lower his blood cholesterol?

REFERENCES

1. Torres MM. Incidence and causes of limb amputations. Phys Med Rehab: State of the Art Rev 1994;8:1–8.

2. U.S. Department of Health and Human Services. Vital and Health Statistics: Detailed Diagnosis and Procedures for Patients Discharged from Short-Stay Hospitals, United States, Series 1994;13(118):130.

3. Pitetti KH. Lower extremity amputees and physical fitness. American Association of Cardiovascular Pulmonary Rehabilitation Annual Meeting Syllabus, 1998:536–540.

4. Mayfield JA, Reiber GE, Maynard C, et al. Trends in lower limb amputation in the Veterans Health Administration, 1989–1999. J Rehabil Res Dev 2000;37(1):32–53.

5. Kald A, Carlson R, Nilsson E. Major amputation in a defined population: incidence, mortality and results of treatment. Br J Surg 1989;76:308–310.

6. Bodily K, Burgess E. Contralateral limb and patient survival after leg amputation. Am J Surg 1983;146:280–287.

7. Hrubec Z, Ryder RA. Traumatic limb amputations and subsequent mortality from cardiovascular disease and other causes. J Chron Dis 1978;33:239–250.

8. Rose HC, Schweitzer P, Charoenkul V, Schwartz E. Cardiovascular disease risk factors in combat veterans after traumatic leg amputation. Arch Phys Med Rehabil 1987;68:20–23.

9. Pitetti KH, Manske RC. Amputation. In: ACSM's Resource Manual for Guidelines for Exercise Testing and Prescription. 3rd Ed. Baltimore: Lippincott Williams & Wilkins, (in press).

10. Roth EJ, Park KL, Sullivan WJ. Cardiovascular disease in patients with dysvascular amputation. Arch Phys Med Rehabil 1000;79:205–215.

11. U.S Department of Health and Human Resources. Physical Activity and Health: A Report of the Surgeon General. Atlanta: U.S. Department of Health and Human Services, Centers for Disease Control and Prevention, National Center for Chronic Disease Prevention and Health Promotion, 1996.

12. Booth FW, Gordon SE, Carlson CJ, Hamilton MT. Waging war on modern chronic disease: primary prevention through exercise biology. J Appl Physiol 2000;88:774–787.

13. Owen N, Leslie E, Salmon J, Fotheringham MJ. Environmental determinants of physical activity and sedentary behavior. Exerc Sport Sci Rev 2000;22:153–158.

14. Huang C-T, Jackson JR, Moore NB, et al. Amputation energy cost of ambulation. Arch Phys Med Rehabil 1979;60:18–24.

15. Ganguli W, Datta SR, Chatterjee BB, Roy BN. Performance evaluation of an amputee prosthetic system in below-knee amputees. Ergo 1973;16:797–810.

16. Pagliarulo MA, Waters R, Hislop HS. Energy cost of walking of below-knee amputees having no vascular disease. Phys Ther 1979;59:538–542.

17. Waters RL, Perry J, Antonelli D, Hislop H. Energy cost of walking of amputees: the influence of level of amputation. J Bone Joint Surg Am 1976;58:42–52.

18. Ward KH, Meyers MC. Exercise performance of lower-extremity amputees. Sport Med 1995;20:207–214.

19. Crouse SF, Lessard CS, Rhodes J, Lowe RC. Oxygen consumption and cardiac response of short-leg and long-leg prosthetic ambulation in a patient with bilateral above-knee amputation: Comparison with able-bodied men. Arch Phys Med Rehabil 1990;71:313–317.

20. American College of Sport Medicine. ACSM's Guidelines for Exercise Testing and Prescription. 6th Ed. Philadelphia: Lea & Febiger, 2000.

21. American College of Sports Medicine. ACSM's Exercise Management for Persons with Chronic Diseases and Disabilities. Champaign, IL: Human Kinetics, 1997:94–100.

22. Huang C-T, Jackson JR, Moore NB, et al. Amputation energy cost of ambulation. Arch Phys Med Rehabil 1979;60:18–24.

23. Pitetti KH, Snell PG, Stray-Gundersen. Maximal response of wheelchair-confined subjects to four types of arm exercise. Arch Phys Med Rehabil 1987;68:10–13.

24. James U. Effect of physical training in healthy male unilateral above-knee amputees. Scand J Rehabil Med Rehabil 1973;5:88–101.

25. Corbin C. Flexibility. Clin Sports Med 1984;3:101–117.
26. Gailey RS, Gailey AM. Stretching and strengthening for lower extremity amputees. Miami, FL: Advanced Rehabilitation Therapy, Inc, 1994.
27. Gailey RS, Gailey AM. Balance, agility, coordination and endurance for lower extremity amputees. Miami, FL: Advanced Rehabilitation Therapy, Inc., 1994.
28. Burgess EM, Rappoport A. Physical Fitness: A Guide for Individuals With Lower Limb Loss. Washington, DC: Department of Veterans Affairs, 1990.
29. ACSM's Resource Manual for Guidelines for Exercise Testing and Prescription. Philadelphia: Lea & Febiger, 1988.
30. Franklin BA. Exercise testing, training and arm ergometry. Sports Med 1985;2:100–119.
31. Wartan SW, Hamann W, Wedley JR, McColl I. Phantom pain and sensation among British veteran amputees. Br J Anaesth 1997;78:652–659.
32. Schmid HJ. Phantom limb after amputation: overview and new knowledge. Schweiz Rundsch Med Prax 2000;89:87–94.
33. Ebert RV. Abstinence from cigarette smoking and pulmonary disease. JAMA 1978;240:2159–2161.
34. Mannond EC. Smoking in relation to the death rates of one million men and women. In: Haensxel W (ed). Epidemiological Approaches to the Study of Cancer and Other Diseases. National Cancer Institute Monograph 19. Bethesda: NIH, 1966, pp 127–204.

SUGGESTED READING

Pitetti KH, Snell PG, Stray-Gunderson J, Gottschalk FA. Aerobic training exercise for individuals who had amputations of the lower limb. J Bone Joint Surg Am 1987;69:914–921.

CHAPTER 16

Multiple Sclerosis

Janet A. Mulcare, Kurt Jackson

Overview

Multiple sclerosis (MS) is a **chronic**, often disabling, disease, characterized by a destruction of the myelin sheath (i.e., **demyelination**) that surrounds the nerve fibers of the **central nervous system (CNS)**. **Lesions** representing areas of inflammatory demyelination can be present in any part of the brain and spinal cord. For a definite diagnosis to be established, two or more areas of demyelination must be de-tected. This usually is accomplished through a careful clinical history. **Magnetic resonance imaging (MRI)** and analysis of **cerebrospinal fluid (CSF)** for oligoclonal bands are used to support the diagnosis. Evoked potentials of the visual systems (**visual evoked potential [VEP]**), the brain stem (**brain stem-auditory evoked potential [BAEP]**), or **somatosensory** (**somatosensory evoked potential [SSEP]**) systems often are obtained to evaluate neurologic function in other systems. These types of clinical tests are extremely important in the diagnosis of MS because they can confirm the presence of a suspected lesion (demyelination) or identify the presence of an unsuspected lesion that has produced no symptoms.

Worldwide, MS occurs at a higher frequency in latitudes further from the equator (40°) than those closer to the equator. In the United States, the MS prevalence rate below the 37th parallel is 57 to 78 cases per 100,000, whereas the prevalence rate above the 37th parallel is 140 cases per 100,000 (1). Estimates from the National Multiple Sclerosis Society indicate there are between 250,000 and 350,000 people in the U.S. with MS (2).

Etiology

The **etiology** of MS is not known; however, much of the scientific research indicates that a combination of factors may be involved. The major scientific theories regarding the etiology of MS are based on immunologic, environmental, viral, and genetic factors.

Immunologic

It is generally accepted that MS involves an **autoimmune** process directed against myelin in the central nervous system, but the exact antigen that the immune cells are sensitized to attack is not known. An in-depth discussion of the immunopathological features of MS is beyond the scope of this chapter; however, comprehensive information on this topic is available from other sources (3).

Environmental

Epidemiologic studies have shown that people who are born in a geographic area with a high risk for MS and move to an area with lower risk acquire the risk of their new home, if the move occurs prior to adolescence (4). Such data suggest that exposure to some environmental agent encountered before puberty may predispose a person to develop MS later in life.

Viral

During childhood most individuals are exposed to a variety of viruses. Because some viruses are known to cause demyelination and inflammation, it has long been hypothesized that a viral infection may be the triggering factor for MS. More than a dozen viruses have been studied, including measles, canine distemper, and herpesvirus (HHV-6) to determine their possible involvement in the development of MS. It has not yet been definitively proven that any one virus triggers MS (5).

Genetic

Although MS itself is not hereditary, siblings of an affected individual are at much higher risk for the disease (6). The importance of genetic factors in accounting for the increased risk has been confirmed by the results of twin and adoption studies. Some neurologists have theorized that MS develops because a person is born with a genetic predisposition to react to an environmental agent that triggers an autoimmune response upon exposure.

Types of Multiple Sclerosis

Each case of MS displays one of several different patterns. Multiple sclerosis is characterized by great variability. It can be divided into asymptomatic (subclinical or pathologic disease) and symptomatic disease. Experts now agree that there are four major clinical subtypes based on disease pattern: relapsing, of which a benign or mild form is seen in 10% to 20% of patients; primary progressive; secondary progressive; and progressive relapsing (7). The course and distribution (%) of each clinical subtype are presented in Figure 16.1.

Relapsing (R) MS is the most common type and is characterized by a series of attacks, each followed by complete or partial remission as **symptoms** mysteriously lessen, only to return later after a period of stability (Figure 16.1A). Among this group are a minority of patients who will have minimal disease activity and little to no disability 25 years into their course. These patients have benign or mild MS, and make up 10% to 20% of symptomatic MS patients (8). **Primary-progressive** (PP) MS is characterized by a gradual clinical decline with no distinct remissions, although there may be temporary plateau or minor relief from the symptoms (Figure 16.1B). **Secondary progressive** (SP) MS begins with a relapsing-remitting course followed by a later primary-progressive subtype 5 to 15 years into the disease course (Figure 16.1C). Rarely, patients may have a **progressive-relapsing** (PR) course in which the disease takes a progressive path punctuated by **acute** attacks (Figure 16.1D). Multiple sclerosis is very rarely fatal, and most people with MS have a fairly normal life expectancy.

Initial Symptoms of Multiple Sclerosis

The most frequent initial symptom of MS is an acute or subacute onset of numbness or tingling in one or more limbs. The symptoms usually begin distally in the limbs and expand proximally. Occasionally the symptoms will migrate from one side to the other, a feature that is believed to represent the transverse expansion of lesions in the spinal cord (9). In some patients, a paroxysmal sensory symptom in the back or lower limbs brought on by flexing the head forward

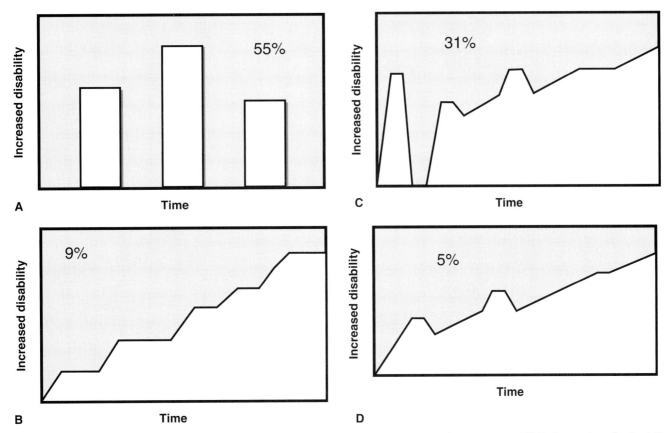

FIGURE 16.1. A. Relapsing-remitting multiple sclerosis (MS). B. Primary progressive MS. C. Secondary progressive MS. D. Progressive relapsing MS. (Adapted from Coyle P [8].)

(**Lhermitte's symptom**) may precede the persistent sensory symptoms or may occur in isolation (9). Symptoms that are less likely to appear initially but are common as the disease progresses are bladder dysfunction, heat intolerance, pain, movement disorders, higher cortical function disorders, and dementia. A summary of the most common symptoms seen at the onset of MS has been derived from a study of 1721 patients in the United Kingdom with clinically definite MS (10) (Table 16.1).

Symptoms of MS

Most individuals with MS experience symptoms that are related to demyelination within the brain and spinal cord, often referred to as "primary symptoms" (11). These can include muscle weakness in the extremities, clumsiness, numbness and tingling, bowel and bladder dysfunction, sexual dysfunction, and visual symptoms. Complications that result from these symptoms often are referred to as "secondary symptoms"; these may include joint contractures, urinary tract infection, osteoporosis, muscle atrophy, and skin breakdown (11). **Spasticity**, the involuntary increased tone in muscles, also is common and can lead to joint stiffness and spasms.

Fatigue is the most common symptom of MS (Box 16.1). Overall, 75% to 90% of persons with MS report having some form of fatigue, with 50% to 60% reporting fatigue as the worst symptom of their disease (12–14). Several studies have shown that fatigue is more common in persons whose disease is progressive in nature (12). It has been proposed that multiple factors probably are involved in the origin of fatigue as experienced by the individual with MS. Electrophysiologic studies have proposed "twitch decline" (15), a decline in central motor drive, and a drop in muscle torque during sustained contraction (16). Abnormalities in periph-

TABLE 16.1. SYMPTOMS COMMON AT ONSET OF MULTIPLE SCLEROSIS

Symptoms	%
Sensory symptoms (arms/legs)	33
Unilateral visual loss	16
Slowly progressive motor deficits	9
Acute motor deficits	5
Diplopia	7
Polysymptomatic onset	14
Others	16

Data from Paty DW (10).

BOX 16.1. Fatigue

Fatigue is the most common and debilitating symptom associated with MS. More than 75% of people with MS report fatigue, and 60% cite it as the worst symptom of their disease (2). Much research has focused on trying to identify the source of fatigue (e.g., central or peripheral), but there have been no conclusive findings. Recent research looking at central mechanisms of fatigue used positron-emission tomography (PET) scanning. Findings revealed a potential association between focal brain dysfunction and fatigue in MS. This study found decreased glucose utilization in the frontal lobes and basal ganglia in patients with MS who were experiencing fatigue. These findings are promising, but their interpretation is limited, and further prospective-type intervention studies are required to truly understand the relationship of this phenomenon to MS fatigue. Research on peripheral muscle metabolism reported a "blunting" of phosphocreatine resynthesis and slower adenosine diphosphate recovery following exercise in MS, which is indicative of impaired oxidative capacity in the skeletal muscle (18). Impaired oxidative capacity may be the result of disuse or inactivity, which is common in this population.

Many common medications used by the average adult may contribute to fatigue in the person with MS, and clinicians should be aware of all the types of medications being taken by their clients. The following types of drugs can contribute to MS fatigue:

Analgesics	Anticonvulsants
Antihistamines	Antihypertensive agents
Antidepressants	Anti-inflammatories
Antipsychotics	Asthma drugs
Cardiac agents	Diabetic agents
Hormone replacement therapy	Carbonic anhydrase inhibitors
Gastrointestinal agents	Immune modulators
Muscle relaxants	Nicotinic agents

---

eral motor function also have been observed. Muscle fatigue has been associated with a decline in tetanic force, phosphocreatine, and intracellular pH in conjunction with intact neuromuscular transmission (17, 18). Still other factors related to neuroendocrine function and cerebral metabolism using positron emission tomography (PET) report a positive correlation between fatigue reported on the Kurtzke Functional Status Scale and cerebral glucose availability (19). Secondary complications of the disease also may be related to the fatigue and should be addressed in the management of this symptom. Excessive energy use during walking associated with muscle weakness, spasticity, and ataxia (20) may contribute to the overall feeling of fatigue. Deconditioning, medication side effects (21, 22), depression (Box 16.2) (23) and **nocturia** (24–26) are other secondary problems that may increase fatigue level in people with MS.

It is generally accepted that 45% to 65% of patients with MS have some cognitive **impairment** (27–29), but such impairments are rarely disabling. Changes in memory are common (30); intellectual and language abilities usually are spared (31–32).

Approximately 80% of people with MS report an adverse effect to heat, whether generated by outside, climatic changes, or internally (e.g., fever, thermogenesis, exercise) (33). In addition, in studies where subjects with MS have been overheated, 60% report signs not previously recognized. However, the elimination of the heat source usually reverses the symptoms. The mechanisms for this sensitivity to heat have been speculated and investigated for more than 100 years using human (34–39), animal (40), and mathematical (41) models. More contemporary research has introduced the element of activity (i.e., exercise) into the search for an answer to this question. Perturbations that include total body surface cooling (42–44), cooling prior to exercise (45), cooling during chronic exercise (46), as well has heating during exercise (47) have all been utilized, and the results are discussed later in this chapter. In spite of recent efforts to solve this mystery, a definitive answer to the origin of this symptom remains unknown. Variables that have been proposed to contribute to this phenomenon are the heat itself, effects of serum calcium, blockade of ion channels, circulatory changes, heat shock proteins, and unidentified humoral substance (33).

The myelinated pathways of the autonomic nervous system (ANS) lying within the brain and spinal cord may be involved in MS; however, the symptoms associated with the somatic nervous system caused by this disease often divert attention away from these disturbances. The ANS plays an important role in cardioacceleration, maintenance of blood pressure, cutaneous vasomotor function, and sudomotor function (48). Research indicates that abnormalities in heart rate and blood pressure occur during autonomic testing (49–51), isometric exercise (52), and incremental dynamic exercise (53, 54). Simple noninvasive tests often are used to document cardiovascular abnormalities that require limited equipment and training. Bannister (55) offers an in-

---

BOX 16.2. Depression and Fatigue

People with MS often experience depression, which can contribute to the perception of fatigue and lead to lack of interest in physical activity. Research focusing on subjects with MS has shown that depression can be reduced significantly by following a program of moderate exercise (15, 16), not unlike the general population.

Sleep disturbances also are common in persons with MS. These disturbances are characterized by increased sleep latency (time to fall asleep) as well as periods of apnea and restless limb movements. This secondary symptom of MS can contribute to the general daily fatigue experienced by these individuals. Although fatigue is a genuine concern for most persons, many individuals who regularly participate in exercise report a reduction in their overall level of fatigue and improved quality of life.

depth description of the underlying anatomy and physiology of each test with specific instructions for performing them and also provides normative values for comparison purposes.

More than 30 years ago Cartlidge (56) reported abnormal sudomotor responses in persons with MS when challenged using hot water immersion. More recently, sudomotor responses were examined during submaximal steady state exercise and found to be abnormal in 50% of the patients examined (47). Central and peripheral vasomotor function has been tested using a technique known as the 133-xenon washout method. Using a small sample of six patients with extreme thermoregulation disturbances Andersen and Nordenbo (57) demonstrated that vasoconstrictor responses in skeletal muscle and subcutaneous tissue remained intact. Other features of autonomic disturbances in MS include postural dizziness (51) and an increased dependence on anaerobic energy substrates in peripheral skeletal muscle (18). Bladder dysfunction may manifest as urgency of micturation or difficulty voiding, depending upon whether the origin is detrusor instability or detrusor-external sphincter dyssynergia, respectively. Bowel dysfunction may present as frequent diarrhea, but more often severe constipation is predominant (58). Many of the medications used in the management of MS symptoms may have side effects on ANS function (Box 16.3.) It is important that a complete history of medications be included prior to patient evaluation and exercise prescription for people with MS. Several of these medications and their side effects related to ANS function are listed in Table 16.2.

Team Approach to the Clinical Management of Multiple Sclerosis

Effective management of the numerous problems associated with MS requires the highly coordinated efforts of a multidisciplinary health care team. The team includes the following members:

- The *primary care provider* usually is involved in the identification of the initial symptoms and referral to a neurologist. He or she manages and coordinates most of the patient's day-to-day health care needs.
- The *neurologist* is involved primarily with testing, diagnosis, and monitoring of the disease as well as the management of symptoms through the use of various medications including immunotherapy.
- A *physiatrist* becomes an important member of the health care team if physical rehabilitation is required. In addition to providing input into various aspects of symptom management, the physiatrist is highly involved in addressing functional issues and management of the rehabilitation team.
- The *physical therapist* evaluates and treats neuromuscular and musculoskeletal impairments, functional

limitations, and disabilities through the use of interventions such as therapeutic exercise, functional training, patient education, and use of assistive and adaptive equipment.
- The *occupational therapist* addresses the patient's ability to perform self-care duties and activities of daily living using numerous interventions such as therapeutic exercise, instruction in energy conservation techniques, and the use of adaptive equipment. Occupational therapists also are involved in home and workplace assessment and modification.
- The *speech pathologist* evaluates and treats disorders that affect communication, swallowing, and cognitive function, all of which are common in MS.
- The *psychologist* works with the patient and family on the emotional and cognitive components of the disease by providing counseling and teaching coping skills.
- The *social worker* assists the client and family by identifying community resources such as support groups, potential income sources, and other benefits available to persons with disabilities. The social worker often complements the psychologist in dealing with the personal and family issues associated with a chronic illness.
- In addition to the disciplines mentioned above, other important health care providers can include a dietitian, rehabilitation nurse, vocational counselor, therapeutic recreation specialist, exercise physiologist, and chaplain or minister.

BOX 16.3. The Autonomic Nervous System and Cardiovascular Dysfunction

Autonomic nervous system (ANS) pathways contribute to central and peripheral cardiovascular adjustments in both heart rate and blood pressure with postural changes and during dynamic activity such as exercise. Research using quiescent as well as dynamic perturbations has reported the presence of abnormalities in heart rate (HR) and blood pressure (BP) responses in approximately 30% to 40% of the MS population. The presence of abnormal cardiovascular reflexes (ACR) in both HR and BP is extremely important when evaluating a patient's aerobic exercise capacity and prescribing workload intensities. For example, diminished cardioacceleration as a result of MS may give the mistaken impression that a patient is not exercising hard enough if HR is used as the index of intensity. These patients should be treated as if they are using a beta-blocker, and an alternate measure of exercise intensity (e.g., Borg Scale) should be used. Furthermore, published submaximal prediction equations based on HR or workload intensity should be used with caution if the patient has a diminished HR response. To determine whether a patient has ACR of either the sympathetic or parasympathetic pathway, several simple, noninvasive tests have been developed that require very little time and equipment (57, 58).

TABLE 16.2. FDA-APPROVED DRUGS FOR TREATMENT OF MULTIPLE SCLEROSIS

Drug	Date of FDA Approval	Dosing	Common Side Effects
Interferon beta-1a (Avonex; Biogen Inc.)	1996	Weekly; intra-muscular injection	Flulike symptoms following injection, which lessen over time Uncommon: mild anemia, elevated liver enzymes
Interferon beta-1b (Betaseron; Berlex Laboratories, Inc.)	1993	Every other day; subcutaneous injection	Flulike symptoms following injection, which lessen over time. Injection site reactions Uncommon: elevated liver enzymes, low white blood cell counts
Glatiramer acetate (Copaxone; Teva Pharmaceutical Industries Ltd.)	1996	Daily; subcutaneous injection	Injection site reactions Uncommon: a reaction immediately after injection, which includes anxiety, chest tightness, shortness of breath, and flushing
Mitoxantrone	2000	Monthly or bimonthly; intravenous	Hemorrhagic cystitis, nausea, vomiting, alopecia, infertility

Medications Used by Patients with MS

Five drugs have been recently approved to safely and effectively modify the course of MS. This is an important milestone for the treatment of MS because up until this point, medications were prescribed to address specific symptoms rather than the disease itself. Interferon beta-1a (Avonex, Rebif) has been effective in reducing the number and severity of **exacerbations** in persons with relapsing-remitting MS. These drugs also have shown promise in slowing the course of the disease in persons with secondary progressive MS (59). Glatiramer acetate (Copaxone) has been shown to be equally effective in the modulation of exacerbations and progression, with fewer reported side effects (60, 61). Glatiramer acetate also has been shown to have sustained efficacy over a 5-year period, reducing the accumulation of disability and relapse rate in patients with relapsing forms of MS (62). A summary of these drugs is presented in Table 16.3.

Most of the other medications that are commonly used with MS are directed at treating symptoms (see Table 16.2).

Based on the mechanism of action of these drugs, special considerations have been suggested related to the use of this drug and how it might affect an MS patient's ability to perform exercise.

Alternative and Complementary Therapy

Various studies of **complementary alternative medicine** (CAM) indicate that between 30% and 67% of persons with MS use some form of alternative medicine (73) in conjunction with conventional medicine. This is termed *complementary* alternative medicine because it is used in conjunction with traditional medicine, not as a replacement. Complementary and alternative medicines that are commonly used by persons with MS are placed in the following categories by the National Center for Complementary and Alternative Therapy (74): (1) specific practices; (2) life-enhancement therapies; (3) ingested or injected substances; (4) toxic removal therapy; (5) special diets; and (6) other therapies (Table 16.4). Unfortunately, there is no scientific evidence to support most of the claims associated with these therapies. Furthermore, there are fundamental risks

TABLE 16.3. MEDICATIONS COMMONLY USED TO TREAT SYMPTOMS RELATED TO MULTIPLE SCLEROSIS

Medication	Symptom	Special Considerations
Amantadine HCl	Fatigue	May cause dizziness, peripheral vasodilation, and orthostatic hypotension
Baclofen	Spasticity	High dosage may cause tachycardia, constipation, bladder dysfunction, muscle weakness, and fatigue
Tricyclic antidepressants	Depression	May cause tremor, dizziness, lightheadedness, hypotension, tachycardia, constipation, bladder dysfunction, and abnormal gait
Prednisone	Acute exacerbation	May cause muscle weakness, loss of muscle mass, hypertension, and osteoporosis (osteoporosis may result from chronic use)
Modafinil	Fatigue (off-label)	May interact with other drugs commonly used by MS patients. Side effects include anxiety, headache, nausea, nervousness, and insomnia
Selective serotonin reuptake inhibitors	Neuropsychological symptoms	May cause hypotension or tachycardia

Data from references 63–72.

TABLE 16.4. COMPLEMENTARY ALTERNATIVE THERAPIES USED BY MULTIPLE SCLEROSIS PATIENTS

Specific Practice
Traditional Chinese medicine
   Acupuncture
   Qigong
Ayurveda
Chiropractic medicine
Homeopathy
Naturopathy

Life-Enhancement Therapies
Yoga
Massage therapy
Tai chi
Reiki
Feldenkrais
Therapeutic touch

Ingested or Injected Substances
St. John's wort
Evening primrose oil
Ginseng
Ginkgo biloba
Melatonin
Pycnogenol
Dehydroepiandrosterone (DHEA)
Beesting therapy

Ingested or Injected Substances (continued)
Noni juice
Herbal energy enhancers
   5-hydroxytripotophane
   Citrus aurantium
   Ephedra
   Guarana
Vitamins
Echinacea and astragalus
Estrogen/progesterone
Procarin

Toxic Removal Therapy
Chelation therapy
Dental amalgam removal

Special Diets
Swank low-fat diet
Aspartame-free diet
Gluten-free diet
MacDougall diet

Other
Cooling
Electromagnetic therapies
Hyperbaric oxygen

Adapted from Bowling AC et al. (75)

in using many of these products without medical supervision, risks that often are not recognized by the patient.

Exercise Response in Persons with Multiple Sclerosis

Measuring Maximal Aerobic Power

Establishing a baseline aerobic fitness level for the patient with MS can help provide a basis for developing goals for a program of regular exercise, as well as for increasing physical activity in general. Depending on the level and nature of the patient's physical impairment, adjustments may be necessary in selecting a mode of testing and training that is both effective and safe. The value most often described from research as a maximal effort in MS patients has been VO_{2peak} (mL/kg/min), rather than VO_{2max}. These values should be construed as the same. Current recommendations by the American College of Sports Medicine (ACSM) support use of bicycle ergometry as the "mode of choice" for evaluating aerobic fitness in this population (76). Peripheral leg fatigue can preempt a true maximal effort when using a bicycle ergometer in the untrained subject; however, most research has also reported corresponding heart rate (HR) maximums that vary between 90% and 96% of the expected age-related maximum, so reporting VO_{2peak} as a substitute for VO_{2max} for pa-

tients with MS is reasonable. Consequently, in the absence of expensive metabolic equipment, an inexpensive HR monitor is sufficient for estimating a maximal effort based on the attainment of at least 90% of age-predicted maximal HR.

Some clinicians may feel uncomfortable stressing the MS patient to such a level and wonder whether submaximal HR can be used with existing prediction equations. Limited research has shown that the use of existing regression models (e.g., the Astrand-Rhyming nomogram) for predicting VO_{2peak} from submaximal values can result in an error greater than 15% (77). One reason for the error may be related to a blunting of the HR response during submaximal exercise that occurs in some patients with MS (54).

Mode of Testing

Most research literature, similar to ACSM recommendations, reports using the bicycle ergometer (e.g., Schwinn Air-Dyne, Monark) as the "mode of choice" for testing (42–45, 54, 78, 79). This choice often has been made out of necessity to standardize a protocol that could accommodate a variety of disability levels but also to reduce the risk of injury. Treadmill walking is acceptable if the patient can perform it safely. Some of the MS-related symptoms that have a direct bearing on the choice of ergometry and special modifications are presented in Table 16.5.

Test Protocol

No single protocol best suits every patient with MS. The choice of continuous vs. discontinuous exercise, intensity of workload, and length of time for each stage differs from patient to patient. Subjective reports from some MS patients show preference for the abbreviated, continuous test; however, providing brief rest periods between progressively more difficult workloads as in the discontinuous-type test may provide psychological benefit to the patient. Research has shown that both continuous and discontinuous methods should elicit similar endpoints.

Beginning the exercise test with an initial stage of "no resistance" pedaling is helpful as a warm-up period and to acquaint the patient with the exercise. A cadence of 50 to 60 RPM is appropriate; individuals with lower extremity spasticity may have difficulty pedaling without resistance, however, because this type of movement often elicits ankle **clonus.** Use of toe clips and heel straps will prevent the foot from slipping off the pedal in this situation, and the addition of resistance in subsequent stages should eliminate the clonus response.

When designing an exercise protocol, one should consider the subject's gender, size, and level of neurologic impairment. For most applications the stages should last from 3 to 5 minutes. This usually is enough time to reach a "steady state" response for the particular workload. Increments for each stage will vary depending on the individual's level of impairment. Most research on patients with MS has reported using increments of 12 to 15 watts. However, for a larger person who is minimally disabled, the workloads may need to be adjusted upward (e.g., 25-watt increments) to prevent the test from becoming overly protracted. Research has shown that people who exhibit more neurologic impairment are capable of lower maximal work intensity and experience less benefit from training (45).

The Borg CR10 is a useful index for tracking the level of physiologic stress experienced during a test of maximal aerobic power (80). This index provides a means for tracking absolute intensity of physiologic response as well as perceptions of exertion that can be related to other factors such as local muscle pain, difficulty breathing, or chest pain. Using an earlier version of the CR10 it was found that most patients with MS rated local leg pain and fatigue (i.e., peripheral category) higher than other sources (i.e., heart rate and breathing) during both submaximal and maximal exercise. It must be noted that the presence of subtle cognitive impairment in some persons with MS may make it difficult to use this scale. Careful explanation and confirmation of understanding before testing is recommended when using the Borg Scale.

Exercise Programming Options

Endurance Training Program

The primary goal of endurance training in patients with MS is the same as that in the general, nondisabled populations—that is, to improve cardiovascular function. Activities such as stationary cycling, walking, and low-impact, chair, or water aerobics are all possible choices depending on personal interest and the level and nature of physical impairment (Table 16.5). For example, a patient with impaired balance or proprioceptive deficits may find that either the buoyancy offered in water aerobics or the stability of an increased base of support in chair aerobics is more accommodating than trying to maintain balance while performing standard low-impact aerobics. Walking in a climate-controlled area such as an indoor track or a mall provides stable temperatures, a level surface, and the opportunity to rest when needed. Stationary cycling is a more appropriate option for the nonambulatory MS patient, offering a controlled environment and standardized workloads. These options should be discussed with the patient when selecting a mode of exercise.

The intensity level of the exercise can be monitored by manually palpating a radial pulse. Several inexpensive telemetry-type monitors are available and occasionally are included with various models of exercise equipment. Exercise HR should be maintained at 60% to 75% of age-predicted maximal HR for most patients, but more severely impaired or elderly individuals may need to be limited to

TABLE 16.5. CHOOSING A MODE OF ERGOMETRY FOR EXERCISE TESTING AND TRAINING

Symptom	Special Consideration
Spasticity	May cause ankle **clonus,** which makes foot stability during cycling difficult.
	Agonist/antagonist cocontraction may impair treadmill walking, appear as muscle weakness of the agonist group.
	Hip adductor and abductor spasticity could interfere with bicycle ergometry.
Incoordination	Combined arm/leg ergometers that are not mechanically synchronized may be difficult to coordinate.
Ataxia	May make treadmill walking difficult without handrail support.
Sensory	Lower extremity sensory or proprioceptive deficits could make treadmill walking difficult.
Muscle weakness	Lower extremity muscle weakness may limit workload increments using a bicycle ergometer.
Foot drop	Weakness in the tibialis anterior muscle group is common and result in "foot drop" as fatigue ensues following continuous walking. If not corrected with an ankle foot orthotic, treadmill walking could be dangerous.
Visual disturbances	Central scotoma and loss of peripheral vision may necessitate modifications during treadmill walking and use of handrails.

between 50% and 65% of age-predicted HR_{max} until they have reached a higher level of fitness.

Ideally, people with MS should try to incorporate some form of moderate physical activity into each day as recommended by the Surgeon General and the Centers for Disease Control and Prevention (81). However, a more realistic and achievable goal for structured exercise is three times per week for a minimum of 30 minutes. The 30 minutes can be divided into three 10-minute or two 15-minute sessions, which is a valuable option for the person with a very low initial fitness level or low resistance to fatigue. The days on which formal exercise is not performed may be reserved for completion of household or leisure activities, tasks that place a fairly high demand on most physically impaired individuals.

When developing an exercise training program for persons with MS, two other important issues that must be addressed are heat sensitivity and hydration.

Heat Sensitivity

There is ample research documenting heat sensitivity in most persons with MS. The exact mechanism of how either external (i.e., environmental) or internal (i.e., metabolic) heat affects these individuals is unknown. It has been reported that as much as 50% of the general MS population may have abnormal or absent sweating, which may contribute to the perception of overheating as capillary skin blood flow increases to dissipate heat generated during exercise.

The use of fans, wet neck wraps, and spray bottles may help reduce the perception of overheating, but does not actually lower core temperature. Surface cooling via water immersion (16–17°C) before exercise (i.e., pre-cooling) has been shown to reduce core temperature significantly, as well as improve aerobic endurance and reduce submaximal exercise HR and perceived level of exertion (45). In addition, the reduction in core temperature that occurs immediately following cooling has been shown to persist for several hours and is associated with significantly less perceived fatigue. Furthermore, this strategy, coupled with exercising early in the day to take advantage of the lower circadian body temperature, might pose less physiologic and psychological stress. Subjective reports from many individuals with MS indicate there is a general decline in energy level during the afternoon hours, with the occurrence of fatigue and other MS-related symptoms. Most individuals in general reach at their highest circadian temperature (i.e., core temperature) in the later afternoon hours.

Hydration

Many people with MS experience symptoms that affect bladder function. These patients may severely limit their daily intake of fluids because of problems with bladder ur-

gency and exertional incontinence. This can result in chronic dehydration and may contribute to the general fatigue experienced by some individuals. Recommendations for proper hydration prior to exercise and rehydration following should be addressed when working with patients with MS (82).

Strength Training (Box 16.4)

Weakness is one of the most common manifestations of MS and often is reported as an initial symptom. It has been estimated that at least half of persons with MS experience muscle weakness and motor fatigue (83). Weakness can have a profound impact on an individual's functional independence. Basic activities such as walking, rising from a chair, and climbing stairs can become difficult over time because residual weakness often increases following repeated exacerbations. Although strengthening will not alter the disease process itself, compensatory strengthening of unin-

---

BOX 16.4. Strength Training Recommendations

- Optimize strength in unaffected muscle groups to allow for effective compensation and stabilization.
- When possible, make exercises functional (e.g., partial squats for working quadriceps as opposed to seated knee extensions).
- Allow 1 to 5 minutes of rest time between exercises, especially when working weaker muscle groups.
- Educate the patient regarding the difference between the temporary fatigue and discomfort associated with exercise and profound fatigue or pain.
- Emphasize larger proximal muscle groups. Distal muscle groups can be worked if time and fatigue levels allow.
- Allow for adequate warm-up before strength training: 5–10 minutes on a stationary bicycle or treadmill followed by stretching of appropriate muscle groups
- Increase the intensity and duration of training slowly but steadily.
- During exacerbations of symptoms focus on stretching and gentle active range of motion rather than strengthening.
- Use weight machines for patients with poor balance and coordination because they allow for more controlled movement and postural stability.
- Emphasis should be placed on slow, smooth, controlled movement to prevent interference of spasticity and ataxia.
- When instructing a patient in a home exercise program, give clear written instructions because short-term memory impairment is common.
- Set realistic goals and expectations with the patient. Emphasize the general wellness aspects of strength training as opposed to absolute increases in strength.

volved muscle groups and prevention of weakness secondary to disuse may improve function.

Before a training program is initiated, it is important to evaluate the patient's baseline strength levels for proper exercise prescription. This evaluation can be done using traditional manual muscle testing, an estimated one-repetition maximum, **isokinetic dynamometry**, or a functional strength assessment. Special modifications to testing procedures may be necessary when an individual presents with significant spasticity or **contracture**. These adaptations should be documented so that follow-up testing can be performed the same way. When testing, it is often useful to perform several repetitions to assess muscular endurance, because strength often can appear normal during the initial test but quickly deteriorate after just a few repetitions. Functional strength testing often provides the most useful information about a person's ability to accomplish various **activities of daily living** (ADLs). For example, sit-to-stand performance has been shown to correlate well with isokinetic measures of lower extremity strength, walking speed, and balance (84, 85). This can be assessed by asking the individual to perform activities such as rising from a chair multiple times, ascending and descending stairs, and repeatedly lifting an object of a given weight onto a shelf.

Following a careful assessment, an individualized resistance training program can be developed. Unfortunately, there is very little research to guide us in this process as it relates to individuals with MS. A pilot study by Kraft et al. (86) investigated the effects of a 3-month, 3 days per week strength training program in persons with mild and severe MS. During the study subjects performed three sets of 10 repetitions of each exercise with 60 seconds of rest between exercises. Following training, subjects demonstrated significant improvements in strength, walking velocity, and stair-climbing ability, with the mildly affected group showing the greatest improvement. In addition, no MS-related exacerbations were reported during the training. In general, it appears that strength training of major muscle groups performed 2 or 3 nonconsecutive days per week using 1 to 3 sets of 10 to 15 repetitions appears relatively safe and effective.

Flexibility

Maintenance of adequate range of motion (ROM) and flexibility is critical to preserving functional mobility in persons with MS. Some persons with MS are at a high risk for contracture formation due to limited mobility and the presence of spasticity. For this reason aggressive flexibility and ROM exercises should be an essential component of any comprehensive fitness program. There has been little research on the effects of stretching in persons with MS, but a study by Brar and associates (87) demonstrated that regular stretching might enhance the effects of Baclofen in the management of spasticity.

The muscle groups most prone to developing tightness and contracture include the iliopsoas, hamstrings, gastrocnemius, and pectoralis major and minor (Table 16.6). These muscle groups are predominantly affected when a person spends prolonged periods of time in a seated position or lying in bed with the head elevated and pillows propped under the knees.

Although the literature provides limited guidelines regarding stretching parameters, it is generally accepted that flexibility exercises should be performed once or twice per day depending on the patient's level of activity and degree of spasticity. Most stretches are held for a period of 30 to 60 seconds and repeated three to five times. Persons with severe spasticity or contracture may require stretching of much longer duration. In these cases, low-load, prolonged stretches of 20 minutes to several hours using dynamic splints or weights may be needed to induce plastic deformation of connective tissue. Use of modalities such as heat and ice may be indicated in certain cases to increase the effectiveness of the stretch.

TABLE 16.6.   MUSCLE GROUPS THAT MAY DEVELOP TIGHTNESS AND CONTRACTURE IN PERSONS WITH MULTIPLE SCLEROSIS

Muscle Group	Motion Restricted	Functional Limitations
Iliopsoas	Hip extension	Inability to achieve trailing limb posture during walking, which shortens stride length and increases energy expenditure. Can cause forward trunk lean, affecting posture and balance.
Hamstrings	Knee extension when hip is flexed	Limits step length during walking, causes difficulty when bending over to dress, pick up objects off floor, or perform household activities such as loading laundry.
Gastrocnemius	Ankle dorsiflexion, especially with knee extended	Limits gait if less than 10 degrees of dorsiflexion. Difficulty with sit-to-stand transfers. Decreased ability to use ankle strategy for balance
Anterior trunk: pectoral, intercostal, rectus abdominis muscles	Trunk extension, rib elevation, shoulder flexion, external rotation	Inability to achieve erect posture. Reduced pulmonary function. Difficulty with dressing and grooming

Balance

Abnormalities in balance and vestibular function have long been recognized as common manifestations of MS. Despite the high incidence of balance impairment and its potential negative impact on functional ability, little attention has been directed toward improving balance through training for this population. Case reports on small samples have shown variable results from training on a computerized balance system for 12 weeks under clinical supervision (88). These findings are somewhat encouraging, but are hardly practical given the current health care environment and lack of availability of such specialized training equipment. Recently, Jackson completed a study based on a home-based exercise model in 13 subjects with MS (89). Overall, there was an average improvement of 12% on the Berg Balance Scale, as well as improvements on various static and dynamic computerized balance assessments between 6% and 33%.

Balance Testing

Although there is currently no universally accepted method for training balance, recent research has led to a greater understanding of how balance is controlled (90). Most of this research supports a "systems" model of postural control in which balance emerges from a complex interaction among the individual, environment, and task. Individual factors affecting balance include a person's musculoskeletal and neurologic systems, as well as their level of motivation and cognition. Environmental conditions such as lighting, support surfaces, and visual distractions also can influence balance strategies. Additionally, the task itself (e.g., taking a leisurely walk vs. running to catch a cab) can impose a wide variety of task-specific postural demands. Principles of motor learning such as "transfer" and "specificity" of training also demonstrate the important relationship between individual, environment, and task. Unfortunately, most balance tests and interventions do not address these theoretical considerations adequately and consequently fail to imitate the various challenges to posture and balance routinely encountered in daily life (89).

Balance Training (Box 16.5)

Whipple (90) suggests that balance training should involve repeated exposures to diverse postural challenges that stimulate multiple sensory systems. Training programs also should involve a wide variety of goal-directed activities (e.g., reaching for an object, walking to the bathroom, picking up an object from the floor) performed under different environmental conditions. If these important theoretical concepts are not considered when designing a training program, limited improvement in functional balance ability will result.

BOX 16.5. Balance Training Considerations

A comprehensive balance training program should include a variety of tasks designed to challenge multiple components of the neurologic and musculoskeletal systems under diverse environmental conditions. As a learned skill, balance training should be performed on a regular basis. A regimen of three sessions per week lasting 20 to 25 minutes has been shown to result in favorable improvements (89–91). Furthermore, based on our current understanding of postural control and motor learning, it is recommended that a patient participate in as aggressive a program as can be safely tolerated. Ideally, such a program would include activities using both self-imposed and externally applied perturbations that destabilize the patient, causing a repeated loss of balance. Safety is the most important element in any type of program, of course, so in a home-based program, it may be necessary to sacrifice the level of challenge to ensure the patient's safety. Consequently, high-functioning individuals may benefit more from clinically based programs in which there is close supervision to prevent injuries and falls. One final consideration when developing a balance program is the time of day at which the training occurs. Research has shown that balance (or, rather, the perception of stability) can be affected by fatigue without a true loss in balance function (92). Because circadian variation in temperature appears to be associated with level of fatigue, it would be prudent to recommend that the patient perform these activities in the morning as opposed to the afternoon or evening. The afternoon may find the patient experiencing the fatigue that is associated with a higher core temperature, and evening fatigue may be related to the total energy expenditure over the course of the day.

Potential Physiologic Adaptations to Training

Very little research is available regarding the effects of training on muscle performance in persons with MS. However, from the research that has been reported, we can conclude that patients with MS have the capacity to improve muscle strength following a supervised program of aerobic exercise training (79) and an unsupervised program of free weights (94). Petajan and colleagues (79) reported a mean improvement of 17% in upper extremity isometric strength (sum of four different muscle groups) and an 11% improvement in lower extremity isometric strength (sum of five different muscle groups) in a group of 21 subjects with MS. Mulcare and coworkers (46) observed a 29% improvement in power output during leg cycling following 24 weeks of supervised aerobic exercise training.

A supervised program of aerobic exercise for as little as 15 weeks can improve aerobic fitness level (i.e., VO_{2max}) in some persons with MS. Petajan and colleagues (79) reported a 22% increase in VO_{2max} and a 48% improvement in physical work capacity. Ponichtera-Mulcare and colleagues (46) found similar improvements (19%) in persons with equivalent impairment level but less dramatic improvement (7%) for those more severely impaired after a 24-week supervised program. This raises an important issue regarding the development of realistic expectations based on the baseline impairment level of the individual. Subtle neurologic changes may not be observable to the clinician. However, small unnoticeable changes may affect exercise training outcomes. It is important to monitor neurologic changes carefully by periodically interviewing the client regarding subjective impressions of his or her disease status. Consideration must also be given to the fact that training outcomes observed under strict supervision may not be similar to those outside of the supervised, controlled program environment, e.g., a home exercise program. Unfortunately, there is no research on a home-based program of aerobic exercise in this population.

What We Would Like to Know
About Exercise and Multiple Sclerosis

Certain aspects of exercise response in the patient with MS have been substantiated by a number of studies. However, numerous other facets regarding exercise response remain a mystery. To fully understand how MS affects physiologic adjustments to exercise the following questions need to be addressed:

1 How does autonomic dysfunction related to MS demyelination affect peripheral circulation in response to exercise?

2 Are peripheral circulatory adjustments during exercise sufficient to sustain aerobic metabolism? If not, is there a relationship between this peripheral circulation and exercise-related fatigue in the patient with MS?

3 Are unsupervised home-based exercise programs as effective in terms of strength, endurance, and flexibility training as supervised programs in this population?

4 Does chronic exercise have any benefit with respect to slowing disease progression in certain types of MS?

5 Are people with MS different from the general population with respect to general health and wellness behaviors such as diet, smoking, physical activity, etc.?

6 How does the neuropsychological impairment associated with the disease affect the various facets of the clinician–patient relationship in providing instruction, motivation, and goal setting?

Summary

Multiple sclerosis remains a mystery in many ways to those who have it and those who treat it. There is a growing body of evidence that exercise can be an important intervention in counteracting the secondary symptoms of the disease that are compounded by reduced physical activity. When prescribing exercise to the patient with MS, careful consideration should be given to the unique symptoms of the individual patient. The presence and magnitude of various symptoms should guide the decision-making process when selecting the mode, intensity, frequency, and duration of exercise. In addition, slight modifications in equipment may be necessary to accommodate symptoms such as muscle weakness, spasticity, **ataxia, foot drop,** and ankle clonus. Heat sensitivity and general fatigue are the most common complaints of this population. Regulation of environmental conditions, providing opportunities for frequent rest periods, and maintaining adequate hydration should counteract some of the effects of these symptoms and improve exercise tolerance.

CASE STUDY

Patient Information

Julie is a single, 52-year-old woman with a 12-year history of MS. She currently works part-time doing secretarial work for a nonprofit organization, and her primary form of recreation is reading. Recently she has noticed increased difficulty with walking long distances. She also complains of right hip pain, dragging the right foot, and poor balance, especially when fatigued. Julie is reluctant to take any medication for her MS and prefers to manage her symptoms "naturally" with supplements and diet. She has never participated in a regular exercise program before and is unsure of her ability to do so now.

Assessment

An assessment of Julie's gait reveals an obvious **Trendelenburg sign.** She drags the right toes during swing approximately 50% of the time, and there is a left lateral trunk shift during swing of the right lower extremity to assist in toe clearance. Mild ballistic hyperextension of the right knee also is present during stance. Julie reports falling at least once a month and scored a 45 out of a possible 56 on the Berg Balance Scale, indicating an increased risk of falls. There is reduced flexibility of the hamstrings, right hip adductors, and ankle plantar flexors, and 5-degree hip flexion contractures are evident bilaterally. She also displays tightness of the shoulder internal rotators including pectoralis major and minor with thoracic kyphosis and a forward head posture. There is mild to moderate spasticity in the lower extremities, primarily involving the extensor muscles, with the right side affected more than the left. Julie also demonstrates 3+/5 strength throughout the right lower extremity, which quickly fatigues after five to 10 repeated contractions. A moderate impairment of proprioception is evident in the right leg. She has no personal or family history of cardiovascular disease; her current resting heart rate is 72 beats per minute, and her blood pressure is 110/64. Her body mass index (BMI) is 29.

Intervention

Based on these findings it was apparent that Julie would benefit from a comprehensive program involving aerobic, strength, balance, and flexibility exercises designed to meet her specific needs.

To increase her aerobic endurance Julie used a Schwinn Air-Dyne. This combination upper- and lower-extremity ergometer allows people with weak extremities to generate more work by reducing the chance that local muscle fatigue will limit exercise time and potential aerobic benefits. Cycling also is a low-impact activity and should not exacerbate the right hip pain she experiences during walking. Julie started with short bouts (about 10 minutes) of exercise and eventually progressed to 30 minutes of continuous cycling. Initial exercise intensity was set at 65% to 70% of peak HR and progressed to 70% to 80% as tolerated or an RPE between 11 and 13 (on the 6–20 scale). Emphasis was placed on a smooth efficient pedal stroke with the use of foot straps to reduce the interference of spasticity. She also was encouraged to do some of her pedaling in the reverse direction to promote greater use of lower extremity flexors.

Strength training focused on larger muscle groups of the lower extremities as well as postural extensors of the trunk. Julie was instructed in the use of a supine leg press machine and a latissimus pull-down machine. At first she performed two sets of 12-25 repetitions to learn the movement and increase muscular endurance, progressing later to two sets of eight to 12 repetitions using a higher weight to increase strength.

Balance training involved a number of exercises designed to challenge the primary sensory systems involved in postural control, including visual, sensory, and vestibular input. Activities such as standing with eyes closed while turning the head, tandem walking, and negotiating an obstacle course were included in her exercise program.

Flexibility training focused on stretching the anterior trunk, hamstrings, hip flexors, adductors, and gastrocnemius. Julie was instructed in daily home stretching program for each of these muscle groups.

Questions

1. Based on your reading in the chapter, identify several additional reasons why a Schwinn Air-Dyne bicycle might be a good choice for Julie's aerobic training.

2. What is the rationale for the choice of strength training exercises and parameters?

3. How might you best address the concerns for Julie's long-term compliance?

4. In addition to the balance exercises that Julie is performing, what other issues are there to consider regarding her balance?

5. Discuss suitable strategies for combating heat sensitivity during exercise in this population.

6. What would be the advantage of Julie exercising in the morning instead of late afternoon?

REFERENCES

1. Kurtzke JF, Wallin MT. Epidemiology. In: Burks JS, Johnson KP, eds. Multiple Sclerosis: Diagnosis, Medical Management and Rehabilitation. New York: Demos Publications, 2000:70.
2. National Multiple Sclerosis Society. Sourcebook—Epidemiology. Available at http://nmss.org.
3. Martin R, Dhib-Jalbut S. Immunology and etiology concepts. In: Burks JS, Johnson KP, eds. Multiple Sclerosis: Diagnosis, Medical Management and Rehabilitation. New York: Demos Publications, 2000:141–165.
4. Rosati G. Descriptive epidemiology of MS in Europe in the 1980's: a critical overview. Ann Neurology1994;36:5164–5174.
5. National Multiple Sclerosis Society. Sourcebook—Etiology. Available at http://nmss.org
6. Sawcer S, Jones HB, Feakes R, et al. A genome screen in multiple sclerosis reveals susceptibility loci on chromosome 6p21 and 17q22. Nat Genet 1996;13:464–468.
7. Lublin FD, Reingold SC. Defining the clinical course of multiple sclerosis: results of an international survey. National Multiple Sclerosis Society (USA) Advisory Committee on Clinical Trial of New Agents in Multiple Sclerosis. Neurology1996;46:907–911.
8. Coyle PK. Diagnosis and classification of inflammatory demyelinating disorders. In: Burks JS, Johnson KP, eds. Multiple Sclerosis: Diagnosis, Medical Management and Rehabilitation. New York: Demos Publications, 2000:84.
9. Paty DW, Noseworthy JH, Ebers GC. Diagnosis of multiple sclerosis. In: Paty DW, Ebers GC, eds. Multiple Sclerosis. Philadelphia: FA Davis, 1997.
10. Paty DW. Initial symptoms. In: Burks JS, Johnson KP, eds. Multiple Sclerosis: Diagnosis, Medical Management and Rehabilitation. New York: Demos Publications, 2000:76.
11. Britell CW, Burks JS, Schapiro RT. Introduction to symptom and rehabilitation management: disease management model. In: Burks JS, Johnson KP, eds. Multiple Sclerosis: Diagnosis, Medical Management and Rehabilitation. New York: Demos Publications, 2000:215.
12. Fisk JD, Pontefract A, Ritvo PG, et al. The impact of fatigue on patients with multiple sclerosis. Can J Neurol Sci 1994;21:9–14.
13. Freal JE, Kraft GH, Coyell JK. Symptomatic fatigue in multiple sclerosis. Arch Phys Med Rehabil 1984;5:135–148.
14. Berganaschi R, Romani V, Versino M, et al. Clinical aspects of fatigue in multiple sclerosis. Functional Neurol 1997;12:247–251.
15. Sheehan GL, Murray NMF, Rothwell JC, et al. An electrophysiological study of the mechanism of fatigue in multiple sclerosis. Brain 1997;120:299–315.
16. Latash M, Kalugina E, Orpet NJ, et al. Myogenic and central neurogenic factors in fatigue in multiple sclerosis. Mult Scler 1996;1:236–241.
17. Sharma KR, Kent-Brown J, Mynhier MA, et al. Evidence of an abnormal intramuscular component of fatigue in multiple sclerosis. Muscle Nerve 1995;18:1403–1411.
18. Kent-Braun J, Sharma KR, Miller RG, Weiner MW. Postexercise phosphocreatine resynthesis is slowed in multiple sclerosis. Muscle Nerve 1994;17:835–841.
19. Roelcke U, Kappos L, Lechner-Scott J, et al. Reduced glucose metabolism in the frontal cortex and basal ganglia of multiple sclerosis patients with fatigue: a 18F-fluorodeoxyglucose positron emission tomography study. Neurology 1997;48:1566–1571.
20. Olgiati R, Jacquet J, DiPrampero PE. Energy cost of walking and exertional dyspnea in multiple sclerosis. Am Rev Respir Dis 1986;134:1005–1010.
21. Quesada JR, Talpaz M, Rios A, et al. Clinical toxicity of interferons in cancer patients, a review. J Clin Oncol 1986;4:234–243.
22. Neilly LK, Goodin DS, Goodkin DE, Hause SL. Side effect profile of interferon beta-1b in MS: Results of an open label trial. Neurology 1996;46:552–554.
23. Archibald CJ, McGrath P, Ritvo PG, et al. Pain in multiple sclerosis: prevalence, severity, and impact on mental health. Pain 1994;58:89–93.
24. Caruso LS, LaRocca NC, Tyron W, et al. Activity monitoring of fatigued and non-fatigued persons with MS. Sleep Res 1001;20:368.
25. Taphoorn MJ, van Someren E, Snoeck FJ, et al. Fatigue, sleep disturbances, and circadian rhythm in multiple sclerosis. J Neurol 1993;240:446–448.
26. Gincarlo T, Kapen S, Saad J, et al. Analysis of sleepiness and fatigue in multiple sclerosis. Ann Neurol 1997;22:1987.
27. Rao SM, Leo GJ, Bernardin L, Unverzagt F. Cognitive dysfunction in multiple sclerosis: I. Frequency, patterns, and prediction. Neurology 1991;41:685–691.
28. LaRocca NG. Cognitive and functional disorders. In: Burks JS, Johnson KP, eds. Multiple Sclerosis: Diagnosis, Medical Management and Rehabilitation. New York: Demos Publications, 2000:405–406.
29. Peyser JM, Rao SM, LaRocca NG, Kaplan E. Guidelines for neuropsychological research in multiple sclerosis. Arch Neurol 1990;47:94–97.
30. Thornton AE, Naftail R. Memory impairment in multiple sclerosis: a quantitative review. Neuropsychology 1997;11:357–366.
31. Pozzilli C, Passfiume D, Bernardi S, et al. SPECT, MRI and cognitive function in multiple sclerosis. J Neurol Neurosurg Psychiatry 1996;54:110–115.
32. Ryan L, Clark CM, Klonoff H, et al. Patterns of cognitive impairment in relapsing-remitting multiple sclerosis and their relationship to neuropathology on magnetic resonance images. Neuropsychology 1991;10:176–193.
33. Guthrie TC, Nelson DA. Influence of temperature changes on multiple sclerosis: critical review of mechanisms and research potential. J Neurol Sci 1995;129:1–8.
34. Berger JR, Sheremata WA. Persistent neurological deficit precipitated by hot bath test in multiple sclerosis. JAMA 1983;249:1751–1753.
35. Guthrie TC. Visual and motor changes in patients with multiple sclerosis. A result of induced changes in environmental temperature. AMA Arch Neurol Psychiatry 1951;65:437–451.
36. Michael JA, Davis FA. Effects of induced hyperthermia in multiple sclerosis: differences in visual acuity during heating and recovery phases. Acta Neurol Scand 1973;49:141–151.
37. Nelson DA, McDowell F. The effects of induced hyperthermia on patients with multiple sclerosis. J Neurol Neurosurg Psychiatry 1959;22:113–116.
38. Namerow NS. Circadian temperature rhythm and vision in multiple sclerosis. Neurology 1968;18:417–422.
39. Hopper CL, Mathews CG, Clelland CS. Symptom instability and thermoregulation in multiple sclerosis. Neurology 1972;22:142–148.
40. Raminsky M. The effects of temperature on conduction in demyelinated single nerve fibers. Arch Neurol 1973;28:287–292.
41. Shauf CL, Davis RA. Impulse conduction in multiple sclerosis: a theoretical basis for modification by temperature and pharmacological agents. J Neurol Neurosurg Psychiatry 1974;37:152–161.
42. Ponichtera-Mulcare JA, Glaser RM, Mathews T, Camaione DN. Maximal aerobic exercise in persons with multiple sclerosis. Clin Kinesiol 1992;46:12–21.
43. Ponichtera JA, Glaser RM, Camaione DN, Mathews T. Physiologic responses to prolonged recumbent cycling of individuals with multiple sclerosis and able-bodied individuals. Med Sci Sports Exerc 1990;20:S123.
44. Mulcare JA, Mathews T, Barrett PJ, Gupta SC. Changes in aerobic fitness of patients with multiple sclerosis during a 6-month training program. Sports Medicine Training and Rehabilitation 1997;7:265–272.
45. White AT, Wilson TE, Davis SL, Petajan JH. Effect of precooling on physical performance in multiple sclerosis. Multiple Sclerosis 2000;6:176–180.
46. Mulcare JA, Webb P, Mathews T, et al. The effect of body cooling on the aerobic endurance of persons with multiple sclerosis following a 3-month aerobic training program. Med Sci Sports Exerc 1997;29:S83.
47. Mulcare JA, Webb P, Mathews T, Gupta SC. Sweat response in persons with multiple sclerosis during submaximal aerobic exercise. Int J MS Care 2001;3(3):33–38.
48. Brodal P. Peripheral autonomic nervous system. In: Brodal P (ed.). The

Central Nervous System: Structure and Function. New York: Oxford University Press, 1998.

49. Drory VE, Nisipeanu PF, Kroczyn AD. Tests of autonomic dysfunction in patients with multiple sclerosis. Acta Neurol Scand 1995;92:356–360.

50. Brinar V, Brzovic ZX, Papa J, et al. Autonomic dysfunction in patients with multiple sclerosis. Coll Antropol 1997;21:493–497.

51. Flachenecker P, Wolf A, Krauser M, et al. Cardiovascular autonomic dysfunction in multiple sclerosis: correlation with orthostatic intolerance. J Neurol 1999;246:578–586.

52. Pepin EB, Hicks RW, Spencer MK, et al. Pressor response to isometric exercise in patients with multiple sclerosis. Med Sci Sports Exerc 1996;28:656–660.

53. Senaratne MP, Carroll D, Warren KG, Kappagoda T. Evidence for cardiovascular autonomic nerve dysfunction in multiple sclerosis. J Neurol Neurosurg Psychiatry 1984;47:947–952.

54. Ponichtera JA, Mathews T, Glaser RM, Ezenwa BN. A test to determine dynamic exercise capacity and autonomic cardiovascular function in individuals with multiple sclerosis. Proceedings of the IEEE 1992;12–14.

55. Bannister R, Mathias C. Testing autonomic reflexes. In: Autonomic Failure: A Textbook of Clinical Disorders of the Autonomic Nervous System. 2nd Ed. Oxford: Oxford University Press, 1988:289–307.

56. Cartlidge NE. Autonomic function in multiple sclerosis. Brain 1972;95:661–664.

57. Andersen EB, Nordenbo AM. Sympathetic vasoconstrictor responses in multiple sclerosis with thermo-regulatory dysfunction. Clin Autonom Res 1997;7:13–16.

58. Eidelman BH. Autonomic disorders. In: Burks JS, Johnson KP, eds. Multiple Sclerosis: Diagnosis, Medical Management and Rehabilitation. New York: Demos Publications, 2000:473.

59. Rudick RA. Contemporary immunomodulatory therapy for multiple sclerosis. J Neuroophthalmol 2001;21:284–291.

60. Khan OA, Tselis AC, Kamholz JA, et al. A prospective, open-labeled treatment trial to compare the effect of IFN beta-1a (Avonex), IFN beta-1b (Betaseron), and glatiramer acetate (Copaxone) on the relapse rate in relapsing-remitting multiple sclerosis. Eur J Neurol 2001;8:141–148.

61. Francis DA. Glatiramer acetate (Copaxone). Int J Clin Pract 2001;55:394–398.

62. Johnson KP, Brooks BR, Ford CC, et al. Sustained clinical benefits of glatiramer acetate in relapsing multiple sclerosis patients observed for 6 years. Copolymer 1 Multiple Sclerosis Study Group. Mult Scler 2000;6:255–266.

63. Hartung HP. Mitoxantrone: Further define its role in MS treatment. Int J MS Care 2000;December (Suppl):3–7, 9.

64. Jain KK. Evaluation of mitoxantrone for the treatment of multiple sclerosis. Expert Opin Investig Drugs 2000;9:1139–1149.

65. Murray TJ. Amantadine therapy for fatigue in multiple sclerosis. Can J Neurol Sci 1985;12:251–254.

66. Cohen RA, Fisher M. Amantadine treatment of fatigue associated with multiple sclerosis. Arch Neurol 1989;45:676–680.

67. Krupp LB, Coyle PK, Doscher C, et al. Fatigue therapy in multiple sclerosis: results of a double-blind, randomized, parallel trial of amantadine, premoline, and placebo. Neurology 1995;45:1956–1961.

68. Rammohan KW. Wake-promoting agent shows benefit in MS-related fatigue. Int J MS Care 2000;October(Suppl):11–12, 14.

69. Duncan GW, Shahani BT, Young RR. An evaluation of baclofen treatment for certain symptoms in patients with spinal cord lesions. Neurol (Minneap) 1976;24:441–446.

70. Bass B, Weinshenker B, Rice GP, et al. Tizanidine versus baclofen in the treatment of spasticity in patients with multiple sclerosis. Can J Neurol Sci 1988;15:15–19.

71. Bes A, Eyssette M, Pierrot-Deseilligny E, et al. A multi-centre, double-blind trial of tizanidine, a new antispastic agent, in spasticity associated with hemiplegia. Curr Med Res Opin 1988;10:709–718.

72. Stewart-Wynne EG, Silbert PL, Buffery S, et al. Intrathecal baclofen for severe spasticity: five years experience. Clin Exp Neurol 1991;28:244–255.

73. Eisenberg DM, Davis RB, Ettner SL, et al. Trends in alternative medicine use in the United States, 1990–1997: results of a follow-up national survey. JAMA 1998;280:1569–1575.

74. National Institutes of Health, National Center for Complementary and Alternative Medicine. Available at http://nccam.nih.gov/nccam/fcp/classify.

75. Bowling AC, Ibrahim R, Stewart TM. Alternative medicine and multiple sclerosis: an objective review from an American perspective. Int J MS Care 2000;2(3):14–21.

76. Mulcare JA. Multiple sclerosis. In: ACSM's Exercise Management for Persons with Chronic Diseases and Disabilities. 2nd Ed. Champaign, IL: Human Kinetics, 2003:267–268.

77. Ponichtera-Mulcare JA, Mathews T, Glaser RM, Gupta SC. Maximal aerobic exercise of individuals with multiple sclerosis using three modes of ergometry. Clin Kinesiol 1995;49:4–12.

78. Shapiro RT, Petajan JH, Kosich D, et al. Role of cardiovascular fitness in multiple sclerosis. J Neurol Rehabil 1988;2:43–49.

79. Petajan JH, Gappmeir E, White AT, et al. Impact of aerobic training on fitness and quality of life in multiple sclerosis. Ann Neurol 1996;39:432–441.

80. Borg G. The Borg CR10 Scale. In: Borg's Perceived Exertion and Pain Scales. Champaign, IL: Human Kinetics, 1998:39–43.

81. United States Department of Health and Human Services. Healthy People 2010. Vol II. Objectives for Improving Health Part B: Focus Areas 15-28. Bethesda: International Medical Publishing, Inc. 2000:22–29.

82. Convertino VA, Armstrong LE, Coyle EF, et al. Exercise and fluid replacement. Med Sci Sports Exerc 1998;28:i–vii.

83. Petajan JH. Weakness. In: Burks JS, Johnson KP, eds. Multiple Sclerosis: Diagnosis, Medical Management and Rehabilitation. New York: Demos Publications, 2000:307–321.

84. Bohannon RW. Sit to stand test for measuring performance of lower extremity muscles. Perceptual and Motor Skills 1995;80:163–166.

85. Csuka M, McCarty DJ. Simple method for measurement of lower extremity muscle strength. Am J Med 1985;78:77–81.

86. Kraft GH, Alquist AD, de Lateur BJ. Effect of resistive exercises on strength in patients with multiple sclerosis. Rehabilitation R&D Progress Reports 1995;33:328–330.

87. Brar SP, Smith MB, Nelson LM, Franklin GM, Cobble ND. Evaluation of treatment protocols on minimal to moderate spasticity in multiple sclerosis. Arch Phys Med Rehabil 1991;72:186–189.

88. Kasser K, Rose D, Clark S. Balance training for adults with multiple sclerosis: multiple case studies. Neurol Report, 1999;23:5–12.

89. Jackson KJ. Effects of balance training on individuals with multiple sclerosis. Unpublished doctoral dissertation. Union Institute and University, 2002.

90. Whipple R. Improving balance in older adults: Identifying the significant training stimuli. In: Masdeu J, Sudarsky L, Wolfson L, eds. Gait Disturbances in the Elderly. New York: Lippincott-Raven, 1997.

91. Wolfson L, Whipple M, Judge J. Training balance and strength in the elderly to improve function. JAGS 1993;3:341–343.

92. Gill-Body K, Popat R, Parker S, Krebs D. Rehabilitation of balance in two patients with cerebellar dysfunction. Phys Ther 1997;77:534–551.

93. Frovic D, Morris M, Vowels L. Clinical tests of standing balance: performance of persons with multiple sclerosis. Arch Phys Med Rehabil 2000;81:215–221.

94. Summers LS, McCubbin JA, Manns PJ. The effects of resistance exercise on balance and gait speed in adults with multiple sclerosis. Med Sci Sports Exerc 2000; S263.

CHAPTER 17

Parkinson Disease

Iris Reuter, Martin K. Engelhardt

Overview

In 1817 James Parkinson (1) first described the condition that now bears his name as "shaking palsy," naming it for the cardinal symptom of the disease. **Parkinson disease** is one of the most common neurodegenerative diseases, with a prevalence of 60 to 187 per 100,000 people worldwide (2). The risk of developing Parkinson disease increases with age. Ten percent of patients become symptomatic before the age of 40, 30% before 50, and 40% between 50 and 60 years. The neuropathologic characteristics are loss of dopaminergic cells in the substantia nigra pars compacta (SNpc) with preference for the ventrolateral part (3). Intraneuronal eosinophilic inclusion bodies (Lewy bodies)

in the substantia nigra, substantia innominata, dorsal vagal nucleus, and locus ceruleus are pathognomic for the disease. Occasionally Lewy bodies can be found in the neocortex and limbic cortex. By the time a patient first visits a physician presenting with symptoms, about 70% on average of the dopaminergic cells are lost. The primary clinical features of PD are motor symptoms such as **akinesia, bradykinesia** and **hypokinesia**, **rigidity**, **postural imbalance**, and **tremor**.

Etiology

The reason for the degeneration of dopaminergic cells is not known. The cytotoxic effect of hydroxyl radicals generated by the dopamine degradation (oxidative stress), deficits in cellular scavengers and in mitochondrial energy metabolism with impaired function of the respiratory chain (complex 1), and a pathological accumulation of Fe^3 ions in nigral neurons have been suggested as possible causes (4).

Environmental factors such as herbicides and pesticides also have been investigated. The strongest evidence for an environmental factor was the discovery that N-Methyl-4-phenyl-1,2,3,6-tetrahydropyridine (MPTP), a piperidine derivative, in heroin caused Parkinsonism in drug addicts. It is now used to induce PD in primates as an animal model for research (5).

For many years genetic factors in PD were dismissed. Recently, however, molecular genetic analysis has identified common genetic factors in families with high incidences of PD. Mutations of the α-synuclein gene on chromosome 4 are associated with an autosomal dominant inherited Parkinson syndrome (6), and mutations of the Parkin gene on chromosome 6 are associated with an autosomal recessive inherited Parkinson syndrome (7). A third locus has been mapped to chromosome 2p13 in PD families with autosomal inherited disease, low penetrance, and typical Lewy body pathology (8). There is further evidence that the same pathogenic mutation on chromosome 4 p haplotype might code for autosomal dominant Lewy body PD, and in some circumstances postural tremor also can be a phenotype of the same mutation (9). However, it is not clear which role genetic factors play in most patients with PD.

Pathophysiology

Parkinson disease is a disorder of the basal ganglia. The principal deficit is a loss of dopaminergic cells in the substantia nigra pars compacta (SNpc). Progressive loss of dopaminergic cells is associated with normal aging but seems to be accelerated in patients with PD. Symptoms of PD occur when the loss of dopaminergic cells exceeds 70% to 80%.

The function of the basal ganglia is still controversial, but they are involved in movement control, motor learning, memory, planning, and motivation (10–12). The basal ganglia consist of the caudate nucleus, putamen, globus pallidum, substantia nigra, subthalamic nucleus, nucleus accumbens, and parts of the tuberculum olfactorium. The caudate nucleus and putamen are called *neostriatum* or *dorsal striatum*. The ventral parts of the ventral caudate nucleus, putamen, nucleus accumbens, and tuberculum olfactorium are called *ventral striatum*. The substantia nigra consists of two main parts, the dopaminergic pars compacta and the GABAergic substantia nigra pars reticulata (SNpr). The SNpr and the globus pallidum internum (Gpi) are the major output system of the basal ganglia.

The basal ganglia are organized in two major output pathways. The direct pathway colocalizes substance P as cotransmitter and projects directly to the SNpr and to the GPi. It is an inhibitory GABAergic pathway, which allows,

via double inhibition (inhibition of the inhibitory effect of globus pallidum on thalamus), an increase of thalamic stimulation of the cortex. The indirect pathway contains enkephalin as cotransmitter and projects via the globus pallidum pars externa (GPe), subthalamic nucleus (STN), and GPi to the thalamus (13). Gerfen (14) suggested that substance P–containing neurons of the **direct pathway** express D_1 **dopamine** receptors, and that the enkephalin-containing neurons of the **indirect pathway** express D_2 dopamine receptors. The main input to the striatum originating from the cortex is glutamatergic excitatory.

Three major loops can be allocated to the different functions of the basal ganglia:

1. *The prefrontal loop.* The lateral orbitofrontal and dorsolateral prefrontal cortex project to the caudate nucleus. Information is then processed in the cortico-striatal-thalamo-cortical loop via the striatum and thalamus back to the cortex. It is thought that high cognitive functions such as attention, planning of sequential movements, and abstract thinking are associated with this loop.
2. *Limbic pathway–integrative associative tasks.* The limbic loop connects the anterior cingulate area, medial orbitofrontal cortex, and temporal cortex with the nucleus accumbens and tuberculum olfactorium. Information from the hippocampus, amygdala, and entorhinal and perirhinal areas is contributed to this loop. Disturbance of this loop is thought to result in deficits of spatial memory, selective attention, emotional affect, and representation of environment.
3. *Motor loop.* The striatum receives via the putamen strictly topographically organized afferents from the primary motor cortex, arcuate premotor area, associative motor cortex, primary sensory cortex, and somatosensory association cortex (10, 15).

Although the motor function of the basal ganglia is the feature that has been most extensively investigated, their exact role is still controversial. Under resting conditions the neurons of the striatum are silent. Only the neurons of the output system—the substantia nigra pars reticulata and the globus pallidum interna—show permanent tonic activity (16, 17). Dopamine (from SNpc) stimulates the D_1 receptors of the direct pathway, which leads via double inhibition to a release of the thalamus from pallidal inhibition. Stimulation of the indirect pathway via D_2 receptors results in reduced inhibition of the GPe, which then results in an increased inhibitory effect of GPe on STN. The reduced excitatory effect of STN on GPi reduces the inhibitory effect on the thalamus and increases stimulation of the cortex (Figure 17.1). Loss of dopamine reduces stimulatory transmission via the direct pathway and leads to a reliance on the indirect striatal system (Figure 17.2). Reduced stimulation of the D_2 receptors increases inhibition of GPe, which results in disinhibition of STN and an increased excitation of the striatal output complex (GPi and SNpr). The result is

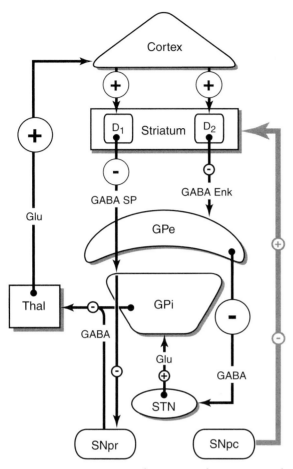

FIGURE 17.1. Dopaminergic pathways: normal state. *Direct pathway:* Stimulation (+) of D$_1$ receptor → inhibition (–) of GPi → disinhibition (+) of thalamus→excitation (+) of cortex. *Indirect pathway:* Stimulation (+) of D$_2$ receptor → reduced inhibition (–) of GPe → inhibition (—) of STN → reduced stimulation (+) of GPi → release of thalamus → excitation of cortex.

GABA Enk, enkephalinergic γ-aminobutyric acid; GABA SP, γ-aminobutyric acid; Glu, glutamic acid; GPe, globus pallidum pars externa; SNpr, substantia nigra pars reticulata; SNpc, substantia nigra pars compacta; STN, subthalamic nucleus; Thal, thalamus.

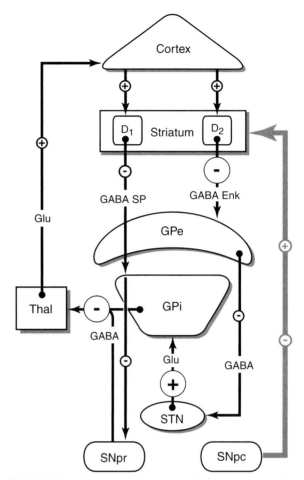

FIGURE 17.2. Dopaminergic pathways: Parkinsonian state. *Direct pathway:* Reduced stimulation (+) of D$_1$ receptor → reduced inhibition (–) of GPi → inhibition of thalamus → reduced excitation (+) of cortex. *Indirect pathway:* Reduced stimulation (+) of D$_2$ receptor → inhibition (—) of GPe → reduced inhibition (–) of STN → stimulation (+) of GPi → inhibition of thalamus → reduced excitation of Cortex.

GABA Enk, enkephalinergic γ-aminobutyric acid; GABA SP, γ-aminobutyric acid; Glu, glutamic acid; GPe, globus pallidum pars externa; Gpi, globus pallidum internum; SNpr, substantia nigra pars reticulata; SNpc, substantia nigra pars compacta; STN, subthalamic nucleus; Thal, thalamus.

an inhibition of the thalamus and reduced activity of thalamofrontal neurons. Although there is strong evidence for segregation of the striatal pathways (18), a remarkable dendric arborization of the interneurons at a cellular level permits information to converge (10, 19).

Electrophysiologic studies support the involvement of the basal ganglia in motor function. Neurons of the basal ganglia increase the fire rate during automatic movements (20). The basal ganglia seem to be more involved in ongoing movement control (20, 21) than in movement initiation, but they may provide movement templates for the motor cortex (22). Some neurons respond to specific joint movements (16), whereas others respond to the amplitude, direction, and velocity of movements (23, 24). The basal ganglia play a role in visuomotor control, especially saccades (15, 25). There are close connections to the limbic

system, and the ganglia seem to be involved in motor learning, especially of sequential or reward-promising tasks, award-predicting behavior, and motivation (26).

The motor disturbance is best described as a combination of impaired movement initiation (akinesia), slowed movement (bradykinesia), and reduction in movement range (hypokinesia). The disturbance is expressed in reduced arm swing during walking, slow gait, shuffling, difficulties in turning around, and difficulties in initiating walking after sitting or to get up from a chair. There is good evidence that self-cued or internally **cued** movements are impaired more severely than externally cued movements (27). The deterioration of motor task performance in PD as a result of reduction of internal cues makes increased dependence on external cues necessary (28–30). Alternating movements, simultaneous movements, and motor sequences also are impaired

(30, 31). Although electrical stimulation of muscle does not reveal any deficit in muscle strength, voluntary strength production is impaired. The extensor muscles are affected more severely than the flexor muscles. The proximal muscles seem to be more severely impaired, and the velocity of force generation is decreased (32, 33). The deficit is medication-dependent (34). In addition to the agonist weakness that is present in most patients, Yangawa (35) found an antagonist activation in some patients.

One result of the reduced movements is the characteristic lack of facial expression (masked face). The hypokinesia of Parkinsonian gait is accompanied by decreased stride length and altered rhythm. The basic deficit seems to be an inability to regulate stride length by using internal cues (27, 28). Reduced range of motion in the hip, knee, and ankle aggravates the hypokinetic gait (36). Patients move at a steady speed and are, in most cases, unable to increase their velocity quickly. Patients with PD tend to walk on their toes and lean forward; they experience difficulties in stopping movement, especially at higher speed. They start running with short, quick steps and cannot stop quickly. Hurrying can be very dangerous for the patient because it often results in a fall. One symptom in advanced PD is *freezing*—a motor block that patients often experience in narrow spaces, for instance when passing through a door. *Rigidity* is an increase of muscle tone to passive range of movements. This increased muscle tone can break down rhythmically; when it happens this is called the *cogwheel phenomenon*. The tremor in PD is characterized electrophysiologically as agonist-antagonist tremor with a frequency of 5 to 7 Hz. Classically it persists during movement; however, action and postural tremor can be observed in PD. The impairment of **postural reflexes** is very disabling for the patient, because it results in instability and falls.

In addition to motor symptoms, autonomous symptoms may occur (37). It is still not known whether these symptoms are related to the disease itself or to medication. The most common autonomous dysfunctions are constipation, bladder problems, seborrhea, sweating, **orthostatic hypotension**, **cardiac arrhythmias**, and swallowing problems (38, 39). Sleep often is disturbed due to off-period symptoms such as dystonia and cramps and sensory symptoms such as paresthesias and restless legs syndrome (40). Respiratory dysfunction including obstructive lung disease is reported (41, 42). Patients with PD often are not able to use their maximal respiratory muscle strength voluntarily. Nonvolitional tests of the inspiratory and expiratory muscles have shown normal results in both the "on" and "off" states, whereas the volitional tests in the same patients were highly abnormal in the "off" state (43). Dopaminergic stimulation with apomorphine improve only the expiratory muscles—the effect on the inspiratory muscles did not reach significance. We saw deterioration in the voluntary use of the respiratory muscles due to disturbed coordination after apomorphine injection in two patients who also responded to apomorphine with truncal dyskinesias.

According to the literature, about 30% of patients with PD develop a cognitive decline, which often is associated with deterioration of motor function, isolation, and withdrawal from social and physical activities (44, 45). Anxiety, apathy, and depression occur early in the disease.

Diagnosis

The disease typically begins asymmetrically. Patients often present with shoulder, hip, or back problems and complain of stiffness or pain. These symptoms are likely to be misdiagnosed as shoulder-arm syndrome, spondyloarthritis, or degenerative joint disease (46). Table 17.3 presents the clinical features suggesting a diagnosis of PD and the red flags for the disorder (47). The clinical manifestation may be of the akinetic-rigid, tremor-dominant, or akinetic-rigid-tremor phenotype. Stages are defined corresponding to the severity of the disease, with Hoehn and Yahr scores from 1 through 4 (Table 17.2) (48). The course of the disease varies among individual patients. Slow progression is seen in elderly patients, and the disease usually manifests in the tremor-dominant form. Rapid progression is seen more often in young patients, in whom it usually presents in the akinetic-rigid clinical manifestation.

Treatment of Parkinson Disease

Drugs

Levodopa

Levodopa (L-dopa) plus decarboxylase inhibitor is still the most effective treatment for PD. The aromatic amino acid levodopa is the precursor for dopamine and is able to cross the blood–brain barrier. It probably is taken up by the neurons and converted to dopamine by the L-amino acid decarboxylase. Dopamine is stored presynaptically. However, the exact location where levodopa is converted to dopamine and dopamine is released is not known. To prevent decarboxylation of levodopa outside the brain, decarboxylase inhibitors (e.g., carbidopa, benserazide) are added to the drug regimen. Levodopa preparations are available in standard preparations with a half-life of 3 to 4 hours, in time-release preparations, and in soluble tablet form for "emergency rescue." Despite its relatively short half-life, levodopa has a long-term effect that provides a stable motor response in early stages of the disease. Patients in early stages of the disease do not notice the onset and wearing off of levodopa, therefore. In advanced stages patients may develop fluctuations of their motor responses because the neurons seem to lose the capacity to store dopamine. This loss may result in a reflection of levodopa plasma concentrations in the brain. Patients experience peak-dose dyskinesias, wearing-off of levodopa, and more complex biphasic dyskinesias. The first symptom of fluctuations is nocturnal stiffness. Some

TABLE 17.1. DIAGNOSIS OF PARKINSON DISEASE

Symptom	Supporting Data	Red Flags
Bradykinesia *plus* Resting tremor (4–7 HZ) *or*	Asymmetric onset Maintenance of symptom asymmetry after years	Early falls Predominant autonomous dysfunction
Rigidity *or*	Progressive course of disease	Early cognitive decline
Postural imbalance	Levodopa response: persistent levodopa response after 2 years Levodopa-induced dyskinesias	Marked truncal rigidity No or poor response to levodopa Oculomotor dysfunction, gaze palsy History of neuroleptic treatment

A CT scan should be performed in all patients to exclude normal pressure hydrocephalus or a tumor.

patients experience "off " periods, which are not dependent on medication. Slow-release preparations with delayed absorption are used for overnight and to level out "on–off" fluctuations. Complex fluctuations and dyskinesias can be difficult to treat with slow-release preparations, however, due to the unpredictability of absorption. Levodopa also ameliorates motor function disorders such as akinesia, bradykinesia, and hypokinesia and improves rigidity. It works reasonably well for tremor. It does not improve postural imbalance, autonomic dysfunction, and cognitive impairment. There is some evidence that levodopa may cause autonomous function to deteriorate (49).

Dopamine Agonists

Dopamine agonists stimulate postsynaptic striatal dopamine receptors directly. Ideally, dopamine agonists should work on both types of dopamine receptors. Ergot-type dopamine agonists work mainly on D_2 receptors. Effects and side effects depend on the subset of dopamine receptors that are stimulated. These were used in the past mainly as adjunctive treatment in advanced stages of PD, but nowadays they are given as monotherapy in early stages of the disease to prevent levodopa–induced dyskinesias.

TABLE 17.2. MODIFIED HOEHN AND YAHR STAGING OF PARKINSON DISEASE

Stage 1	Unilateral symptoms; mild tremor in one limb
Stage 1.5	Unilateral symptoms plus axial symptoms
Stage 2	Bilateral symptoms, minimal disability, gait impaired, posture not affected
Stage 2.5	Bilateral symptoms, minimal disability, gait impaired, posture affected but does not fall
Stage 3	Significant slowing of body movements, generalized dysfunction, moderately severely disturbed posture, loss of postural reflexes
Stage 4	Unable to live independently, can still walk to a limited extent, severe rigidity and bradykinesia
Stage 5	Confined to bed or wheelchair, cannot walk or stand, needs permanent nursing care, invalidism

Data from (48).

However, only about one third of patients can cope with dopamine agonist monotherapy for longer than 2 years before levodopa has to be added. The side effects of dopamine agonists are nausea, constipation, vomiting, orthostatic hypotension, cardiac arrhythmias, nasal congestion, peripheral circulation problems, vertigo, dizziness, sedation, hallucinations, increased libido, increased appetite, weight gain, headaches, erythromelalgia, and lung fibrosis. Orthostatic hypotension is mediated primarily by stimulation of peripheral dopamine receptors. Dopamine agonists are less potent than levodopa, and they have a good effect on akinesia and rigidity. Tremor responds less, although pramipexole and ropinirole are considered more potent for treatment of tremor than the other dopamine agonists. Carbergoline is another dopamine agonist of interest because of its long half-life. It is taken once per day and usually produces a stable motor response.

Selegiline

Selegiline is a monoamine oxidase type B (MAO-B) inhibitor that reduces cerebral dopamine degradation and extends the duration of action of levodopa. Its neuroprotective effect lasts for 1 to 2 years. It has a weak symptomatic antiparkinsonian effect. Potential side effects are hypertension, arrhythmia, and sleeplessness. Olanow and coworkers (50) conducted a meta-analysis on selegiline treatment in combination with levodopa and without levodopa. The results of this study refuted the finding of increased mortality with combined selegiline/levodopa treatment that was reported by the Parkinson's Disease Research Group of the United Kingdom (51, 52).

Amantadine

Amantadine is an antiviral drug that was discovered to have an antiparkinsonian effect. It is an N-methyl D-aspartate (NMDA) receptor antagonist and blocks glutamate (i.e., projection from STN to GPi.) It is absorbed more readily when given intravenously rather than orally. The effect is mainly anti-akinetic.

Anticholinergic Drugs

Anticholinergic drugs suppress central cholinergic activity. The main indication is treatment of tremor—the effect on akinesia is weak. Side effects are considerable, especially in elderly persons, and include dry mouth, glaucoma, bladder disturbance, confusion, accommodation difficulties, and memory deficits.

Surgical Treatment

Deep Brain Stimulation

The study group working with Benabid performed the first deep brain stimulations in the 1980s. At the beginning the ventral intermedius nucleus (VIM) of the thalamus was the target of choice. Since that time the method has developed further, and the main target today is the STN (53). Stimulation of the STN leads to improvement in all modalities of PD. This type of treatment is indicated when dyskinesias are resistant to medical treatment or when the threshold between motor response and onset of dyskinesias is too small to attain a clinical benefit. An additional indication is severe "off" periods. Subthalamic stimulation can improve akinesia and tremor.

Ablative Surgery

Ablative intervention experienced a renaissance in the form of ventrolateral pallidotomy but now is used mainly for treatment of medication-resistant dyskinesias. Bilateral procedures can result in severe cognitive impairment.

Neural Transplantation

Transplantation of mesencephalic dopaminergic cells is an experimental treatment. The rationale behind this procedure is essentially to install an internal dopamine pump (i.e., the transplanted cells), thereby restoring the nigrostriatal pathways. The results so far are controversial, and graft survival continues to be a problem.

Interaction of Exercise and Medication

Effect of Medication on Exercise

There are no systematic data available in the literature on the effect of dopaminergic medication on exercise performance. Dopaminergic medication has the potential to produce cardiac side effects such as arrhythmias and tachycardia. Because exercise often reveals ischemic heart disease with an increased risk of arrhythmia, dopaminergic medication has the potential to cause deterioration of the cardiac situation in these patients under exercise.

Patients taking levodopa are prone to postural hypotension (and, rarely, labile hypertension), tachycardia, and arrhythmias. Levodopa can increase sweating, at times profusely. When patients exercise, they should take care to maintain adequate hydration, because dehydration increases the likelihood of arrhythmia. Dopamine agonists sensitize patients for postural hypotension; patients should be monitored after completion of the exercise for drops in blood pressure. Dopaminergic medications with postural hypotension as a side effect may lower the blood pressure during exercise. We have often observed that patients with PD tend to have slightly lower blood pressure under exercise than healthy people (54). The clinical impact of this finding has not yet been analyzed. The side effects of individual dopamine agonists differ slightly. Pergolide can provoke arrhythmia, tachycardia, and atrial premature contractions. Ropinirole can induce bradycardia. Exercise produces an increase in blood pressure, and selegiline per se has the potency to elevate blood pressure; the effects can be additive. People doing vigorous exercise sometimes report bowel problems, and entacapone can exacerbate such a condition by provoking diarrhea.

However, most patients with PD are not capable of exercising without medication. For instance, patients with "on-off" fluctuations will not be able to exercise during an "off" period and will not enjoy doing so. Therefore, patients are advised to keep a diary to record their "on-off" fluctuations and times of good and poor mobility so they can optimize medical treatment and adjust medication use to sports activity.

Effect of Exercise on Medication

Some patients report quick exhaustion under physical therapy, whereas others say they need the physical exercise to remain mobile. These reports raise the question of whether physical activity may have an influence on the pharmacokinetics and pharmacodynamics of levodopa. One might argue that patients feel the lack of dopamine more intensively while exercising, but this explanation does not seem to be sufficient. Mouradian and coworkers (55) found that exercise did not alter patient response to a constant infusion of levodopa, nor did it change plasma levels of levodopa during infusion. These observations suggest that neither the volume of distribution of levodopa nor the requirement for levodopa changes markedly during exercise. Two clinical studies reported no significant effect of exercise on levodopa absorption (56, 57).

A more recent study (58) did not show a significant net effect of exercise on the pharmacokinetics and dynamics of levodopa, but it did reveal two counteracting trends. The levodopa absorption improved under physical activity, whereas the EC_{50}, which can be used as a measure of the amount of levodopa to attain a certain motor response, increased. In some patients, the tendency to a higher demand on levodopa outweighed the trend to better levodopa absorption; in other patients, however, the effects were balanced.

Maximal Exercise Test

Pretest Considerations

Most patients with PD are elderly, and elderly persons are most likely to suffer from cardiovascular disease. Sympathetic and parasympathetic cardiovascular reflexes are more often pathologic in patients with PD than in an age-matched control group of healthy people (38, 54). The deep breathing test and the Ewing test are the most relevant to exercise performance: the deep breathing test evaluates the adaptation to increased breathing work, and the Ewing test evaluates the activation of the sympathetic nervous system. Patients with a fixed **heart rate** may be at risk for cardiac problems during exercise, because it will not be possible for the heart rate to change adequately in response to exercise. There also is a risk of **exercise-induced hypotension**, which can occur at the end of an intensive workout or shortly after completion of exercise (54, 59). Although it is difficult to predict the occurrence of exercise-induced hypotension in the individual patient, those with an akinetic-rigid phenotype of PD and known orthostatic or postprandial hypotension are at greater risk. Blood pressure should be measured and recorded at regular intervals, and the patient should be observed for at least 20 minutes after completion of the exercise test. A high rate of obstructive pulmonary dysfunction is reported in PD, and it can become obvious with the stress of exercise. In addition, dyspnea and stridor are observed with exercise, at least partially due to impaired muscle coordination. The effect of exercise on pulmonary symptoms is not clear.

Patients who are scheduled to have a maximal exercise test first should undergo an electrocardiogram (ECG); an assessment of cardiovascular reflexes, to reduce the risk of unwanted cardiovascular problems; and a lung function test. Rigidity, akinesia, and instability should be known, and a history of "on-off" fluctuations, occurrence of dyskinesia, and severity of dyskinesia should be recorded. These data are important because they must be taken into consideration when analyzing the results of the patient's exercise performance.

Some technical issues must be mentioned. Patients with PD suffer from seborrhea and tend to sweat profusely around the head and upper thorax, which may make it difficult to fix the ECG electrodes to the skin. Rubbing the skin with Omniprep and degreasing the skin with an alcohol patch helps to obtain a better signal. It also is useful to check first to find out if the patient suffers from dyskinesia and which limb is most affected. The blood pressure cuff should always be placed on the limb with less dyskinesia to avoid disturbances of the device.

Test Protocol

Cardiovascular disease is the leading cause for death in patients with PD. Data generated from maximal exercise tests provide important information about cardiovascular function. Only a few studies have been published employing a maximal exercise test in patients with PD, and there is no generally agreed-upon test protocol for conducting a maximal exercise test in PD. However, most of the authors who have reported on such exercise testing took a similar approach.

The following protocol was the one most often used (60, 61). The exercise test, using a **bicycle ergometer**, started at a workload of 40 W, increasing every 2 minutes at the end of each stage by 20 W. Exercise was considered maximal if two of the following three criteria were met: (1) age-predicted maximal HR $\pm$ 10 beats per minute; **respiratory exchange ratio (RER)** > 1.1; and subjective exhaustion. Heart rate was monitored continuously and was recorded for at least 10 seconds at the end of each 2-minute stage. Oxygen consumption and RER were measured every 20 seconds. Caning and coworkers (62) used a slightly different protocol, starting at 20 W and increasing every minute by 10, 20, or 30 W to reach maximum workload within 6 to 12 minutes. They measured peak work rate, peak ventilation, peak heart rate, peak respiratory exchange rate, and peak oxygen consumption. Dyspnea was recorded during the last 30 seconds of the test.

Exercise Responses

The studies on maximal exercise responses agree on some parameters but not on all of them. There was no difference in VO_{2max} (mL/min) and relative VO_{2max} (mL/kg/min) values between healthy people and patients with PD. Peak heart rate did not differ. The studies agreed that the submaximal heart rate and oxygen consumption were higher in the patients with PD. The relative workload (W/kg) was lower in patients with PD than in healthy subjects in one study (61), but did not differ in the other studies (60, 62). Protas (61) found a higher RER in patients with PD, which indicated anaerobic work and increased carbohydrate metabolism. In one study, patients with PD reached a higher percentage of their predicted VO_{2max} (mL/kg/min) (60). The time to reach maximal exercise was shorter in males with PD than in healthy male subjects, in keeping with the high submaximal heart rate and increased submaximal oxygen consumption. The arterial oxygen saturation was normal.

Rigidity or dyskinesias might have caused mechanical insufficiency (63) and resulted in a higher energy requirement and a higher energy expenditure during the task. This was reflected in a higher submaximal heart rate and submaximal oxygen consumption in patients with PD. Rigidity and dyskinesia can already produce a higher resting energy expenditure in the setting of PD. Dyskinesias during the exercise test might increase the VO_{2max} (mL/kg/min) in patients with PD as well. Patients with PD tend to express dyspnea more often than do healthy subjects, which can lead to premature termination of the exercise test. Although VO_{2max} was not different between patients with PD and healthy controls, suggesting normal cardiovascular adaptation to exercise, detailed analysis including submaximal heart rate and oxygen consumption revealed some significant differences of patients with PD in response to exercise. The power of all studies was low, which might have masked more statistically significant differences.

Maximal Exercise Testing

Researchers have asked whether it is necessary to perform a maximal exercise test in patients with PD and whether those patients achieve true VO_{2max} values. It might be better to use $VO_{2\ peak}$ values instead. In Stanley's (60) study, a high percentage of patients did not meet the criteria for VO_{2max}. In another study, patients complained more often about dyspnea (62), which can lead to premature termination of the exercise test. Because of autonomous impairments, motor deficits, and increased muscle tone in PD it is questionable whether the exercise tests truly were maximal regarding cardiovascular function, and it might be better to use VO_{2peak} values (maximal oxygen consumption during the experiment). Absolute and relative VO_{2peak} values should be recorded. Relative VO_{2peak} includes the body weight. This approach has one drawback: if the patient is extremely overweight, the VO_{2peak} result indicates a lower level of cardiovascular fitness than is actually the case, and if a person is very slim, the results overestimate his or her cardiovascular fitness. Patients with PD, especially those with akinetic-rigid disease and dyskinesias, tend to have a lower body weight than the average population. Therefore, it is useful to calculate the relative workload (W/kg). In addition, analysis of the submaximal oxygen consumption and heart rate are useful for targeting an appropriate exercise level. It might be useful to choose lower exercise intensity than the usual suggested heart rate of 60% to 85% of VO_{2max} (64) to avoid too much anaerobic work.

Although treadmill exercises with a moving belt place more stress on the individual, cycle ergometry is preferable considering the postural instability and motor dysfunction in PD. Motor blocks occur during walking and running, and dyskinesias, if present, interfere with normal forward movement, which can result in falls. Hurrying can provoke a dangerous situation on a moving belt. Apart from safety considerations, there are additional reasons for using a bicycle ergometer. Many patients would not be able to increase their running speed to a level at which they would attain a maximal or even near-maximal workout. Poor performance on the treadmill test would be used as the basic measure for cardiovascular fitness and would give misleading guidelines for training. The disadvantage of a cycle ergometer is that fewer muscles are involved in exercise, and the VO_{2max} therefore is lower. A further problem occurs when subjects are not used to cycling. Local fatigue of the quadriceps muscle can make it necessary to end the exercise test early. This problem can be circumvented if patients are allowed to become acclimated to bicycle ergometer exercise before the actual test.

Another alternative, the arm-crank ergometer, did not prove to be as useful as the bicycle ergometer. In one study reported in the literature the arm-crank ergometer was used, but the achieved heart rates and $VO_{2\ peak}$ values were low (61). Our own experience has been that patients, especially women complain early about local muscle fatigue and hardly reach an intensity level that provokes a cardiovascular response.

In summary, a maximal exercise test in patients with PD is desirable, but it will not be possible to attain one in all patients with PD, especially those in a more advanced stage of the disease. All of the maximal exercise tests that have been reported in the literature were performed in patients with slight to moderate PD.

Submaximal Exercise Test

We performed a submaximal exercise test with an upper intensity workload limit of 175 W (54). We included patients in more advanced stages of PD, who experienced difficulties in maintaining the revolutions per minute at the beginning of each new workload level. Because these patients needed more time to adapt to a new stage than healthy controls, we had chosen a 4-minute interval at each intensity level. One might argue that patients with PD do not have enough endurance to stand such a test. However, more advanced patients pulled out of the test on low levels when a program with rapid increases in intensity levels (every 1 or 2 minutes) was applied. The influence of pretest training on test results was greater for patients in more advanced stages of the disease.

There is speculation that patients with PD might have disturbances in the **respiratory chain**, especially complex 1 and 4 (65–67). Impairment of the respiratory chain should lead to increased lactate levels compared to healthy controls. This exercise test was focused on cardiovascular performance and metabolic response to the exercise test in patients with PD. At rest and at the end of each interval blood pressure and capillary lactate samples were taken. Heart rate was monitored continuously. Patients with PD achieved a lower absolute workload, but performance, expressed as W/kg, did not differ significantly between patients with PD and controls. We did not find a statistically significant difference in heart rate increase between patients with PD and healthy subjects. At higher intensity levels, the controls showed a tendency to higher lactate concentrations in blood than the patients with PD. Furthermore, the lactate level of the controls decreased more slowly than that of patients with PD. The results did not reach statistical significance, but the trend was the opposite of what we had expected. The systolic blood pressure rose significantly higher in controls than in patients with PD at high intensity levels. During the recovery period the drop in blood pressure was greater in patients with PD and was sustained at 8 minutes after the exercise test. In summary, we did not find striking differences in **cardiovascular endurance** based on graded exercise test between patients with PD and controls. These results might suggest that either there is no defect of the respiratory chain in skeletal muscles resulting in impaired metabolism or the defect is mild and insufficient to raise lactic acid. Although the data imply some limitations, it is justified to conclude that patients with PD are capable of performing endurance training. A submaximal exercise test seems to be sufficient for pretraining testing and planning of training intensity.

Training Options

The goals of a training program must be attainable for the patients. Training programs in PD do not target improvement of cardiovascular performance as a first aim. In general patients need to ameliorate motor function to gain the capacity to perform exercise at an intensity level that increases their cardiovascular endurance.

The first aim of physical treatment is to keep the patient as functional as possible. Exercise treatment will not stop the progress of PD, but it should prevent secondary complications such as loss of muscle strength, decrease of movement range with subsequent contractures, orthostatic hypotension, inactivity osteoporosis, and pneumonia. To our knowledge there is no literature available regarding specific cardiovascular endurance training or anaerobic training in PD. There are currently no data available that provide information on pre- and posttraining exercise test results. After exclusion of contraindications for physical training and with exercise responses in the normal range a training program can be established. Most training programs consist of a mixed program to improve motor function, i.e., flexibility, balance, muscle strength, and coordination. Improvement of these parameters often results in improvement of the cardiovascular parameters. There is still considerable debate about the pathophysiology of movement impairment in PD. Therefore, it is difficult to develop a training program that specifically tackles the motor disability impairment in PD.

Comella and coworkers (68) found significant improvement in activities of daily living and motor scores using a PD-specific rating scale after regular physical training for 4 weeks (three times per week) in a randomized single-blind crossover study evaluating physical disability in medium-staged parkinsonian patients. All of these factors returned to baseline, however, after 6 months without participation in a formal exercise program. The exercise program was tailored to improve range of motion, endurance, balance, and gait (69). Passive and active mobilization exercises performed over 4 months significantly improved some aspects of motor disability in patients with PD (70). Palmer and coworkers (71) compared the effects of karate training with

a special stretching program of the United Parkinson Foundation (72). After a training period of 12 weeks with three sessions per week of 1 hour each the outcomes in both groups were similar. Functional improvement was observed in gait, arm tremor, and coordination, but not in active movements involving both arms and trunk.

In two further studies (73, 74), patients participated in a 10-week training program with three sessions per week. The studies aimed to improve spinal flexibility, axial mobility, time to stand up, and functional reach. Strategies using external cues were taught. Axial mobility and spinal flexibility improved.

In one of the first studies comparing the effect of **physiotherapy** using proprioceptive neuromuscular facilitation, Bobath and Peto's technique with the effect of occupational therapy failed to show any benefit of these treatments (75).

Our study group combined a program designed to improve muscle strength, flexibility, balance, and respiratory function with a mild cardiovascular endurance program. Regular exercise training was performed twice weekly for 14 weeks. Each training session lasted 1 hour. Once per week the training took place in warm water to increase muscle strength against water resistance and to reduce trunk stiffness and rigidity. The second training session of the week was held in the gymnasium to improve initiation of movements, gait, flexibility, and coordination of motor skills. Balance exercises were performed on Pezzi balls. Exercise can improve balance and together with improved motor function may reduce the likelihood of falls (76). Music was used as an external stimulus to initiate movements, because in the basal ganglia different pathways are involved in externally and internally cued movements (77, 78). Circuits of externally cued movements are less disturbed in PD and have proved to be of benefit in gait training and **motor sequences** (79). There is evidence that exercises using external cues as well as exercises that develop sequential or simultaneous movements from simple movements are specific to the pathophysiology of PD (Table 17.3). For cardiovascular improvement we used quick walking to increase the heart rate to 130 beats per minute (maximal up to 100 + age − 20%) accompanied by music indicating different walking speeds. In the swimming pool we encouraged patients to swim 20 meters without stopping. At the beginning of the exercise training only three patients managed this task. The other patients initially needed to improve their swimming and breathing technique and to gain muscle strength. The target was to swim for 10 minutes without pausing by the end of the training period (Table 17.4).

It is more difficult to assess objective improvement of motor function than cardiovascular endurance. There is always the risk that subjective judgment, self-ratings by patients, and improvement of psychological parameters confound the assessment. The PD typical rating scales often are not sensitive enough to measure training improvement or do not test the parameters that were trained. Therefore,

TABLE 17.3. EXERCISE PROGRAM: TRAINING OF MOTOR FUNCTION

Mode	Type of Training
Resistance training	*Static strength training:*
	Contraction of arm and leg flexor/extensor muscles with 60% to 70% of maximal strength for 5 seconds, 5 repeats
	Lifting of trunk from supine position 5 times for 5 seconds, lifting of trunk from front position 5 times for 5 seconds
	Theraband training:
	Sling a Theraband around the foot and stretch the leg against the resistance provided by the band
	or
	Sling a Theraband around the hand and stretch the arm against the resistance of the band 10 times, then extend and flex the hand against the resistance.
	Dynamic force:
	Ball exercise: 500- to 1000-g balls are lifted with both hands over the head 20 times. Rhythmic movements are attempted.
	Quadruple position: lowering body up and down
	Sitting position: Ball between feet, stretching and flexing of legs.
	Water: leg and arm movements against water resistance with and without paddles
	Flexibility
	Antagonistic action to tendency of patients with PD to sit, stand, and walk in a flexed posture
	Nondynamic stretching of Achilles' tendon, hamstrings, flexor femoris, quadriceps muscle, pectoral muscle, triceps muscle
	Stretching exercises on Pezzi ball
	Water: backstroke
	Training of large-scale movements
Balance	Roll exercises on Pezzi ball
	One-legged stand for 10 seconds alternating on right and left leg.
	Walking on soft ground and varying ground (artificial lane with sand, pebbles, water)
	Water: exercise with paddles, swim boards and so called "swim noodles," patients should keep a horizontal posture in water
Coordination	Preparing gait exercises:
	Training of simple movements that will combine to form a compound movement. After simple movements have been mastered, performance of two simple movements at the same time or in sequence.

we combined a sport-specific scale (basic motor test [80]) with the **Unified Parkinson's Disease Rating Scale (UPDRS)** (69). The sport-specific Basic Motor Test (BMT) (80) included subscores measuring strength, flexibility, and coordination of motor skills (performing two different movements simultaneously, for example balancing on a line and bouncing a ball). The UPDRS consists of measurement of cognitive function (subscore 1), activities of daily living (subscore 2), motor scores (subscore 3), complications of

TABLE 17.4. ENDURANCE TRAINING

Respiratory exercise
Strengthening of auxiliary respiratory muscles
Blowing up balloons
Blowing ping-pong balls in the pool to a designated target

Endurance training
Quick walking with increase of heart rate to 130 beats per minute, maximal 100 plus age − 20% for 10 minutes
Swimming: 10 minutes swimming without a break

treatment (subscore 4), modified stage rating according to Hoehn and Yahr (subscore 5), and rating of independence in daily living (subscore 6). In addition, all patients performed a walking test (2 × 10 m walking with two 180-degree turns). Psychometric data were registered using the Mini Mental Status Examination (MMSE) for dementia and Zeersen's Adjective Mood Questionnaire and the Sickness Impact Profile (SIP) for subjective well-being. The complete test battery was performed on all patients.

Patients improved clearly on the UPDRS scale in motor function and activities of daily living and showed reduced duration and severity of dyskinesia. Walking time decreased significantly during the training period. The basic motor test, which assessed strength, coordination, and flexibility without the risk of being contaminated by improvement in mood, showed a significant improvement. At the beginning of the training period only three patients were able to rise from a chair with one leg support, whereas by the end of the training period 10 patients were able to perform the task. All patients were able to stand up from a supine position. All patients could keep their balance on a Pezzi ball. All patients managed 10 minutes of quick walking, and 80% of the patients managed 10 minutes of swimming. There was only a minimal loss of regained motor skills 6 weeks after termination of intensive exercise therapy focused on sports activity. A sustained ongoing effect outlasting the active training period for at least 6 weeks could be achieved.

As expected, due to the increased social activity of the exercise sessions, the patients felt better emotionally. However, results of the motor assessment with the BMT makes us confident that the improvement of motor function was not only due to psychological aspects. Three of our patients with PD were able to perform exercises on a higher intensity level and were able to manage cardiovascular endurance training. One patient played tennis with a healthy partner twice a week for about 1 hour, and two patients were able to run at a speed of 5 min/km for 10 km twice a week. All three patients were very well controlled with medication and did not experience fluctuations of motor disability. In this study patients with PD exercised twice per week. For improvement of cardiovascular endurance one should aim for at least three training sessions per week (Box 17.1).

Neurons of the striatum and the substantia nigra pars compacta change their firing patterns during sensory motor learning. To study the role of dopamine and dopamine depletion for learning and memory of motor sequences macaque monkeys were subjected to unilateral lesions using N-Methyl-4-phenyl-1,2,3,6-tetrahydropyridine (MPTP). Two groups of monkeys were compared, one of which learned the sequential push button task before the lesion was inflicted and the other group after lesioning. Performances of the task first with the arm ipsilateral and then with the one contralateral to the lesion were compared. Reaction time, single and serial movement times for the push button movements, electromyographic activity of the arm, orofacial movements, and reward licking and saccadic eye movements during movement were recorded. Monkeys that learned the motor sequence after lesioning showed progressive shortening of movement times and performed the motor sequences after some trial with perfect hand–orofacial and hand–eye coordination. The movement became automatic and predictive. Task performance with the arm contralateral to the lesion showed clear motor and coordination deficits. The monkey did not develop automatic movements with this arm. Monkeys that were trained on this task before lesioning were skilled on this task with both arms before lesioning. The unilateral MTPT lesion produced severe movement impairment of the arm contralateral to the lesion. However, in contrast to the monkeys that learned the task after lesioning, their performance with the contralateral arm improved greatly with time. This finding suggests that the striatum and nigrostriatal system are more involved in the initial learning of movement than in remembering movements. If these results are applicable to human patients with PD, those with highly developed motor skills should be able to cope better with the motor deficits, and motor training started at an early stage of the disease should improve motor function (85).

draw the attention of the patient to the gait performance are of additional help. Patients learn to be more aware of using compensatory strategies to manage tasks and to overcome slowness by using external cues. This does not improve self-cued movement, however—the withdrawal of external cues will always result in deterioration of the performance (29, 81).

Improvement of axial flexibility and truncal muscle strength helps patients to get an upright posture, which helps respiratory function. In a second step, increase of cardiovascular endurance can be targeted. A recent study showed improvement of pulmonary function after an exercise program in patients with PD (82). Because the test results have shown that patients with PD have a response to exercise similar to that of healthy controls, the same pathophysiological consideration can be applied. Improvement of motor function and optimization of medication should normalize the increased submaximal heart rate, oxygen consumption, and increased RER. Improvement of cardiovascular performance depends on regular exercise at an appropriate intensity level to decrease resting heart rate and to increase peak aerobic capacity. The increase in daily physical activity encouraged by better motor function will contribute to increase of cardiovascular performance, but regular endurance training will be essential. The effect of chronic exercise on central levodopa storage in humans is not known. Chaouloff (83) found in rats an increase of dopamine release and turnover during exercise and a decreased **dopamine turnover** after exercise due to D_2-receptor hypersensitivity. A reduced dopamine turnover decreases the production of hydroxyl radicals and, consequently, the oxidative stress. If Chaouloff's results were applicable in human beings, one might speculate that exercise had neuroprotective potency.

Mechanism of Exercise Benefit in Parkinson Disease

Several peripheral parameters lead to improvement in motor performance in PD. Improvement of muscle strength and range of movements enabled patients to move more smoothly and quickly. Reduction of muscle rigidity and dyskinesias and better muscle coordination increases economy of movement and reduces energy expenditure. The decrease in walking time shown in the Webster Second Step Test indicates that the sequences of complex movements such as gait are not primarily destroyed, but range and speed of movement and movement sequence are disturbed. Improvement in movement range of the hip, knee, and ankle and increase of quadriceps strength and heel strike provide the prerequisites for gait normalization. Improvement in balance enables patients to increase the time of one-leg support in the gait cycle. External cues that

Clinical Tips

Patients with PD often are very anxious at the beginning of exercise training. Many patients feel more secure if their spouse accompanies them and takes part in the program. A secondary advantage is that the spouse then can perform some of the exercises with the patient at home between the sessions. The partner's presence is especially important for patients with cognitive decline or psychiatric symptoms. The exercise area should not be too far from the changing rooms and the bathrooms, because patients with PD need more time for changing and often need to use the toilet during the training session. Ideally a physiotherapist or sports therapist and a physician are present during the sessions. For good supervision, especially in water, and for help with the exercises a ratio of one therapist to six patients is recommended. There should be no spot in the swimming pool where the water is too deep for patients to stand, and a railing should be in place. Factors for further consideration are listed in Table 17.5.

TABLE 17.5. GUIDELINES FOR EXERCISE IN PARKINSON DISEASE

Category	Guidelines
Frequency of exercise training	At least two times per week, preferably 3-4 times per week
Duration	45 to 60 minutes
Intensity	50% to 70% of peak heart rate—if VO_{2max} is measured, 50% to 70% of VO_{2max}, according to own experience
	Begin with about 50% to 60% of maximal heart rate or VO_{2max}
Special considerations	Medication optimized
	Dopaminergic medication available during training for sudden "off" state
	Sufficient fluid intake to avoid dehydration
	Appropriate sweat-absorbing training suit
	Temperature in gymnasium about 20°C: if too hot, patient will have impaired if too cold, patient will experience increased muscle tone
	Water temperature in pool 25–30°C to avoid increase of rigidity
Preferable exercise activity	Gymnastics, walking, dancing, bicycle ergometry, swimming
	Ball games, mountain or racing bicycle

What We Know
About Parkinson Disease

1 Parkinson disease is the most common neurodegenerative disease, and the risk of PD increases with age.

2 The main clinical features of PD are tremor, rigidity, bradykinesia, and loss of postural reflexes, but there is also an involvement of the autonomous nervous system. Impaired cardiovascular reflexes can cause abnormal cardiac response to exercise.

3 Initiation and maintenance of movements as well as complex movements such as sequential and simultaneous movements are impaired in PD.

4 Dopaminergic medication can cause deterioration in cardiac function.

5 The cardiovascular response of patients with PD to exercise is similar to that of healthy subjects in terms of maximal oxygen consumption and maximal heart rate. However, thorough analyses of test results have shown that patients with PD have higher submaximal VO_2 values and higher submaximal heart rates.

6 The aim of exercise therapy in PD is to keep the patients on a high functional level, to avoid secondary deficits, and to improve motor function.

7 The approach to physical treatment in PD must be comprehensive and should include assessment of motor disability, general health, mental state, and drug treatment.

8 Exercise treatment can improve flexibility, balance, strength, coordination, and cardiovascular endurance. Social isolation decreases and patients improve in mood.

What We Would Like to Know
About Parkinson Disease

1 Why do patients with PD reduce physical activity significantly, even in early stages of the disease?

2 Is there any long-term effect of physical exercise on levodopa pharmacokinetic data or an effect on storage capacity in the central compartment?

3 Does long-term exercise treatment influence the central dopamine turnover?

4 Morris (27, 28) showed that patients with PD maintained their improved gait for 2 hours after gait training using external cues. Is it possible to develop a training program that provides a long-term improvement of gait and complex movements?

5 Are there any strategies to replace internal cueing?

6 How specific to PD pathophysiology are the so-called PD-specific exercises?

7 What level of physical fitness could patients with PD attain if they exercised three to four times per week and if they began exercise training early in the course of the disease?

8 Could cardiovascular side effects of dopaminergic medication become a risk to the health of patients with PD when they exercise at a high intensity level?

Summary

Exercise treatment and sports therapy cannot cure PD and cannot overcome the central dopamine deficit. However, secondary complications can be avoided and motor symptoms ameliorated so that patients with PD are able to use the full range of remaining motor function. Physical treatment in PD requires a comprehensive approach (84). Patients with PD need assessment of their motor disability; their general health, including concomitant diseases; their autonomic nervous system function; and their medications. The physical treatment must be supported by optimization of dopaminergic medication. Cognitive and psychiatric status have to be considered. Psychological factors, general (i.e., nonspecific to the pathophysiology of PD), and PD-specific exercises contribute to improvement of motor function. Cardiovascular endurance can be improved in a second step based on improved motor function. A decrease in mortality with increase of physical activity in PD is reported (84).

DISCUSSION QUESTIONS

1 Should exercise training for patients with PD be hospital- or community-based? Should it be arranged by patient support groups or privately?

2 How should the funding be provided—by public health system or privately?

3 When should exercise training be started—in an early or in a more advanced stage of the disease? Who should be treated: patients with PD who are stable, patients who are deteriorating, patients with concomitant diseases, young or elderly, patients with family support, or only those without family support?

4 Would it be useful for patients with PD to receive an intensive 2- to 4-week treatment course in a rehabilitation unit each year?

5 What implications does PD have for the patient's family?

6 How do PD patients cope with a disease that is so treatment-intensive and disabling?

7 Which trials are necessary and how should they be designed to develop an exercise training that is specific to motor deficits in PD?

CASE STUDY

Patient Information

Mr. S. is a 57-year-old man who was diagnosed with Parkinson disease 5 years ago. He had difficulties in accepting the diagnosis and gave up his previous very active lifestyle. He is no longer engaged in physical exercise and has put on some weight. He has reduced his working hours to 30 hours per week and is considering retiring. His medication is Sinemet-Plus (a combination of carbidopa and levodopa), 4 tablets per day plus pergolide, 4 mg/day. He complains about stiffness in the morning, difficulties in rising from a chair, and one severe "off" period in the early afternoon. Sometimes he cannot do anything from 2 PM to 7 PM. He complains of a lot of pain and no longer feels like his normal self. His physician suggested that he join a PD group and try some physical training.

Assessment

On examination Mr. S. was slightly overweight. His blood pressure was normal, and his heart rate was slightly tachycardic with 100 bpm and some irregularity. Blood tests were normal. Neurologic assessment showed a bent-forward posture, slow gait with difficulty in turning around, and rigidity more right than left, moderate to severe. Mild tremor, predominant on the right side more than left, persists on movements. The stage of the disease was rated as Hoehn & Yahr stage 3. Psychological assessment reveals mild depression.

On exercise testing, Mr. S. had an increased heart rate (170 bpm) in response to exercise, a blood pressure response slightly lower than expected, and high submaximal VO_2. He sweated profusely during the test and felt lightheaded and rather faint. In addition, he complained of burning thigh muscles. The test was stopped at 80 W.

*About 30% of patients with PD suffer from autonomous disturbances, which can influence adaptation to exercise. Autonomic impairment can manifest as impaired cardiovascular reflexes; faulty temperature regulation including sweating; arrhythmias; and impaired blood pressure regulation. Impaired blood pressure regulation can result in exercise-induced hypotension. Patients are more likely to suffer from autonomous disturbances in the more advanced stages of PD. Some patients diagnosed with PD suffer from a different type of neurodegenerative disease called **multisystem atrophy, Parkinsonian type (MSA-P)**. These patients present with parkinsonian features, but respond less to medication and show severe autonomous disturbances early in the course of the disease. Treatment of these patients is difficult because they often cannot tolerate the dosage of dopaminergic medication that they would need for motor improvement. Remember: dopaminergic medication can worsen cardiac function and provoke arrhythmias.*

Some patients with PD suffer cognitive impairment. They may not remember exercise instructions or how to use an exercise machine. Therefore, if patients with cognitive impairment participate in training, a person should be allocated to these patients to repeat instructions, to operate the exercise machines, and to check the workload. Patients with cognitive impairment tend to be anxious, especially in new environment, are prone to panic, and get lost easily in less familiar surrounding. The presence of a familiar person like the spouse or a friend is often helpful.

Questions

1. How do you interpret Mr. S.'s exercise test results and what happened during the test?

2. Are there any considerations to be taken in account before beginning an exercise program for Mr. S., or do you think that the patient could start an exercise program immediately?

3. Which exercise program do you suggest?

REFERENCES

1. Parkinson J. An essay on the shaking palsy. London: Sherwood, Neely and Jones, 1817.
2. Tanner CM. Epidemiological clues to the cause of Parkinson's disease. Mov Dis 1993;3:124–146.
3. Gibb WR, Lees AJ. Pathological clues to the cause of Parkinson's disease. Mov Dis 1994;3:147–166.
4. Seidler A, Hellenbrand W, Robra BP, et al. Possible environmental, occupational, and other etiologic factors for Parkinson's disease: a case control study in Germany. Neurology 1996;46:1275–1284.
5. Mitchell IJ, Boyce MA, Sambrock MA, Crossman AR. A 2-desoxyglucose study of the effects of dopamine agonists on the Parkinsonian primate brain. Implications for the neural mechanism that mediate dopamine agonist induced dyskinesia. Brain 1992;115:809–824.
6. Polymeropoulos MH. Autosomal dominant Parkinson's disease. J Neurol 1998;245 (11 suppl 3):1–3.
7. Kitada T, Asakawa S, Hattori N, et al. Mutations in the Parkin gene cause autosomal recessive juvenile parkinsonism. Nature 1998;392:605–608
8. Gasser T, Müller-Myhsok B, Wszolek ZK, et al. A susceptibility locus for Parkinson's disease maps to chromosome 2p13. Nat Genet 1998;18:262–265.
9. Farrer M, Gwinn-Hardy K, Muenter M, et al. A chromosome 4p haplotype segregating with Parkinson's disease and postural tremor. Hum Mol Genet 1999;1:81–85.
10. Parent A, Hazrati LN. Functional anatomy of the basal ganglia. I The cortico-basal-ganglia-thalamo-cortical loop. Brain Res Rev 1995;20:91–127.
11. Parent A, Hazrati LN. Functional anatomy of the basal ganglia. II The place of the subthalamic nucleus and external pallidum in basal ganglia circuitry. Brain Res Rev 1995;20: 128–154.
12. Marsden CD, Obeso JA. The functions of the basal ganglia and the paradox of stereotaxic surgery in Parkinson's disease. Brain 1994;117: 877–897.
13. Gerfen CR. The neostriatal mosaic: multiple levels of compartmental organization. Trends Neurosci 1992;15:133–139.
14. Gerfen CR, Engber TM, Mahan LC, et al. D1 and D2 dopamine receptor regulated gene expression of striatonigral and striatopallidal neurons. Science 1990;250:1429–1432.
15. Alexander GE, Crutcher MD, DeLong MR. Basal ganglia-thalamocortical circuits: parallel substrates for motor, oculomotor, prefrontal and limbic functions. Prog Brain Res 1990;85:119–146.
16. DeLong MR, Georgopoulos AP, Crutcher MD, et al. Functional organization of the basal ganglia: contribution of single cell-recording studies. Ciba Found Symp 1984;107:64–82.
17. Mitchell SJ, Richardson RT, Baker FH, DeLong MR. The primate globus pallidus: neuronal activity related to direction of movement. Exp Brain Res 1987;68:491–505.
18. Alexander GE, Crutcher MD. Functional architecture of basal ganglia circuits: neural substrates of parallel processing. Trends Neurosci 1990;13:266–271.
19. Gerfen CR. The neostriatal mosaic: compartmentalization of corticostriatal input and striatonigral output system. Nature 1984;311:461–469.
20. Brotchie P, Iansek R, Horne MK. Motor function of the monkey globus pallidus. 2. Cognitive aspects of movement and phasic neuronal activity. Brain 1991;114:1685–1702.

21. DeLong MR, Alexander GE, Georgopoulos AP, et al. Role of the basal ganglia in limb movements. Human Neurobiology 1984;2:235–244.

22. Chevalier G, Deniau JM. Disinhibition as a basic process in the expression of striatal functions. Trends Neurosci 1990;13:277–280.

23. DeLong MR, Crutcher MD, Georgopoulos AP. Primate globus pallidus and subthalamic nucleus: functional organization. J Neurophysiol 1985;53:530–543.

24. Georgopoulos AP, DeLong MR, Crutcher MD. Relations between parameters of step-tracking movements and single cell recording in the globus pallidus and subthalamic nucleus of the behaving monkey. J Neurosci 1983;3:1586–1598.

25. Hikosaka O, Wurtz RH. Visual and oculomotor functions of monkey substantia nigra pars reticulata. IV Relation of substantia nigra to superior colliculus. J Neurophysiol 1983;49:1285–1301.

26. Lungberg T, Apicella P, Schultz W. Response of monkey dopamine neurons during learning of behavioural reactions. J Neurophysiol 1992;67:145–163.

27. Morris ME, Iansek R, Matyas TA, Summers JJ. The pathogenesis of gait hypokinesia in Parkinson's disease. Brain 1994;117:1169–1181.

28. Morris ME, Iansek R, Matyas TA, Summers JJ. Stride length regulation in Parkinson's disease. Normalization strategies and underlying mechanism. Brain 1996;119:551–568.

29. Georgiou N, Bradshaw JL, Iansek R, et al. Reduction in external cues and movement sequencing in Parkinson's disease. J Neurol Neurosurg Psychiatry 1994;57:368–370.

30. Martin KE, Phillips JG, Iansek R, Bradshaw JL. Inaccuracy and instability of sequential movements in Parkinson´s disease. Exp Brain Res 1994;102:131–140.

31. Phillips JG, Martin KE, Bradshaw J, Iansek R. Could bradykinesia in Parkinson's simply be compensation. J Neurol 1994;241:439–447.

32. Bridgewater KJ, Sharpe MH. Trunk muscle performance in early Parkinson's disease. Physical Therapy 1998;78:566–576.

33. Corcos DM, Chen C-M, Quinn NP, et al. Strength in Parkinson's disease: relationship to rate of force generation and clinical status. Ann Neurol 1996;36:76–88.

34. Pedersen SW, Oberg B. Dynamic strength in Parkinson's disease: quantitative measurements following withdrawal of medication. Eur Neurol 1993;33:97–102.

35. Yanagawa S, Shindo M, Yanagisawa N: Muscular weakness in Parkinson's disease. Adv Neurol 1990;53:259–269.

36. Knutsson E. An analysis of Parkinsonian gait. Brain 1972;95:475–486.

37. Koike Y, Takahashi A. Autonomic dysfunction in Parkinson's disease. Eur Neurol 1997;38(suppl 2):8–12.

38. Mastrocola C, Vanacore W, Giovani A, et al. Twenty-four-hour heart rate variability to assess autonomic function in Parkinson's disease. Acta Neurol Scand 1999;99:245–247.

39. Braune S, Reinhardt M, Bathmann J, et al. Impaired cardiac uptake of meta [123J] iodobenzylguanidine in Parkinson's disease with autonomic failure. Acta Neurol Scand 1998;97:307–314.

40. Reuter I, Ellis CM, Ray Chaudhuri K. Nocturnal subcutaneous apomorphine infusion in Parkinson's disease and restless legs syndrome. Acta Neurol Scand 1999;100:163–167.

41. Yamada H, Murahashi M, Takahashi H, et al. Respiratory function impairment in patients with Parkinson's disease—a consideration on the possible pathogenetic relation to autonomic dysfunction. Rinsho Shinkeigabu-Clinical Neurology 2000;40:125–130.

42. Neu HC, Connolly JJ, Schwertley FW, et al. Obstructive respiratory dysfunction in Parkinson's patients. Am Rev Respir Dis 1967;95:33–47.

43. Lyall RA, Reuter I, Mills J, et al. Effects of acute subcutaneous apomorphine in Parkinson's disease [abstract]. Mov Dis 1998;13(suppl 2):177.

44. Levy G, Tang MX, Cote LJ, et al. Motor impairment in PD: relationship to incident dementia. Neurology 2000;55(4):539–544.

45. Hughes TA, Ross HF, Musa S, et al. A 10-year study of the incidence of and factors predicting dementia in Parkinson's disease. Neurology 2000;54:1596–1602.

46. Riley DE, Lang AE, Blair RDG, et al. Frozen shoulder and other shoulder abnormalities in Parkinson's disease. J Neurol Neurosurg Psychiatry 1988;52:63–66.

47. Hughes AJ, Daniel SE, Kilford L, Lees AJ. Accuracy of clinical diagnosis of idiopathic Parkinson's disease: a clinico-pathological study of 100 cases. J Neurol Neurosurg Psychiatry 1992;55:181–184.

48. Fahn S, Elton RL. Members of the UPDRS Development Committee: Unified Parkinson's Disease Rating Scale. In: Fahn S, Marsden CD, Calne DB, Goldstein M (eds). Recent Developments in Parkinson's Disease. Florham Park, NJ: Macmillan, 1987:2:153–163, 293–304

49. Matsui TA, Nishikawa S, Saigo K, et al. Problem in prolonged levodopa administration of Parkinson's disease patients-from the standpoint of the autonomic nervous function. Rinsho Shinkeigaku-Functional Neurology 1998;38:295–300.

50. Olanow CW, Myllyla VV, Sotaniemi KA. Effect of selegiline on mortality in patients with Parkinson's disease. A meta analysis. Neurology 1998;51:825–830.

51. Lees AJ. Comparison of therapeutic effects and mortality data of levodopa combined with selegiline in patients with early, mild Parkinson's disease. Br Med J 1995;311:1602–1607.

52. Ben Shlomo Y, Churchyard A, Head J, et al. Investigation by Parkinson's disease research group of United Kingdom into excess treatment seen with combined levodopa and selegiline treatment in patients with early, mild Parkinson's disease: Further results of randomised trial and confidential inquiry. Br Med J 1998;316:1191–1196.

53. Benabid AL, Koudsie A, Pollak P, et al. Future prospects of brain stimulation. Neurol Res 2000;22:237–246.

54. Reuter I, Engelhardt M, Freiwaldt J, Baas H. Exercise test in Parkinson's disease. Clin Autonom Res 1999;9:129–134.

55. Mouradian MM, Juncos JL, Serrati C, et al. Exercise and antiparkinsonian response to levodopa. Clin Neuropharmacol 1987;10:351–355.

56. Carter JH, Nutt JG, Woodward WR. The effect of exercise on levodopa absorption. Neurology 1992;42:2042–2045.

57. Goetz CG, Thelen JA, Macleod CM, et al. Blood levodopa levels and Unified Parkinson's Disease Rating Scale function: with and without exercise. Neurology 1993;43:1040–1042.

58. Reuter I, Harder S, Engelhardt M, Baas H. Pharmacodynamics and pharmacokinetics of levodopa under rest and exercise. Mov Dis 2000;15:862–868.

59. Smith GDP, Watson LP, Pavitt DV, Matthias CJ. Abnormal cardiovascular and catecholamine responses to supine exercise in human subjects with sympathetic dysfunction. J Physiol 1995;484:225–265.

60. Stanley RK, Protas EJ, Jankovic J. Exercise performance in those having Parkinson's disease and healthy normals. Med Sci Sports Exerc 1999;31:761–766.

61. Protas EJ, Stanley RK, Jankovic J, MacNeal B. Cardiovascular and metabolic responses to upper and lower extremity exercise in men with idiopathic Parkinson's disease. Phys Ther 1996;76:34–40.

62. Canning CG, Alison JA, Allen NE, Groeller H. Parkinson's disease: an investigation of exercise capacity, respiratory function, and gait. Arch Phys Med Rehabil 1997;78:199–207.

63. Shephard RJ. Physical Activity and Aging. Rockville: Aspen Publishers, 1987:97;16–29.

64. American College of Sports Medicine. Position stand: The recommended quantity and quality of exercise for developing and maintaining cardiorespiratory and muscular fitness, and flexibility in healthy adults. Med Sci Sports Exerc 1998;30:975–991.

65. Bindoff LA, Birch Machin MA, Cartlidge NEF, et al. Respiratory chain abnormalities in skeletal muscle from patients with Parkinson's disease. J Neurol Sci 1991;104:203–208.

66. Nakagawa-Hattori Y, Yoshino H., Kondo T, et al. Is Parkinson's disease a mitochondrial disorder? J Neurol Sci 1992;107:29–33.

67. Schapira AHV. Evidence for mitochondrial dysfunction in Parkinson's disease—a critical appraisal. Mov Dis 1994;9:125–138.

68. Comella CL, Stebbins GT, Brown-Toms N, Goetz CG. Physical therapy and Parkinson's disease. Neurology 1994;44:376–378.

69. Wroe M, Greer M. Parkinson's disease and physical therapy management. Phys Ther 1973;53:849–854.

70. Formisano R, Pratesi L, Modarelli FT, et al. Rehabilitation and Parkinson's disease. Scand J Rehab Med 1992;24:157–160.

71. Palmer SS, Mortimer JA, Webster DD, et al. Exercise therapy for Parkinson's disease. Arch Phys Med Rehabil 1986;67:741–745.

72. United Parkinson Foundation: Exercise Program. Chicago: United Parkinson Foundation, 1984

73. Schenkman M, Cutson TM, Kuchibhatla M, et al. Exercise to improve spinal flexibility and function for people with Parkinson's disease: a randomized, controlled trial. J Am Geriatr Soc 1998;46:1207–1216.

74. Viliani T, Pasquetti P, Magnolfi S, et al. Effects of physical training on straightening-up process in patients with Parkinson's disease. Disability and Rehabilitation 1999;21:68–73.

75. Gibberd FB, Page NGR, Spencer KM, et al. Controlled trial of physiotherapy and occupational therapy for Parkinson's disease. Br Med J 1981;282:1196.

76. Shumway-Cook A, Gruber W, Baldwin M, Liao S. The effect of multidimensional exercises on balance, mobility, and fall risk in community-dwelling older adults. Phys Ther 1997;77:46–57.

77. Thaut MH, McIntosh GC, Rice RR, et al. Rhythmic stimulation in gait training for Parkinson's disease patients. Mov Dis 1996;11:193–200.

78. McIntosh GC, Brown SH, Rice RR, Thaut MH. Rhythmic auditory motor facilitation of gait patterns in patients with Parkinson's disease. J Neurol Neurosurg Psychiatry 1997;62:22–26.

79. Burleigh-Jacobs A, Horak FB, Nutt JG, Obeso JA. Step initiation in Parkinson's disease: influence of levodopa and external sensory triggers. Mov Disord 1997;12:206–215.

80. Bös K, Wydra G, Karisch G. Motorische Basisdiagnostik. In: Gesundheitsförderung durch Bewegung, Spiel und Sport. Ziele und Methoden des Gesundheitssports in der Klinik. Erlangen: Perimed-Fachbuch-Verlagsgesellschaft mbH, 1992:122–136.

81. Azulay JP, Mesure S, Amblard B, et al. Visual control of locomotion in Parkinson's disease. Brain 1999;122:111–120.

82. Köseoğlu F, İnan L, Özel S, et al. The effects of a pulmonary rehabilitation program on pulmonary function tests and exercise tolerance in patients with Parkinson's disease. Funct Neurol 1997;12:319–325.

83. Chaouloff F. Physical exercise and brain monamines: a review. Acta Physiol Scand 1989;137:1–13.

84. Kuroda K, Tatara K, Takatorige T, Shinsho F: Effect of physical exercise on mortality in patients with Parkinson's disease. Acta Neurol Scand 1992;86:55–59.

85. Matsumoto N, Hanakawa T, Maki S, et al. Role of [corrected] nigrostriatal dopamine system in learning to perform sequential movement tasks in a predictive manner. J Neurophys 1999;82:978–998.

CHAPTER 18

Polio

Thomas J. Birk, Edward C. Nieshoff

Overview

Poliomyelitis is an acute infectious disease caused by an enteric virus that was prevalent in epidemic proportions during the 1940s and 1950s in North America (1, 2). Once ingested the virus crosses the blood–brain barrier, and central nervous system damage can be expected. In addition to having devastating effects on the motor neurons in the spinal cord, the infection and subsequent inflammatory response also injure **motor cortex** and **premotor corticol** sections in the brain (3). During an acute 2-week period fever, headache, sore throat, severe muscle pain sensitive to touch and stretch, and flaccid muscle paresis or paralysis are common. Progressive weakness and fatigue of muscle fibers abandoned by destroyed

motor neurons as a result of **wallerian degeneration** became increasingly evident. In most cases, by the end of this 2-week period ventral horn cells either have been destroyed or appear normal on microscopic examination (2).

Motor neurons that survive the acute phase, either partially or fully, eventually help to produce an increase in muscle strength during the recovery period. Some of the abandoned or "orphaned" muscle fibers eventually become reinnervated by surviving motor neurons over a period of several years (4). This **terminal sprouting** process results in increased numbers of myofibers being reinnervated by each motor neuron, with surviving motor units increasing in size as much as seven-fold (4). The degree of recovery is related to the percentage of motor neurons affected. If 50% or fewer of the total motor neurons are damaged, either partially or completely, recovery is more rapid and sustained.

At some point years after the acute bout, myofiber hypertrophy and transformation are likely to occur. Muscle fibers increase in size to more than twice that of normal muscle tissue. **Type II fibers** (**fast-twitch**) become almost nonexistent, as they eventually transform into **type I fibers** (**slow-twitch**). These adaptations occur secondary to severe demands placed on the muscle, both by extreme weakness and prolonged use for activities of daily living (ADLs) (1).

The virus did not have the same acute impact on everyone who contracted it. Clinically, polio is classified into four forms or types: paralytic, nonparalytic, subclinical, and abortive.

The most severe form, paralytic polio, inflicts the most severe damage to the ventral horn of the lower motor neurons of the spinal cord and results in **muscle tremors**, **flaccid paresis**, paralysis, weakness, subsequent **atrophy**, fatigue, and pain (5). In most survivors of paralytic polio who had these symptoms, more than 50% of the motor neurons were damaged or destroyed (6).

A second clinical presentation is nonparalytic polio. Despite the name, muscle paralysis and weakness do occur in this type, both early in the course of the disease and again many years after the acute infection. The acute clinical signs and symptoms include pain in the back, abdomen, neck and limbs, along with fever, lethargy, vomiting, and irritability. However, these symptoms resolve rapidly, except for some muscle sensitivity and spasm, and there is no prolonged weakness or atrophy immediately following the illness as in the paralytic type. The transient nature of the symptoms probably has led to an underestimation of the severity of the underlying disease (7); however, greater neuronal damage than initially suspected has been shown in affected survivors (8, 9).

Two other less severe forms of polio are the subclinical and abortive types. A person with subclinical polio is unaware of the infection. This form usually occurs in very young children, and there are no physical signs or symptoms of the disease. Abortive polio primarily affects the respiratory and gastrointestinal systems. Symptoms include sore throat and fever, vomiting, diarrhea, and constipation. However no physical or skeletal muscle problems other than these short-lived symptoms are reported.

For most survivors of paralytic polio and probably some of the survivors of the more severe nonparalytic type, the approximately 15-year recovery period generally is clinically uneventful. These survivors can perform ADLs and most physical activities without undue strain or fatigue. However, at some point the remaining motor neurons are unable to generate new sprouts and denervation exceeds reinnervation (Figure 18.1). What follows is a slow but progressive loss in muscle strength that is disproportionate to that seen with normal aging (10, 11). Symptoms such as fatigue, weakness, pain, muscle atrophy, cold intolerance, and difficulty in completing ADLs become evident. **Muscle fasciculations**, spasms, and cramps are experienced as well. These

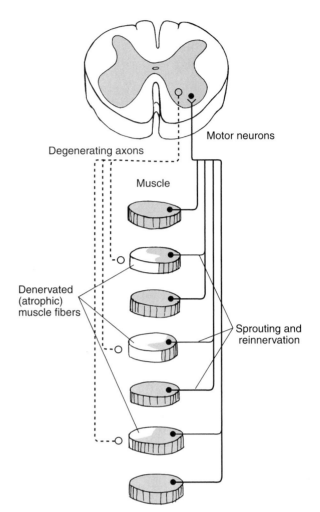

FIGURE 18.1.   Denervation and reinnervation of muscle fibers.

clinical manifestations return for many survivors of paralytic polio anywhere from 15 to 40 years after acute infection (1).

A greater incidence of late symptoms has been documented in paralytic polio survivors (7). However, even in nonparalytic cases, especially in those patients whose motor neuron level has dropped below 50%, symptoms of muscle pain, weakness, and fatigue may appear. This return of clinical signs and symptoms has been termed *post-polio syndrome* (PPS) (12). Not every polio survivor experiences the return of the original symptoms many years after virus onset, and the factors that lead to development of PPS have not been fully elucidated. However, speculation regarding the etiology has led to the proposal of several possible mechanisms.

Pathophysiology of Post-Polio Syndrome

Post-polio syndrome may result from premature aging and the death of motor neurons originally damaged by the polio virus. A distal degeneration and gradual loss of muscle fibers may occur within motor units. Premature destruction of the motor neurons of surviving motor units also may be a consequence of excessively elevated metabolic demand (2, 10). Evidence suggests that although abandoned muscle fibers are incorporated into surviving motor units, a critical juncture is reached at which motor units no longer can exert their trophic influence on all of the muscle fibers. The result is diminished motor unit capacity due to death of muscle fibers (10).

The symptoms of PPS vary depending on the initial magnitude and subsequent rate of muscle fiber orphaning. For example, a recently diagnosed patient may have considerable initial muscle fiber loss but in the future exhibit a much slower muscle fiber reduction. Another patient may have only a moderate initial reduction in muscle fibers (but still lower than 50% of total motor neurons) where weakness becomes symptomatic, however, but later show a rapid loss and deterioration of muscle fibers.

Two subtypes of PPS have been recognized. Post-poliomyelitis progressive muscular atrophy (PPMA) usually is regarded as encompassing neurologic symptoms. In contrast, the symptoms of musculoskeletal post-poliomyelitis (MPPS) do not include weakness and atrophy from neurologic decline; consequently, this form has been less recognized as PPS. It may be that the wide variability in reported incidence of PPS is secondary to greater recognition of MPPS in some studies, in which the associated functional capacity deterioration is considered secondary to "wear and tear" on joints rather than to adverse neurologic changes (1).

Epidemiology and Risk of Post-Polio Syndrome

Post-polio syndrome appears to affect from 22% to 90% of the almost 1.8 million survivors of polio (Box 18.1) (13–15). As many as 40% of these individuals have indicated that fatigue has interfered significantly with work performance and completion (Figure 18.2). At least 25% have reported that fatigue also has interfered with performance

BOX 18.1.	**Relevant Statistics**

Did you know?
- The prevalence of post-polio syndrome (PPS) varies according to diagnostic process.
- Conservatively, it is estimated that there are approximately one-half million people in North America with PPS.
- Women with PPS have more symptoms in more bodily locations.
- The greatest risk of PPS is for those who had paralytic polio, especially when all four limbs were affected and the infection occurred after the age of 10.
- Neurologic symptoms appear first in the weakest limbs or bodily areas.

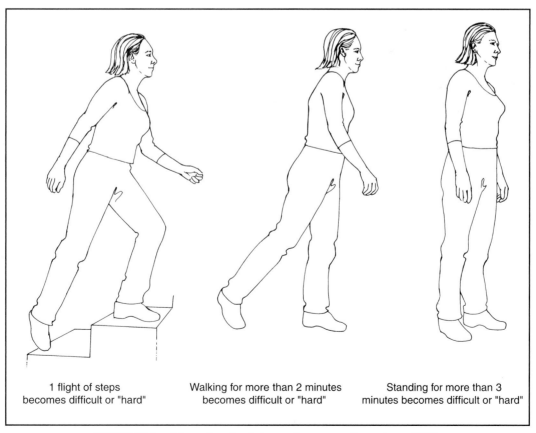

1 flight of steps becomes difficult or "hard"   Walking for more than 2 minutes becomes difficult or "hard"   Standing for more than 3 minutes becomes difficult or "hard"

FIGURE 18.2.   Adverse functional changes from post-polio syndrome (PPS).

of self-care activities (16). As polio survivors age, these problems become more pronounced.

The broad range of reported prevalence of PPS may be the result of variations in the diagnostic process. Some clinicians have defined the syndrome as any type of excessive fatigue and pain along with new weakness precipitating reduced function and quality of life (14). Others have proposed more specific criteria and included a requirement for atrophy coupled with new and increasing pain, fatigue, and weakness (15). Some clinicians have given the PPS designation only to limbs that develop muscular instability reflected in abnormal electromyography findings and weakness on physical examination (16). The more conservative estimates indicate that PPS affects up to approximately half a million survivors, beginning 15 to 40 or more years after the acute infection (1, 14).

Symptoms may vary with gender—women seem to have experienced pain for greater number of years and at more locations than men (13). In general, PPS-related pain is greatest in prevalence and intensity in the legs, back, and arms (15) (Figure 18.3). The pain usually is described as constant and throbbing in character with varying levels of intensity.

Post-polio syndrome occurs earlier when the original paralysis affected all four limbs, a ventilator is required due to breathing problems, hospitalization is necessary, and the original polio infection occurred after the age of 10 years (1). These risk factors are associated with the severity of acute poliomyelitis, and hypoventilation and breathing problems often are experienced as well. Neurologic symptoms often manifest themselves first in the areas that were most severely affected during the acute illness.

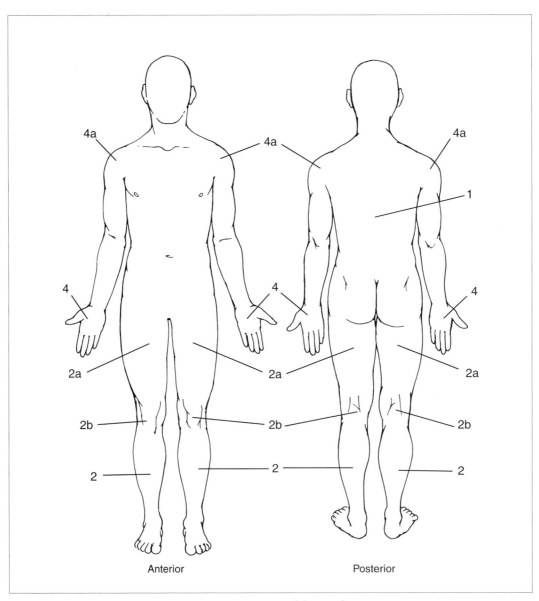

FIGURE 18.3.   Most painful areas of PPS.

The fatigue common to both paralytic and nonparalytic polio may be a result of injury to structures other than the ventral horn of the spinal cord. Changes in **reticular formation**, **hypothalamic** and **thalamic nuclei**, and **dopaminergic neurons** have been reported (14). These findings have contributed to development of a brain fatigue generator model (BFG), to explain not only the physical fatigue and weakness, but also the difficulties with concentration, memory, and attention that have been reported (14). The BFG model suggests that viral damage to reticular formation, hypothalamic and thalamic nuclei, and dopaminergic neurons diminishes cortical activity, thereby reducing information processing and impairing motor activity. Lower levels of dopamine have been found in PPS and added to the support for BFG model. Additional credence for the theory that depleted dopamine plays a part was gained when fatigue and diminished attention and memory in persons with PPS were improved with a dopamine receptor agonist medication (14).

Medications That May Be Useful for Post-Polio Syndrome

Several different types of medications have been prescribed and used for PPS. This section reports on the results of medications in reducing symptoms and the effects of these medications on exercise (Table 18.1).

Medications for Amelioration of Symptoms

Most of the medications prescribed for persons with PPS have been used for symptom reduction. Pain in soft tissue and joints has been addressed with nonsteroidal anti-inflammatory drugs (NSAIDs) and muscle relaxant medications. Other medications that have been prescribed for reduction of pain and fatigue include heterocyclic antidepressants (HA) and serotonin-specific reuptake inhibitors (SSRIs). These medications are used not only to reduce pain but also to facilitate anxiety reduction, thus enhancing overall relaxation and restful sleep. Additional medications such as prednisone, amantadine, pyridostigmine, and bromocriptine mesylate have been used in attempts to diminish fatigue and weakness and enhance physical performance.

It had been thought that prednisone, a corticosteroid, would be able to increase muscle strength in PPS, but follow-up results have been disappointing. Similarly, amantadine was purported to decrease muscle fatigue but was found to be ineffective after more rigorous evaluation (17). Results with pyridostigmine, an anticholinesterase drug that was touted to be able to improve neuromuscular transmission and reduce fatigue, also have been disappointing (18). Bromocriptine mesylate, a postsynaptic dopamine re-

ceptor agonist, has been studied regarding its effects on diminishing fatigue (14) and has been found to enhance attention, cognition, and memory. Although the variables studied were not physical parameters, there was improvement in fatigue at awakening and staying awake during the day. The reduced feeling of fatigue, common in some with PPS, may suggest less physical fatigue, at least during the morning hours after awakening.

Impact of Medications on the Exercise Response

Nonsteroidal anti-inflammatory medications and muscle relaxant drugs usually do not restrict acute or chronic exercise performance. Whereas the new SSRIs have relatively little overall effect on exercise performance, HA (also called tricyclic) antidepressants have been shown to increase heart rate and decrease blood pressure during both rest and exercise. Abnormalities on electrocardiogram (ECG) have included false-positive and false-negative exercise test results, T-wave changes. In addition, dysrhythmias have been reported with the use of HA antidepressants, especially in patients with a cardiac history. Pyridostigmine, amantadine, and bromocriptine would not be expected to significantly affect exercise performance. However, chronic use of prednisone can result in muscle atrophy, increased adipose tissue, and edema.

The Exercise Response

Acute physiologic responses to aerobic exercise have been varied and typically diminished for persons with PPS. This section discusses chronic exercise responses and training as well as resistive training responses and includes maximal and submaximal exercise testing guidelines for persons with PPS.

Typical Aerobic Responses to Exercise

The aerobic capacities of persons with PPS have been found to be lower than those of healthy controls matched for age and gender (1, 19). Exercise intensity levels may range from 2 to 9 METs, depending on peripheral limitations. Acute maximal or symptom-limited exercise can increase heart rate from 120 bpm to 180 bpm, depending on age and muscle mass utilization. Blood pressure responses during exercise generally have been similar to those of persons without PPS. Blood lactate responses have ranged from 2 to 8 mmol/L during maximal and symptom-limited exercise. Ventilatory responses generally have been up to 20% lower compared with persons without PPS (1). The **differentiated rate of perceived exertion** (RPE) also was found to be disproportionately ele-

TABLE 18.1. ACTIONS AND EFFECTS OF MEDICATIONS COMMONLY PRESCRIBED FOR PERSONS WITH POST-POLIO SYNDROME

Drug (generic/brand)	Actions	Indications	Exercise effects
HA Amitriptyline/Elavil, Endep, Vanatrip; Nortriptyline/ Aventyl, HCl, Pamelor; Doxepin/ Adapin, Sinequan	Blocks reuptake of norepinephrine and serotonin	Clinical depression; pain	No increase and in some cases a decrease in strength or endurance
NSAIDs Piroxicam/Feldene; ibuprofen/ Motrin; Naproxen/Naprosyn; Sulindac/Daypro; Aspirin	Inhibits prostaglandin synthesis	Muscle or joint pain	May increase if pain reduced; generally no effect
Muscle relaxants Metaxalone/Shelaxin; Methocarbamol/Robaxin;	Suppress nociceptive nerve impulses	Muscle stiffness, pain	No significant increases or decreases
SRRI Fluoxetine/Prozac, Sarafem	Blocks reuptake of serotonin	Clinical depression and bipolar disorders; bulimia; premenstrual dysphoric disorder	No increase and in some cases mild decrease in strength or endurance
Sertraline/Zoloft	Blocks reuptake of serotonin	Clinical depression and anxiety disorders; posttraumatic stress disorder	No increase and in some cases mild decrease in strength or endurance
Bromocriptine/Parlodel	Dopamine agonist	Muscle stiffness, tremors, spasms and poor control	No significant increase in strength or endurance
Amantadine/Symmetrel	Impairs ability of virus to uncoat RNA in host cells	Stiffness and shaking	No significant increase in strength or endurance
Prednisone/Deltasone	Inhibit inflammatory and immunologic responses and protein synthesis; stimulate formation of glucose	Reduce inflammation or block immunologic actions	Short-term: no decrease in strength or endurance, may be some increase in strength from relief of inflammation; long-term: use decreases strength and endurance
Pyridostigmine/no brand	Stimulates nicotinic receptors at neuromuscular junction and inactivate cholinesterase	Weakness of skeletal muscle	No significant, consistent increase in strength or endurance

PAC, premature atrial contraction; BP, blood pressure; CNS, central nervous system; HR, heart rate; MAOI, monoamine oxidase inhibitors; NSAIDs, nonsteroidal anti-inflammatory drugs; OTC, over-the-counter; PVC, premature ventricular contraction.

vated and inverse to exercise heart rate during stationary bicycling, suggesting peripheral limitation (20). The RPE focus has been on peripheral pain and fatigue and less on central cues such as dyspnea. Peak power outputs during four-limb ergometry have ranged from 15 to 200 watts (W) (21).

Measurements of combined central and peripheral responses have revealed that oxygen uptake was decreased and correlated with reduced muscle strength of the lower extremities when stationary bicycle exercise was used (22, 23). The correlation was particularly strong between muscle strength of legs and oxygen uptake (22), but the anaer-

obic threshold was not abnormally low compared to reduced maximal oxygen uptake. Together these data suggest that the reduced level of oxygen uptake was secondary to weak muscle function rather than a cardiorespiratory limitation: the diminished performance on the bicycle was limited by leg muscle weakness, thus keeping the oxygen uptake level lower and closer to the anaerobic threshold.

Further evidence of a relationship between lower extremity muscle strength and aerobic capacity also was found (22) when muscle strength was correlated (but not as strongly) with maximal walking speed. Indirect support for this idea has been suggested by the finding that persons

Side effects	Exercise heart rate and blood pressure	Exercise ECG	Interactions
Possible tachycardia, arrhythmia, hypotension, muscle stiffness and weakness	Increase to no effect for HR; decrease to no effect for BP	May result in false-positive or false-negative test through T-wave changes; possible ectopy	MAOI use can result in significant hypertension; use of other sedatives increases sedative effect
Possible muscle cramps, weakness, fluid retention	No effect	No effect	Other NSAIDs, anticoagulants, diuretics will increase effects; will decrease effects of ACE inhibitors
GI distress, headache, dizziness	No effect	No effect	Increased effects with antihistamines, codeine, narcotics, antidepressants
Possible arrhythmia, hyper- or hypotension, weakness	Possible increase in HR and BP or decrease in BP	May result in false-positive test; PACs, PVCs	MAOI use could result in dangerous arrhythmia; alcohol enhances hypotension
Possible arrhythmia, hyper- or hypotension, weakness	Possible increase in HR and BP or decrease in BP	May result in false-positive test; PACs, PVCs	MAOI use could result in dangerous arrhythmia or hypertension; alcohol enhances hypotension
Occasional orthostatic hypotension	May decrease BP	No effect	Albuterol and terbutaline use could increase hypotension
Orthostatic hypotension, possible muscle stiffness	May decrease BP	No effect	Phenothiazines and caffeine, decongestants may increase tremor
Short term: none; long-term: osteoporosis, edema, weight gain, decalcification of bone, loss of strength, increased blood pressure	May increase BP	No effect	Other immunosuppressive drugs could significantly depress immune function; OTC cold drugs could decrease effects
GI distress, cramps, salivation, sweating	No effect	No effect	If drug crosses blood-brain barrier can increase anxiety and tremor; these effects can be elevated by use of CNS stimulants

with PPS feel less fatigued and stronger after undertaking a walking program (24). Apparently walking, although more painful for some patients with osteoarthritis, was less symptomatic in this study.

Typical Aerobic Training Responses

Aerobic exercise training has resulted in significant increases in oxygen uptake during programs of stationary bicycling, walking, and arm cranking (1, 25, 26). These increases, which are similar to those found for persons who

had not had polio, occurred in aerobic exercise programs ranging in length from 8 to 22 weeks. No adverse effects from aerobic exercise training were reported.

Typical Resistive Training Responses

Lower extremity muscle strength, particularly loss of knee extensor strength, has been investigated extensively (1). There was concern about instituting resistive training, because of the fear that if it was too intensive it could result in quadriceps weakness when the already overextended motor neurons were overworked. However, significant increases in knee extensor strength without deleterious effects have been found after resistive training (26–28). These strength gains were seen over a period of 6 to 12 weeks, although in one study (27) the subjects appeared to be much stronger from the onset and less symptomatic. No increased muscle or joint pain or evidence of weakness was seen in these three studies using intensities that could be classified as a "moderate to hard" level of differentiated RPE.

Although most resistive training has not been detrimental, new lower extremity weakness and unstable skeletal muscle conditions have been found (20). Knee extension performance reductions were greater than expected after 4 years of follow-up assessment. In this study muscle volume of the legs also was found to be reduced in some but not all persons with PPS, and muscle strength losses were in greater proportion as compared to volume. For those with new or increased weakness, the muscle volume of the legs was consistently reduced.

Upper extremity strength and lower extremity flexor muscles also have shown to have decreased more than expected after 9 months (11). Although strength was measured with a dynamometer, which raises the question of the reliability of the results, the results suggest that there may be greater losses in lower extremity flexor musculature than originally expected. It may be that renewed effort should be directed to assessing and training flexor muscle groups rather than extensor groups of the lower extremity.

Is Maximal Exercise Testing Recommended?

Maximal or symptom-limited aerobic exercise testing is not necessary and is contraindicated in polio survivors with new weakness and unstable musculature. Although there are no published reports, maximal exercise testing conceivably could reduce the number of motor neurons. Fragile motor neurons already overburdened with excessive fiber sprouting could degenerate more rapidly in response to the large demand of high-intensity exercise (1). Unless cardiac disease is suspected and symptom-limited performance is necessary to determine coronary artery compliance to high levels of exercise, maximal exercise testing contributes more risk than benefit.

For some polio survivors without symptoms of weakness, pain, or fatigue, however, maximal exercise may be considered. Workloads of 10 to 25 W are suggested for the initial stage, with increases of 10 to 25 W for subsequent stages depending whether arm or leg ergometry is used. Workload stages of 2 to 4 minutes are recommended with a 2- to 4-minute recovery between each stage. A discontinuous graded or ramped protocol is suggested to maximize cardiopulmonary demand and minimize early skeletal muscle fatigue limitations. Peak power of up to 200 W, constituting low aerobic capacities, has been reported (21). Standard leg or arm ergometry can be used to obtain valid and reliable data (21). However, if the only objective for the test is to develop an exercise prescription or determine fitness program progress, a submaximal protocol is advised.

Submaximal testing protocols should follow the same initial workload and stage levels, but conclude at a predesignated point. The termination of the test could be based on a submaximal heart rate or RPE response. It also could be concluded by achievement of a predesignated workload. For efficiency, the length of the test should be restricted to approximately 6 continuous minutes over two to three graded or ramped stages. Walking tests, for those able, of up to 6 minutes could be used to estimate aerobic capacity (Box 18.2).

Muscle strength testing has included **isometric**, **isotonic**, and **isokinetic** techniques. Dynamometer isometric strength assessment of knee extensors is not able to detect small differences (29). However, isometric assessment was sensitive enough to find reduced hip abductor strength when compared to the asymptomatic leg (30). **Manual muscle testing** (MMT) and isometric testing with a dynamometer should include several repetitions, with each contraction being held for up to 10 seconds. **Open chain** isotonic and isometric testing of the quadriceps usually has been administered with the patient in a seated position (1). Isotonic assessment has included 5 to 10 RM, avoiding the excessive overexertion of testing with 1RM. Isokinetic testing, although done at low to high speeds, probably is more safely and practically conducted at speeds greater than 60 degrees per second. Limbs and muscle groups with a muscle grade less than 3/5 should not be assessed. A 3/5 grade is assigned when the person can move the limb only against gravity (Box 18.3).

Proper frequency of strength testing also must be considered. Testing sessions should be separated by more than 2 days, particularly if there were initial symptoms in unsta-

---

BOX 18.2. Aerobic Exercise Testing Guidelines

1. Maximal testing is contraindicated in persons with new weakness and unstable limbs or musculature.

2. Non–weight-bearing exercise (arm and/or leg ergometry) is advised for all modalities.

3. Maximal tests on asymptomatic persons with PPS should be discontinuous to maximize central and peripheral endurance. The preferred total exercise duration is 8 to 12 minutes.

4. Initial workloads of 10 to 25 W depending on the age and fitness of the patient are recommended, with increases of up to 25 W every 2 minutes until fatigue.

5. Submaximal tests should stop at a predetermined heart rate or RPE, and generally use the same modalities and follow the same initial workloads as maximal testing.

6. The duration of submaximal test should be approximately 6 minutes.

7. A 6-minute walking test can be administered for those with sufficient lower extremity function.

1. Manual muscle testing and isometric techniques are preferred if there is a history of weakness of limbs and musculature.
2. Several repetitions for up to 10 seconds should be included when using MMT and isometric techniques, which also will facilitate greater reliability and taxing of local endurance.
3. Isotonic assessment should be done if there is no history of weakness and the patient had a full recovery. This should include 5 to 10 RM to avoid overexertion of 1 RM.
4. Musculature with less than 3/5 should not be tested.

Intensity
50–80% of MHHR if no history or full recovery from weakness
  40–60% of MHHR if history of variable recovery from weakness and currently stable, but up to 40% of MHRR if recent new weakness

Duration
30–40 continuous minutes, with intervals for the first few weeks if needed, if no history or full recovery from weakness
  15–20 minutes divided into intervals of approximately 3 minutes if history of variable recovery from weakness, and up to 15 minutes if recent new weakness

Frequency
3–5 days per week, with only 3 nonconsecutive days if history of variable recovery from weakness and currently stable or especially if new recent weakness

Mode
Non–weight-bearing activities preferred (arm or leg cycling, or both; swimming and water walking/exercises)
  Walking advised only if lower extremities are functional and capable of up to 2–3 minutes duration without symptoms

Special Considerations
Must determine extent of limb function prior to prescribing aerobic exercise
  Even if no history of weakness, some of the exercise session should consist of non–weight-bearing activities
  The patient must not exercise beyond RPE of "hard" even if no history of weakness
  The patient must stop and modify exercise amounts if increased fatigue, weakness, or pain results
  Adequate hydration is encouraged, especially in warmer than usual temperatures

ble musculature. Excessive muscle fatigue has been reported at least 2 days after isometric quadriceps testing (31). This suggests that when unstable (symptomatic) musculature is being tested, at least 3 days should be allowed between repeated tests.

Clinically if the participant has new weakness and appears overly fatigued with minimal exercise, postponing the muscle strength and endurance assessment is advised. Not only will the patient's performance suffer, but symptomatic motor neurons could be unduly loaded and irreversibly damaged.

Exercise Programming Options

Exercise training reports have included the results of aerobic and resistive strength training for polio survivors. The following sections of this chapter review the literature and include recommendations on safe and effective exercise prescription and programming for aerobic and resistive training.

Endurance Training

The primary technique for improving endurance has been aerobic exercise (21). Aerobic exercise prescription and programming for polio survivors should be individualized based on the patient's medical history and current clinical status (Box 18.4). Safer and more effective exercise can be prescribed by accurately classifying the polio survivor based on his or her symptoms and clinical findings in the most affected muscles of a limb (32). If a polio survivor is incorrectly assessed and classified, the prescribed exercise program may be ineffective—or worse, injurious to unstable motor units.

The highest functioning and least symptomatic polio survivors include those with no history of neurologic symptoms, regardless of documented infection with the virus. The physical examination finds include good to normal strength, sensation, and reflexes and no muscle atrophy. **Electromyography** (EMG) and **nerve conduction velocity**

(NCV) results are normal. Individuals in this classification should be able to exercise aerobically at moderate intensities of 60% to 0% of heart rate reserve (HRR), RPE at 12 to 14, or MET levels in the range of 7 to 10. Exercise duration of up to 40 minutes, 3 to 5 days per week, is recommended. Modalities include typical gross motor activities such as swimming, walking, and bicycling.

Subclinical polio is the second classification. People with subclinical polio have no new symptoms of weakness, but do have a past history of weakness with full recovery. The physical examination results should be similar to those of patients with no history of neurologic symptoms, but EMG and NCV testing exhibit chronic denervation or large **polyphasic motor unit** action potentials but no acute denervation. Exercise recommendations include 50% to 70% of HRR, RPE at 12 to 14, and MET levels in the 6 to 9 range. Exercise should include intervals of up to 5 minutes with a "rest" period of up to 1 minute for a total of 30 exercise minutes, at least for the first 2 to 4 weeks. A frequency of 3 or 4 alternate days is recommended. Modalities suggested are similar to those described for the least affected survivors.

A third classification, *clinically stable polio*, is defined by a history of weakness with variable recovery but no new weakness. Physical examination findings include poor to good strength, normal sensation, normal to decreased reflexes, and possibly some atrophy. The EMG and NCV results indicate chronic denervation and possibly acute denervation. Exercise intensity should include HRR of 40% to 60%, RPE of 11 to 13, with MET levels of 4 to 5. Exercise duration should be up to 20 minutes total with intervals of no more than 3 minutes, with recovery of up to 1 minute. The recommended frequency and modalities are similar to those previously prescribed.

The fourth classification, *clinically unstable polio,* is defined by a history of weakness with variable recovery and a recent history of new weakness. The physical examination and EMG and NCV show results similar to those seen in clinically stable polio. For these patients, the bulk of aerobic exercise should consist of ADLs. These activities should be done for 2 to 3 minutes followed by a 1- to 2-minute recovery for a total exercise time of 15 minutes per day. The recommended frequency is three times per week. For most patients 3 or fewer METs, a HRR of 40% to 50%, and RPE of 11 are suggested for intensity, and then for asymptomatic regions for the first 2 to 3 weeks.

A final classification, *severely atrophic polio,* accounts for the lowest functioning and most symptomatic group. History reveals weakness with little recovery, and current symptoms of new weakness. The physical examination results include trace to poor muscle strength, normal sensation, and areflexic and severe limb atrophy. The EMG and NCV studies show decreased insertional activity with few to no motor unit action potentials and most likely acute denervation. Exercise is generally contraindicated. Activities of daily living, spaced apart throughout the day, should be the extent of exercise programming. For most patients LE **orthotic** use and bracing are indicated, usually with a wheelchair or motorized scooter for mobility.

Resistance Training Program

Resistive training has centered on isolated muscle groups in the lower and upper extremities (Box 18.5). Muscle strength of the elbow and knee extensors, using concentric contraction and training three nonconsecutive times/week with three sets of 20, 15, and 10 repetitions, has yielded significant improvement (27). Eccentric contractions were minimized in this study to avoid overstraining. Resistance intensity was 75% of 3 RM with 90 seconds recovery between sets and 3 minutes rest between exercises. Isotonic training consisting of three sets of 12 repetitions on Tuesdays and Fridays, together with isometric training consisting of four maximal static contractions for 5 seconds using differentiated RPE as a means of safely and effectively monitoring resistance, has been successfully implemented (29) for some post-polio patients. Initial resistance was determined by placing weights on the ankle (for knee extension) until an RPE of 13-14 on the Borg 15-grade scale was perceived. The weight or resistance for each set was increased gradually during the first 2 weeks. If, by the end of the third set, the RPE was less than 19, weight or resistance was increased for the next session. A 1-minute rest was given at the end of each set. Although the differentiated RPE appears to be too high in this protocol, especially by the third set, no histopathologic or serologic deleterious effects were found in subjects performing at this level.

Prescription of muscle strength exercise also should be based on a limb assessment/classification procedure similar to the one that was detailed in the preceding section on endurance training programs. Polio survivors with no clinical or subclinical polio should be able to perform muscle strength exercise safely at an intensity or resistance that is perceived differentially up to at least 14 RPE. Sensations and perceptions of "hard" or more, especially over long pe-

---

BOX 18.5. Muscle Strength Resistive Training Prescription Summary

Intensity
- Differentiated RPE of 14 if no history of or full recovery from weakness
- Differentiated RPE of 11–13 if variable recovery from weakness, and 11 if new weakness

Duration
- 1 to 15 repetitions per set for 3 to 6 sets if no history of or full recovery from weakness
- 1 to 15 repetitions per set for 1 to 3 sets if variable recovery from weakness, and up to 10 repetitions for 1 set if new weakness

Frequency
- 3 alternate days per week

Mode
- Isometric (multiangle) if weak in any part of range initially, but isotonic preferred with free weight, machine weight, or Thera-Band resistance if no history of or full recovery from weakness
- Multiangle isometric exercise, at least initially, if variable recovery from weakness or recent new weakness

Special considerations
- Recovery periods of 1 to 3 minutes between sets, depending on resistance and number of repetitions performed
- Total exercise time for recent new muscle weakness is up to 10 minutes per day
- Isometric intensities should not exceed two thirds of maximum effort, especially for variable recovery or recent new muscle weakness
- Exercise amounts or mode should be modified and reduced if increased weakness or pain results

riods, could expose undetected fragile motor units to unnecessary overload. Depending on goals, repetitions can range from low (3 to 6 per set) to high (<15 per set), without significant risk of overburdening motor neurons. One to three or more sets per exercise are suggested, with the total time of the session ranging from 20 to 30 minutes, depending on the goals of the program. Recovery periods of at least 1 minute between sets are suggested, with up to 1 to 3 minutes between exercises depending whether the program is oriented more toward endurance or strength. Isotonic or isometric exercise can be equally effective, with initial status and functional goals determining which is emphasized. It is recommended that the exercise be done on no more than 4 nonconsecutive days per week. These guidelines are similar to those recommended for apparently healthy adults by the American College of Sports Medicine (ACSM) (33).

Polio survivors with no new weakness but a variable recovery history of weakness and fatigue should use perceptive muscle sensations of up to only 12-13 differentiated RPE for muscle strength and endurance. From one to a maximum of three sets with up to 15 repeats per set are recommended. The session should be limited to no more than 20 minutes. A frequency of 3 nonconsecutive days per week is suggested to avoid exposing potentially problematic motor units to excessive stimulation. Multiangle isometric exercise may provide equally effective strength enhancement throughout the range of motion and reduce the chance of overtraining. Isometric exercise at two thirds of maximum exertion may offer less chance of injury but still provide adequate overload, particularly if done every 20 degrees of motion throughout the range of the particular joint.

Polio survivors with new weakness, fatigue, and atrophy should not exercise the symptomatic muscle groups beyond "light" or a score of 9 on the differentiated RPE. Because the intensity of isometric exercise is more easily controlled, multiangle isometrics are suggested at intensities not to exceed one half of maximum. Again, excessive exercise intensity could hasten the axonal degeneration process and curtail sprouting and regeneration of orphaned fibers. Up to five repeats per set with total time not exceeding 5 minutes are recommended. A frequency of two to three nonconsecutive sessions per week is suggested to promote adequate recovery. Rest and adequate recovery are paramount to facilitating healthy protein levels of reinnervating muscle fibers (34).

The most symptomatic polio survivors, those with recent weakness and fatigue, as well as those with severe atrophy, should not perform any strength or endurance exercise on the limbs in question. If the original viral polio bout was severe, even the remaining asymptomatic regions are at risk if overexercised. Instead, doing ADLs with frequent recovery periods and conserving energy is recommended.

For muscle groups that were never affected by the polio virus, have no history of weakness, and currently are asymptomatic, exercise (for these muscle groups only) may be done at the same levels recommended for patients with

no clinical or subclinical polio. However, during periods during which other muscle groups are symptomatic, excessive intensity from asymptomatic musculature could affect and further damage symptomatic motor units. Any polio survivor should note symptoms including overuse weakness, pain, or fatigue when exercising and modify the amount or type of exercise being performed. Polio survivors with a variable history but no recent weakness, as well as those with new weakness, may be most susceptible to new symptoms. Individuals with severe symptoms should be evaluated carefully, with consideration given to the use of orthotic devices for ankle and knee if muscle or structural support is insufficient for some weight-bearing activities. Occasionally a motorized scooter may be needed when traveling for long distances or times will be required.

Potential Physiologic Adaptations and Associated Mechanisms

Exercise training effects have been reported, but the literature has focused primarily on whether additional muscle weakness has been incurred rather than training effects. This section discusses the results of investigations in central (cardiac, pulmonary) and peripheral (skeletal muscle) mechanisms to exercise adaptation.

Central Mechanisms

Maximum oxygen consumption does exhibit similar improvement compared to persons with no symptoms of PPS. Although absolute maximum oxygen consumption for those with PPS generally is about 20% lower than that in age- and gender-matched persons without PPS, some mechanisms need to be considered to achieve relatively equal improvement (21). These mechanisms, which facilitate increases in cardiopulmonary performance, include bradycardia at rest and with any given workload, increases in stroke volume (SV) at any given workload through greater **myocardial contractility**, and central venous pressure via augmented **venous return**. Other suspected improvements from exercise include blood volume and **blood shunting** through sympathetic rerouting. In the studies reported (1,10) only heart rate was measured; thus myocardial change, SV, and blood volume are speculative, but it is reasonable to consider these because they have been documented in studies where maximum oxygen uptake increased in persons without prior polio (35).

Pulmonary mechanisms contributing to increased oxygen consumption include an increase in maximum minute volume (1). Increased ventilation probably was mediated through an increased **tidal volume** at any given workload with subsequent decrease in respiratory frequency. Greater pulmonary diffusion, although not documented, is another favorable change that may be expected.

Peripheral Mechanisms

Favorable morphologic and biochemical changes as a result of exercise training have not been the primary focus of most PPS investigations. Instead, most reports have focused on the lack of further abnormal skeletal muscle changes (25–30). The result has been that indirect evidence at least partially attests to the functional value of exercise training. Several peripheral variables have been assessed after exercise training and thus used as a standard for exercise training efficacy.

Appropriate resistive exercise training has not resulted in further weakening of already weak, hypertrophied motor neurons (10). However, further type I muscle fiber hypertrophy has been reported with excessive use (36). Fortunately, jitter and fasciculations have not increased and further orphaned more muscle fibers (10). It is presumed that increased **myoglobin** stores may have been at least partially responsible for preventing additional unfavorable changes, because blood lactates measured after exercise in a small PPS sample did not consistently show anaerobic acidosis (1). Exercise metabolic overload and subsequent blood acidosis have been cited as possible causes of oversized motor neurons and new weakness and atrophy (2,10).

Muscle type changes from type II to type I have been found (36) (Figure 18.4). Presumably the morphologic adaptation was the result of overuse, because elevated **creatine kinase** also has been demonstrated (37). However, increased muscle endurance, which usually is associated with increased type I muscle fibers, has not resulted. Most likely, lack of local vascularization and diminished levels of oxidative enzymes reduce the metabolic endurance potential of increased type I fibers (1). It may be that one of the local training effects is an increase in capillary density, because muscle endurance has been reported, but the mechanism remains undocumented in PPS. All of these changes have been reported as a result of exercise training in persons without PPS (35).

Another possible local mechanism is enhanced efficiency. Muscle strength and endurance increases in force have been reported (1,10). Usually increased motor unit recruitment results in greater performance. However, because it is likely that all motor units are activated, increased activation appears unlikely and potentially injurious. Greater demands on overburdened and oversized motor neurons could prematurely orphan muscle fibers. Greater motor efficiency and coordination may explain the increased local endurance.

Changes in body composition through exercise training have been associated with increases in oxygen consumption (35). Body weight decreases have facilitated increases in oxygen consumption distribution. It is likely that diminished body weight also reduces the load on lower extremity musculature and joints during weight-bearing activity, adding to a greater endurance effect. However, specific fat to fat-free tissue measurements and aerobic capacity changes have not been reported to confirm these suspicions.

Clinical Tips

Although periods of new weakness and fatigue require that exercise be contraindicated or at least significantly reduced for the involved muscle groups, the symptoms eventually may diminish in frequency and intensity. When the symptomatic period has decreased, exercise should be very carefully increased, first in duration and then gradually in intensity. However, the weakened musculature probably will not be able to exercise as intensely as previously.

What We Know
About Post-Polio Syndrome

1 Includes symptoms of pain, weakness, fatigue, and atrophy in limb and muscle areas once affected by polio virus.

2 Symptoms often occur up to 35 to 40 years after initial infection with polio virus.

3 Neurologic changes accompany symptoms. Without abnormal motor neuron changes symptoms may be due to soft tissue and joint overuse.

4 More than 50% of the motor neurons must be depleted before symptoms of significant weakness and fatigue occur.

5 Some muscle strength and aerobic endurance programs have shown improvements while not furthering motor neuron loss.

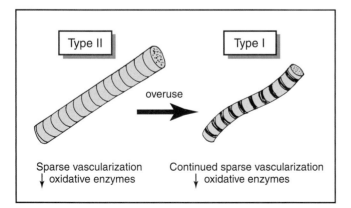

FIGURE 18.4.   Muscle fiber changes in PPS overuse.

What We Would Like to Know
About Post-Polio Syndrome

1 Why do motor neurons die sooner than expected in patients with PPS?

2 Does excessive exercise or physical exertion contribute to the death of the motor neurons in PPS?

3 Will nonparalytic polio survivors incur the same amount of motor neuron loss as paralytic polio survivors?

4 Will proper type or amount of exercise contribute to motor neuron retention?

5 Can nonsymptomatic muscle fibers that never were affected by the polio virus exercise at high intensities and durations without fear of premature motor unit loss?

6 Does the original polio virus become reactivated, and is it responsible for some of the return of symptoms?

Summary

Post-polio syndrome includes fatigue, pain, and weakness of skeletal muscle groups. These symptoms may arise from premature aging and death of motor neurons originally damaged by the polio virus. Although these symptoms usually do not manifest until almost 40 years after the initial infection, they generally are chronic.

Diagnosis of PPS is critical not only to treatment but also for determination of prevalence. Anywhere from 22% to 90% of the almost 1.8 million polio survivors appear to be affected by PPS. In addition to symptom identification, more specific criteria, including atrophy associated with new and increasing pain, must be present. Abnormal EMG findings also should be apparent before the diagnosis of PPS is established. Risk factors such as original paralysis of all four limbs, ventilator necessary for breathing during hospi-

talization, and polio virus contracted after the age of 10 years also should be considered in determining PPS.

Treatment has included NSAIDs and antidepressant medications for pain modification. Other medications generally have been unsuccessful in decreasing fatigue and weakness. Moderate amounts of exercise have been successful in most patients in increasing muscle strength and endurance and aerobic capacity without resulting in adverse effects. Adverse effects could result from exercise that is too intense, because such exercise could further hasten the damage to fragile, surviving motor neurons. Persons with new weakness and pain associated with atrophy should not exercise the symptomatic limb or muscle group(s).

Further research is needed to determine whether exercise can save motor neurons and muscle fibers. More importantly, research is needed to establish whether exercise significantly improves the day-to-day function of persons with PPS and thus becomes an integral part of the treatment process.

DISCUSSION QUESTIONS

1 What pathology and symptoms are similar in presentation and can be confused with PPS?

2 When should assistive devices and power chairs or scooters for mobility be considered?

3 What recreational and leisure activities should be recommended for a person who has PPS?

4 Many of those afflicted with PPS are "baby boomers" who tend to overachieve using the "no pain-no gain" philosophy. Why is this more potentially physically harmful than beneficial?

5 Not everyone who has had polio will eventually come down with PPS. What can be done for the person who refuses to exercise for fear of "overworking" yet has no adverse history or risk factors and currently has no apparent clinical signs or symptoms of PPS?

CASE STUDY 1

Patient Information

Ms. H. is a 52-year-old divorced mother of two grown children. She was diagnosed with paralytic polio at the age of 4 years. She uses Lofstrand crutches for ambulation (walking) assist secondary to left lower extremity (LLE) weakness and atrophy. The LLE becomes significantly weaker after about 3 minutes of walking. Ms. H. did not use an assistive device for walking until 2 years ago, when balance and ambulation became more difficult. She has gained 30 pounds over the past 12 months. Ms. H. does not exercise regularly. She has experienced recent sleep difficulties. Ms. H. currently is unemployed. She takes NSAIDs for lower extremity pain, with 6/10 being the worst and 2/10 to 3/10 the best after rest. She has been referred to the clinic for gait and balance problems.

Assessments

After reviewing the EMG of Ms. H.'s LLE, which indicated significant motor unit amplitude and duration with increased fasciculations, a physical examination and evaluation followed. Findings of the examination were as follows:

Height: 157.5 cm
Weight: 88.6 kg
Body fat percentage: 41%
Resting blood pressure: 154/90
Heart rate: 90 bpm.

Her appearance was obese. Postural analysis while standing indicated moderate lumbar hyperextension, severe anterior pelvic tilt, moderate to severe atrophy for a moderately flaccid LLE mid-thigh to ankle, left knee recurvatum, mild C-shaped right lumbar scoliosis, and the majority of body weight on the RLE. Neurologic findings indicated a flat affect but not depressed mood; diminished LLE of L 4-5 to light touch, vibration, sharp-dull, and temperature sensations; significantly diminished to absent deep tendon reflexes of knee and ankle of LLE. Active range of motion for the LLE was significantly reduced for hip flexion, extension, abduction, and internal rotation; knee flexion; and ankle dorsiflexion. Dynamic standing balance with crutches included functional reach of 4 inches and mild perturbation-induced step strategy. During sit-stand and stand-to-sit, Ms. H. completed three repetitions in 45 seconds safely before becoming fatigued. Her 2-minute self-selected pace gait (with Lofstrand crutches) was ataxic with moderately excessive left pelvic rotation, minimal left hip extension/flexion, left knee flexion/extension and severe left plantar flexion (foot-drop). Efficiency of gait was reduced by 75% secondary to lack of step and stride length, and after 1 minute there was an additional 15% reduction in step and stride length. Manual muscle testing (MMT; 3 repetitions) indicated all left hip movements were 2-2+/5; left knee and plantar flexors were 3/5, while dorsiflexors were 1/5. Pain increased from 2/10 to 4/10 by the third repetition for all MMT. The RLE was 4/5 for all movements. Submaximal aerobic capacity test on a Schwinn AirDyne (without use of LLE) revealed a "low" fitness rating (predicted maximum, 4 METs) based on gender and age comparisons.

Questions

1. What clinical considerations must be made in developing an exercise program for Ms. H?

2. Develop a safe and effective aerobic exercise program for Ms. H., specifying intensity, duration, frequency, and mode.

3. What other health care professionals should be involved, especially in development of a muscle strength-resistive program?

4. How and when would you assess Ms. H.'s progress?

CASE STUDY 2

Patient Information

Mr. Y. is a 44-year-old married man with no children. He was diagnosed with paralytic polio at age 7. He is employed as an administrator at a local bank. He does not use any assistive devices for ambulation, mobility, or balance, and he is physically active and exercises regularly. However, he is beginning to have periodic problems with stumbling during gait. The stumbling appears to be caused by reduced dorsiflexion of the right LE during the end of swing phase. Apparently the toe or front portion of his right shoe hits the floor, especially carpeting, resulting in a stumbling motion, especially after he has been walking for at least 2 minutes. He notes that he experiences pain at about 4/10 at about the same time that he begins to have a stumbling motion. This abnormality has become more evident over the past 6 weeks. Mr. Y. also reports a "weakness" in the right anterior LE that he did not have 2 months ago. He reports no other problems. Over the past year his body weight has been stable. He is not taking any prescription or over-the-counter medications. He is referred to the clinic for evaluation and treatment of gait problems associated with the right LE.

Assessments

Mr. Y. underwent EMG and NCV assessment of the lower portion of his RLE. Results included moderate motor neuron amplitude and duration, erratic fasciculations increased with exercise, and slowed NCV of the tibialis anterior with exercise. Findings on physical examination were:

Height: 180.3 cm
Weight: 77.1 kg
Body fat percentage: 19%
Resting blood pressure:122/76 mm Hg
Heart rate: 68 bpm

His appearance is moderately lean and rather fit. A standing postural analysis found only slight right knee recurvatum and right eversion deviation of the transverse tarsal (midtarsal) joint. The circumference of the right calf is 2 inches less than that of the left, but Mr. Y is not sure whether that atrophy is new or has been present for some time. Pulses were 2+ for all LE anterior and posterior arteries. Neurologic findings were generally unremarkable except for erratic light touch of L5 and diminished ankle DTR. The active range of motion for both LEs was WNL except for right dorsiflexion (DF), which was impaired by 20%. Dynamic standing balance was 8 inches for functional reach, and it took greater than moderate perturbation to induce step strategy. Mr. Y. had no functional endurance deficits such as transferring (sit-to-stand, supine-to-sit). During gait the chief complaint of decreased RDF after 2 minutes became apparent and resulted occasionally in a stumbling type of motion, which although not falling increased susceptibility. Stride and step length of gait shortened by 25% after 2 minutes of self-paced walking, and was concomitant with decreased right DF. There also was a "softer" heel strike on the RLE during initiation of the stance phase, probably secondary to decreased RDF. A manual muscle test (MMT) using 3 repetitions indicated a 3+/5 before self-paced gait for the RDFs, but only a 2/5 after 2 minutes of walking. The LLE for DF was 4+/5 and 5/5 for hip and knee motions. Pain increased in the right lower leg during gait, to a 5/10. At rest the right lower leg generally has no pain. A submaximal aerobic capacity test on a Schwinn AirDyne with the use of all limbs, including the RLE because DFs are not overly active during pedaling, gave an "above average" fitness rating (predicted maximum was 11 METs), based on gender and age comparisons.

Questions

1. What clinical considerations need to be made before developing an exercise program for Mr. Y.?

2. Develop a safe and effective aerobic exercise program specifying intensity, duration, frequency, and mode.

3. Develop a safe and effective muscle strength-resistive program for the LEs, particularly the right lower leg. Should other health care professional be consulted before implementing the program?

4. When would you reassess Mr. Y.'s progress? What type of assessments would you administer?

REFERENCES

1. Birk TJ. Poliomyelitis and the post-polio syndrome: exercise capacities and adaption—current research, future directions, and widespread applicability. Med Sci Sports Exerc 1993;25:466–472.
2. Smith LK, Mabry M. Poliomyelitis and postpolio syndrome. In: Umphred DA, ed. Neurologic Rehabilitation. 3rd Ed. St. Louis: Mosby, 1995:571–587.
3. Bodian D. Poliomyelitis: neuropathologic observations in relation to motor symptoms. JAMA 1947;134:1148–1154.
4. Agre JC, Rodriquez AA, Tafel JA. Late effects of polio: critical review of the literature on neuromuscular function. Arch Phys Med Rehabil 1991;72:923–931.
5. Falconer M, Bollenbach E. Late functional loss in nonparalytic polio. Am J Phys Med Rehabil 2000;79:19–23.
6. Sharrard WJW. The distribution of the permanent paralysis in the lower limb in poliomyelitis. J Bone Joint Surg Br 1955;37:540–558.
7. Dalakas MC. Pathogenetic mechanisms of post-polio syndrome: Morphological, electrophysiological, virological and immunological correlations. Ann NY Acad Sci 1995;753:167–185.
8. Bodian D, Howe HA. Experimental nonparalytic poliomyelitis: frequency and range of pathological involvement. Bull Johns Hopkins Hosp 1945;76:1–10.
9. Bodian D, Howe HA. Non-paralytic poliomyelitis in the chimpanzee. J Exp Med 1945;81:255–274.
10. Agre JC, Sliwa JA. Neuromuscular rehabilitation and electrodiagnosis. 4. Specialized neuropathy. Arch Phys Med Rehabil 2000;81:S27–S44.
11. Klein MG, Whyte J, Keenan MA, et al. Changes in strength over time among polio survivors. Arch Phys Med Rehabil 2000;81:1059–1064.
12. Dalakas MC, Hallett M. The post-polio syndrome. In: Plum F, ed. Advances in Contemporary Neurology. Philadelphia: FA Davis, 1988:51–94.
13. Widar M, Ahlstrom G. Pain in persons with post-polio. Scand J Caring Sci 1999;13:33–40.
14. Bruno RL, Creange SJ, Frick NM. Parallels between post-polio fatigue and chronic fatigue syndrome: a common pathophysiology? Am J Med 1998;105:66S–73S.
15. Aurlien D, Strandjord RE, Hegland O. The postpolio syndrome—a critical comment to the diagnosis. Acta Neurol Scand 1999;100:76–80.
16. Thornsteinsson G. Management of postpolio syndrome. Mayo Clin Proc 1997;72:627–638.
17. Dalakas MC, Bartfeld H, Kurland LT. The postpolio syndrome: advances in the pathogenesis and treatment. Ann NY Acad Sci 1995;753:1–411.
18. Trojan DA, Collet JP, Shapiro S, et al. A multicenter, randomized, double-blinded trial of pyridostigmine in postpolio syndrome. Neurology 1999;53:1225–1233.
19. Stanghelle JK, Festvag LV. Postpolio syndrome: a 5 year follow-up. Spinal Cord 1997;35:503–508.
20. Grimby G, Kvist H, Grangard U. Reduction in thigh muscle cross-sectional area and strength in a 4-year follow-up in late polio. Arch Phys Med Rehabil 1996;77:1044–1048.
21. Birk TJ. Polio and post-polio syndrome. In: ACSM's Exercise Management for Persons with Chronic Diseases and Disabilities. Champaign, IL: Human Kinetics, 1997: 194–199.
22. Willen C, Cider A, Sunnerhagen KS. Physical performance in individuals with late effects of polio. Scand J Rehabil Med 1999;31:244–249.
23. Stanghelle JK, Festvag L, Aksnes A. Pulmonary function and symptom-limited exercise stress testing in subjects with late sequelae of postpoliomyelitis. Scand J Rehab Med 1993;25:125–129.
24. Jones DR, Speier K, Canine R, et al. Cardiorespiratory responses to aerobic training by patients with post-poliomyelitis sequelae. JAMA 1989;261:3255–3258.
25. Kriz JL, Jones DR, Speier JL, et al. Cardiorespiratory responses to upper extremity aerobic training by post-polio subjects. Arch Phys Med Rehabil 1992;73:49–54.
26. Agre JC, Rodriquez AA, Franke TM. Strength, endurance, and work capacity after muscle strengthening exercise in postpolio subjects. Arch Phys Med Rehabil 1997;78:681–686.
27. Spector SA, Gordon PL, Feuerstein IM, Sivakumar K, Hurley BF, Dalakas MC. Strength gains without muscle injury after strength training in patients with postpolio muscular atrophy. Muscle Nerve 1996;19:1282–1290.
28. Einarsson G, Grimby G. Strengthening exercise program in postpolio subjects. In: Halstead LS, Wiechers DO, eds. Research and Clinical Aspects of the Late Effects of Poliomyelitis. White Plains, NY: March of Dimes Birth Defects Foundation, 1987:275–283.
29. Agre JC, Rodriquez AA, Franke TM. Subjective recovery time after exhausting muscular activity in postpolio and control subjects. Am J Phys Med 1998;77:140–144.
30. Nollet F, Beelen A, Prins MH, et al. Disability and functional assessment in former polio patients with and without postpolio syndrome. Arch Phys Med Rehabil 1999;80:136–143.
31. Einarsson G, Grimby G. Disability and handicap in late poliomyelitis. Scand J Rehabil Med 1990;22:113–121.
32. Halstead L, Gawne AC. NRH proposal for limb classification and exercise prescription. Disabil Rehabil 1996;18:311–316.
33. ACSM's Guidelines for Exercise Testing and Prescription. 6th Ed. Philadelphia: Lippincott Williams & Wilkins, 2000.
34. Herbison GJ, Jaweed MM, Ditunno JF, Scott CM. Effect of overwork during reinnervation of rat muscle. Exp Neurol 1973;41:1–14.
35. Astrand PO, Rodahl K. Work Physiology: Physiological Bases of Exercises. St. Louis: CV Mosby, 1986.
36. Grimby G, Einarsson G, Hedberg M, Aniansson A. Muscle adaptive changes in post-polio subjects. Scand J Rehab Med 1989;21:19–26.
37. Waring WP, Davidoff G, Werner R. Serum creatine kinase in the postpolio population. Am J Phys Med Rehabil 1989;68:86–90.

SUGGESTED READINGS

Dalakas MC. New neuromuscular symptoms after old polio ("post-polio syndrome"): Clinical studies and pathogenic mechanisms. Birth Defects 1987;23:241–264.

Dalakas MC, Bartfield H, Kurland LT. The postpolio syndrome: advances in the pathogenesis and treatment. Ann NY Acad Sci 1995;753:1–411.

CHAPTER 19

Pediatric Cerebral Palsy

Viswanath B. Unnithan, Désirée Maltais

Overview

Cerebral palsy (CP) is an umbrella term covering a group of non-progressive, but often changing; motor **impairment** syndromes secondary to **lesions** or anomalies of the brain arising early in development (1) (Box 19.1). Cerebral palsy may be the most common pediatric physical disability (2). In developed countries, CP occurs in 2 to 2.5 per 1000 live births, a rate that has remained fairly stable since the 1960s (3). The effect of changes in **obstetric** and **neonatal** medical practice that have occurred during this period are reflected in the rates of CP when they are considered in relation to **gestational age** and birth weight (Box 19.2). Because many factors, which result in varying amounts of brain damage, can lead to CP, the cause and the ensuing degree of motor dysfunction vary widely. This makes "cerebral palsy" an imprecise term, although it remains in use, probably because it continues to be a convenient way to group children for health care and other services (4, 5). Cerebral palsy is a life-long condition; this chapter, however, focuses on the child and adolescent with CP. Most exercise-related research has been done with these younger age groups, and this is where our own research and clinical expertise lie.

Because the term "cerebral palsy" refers to such a heterogeneous group of conditions, it is important to distinguish among the different kinds of CP. Classification is based on clinical descriptions of the motor impairment: its type, topographic distribution, and severity as determined by the **functional ability** of the child (6, 7). Although intraobserver agreement on classification can be quite low, it improves greatly when classification criteria are clear and standardized and the observers are trained in their use(8).

BOX 19.1. What Is and Is Not Cerebral Palsy

- The term *cerebral palsy (CP)* describes many conditions arising from different causes (1) that result in abnormal movement (5, 6).
- Movement is abnormal because these causal factors damage the immature brain, or result in its developing abnormally, or both (1, 5, 6).
- Brain damage in adults or older children (usually >5 years[7]) that results in movement abnormalities, is referred to as *acquired brain injury* (or a similar term), not CP.
- Brain damage in CP is static; typically it does not improve or worsen, but the damage is permanent. Cerebral palsy is a permanent condition (1, 6).
- Brain damage that is progressive, or due to a recognized syndrome or disease, or both, is not called CP (7).
- Although the brain damage in CP is static, its effect on motor abilities can change over time (1); most interventions are targeted at these effects, not at the brain damage itself.

BOX 19.2. How Often Does Cerebral Palsy Occur?

Stanley and coworkers (4) drew the following conclusions from a review of several population-based CP registers from developed countries:

1. The rate of occurrence of CP, 2 to 2.5 times per 1000 live births, has not changed markedly from the 1960s to the early 1990s (the most recent years for which data are available since a definitive diagnosis of CP cannot be made in very young children).

2. Changes in obstetric and neonatal medical practice during that same period have resulted in increased survival of low-birthweight (< 1500 g) and very premature (<32 complete weeks' gestation) infants.

3. The risk of CP increases as either birthweight or gestational age decreases. The risk of CP for a very pre-term birth, for example, is about 100 times higher than for a term birth (12).

4. The increased survival of the high-risk infants in this study was reflected by increases in the rates of CP in these particular groups. The rate of CP per 1000 neonatal survivors in babies born at < 28 weeks' gestation reported in the Western Australia CP register, for example, increased from 33.1% for those born in 1980–1982 to 94.2% for those born in 1991–1992.

5. Preterm and low-birthweight infants made up a greater proportion of the total CP population as time went on. In 1980, 10% of children in Western Australia with CP had been born at less than 32 weeks' gestation; by 1991, this proportion had doubled.

The category *type of motor impairment* refers to certain aspects or attributes of muscle function. In **spastic CP**, the muscles appear stiff, especially during movement. Movements themselves also look stiff and lack fluidity, often because there is excessive **coactivation** of **antagonist** muscles. About 80% of children with CP are predominantly spastic, making this the most common type of CP motor impairment (7). Spasticity in CP results from lesions or abnormalities to the nerve cell bodies in the **motor cortex**, or to the **axons** projecting to and from the **sensorimotor cortex**. Children with **dyskinetic CP** also often are spastic, but they demonstrate chiefly involuntary, writhing movements (athetosis), or rigidity (dystonia), or both (7). With dyskinesia, the basal ganglia, collections of nerve cell bodies deep within the brain, are involved. **Ataxic CP** often is associated with the previously mentioned types of motor impairment (7) and is characterized by poor coordination, instability, and jerky or shaky movements. Ataxia is caused by problems with **cerebellar** structures.

Classification by topography refers to the area of the body where the motor impairment is seen. Children with **quadriplegic CP** (also known as **tetraplegic** CP) demonstrate one or more of the previously discussed motor impairments (e.g., spasticity, dyskinesia, ataxia) in the arms and legs, with about equal involvement of both (9). A child who has quadriplegic CP has bilateral brain lesions or abnormalities. Individuals with **diplegic** CP demonstrate spasticity in all four limbs, but the spasticity is much more significant in the legs than in the arms (9). Children can be classified as having diplegia, for example, with very little involvement of the arms, as long as spasticity is found in both legs. Diplegia also is the result of bilateral brain involvement, but it typically is more focal than in quadriplegia. In **hemiplegic CP** there is spasticity on one side of the body only (9). Right hemiplegia is more common than left hemiplegia (7). Brain damage in hemiplegia is unilateral, but because of the pathway of the motor tracts, the abnormality in the brain is on the side opposite the side of the body on which hemiplegia occurs. The most common topographic distributions are hemiplegia and diplegia; together these types of CP account for 50% to 60% of cases of CP in industrialized countries (7). Most of what we know about exercise in young people with CP pertains to those with spastic diplegia and hemiplegia.

As noted, classification by severity of CP usually refers to the functional motor abilities of the child. According to Gage (10), children are classified as having mild CP when they have very good functional movement with little limitation. They have moderate CP when they have some function but have definite difficulties with activities requiring motor ability. Those with severe CP have minimal function and are very dependent on others or on technology for care and mobility. Available information on exercise in CP relates for the most part to those with mild and moderate CP. Recently, a more standardized classification system based on **gross motor function** has been developed (11) (Table 19.1). In general, levels I and II in this classification system would be considered mild CP, level III would be moderate, and levels IV and V would be severe, although this is not absolute.

Although impairment of the motor system is the main distinguishing feature of CP, the areas of the brain relating to various other functions are interconnected with those of the motor system, and brain lesions and abnormalities seldom restrict themselves to following a single functional pathway. Individuals with CP often have other impairments, which may add to their problems managing in various environments (e.g., home, school or work, and community) and affect rehabilitation, including exercise testing and exercise-based interventions. The most common associated impairments are sensory deficits such as blindness or deafness, learning disability, mental retardation, behavioral disorders, and seizure disorders (7). Children with more severe CP are more likely to have other impairments, and the severity of these other impairments increases as the severity of the motor problem increases. Using the data from the population-based (i.e., all children with CP in a given area are taken into consideration) CP register of Western Australia, Stanley et al. (7), for example, found that only 4.4% of children with mild CP had

TABLE 19.1. GROSS MOTOR FUNCTION CLASSIFICATION SYSTEM

Level	Gross Motor Ability at 6–12 Years of Age
I	Children walk indoors and outdoors, and climb stairs without limitations. Children perform gross motor skills including running and jumping, but speed, balance, and coordination are reduced.
II	Children walk indoors and outdoors and climb stairs holding onto a railing but experience limitations walking on uneven surfaces and inclines and walking in crowds or confined spaces. Children have at best only minimal ability to perform gross motor skills such as running and jumping.
III	Children walk indoors and outdoors on a level surface with an assistive mobility device. Children may climb stairs holding onto a railing. Depending on upper limb function, children propel a wheelchair manually or are transported when traveling for long distances or outdoors on uneven terrain.
IV	Children at best walk short distances with a walker and adult supervision but have difficulty turning and maintaining balance on uneven surfaces, or they rely more on wheeled mobility at home, school, and in the community. Children may achieve self-mobility using a power wheelchair.
V	Children have no means of independent mobility and are transported. Some children achieve self-mobility using a power wheelchair with extensive adaptations.

Adapted from Palisano R, Rosenbaum P, Walter S, et al (11).

marked cognitive impairment (IQ <35), whereas over half (52%) of those with severe CP had significant cognitive impairment.

Pathophysiology

The motor impairments in CP result from damage to the structures concerned with movement: the motor cortex, basal ganglia, and cerebellum, and the connections to and from them. **Congenital anomalies**, prematurity, low birth weight, and multiple pregnancy are associated with an increased rate of CP, although it is still unknown if these factors *cause* CP (12, 13). Recently, intrauterine infection also has been seen as a significant risk factor, but one for which there is stronger evidence for causality. Although their study concluded before a definitive diagnosis of CP could be made, Alexander and coworkers (14) found the risk for brain damage highly indicative of CP to be about three times greater than average in low-birthweight (500–1500 g) infants whose mothers were diagnosed with **chorioamnionitis**. It has been suggested that CP occurs from destruction of **white matter** during the neonatal period due to a fetal **proinflammatory cytokine response** to infection (15). Although it is popularly believed that CP usually is due to **birth asphyxia**, the death of nerve cells as a result of the lack of oxygen is the underlying cause in only 8% to 10% of cases of CP in developed countries (16, 17). In a recent review, Stanley and coworkers (18) concluded that CP rates are reduced by interventions that address the various risk factors. Among the interventions they considered highly efficacious were delivery of premature infants in a specialized care facility; limiting the number of embryos implanted in fertility therapies to no more than three; and aggressive treatment for infections in newborns.

In developed countries, about 90% of children with CP survive to adulthood (19–21). Life expectancy is limited by severe deficits in mobility, feeding, and cognitive abilities (19, 21). The child's potential for independent mobility (walking) is best predicted by his or her sitting balance. Children with CP who sit independently by 24 months are most likely to walk independently by about 8 years, at least for short distances indoors with assistive devices (22, 23).

Most of the research on motor impairment in CP pertains to the spastic subtype; therefore, the information presented here applies more directly to this form than to the other subtypes. Spastic muscle is stiff: the muscle "resists" being stretched passively at a shorter length than nonspastic muscle (24). This resistance may occur because of changes in the mechanical properties of muscle fibers (25), or because the muscle is shorter than normal, a condition that has been found to be related to a decreased number of **sarcomeres** in animal models of spastic CP (26). Movements also appear stiff because of increased coactivation of antagonist muscles (27, 28). Increased coactivation in spastic CP has many possible causes (29–31), but most are related to a lack of inhibitory **supraspinal** input to the motoneuron pool in the spinal cord as a result of the brain damage (29, 32). Spastic muscle also is weaker than that of healthy children (33). This weakness may be related to any of the following factors: decreased excitatory supraspinal input due to the brain damage (fewer motor units are activated); increased coactivation (33) (the muscle is functionally weaker since a portion of the force it produces is expended overcoming the antagonist); or an increase in the ratio of low-force–producing type I fibers to high-force–producing type II fibers (34–36).

Balance challenges performed with children with CP result in excessive sway, indicating that balance is compromised in this population (37). Some suggested causes of balance deficits are as follows: (1) the spastic muscles that affect balance strategies are weak; (2) the sequencing of muscles for balance strategies is abnormal; and (3) the anticipatory balance strategies that minimize the amount of displacement during a balance challenge are greatly decreased (37).

The end results of stiff muscles and movements, weak muscles, and poor balance are seen in most motor activities of those children with spastic CP, but are especially noticeable when they walk. Although there is much variability among the gait patterns of children with CP due to both the variability within the condition and the interventions a particular child could undergo, there are some common gait patterns (38). One such pattern, crouch gait, is described in Box 19.3

BOX 19.3. Crouch Gait Pattern in Children With Spastic Cerebral Palsy

- Spasticity and shortening of the hip and knee flexor and the ankle plantar flexor muscles result in increased flexion of the hips and knees and increased plantar flexion of the ankles as the child walks.

- Spasticity and shortening of the ankle plantar flexors limit the smooth progression of the body forward over the feet; there is increased excursion in the vertical plane and the child's gait appears to have a "bouncing" quality.

- Spasticity and shortening of the hamstring muscles restrict forward placement of the advancing leg, both by limiting the amount of forward hip flexion and by limiting knee extension; the child takes small steps with the anterior portion of the foot often being the initial point of contact.

- Spasticity and shortening of the hip flexors limit hip extension in the stance (weight-bearing) leg as the swing leg progresses forward to make initial contact with the ground; this contributes both to the increased excursion in the vertical place and to the short steps.

- Movement in all planes is increased because balance strategies, which minimize excessive movement, are compromised.

Adapted from Perry (38).

Exercise Responses

Typical Aerobic Responses

Peak $\dot{V}O_2$ Testing

To obtain valid **peak $\dot{V}O_2$** data in children with CP, the child must first become accustomed to the laboratory environment and especially to the ergometer being used for the testing, a process known as **habituation**. The importance of habituation and standardization of exercise protocols for children with CP was demonstrated by Hoofwijk et al. (39). Insufficient habituation results in lower peak $\dot{V}O_2$ responses, and the usefulness of some studies (40, 41) has been limited by a lack of information on habituation. Arm (42) or leg (43) ergometry and treadmill testing can be achieved in children with CP if extensive familiarization and habituation procedures are followed before the testing is done (39).

Specific protocols have been developed for peak $\dot{V}O_2$ testing on the treadmill (39) and for both arm (42) and leg (43) ergometry. In general, when habituating children with CP (those with hemiplegia, diplegia and quadriplegia) to the treadmill, the emphasis is on ensuring they can walk comfortably and independently. To walk independently (without support) on the treadmill, the child must have some independent overground walking ability, and, typically, no severe cognitive impairment. It is our experience that many children who prefer crutches and orthoses as their normal walking aids, but who walk overground by themselves to even a limited extent, can be trained to walk independently on the treadmill using a standardized habituation protocol. When habituating the child to the cycle or arm ergometer, the emphasis should be on helping the child attain the appropriate pedal cadence. A metronome or flashing light system can be very helpful.

If serial peak $\dot{V}O_2$ data are being collected, it is important to establish the natural, day-to-day variability of the measurement (reproducibility). Knowing the reproducibility of peak $\dot{V}O_2$ allows practitioners to establish whether any improvement in performance over time is a product of treatment or merely a reflection of the natural variability of peak $\dot{V}O_2$. The reproducibility (Spearman rank correlations) of peak aerobic power in children with CP (0.72–0.84) (44) is less than that of able-bodied children (0.90) (44), although the measure generally is considered sufficiently reliable for use as an outcome measure in intervention studies.

Children and adolescents with CP have a lower peak $\dot{V}O_2$ than do their able-bodied peers (39, 40, 42, 43). Most of the research has focused on cycle (41) or arm ergometry (42) assessments of peak $\dot{V}O_2$, primarily due to the practical problems associated with testing on a treadmill. Only two studies have attempted to measure peak $\dot{V}O_2$ of children with CP on a treadmill (39, 40). Table 19.2 summarizes the literature on peak $\dot{V}O_2$ values in children with CP.

Many mechanisms could account for the lower peak $\dot{V}O_2$ values seen in children with CP compared with able-bodied controls. It might be due to lower efficiency of breathing—children with CP have higher than normal ventilatory equivalent values for oxygen (39, 41). This inefficiency may result from chest wall distortion due to respiratory muscle spasticity. In addition, there are several factors that could lower peak $\dot{V}O_2$ by increasing local muscle fatigue. High muscle tone (which could cause local fatigue by reducing venous return and inhibiting muscle lactate clearance during exercise) is one possibility (43). A second possible cause of local muscle fatigue would be involuntary movements (43, 45) that cause the child to work harder than otherwise would be necessary. A third possibility is the high level of coactivation (simultaneous activation of agonist and antagonist muscles) found in the lower limbs of these children during movement. Increased coactivation is, for example, highly related to the elevated energy cost of walking at submaximal speeds in children with CP (28). Because these young people also complain of fatigue at speeds that would be considered slow for able-bodied individuals (46), it may be that at peak exercise intensity these high levels of coactivation cause early fatigability of the leg muscles. The level of motor impairment and the reduced muscle mass seen in children with CP also might prevent them from achieving peak exercise intensities.

In children with CP, assessment of maximal aerobic power often is used to determine the outcome of aerobic training (47, 48) and also has been used to measure the efficacy of orthopaedic surgery (46). A child's maximal aerobic power does give some indication of his or her functional capacity, because it is likely that factors that limit aerobic performance also may limit function. The interpretation of a low peak $\dot{V}O_2$ is difficult and by itself is of little value to the clinician. Peak $\dot{V}O_2$ should be considered a useful adjunct to other types of exercise and orthopaedic and functional testing for the child with CP.

Submaximal $\dot{V}O_2$ Testing

Issues of protocol and technology become even more important for **submaximal** $\dot{V}O_2$ testing than for peak $\dot{V}O_2$ testing in children with CP. The technology and protocols employed with the former must allow the attainment of a cardiorespiratory **steady state**. Failure to achieve steady state makes the interpretation of submaximal data problematic.

Three major issues must be considered when developing a submaximal steady state test for a child with CP:

1. *Mode of testing.* Consideration should be given to whether the test would be best conducted overground, with a treadmill, or with an arm or leg ergometer.

TABLE 19.2. PEAK $\dot{V}O_2$ TESTS IN CHILDREN WITH CEREBRAL PALSY

Study	Type of Ergometry	No. Participants	Form of CP	Age (y)	$\dot{V}O_2$(mL/ kg/min)	Comments
Bar-Or et al., 1976 (42)	Arm	10 M+F	di	15–22	21.3	Active
		6 M+F	di	15–22	20.9	Inactive
Lundberg, 1978 (43)	Cycle	4 F	di	7–9	28	
		5 M	di	11–12	48	
Rieckert et al., 1977 (40)	Treadmill	8 M+F	3 t, di[a]	7–19	28	Walk, usually with supports
		8 M+F	4 h, 2t[a]	14–18	34.7	Walk, usually without supports
Hoofwijk et al., 1995 (39)	Treadmill	9 M+F	1h, 7di, 1q	10–16	32.7	Walk, always without supports

h, spastic hemiplegia; di, spastic diplegia; t, spastic tetraplegia; q, spastic quadriplegia; M, males; F, females.

[a]Remaining children had other handicaps such as ataxia, spina bifida, or myelodysplasia.

Reproduced with permission from Unnithan VB, Clifford C, Bar-Or O. Evaluation by exercise testing of the child with cerebral palsy. Sports Med 1998;26:239–251.

2. *Habituation to the equipment and testing environment.* Habituation is crucial to obtaining stable (and hence valid), submaximal, steady state data. The guidelines for habituation previously described for peak $\dot{V}O_2$ testing should be employed.

3. *Measurement reproducibility.* As with peak $\dot{V}O_2$, if serial submaximal oxygen consumption measures are used to assess the efficacy of rehabilitation or to monitor physical status, then the reproducibility of these measurements needs to be established.

The overground walking energy expenditure ($\dot{V}O_2$) can be up to three times higher in children with CP than that in healthy children (49–51). Children with CP also require more energy to walk on the treadmill than do their able-bodied counterparts (28, 52–54) (Table 19.3). Although the magnitude of difference (27%) in the energy cost of treadmill walking between CP and able-bodied groups appears to be less than for overground walking, it cannot be determined to what extent these differences are due to the walking surface, walking speed, or level of disability because neither the walking speed nor the level of disability were standardized among all studies. One possible consequence of the increased energy cost walking in CP, regardless of the walking surface, is that children with CP fatigue at low walking intensities (28, 46, 55). This "early fatigue" has the potential to affect the ability of children with CP to keep up with peers at school and on the playground. In our clinical experience, excessive or early fatigue while walking is one of the primary reasons why children with CP require a manual or powered wheelchair at least part of the time.

TABLE 19.3. SUBMAXIMAL OXYGEN CONSUMPTION VALUES IN THREE TREADMILL STUDIES IN CHILDREN WITH CP COMPARED WITH ABLE-BODIED CONTROL SUBJECTS

	CP	Able-bodied
Unnithan et al. (28): 50 m/min		
$\dot{V}O_2$ net (L/min)	0.55 ± 0.30	0.30 ± 0.11
$\dot{V}O_2$ (mL/kg/min)	16.6 ± 5.9	10.2 ± 0.84
% peak $\dot{V}O_2$	53.5 ± 26.0	22.5 ± 4.93
Rose et al. (52): 51 m/min		
$\dot{V}O_2$ (mL/kg/min)	18 ± 5.00	10 ± 0.5
Rose et al. (54): 21.5 m/min		
$\dot{V}O_2$ (mL/kg/min)	14.25 ± 3.67	8.63 ± 1.27
Rose et al. (54): @37.6 m/min		
$\dot{V}O_2$ (mL/kg/min)	19.08 ± 7.20	10.55 ± 1.24

$\dot{V}O_2$ net, exercise minus pre-exercise sitting $\dot{V}O_2$ value

Reproduced with permission from Unnithan VB, Clifford C, Bar-Or O. Evaluation by exercise testing of the child with cerebral palsy. Sports Med 1998;26:239–251.

Limited evidence gathered by the Children's Exercise and Nutrition Centre at McMaster University in Canada suggests that the level of disability, as estimated by topographic classification, is related to the energy cost of treadmill locomotion (see Figure 19.1). Duffy and coworkers (51), Bowen and coworkers (50), and Boyd and coworkers (55) showed that the energy cost of overground walking also is likely to be related to the level of disability. Further work is required using standardized and valid classifications of disability.

Assessment of the high oxygen cost of walking in children with CP is an important outcome measure but does not provide any information on the mechanisms that give rise to this phenomenon. A multidisciplinary approach using **kinetic, kinematic,** and **electromyographic techniques** may help identify potential mechanisms responsible for the elevated energy cost of walking seen in children with CP. Such information could guide the clinician in proper selection of type of intervention and evaluation.

Mechanical power and work, including changes between kinetic and potential energy, can be obtained using computer analysis of cinematographic or optoelectronic markers. In this approach, the body is divided into segments whose mass and moment of inertia are estimated. The velocity of each part is calculated from the motion data, and the kinetic and potential energy changes of each part are calculated for each instant in time (56).

Phasic activity as measured by electromyography (EMG) demonstrates when a muscle is electrically active and inactive. This type of assessment is a purely qualitative means of measuring muscle electrical activity, i.e., one cannot say by how much a muscle is more active or less active (or exerting more or less force) than in another situation or another muscle. Simply measuring phasic activity alone

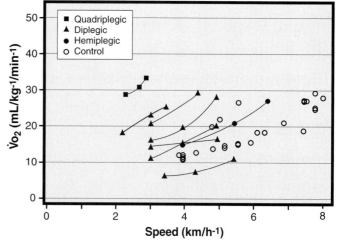

FIGURE 19.1. Relation between O_2 uptake and speed of walking in children with spastic CP versus able-bodied controls. (Reprinted with permission from Unnithan VB, Clifford C, Bar-Or O. Evaluation by exercise testing of the child with cerebral palsy. Sports Med 1998;26:239–251.)

may not be an adequate marker of the efficacy of a surgical intervention (57).

A coactivation index is one way to quantify muscle activity. Unnithan and coworkers (28) studied seven boys and two girls with a median age of 12 years and demonstrated that increased coactivation of the lower leg (tibialis anterior/soleus) and thigh (vastus lateralis/hamstrings) was related to the metabolic cost of walking in children with CP in that the higher the coactivation, the higher the energy cost of walking (see Figures 19.2 and 19.3). The effect of interventions theoretically designed to decrease lower limb coactivation on the energy cost of walking and on lower limb cocontraction index (CI) is currently under investigation at our laboratory at the Children's Exercise and Nutrition Centre (McMaster University, Ontario, Canada).

Although coactivation explains some of the variability in the oxygen cost of walking in children with CP, much of the variability is not accounted for. Unnithan et al. (58) studied other factors that could influence the submaximal O_2 cost of treadmill walking using a kinematic or biomechanical approach that allowed the researchers to estimate mechanical power from the acceleration (and estimates of the mass) of various body segments without directly measuring it using a force platform, which is problematic in treadmill protocols.

Results from this study demonstrated that mechanical power helped to explain 87.2% of the variability seen in the oxygen cost of walking in children with cerebral palsy (see Figure 19.4). In other words, the increased energy cost of treadmill walking in children with CP is closely related to how hard or how much they are working while walking.

Adolescents and young adults with spastic CP are less efficient in leg cycling than their able-bodied counterparts (CP, 12%; control, 22% [45]). Cycle ergometry is difficult

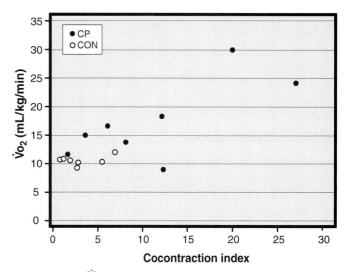

FIGURE 19.3. $\dot{V}_{O_2}$ versus thigh (vastus lateralis and hamstrings) coactivation index at 3 km/h: children with CP versus controls. (Reprinted with permission from Unnithan VB, Dowling JJ, Frost G, Bar-Or O. Role of cocontraction in the O_2 cost of walking in children with cerebral palsy. Med Sci Sports Exerc 1996;28:1498–1504.)

for many children with CP, however. Depending on the level of disability, a child with CP may not be able to complete even a single pedal revolution, possibly due to the high levels of lower limb coactivation (59). Consequently, arm cranking protocols may be preferable in many instances. The **mechanical efficiency** of arm cranking also is lower in adolescents with spastic diplegia (15%, Bar-Or et al. [42]; 12%, Maltais et al. [60]) and in children with quadriplegia and diplegia (8.4%, Emons [44]) compared to healthy adults (28%, Powers et al. [61]). No data are avail-

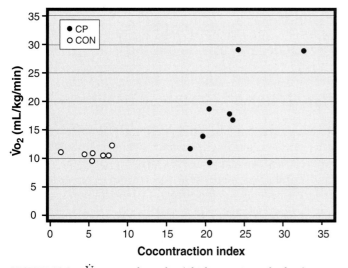

FIGURE 19.2. $\dot{V}_{O_2}$ versus lower leg (tibialis anterior and soleus) coactivation index at 3 km/h: children with CP versus controls. (Reprinted with permission from Unnithan VB, Dowling JJ, Frost G, Bar-Or O. Role of cocontraction in the O_2 cost of walking in children with cerebral palsy. Med Sci Sports Exerc 1996;28:1498–1504.)

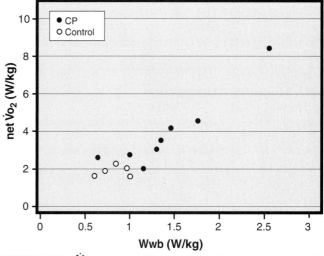

FIGURE 19.4. $\dot{V}_{O_2}$ versus total body mechanical power estimates at 3 km/h: children with CP versus control subjects. (Reprinted with permission from Unnithan VB, Dowling JJ, Frost G, Bar-Or O. Role of mechanical power estimates in the O_2 cost of walking in children with cerebral palsy. Med Sci Sports Exerc 1999;31:1703–1708.)

able for mechanical efficiency of arm cranking in healthy children. Thus, as with walking, children with CP appear to require more energy to cycle or to arm crank than do able-bodied individuals.

Typical Anaerobic Responses

Wingate Anaerobic Testing

In children with CP anaerobic power typically is measured using the **Wingate Anaerobic Test (WAnT)**, which gives information on **peak** and **mean muscle power** and **local muscle endurance**. Intertest leg WAnT (Spearman rank) correlations ranging from 0.90 to 0.94 for peak power (PP) and 0.92 to 0.95 for mean power (MP) have been noted in children with CP (44). These values are in line with the test–retest values seen in able-bodied children (PP, 0.96, and MP, 0.92).

The WAnT is fairly easy to perform with this population, but some general practical issues need to be addressed to ensure a successful test, such as taping the legs or hands to the pedals or handles, respectively. Specific details regarding the optimal protocols to follow have been well described by Parker and coworkers (62). Body mass has been used to select the optimal braking force in the WAnT, because anaerobic muscle power is highly related to lean limb mass. In individuals in whom the lean mass to total body mass ratio is normal, this approach is satisfactory. A more individualized approach is required, however, for children with CP (63, 64)

Research to date suggests that for children with neuromuscular disabilities, including CP, motor performance is very much limited by both peak muscle power and local muscle endurance (65–67). Anaerobic power is considered a better measure of functional ability than maximal aerobic power, at least maximal aerobic power as measured by arm ergometry. Parker and coworkers (66) found that mean muscle power (leg), but not maximum aerobic power significantly correlates with gross motor function as measured by the Gross Motor Function Measure, a reliable and valid assessment of gross motor function in children with CP (68). When only the subsections of this gross motor assessment that relate to standing and walking, running, and jumping were considered, mean lower limb muscle power accounted for 64% of the variability in gross motor function (66). When compared to normal data derived from healthy controls, children with CP scored between 2 and 4 standard deviations below the expected average for mean power (69).

Differences in anaerobic power can be demonstrated not only between groups of children with CP and able-bodied children, but also with respect to the level of disability in children with CP. Parker and colleagues (62) compared 19 quadriplegics, 16 diplegics, and 14 hemiplegics in terms of peak and mean power. Absolute peak power and mean muscle power in the arms were significantly greater

($P<0.05$) in diplegics whose lower limbs were predominantly affected than in hemiplegics and quadriplegics (who also have upper limb involvement). Also, peak and mean power in the lower limbs were significantly lower ($P<0.05$) in quadriplegics than in diplegics and hemiplegics.

Impairment of the motor control system can reduce optimal anaerobic performance. Maximizing short-term power in cycle ergometry tests depends on the nature of the force application on the pedal and the skill and coordination required for the task (62), both of which are likely to be problematic in children with CP. As summarized by Parker and coworkers (62) and by Emons and colleagues (65), there are several possible mechanisms for the low anaerobic performance in these children. Firstly, the normal reciprocal synchronization between agonist and antagonist muscle groups during voluntary movement is compromised, i.e., children with CP have increased coactivation, which limits their ability to pedal or arm crank, especially at high degrees of muscular power. Spasticity, which can be considered a velocity-dependent increase in resistance to muscle stretch, has the long-term effect of inhibiting muscle growth and reducing muscle mass, which can exacerbate the inability of the child with CP to produce high power, consequently affecting anaerobic performance (64). A low anaerobic power also may be due to an increase in the ratio of low-force–producing slow-twitch fibers (type I) to high-force–producing fast-twitch fibers (type II). Upper motor lesions have been demonstrated to cause atrophy of type II muscle fibers, resulting in a greater proportion of type I fibers (70).

In summary, the upper (67) and lower (44) limb WAnT are logistically possible to implement and demonstrate good reproducibility. On this basis the test should be considered a central component of any exercise evaluation of the child with CP. To date the WAnT has been used in only one published intervention study with CP (69), possibly because most rehabilitation professionals who are involved with intervention studies in this population do not have the necessary equipment readily available in their clinics.

Typical Strength Responses

Recently there has been increased interest in the relationship between muscle strength (defined as the ability of a muscle group to exert maximum contractile force against a resistance) and gross motor function in young people with CP and, consequently, on the effects of strength training on function in this population (71, 72). Previously, children with CP were not encouraged to strength train because it was felt this would increase spasticity and reduce flexibility, which would lead to worsening of deformities and walking problems.

Isokinetic muscle strength of knee flexors and extensors can be measured reliably in children with CP. Ayalon and coworkers (73) reported within- and between-session intraclass correlation coefficients (estimates of reliability) of

0.90 to 0.99 and 0.95 to 0.98, respectively. In addition, the handheld dynamometer has been found to give reliable isometric strength values in children and in adults with spasticity (intraclass correlation coefficients ranging from 0.91 to 0.96 for test–retest reliability [74]).

The affected limbs of children with CP are weak, and the level of weakness is related to the child's motor abilities, including walking. The strength of knee extensors in subjects with CP correlates positively with both gross motor function (75) and walking speed (76), and negatively with economy of locomotion as measured by HR (75) and with crouch (excessive knee flexion during the stance or weight-bearing phase of gait). Daminano and coworkers (76) showed that quadriceps strength at the weakest position (30 degrees from full knee flexion), in the weakest leg correlates with gait velocity in children with mild spastic cerebral palsy ($r = 0.62$) (Figure 19.5).

The feasibility of strength training for children and adolescents with CP depends on the extent of their motor involvement or, more specifically, on their ability to activate and generate muscle force and their ability to isolate a muscle or muscle group. Thus, most studies (72, 76–78) have looked at mild and moderately involved individuals with CP. Most protocols had the young people train three times weekly for 6 to 8 weeks (72, 76, 77). Unfortunately, most of these studies did not include a control group (72, 76, 77). However, despite the small number of subjects, lack of control groups, and the short duration of the training period, the children studied did demonstrate comparatively large increases in muscle strength. The short time over which these changes were obtained also seems to indicate that these improvements could not stem from improvements in strength that resulted from normal growth and development.

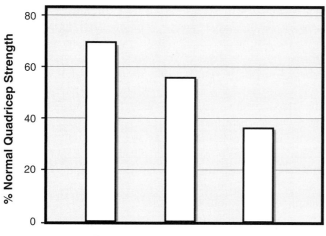

FIGURE 19.5. Strength deficits in children with CP with respect to limb position. (Adapted from Daminano et al. Muscle response to heavy resistance exercise in children with spastic cerebral palsy. Dev Med Child Neurol 1995;37:731–739.)

The quadriceps muscle group has been investigated most often in children with CP, probably because of ease of testing and training as well as because of the previously mentioned relation between knee extensor muscle group strength and function. Isometric (79), isokinetic (77), and isotonic protocols (72, 76, 79, 80) have been employed. All studies showed improvements in muscle strength. MacPhail and Kramer (77) found the magnitude of strength gain for mildly involved young people with CP to be similar to that of healthy children— a 25% increase in peak torque and a 21% increase in work in knee flexors and extensors (isokinetic program, training, and measurement with a Kin-Com AP active dynamometer [Chattecx Corporation]). One possible limitation of this study design was that the subjects trained and were tested on the same machine. Consequently, the improvements seen may reflect a learning curve rather than a true training response. The magnitude of improvement, however, seems to indicate that a true training response was seen. Spasticity has not been found to increase with strength training (76–78). Although muscle strength is related to function in these children, as noted earlier, the relation between training-induced improvements in strength and improvements in function is not clearcut (i.e., there is no substantial evidence to link improved quadriceps strength with increased independent mobility).

Training Responses

Aerobic and Anaerobic

Aerobic training of the child with CP has been well documented (42, 48, 81–83). Unfortunately, many of these studies have design problems that make it impossible to reach any definitive conclusions about the efficacy of aerobic training in these children. One common limitation is failure to include a control group carefully matched to the training group for the motor impairment by type (e.g., spasticity), topographic distribution (e.g., diplegia), and severity (e.g., moderate). However, such an approach would raise the question of whether it would be unethical to withhold "treatment" from the control group. One solution would be to use a nonexercise intervention with the control group, such as life skills sessions or other types of interventions aimed at factors different from those directly related to exercise. A second solution would be to offer the exercise intervention to the control group after they have completed the initial formal study.

Although there is considerable evidence to suggest that children with CP are aerobically trainable (69, 84–86), only Emons and Van Baak (69) included properly matched control subjects in their study. These researchers used a 9-month aerobic exercise training program that consisted of four sessions for 45 minutes per week and demonstrated significant improvements (32%) in peak aerobic power in nine children with CP. The effect of this same training program on anaerobic power also was examined. No change in local muscle endurance (mean power in the Wingate test) was observed. As noted, to the best of our knowledge, no other studies have investigated the effects of exercise training on anaerobic power.

Medications and Other Interventions

The nature of the interventions required for young people with CP varies according to their impairments, level of involvement, and family needs. Children may require some or all of the following: specialized education services; speech and language therapy; hearing, visual or communication aids; and social support services. Many children also need assistive devices for written output (e.g., computer) and for mobility (e.g., walker, canes, or wheelchair). This section, however, focuses on common interventions for those with mild and moderate involvement that address physical (and hence exercise-related) issues in orthopaedic surgery, neurosurgery (e.g., selective dorsal rhizotomy), medication (botulinum toxin A), orthoses, and physical therapy.

Orthopaedic Surgery

In children who are able to walk, orthopaedic surgery usually is done when they are 6 to 8 years old (87). These surgeries are performed to correct muscle and joint contractures, which are due to shortened muscles (usually because of excessive spasticity) that limit the range of motion at the joints they cross (87). Children with shortened, spastic calf muscles, for example, have decreased ankle dorsiflexion and often walk on their toes, which compromises balance. Orthopaedic surgery also is done at this time to correct any torsional deformities of the long bones of the legs (87), which can cause the child to walk with his or her legs excessively turned in or out. Multilevel surgery (surgery at two or more sites, e.g., the hips, knees, ankles and feet) is preferred, because only rarely is a single muscle, muscle group, or site involved. This approach also means that only one surgery rather than a succession of surgeries (and time away from school) is required to correct each problem (87). One study (88) found that orthopaedic surgery reduced the oxygen cost of treadmill walking by about 5%; it was thought this reduction was due to improvement in gait mechanics, although gait was not specifically assessed in the study.

Selective Dorsal Rhizotomy

Selective dorsal rhizotomy (SDR) is commonly used for ambulatory children with spastic diplegia in whom lower limb spasticity is the primary impairment affecting gross motor abilities (89, 90). Spasticity in the lower limbs is greatly reduced by cutting and removing about 50% of each dorsal

nerve root from L1 to S1 (90). Although SDR is found to reduce spasticity (89–91), it is unclear which children receive the greatest degree of functional benefit. Two randomized, controlled clinical trials (90, 91) found greater improvements in gross motor function in children who had this surgery and received postoperative physical therapy (which is very necessary following SDR because the children who require this procedure are very weak) compared with children who received physical therapy only. Two other randomized, controlled clinical trials (89, 92), however, found similar improvements in gross motor function in those who had SDR with physical therapy afterward and those who received only physical therapy, although children who had the surgery had better ankle dorsiflexion and hip and knee extension in the stance phase of gait 1 year later compared with those who did not have the surgery (92). Better standardization among clinical trials of both the selection criteria for who receives SDR and the intensity of physical therapy is required before it can be determined which children benefit most from this intervention.. To date the effects of selective dorsal rhizotomy on walking economy or on any physiologic response to exercise are unknown.

Botulinum Toxin A

Most medications used in the physical management of children with CP are used to reduce spasticity, especially in very involved children whose spasticity is such that it affects their ability to sit and causes difficulties with hygiene. In the last several years, however, botulinum toxin A (BTA) was introduced and has become frequently used in the physical management of mild and moderately involved ambulatory children (93–95). Botulinum toxin A reduces spasticity by partially paralyzing the muscle into which it is injected, which it does by preventing the release of the neurotransmitter acetylcholine at the neuromuscular junction (96). Following one treatment with BTA, clinically relevant muscle relaxation lasts for about 12 to16 weeks. The functional improvements, however, last much longer—up to 6 months and even longer in some children. Recovery of muscle contraction ability and relief of spasticity results from the reinnervation of the affected muscle via the sprouting of new motor nerve terminals that are able to release acetylcholine. The main effects of BTA on walking are an increased stride length (93) and improvements in ankle dorsiflexion and knee extension in the stance and swing phases of gait (97). It also appears to have a negligible effect on reducing the energy cost of walking in children with CP (94, 95), although further research is required before definitive conclusions can be made.

Orthoses

The most commonly used orthoses in children with mild to moderate CP who are able to walk probably are ankle–foot orthoses—either a rigid brace, which holds the ankle at 90 degrees, or a hinged brace, which allows for some degree of dorsiflexion (87). These braces are used mainly to control the tendency to walk up on the toes due to excessive plantar flexion from stiff and spastic plantar flexors (87). In addition, hinged ankle–foot orthoses have been shown to reduce the energy cost of walking in children with CP at both absolute and relative exercise intensities (98).

Physical therapy is not one single intervention but a variety of interventions. Stretching, strength training, and aerobic training are all physical therapy, as is the education of the parents on the easiest ways to hold and move their children and selection of the most appropriate assistive devices for enhancing mobility (87). Physical therapy is considered essential after both orthopaedic surgery (87) and selective dorsal rhizotomy (89) to improve the strength and the range of motion of children who have been weakened and immobilized while recovering from these surgeries.

What We Know
About Pediatric Cerebral Palsy and Exercise

1 The energy cost of walking in children with CP can be up to three times greater than that of able-bodied control subjects.

2 Children with CP complain of fatigue at very low exercise intensities.

3 Excessive coactivation and transfers of energy within and between adjacent body segments could be responsible for the high energy cost of walking in children with CP.

4 Children and adolescents with CP demonstrate lower peak $\dot{V}o_2$ values compared to able-bodied control subjects.

5 A lower efficiency of breathing, high muscle tone, involuntary movements, and excessive coactivation could all be responsible for this deficit in peak $\dot{V}o_2$.

6 Mean muscle power of the leg derived from the Wingate Anaerobic Test is significantly associated with gross motor function in children with CP.

7 There also appears to be a significant association between the level of disability and peak and mean power generated by both arm and leg Wingate Anaerobic Tests.

8 There is evidence of a limited relationship between lower limb strength values and motor abilities.

What We Would Like to Know
About Pediatric Cerebral Palsy and Exercise

1 Data are few with regard to aerobic and anaerobic responses to training in children with CP. We would like to see well designed intervention studies in these two areas.

2 More work is needed with regard to the relationship between the level of disability (using standardized classification systems) and the energy cost of walking in children with CP.

3 Further work is needed with regard to identifying the physiologic mechanisms that give rise to the high energy cost of walking in children with CP and to see whether techniques such as biofeedback could reduce the energy cost of walking.

4 More work is required in identifying the mechanisms responsible for the lower peak and mean power values seen in children with CP.

5 Even though muscle strength is related to function in children with CP, the relation between improvements in strength and function is not clear, and significant further investigation is warranted.

Summary

There are four major reasons for performing exercise testing in children with CP:

1. Repeated tests of physiologic function over time can provide information on the improvement or decline in the child's condition.
2. The child's muscle function can be evaluated through the application of certain physiologic tests.
3. Results from various exercise tests can assist the clinician in determining the intensity, frequency, duration, and mode of exercise best tolerated by the client.
4. Just as for nondisabled children, feedback in the form of physiologic fitness data can aid the coach and child-athlete with CP in judging the effectiveness of training programs. With major sporting events for the physically disabled such as the Para-Olympics gaining public recognition and support, such information has the potential to become increasingly more relevant as children with CP see themselves as potential athletes.

Each of these four reasons for exercise testing in this population explores an area with many unknowns. Children with CP, for example, fatigue at very low exercise intensities, and it is suspected that this is due to their increased energy expenditure during exercise. Although we are aware of some of the mechanisms (coactivation/energy transfers) that are responsible for this during walking activities, it is unclear whether any type or degree of exercise training could reduce the energy cost of ambulation. Furthermore, although we know that young people with CP generate lower peak and mean power values and demonstrate deficits in strength compared to their able-bodied peers, we require more information about the effects of various training programs and other interventions on anaerobic power and strength. More importantly, we require more information about how improvements in any physiologic parameter measured during exercise, relate to the functional needs and concerns of the child with CP and their family.

DISCUSSION QUESTIONS

1 What type of exercise evaluation(s) should a practitioner use for identifying the functional ability of a child with CP?

2 Children with CP complain of fatigue at very low exercise intensities. Explain the potential physiologic mechanisms responsible for this fatigue.

3 List the major effects of the medications used in the management of children with CP and discuss the evidence for any gait or exercise-related effects.

CASE STUDY

Patient Information

Raj is an 8.7-year-old boy diagnosed with mild spastic diplegic CP. He has been wearing ankle–foot orthoses (AFO) since he was 2 years old because of spastic ankle plantar flexors that cause him to walk up on his toes (equinus) and result in an increased tendency to fall when he is walking outside on uneven ground. The braces correct these problems. Originally, he wore solid AFO. At 4 years of age, he received his first pair of hinged AFO. His present orthoses, which are 3 months old, allow 20 degrees of ankle dorsiflexion, but prevent any plantar flexion beyond neutral (i.e., ankle at 90 degrees). His physical therapist recently measured his passive range of motion at the ankles. He has 5 degrees of dorsiflexion beyond neutral, bilaterally, with the knee flexed; and 0 degrees, bilaterally, with the knee fully extended. He has not had any orthopaedic surgery, nor is any planned for him in the near future. His parents are not interested in having him take any medication for spasticity at this time. Raj usually wears his braces at school and for outings, but generally does not wear them around the house. He does not use any other assistive devices to walk. Lately, Raj has been complaining of being teased at school because he "walks funny." Raj does not like to wear his braces, and his parents are wondering if his dislike of the braces stems from the orthoses making it harder for him to walk because of the added weight, or if the dislike might be due to the teasing. They are willing to increase his exercise level if the problem is due to the added weight of the braces. Their pediatrician at the local children's rehabilitation center referred them to the center's exercise testing and gait laboratory for a walking economy study.

Assessments

Raj weighs 22.3 kg, has a sum of four skinfolds (biceps, triceps, subscapular, suprailiac) of 21 mm, and a height of 129.0 cm. Compared to same-aged healthy children, he is in the 5th percentile for mass, 30th for sum of four skinfolds, and 1 standard deviation below the mean for height. Thus, he is somewhat short and slight, which is not uncommon for children with CP (99). Raj's gross motor skills related to walking are similar both with and without his AFOs. His comfortable and fast walking speeds on the ground with braces off are 65 and 82 m/min, respectively. With braces on, his comfortable and fast walking speeds are slightly faster, at 66 and 85 m/min, respectively. Because the mean comfortable and fast walking speeds for children his age are about 70 and 88 m/min, respectively, he probably has to walk faster than his comfortable speed to keep up with his classmates at school, even with his braces on. Wearing AFO reduces the oxygen cost of walking by 20% at his fast walking speed, but the oxygen costs at the comfortable speed are similar with braces on and off.

> ## Questions
>
> 1. Do you think that wearing his braces at school would inhibit Raj in his activities with his peers?
> 2. Would wearing the braces at home confer any physiologic or functional benefits for Raj?
> 3. What specific strategies could be employed to identify the cause of Raj's reluctance to wear his braces?
> 4. What specific type of training might increase Raj's comfortable walking speed?

REFERENCES

1. Mutch L, Alberman E, Hagberg B, et al. Cerebral palsy epidemiology: where are we now and where are we going? Dev Med Child Neurol 1992;34:547–551.
2. Pharoah POD. The epidemiology of chronic disability in childhood. Int Rehabil Med 1985;7:11–17.
3. Stanley F, Blair E, Alberman E. Cerebral Palsies: Epidemiology and Causal Pathways. London: MacKeith Press, 2000:22–39.
4. Stanley F, Blair E, Alberman E. Cerebral Palsies: Epidemiology and Causal pathways. London: Mac Keith Press, 2000:8–13.
5. Bax MCO. Terminology and classification in cerebral palsy. Dev Med Child Neurol 1964;6:295–297.
6. Nelson KB, Ellenburg JH. Epidemiology of cerebral palsy. In: Schoenberg BS, ed. Advances in Neurology. New York: Raven Press, 1978:421–435.
7. Stanley F, Blair E, Alberman E. Cerebral Palsies: Epidemiology and Causal Pathways. London: Mac Keith Press, 2000:14–21.
8. Blair E, Stanley F. Interobserver agreement in the classification of cerebral palsy. Dev Med Child Neurol 1985;27:615–622.
9. Minear WL. A classification of cerebral palsy. Pediatrics 1956;18:841.
10. Gage JR. Gait analysis in cerebral palsy. London: MacKeith Press, 1991:1–11.
11. Palisano R, Rosenbaum P, Walter S, et al. Development and reliability of a system to classify gross motor function in children with cerebral palsy. Dev Med Child Neurol 1997;39:214–223.
12. Cummins SK, Nelson KB, Grether JK, Velie EM. Cerebral palsy in four northern California counties, births 1983 through 1985. J Pediatr 1993;123:230–237.
13. MacLennan A. A template for defining a causal relation between acute intrapartum events and cerebral palsy: international consensus statement. BMJ 1999;319:1054–1059.
14. Alexander JM, Gilstrap LC, Cox SM, et al. Clinical chorioamnionitis and the prognosis for very low birth weight infants. Obstet Gynecol 1998;91:725–729.
15. Gilstrap LC, Ramin SM. Infection and cerebral palsy. Semin Perinatol 2000;24:200–203.
16. Blair E, Stanley FJ. Intrapartum asphyxia: a rare cause of cerebral palsy. J Pediatr 1988;112:515–519.
17. Yudkin PL, Johnson A, Clover LM, Murphy KW. Assessing the contribution of birth asphyxia to cerebral palsy in term singletons. Paediatr Perinat Epidemiol 1995;9:156–170.
18. Stanley F, Blair E, Alberman E. Cerebral Palsies: Epidemiology and Causal Pathways. London: MacKeith Press, 2000:138–175.
19. Evans PM, Evans SJ, Alberman E. Cerebral palsy: why we must plan for survival. Arch Dis Child 1990;65:1329–1333.
20. Hutton JL, Cooke T, Pharoah PO. Life expectancy in children with cerebral palsy. BMJ 1994;309:431–435.
21. Strauss DJ, Shavelle RM, Anderson TW. Life expectancy of children with cerebral palsy. Pediatr Neurol 1998;18:143–149.
22. Paz AC Jr, Burnett SM, Braga LW. Walking prognosis in cerebral palsy: a 22-year retrospective analysis. Dev Med Child Neurol 1994;36:130–134.
23. Watt JM, Robertson CM, Grace MG. Early prognosis for ambulation of neonatal intensive care survivors with cerebral palsy. Dev Med Child Neurol 1989;31:766–773.
24. Tardieu C, Huet de la Tour E, Bret MD, Tardieu G. Muscle hypoextensibility in children with cerebral palsy: I. Clinical and experimental observations. Arch Phys Med Rehabil 1982;63:97–102.
25. Berger W, Quintern J, Dietz V. Pathophysiology of gait in children with cerebral palsy. Electroencephalogr Clin Neurophysiol 1982;53:538–548.
26. Ziv I, Blackburn N, Rang M, Koreska J. Muscle growth in normal and spastic mice. Dev Med Child Neurol 1984; 26:94–99.
27. Crenna P, Inverno M, Frigo C, et al. Pathophysiological profile of gait in children with cerebral palsy. In: Forssberg H, Hirschfeld H, eds. Movement Disorders in Children. Basel: Karger, 1992:186–198.
28. Unnithan VB, Dowling JJ, Frost G, Bar-Or O. Role of cocontraction in the O₂ cost of walking in children with cerebral palsy. Med Sci Sports Exerc 1996;28:1498–1504.
29. Burke D. Spasticity as an adaptation to pyramidal tract injury. Adv Neurol 1988;47:401–423.
30. Brouwer B, Ashby P. Altered corticospinal projections to lower limb motoneurons in subjects with cerebral palsy. Brain 1991;114:1395–1407.
31. Leonard CT, Herschfeld H, Moritani T, Forssberg H. Myotatic reflex development in normal children and those with cerebral palsy. Exp Neurol 1991;111:379–382.
32. Leonard CT, Moritani T, Hirschfeld H, Forssberg H. Deficits in reciprocal inhibition of children with cerebral palsy as revealed by H reflex testing. Dev Med Child Neurol 1990;32:974–984.
33. Wiley ME, Damiano DL. Lower-extremity strength profiles in spastic cerebral palsy. Dev Med Child Neurol 1998;40:100–107.
34. Castle ME, Reyman TA, Schneider M. Pathology of spastic muscle in cerebral palsy. Clin Orthop 1979;142:223–232.
35. Romanini L, Villani C, Meloni C, Calvisi V. Histological and morphological aspects of muscle in infantile cerebral palsy. Ital J Orthop Traumatol 1989;15:87–93.
36. Rose J, Haskell WL, Gamble JG, et al. Muscle pathology and clinical measures of disability in children with cerebral palsy. J Orthop Res 1994;12:758–768.
37. Nashner LM, Shumway-Cook A, Marin O. Stance posture control in select groups of children with cerebral palsy: deficits in sensory organization and muscular coordination. Exp Brain Res 1983; 49:393–409.
38. Perry J. Gait Analysis: Normal and Pathological Function. Thorofare, NJ: Slack Inc., 1992:327–342.
39. Hoofwijk M, Unnithan V, Bar-Or O. Maximal treadmill performance of children with cerebral palsy. Ped Exerc Sci 1995;7:305–313.
40. Rieckert H, Bruhn U, Schwalm U, Schnitzer W. Endurance training within a program of physical education in children predominantly with cerebral palsy. Med Welt. 1977;28:1694–1701.
41. Lundberg A. A longitudinal study of physical working capacity of young people with spastic cerebral palsy. Dev Med Child Neurol 1984;26:328–334.
42. Bar-Or O, Inbar O, Spira R. Physiological effects of a sports rehabilitation program on cerebral palsied and post-poliomyelitic adolescents. Med Sci Sports 1976;8:157–161.

43. Lundberg A. Maximal aerobic capacity of young people with spastic cerebral palsy. Dev Med Child Neurol 1978;20:205–210.

44. van den Berg-Emons RJG, van Baak MA, de Barbanson DC, et al. Reliability of tests to determine peak aerobic power, anaerobic power and isokinetic muscle strength in children with spastic cerebral palsy. Dev Med Child Neurol 1996;38:1117–1125.

45. Lundberg A. Oxygen consumption in relation to work load in students with spastic cerebral palsy. J Appl Physiol 1976;40:873–875.

46. Dahlback GO, Norlin R. The effect of corrective surgery on energy expenditure during ambulation in children with cerebral palsy. Eur J Appl Physiol 1985;54:67–70.

47. Fernhall B, Millar AL, Tymeson GT, Burkett LN. Maximal exercise testing of mentally retarded adolescents and adults: Reliability study. Arch Phys Med Rehabil 1990;71:1065–1068.

48. Dresen MHW, de Groot G, Mesa Menor JR, Bouman LN. Aerobic energy expenditure of handicapped children after training. Arch Phys Med Rehabil 1985;66:302–306.

49. Campbell J, Ball J. Energetics of walking in cerebral palsy. Orthop Clin North Am 1978;9:374–377.

50. Bowen TR, Miller F, Mackenzie W. Comparison of oxygen consumption measurements in children with cerebral palsy to children with muscular dystrophy. J Pediatr Orthop 1999;19:133–136.

51. Duffy CM, Hill AE, Cosgrove AP, et al. Energy consumption in children with spina bifida and cerebral palsy: a comparative study. Dev Med Child Neurol 1996;38:238–243.

52. Rose J, Gamble JG, Medeiros J, et al. Energy cost of walking in normal children and in those with cerebral palsy: comparison of heart rate and oxygen uptake. J Pediatr Orthop 1989;204:276–279.

53. Rose J, Gamble JG, Burgos A, et al. Energy expenditure index of walking for normal children and for children with cerebral palsy. Dev Med Child Neurol 1990;32:333–340.

54. Rose J, Haskell WL, Gamble JG. A comparison of oxygen pulse and respiratory exchange ratio in cerebral palsied and nondisabled children. Arch Phys Med Rehabil 1993;74:702–705.

55. Boyd R, Fatone S, Rodda J, et al. High- or low-technology measurements of energy expenditure in clinical gait analysis? Dev Med Child Neurol 1999;41:676–682.

56. Olney SJ, MacPhail A, Hedden DM, Boyce WF. Work and power in hemiplegic cerebral palsy gait. Phys Ther 1990;70:431–438.

57. Lee EH, Goh JCH, Bose K. Value of gait analysis in the assessment of surgery in cerebral palsy. Phys Med Rehabil 1992;73:642–646.

58. Unnithan VB, Dowling JJ, Frost G, Bar-Or O. Role of mechanical power estimates in the O_2 cost of walking in children with cerebral palsy. Med Sci Sports Exerc 1999;31:1703–1708.

59. Kaplan SL. Cycling patterns in children with and without cerebral palsy. Dev Med Child Neurol. 1995;37:620–630.

60. Maltais D, Kondo I, Bar-Or O. Arm cranking economy in spastic cerebral palsy: effects of different speed and force combinations yielding the same mechanical power. Ped Exerc Sci 2000;12:258–269.

61. Powers SK, Beadle RE, Mangum M. Exercise efficiency during arm ergometry: effects of speed and work rate. J Appl Physiol 1984;56:495–499.

62. Parker DF, Carriere L, Hebestreit H, Bar-Or O. Anaerobic endurance and peak muscle power in children with spastic cerebral palsy. Am J Dis Child 1992;146:1069–1073.

63. Bar-Or O. The Wingate Anaerobic Test. An update on methodology, reliability and validity. Sports Med 1987;4:381–394.

64. Van Mil GAH, Schoeber N, Calvert RE, Bar-Or O. Optimization of braking force in the Wingate test for children and adolescents with a neuromuscular disease. Med Sci Sports Exerc 1996;28:1087–1092.

65. Emons HJG, Groenenboom DC, Burggraaff YI, et al. Wingate Anaerobic Test in children with cerebral palsy. In: Coudert J, Van Praagh E, eds. Children and Exercise XVI. Paris: Masson, 1992:187–189.

66. Parker DF, Carriere L, Hebestreit H, et al. Muscle performance and gross motor function of children with spastic cerebral palsy. Dev Med Child Neurol 1993;35:17–23.

67. Tirosh E, Rosenbaum P, Bar-Or O. A new muscle power test in neuromuscular disease: feasibility and reliability. Am J Dis Child 1990;144:1083–1087.

68. Russell DJ, Rosenbaum PL, Cadman DT, et al. The gross motor function measure: a means to evaluate the effects of physical therapy. Dev Med Child Neurol 1989;31:341–352.

69. Emons HJG, Van Baak MA. Effect of training on aerobic and anaerobic power and mechanical efficiency in spastic cerebral palsied children. Pediatr Exerc Sci 1993;5:412.

70. Brooke MH, Engel WK. The histographic analysis of human muscle biopsies with regard to fibre types. Neurology 1969;19:591–605.

71. Darrah J, Fan JSW, Chen LC, et al. Review of the effects of progressive resisted muscle strengthening in children with cerebral palsy: A clinical consensus exercise. Pediatr Phys Ther 1997;9:12–17.

72. Damiano DL, Vaughan CL, Abel MF. Muscle response to heavy resistance exercise in children with spastic cerebral palsy. Dev Med Child Neurol 1995;37:731–739.

73. Ayalon M, Ben-Sira D, Hutzler Y, Gilad T. Reliability of isokinetic strength measurements of the knee in children with cerebral palsy. Dev Med Child Neurol 2000;42:398–402.

74. Riddle DL, Finucaine SD, Rothstein JM, Walker ML. Intrasession and intersession reliability of hand-held dynamometer measurements taken on brain-damaged patients. Phys Ther 1989;69:182–194.

75. Kramer JF, MacPhail HEA. Relationships among measures of walking efficiency, gross motor ability and isokinetic strength in adolescents with cerebral palsy. Pediatr Phys Ther 1994;6:3–8.

76. Damiano DL, Kelly LE, Vaughn CL. Effects of quadriceps femoris muscle strengthening on crouch gait in children with spastic diplegia. Phys Ther 1995b;75:658–671.

77. MacPhail HEA, Kramer JF. Effect of isokinetic strength-training on functional ability and walking efficiency in adolescents with cerebral palsy. Dev Med Child Neurol 1995;37:763–775.

78. Holland LJ, Steadward RD. Effects of resistance and flexibility training on strength, spasticity/muscle tone, and range of motion of elite athletes with cerebral palsy. Palaestra 1990 (Summer):27–31.

79. Healy A. Two methods of weight-training for children with spastic cerebral palsy. Res Q 1958;29:389–395.

80. Horvat M. Effects of a progressive resistance training program on an individual with spastic type of cerebral palsy. Am Corr Ther J 1987;41:7–11.

81. Spira R, Bar-Or O. An investigation of the ambulation problems associated with severe motor in adolescents: influence of physical conditioning and adapted sports activities. Final report (Project number: 19-P: 58065-F-01). Washington, DC: Department of Health Education and Welfare SRS, 1975:1–81.

82. Berg K. Effect of physical training of school children with cerebral palsy. Acta. Paediatr Scand Suppl 1970;204:27–33.

83. Sommer M. Improvement of motor skills and adaptation of the circulatory system in wheelchair-bound children in cerebral palsy. Lecture No. 11. In Simon U (ed.). Sports as a Means of Rehabilitation. Netanya, Israel: Wingate Institute, 1971:1–11.

84. Ekblom BB, Lundberg A. Effects of physical training on adolescents with severe motor handicaps. Acta Paediatr Scand 1968;57:17–23.

85. Lundberg A, Ovenfors CA, Saltin B. Effect of physical training on school-children with cerebral palsy. Acta Pediatr Scand 1967;56:182–188.

86. Lundberg A, Pernow B. The effect of physical training on oxygen utilization and lactate formation in the exercising muscle of adolescents with motor handicaps. Scand J Clin Invest 1970;26:89–96.

87. DeLuca PA. The musculoskeletal management of children with cerebral palsy. Pediatr Clin North Am 1996;43:1135–1150.

88. Dahlbäck GO, Norlin R. The effect of corrective surgery on energy expenditure during ambulation in children with cerebral palsy. Eur J Appl Physiol 1985;54:67–70.

89. McLaughlin JF, Bjornson KF, Astley SJ, et al. Selective dorsal rhizotomy: efficacy and safety in an investigator-masked randomized clinical trial. Dev Med Child Neurol 1998;40:220–232.

90. Wright FV, Sheil EMH, Drake JM, et al. Evaluation of selective dorsal rhizotomy for the reduction of spasticity in cerebral palsy: a randomized controlled trial. Dev Med Child Neurol 1998;40:239–247.

91. Steinbock P, Reiner AM, Beauchamp R, et al. A randomized clinical trial to compare selective posterior rhizotomy plus physiotherapy with physiotherapy alone in children with spastic diplegic cerebral palsy. Dev Med Child Neurol 1997;39:178–184.

92. Graubert C, Song KM, McLaughlin JF, Bjornson KF. Changes in gait at 1 year post-selective dorsal rhizotomy: Results of a prospective randomized study. J Pediatr Orthop 2000;20:496–500.

93. Sutherland D, Kaufman K, Wyatt M, Chambers H. Injection of botulinum A toxin into the gastrocnemius muscle of patients with cerebral palsy: a 3-dimensional motion analysis study. Gait 1996;4:269–279.

94. Corry IS, Cosgrove AP, Duffy CM, et al. Botulinum toxin A in hamstring spasticity. Gait Posture 1999;10:206–210.

95. Massin M, Allington N. Role of exercise testing in the functional assessment of cerebral palsy children after botulinum A toxin injection. J Ped Orthop 1999;19:362–365.

96. Graham HK, Aoki RK, Autti-Ramo I, et al. Recommendations for the use of botulinum toxin type A in the management of cerebral palsy. Gait Posture 2000;11:67–69.

97. Cosgrove AP, Graham HK. Botulinum toxin A prevents the development of contractures in the hereditary spastic mouse. Dev Med Child Neurol 1994;36:379–385.

98. Maltais D, Bar-Or O, Galea V, Pierrynowski M. Use of orthoses lowers the O_2 cost of walking in children with spastic cerebral palsy. Med Sci Sports Exerc 2001;33:320–325.

99. Stallings VA, Charney EB, Davies JC, Cronk CE. Nutritional status and growth of children with diplegic or hemiplegic cerebral palsy. Dev Med Child Neurol 1993;35:997–1006.

SUGGESTED READINGS

Bar-Or O. Pediatric Sports Medicine for the Practitioner: From Physiologic Principles to Clinical Applications. Hamburg, Germany: Springer-Verlag, 1983.

Unnithan VB, Clifford C, Bar-Or O. Evaluation by exercise testing of the child with cerebral palsy. Sports Med 1998;26:239–251.

METABOLIC
DISEASES
AND DISORDERS

CHAPTER 20

Obesity

Paul J. Arciero, Bradley C. Nindl

Overview

Recent statistics estimate that one of every two adults in the United States is overweight or obese, defined as having a **body mass index (BMI)** (calculated as weight in kg divided by the square of the height in meters [kg/m²]) greater than 25 (1). These staggering numbers are even more disturbing in light of the fact that over the past three decades the prevalence of **obesity** (BMI ≥30) in the United States has increased by over 50%. Obesity is a condition of excess body fat accumulation resulting from a state of positive energy balance due to energy intake exceeding **energy expenditure** over extended periods of time. In other words, obe-sity results from either chronic excessive food intake or sig-nificantly decreased energy expenditure due to low levels of physical activity or reduced **resting energy expenditure** with no corresponding drop in food intake (Figure 20.1).

Pathophysiology of Obesity

The pathophysiology of obesity appears to be a dysregula-tion of the body's ability to control weight either because energy intake is chronically excessive or energy expenditure is inappropriately low. The etiology is undoubtedly multi-factorial, consisting of a complex interaction between an in-

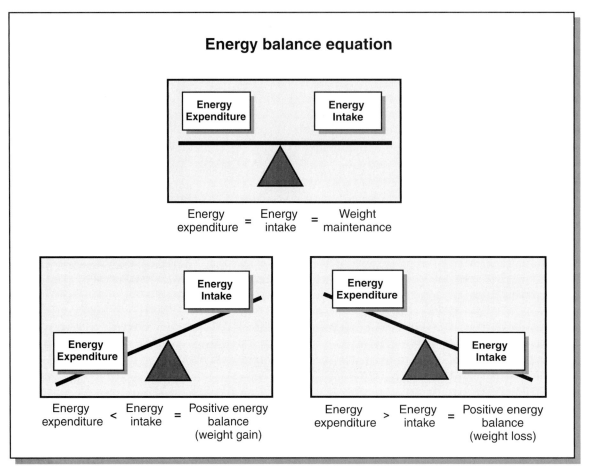

FIGURE 20.1.   Energy balance equation.

dividual's genotype and his or her environment. Our current understanding of obesity is incomplete, but it appears to involve a combination of metabolic, genetic, and social components. An individual's total energy expenditure on a daily basis is based on three major components: the resting metabolic rate, the thermic effect of food, and the thermic effect of physical activity (see Figure 20.2).

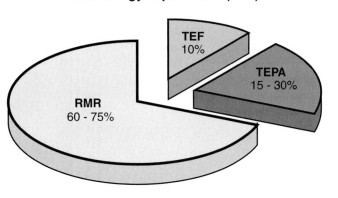

FIGURE 20.2.   Components of daily energy expenditure.

Resting metabolic rate (RMR), defined as the energy expenditure required to maintain normal physiologic functions of the body at rest in a fasted state, represents the largest component (50–75%) of total energy expenditure, and therefore is important in the regulation of energy balance and body composition. Specifically, these processes include the energy required to maintain body temperature and electrolyte gradients, sustain cardiovascular and pulmonary work at rest, and supply energy for the central nervous system and other chemical reactions. The RMR usually is measured in the early morning following a 10- to 12-hour overnight fast and at least 36 hours after the most recent bout of exercise. The measurement of energy expenditure at any other time of the day under resting conditions is termed "resting energy expenditure" and may or may not include the increase in energy expenditure associated with the individual's level of physical activity or food ingestion. The RMR is determined in the laboratory setting by the collection and analysis of oxygen and carbon dioxide respiratory gases and their subsequent conversion to **caloric equivalents**. Resting metabolic rate is influenced by factors such as age, gender, heredity, body size and composition, body temperature, physical activity, nutritional status, and various hormones. The quantity of fat-free mass is the major determinant of RMR, but physical activity status, gender, and nutrient intake also play a part (2,3).

The **thermic effect of food (TEF)** is the energy expended above RMR following food intake and accounts for approximately 10% of an individual's total energy expenditure. The increase in energy expenditure following food ingestion is due primarily to the metabolic cost of absorbing, transporting, and converting the ingested nutrients into their respective storage forms. For example, fat digestion and storage requires the least amount of energy to metabolize (0–3%), whereas protein (20–30%) and carbohydrate (5–10%) metabolism are the most energetically expensive (4). The TEF is made up of two components: obligatory and facultative thermogenesis. **Obligatory thermogenesis** is the energy cost of the absorption, transport, and synthesis of protein, fat, and carbohydrate for subsequent use by the body. However, evidence has shown that the actual measured energy expenditure following food ingestion is higher than the value expected due to the obligatory component of nutrient disposal and storage. This excess energy expenditure above obligatory thermogenesis is termed **facultative thermogenesis** and is thought to be partially mediated by sympathetic nervous system activity and increased substrate cycling. The magnitude and duration of the thermic effect of food is influenced by the caloric content and composition of the food eaten, as well as the nutritional state (e.g., energy surplus or deficit) of the individual. For example, under conditions of caloric underfeeding, RMR decreases as a protective mechanism to conserve body energy stores from excessive depletion and thus causes the body to be more energy efficient. Conversely, during periods of overeating, RMR increases in proportion to the magnitude and duration of the food surplus condition (5).

The **thermic effect of physical activity** is the most variable component of an individual's total daily energy expenditure. It consists of the energy expended above RMR and TEF due to physical and muscular activity. The thermic effect of physical activity ranges from 15% of daily energy expenditure in sedentary persons to as much as 50% or more in individuals who regularly engage in vigorous exercise regimens. In addition to the direct energy cost of physical activity, exercise also may influence RMR by any of the following: (1) a prolonged increase in postexercise metabolic rate following an acute bout of exercise; (2) a chronic increase in resting metabolic rate due to an exercise training effect; and (3) a potentiating effect on metabolic rate due to its influence on dietary thermogenesis.

Central Regulatory Signals

The brain plays a major role in energy homeostasis and the regulation of body weight.

Its functions include hunger control, control of energy expenditure, and secretion of hormones involved in the control of energy stores. The **hypothalamus** serves to both integrate afferent signals related to energy homeostasis and produce efferent signals to regulate energy stores properly (6).

Experimentation has suggested a primary role for the hypothalamus in controlling food intake. In one study, when the ventromedial hypothalamic (VMH) nucleus was stimulated in animals, food intake was inhibited. Destruction of this nucleus resulted in hyperphagia and obesity (7). Conversely, stimulation and destruction of the lateral hypothalamic (LHA) nucleus resulted in hyperphagia and weight loss, respectively (8). Thus, it was proposed that the VMH represented the satiety center and the LHA represented the hunger center. Further evaluation of the role of the hypothalamus in energy homeostasis has focused on the particular neurotransmitters that are its molecular mediators.

Serotonin is one such neurotransmitter that has received attention because serotonergic neurons have been shown to regulate appetite (9). Injection of serotonin directly into the hypothalamus inhibits food intake. Furthermore, agents that increase the concentration of serotonin at neural synapses decrease food intake and body weight (10).

Other neuropeptides that may participate in the regulation of food intake include **neuropeptide Y (NPY)** and corticotropin-releasing hormone (11, 12). Starvation induces an increased expression in NPY mRNA in the paraventricular nuclei that are dorsal and rostral to the VMH (13). When NPY is injected directly into the cerebral ventricles of rodents, increased food intake is observed (11). The anabolic effects of NPY also include stimulation of both insulin secretion and lipoprotein lipase in adipose tissue (14). Corticotropin-releasing hormone appears to play a central catabolic role (12): when it is injected directly into the paraventricular nuclei, reduced food intake is observed (15).

Peripheral Regulatory Signals

The peripheral satiety signals include both short-term factors, which are related to the size of an individual meal, and long-term factors, which are concerned with overall energy stores and balance. **Cholecystokinin (CCK)** has emerged as a key short-term regulator of satiety with peripheral administration reducing individual meal size (16); however, it also leads to greater meal frequency (17) and therefore does not appear to contribute to long-term regulation of body weight. Such a role does appear to be served by **leptin**, an **adipocyte**-derived peptide that plays an important role in the pathogenesis of obesity and may mediate the neuroendocrine response to food deprivation. Work with *ob/ob* mice has helped to discern leptin's role in regulation of weight.

The *ob* gene is expressed in adipocytes to produce leptin. A total deficiency of this peptide can be realized in *ob/ob* mice, which have two mutant alleles of the gene preventing the synthesis of leptin. Such mice display hyperphagia and decreased energy expenditure, resulting in massive obesity (18,19). When leptin is administered peripherally to these mice, the disorder is reversed (18,19). Leptin activates specific centers in the brain, including the hypothalamus, to decrease food intake; increase energy expenditure through activation of the sympathetic nervous system; affect glucose and fat metabolism; and alter neuroendocrine function (20).

The dramatic effects of leptin administration in leptin-deficient *ob/ob* mice spurred investigators to ascertain whether human obesity also was the result of leptin deficiency. Although a few individuals with extreme, early-onset obesity due to a mutation of the leptin gene have been identified, several population studies have failed to demonstrate mutations in the leptin gene across human populations; instead, leptin levels actually are increased in most obese people (21). As in rodents, the levels of leptin in the circulation reflect the size of adipose storage (22). Levels decline with weight loss (23). This suggests that obesity may be a leptin-resistant state and has prompted research for identifying receptor and postreceptor defects that could explain this resistance.

The functions of adipocytes include **triglyceride** synthesis for energy storage, triglyceride degradation for energy release, and signal transmissions to the brain concerning energy storage in the form of leptin. In addition to the secretion of leptin, adipocytes also secrete lipoprotein lipase (LPL), which hydrolyzes triglycerides in chylomicrons and very-low-density lipoproteins to free fatty acids for eventual uptake by the adipocyte for triglyceride synthesis (24). The activity of LPL has been shown to be greater in obese individuals than in lean ones (25). Furthermore, the activity of the LPLs increases with weight loss, thus subjecting the individual to a regaining of the weight through triglyceride production and adipocyte filling (26). It is not known whether increased LPL activity precedes obesity or is a consequence of it. Further elucidation of how LPLs are regulated would certainly shed light on its role in obesity.

Role of the Sympathoadrenal System

The sympathoadrenal system appears to play a role in controlling energy expenditure through secretion of catecholamines. Catecholamines stimulate lipolysis in triglycerides and thermogenesis in brown adipose tissue and skeletal muscle, whereas low adrenal sympathoadrenal activity may predispose an individual to obesity (27). This notion has been reinforced by longitudinal studies in both Pima Indians and Caucasians that show a relation between low urinary noradrenaline excretion and weight gain (27).

The contribution of the sympathoadrenal system to 24-hour energy expenditure has been addressed using measurements in whole-body calorimeters. Propranolol, a β-antagonist, causes only some inhibition of the β-adrener-

gically mediated component. Administration of propranolol results in a 2% to 4% decrease in the 24-hour energy expenditure, suggesting that complete blockade of the sympathoadrenal system could reduce 24-hour energy expenditure by as much as 4% to 6%—approximately 50 to 150 kcal per day (27).

In addition to energy expenditure, the sympathoadrenal system also appears to influence the type of substrate oxidized. An inverse relationship has been observed between the 24-hour respiratory quotient and basal muscle sympathetic nerve activity; this suggests that low **sympathetic nervous system (SNS)** activity is associated with decreased lipid oxidation (27). Individuals with low intrinsic SNS activity therefore will display decreased sympathetic-induced lipolysis, predisposing them to triglyceride retention and weight gain.

Further elucidation of the role of the sympathoadrenal system has focused on the β_3-adrenergic receptor. The β_3 receptor is responsible for mediating catecholamine-stimulated thermogenesis in brown adipose tissue and lipolysis in white fat cells in humans (28). Interestingly, studies of adipose tissue in genetically obese mice show a decreased expression of β_3-adrenergic receptors (29). Recent studies have revealed a mutation in the gene for the β_3-adrenergic receptor in humans (30). This mutation has been associated with an increased capacity to gain weight in some morbidly obese persons (30).

It is postulated that low β_3-adrenergic receptor activity could promote obesity in different ways. Low receptor activity would result in decreased thermogenesis in brown adipose tissue; in addition, lipolysis would be inhibited in white adipose tissue, causing retention of lipids in adipocytes (28). This theory has stimulated the development of agonists to the receptor as potential weight-loss agents.

Genetic and Environmental Influences on Obesity

In humans, obesity is not thought to be inherited in a simple mendelian fashion. However, there is a genetic component that cannot be overlooked. Studies of obese children show that in 72% of cases at least one parent was obese (31). Perhaps the best evidence of a genetic influence comes from studies in Denmark using adoptees and in Sweden using twins who were reared apart (32). Adoptees were found to have a BMI similar to that of their biologic parents rather than their cultural parents (33). Similarly, the BMIs of monozygotic twins resembled each other more closely than those of dizygotic twins, regardless of their rearing (32).

It seems likely that obesity results from an interaction between multiple genes and the environment. Obesity is more prevalent at lower socioeconomic levels and has been correlated directly to television watching in children (34).

Women in the United States with low incomes or a lower level of education are more likely to be obese than those of higher socioeconomic status; this association is weaker in men (35). Cultural factors also probably play a role. For example, in households where both parents work, consumption of fast food and microwave meals is increased (36). These foods tend to be high in fat, and studies confirm that adiposity in humans is directly associated with fat content of the diet (37).

Medical Causes of Obesity

Occasionally, obesity can be classified as secondary. In secondary obesity, an underlying primary disease state is considered responsible for the obesity. In adults, **Cushing syndrome** and **hypothyroidism** are possible causes; in children, one should consider lesions of the hypothalamus (e.g., craniopharyngioma).

In Cushing syndrome, excess cortisol is produced from either iatrogenic causes (e.g., chronic use of prednisone for rheumatologic disorders), pituitary tumors, or tumors of the adrenal gland. This state of cortisol excess favors lipogenesis and creates a classic clinical picture characterized by central obesity, thinning skin, glucose intolerance, and proximal myopathy.

Hypothyroidism is fairly prevalent in the general population, especially in women older than 50 years of age. In hypothyroidism, the patient often presents with vague complaints such as fatigue, dry skin, cold intolerance, weight gain, and constipation. Most cases are secondary to Hashimoto thyroiditis, an autoimmune disease that results in inflammation, fibrosis, and eventual failure of the thyroid gland.

As discussed earlier, lesions of the hypothalamus, specifically the ventromedial nucleus, can result in hyperphagia and obesity in rats. A similar effect is observed in children with craniopharyngioma, a central nervous system tumor that has a propensity to compress and inhibit this region of the hypothalamus.

Clinical Complications of Obesity

Second only to cigarette smoking as the leading cause of preventable death in the United States, obesity contributes to approximately 300,000 deaths annually (38, 39). In morbidly obese men between the ages of 25 and 34, mortality is increased 12-fold (40), and a similar effect is seen in women (41). Cardiovascular disease is the greatest risk, but increased mortality from cancer of the colon, rectum, prostate, breast, and uterus also occurs (41, 42).

The clinical complications are far-reaching, involving almost every physiologic system. Weight loss improves or reverses most of these complications. For example, even modest weight loss can significantly improve glucose toler-

ance and insulin action in **type 2 diabetes mellitus** (43). The clinical complications of obesity are addressed in the following sections and are summarized in Table 20.1. All overweight and obese adults with a BMI greater than 25 are considered at risk for developing the morbidities of obesity discussed in the following sections.

Diabetes Mellitus

Obesity induces an insulin-resistant state, placing the individual at risk for type 2 diabetes mellitus. In fact, over 80% of individuals with this disorder are obese (44). Insulin resistance usually does not develop until his or her body weight has passed 120% of normal (45). The risk for developing diabetes increases as the degree of obesity and the person's age increase (46). The underlying reason for the resistance in obesity probably is multifactorial and may include a decline in the number and function of insulin receptors as well as postreceptor defects (47,48).

The increased levels of circulating free fatty acids may mediate the insulin resistance in obesity (49). Free fatty acids have been shown to inhibit insulin-stimulated glucose utilization in the muscles and stimulate hepatic gluconeogenesis (50, 51). In addition, pharmacologic reduction in the level of free fatty acids, a low-calorie diet, or exercise training is associated with improved glucose utilization and insulin action (43, 52).

Cardiovascular System

Most studies indicate that obesity increases the risk for cardiovascular disease even when confounding variables are taken into account. In the Framingham Heart Study, abdominal obesity was associated with an increase incidence of coronary heart disease, congestive heart failure, and stroke (53). Whether obesity is an independent risk factor

TABLE 20.1.   MEDICAL COMPLICATIONS OF OBESITY

Type 2 diabetes mellitus
Hypertension
Dyslipidemia ($\uparrow$ LDL $\uparrow$ TG $\downarrow$ HDL)
Macrovascular disease (coronary artery disease, stroke)
Pickwickian syndrome
Sleep apnea
Gallstones (cholecystitis, pancreatitis)
Nonalcoholic steatohepatitis
Polycystic ovarian syndrome
Osteoarthritis
Stress incontinence
Lower back pain
Pseudotumor cerebri
Intertrigo
Cancer (endometrial, breast, colon, prostate, gallbladder)

and has a direct effect on cardiovascular disease has not been determined. It may be that the effects of obesity on cardiovascular risk are indirect, because obesity often is associated with proven risk factors such as diabetes mellitus, **hypertension**, and **hyperlipidemia**.

Although the connection remains uncertain, obesity appears to be associated with hypertension (54). This effect has even been observed in obese adolescents (55). A cross-sectional study in Norway revealed that an increase of 3 mm Hg each in systolic and diastolic pressures was observed with every 10-kg increase in body weight (46). Increased levels of norepinephrine may account for the hypertension (55). Some argue that it may be a consequence of insulin resistance. Regardless of the underlying mechanism, it is certain that the hypertension improves or reverses with weight loss (56).

Obesity induces an atherogenic lipid profile with increased low-density lipoprotein (LDL) cholesterol, increased triglycerides, and decreased high-density lipoprotein (HDL) cholesterol (46). It is proposed that high circulating levels of free fatty acids in obese persons travel to the liver, leading to the overproduction of very-high-density lipoproteins (VLDL), the precursor to LDL. In addition to its atherogenic lipid profile, obesity further increases the chance for an acute coronary event by its inhibition of tissue plasminogen activator, a potent inhibitor of thrombosis (57).

The effect of obesity on circulatory demands predisposes the individual to congestive heart failure. These effects include an increased **cardiac output** to perfuse the enlarged body mass and an increased systemic vascular resistance in the setting of hypertension (58). This increased workload induces cardiac dilatation and hypertrophy. Obesity can result in alterations of cardiac structure and function, even in the absence of hypertension (35). The diastolic dysfunction from eccentric hypertrophy and systolic dysfunction from excessive wall stress results in "obesity cardiomyopathy" (35).

The relation of obesity to cerebrovascular disease has not been evaluated as thoroughly as its relation to coronary heart disease. However, recent prospective studies indicate that the risk of stroke increases as the BMI rises. Specifically, compared to women with a BMI below 21, the risk of ischemic stroke is 75% higher in women whose BMI is higher than 27 and 137% higher in women whose BMI is greater than 32 (35).

Pulmonary Effects

Obese individuals are at risk for hypoventilation, characterized by an elevated P_{CO_2} on arterial blood gas measurement. The increased girth of the chest wall and abdomen decrease the compliance of the respiratory system, thereby altering the respiratory pattern (46). Due to an increased ventilation perfusion mismatch, they are predisposed to hypoxia as well (59). This combination of hypoxemia and carbon dioxide retention in obese patients is referred to as the Pickwickian syndrome.

Obese individuals also are at increased risk for obstructive and central **sleep apnea** (60). The combination of a large neck girth, defined as a neck circumference larger than 17 inches in men and 16 inches in women, and snoring is highly predictive of sleep apnea (35). Chronic fatigue, sluggishness, morning headaches, hypertension, and increased pulmonary resistance characterize this disorder. Treatment for these patients includes weight loss and avoidance of alcohol and sedatives (60). Continual positive airway pressure can be beneficial. Uncontrolled sleep apnea can lead to pulmonary hypertension, polycythemia, and cor pulmonale, which can predispose the individual to sudden cardiac death from ventricular arrhythmias. Such patients may require a tracheotomy for definitive treatment (60).

Hepatic and Gastrointestinal Effects

In recent years, **nonalcoholic steatohepatitis (NASH)** has been increasingly recognized as a complication of obesity (61). In the obese patient, this disorder is marked by elevated liver enzymes, hypertriglyceridemia, hepatomegaly, and hepatic histologic changes similar to those of alcoholic hepatitis (61). Data suggest that NASH is progressive in approximately 40% of patients, leading to cirrhosis in about 10% (61).

The pathophysiology of NASH may be secondary to interactions between insulin and leptin, both of which are elevated in obesity. It is postulated that leptin promotes both insulin secretion and resistance, which together enhance delivery of free fatty acids to the liver. Accumulation of free fatty acids in the liver increases the chance for lipid peroxidation, a mediator of inflammation and subsequent fibrosis (61).

Gallstones are a well-established consequence of obesity, especially in women. Gallstones occur approximately four times more often in obese than in nonobese persons. The prevalence of this disorder increases with age and with increasing obesity (46). Gallstones in obese women appear to be the result of an increased lithogenic bile composition (cholesterol supersaturation of the bile) and decreased gallbladder emptying (61). Interestingly, the incidence of gallstone formation increases significantly during dieting. This risk is correlated directly with the patient's BMI and the severity of calorie restriction; it is inversely related to the amount of dietary fat (62). Gallstones can lead to cholecystitis and pancreatitis and are a risk factor for gallbladder carcinoma.

Endocrine Effects

In obese men, the presence of excess adipose tissue leads to the increased production of estrogen. Adipose tissue is capable of converting androstenedione into estrone. The increased estrogen levels in men are usually clinically silent but occasionally may manifest as gynecomastia or impotence. In women, this hyperestrogenic state actually protects against osteoporosis.

Gynecologic Effects

Peripheral overproduction of estrogen in obese postmenopausal women is suspected of promoting uterine cancer. The risk is three times higher among obese women (BMI >30 kg/m²) compared to women of normal weight (35). In premenopausal women, obesity plays an unclear role in the constellation of changes observed in **polycystic ovarian syndrome** (PCOS), including infertility, abnormal vaginal bleeding, and hirsutism. Polycystic ovarian syndrome results from a dysregulation of the pituitary-gonadal axis in which increased secretion of luteinizing hormone (LH) leads to increased ovarian production of androstenedione and subsequent adipose production of estrone; the increased estrogen, in turn, drives further LH secretion, thus establishing a dysregulated cycle.

Musculoskeletal Effects

A few studies indicate that obesity, especially when central in distribution, is a risk factor for development or aggravation of existing lower back pain (63). The excessive abdominal girth places an unnecessary stress on the musculature of the lower back when the individual stands.

Obesity is a well-established risk factor for osteoarthritis, with a particularly strong association for bilateral knee disease in women (63). Prospective data in women reveal that the risk for osteoarthritis in the knee is increased by approximately 15% for each additional kg/m² of BMI greater than 27 (64). The excess weight in obesity increases the amount of force across a weight-bearing joint, thereby predisposing it to premature degeneration.

Dermatologic Effects

Intertrigo is characterized by pruritic erythematous plaques with small peripheral pustular lesions. This condition is a form of cutaneous candidiasis and often appears in regions of increased moisture such as the inframammary or axillary areas or the groins. The excess skin folds in obesity offer a moist, occluded environment that is ideal for the proliferation of *Candida albicans*.

Neurologic Effects

Pseudotumor cerebri (also known as benign intracranial hypertension) usually is seen in obese women younger than 40 years of age. Secondary to an idiopathic increase in intracranial pressure, the patient complains of headache and occasionally, transient visual obscurations. It is uncertain how obesity increases the risk for this disorder.

Clinical Approach to the Obese Patient

The health care provider's approach to the obese patient consists of the same three components applied for all chronic care patient encounters: history, physical examination, and laboratory and diagnostic tests. Only after the health care provider performs these steps can a proper risk assessment and therapeutic regimen, including exercise training, diet, and, if needed, pharmacologic therapy be considered.

Taking an Obesity-Focused History

A thorough history remains the most important element of the patient encounter. The following areas should be explored: chronological history of weight gain, possible precipitating events (e.g., smoking cessation), prior weight loss attempts, occupation, family history, diet, physical activity, and medication use (65). Medications associated with weight gain include antipsychotics (phenothiazines and butyrophenones), antidepressants (amitriptyline and lithium), antiepileptics (valproate and carbamazepine), corticosteroids (glucocorticoids, estrogen, and megestrol acetate), and antidiabetic agents (insulin, sulfonylureas, and thiazolidinediones) (65).

A review of systems with attention to those clinical conditions described in the previous section is essential. A history of early morning headache and daytime fatigue suggests obstructive sleep apnea, whereas right upper abdominal discomfort, particularly after fatty meals, suggests the presence of gallstones. The patient should be queried about dyspnea, angina, or edema that may reflect underlying coronary artery disease or cor pulmonale. In premenopausal women, a history of amenorrhea, hirsutism, and menorrhagia should be probed. In postmenopausal women, any history of vaginal bleeding should be noted.

Finally, the patient's understanding of how body weight is regulated should be explored. For any treatment program to be effective, the patient must understand that weight loss will result only if energy in is less than energy out.

Physical Examination of the Obese Patient

Accurate measurement of height and weight is the initial step in the physical examination of the obese patient. The best method for assessing the degree of obesity is the BMI, which is calculated as the body weight (kg) divided by the square of the height (m²) (65). The BMI is well correlated with body fat and shows a curvilinear relation to risk. A BMI of 30 kg/m² defines obesity (65). A BMI between 25 kg/m² and 30 kg/m² is considered overweight; a BMI less than 25 kg/m² is desirable (65). It is important to remember that individuals who are muscular or of short stature may have BMIs that seem high but do not, in those cases, indicate obesity (35).

The waist circumference also is an indicator of abdominal fat. This value is recorded with a flexible tape placed horizontally at the superior aspect of the iliac crests (65). A waist circumference greater than 40 inches in men and 35 inches in women is an independent risk factor for obesity-related complications in adults with a BMI of 25 to 34.9 kg/m² (65). For patients with BMI higher than 35 kg/m², waist circumference measurements are not necessary because this value loses its predictive power at very high BMIs (35).

The remainder of the physical examination for obese patients is similar to that for other adult patients. Special considerations are necessary in certain instances, however. For instance, use of a cuff that is too small when measuring blood pressure can lead to an overestimation of blood pressure and a false diagnosis of hypertension. To ensure accurate measurement the bladder width of the cuff should be approximately 50% of the upper arm circumference (65). A thigh cuff is needed for patients with severe obesity and arm circumferences greater than 16 inches.

Obesity-related complications often have corresponding findings on physical examination, providing a clue to the underlying diagnosis. On cardiac examination, a prominent P2 component of the second heart sound may be heard in patients who have cor pulmonale from long-standing obstructive sleep apnea or pickwickian syndrome. Other manifestations of cor pulmonale and right-sided heart failure include hepatomegaly, venous jugular distention, and bilateral lower leg edema.

On the abdominal examination, hepatomegaly may suggest nonalcoholic steatohepatitis, and the presence of right upper quadrant pain on palpation may be a manifestation of gallbladder complications (e.g., cholecystitis). Choledocholithiasis, obstruction of the common bile duct by a gallstone, can manifest with jaundice, icteric sclerae, and fever.

On examination of the integument, erythematous plaques that indicate *Candida albicans* infections may be observed in intertriginous areas such as the groin or beneath pendulous breasts. Obese patients with severe hypertriglyceridemia (>1000 mg/dl) may present with eruptive xanthomas, which are yellowish, dome-shaped papules that tend to appear suddenly on the back, elbows, or buttocks. Women with polycystic ovarian syndrome often display hirsutism, excessive hair growth in androgen-dependent regions (e.g., the face, chest, areolae, lower back, and inner thighs).

The physical examination sometimes provides clues to an underlying medical cause for the obesity. Cushing syndrome manifests as thin skin with purple striae, facial plethora, hirsutism, and central obesity. Due to the central distribution of fat, the patient often displays a "moon face" and a "buffalo hump" but has relatively thin limbs. The hypothyroid patient can present with nonpitting edema, usually on the hands and eyelids, goiter, and delayed relaxation phases of the peripheral reflexes.

Laboratory Evaluation of the Patient

All obese patients should have an initial serum thyroid-stimulating hormone (TSH) and a fasting blood glucose and lipid panel drawn annually. The higher incidence in this group of nonalcoholic steatohepatitis also warrants routine liver function testing. Obese patients should undergo the same preventive measures as the middle-aged adult patient such as annual mammograms for women and prostate-specific antigen (PSA) levels for men.

Certain clues on history or physical examination may warrant particular tests. For the patient suspected of sleep apnea, a sleep study should be performed to confirm that diagnosis. In patients suspected of having the pickwickian syndrome, a complete blood count (to rule out polycythemia), arterial blood gas (to screen for elevated P_{CO_2}), and electrocardiogram and chest x-ray to assess the degree of right heart strain and cor pulmonale should be ordered. Suspected gallstones can be ascertained with ultrasonography of the right upper quadrant. An LH-to-FSH ratio should be obtained in females with suspected polycystic ovarian disease (LH/FSH >2.5). If underlying Cushing disease is suspected as the cause of the obesity, a 24-hour urine screen for free cortisol (a finding of >150 μg/24h should be considered abnormal) and an overnight dexamethasone suppression test should be performed.

Risk Stratification of the Obese Patient

Once the history, physical examination, and laboratory workup are complete, the health care provider can risk-stratify the obese patient properly and design an appropriate treatment regimen. The health care provider should be able to identify factors contributing to the patient's weight gain; identify resultant medical conditions that may benefit from weight loss; and develop a safe and effective weight loss program for the patient.

The primary classification of obesity is based on the measurement of BMI. Individuals with a BMI below 25 kg/m² are deemed a low risk for clinical complications; a significant rise in risk is seen when the BMI is greater than 25 kg/m² (66). This risk is further increased by the presence of comorbid risk factors (66). For individuals with a BMI higher than 30 kg/m², mortality rates from all causes are increased by 50% to 100% above that of persons with a BMI between 25 and 30 kg/m² (35).

TABLE 20.2. BRAY AND RYAN RISK STRATIFICATION OF OBESE PATIENTS

BMI	No. of Risk factors	High Waist Circumference	Risk Category	Treat Risk Factors	Diet	Exercise	Behavior	Drugs	Surgery
<25	0	N	Very low	N					
	0	Y	Low	N	+	+	+	–	–
	>1	Y or N	Moderate	Y	+	+	+	+	–
25–29.9	0	N	Low	N	+	+	+	–	–
	0	N	Moderate	N	+	+	+	±	–
	>1	Y or N	Moderate	Y	+	+	+	+	–
30–34.9	0	Y or N	Moderate	No	+	+	+	+	–
	>1	Y or N	High	Yes	+	+	+	+	–
>35	0	Y or N	High	No	+	+	+	+	±
	>1	Y or N	Very high	Yes	+	+	+	+	+

(Header spanning Diet–Surgery: CONSIDER AS TREATMENT FOR OVERWEIGHT)

Bray and Ryan have stratified the medical risk of obese patients, taking into account these risk factors, the BMI, and the waist circumference (66). Risk factors include diabetes or impaired glucose tolerance (FBG >110–126), hyperlipidemia (HDL-cholesterol <35 mg/dL in men and <45 in women or TG >200), and hypertension (treated, or BP >140/90) (66). A high waist circumference is defined as larger than 102 cm in men and 88 cm in women (66).

Based on these parameters, five categories of risk are delineated (see Table 20.2). Each category of risk dictates a possible treatment regimen for the patient. For example, a patient with a BMI of 33 and high waist circumference but no other coexisting risk factors would be classified as moderate risk. Such a patient would benefit from a therapeutic regimen of diet, exercise, behavior therapy, and pharmacotherapy.

According to the guidelines on obesity from the National Institutes of Health (NIH), high-risk concomitant diseases include coronary heart disease or other atherosclerotic diseases, type 2 diabetes mellitus, and sleep apnea (35). Patients with these disorders should be classified as being at very high risk for disease complications and mortality (35). The NIH guidelines classify obesity by BMI, waist circumference, and associated disease risk (Table 20.3).

Treatment of the Obese Patient

The foundation for any weight loss regimen includes exercise, diet, and behavioral therapy. Obese patients with comorbid risk factors are candidates for pharmacologic intervention. For morbidly obese patients who are recalcitrant to these measures, surgery can be considered. It is essential that the physician establish reasonable goals for the weight loss. Initially, a 10% reduction in weight over the first 6 months would be considered appropriate (67).

Acute Exercise Response

It is generally accepted that a sedentary lifestyle promotes accumulation of excess body fat. Exercise, on the other hand, leads to a healthy body weight and composition due to an increase in total daily energy expenditure because of the direct caloric cost of the exercise bout and the elevation in energy expenditure during the immediate postexercise period. Following a single bout of exercise, oxygen consumption and, therefore, the metabolic rate, remains elevated above the resting level for a period of time and is

TABLE 20.3. NIH OBESITY CLASSIFICATION AND RISK STRATIFICATION

	BMI (kg/m²)	Obesity Class	Men < 40 in, Women < 35 in	Men > 40 in, Women > 35 in
Underweight	<18.5		–	–
Normal	18.5–24.9		–	–
Overweight	25.0–29.9		Increased	High
Obese	30.0–34.9	I	High	Very high
	35.0–39.9	II	Very high	Very high
Extremely Obese	>40	III	Extremely high	Extremely high

(Spanning header over last two columns: DISEASE RISK (CVD, HTN, DIABETES) BASED ON WAIST CIRCUMFERENCT)

BMI, body mass index; CVD, cardiovascular disease; HTN, hypertension.

termed excess postexercise oxygen consumption (EPOC). The increased metabolic rate during the postexercise period is due to the rephosphorylation of creatine and adenosine diphosphate (ADP), replenishment of glycogen stores, elevated catecholamine concentrations, triglyceride–fatty acid recycling, and elevation of core body temperature. It has been reported that acute bouts of resistance exercise may elicit greater EPOCs than comparable bouts of endurance exercise (68). From a practical standpoint, the intensity and duration of a single exercise bout prescribed for the obese patient would produce an increase in postexercise metabolic rate of approximately 10 to 30 kcal. Whether EPOC following acute exercise bouts may play a significant role in weight reduction in obese individuals has not been determined.

Exercise Training Response

Exercise training and an active lifestyle are consistently cited as important factors of long-term success in weight management as a result of inducing a negative caloric balance. A recent study among obese women who had lost weight following a 16-week treatment program demonstrated that over a 1-year follow-up the most active third of subjects continued to lose weight, and the middle third maintained their end-of-treatment weight loss, whereas the least active third gained weight steadily throughout the year (69). It has been proposed that the higher energy expenditure, specifically RMR, associated with a higher level of physical activity (or endurance training) is partly responsible for weight stability among active individuals of normal weight, possibly because the energy demands of the "active metabolic tissue" are increased with high levels of exercise training. These findings highlight the importance of daily physical activity in reducing obesity.

Exercise training also is beneficial for obese people even if no weight is lost. A negative caloric balance induced by exercise training is known to influence energy expenditure, glucose tolerance, and insulin action long before there is a major reversal of obesity and changes in body composition. Whatever the mechanism, it appears that reversal of insulin resistance in obese subjects occurs rapidly in response to negative energy balance, probably as a result of fat loss instead of storage in adipocytes, before any significant reversal of the obese state occurs. Clinical trials consistently verify that diet and physical activity interventions are effective strategies for eliciting a negative caloric balance. A low-calorie diet is clearly more effective in causing a negative fat balance than is exercise training for sedentary obese people with a low exercise capacity. However, recent findings by Arciero and colleagues (43) demonstrated that even a moderate exercise training program (about 50 minutes at 60% to 65% $\dot{V}_{O_{2max}}$) for 10 days in obese people results in a significantly greater improve-

ment in glucose disposal than did a low-calorie diet that induced more than 2.5 times the negative energy balance. The authors concluded that even an exercise training program that is practical for obese individuals has a major beneficial effect on insulin action above and beyond that induced by negative energy balance. These results provide strong support for the commonly made recommendation that a combination of diet and exercise should be used for the prevention and treatment of insulin resistance associated with obesity.

Diet

For weight to be lost, the obese patient has to grasp that energy intake must be less than energy expenditure. Because total energy requirements increase with increasing weight, obese patients will lose more weight for a given amount of fixed calorie restriction than their thinner counterparts (6). In general, a loss of 1 kg of weight requires a negative balance of approximately 7500 kcal (6). Therefore, by reducing dietary intake by 250 kcal/d, one can expect to lose approximately 1 kg (2.2 lbs) per month, or 12 kg (26.4 lbs) per year. The process often is slow, and patients tend to relapse when results are not immediately appreciated. Such patients are easily drawn to one of the numerous fad diets that promise instant results.

High-protein, low-carbohydrate diets (e.g., the Atkins diet, the Sugar Busters diet, and the Zone diet) are examples of such diets. These diets claim that the dieter can eat as much as he or she wants and lose weight as long as carbohydrate intake is restricted. Although patients will experience immediate weight loss with these diets (1 kg in the first week), the loss is secondary to diuresis, not to increased fat catabolism (70).

Restriction of carbohydrate intake induces diuresis in two different ways. First, a state of relative glucagon excess is created, favoring mobilization of glycogen stores in the liver and muscle. Each gram of glycogen is bound to approximately 2 g of water, so total mobilization of body glycogen stores (500 g) produces a weight loss of about 1 kg (70). Generation of ketone bodies from catabolism of dietary and endogenous fat is the second means of diet-induced diuresis. After being filtered by the kidney as nonresorbable anions, ketone bodies increase distal sodium secretion into the lumen, creating a net loss of sodium and water (70). This diuretic effect is limited to the first week of the diet (70).

High-protein, low-carbohydrate diets actually can have untoward metabolic effects. These diets are associated with increases in total cholesterol and LDL cholesterol and can lead to deficiencies in micronutrients secondary to the exclusion of fruits, vegetables, and grains (70). Furthermore, they promote a physiologic environment favorable for osteoporosis and nephrolithiasis (70).

Long-term weight loss is influenced by restriction of caloric, not carbohydrate, intake. In one study, patients adhering to the Atkins diet reduced their caloric intake by 500 kcal/day (71). After 8 weeks, the average weight loss was 7.7 kg, no greater than what would be expected from caloric restriction alone (71). The health care provider should design a diet that the patient will tolerate and will be able to adhere to for a lifetime. Simple suggestions include eating three meals a day; eating only at mealtimes; and eating only one serving. Ideally, diets should limit fats to no more than 30% of the total energy intake and should be rich in fruits and vegetables.

The low-calorie diet recommended should be consistent with the NCEP's Step I or Step II Diet, consisting of 1000 to 1200 kcal/day for women and 1200 to 1500 kcal/day for men (35). Low-calorie diets can reduce total body weight by an average of 8% over 3 to 10 months (35). The patient must get rid of the concept that diets are a temporary treatment and come to understand that effective dietary practice is a lifelong commitment.

Behavioral Therapy

Behavioral therapy attempts to alter eating habits through guided training (72). This therapy requires extensive self-monitoring of dietary behaviors and attempts to identify stimuli for eating behavior. Behavioral therapy changes habits to reduce energy intake by slowing food intake (e.g., putting utensils down between bites); separating eating from triggering stimuli (e.g., not eating while watching television); replacing maladaptive habits (e.g., reading a book instead of snacking when bored); substituting low-calorie foods for high-calorie foods (e.g., drink water with meals instead of soda); and increasing exercise. Behavioral therapy increases the patient's awareness of bad habits and empowers the obese patient in the struggle to reduce energy intake.

Behavioral therapy, when used in conjunction with other weight loss modalities, provides additional benefits in assisting the patient to lose weight short-term (35). Behavioral therapy can be particularly helpful for individuals who exhibit binge-eating tendencies (72). Binge eating is reported in about 30% of all obese patients; it is essential for this behavior to be abolished as an initial step in the weight loss program (72).

Pharmacologic Therapy

Pharmacologic treatment should be considered for any patient with a BMI higher than 30, regardless of attendant risk factors, and for patients with a BMI above 27 who have concomitant risk factors or diseases such as hypertension, dyslipidemia, coronary artery disease, type 2 diabetes, and sleep apnea (35). In general, lifestyle therapy directed toward diet, behavioral modification, and exercise should be tried for at least 6 months before pharmacotherapy is considered (35).

Currently available medications can effectuate weight loss by one of three mechanisms: decreasing energy intake, decreasing gastrointestinal absorption of nutrients, or increasing energy expenditure. Medications should supplement, not replace, diet, behavior, and exercise interventions.

Agents That Reduce Energy Intake

Two classes of drugs that reduce energy intake are available: **noradrenergic agents** and **serotonergic agents**. The noradrenergic class includes diethylpropion (Tenuate), mazindol (Sanorex), phenylpropanolamine (Dexatrim), phentermine (Fastin), and phendimetrazine (Bontril) (73). The adrenergic drugs induce anorexia through a centrally mediated pathway in the hypothalamus. While preserving the anorectic effect of amphetamines, these drugs do possess weak abuse potential (73). Side effects include insomnia, anxiety, irritability, and headache. Sanorex and Fastin can increase blood pressure and may precipitate angina in patients with underlying coronary artery disease (74).

Fenfluramine (Pondimin) and dexfenfluramine (Redux) were the first two available serotonergic medications. These agents enhance presynaptic release of serotonin and increase its concentration at the synapse (73). The anorectic effects of serotonin have been previously addressed. Although these two drugs effectuated weight loss, they were withdrawn from the market after a combination of fenfluramine and phentermine (Phen-Fen) was found to be associated with valvular heart disease and pulmonary hypertension (75).

Sibutramine (Meridia), an agent that blocks the reuptake of serotonin, norepinephrine, and dopamine, produces weight loss by an anorectic effect and by stimulating thermogenesis (73). Studies reveal that 40% of patients lost at least 5% of their initial weight after 6 months; the weight loss appears to be dose-dependent (76, 77). Results should be appreciated within the first month. Unfortunately, weight gain often recurs after the drug is discontinued (77). Sibutramine can cause headache, insomnia, dry mouth, and increased blood pressure; it should be avoided in patients with cardiac or hepatic disease. Currently, there is no evidence suggesting an association with cardiac valve disease (73). If patients do not experience weight loss within the first month, sibutramine should be withdrawn.

Fluoxetine (Prozac), a selective serotonin reuptake inhibitor (SSRI), has been studied as a potential obesity agent. A 3-month study failed to show a significant reduction in weight when compared to placebo (78). Fluoxetine has been approved for depression and bulimia, but it has not been approved by the FDA for weight loss therapy.

Agents That Inhibit Nutrient Absorption

Orlistat (Xenical) is a lipase inhibitor that acts in the gastrointestinal tract to decrease fat absorption. It inhibits pancreatic and gastric lipases, thereby preventing triglyceride hydrolysis and, thus, absorption of free fatty acids. It is reported to increase fecal fat from 5% to 30% (79). Randomized, placebo-controlled studies indicate that significant weight loss occurs with treatment with orlistat for 12 months—8.8 kg in the treated group versus 5.8 kg in the placebo group (79). Reductions in LDL and total cholesterol also are observed (79). Side effects include flatus and steatorrhea. This drug should be avoided in patients with cholestasis and in patients using warfarin (Coumadin) because it prevents vitamin K absorption (73).

Agents That Increase Energy Expenditure

Compounds that stimulate thermogenesis are attractive options for weight loss. Several agents, including leptin and thyroid hormone, have been investigated, but the results thus far have been somewhat disappointing. Currently, no agents in the thermogenic class have been approved by the FDA for weight loss.

Ephedrine and caffeine have been shown to increase metabolic weight and are effective for short-term weight loss (27). Ephedrine stimulates the release of norepinephrine from sympathetic nerve endings and is a direct agonist on β-receptors (β_1, β_2, and β_3) (27). Caffeine is believed to potentiate the thermogenic effects of ephedrine (27).

In a randomized, double-blind, placebo-controlled study, the effects of a combination of 20 mg of ephedrine and 200 mg of caffeine three times per day as an adjuvant to a hypocaloric diet on weight loss were observed (27). The ephedrine/caffeine combination proved to be superior to placebo, promoting a weight loss of 16.6 kg versus 13.2 kg in the placebo group after 24 weeks (27). Another study suggested that the increased fat loss seen in a group receiving ephedrine and caffeine was secondary to enhanced thermogenesis and fat oxidation. Despite clinical studies that strongly support the effectiveness of an ephedrine/caffeine combination as a therapeutic agent for obesity, the limited number of patients treated in the trials fails to meet the requirements of the FDA for licensing as a prescription compound (27). Various herbal combinations of ephedrine and caffeine are available over the counter, netting $950 million in total sales in 1999 (27).

Other attempts to enhance thermogenesis have not been as successful as the ephedrine/caffeine combination in effectuating weight loss. Despite increasing the metabolic rate, thyroid hormone has only a modest effect on weight loss and causes a disproportionate loss of lean body mass (80).

Observational studies in humans suggest that leptin stimulates SNS and energy expenditure (27). Because obesity is a leptin-resistant state in which actual levels tend to be increased, it is unclear whether exogenous leptin administration can bypass this resistance and produce its effects. In both normal-weight and obese subjects, recombinant subcutaneous leptin injections produced only a modest weight loss over 6 months (27). Further work concerning optimal leptin dosages and route of administration is necessary.

Other Potential Agents

Several other agents are under consideration for use as antiobesity medications. Produlestan (Genaera Pharmaceuticals) is an aminosterol compound that has been shown to produce appetite suppression and weight loss in mice (81). It is believed that specific brain mechanisms are responsible for the appetite suppressant effects of the compound (81).

Subcutaneous growth hormone (GH) injections are also postulated to enhance loss of body fat, while building lean body mass (82). However, fears concerning its potential side effects and limited clinical studies have prevented its clinical application in obesity.

Selective β_3 **agonists** currently are being investigated as potential stimulators of thermogenesis. The role of the β_3-adrenergic receptor in obesity has been previously described. These agents have displayed excellent antiobesity effects in rodents; however, pharmaceutical problems including low bioavailability, a short half-life, and failure of the prodrugs to be metabolized to selective β_3 agonists have hindered their clinical development (27). One compound from Lilly Pharmaceuticals, LY-377604, is reported to have a 20% oral bioavailability and increases the resting metabolic rate by approximately 17.5% in normal and obese subjects (27). Further clinical studies are needed to determine whether these agents produce meaningful weight loss in humans.

Surgery

Some morbidly obese patients fail to lose weight despite regimens of diet, exercise, and medications. For such patients, especially those with comorbid conditions, surgical intervention should be considered. Surgical approaches can result in substantial weight loss, with losses of 110 to 220 pounds within a year reported by some subjects. The National Institutes of Health consensus conference on obesity surgery stated that individuals with a BMI higher than 40 kg/m² or with a BMI higher than 35 kg/m² concomitant with serious medical conditions are appropriate candidates for surgery (83).

The **jejunoileal bypass** was one of the original surgical attempts to reverse obesity. This procedure, which con-

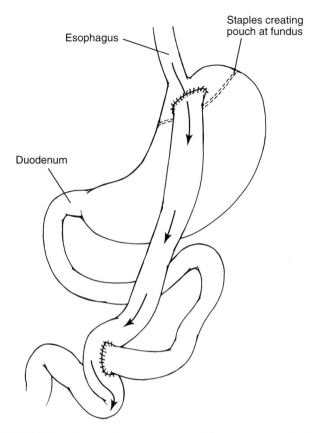

FIGURE 20.3. Roux-en-Y gastric bypass. In this procedure a vertically constructed, small (15–30 mL) gastric pouch and 1-cm gastrojejunal stoma are created using three superimposed applications (not shown) of a 90-mm stapling device. (Courtesy of George A. Bray, MD.)

nected 35 cm of proximal jejunum to the distal 10 cm of the terminal ileum, produced weight loss of approximately one third the patient's preoperative weight (84). The weight loss was effectuated by inducing a state of malabsorption, allowing calories to be passed in the stool. Unfortunately, the procedure resulted in several complications, including hepatic steatosis and cirrhosis; calcium and vitamin D deficiencies leading to osteomalacia; hyperoxaluria and secondary nephrocalcinosis; and diarrhea (84).

In light of these complications, alternative procedures, such as the **roux-en-Y gastric bypass** procedure and the vertical banded gastroplasty, have emerged. In the gastric bypass procedure, a loop of proximal jejunum is attached to the stomach. The mortality of the procedure is significantly less than that seen with the jejunoileal bypass, but the procedure is associated with deficiencies of iron, thiamine, and B_{12}, so that constant supplementation is required (84). The roux-en-Y gastric bypass procedure appears to induce weight loss through creation of a dumping syndrome and has been shown to maintain a weight loss of approximately 33% after 10 years (84).

The vertical banded gastroplasty procedure creates a 15-mL gastric reservoir through stapling, thereby decreasing gastric volume and subsequent food intake (84). Because continuity of the stomach and duodenum is preserved, there is little potential for malabsorption. Because late weight gain and need for revision tend to be more problematic with this procedure, however, most surgeons prefer the roux-en-Y gastric bypass. Both procedures have cured some of the comorbid complications such as diabetes mellitus, hypertension, sleep apnea, and the obesity hypoventilation syndrome in some patients (85).

Other unproven techniques have been espoused as potential surgical treatments. Insertion of silicone gastric balloons has had conflicting results. One study employing a 500-mL balloon in massively obese patients showed no effect on weight loss after 2 months (85), but another study using a 300-mL gastric balloon produced more weight loss in the balloon group than the control group (86). Further clinical trials are necessary to define the proper balloon size needed for optimal weight loss.

Liposuction has produced disappointing long-term weight loss results. It is postulated that a feedback mechanism is in place whereby following this procedure adipose tissue hypertrophies under the direction of leptin (27). Liposuction can produce transient cosmetic effects but should not be considered as a potential medical treatment for the obese individual.

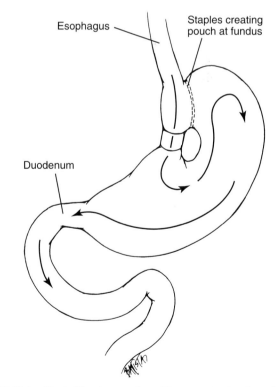

FIGURE 20.4. Vertical band gastroplasty. This operation involves elongation of the esophagus with a fixed termination midway along the lesser curvature of the stomach. (Courtesy of George A. Bray, MD.)

CASE STUDY

Patient Information

J. D. is a 46-year-old white man who presents to his primary physician with concerns over his increasing body weight. He states that he has always been considered "overweight" but has noticed a steady weight gain over the last few years—approximately 20 pounds over the last 3 years. He also expresses distress about "constantly feeling tired." Of note is the fact that he has not been seen by a physician "for several years."

J. D.'s past medical and surgical histories are negative. His family history is significant for obesity and type 2 diabetes mellitus in his mother. He has no siblings. He drinks alcoholic beverages on weekends—about 1 six-pack—and has a 25 pack-year history of cigarette abuse. He denies any history of drug use and currently does not take any prescription or over-the-counter medications. He is married with two adolescent daughters. A high school graduate, he has worked at the local post office for almost 20 years. Review of systems is significant for occasional early morning headaches and chronic fatigue. He admits to frequently nodding off while at work. He states that he often wakes up during the night and has been told by his wife that he snores very loudly. He denies a history of angina or dyspnea on exertion.

He states that he has been overweight since childhood. He does not currently participate in any type of exercise program and has never really been physically active. He reports a poor knowledge of fundamental nutrition and basically eats whatever he wants. In particular, he frequents fast food establishments a couple of times a week. His hobbies include watching sports on television and going to the movies. He has attempted the Atkins diet a few times but was not compliant due to its restriction of carbohydrates.

On physical examination, the patient is an obese middle-aged white male in no apparent distress. Vital signs are as follows:

Temperature: 98.7°F
Blood pressure: 136/88 mm Hg
Pulse rate: 92 bpm
Respiratory rate: 12
Height: 69 inches
Weight: 228 lbs
Waist circumference: 42 inches

The physical examination is remarkable for a short neck with increased girth (his neck circumference is 18 inches). Palpation of the thyroid gland is normal. Cardiac and pulmonary examinations are unremarkable. The abdomen was remarkable for increased girth. The neurologic examination is completely normal. Integument is within normal limits.

Questions

1. How would you risk-stratify J. D.'s obesity based on the history and physical examination?

2. What other laboratory or diagnostic tests are warranted to classify further his obesity?

3. J. D.'s fasting blood glucose is elevated between 155 and 170 on three consecutive occasions. A fasting lipid panel reveals total cholesterol of 290, LDL of 192, HDL of 38, and triglyceride level of 300. A sleep study is remarkable for about six apneic episodes per hour. How do these findings alter the risk stratification for J. D.?

4. What obesity treatment options are suitable for J. D.?

5. What other medical issues need to be addressed for J. D.?

6. How does J. D.'s history of smoking complicate the treatment of obesity?

7. What special considerations need to be taken into account before designing an exercise prescription for J. D.?

8. What specific exercise prescription would be best for J. D.?

REFERENCES

1. Flegal KM, Carroll MD, Kuczmarski RJ, Johnson CL. Overweight and obesity in the United States: prevalence and trends, 1960–1994. Int J Obesity 1998;22:39–47.
2. Arciero PJ, Smith DL, Calles-Escandon J. Effects of short-term inactivity on glucose tolerance, energy expenditure, and blood flow in trained subjects. J Appl Physiol 1998;84:1365–1373.
3. Arciero PJ, Goran MI, Poehlman ET. Resting metabolic rate is lower in women than in men. J Appl Physiol 1993;75:2514–2520.
4. Flatt JP. The biochemistry of energy expenditure. In: Bray G, ed. Recent Advances in Obesity Research II. London: Newman, 1978:211–228.
5. Poehlman ET, Tremblay A, Fontaine E, et al. Genotype dependency of the thermic effect of a meal and associated hormonal changes following short-term overfeeding. Metabolism 1986;35:30–36.
6. Wilson JD, Foster DW, Kronenberg HM, Larsen PR. Williams Textbook of Endocrinology. 9th Ed. 1996;1062–1083.
7. Hetherington A, Ranson SW. Hypothalamic lesions and obesity in the rat. Anat Rec 1940;78:149–172.
8. Anand BK, Brobeck JR. Localization of a "feeding center" in the hypothalamus of the rat. Proc Soc Exp Biol Med 1951;77:323–324.
9. Silverstone T, Goodall E. Serotonergic mechanisms in human feeding: the pharmacological evidence. Appetite 1986:7(Suppl):85–97.
10. Blundell JE. Serotonin and appetite. Neuropharmacology 1984;23:537–1551.
11. Stanley BG, Kyrkouli SE, Lampert S, et al. Neuropeptide Y chronically injected into the hypothalamus: a powerful neurochemical inducer of hyperphagia and obesity. Peptides 1986;7:1189–1192.
12. Arase K, York DA, Shimizu H. Effect of corticotropin releasing factor on food intake and brown adipose tissue thermogenesis in rats. Am J Physiol 1988; 255:E255–E259.
13. Marks JL, Schwartz M, Porte DJ. Effect of fasting on regional levels of neuropeptide Y mRNA and insulin receptors in the rat hypothalamus: an autoradiographic study. Mol Cell Neurol 1992;3:199–205.
14. Zarjevski N, Cusin I, Vetter F, et al. Chronic intracerebroventricular injection of neuropeptide Y on energy metabolism. Am J Physiol 1991;260:R321–R327.
15. Krahn DD, Gosnell BAD. Behavioral effects of corticotrophin releasing factor: localization and characterization of central effects. Brain Res 1988;443:63–69.
16. Gibbs J, Young RC, Smith GP. Cholecystokinin decreases food intake in rats. J Comp Physiol Psychol 1973;84:488–495.
17. West DB, Fey D, Woods SC. Cholecystokinin persistently suppresses meal size but not food intake in free-feeding rats. Am J Physiol 1984;246:R776–R787.
18. Halaas J, Gajiwala K, Maffei M, et al. Weight reducing effect of the plasma protein encoded by the gene. Science 1995; 269:543–546.
19. Campfield L, Smith F, Guisez Y, et al. Recombinant mouse OB protein: evidence for a peripheral signal linking adiposity and central neural networks. Science 1995;269:546–548.
20. Mantzoros C. The role of leptin in human obesity and disease: a review of current evidence. Ann Intern Med 1999;130:671–680.
21. Maffei M, Stoffel M, Barone M, et al. Absence of mutations on the human ob gene in obese Helsinki subjects. Diabetes 1996;45:679–682.
22. Fredrich RC, Hamann A, Anderson S, et al. Leptin levels reflect body lipid content in mice: evidence for diet induced resistance to leptin action. Nature Med 1995;1:1311–1314.
23. Tritus N, Mantzarus CS. Leptin: its role in obesity and beyond. Diabetologia 1997;40:1371–1379.
24. Eckel RH. Lipoprotein lipase: a multifunctional enzyme relevant to common metabolic diseases. N Engl J Med 1989;320:1060–1068.
25. Ong JM, Kern PA. Effect of feeding and obesity on lipoprotein lipase activity, immunoreactive protein, and messenger RNA levels in human adipose tissue. J Clin Invest 1989;84:305–311.
26. Scwartz RS, Brunzell JD. Increased adipose-tissue lipoprotein-lipase activity in moderately obese men after weight reduction. Lancet 1978;1:1230–1231.
27. Astrup A. Thermogenic drugs as a strategy for treatment of obesity. Endocrine 2000;17:207–212.
28. Arner P. The beta₃ adrenergic receptor—a cause and cure of obesity? N Engl J Med 1995;333:382–383.
29. Giaobino J-P. Beta₃-adrenergic receptor: an update. Eur J Endocrinol 1995;132:377–385.
30. Clement K, Vaisse C, Manning B, et al. Genetic variation in the beta 3-adrenergic receptor and an increased capacity to gain weight in patient with morbid obesity. N Engl J Med 1995;333:352–354.
31. Gray GA. The inheritance of corpulence. In: Cioffi LA, James WPT, Itallie TB, eds. The Body Weight Regulatory System: Normal and Disturbed Mechanisms. New York: Raven, 1981:185–195.
32. Stunkard AJ, Sorensen TIA, Hanis C, et al. An adoption study of human obesity. N Engl J Med 1986; 314:193–198.
33. Stunkard AJ, Harris JR, Pedersen NL, et al. The body-mass index of twins who have been reared apart. N Engl J Med 1990;322:1483–1487.
34. Dietz WH, Gortmaker SL. Do we fatten our children at the television set? Obesity and viewing in children and adolescents. Pediatrics 1985;75:807–809.
35. National Heart, Lung, and Blood Institute. Clinical Guidelines on the Identification, Evaluation, and Treatment of Overweight and Obesity in Adults: The Evidence Report. NIH Publication No. 98-4083. Washington, DC: National Institutes of Health, 1998.
36. Cassell JA. Commentary: American food habits in the 1980s. Top Clin Nutr 1989;4:47–58.
37. Dreon DM, Frev-Hewitt B, Ellsworth N. Dietary fat: carbohydrate ratio and obesity in middle-aged men. Am J Clin Nutr 1988;47:995–1000.
38. McGinnis JM, Foege WH. Actual causes of death in the United States. JAMA 1993;270:2207–2212.
39. Allison DB, Fontaine KR, Manson JE, et al. Annual deaths attributable to obesity in the United States. JAMA 1999;282:1530–1538.
40. Drenick EJ, Bale GS, Seltzer F. Excessive mortality and causes of death in morbidly obese men. JAMA 1980;243:443–446.
41. Heald FP. The natural history of obesity. Adv Psychsom Med 1972;7:102–115.
42. Black D, James WPI, Besser GM. Obesity. J R Coll Physicians Lond 1983;17:5–65.
43. Arciero PJ, Vukovich MD, Holloszy JO, et al. Comparison of short-term diet and exercise on insulin action in individuals with abnormal glucose tolerance. J Appl Physiol 1999;86:1930–1935.
44. National Diabetes Data Group. Classification and diagnosis of diabetes mellitus and other categories of glucose intolerance. Diabetes 1979;28:1039–1057.
45. Campbell PJ, Gerich JE. Impact of obesity on insulin resistance in normal subjects and patients with NIDDM. Diabetes 1995;44:1121–1125.
46. Pi-Sunyer FX. Medical hazards of obesity. Ann Intern Med 1993;119:655–660.
47. Kolterman OG, Insel J, Saekow T, et al. Mechanisms of insulin resistance in human obesity: evidence for receptor and post receptor defects. J Clin Invest 1980;65:1272–1273.
48. Kahan CR, White MF. The insulin receptor and the molecular mechanism of insulin action. J Clin Invest 1988;82:151–156.
49. Ferrannini E, Barrett EJ, Bevilacqua S. Effect of fatty acids on glucose production and utilization in man. J Clin Invest 1983;72:1737–1740.
50. Randle PJ, Kerbey AL, Espinal J. Mechanisms decreasing glucose oxidation in diabetes and starvation: role of lipid fuels and hormones. Diabetes Metab Rev 1988;4:623–638.
51. Rebrin K, Steil GM, Mittelman SD, et al. Causal linkage between insulin suppression of lipolysis and suppression of liver glucose output in dogs. J Clin Invest 1996;98:741–749.
52. Meylan M, Henny C, Temier E. Metabolic factors in the insulin resistance in human obesity. Metabolism 1987;36:256–260.
53. Hubert HB, Feinleib M, McNamara PM, et al. Obesity as an independent risk factor for cardiovascular disease: a 26 year follow-up of participants in the Framingham Heart Study. Circulation 1983;67:968–977.
54. Goldring D, Hernandez A, Choi S. Blood pressure in a high school

population. II: Clinical profile of the juvenile hypertensive. J Pediatr 1979;95:298–304.

55. Sowers JR, Whitfield LA, Beck FW. Role of enhanced sympathetic nervous system activity and reduced Na, K-dependent adenosine triphosphatase activity in maintenance of elevated blood pressure in obesity: effects of weight loss. Clin Sci 1982;63(Suppl):121–124.

56. Nehus SJ, Heyden S, Hansen JP. Lipoprotein and blood pressure changes during weight reduction at Duke's Dietary Rehabilitation Clinic. Ann Nutr Metab 1982;26:384–392.

57. Vague P, Juhan-Vague I, Chabert V. Fat distribution and plasminogen activator inhibitor activity in nondiabetic obese women. Metabolism 1989;38:913–915.

58. Vaughan RW, Conahan TJ. Cardiopulmonary consequences of morbid obesity. Life Sci 1980; 26:2119–2127.

59. Luce JM. Respiratory complications of obesity. Chest 1980;78:626–631.

60. Block AJ, Boysen PG, Wynne JW. Sleep apnea, hypopnea and oxygen desaturation in normal subjects: a strong male predominance. N Engl J Med 1979;300:513–517.

61. Halsted CH. Obesity: effects on the liver and gastrointestinal system. Curr Opin Clin Nutr Metab Care 1999;2:425–429.

62. Grundy SM. Mechanism of cholesterol gallstones formation. Semin Liver Dis 1983;3:97–111.

63. Stevenson JM, Weber CL, Smith JT, et al. A longitudinal study of development of lower back pain in an industrial population. Spine 2001;26:370–377.

64. Sower SM. Epidemiology of risk factors for osteoarthritis: systemic factors. Curr Opin Rheumatol 2001;13: 447–451.

65. Kushner RF, Weinsier RL. Evaluation of the obese patient: practical considerations. Med Clin North Am 2000; 84:387–399.

66. Bray G, Ryan D. Clinical evaluation of the overweight patient. Endocrine 2000;13:167–186.

67. Collazo-Clavell M. Safe and effective management of the obese patient. Mayo Clin Proc 1999;74:1255–1260.

68. Melby C, Scholl C, Edwards G, et al. Effect of acute resistance exercise on postexercise energy expenditure and resting metabolic rate. J Appl Physiol 1993;75:1847–1853.

69. Andersen RE, Wadden TA, Bartlett SJ, et al. Effects of lifestyle activity vs structured aerobic exercise in obese women: a randomized trial. JAMA 1999;281:335–340.

70. Denke M. Metabolic effects of high protein, low carbohydrate diets. Am J Cardiol 2001;88:59–61.

71. LaRosa JC, Fug TG, Muesing R, Rosing DR. Effects of high-protein low-carbohydrate diets on plasma lipoproteins and body weight. J Am Diet Assoc 1980;77:264–270.

72. Rodin J, Wing RR. Behavioral factors in obesity. Diabetes Metab Rev 1988 4:701–725.

73. Burke E, Morden N. Clinical pharmacology: medical management of obesity. American Family Physician 2000; 62.

74. Weiser M, Fushman WH, Michaelson MD, Abdeen MA. The pharmacological approach to the treatment of obesity. J Clin Pharmacol 1997;37:453–472.

75. Aronne LJ. Modern medical management of obesity: the role of pharmaceutical intervention. J Am Diet Assoc 1998;98(10 Suppl 2): S23–26.

76. Van Goal LF, Waiters MA, DeLee VW. Antiobesity drugs: what does sibutramine offer? An analysis of its potential contribution to obesity treatment. Exp Clin Endocrinol Diabetes 1998;106(suppl 2):35–40.

77. Bray GA, Ryan DH, Gordon D, et al. A double blind randomized placebo-controlled trial of sibutramine. Obesity Res 1996;4:263–270.

78. Fernandez-Soto ML, Gonzalez-Jimenez A, Barredo-Acedo F, et al. Comparison of fluoxetine and placebo in the treatment of obesity. Ann Nutr Metab 1995;39:159–163.

79. Davidson MH, Hauptman J, DiGirolamo M, et al. Weight control and risk factor reduction in obese subjects treated for 2 years with orlistat: a randomized controlled trial. JAMA 1999;281:235–242.

80. Carlson HF, Drenick EJ, Chopra IJ. Alterations in basal and TRH-stimulated serum levels of thyrotropin, prolactin, and thyroid hormones in starved obese men. J Clin Endocrinol Metab 1977;45:707–713.

81. Genaera Int J Obesity May 2001.

82. Richelsen B, Pedersen SB, Borgulum JD, et al. Growth hormone treatment of obese women for 5 weeks: effect on body composition and adipose tissue LPL activity. Am J Physiol 1994;266:E211–E216.

83. NIH conference. Gastrointestinal surgery for severe obesity. Consensus Development Conference Panel [review]. Ann Intern Med 1991;115:956–961.

84. Greenway F. Surgery for obesity. Endocrinol Metab Clin North Am 1996;25:1005–1027.

85. Geliebter A, Melton PM, McCray RS, et al. Clinical trial of silicone rubber gastric balloons to treat obesity. Int J Obes 1991;15:259–266.

86. Pasquali R, Besteghi L, Cosimiri F, et al. Mechanisms of action of the intragastric balloon in obesity: effects on hunger and satiety. Appetite 1990;15:3–11.

87. American College of Sports Medicine. ACSM's Guidelines for Exercise Testing and Prescription. 6th Ed. Philadelphia: Lippincott Williams & Wilkins, 2000:24–28.

CHAPTER 21

Diabetes

Donald R. Dengel, Thomas H. Reynolds

Overview

Relevant Statistics

Diabetes mellitus affects approximately 6% of the population in the United States and involves perturbations in **insulin** secretion or action. In 1997 the direct and indirect health care costs of diabetes in the United States were estimated by the American Diabetes Association to be almost $100 billion (1). Over the past decade researchers have made great strides in understanding the causes of diabetes; these advances eventually will lead to prevention and better management of the disease and lower the overwhelming associated health care costs. One fertile area of research is the impact of physical activity on diabetes mellitus. The primary focus of this chapter is to review the role that physical activity plays in the treatment and prevention of diabetes mellitus.

There are four types of diabetes mellitus: type 1, type 2, gestational, and "other specific types" of diabetes (1). This chapter focuses on the two primary types of diabetes mellitus, type 1 and type 2. **Type 1 diabetes mellitus**, or **insulin-dependent diabetes**, accounts for approximately 5% to 10% of all diabetes and is caused by a failure of the beta cells of the **pancreas** to secrete insulin. Type 1 diabetes is sometimes referred to as **juvenile diabetes** due to its onset early in life. **Type 2 diabetes mellitus** or **non–insulin-dependent diabetes** accounts for approximately 90% to 95% of all diabetes and it is associated with **hyperinsulinemia** due to a reduction in insulin action in the liver and skeletal muscle (i.e., insulin resistance). The precise cause of type 2 diabetes is unknown but it is associated with several risk factors, which include obesity, a sedentary lifestyle, a family history of type 2 diabetes mellitus, age, and race or ethnicity. Regardless of the type of diabetes mellitus, serious complication can occur if the condition is not managed appropriately. Diabetes is the seventh leading cause of death in the United States. However, deaths due to diabetes mellitus probably exceed the statistics from United States death certificates because heart disease is a common pathology in diabetics. In fact, the incidence of heart disease deaths is two- to four-fold higher in diabetics than in nondiabetics (1). Although the diabetes mellitus statistics are overwhelming, proper management of types 1 and 2 diabetes can offset many of the complications that can occur with diabetes mellitus. Regular physical exercise is an intervention that can improve the health of diabetics, particularly those with type 2 diabetes mellitus.

Classification of Diabetes Mellitus

In 1997 the Expert Committee on the Diagnosis and Classification of Diabetes Mellitus modified the previous criteria recommended by the National Diabetes Data Group (NDDG) (2) and the World Health Organization (WHO) (3). The revised criteria recommended three possible methods to diagnose diabetes. Each of the three criterion methods of diagnosis must be confirmed on a subsequent day by any of the other two methods of diagnosis. The Expert Committee recommended that diabetes be confirmed by: (1) symptoms of diabetes (i.e., polyuria, polydipsia, unexplained weight loss) plus a plasma glucose level ≥200 mg/dl (11.1 mmol/L); (2) a fasting (i.e., no caloric intake for at least 8 hours) plasma glucose concentration ≥126 mg/dl (7.0 mmol/L); or(3) a ≥200 mg/dl plasma glucose concentration 2 hours into a 75 g oral glucose tolerance. In addition, the Expert Committee also recommended a criterion to classify an intermediate group of individuals who do not meet the criteria for diabetes mellitus, but whose levels are too high to be classified as normal. Individuals with a fasting plasma glucose level higher than 110 mg/dl but less than 126 mg/dl or a plasma glucose concentration greater than140 mg/dl but less than 200 mg/dl 2 hours into a 75-g oral glucose tolerance test are classified as having **impaired fasting glucose** or **impaired oral glucose tolerance**. Although these individuals do not have diabetes mellitus they are at greater risk for developing the disease.

Pathogenesis of Type 1 Diabetes

Type 1 diabetes is an autoimmune disease that involves the immunologic destruction of pancreatic beta cells, the insulin-secreting cells of the pancreas. It is thought that autoimmune beta cell destruction is a factor in type 1 diabetes, a theory that is supported by the detection of beta cell antibodies in the blood of prediabetics and newly diagnosed diabetics. Furthermore, immunosuppressant therapy can preserve beta cell function in newly diagnosed diabetic patients (4). The autoimmune destruction of beta cells is thought to be caused by "environmental factors" such as enterovirus,

nutritional factors, interactions between enterovirus and nutritional factors, and chemical toxins (5). In addition to environmental factors, evidence indicates that type 1 diabetes has a genetic component. In monozygotic twins, if one twin develops type 1 diabetes mellitus the other twin has 30% to 70% greater chance of developing type 1 diabetes mellitus, a rate several times higher than that for dizygotic twins and non-twin siblings (6, 7). The genetic basis for type 1 diabetes appears to be primarily human histocompatible leukocyte antigen (HLA) complexes (8), a group of approximately 128 genes (9) that explains 30% to 50% of familial clustering of type 1 diabetes (10). In summary, it is obvious that the etiology of type 1 diabetes is multifactorial, involving several genes and environmental factors that lead to the destruction of pancreatic beta cells and insulin deficiency. Although there is no cure for type 1 diabetes, tight control of blood glucose by exogenous insulin therapy and a healthy and physically active lifestyle may help delay or even prevent diabetic complications.

Pathogenesis of Type 2 Diabetes

Type 2 diabetes involves the improper regulation of glucose metabolism by insulin. Unlike the insulin deficiency of type 1 diabetes, type 2 diabetes is associated with profound insulin resistance. Insulin resistance is defined as a decline in the ability of insulin to increase glucose uptake, primarily in skeletal muscle, and is associated with aging, obesity, a sedentary lifestyle, and genetic predisposition. In response to insulin resistance, the beta cells of the pancreas compensate by increasing insulin secretion. If the peripheral insulin resistance is not overcome by increased insulin secretion, hyperinsulinemia will ensue until the beta cells fail to compensate for the inability to stimulate glucose uptake by skeletal muscle and suppress glucose production by the liver.

The development of insulin resistance and the resulting hyperinsulinemia is multifactorial, involving defects in the ability of glucose to suppress insulin secretion, an inability of insulin to suppress glucose production by the liver, and a defect in the ability of insulin to stimulate glucose uptake into skeletal muscle. Because skeletal muscle is the primary site for postprandial glucose disposal, it is thought that insulin resistance may result from a defect in the ability of insulin to stimulate skeletal muscle glucose uptake. The rate-limiting step in skeletal muscle glucose disposal is thought to be glucose transport. Glucose is transported into skeletal muscle by the glucose transporter proteins GLUT1 and GLUT4. GLUT1 resides in the plasma membrane and mediates basal rates of glucose transport, whereas GLUT4 is housed intracellularly and is translocated to the cell surface in response to insulin. Most experimental evidence indicates that insulin resistance is due to perturbation(s) in the GLUT4 translocation process—total levels of GLUT1 and GLUT4 are not reduced in skeletal muscle of type 2 diabetics. In fact, recent evidence indicates that skeletal muscle insulin resistance is due to a reduced ability to recruit GLUT4 to the cell surface (11, 12). Despite extensive investigation, the precise defect in the insulin signaling pathway or protein trafficking responsible for impaired GLUT4 translocation in insulin resistant skeletal muscle is unclear.

Although a genetic predisposition for type 2 diabetes does exist, lifestyle can be a critical factor in the development and progression of the disease. A preponderance of evidence indicates that type 2 diabetes is strongly related to a sedentary lifestyle and obesity (13). Therefore, increasing physical activity is an ideal intervention for treating and preventing type 2 diabetes. The mechanism linking obesity to diabetes has been an area of intense investigation. Several investigators have established that free fatty acids may play a causative role in the development of type 2 diabetes, because the infusion of lipids produces insulin resistance (14). Other evidence implicates the adipocytes (fat cells) in the development of insulin resistance and type 2 diabetes. Obesity has been associated with an increase in the secretion of tumor necrosis factor-α (TNF-α) from adipocytes. TNF-α is a proinflammatory cytokine that has been shown to inhibit insulin signaling (15), reduce GLUT4 levels (16), and produce insulin resistance that is reversed by the insulin sensitizer troglitazone (17). Furthermore, weight loss decreases TNF-α levels and enhances insulin sensitivity (18). The recently cloned adipocyte-derived hormone resistin also appears to "link" obesity to insulin resistance and type 2 diabetes. Like TNF-α, resistin is secreted from adipocytes and has been shown to induce insulin resistance. Plasma resistin levels are shown to increase in diet-induced insulin resistance and decrease with rosiglitazone therapy. Furthermore, treatment with an anti-resistin antibody improves diet-induced insulin resistance (19). Because exercise and weight loss are primary interventions used to treat insulin resistance and type 2 diabetes, their respective effects on resistin and TNF-α levels are of great interest; no studies have yet been done in this area, however.

Medications

No drugs are currently available to cure diabetes mellitus. However, drugs are available to manage blood glucose levels and help control the disease. The three major classes of medication regimes are insulin replacement therapy; oral hypoglycemic agents; and insulin-sensitizing antihyperglycemic agents.

Insulin Replacement Therapy

About 30% of all people with diabetes in the United States require insulin for the treatment of their disease (4). Patients with type 1 diabetes require daily insulin replacement to treat or avoid ketoacidosis and for glycemic control. Patients with type 2 diabetes also use insulin replacement therapy for glycemic control. In general, insulin is classified by the duration of its action and can be either short-, intermediate-, or long-lasting. The longer-lasting insulin preparations contain additives that prolong their pharmacologic activity in order to reduce the number of injections required during a day.

Diabetic individuals who use insulin therapy to control their blood glucose levels lack the ability to automatically regulate insulin delivery. Therefore diabetic individuals using insulin need to anticipate their exercise and adjust their insulin therapy accordingly. When too much circulating insulin is available, blood glucose is lowered below normal levels, resulting in a condition called **hypoglycemia**. This is a common problem in insulin dependent diabetics, and a major concern when an exercise program is initiated. The risk of hypoglycemia is particularly high in people who take large doses of insulin or have asymptomatic hypoglycemia (20). Decreasing insulin doses by 30% to 50% before exercise is an effective method of preventing hypoglycemia, especially in the postprandial state (21). In type 1 diabetics who are not concerned about weight loss, supplemental carbohydrate feedings may be another way to prevent hypoglycemia during exercise (20). If the planned exercise bout is going to last longer than 60 minutes, it may be necessary to take additional supplemental carbohydrates and less insulin.

Another problem that may be encountered with individuals on insulin therapy is **hyperglycemia**, which occurs when insulin levels are insufficient and glucose disposal is impaired. To avoid this condition individuals on insulin therapy should test their blood glucose levels before exercise. If the blood glucose levels are higher than 250 mg/dl, the urine should be tested for ketones to determine if blood glucose control is still effective. The presence of ketones in the urine suggests that the body's energy demands are being met by lipolysis. Exercising during this condition would only exacerbate it.

Oral Hypoglycemic Agents

Approximately 40% of diabetic patients in the United States take some type of oral hypoglycemic agents (22). Most of the oral hypoglycemic agents prescribed are sulfonylurea derivatives (e.g., chlorpropamide, glyburide, glipizide). These drugs stimulate the pancreatic beta cells to release more insulin by increasing their sensitivity to glucose (4). Metformin (biguanide) is an oral hypoglycemic drug that can be used alone or in combination with sulfonylureas. This drug improves cell insulin sensitivity by decreasing hepatic glucose output (22). In addition, Metformin appears to promote muscle glycogen formation and adipose tissue lipogenesis (22). Little is know about the interaction between exercise and oral hypoglycemic drugs or the effect of these oral hypoglycemic drugs on the metabolic response to exercise.

Insulin-Sensitizing Antihyperglycemic Agents (Thiazolidinedione)

Thiazolidinedione antidiabetic agents are a new class of drugs that enhance insulin sensitivity and therefore are used only for the treatment of type 2 diabetes. These drugs decrease insulin resistance in the periphery and in the liver, resulting in increased insulin-dependent glucose uptake and decreased hepatic glucose output. The precise mechanism of action of thiazolidinediones is currently unknown. Similar to oral hypoglycemic drugs, little is known about the interaction between exercise and insulin sensitizing antihyperglycemic drug or the effect of these drugs on the metabolic response to exercise.

Exercise

Metabolic Responses to Exercise

During physical activity contracting muscles require the delivery of fuels for energy. A number of factors such as age, nutritional status, and work capacity can influence an individual's metabolic responses to exercise. The main determinant of which fuels are used during exercise is primarily a function of the intensity and duration. During the first few minutes of exercise muscle glycogen is the main source of energy utilized by the contracting muscles. As the duration of exercise increases muscle glycogen stores are depleted, and blood glucose and free fatty acids become the main source of energy for the exercising muscles. This process is regulated by changes in hormone levels as well as changes in the sympathetic nervous system. Circulating insulin levels usually decline during exercise as levels of glucagon, cortisol, epinephrine and norepinephrine increase. During prolonged exercise the reduction in circulating levels of insulin and increasing levels of glucagon result in stimulation of hepatic glycogenolysis and gluconeogenesis, thereby increasing glucose release by the liver. Diabetic individuals who are on insulin replacement therapy do not experience this decline in circulating insulin levels in the blood during prolonged exercise. In addition, some type 1 diabetics are unable to produce glucagon and as a result are not able to stimulate glucose production by the liver. The end result is that type 1 diabetics are a greater risk for hypoglycemic episodes during exercise.

Is Maximal Exercise Test Recommended?

The American Diabetes Association recommends that anybody who is at high risk for underlying cardiovascular disease undergo a graded exercise test before beginning a moderate to high-intensity exercise program (13). These high risk factors include age older than 35 years; type 2 diabetes for more than 10 years; type 1 diabetes for more than 15 years; presence of any additional risk factor for coronary artery disease; presence of microvascular disease (retinopathy or nephropathy); peripheral vascular disease; or autonomic neuropathy. In those patients who are planning on participating in a low-intensity (<60% of maximal heart rate) exercise program the American Diabetes Association recommends that the physician should use clinical judgment in deciding whether to recommend an exercise stress test (13).

Exercise Programming

Endurance exercise training has been recommended for use primarily in individuals with diabetes mellitus. However, because the prevalence of type 2 diabetes mellitus increases with advancing age and there also is an age-associated decline in muscle mass, exercise programs designed to increase muscle mass (e.g., resistance training) may prove to be beneficial in this population. Because diabetes mellitus also is linked to a number of cardiovascular risk factors, an exercise training program that combines both endurance and resistance training may be the optimal exercise program for people with diabetes mellitus. Although this will ultimately increase the time required to devote to the exercise training program, the addition of resistance training to endurance training would provide variety and could enhance participation.

Endurance Training Program

To improve one's cardiovascular or cardiorespiratory fitness level, aerobic exercise training must be performed at a particular intensity, duration, and frequency. The aerobic activity needs to be performed at an intensity of approximately 60% to 80% $\dot{V}O_{2max}$ or 70% to 85% maximal heart rate. This intensity must be maintained for 20 to 30 minutes (duration) and should be done three to four times per week (frequency). Although a certain intensity of aerobic exercise is necessary to elicit an improvement in fitness, recent evidence indicates that even regularly performed low-intensity exercise can produce health benefits even if it does not improve cardiovascular fitness (23). However, the exact exercise training intensity necessary to elicit an improvement in either type 1 or type 2 diabetes mellitus is unknown.

Resistance Training Program

Designing a safe and effective resistance training program involves principles similar to those of aerobic exercise but with somewhat different terminology. The intensity of resistance exercise is expressed as a percentage of an individual's one-repetition maximum (1RM). A 1RM is the amount of weight that can be lifted one time. Resistance training programs for individuals who are not competitive athletes typically use an intensity of approximately 60% to 80% of 1RM, which corresponds to roughly 8 to 12 repetitions. Repetitions is defined as the number of times a resistance is moved through a defined range of motion; the number of repetitions completed during a specific resistance exercise constitutes a set. The number of repetitions per set and the number of sets completed is defined as the training volume (volume = number of repetitions $\times$ number of sets). Resistance training programs designed for the general public typically use a high training volume (two to three sets of 8 to 12 repetitions). The training duration for resistance training is determined by the length of rest period between sets and the number of exercises performed per training session. Some evidence indicates that performing more exercises per training session and taking brief rest periods between sets can improve cardiovascular health (24). As with aerobic exercise training, resistance training frequency is the number of exercise sessions completed per week. Typical resistance training programs consist of two to three training sessions per week. It is important that adequate recovery time be allowed between resistance training sessions, so most programs incorporate an every-other-day training regime.

In designing exercise programs for individuals with diabetes mellitus one should consider developing a program that consists of both resistance and endurance training. One could alternate endurance training (3–4 times/week) with resistance training (2–3 times/week).

Physiologic Adaptations to Exercise

Type 1 Diabetes Mellitus

Exercise training has been used for the treatment of diabetes mellitus since ancient times. It has been well documented that aerobic exercise training can improve insulin sensitivity in individuals with normal or impaired glucose tolerance (25–27). The effects of exercise in people with type 1 diabetes is less clear, however. Few long-term studies have examined the effect of aerobic exercise training on glucose control in those individuals with type 1 diabetes. The results of these studies are listed in Table 21.1. In one of the first studies to examine the effects of aerobic exercise training in type 1 diabetics, Peterson and coworkers (28) studied 10 patients over an 8-month period. Patients were enrolled in an exercise program and were encouraged to exercise three times per week for 35 minutes per session at an intensity of 70% of their heart rate reserve. Patients were encouraged to alter their dietary intake to assist in the control of blood glucose. After only 3 months there was a decline in glycosylated hemoglobin. In addition, the authors report that after 8 months of this program the daily insulin requirement was reduced (28). Because the subjects also

were encouraged to alter their diet, it is difficult to separate the specific effects of aerobic exercise from the combined effects of diet and exercise.

Wallberg-Henriksson and coworkers (29) examined the effects of 16 weeks of aerobic exercise training on insulin sensitivity and blood glucose control in nine men with type 1 diabetes. The exercise training program consisted of 1 hour of jogging, running, ball games, and gymnastics performed two or three times per week with no change in dietary habits. The training program resulted in an 8% increase in maximal oxygen uptake. Insulin sensitivity increased by an average of 20%; glycosylated hemoglobin was unchanged, however. In addition, the 24-hour urinary glucose excretion was not reduced, and the frequency of hypoglycemic attacks did not change during the training period. No changes in insulin dose were made during the course of the training program.

In a similar study Zinman and coworkers (30) examined the effects of aerobic exercise training on 13 type 1 diabetics and 7 controls. Patients performed 45 minutes of cycle exercise three times per week for a total of 12 weeks. Heart rate response achieved during each exercise session was 60% to 85% of each individual's predicted maximum. Subjects were instructed to continue with their usual diets during the length of the study. Following the 12-week training program there was a 28% increase in maximal aerobic uptake with no significant change in body weight or in glycosylated hemoglobin levels. In addition the total insulin dose was unchanged after training and the occurrence of hypoglycemic episodes was similar.

Landt and coworkers (31) examined the effects of exercise training on insulin sensitivity in adolescents with type 1 diabetes. Nine adolescents (mean age, 16 years) took part in an aerobic exercise training program three times per week for 12 weeks. Each exercise session lasted for 45 minutes, and patients exercised at a heart rate that represented 80% to 85% of their maximum heart rate. Another six adolescents (mean age, 15.9 years) served as controls. There was no change in the dietary habits of the patients during the study period. Despite an increase in insulin sensitivity following the 12-week aerobic exercise training program there was no change in glycosylated hemoglobin levels. In addition, there were no changes in the average daily insulin dose or the number of hypoglycemic reactions following the training program

In a cross-sectional study, Ligtenberg and coworkers (32) examined the relation between long-term physical activity and glycemic control in 221 patients with type 1 diabetes mellitus. Patients were between 18 and 45 years of age, and a self-report questionnaire was used to determine their degree of physical activity. The authors reported that glycemic control was not associated with long-term physical activity in type 1 diabetes; however physical activity did not negatively affect long-term glycemic control.

Based on studies to date in type 1 diabetics it appears that although endurance training can increase insulin sen-

TABLE 21.1.   EFFECTS OF PHYSICAL ACTIVITY ON GLUCOSE HOMEOSTASIS IN TYPE 1 DIABETES MELLITUS

Study	No. Subjects	Mean Age (y)	Duration of Study (mos)	Exercise Program	Glycemic Control	Insulin Sensitivity	Insulin Requirement
Wallberg-Henriksson et al., 1982 (29)	9	35	4	Intensity? 60 min, 2–3 times/wk	No change in HbA1$_c$	Increase in GDR	No change
Zinman et al., 1984 (30)	20	?	3	60–85% HR$_{max}$ 45 min, 3 times/wk	No change in HbA1$_c$, no change in FPG	NA	No change
Landt et al., 1985 (31)	15	16	3	Intensity? 45 min, 3 times/wk	No change in HbA1$_c$	Increase in GDR	No change
Mosher et al., 1998 (49)	10	17	3	Aerobic circuit 45 min, 3 times/wk	Decrease in HbA1$_c$, no change in FPG	NA	NA

HbA1$_c$, glycosylated hemoglobin; FPG, fasting plasma glucose; GDR, glucose disposal rate; NA, not measured

sitivity in this population there is little or no effect on glycosylated hemoglobin levels. In addition, it appears that endurance training does not result in lower insulin doses or hypoglycemic events in patients with type 1 diabetes.

Type 2 Diabetes Mellitus

Studies that have examined the effect of exercise on improved glycemic control in individuals with type 2 diabetes have produced mixed results (Table 21.2). Some studies reported no improvements in glucose tolerance (33, 34), glycosylated hemoglobin (34), or insulin action (35, 36), whereas other studies have reported improvements in glu-

cose tolerance (35, 37–39), glycosylated hemoglobin (38) and insulin action (37, 40). A number of factors may be responsible for these differences in results. One factor may be the differences in training intensity and frequency. Leon and coworkers (34) had subjects exercise for either 30 or 60 minutes either two or four times per week. When the data were pooled together there was no improvement in glycosylated hemoglobin or glucose tolerance. However, there was a decline in glycosylated hemoglobin in the group that exercised for 60 minutes per exercise session four times a week. Another factor is the length of time between the last bout of exercise and the evaluation of glucose tolerance or insulin action. If glucose tolerance or insulin action is evaluated more than 48 hours after the last bout of exercise lit-

TABLE 21.2.   EFFECTS OF PHYSICAL ACTIVITY ON GLUCOSE HOMEOSTASIS IN TYPE 2 DIABETES MELLITUS (1985–2000)

Study	No. Subjects	Mean Age (y)	Duration of Study (mos)	Type of Exercise Program	Glycemic Control	Insulin Sensitivity	Insulin Secretion
Krotkiewski et al., 1985 (37)	46	50	3	80–90% $\dot{V}O_{2max}$ 50 min, 3 times/wk	No change in FPG	Increase in GDR, decrease in glucose area	No change in FPIns, no change in insulin area
Ronnemaa et al., 1986 (38)	25	52	4	~70% $\dot{V}O_{2max}$ 45 min, 5–7 times/wk	Decrease HbA1$_c$, no change in FPG	Decrease in 2h-PG	No change in FPIns
Segal et al., 1991 (36)	6	36	3	~70% $\dot{V}O_{2max}$ 70 min, 4 times/wk	No change in FPG	No change in GDR, no change in glucose area	No change in FPIns, no change in insulin area
Eriksson et al., 1991 (47)	41	48	72	Intensity? Duration? 3 times/wk		Increase in OGTT	
Schneider et al., 1992 (50)	111	55	3	60–75% HR$_{max}$ 40–60 min, 4 times/wk	Decrease in HbA1$_c$, Decrease in FPG	NA	NA
Dela et al., 1995 (41)	7	58	2.5	~70% $\dot{V}O_{2max}$ 30 min, 6 times/wk	No change in FPG	Increase in GDR	Decrease in FPIns

FPG, fasting plasma glucose; FPIns, fasting plasma insulin; GDR, glucose disposal rate; glucose area, the area under the curve for glucose values during a 2-hour oral glucose tolerance test; 2h-PG, 2 hour oral glucose tolerance test plasma glucose; HbA1$_c$, glycosylated hemoglobin; insulin area, the area under the curve for insulin values during a 2-hour oral glucose tolerance test; NA, not measured

tle change will be observed. Finally, the duration of disease or severity of insulin deficiency may factor into the effect of exercise on improvements in glucose control.

In a very well-controlled study, Krotkiewski and coworkers (37) had patients with type 2 diabetes exercise for 3 months, three times a week for 50 minutes. After this exercise training program, their oral glucose tolerance improved despite no change in the insulin response to oral glucose. These results are supported by Holloszy and coworkers (39), who reported that 1 year of exercise training in type 2 diabetics improved both glucose and insulin responses to an oral glucose challenge.

Recently, Dela and coworkers (41) examined the effects of 10 weeks of one-legged training on insulin-mediated glucose disposal in type 2 diabetics and healthy controls. Insulin-mediated glucose disposal was measured in the whole body and in both legs before, 1 day after, and 6 days after training. Whole body glucose disposal rates were lower in type 2 diabetic patients than in healthy controls. Training significantly increased insulin-mediated glucose disposal in both controls and type 2 diabetics. However, an acute bout of exercise did not increase insulin-mediated glucose disposal in the patients with NIDDM. This would support the idea that improvements in insulin action are due to training adaptations rather than the effect of a single bout of exercise. After 6 days without exercise training insulin-mediated glucose disposal returned to baseline, suggesting that the enhancement in glucose disposal is short-lived.

Although not totally conclusive, studies to date indicate that endurance training in type 2 diabetics results in an improvement in insulin sensitivity. However, this enhanced insulin sensitivity does not always lead to an improvement in glycemic control.

Prevention of Type 2 Diabetes Mellitus

A number of cross-sectional as well as epidemiologic studies have provided strong evidence for the role of aerobic exercise in the prevention of type 2 diabetes mellitus (Table 21.3). Although these studies clearly demonstrate an association between physical activity and the prevention of type 2 diabetes it is difficult to determine whether habitual physical activity is responsible for delaying the development of type 2 diabetes.

A number of prospective studies on the association between physical activity and the prevention of diabetes have been conducted. Manson and coworkers (42) examined the association between regular vigorous exercise and the subsequent incidence of NIDDM in 87,253 female nurses in the United States aged 34 to 59 years of age, who were initially free of diagnosed diabetes, cardiovascular disease, and cancer. After 8 years those women who engaged in vigorous exercise at least once per week had an age-adjusted decrease in the incidence of diabetes. Among the women who exercise at least once per week the authors did not observe a dose-response effect of the exercise on preventing the development of diabetes. The results remained significant even when the data were adjusted for body mass index. In a similar study in 21,271 male physicians in the United States aged 40 to 84 years of age, Manson and coworkers (43) observed that men who exercised at least once per week had an age-adjusted decrease in the risk of developing diabetes. Unlike the study in female nurses a dose-response gradient of increased frequency of exercise and reduced risk of developing diabetes was observed. Vigorous exercise five or more times per week was associated with a 42% reduction in the age-adjusted risk of developing type 2 diabetes mellitus compared with those who exercised less than once

TABLE 21.3.   PHYSICAL ACTIVITY AND THE PREVENTION OF TYPE 2 DIABETES MELLITUS

Study	Age Range (y)	Gender	No. Subjects	Duration of Study (yrs)	Comparison Groups	RR[a]	Potential Confounding Factors Controlled in Analysis
Helmrich et al., 1991 (44)	39–68	Males	5,990	14	Each 500 kcal/week increase in physical activity index	0.94	Age, BMI, history of hypertension, parental history of diabetes
Manson et al., 1991 (42)	34–59	Females	87,253	8	Exercised at least once per week	0.84	Age, BMI
Manson et al., 1991 (43)	40–84	Males	21,271	5	Exercised at least once per week	0.71	Age, BMI
Pan et al., 1997 (48)	42–60	Males and females	1,038	4	>5.5 METs and durations longer than 40 min/wk	0.44	Age, FPG, BMI, triglycerides, parental history of diabetes, alcohol
James et al., 1998 (51)	30–55	Males and females	916	5	Participate in physical activity	0.51	Age, sex, education, BMI, WHR

[a]RR, adjusted for variables in the right column (Potential Confounding Factors Controlled In Analysis), is the ratio of the incidence of NIDDM in those who are most active divided by the incidence of NIDDM in those who are the most inactive.

BMI, body mass index; FPG, fasting plasma glucose; METs, the rate of energy expended above resting metabolic rate; WHR, waist-to-hip ratio.

per week. These benefits remained even when the data were adjusted for body mass index.

The ability of exercise to prevent the development of type 2 diabetes mellitus may be a function of the frequency of exercise. Helmrich and coworkers (44) examined the patterns of physical activity and the incidence of diabetes in 5990 college alumni over a 14-year period. The authors reported a 6% decrease in the age-adjusted risk for the development of diabetes for each 500 kcal increase in energy expenditure during weekly leisure time physical activity. Similarly, Lynch and colleagues (45) reported that in a group of 897 middle-aged Swedish men who participated in at least 40 minutes of exercise per week at an intensity of at least 5.5 METS had a reduced risk for the development of diabetes. This decreased risk persisted after adjusting for age, baseline glucose values, body mass index, serum triglyceride levels, parental history of diabetes, and alcohol consumption. In addition, the obese men in this study who exercised at this duration and intensity reduced their risk of developing diabetes by 64%.

Recently Wannamethee and coworkers (46) conducted a prospective study of 5159 men from Great Britain ranging from 40 to 59 years of age with no history of coronary heart disease, type 2 diabetes, or stroke. At screening, the men were asked to indicate their pattern of physical activity as regular walking or cycling, recreational activities (gardening, pleasure walking and do-it-yourself jobs), or sporting (running, golf, swimming, tennis, sailing and digging). A total physical activity score was calculated for each man based on frequency and intensity of the physical activities. The men were followed up 15.5 to 18 years later. The age-adjusted relative risk decreased progressively with increasing levels of physical activity. After adjusting for age, lifestyle characteristics, and preexisting cardiovascular disease, physical activity remained significantly and inversely associated with type 2 diabetes.

In the first study population diabetes prevention study to examine the effect of physical activity on diabetes prevention, Eriksson and Lindgarde (47) assigned men with impaired glucose tolerance to either an intervention or a control group. The intervention group exercised two times per week for 60 minutes each session. Exercise consisted of walking, jogging, and other recreational activities. The intervention also included dietary manipulation so it was not possible to examine the effects of exercise or diet separately. At the 6 year follow-up there was an improvement in glucose tolerance in 75.8% of the cases, and only 10.6% of the cases developed diabetes. However, in the control group glucose tolerance had deteriorated in 67.1% of the cases and diabetes was found in 28.6% of the participants.

In a true randomized control study to examine the effect of aerobic exercise on the development of type 2 diabetes, Pan and associates (48) screened over 110,000 men and women from 33 health care clinics in the city of Da Qing, China, for impaired glucose tolerance and type 2 diabetes. Of this cohort 577 were classified (using the WHO criteria) as having impaired glucose tolerance. Subjects were randomized by the clinic into either a control group or one of three active treatment groups: diet only, exercise only, or diet plus exercise. Follow-up evaluations were conducted at 2-year intervals over a 6-year period. The incidence of diabetes at 6 years was as follows:

> Control group: 67.7% (95% CI, 59.8–-75.2)
> Diet only group: 43.8% (95% CI, 35.5–52.3)
> Exercise only group: 41.1% (95% CI, 33.4–49.4)
> Diet plus exercise group: 46.0% (95% CI, 37.3–54.7)

All three of the interventions differed significantly from the control group. This large-scale study clearly demonstrates that physical activity can reduce the development of type 2 diabetes in those individuals with impaired glucose tolerance.

Summary

Exercise should be encouraged in individuals with either type 1 or type 2 diabetes mellitus. Like nondiabetic individuals, people with diabetes can decrease risk factors for cardiovascular disease and also may improve their quality of life. Evidence that regular exercise can improve glycemic control in type 1 or type 2 diabetics is still lacking, as is evidence that regular exercise can lower insulin dose levels or the number of hypoglycemic events in individuals with type 1 diabetes. Diabetic individuals using insulin to control their blood glucose levels are faced with a number of challenges in regards to exercise. Because individuals with type 1 diabetes lack normal endocrine responses to exercise they are at a greater risk for hypoglycemia. Therefore, these individuals need to closely monitor their blood glucose levels before, during, and after exercise and make changes in their insulin doses accordingly.

Finally, evidence for regular exercise in preventing the development of type 2 diabetes is fairly convincing. Cross-sectional as well as longitudinal studies provide evidence that regular exercise can prevent the development of type 2 diabetes in individuals with normal as well as impaired glucose tolerance.

What We Know
About Diabetes Mellitus

1 Diabetes mellitus is a heterogeneous cluster of metabolic disease characterized by hyperglycemia, caused by a defect in insulin secretion or insulin action.

2 Diabetes mellitus is a major risk factor for premature cardiovascular disease, including stroke, peripheral vascular disease, and heart attacks.

What We Would Like to Know
About Diabetes Mellitus

1 Several pharmacologic agents currently are used in the treatment of type 2 diabetes mellitus; however, very few data exist concerning the interaction between exercise (acute and chronic) and these medications. Whether exercise can enhance the action of these medications is not known. It is possible that exercise may pose some safety concerns when used in conjunction with various drugs.

2 Epidemiologic studies have reported on the effects of physical activity to reduce mortality, but the exact mechanisms responsible for this improvement in mortality are not known.

CASE STUDY 1

Patient Information

John is a 50-year-old lawyer who is 45 pounds overweight. Although he golfs occasionally on weekends he has not been involved in a regular exercise program since high school. His job demands many long hours and he is under constant pressure. John has not seen a doctor in over 10 years. At his wife's urging John schedules an appointment with the family physician.

Assessments

The doctor's examination revealed that John had a fasting cholesterol count of 295 mg/dl, with a low concentration of high-density lipoprotein (HDL) cholesterol. In addition to elevated cholesterol, John's blood pressure also was high (146/98 mm Hg), and his fasting blood glucose was 180 mg/dl. John's doctor explained to him that he was a type 2 diabetic.

Questions

1. What factors must you take into consideration before you develop an exercise program for John?

2. Will a program of daily physical activity reverse the symptoms of type 2 diabetes and ensure that John will not have to take any medications to control his type 2 diabetes?

3. What other health care professionals should be included in developing John's exercise and weight loss program?

CASE STUDY 2

Patient Information

Julie is a 28-year-old woman who is a type 1 diabetic. She has been taking daily insulin injections since she was diagnosed with type 1 diabetes at the age of 14 years. There is a history of heart disease in her family. For the first 8 years after being diagnosed with type 1 diabetes she was on conventional insulin therapy. Four years ago she switched to intensive insulin therapy, which involves monitoring blood sugar levels and injecting appropriate amounts of regular insulin before each meal.

Assessments

Julie meets with her physician and expresses her desire to start a program of regular physical activity. Julie's physician tells her that although exercise can help a person with type 2 diabetes achieve better glycemic control this cannot be said for an individual with type 1 diabetes. In addition, the doctor informed Julie that exercise would make controlling her blood glucose more challenging, but that he was in favor of her exercising.

Questions

1. What dangers would Julie face by implementing a regular exercise program?

2. What health care professionals should be included in developing Julie's exercise program?

3. Although Julie may not see an improvement in her glycemic control due to regular physical activity, can she expect some health benefits?

REFERENCES

1. NIDDK. Diabetes Overview. Bethesda: National Diabetes Information Clearinghouse, NIH Publication No. 01-3873, November 1998.
2. American Diabetes Association. Report of the Expert Committee on the Diagnosis and Classification of Diabetes Mellitus (Committee Report). Diabetes Care 1998;21(Suppl 1):S5–S19.
3. World Health Organization. WHO Expert Committee on Diabetes Mellitus. In: World Health Organization Technical Report Series 646. Geneva: World Health Organization,1980:6–80.
4. Haire-Joshv D. Management of Diabetes Mellitus: Perspectives of Care Across the Life Span. St. Louis: Mosby, 1996:1–894.
5. Haverkos HW. Could the aetiology of IDDM be multifactorial? Diabetologia 1997;40:1235–1240.
6. Kyvik KO, Green A, Beck-Nielsen H. Concordance rates of insulin dependent diabetes mellitus: a population based study of young Danish twins. Br Med J 1995;311:913–917.
7. Thomson G, Robinson WP, Kuhner MK, et al. Genetic heterogeneity, modes of inheritance, and risk estimates for a joint study of Caucasians with insulin-dependent diabetes mellitus. Am J Hum Genet 1988;43:799–816.
8. Undlien DE, Lie BA, Thorsby E. HLA complex genes in type 1 diabetes and other autoimmune diseases. Which genes are involved? Trends Genet 2001;17:93–100.
9. Complete sequence and gene map of a major histocompatibility complex. The MHC Sequencing Consortium. Nature 1999;401:921–923.
10. Risch N. Assessing the role of HLA-linked and unlinked determinants of disease. Am J Hum Genet 1987;40:1–14.
11. Etgen GT, Wilson CM, Jensen J, et al. Glucose transport and cell surface GLUT-4 protein in skeletal muscle of the obese Zucker rat. Am J Physiol 1996;271:E294–E301.
12. Garvey WT, Mainu L, Zhu JH, et al. Evidence for defects in the trafficking and translocation of GLUT4 glucose transporters in skeletal muscle as a cause of human insulin resistance. J Clin Invest 1998;101:2377–2386.
13. American Diabetes Association. Physician's Guide to Non-insulin Dependent (Type II) Diabetes: Diagnosis and Treatment. 2nd Ed. Alexandria, VA: American Diabetes Association, 1988:1–93.
14. Boden G. Free fatty acids, insulin resistance, and type 2 diabetes mellitus. Proc Assoc Am Physicians 1999;111:241–248.
15. Hotamisligil GS, Spiegelman BM. Tumor necrosis factor α: a key component of the obesity-diabetes link. Diabetes 1994;43:1271–1278.
16. Stephens JM, Pekala PH. Transcriptional repression of the GLUT4 and C/EBP genes in 3T3-LI adipocytes by tumor necrosis factor-alpha. J Biol Chem 1991;266:21839–21845.
17. Miles PD, Romeo OM, Higo K, et al. TNF-alpha induced insulin resistance in vivo and its prevention by troglitazone. Diabetes 1997;46:1678–1683.
18. Halle M, Berg A, Northoff H, Keul J. Importance of TNF-alpha and leptin in obesity and insulin resistance: a hypothesis on the impact of physical exercise. Exerc Immunol Rev 1998;4:77–94.
19. Steppan CM, Bailey ST, Bhat S, et al. The hormone resistin links obesity to diabetes. Nature 2001;409:307–312.
20. Maynard T. Exercise: Part I. Physiological response to exercise in diabetes mellitus. Diabetes Educator 1991;17:196–206.
21. Zinker BA. Nutrition and exercise in individuals with diabetes. Clin Sports Med 1999;18:585–606.
22. Leon AS. Exercise in the prevention and management of diabetes mellitus and blood lipid disorders. In: Shephard RJ, Miller HS, eds. Exercise and the Heart in Health and Disease. New York: Marcel Dekker, Inc., 1999.
23. Blair SN, Kohl HW, Gordon NF, Paffenbarger RS. How much physical activity is good for health? Annu Rev Public Health 1992;13:99–126.
24. Harris K, Holly R. Physiological responses to circuit weight training in borderline hypertensive subjects. Med Sci Sports Exerc 1987;19:246–252.
25. Kahn SE, Larson VG, Beard JC, et al. Effect of exercise on insulin action, glucose tolerance, and insulin secretion in aging. Am J Apply 1993;264:E937–E943.
26. Hughes VA, Fiatarone MA, Fielding RA, et al. Exercise increases muscle GLUT-4 levels and insulin action with impaired glucose tolerance. Am J Physiol 1993;264:E855–E862.
27. Dengel DR, Pratley RE, Hagberg JM, et al. Distinct effects of aerobic exercise training and weight loss on glucose homeostasis in obese sedentary men. J Appl Physiol 1996;81:318–325.
28. Peterson CM, Jones RL, Dupuis A, et al. Feasibility of improved blood glucose control in patients with insulin-dependent diabetes mellitus. Diabetes Care 1979;2:329–335.
29. Wallberg-Henriksson H, Gunnarsson R, Jenriksson J, et al. Increased peripheral insulin sensitivity and muscle mitochondrial enzymes but unchanged blood glucose control in type I diabetics after physical training. Diabetes 1982;31:1044–1050.
30. Zinman B, Zuniga-Guajardo S, Kelly D. Comparison of the acute and long-term effects of exercise on glucose control in type I diabetes. Diabetes Care 1984;7:515–519.
31. Landt KW, Campaigne BN, James FW, Sperling M. Effects of exercise training on insulin sensitivity in adolescents with type I diabetes. Diabetes Care 1985; 8:461–465.
32. Ligtenberg PC, Balns M, Hoekstra JBL, et al. No effect of long-term physical activity on the glycemic control in type 1 diabetes patients: a cross-sectional study. Netherlands Journal of Medicine 1999;55:59–63.
33. Ruderman NB, Granda OP, Johansen K. The effect of physical training on glucose tolerance and plasma lipids in maturity onset diabetes. Diabetes 1979;28:89–92.
34. Leon AS, Conrad JC, Casal DC, et al. Exercise for diabetics: effects of conditioning at constant body weight. J Cardiac Rehab 1984;4:278–286.
35. Reitman JS, Vasquez B, Klimes I, Nagulesparan M. Improvement of glucose homeostasis after exercise training in non-insulin-dependent diabetes. Diabetes Care 1984;7:434–441.
36. Segal KR, Edano A, Abalos A, et al. Effect of exercise training on insulin sensitivity and glucose metabolism in lean, obese, and diabetic men. J Appl Physiol 1991;71:2402–2411.
37. Krotkiewski M, Lonnroth P, Mandroukas K, et al. The effects of physical training on insulin secretion and effectiveness and on glucose metabolism in obesity and type 2 (non-insulin-dependent) diabetes mellitus. Diabetologia 1985;28:881–890.
38. Ronnemaa T, Mattila K, Lehtonen A, Kallio V. A controlled randomized study on the effect of long-term physical exercise on the meta-

bolic control in type 2 diabetic patients. Acta Med Scand 1986;220: 219–224.

39. Holloszy JO, Schultz J, Kusnierkiewicz J, et al. Effects of exercise on glucose tolerance and insulin resistance: brief review and some preliminary results. Acta Med Scand 1986;711(Supplement):55–65.

40. DeFronzo RA, Ferrannini E, Koivisto V. New concepts in the pathogenesis and treatment of non-insulin-dependent diabetes mellitus. Am J Med 1983;75:52–81.

41. Dela F, Larsen JJ, Mikines KJ, et al. Insulin-stimulated muscle glucose clearance in patients with NIDDM: effects of one-legged physical training. Diabetes 1995;22:221–226.

42. Manson JE, Rimm EB, Stampfer MJ, et al. Physical activity and incidence of non-insulin-dependent diabetes mellitus in women. Lancet 1991;338:774–778.

43. Manson JE, Nathan DM, Krolewski AS, et al. A prospective study of exercise and incidence of diabetes among U.S. male physicians. JAMA 1992;268:63–67.

44. Helmrich SP, Bourney RE, Rodnick KJ, et al. Physical activity and reduced occurrence of non-insulin-dependent diabetes mellitus. N Engl J Med 1991;325:147–152.

45. Lynch J, Helmrich SP, Lakka TA, et al. Moderately intense physical activities and high levels of cardiorespiratory fitness reduce the risk of non-insulin-dependent diabetes mellitus in middle-aged men. Arch Intern Med 1996;156:1307–1314.

46. Wannamethee SG, Shaper AG, Alberti GMM. Physical activity, metabolic factors, and the incidence of coronary heart disease and type 2 diabetes. Arch Intern Med 2000;160:2108–2116.

47. Eriksson K-F, Lindarde E. Prevention of type 2 (non-insulin-dependent) diabetes mellitus by diet and exercise. The 6-year Malmo feasibility study. Diabetologia 1991;34:891–898.

48. Pan XR, Li GW, Hu YH, et al. Effects of diet and exercise in preventing NIDDM in people with impaired glucose tolerance. The Da Quing IGT and Diabetes Study. Diabetes Care 1997;20:537–544.

49. Mosher P, Nash M, Perry A, et al. Aerobic circuit exercise training: effect on adolescents with well-controlled insulin-dependent diabetes mellitus. Arch Phys Med Rehabil 1998;79:652–657.

50. Schneider SH, Khachadurian AK, Amorosa LF, et al. Ten-year experience with an exercise-based outpatient lifestyle modification program in the treatment of diabetes mellitus. Diabetes Care 1992;15(Suppl 4):1800–1810.

51. James SA, Jamjoum L, Raghunathan TE, et al. Physical activity and NIDDM in African-Americans. The Pitt County Study. Diabetes Care 1998;21:555–562.

SUGGESTED READINGS

American Diabetes Association. The Health Professional's Guide to Diabetes and Exercise. American Diabetes Association, 1995.

Gordon NF. Diabetes: Your Complete Exercise Guide. Champaign, IL: Human Kinetics Publishers, 1993.

CHAPTER 22

Renal Disease

Jacques R. Poortmans, Patricia Painter

Overview

It is well established that active physical behavior has numerous advantages for healthy subjects, which lead them to more professional disponibility and social activities throughout their lifetime. Life expectancy is increasing in industrial countries, but the process of aging affects many organs, including the kidney. **Renal blood flow, glomerular filtration rate (GFR)**, renal sodium handling, and renal concentrating ability have been shown to decline with advancing age in humans (1, 2). It has been reported that aging induces a delayed ability to restore body fluid homeostasis after a volume-depleting stimulus, rendering older individuals susceptible to chronic hypohydration (3, 4). However, when individuals over 60 years old are submitted to 4 successive days at 50% maximal oxygen consumption for 90 minutes in a warm environment (24°C wet bulb),

there was no significant effect on the healthy older subject's ability to retain body fluid and electrolytes in response to acute dehydration (5).

Diseases involving the renal glomeruli are encountered frequently in clinical practice and are the most common causes of **end-stage renal disease** worldwide. In the United States of America, **glomerular diseases** accounted for 51% of treated end-stage renal disease reported to the U.S. Renal Data System between 1991 and 1995, including 38% of diabetic nephropathy and 13% of nondiabetic glomerular disease (6).

During the past decade, **proteinuria** has assumed new importance, and recent clinical and experimental results have also suggested that proteinuria is an independent risk factor for the progression of **renal disease** (7). The persistence of proteinuria is associated with increased renal mortality. Specifically, urinary albumin excretion >30 mg/24 h

(>20 μg/min) has been identified as a risk factor for the progression of renal disease.

It is a common view that the number of nephropathies has increased over the last decades; besides specific renal diseases, this may be due to the increasing proportion of older individuals requiring a large amount of medical supervision and expenditure. When an individual is diagnosed with end-stage renal disease, a significant period of reduced activity or bed rest often follows. Physical inactivity probably results due to symptoms associated with progressive renal failure, specifically fatigue and weakness. However, precise information is lacking about this specific aspect of renal diseases and how much physical activity should be taken to overcome the low-functioning patient.

Chronic renal failure that slowly progresses to **end-stage renal disease (ESRD)** will require dialysis or kidney transplantation. The role of exercise in uremic patients has been reviewed by Painter (8) and Clyne (9). The goal of this chapter is to summarize previous works on acute performance and **exercise training** in the population with renal impairment, to extend the analysis to kidney recipients after transplantation, and to foster interest in involving these subjects in regular exercise to enhance their physical capacity and capability for professional purposes.

Limitations of Moderate Renal Failure to Exercise

Patients With Kidney Disease

Kidney disease affects more than 3.5 million Americans, resulting in annual health care costs that exceed $10 billion (10). **Hypertension** and **diabetes** are the cause of most renal failure in the United States, and autosomal dominant **polycystic kidney disease (PKD)** is the most inherited nephropathy affecting over 600,000 people in the United States and 12 million people worldwide (11).

The effects of exercise on renal function in patients with moderate impairment of renal function (e.g., chronic glomerulonephritis, PKD) have been investigated (12). Individuals with impaired renal function showed a significant decrease in GFR on exertion compared with healthy subjects. The diseased kidney appeared unable to maintain GFR or conserve water under the stress of 30 minutes of sustained exercise at 110 beats/min.

Poortmans and Vanderstraeten investigated the impact of maximum exercise (mean 125 watts) on proteinuric patients with different etiology (13). The results from this limited number of patients are rather scattered (Figure 22.1). The responses to exercise may depend on the etiology of renal failure. It may be observed that 4 patients (with glomerulonephritis, pyelonephritis, nephrotic syndrome) had a higher postexercise plasma albumin clearance, while the other patients (asymptotic proteinuria) did not show major modifications.

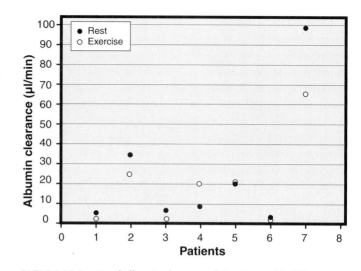

FIGURE 22.1.   Renal albumin clearance of 7 patients with different nephropathies at rest and at maximal exercise on cycle ergometer (mean 125 watts). Patients 1, 2, 3, and 7 with glomerulopathy showed a higher clearance under exercise condition. The albumin clearance in healthy subject at rest should be under 0.3 μL/min.

Patients With Diabetes Nephropathy

The American National Commission on Diabetes reports that the risk of renal insufficiency is 17 times higher in diabetic patients than in the normal population. An important step in the diagnosis of nephropathy was the development of sensitive methods for urine albumin determination. This allowed the detection of weak protein excretion in the stage of functional renal dysfunction that seems to precede the irreversible anatomical lesions.

Mogensen and colleagues demonstrated that light exercise (100 watts) on a bicycle ergometer could reveal functional renal abnormalities early in the course of diabetes and in patients with normal baseline albumin excretion many years before nephropathy is clinically evident (14). In healthy individuals, no increase in albumin excretion was found at this load when maintained for 30 minutes. No increase was obtained in patients with diabetes of 1 year or less. A significant increase in albumin excretion was recorded in juvenile patients with type 1 diabetes of at least 2 years' duration. Jefferson and associates confirmed these observations with a group of 40 diabetic children who performed a moderate exercise test (15 minutes at 2 W/kg body weight) on a bicycle ergometer (15).

Poortmans and colleagues suggested that maximal performance does not give any additional information about discrepancies between normal and diabetic individuals (16). No difference appeared between diabetic individuals with early retinal vascular changes and those free from all retinopathy. From these results, it may be concluded that, in diabetic patients, exhaustive physical exercise does not provoke an enhanced dysfunction of the kidney compared with that already found in nondiabetic people. This conclusion is reinforced by later results obtained by Johansson and associates in insulin-dependent (type 1) diabetic children and adolescents (17) and adults (18, 19). These results suggest that previously observed differences in exercise-induced proteinuria in patients with type 1 diabetes might be related to inappropriate standardization of submaximal exercise intensities. Ala-Houhala investigated the glomerular permeability in patients with diabetic nephropathy by performing fractional clearance of neutral dextrans at rest and after exercise (20). Following exercise (30 minutes with a heart rate of 120 to 130 beats/min), an increased fractional clearance of molecules was observed with a radius >4.8 nm. These findings support the concept of exercise-induced permeability changes in insulin-dependent diabetic patients. As in healthy individuals, noradrenaline appears to contribute to the exercise-induced changes in renal protein handling in patients with microalbuminuria and type 1 diabetes (21).

Heart Transplant Patients

Patients treated with cyclosporine may have altered renal function. Niset and colleagues followed a heart transplant patient (42 years of age) who decided to perform a 20-km run (22). At rest, this patient had a creatinine clearance of 17 ml/min (as compared with 123 ml/min for a healthy population); this rate went down to 4 ml/min at the end of the 20 km performed in minutes. The total protein excretion increased to 288 μg/min (147 μg/min in the control group). Considering these absolute values, the effects are far more pronounced in the heart transplant patient. The use of cyclosporine explains the discrepancy from the normal population; moreover, the immunosuppressive drug had an added effect on the exercise condition. Thus, nephrotoxic drug effects should also be considered in the pathogenesis of acute renal failure that might accompany prolonged exercise, especially when performed in a hot environment under dehydrating conditions.

Since this first work, there have been 2 publications on renal responses to exercise after heart transplantation. Haywood and associates showed that short-term, maximum supine bicycle exercise induced a 44% decrease in renal blood flow in heart transplant recipients, as compared to a 4% decrease in a healthy control group (23). These authors suggested that the surgical division of the cardiac ventricular afferent fibers resulted in an increased vasoconstriction drive to the kidney and nonexercising muscle during exercise. They added that this mechanism might contribute to persistent exercise limitations and renal impairment after heart transplantations. Poortmans and colleagues showed that despite the greater reduction in renal blood flow suggested by Haywood and associates, there was a moderate increase of protein and albumin excretion rates (twofold) in the heart transplant recipients as compared to a control group submitted to the same absolute load (115 watts) (24) (Figure 22.2).

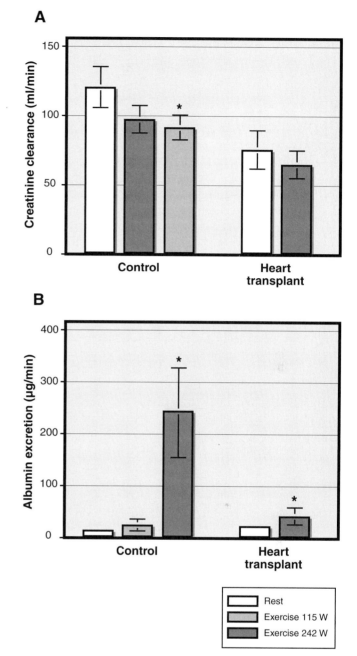

FIGURE 22.2. Glomerular filtration rate (A) and albumin excretion rate (B) in heart transplant recipients and healthy controls at rest and at maximal exercise on cycle ergometer. The heart transplant patients reached a power output of 115 watts while the healthy controls attained 242 watts. The upper limit of albumin excretion under resting condition in a healthy population should be under 20 μl/min.

* $P = 0.05$ between exercise and rest.

The estimated GFR was not modified by the maximum exercise test in the heart transplant patients. The higher urinary albumin clearance after exercise in the patient group could be related to the higher increase of plasma lactate (8.3 mmol/l) as compared to the control group (3.4 mmol/l). The lactate itself does not affect the glomerular membrane permeability, but gives indirect evidence of the relative intensity of exercise anaerobic metabolism. Indeed, the exercise stress might induce a higher response of the renal sympathic nerve activity in the heart transplant recipients, leading to more protein excretion in urine.

Limitations of Chronic Renal Failure to Exercise

Metabolic Consequences in Uremic Patients

Initially, a damaged kidney reacts by increasing its GFR and excretion rate per nephron to compensate for the progressive loss of functional glomeruli. Histological changes occur in the aging nephron (25). The basement membranes of glomeruli become thicker, and glomeruli later collapse or are replaced by hyaline material. Tubule cells undergo fatty degeneration and become relatively ischemic. Progressive renal failure results in inefficient excretion of waste substances, leading to uremia. The accumulation in the blood of substances normally excreted by the kidney (i.e., urea and creatinine) is responsible for the many disturbances associated with renal failure. Blachney and Knochel have focused their attention on the biochemical implications of uremia on cell functions (26). Moreover, Painter described biochemical abnormalities, cardiovascular consequences, and neuromuscular dysfunction of ESRD (8). Recently, Wayand and colleagues observed that sporadic or persistently increased cardiac troponin T (cTnT) and troponin I (cTnI) appear to predict cardiac impairment in patients suffering from ESRD (27).

Significant abnormalities of cellular functions occur in ESRD. The most prevalent symptoms in uremic patients are weakness, hypertension, myocardial dysfunction, anorexia, anemia, fatigue, and psychological and social waning (Table 22.1).

TABLE 22.1. METABOLIC CONSEQUENCES OF UREMIA

Systems	Consequences
Left ventricular hypertrophy	Intolerance to exercise
Myopathy	Reduction in blood flow
	Atrophy of type II fibers
	Limitation in oxidative metabolism
Carbohydrate metabolism	Glucose intolerance
	Hyperinsulinemia, reduced insulin sensitivity
	Hyperglucagonemia
	Decreased activity of key glycolytic enzymes
Lipid metabolism	Hypertriglyceridemia
	Defective removal of VLDL particles
	Decreased lipase activity
	Impaired fatty acid oxidation
Protein metabolism	Increased protein breakdown

Numerous endocrine metabolic disorders are associated with uremia (insulin, glucagon, catecholamines, thyroid, parathyroid). They affect muscle metabolism, leading to impaired exchange of oxygen between blood and muscle as well as protein breakdown, abnormal protein structure, and contractile protein dysfunction.

Physical Work Capacity of Uremic Patients

Clyne reviewed the capability of end-stage renal patients to perform exercise or, more generally, to maintain an active life (9). When predialysis uremic patients underwent an exercise test on a bicycle ergometer, a decrease in working capacity was correlated to the decrease in total hemoglobin (28–31). However, several reports pointed out the lack of correlation between hemoglobin levels and exercise capacity in hemodialysis patients (32–35). These results suggested cardiovascular and/or muscular limitations to strenuous exercise. Indeed, the impaired chronotropic responses observed during exercise in dialysis patients could predict a lower maximal heart rate compared to a healthy population.

Most authors showed reduction in $\dot{V}O_2$ peaks that were only between 50% and 60% of the predicted values for age and sex. Clyne (29) also observed in predialysis patients a statistical relationship between the decrease in GFR and work capacity although the correlation coefficient is rather low ($r = 0.30$). Additionally, there was a significant correlation between the increase in total hemoglobin and the increase in maximal exercise capacity ($r = 0.81$) (36). As the maximal aerobic capacity is related to the total content of hemoglobin in healthy subjects, one may argue that renal anemia may be an important factor in restricting physical work capacity in uremic patients.

Muscle weakness appears to be a common complaint in patients with ESRD (37). Indeed, a characteristic feature of chronic renal failure is the associated myopathy. A few authors investigated muscle strength using either some myometer and programmed electrical stimulation of specific muscles (38), or isokinetic dynamometer (39) and cycle ergometer (40). There was a significant correlation between isokinetic muscle strength and peak $\dot{V}O_2$ for different muscle groups (quadriceps, biceps, triceps, and deltoid muscles). The correlation between muscle strength and peak $\dot{V}O_2$ was stronger than peak $\dot{V}O_2$ and hemoglobin concentrations (40). Following **recombinant human erythropoietin (rHu-EPO) therapy** (see below), there are increases in isometric and isokinetic muscle strength (38, 39). Nevertheless, despite this improvement in muscle strength, the rHu-EPO group did not perform as well as healthy control subjects (38).

The previous lines of evidence suggest that local muscular fatigue may be involved in the limitation of work capacity. Thus, skeletal muscle disorders will also impair end-stage renal patients to perform physical exercise.

Renal Anemia and Acute Effect on Exercise

Since the discovery by Winearls and colleagues (41) and Eschbach and associates (42), nephrologists have recognized that recombinant human erythropoietin (rHu-EPO) therapy is the best method to overcome anemia in ESRD. The benefits and risks of anemia correction with rHu-EPO have been characterized in children (43) and in adults (44). As early as 1988, Mayer and colleagues showed that maximal physical capacity was improved in hemodialysis patients (45). Several studies have confirmed this first observation in predialysis patients (36, 46, 47) and in hemodialysis patients (34, 39, 48–56). An extended Canadian survey (57) of 118 hemodialysis patients, in which 67 individuals received an erythropoietin injection at the end of each session of dialysis (3 times a week), pointed out the association among rHu-EPO, quality of life, and exercise capacity of patients receiving hemodialysis during a 6-month period. The patients who received rHu-EPO had a moderate (10%) improvement in exercise performance (treadmill run with increasing speed and slope, and 6-minute walk test). The high rHu-EPO receiver group had better results than the low rHu-EPO receiver group. Although exercise capacity improves following rHu-EPO treatment, the improvement is not what would be expected, nor is it in proportion to the increase in hemoglobin resulting from EPO therapy. The response in $\dot{V}O_2$ in patients on dialysis following correction of anemia is much less than the response observed in healthy individuals when the hematocrit is manipulated (58, 59). Painter reported that in healthy individuals, the fractional change in peak $\dot{V}O_2$ per change in hemoglobin (following phlebotomy and/or reinfusion of packed red blood cells) ranges from 0.5 to 0.9. In patients on hemodialysis, the fractional change in peak $\dot{V}O_2$ per change in hemoglobin following rHu-EPO therapy ranges from 0.03 to 0.45.

As uremia progresses, a gradual decline occurs in maximal exercise capacity, which is related to hemoglobin concentration (29). This relationship is not well established, since only 2 publications have reported that successful renal transplantation increases maximal aerobic perfor-mance (Table 22.2) (35, 60). However, hemoglobin levels were not normalized at the time of posttransplant testing, and the correlation between changes in peak $\dot{V}O_2$ and hemoglobin was only 0.27 (61). The increase in maximum capacity was not significantly correlated with changes in hemoglobin ($r = 0.27$) (61). One has to conclude that this improvement does not lead the patient to the level of healthy individuals, since the kidney recipients attain about 80% to 90% of maximal aerobic capacity of a normal population, suggesting that other factors affect aerobic capacity following transplant (62). A report from Nyberg and colleagues even pointed out that vital capacity and forced expiratory volume do not improve in patients over 60 years of age following successful kidney transplantation (63). These authors concluded that the general condition of these patients does not vary in the first posttransplant year, and that patients whose condition does improve cannot be identified in advance.

Peripheral Metabolism During Exercise in Patients With ESRD

Increasing exercise intensity in healthy subjects leads to increasing muscle lactate production and accumulation in blood. Barnea and colleagues (32) showed that arterial lactate concentration reached practically the same level after maximal bicycle exercise in dialysis patients (4.8 mmol/L) as compared to healthy controls (4.1 mmol/L) although peak exercise represented only 51% of normal in patients. In contrast, Parrish and Ostapenko (64) reported that dialysis patients had 65% higher lactate levels at submaximal exercise (2.5 mmol/L) than healthy controls (0.9 mmol/L). These two groups of researchers suggested that early muscular fatigue found in dialysis patients during low-level exercise might be caused by an impaired maximal oxygen uptake associated with a rapid onset of anaerobic metabolism. Nevertheless, these authors failed to give precise information on the intensity of work relative to the maximal capacity of the subjects. To solve this problem, Kettner and colleagues submitted hemodialysis patients

TABLE 22.2. MAXIMAL WORK CAPACITY OF KIDNEY TRANSPLANT PATIENTS (KTP) AND HEALTHY CONTROLS (C)

Population (n subjects)	Age (mean, y)	Time of transplant (months)	$\dot{V}O_2$ peak (ml/kg/min)	Power (W)	Authors
KTP (20)	35	40	31.7 ± 7.0	150	(35)
KTP (10)	36	44		150	(153)
KTP (20)	29	2	29.3 ± 4.6	160	(61)
KTP (12)	41	6		148	(60)
KTP (12)	33	62	29.0 ± 7.8		(62)
KTP (83)	33	12	22.0 ± 5.0	114	(154)
C (10)	32		36.7 ± 6.7	258	(154)

and healthy controls to bicycle ergometer exercise at a workload selected to elicit approximately 50% of their respective peak $\dot{V}O_2$ for 60 minutes (65). They showed that plasma lactate levels were similar (1.3–1.9 mmol/l) after 30 and 60 minutes of exercise in both populations. However, $\dot{V}O_2$ reached an average of 0.7 l/min in the hemodialysis patients and 1.3 l/min in the controls. Thus, one may expect that the aerobic capacity of hemodialysis subjects might be less performant than healthy controls even during moderate exercise.

Some authors followed the acid-base and electrolyte changes following maximal (66, 67) and submaximal (66) exercises. These studies showed that maximal and prolonged submaximal exercise (60% peak $\dot{V}O_2$ during 30 minutes) elicited modest changes in pH (not lower than 7.26) and potassium accumulation (around 5 mmol/l).

The correction of the anemia by administering rHu-EPO has been recognized to have an impact on the blood and hemodynamic parameters analyzed during exercise. A mean 20% increase of the lactate threshold (49, 52–54, 56) and ventilation threshold (68) during exercise have been found as soon as 2 months after rHu-EPO treatment. Furthermore, Meierhenrich and colleagues (69) reported a reduction of excess lactate after rHu-EPO therapy during short-term moderate exercise (0.7 W/kg body weight) on cycle ergometer. This suggests that the rHu-EPO treatment improved the oxygen transport in the blood and its tissue uptake, leading to a better aerobic metabolism in skeletal muscle (48, 51). Horina and colleagues (49) investigated the influence of improved oxygen transport capacity on physical performance of patients treated with rHu-EPO. They reported a higher level of red cell 2,3-bisphosphoglycerate after treatment, and as the maximal working capacity and maximal oxygen uptake of their subjects increased by about 20%, they presumed that there was an improved oxygen delivery to skeletal muscles per unit of hemoglobin. However, Marrades and associates observed that muscle blood flow decreases following rHu-EPO administration, suggesting that there may be an increase in peripheral vascular resistance with the increase in hemoglobin (70).

Cardiovascular Responses to Exercise in Uremic Patients

The most common cardiovascular abnormality observed in dialyzed patients is myocardial dysfunction, especially left ventricular hypertrophy, leading to reduced exercise tolerance. Correction to anemia in these patients by rHu-EPO treatment improved the cardiac index (34), reduced the exercise-induced myocardial ischemia (55), and had a normalized left ventricular function in response to exercise (50). Other conditions (e.g., chronic metabolic acidosis; increased preload associated with arteriovenous fistula) may also affect myocardial contractility and the cardiac response to exercise.

Muscle Blood Flow and Oxygen Transport in Patients With ESRD

The limited aerobic exercise capacity of patients with chronic renal disease could be dependent on impaired nutritive skeletal muscle blood flow, reduced oxygen delivery to muscle, and restricted muscle oxygen conductance to mitochondria. Bradley and associates (71) reported that these patients had calf blood flow comparable to that of healthy control subjects at rest. However, after submaximal and maximal bicycle exercise, the patients with ESRD had 33% reduced skeletal muscle blood flow. Decreased blood flow could lead to reduced oxygen delivery to skeletal muscle, thus inducing early onset of anaerobic metabolism. The authors pointed out that the cause of impaired skeletal muscle blood flow during exercise in patients with ESRD remains unclear.

Marrades and colleagues (72) investigated why, despite near normalization of hemoglobin content, patients treated with rHu-EPO fail to significantly improve aerobic capacity. They submitted ESRD patients, before and after rHu-EPO therapy, to submaximal (30%, 60%, and 80% of peak workload) and maximal exercises on bicycle ergometer. Femoral blood flow, leg oxygen uptake, and extraction ratio were calculated. They showed that while rHu-EPO therapy enhanced aerobic capacity by 30% and leg oxygen uptake by 33%, the relative increase compared to pretreatment was much less than that of arterial oxygen content (59%). Their results support that abnormal muscle transport is the key factor limiting increases in oxygen consumption in patients with ESRD even after rHu-EPO treatment. This suggests a myopathy alteration, possibly of the microcirculation, due to renal failure that compromises exercise capacity more than anemia and inactivity alone would predict (72).

Muscle Metabolism in Patients With ESRD

The previous analyses from the literature clearly demonstrate that the reduction in exercise capacity of patients with ESRD affects the muscle itself. Thus, where are the limitations? Are they structural or metabolic? A thorough survey could lead us to the basic principles that still impair these patients in their abilities or willingness to remain as active as possible.

Muscle Morphology

Many patients with ESRD complain of muscle weakness and easy tiring, supported by skeletal myopathy (73). These uremic patients were found to have atrophy of the type II fibers (74, 75), marked variability of fiber area (38, 75), lower proportion of type IIB fibers (76), fiber splitting (38, 77), and degenerative changes including multiple mitochondrial abnormalities (74, 77). Some authors also reported an increased (38, 77, 78) or normal glycogen content (79) together with lipid droplet accumulation (77). After rHu-EPO treatment, Davenport (38) reported a marked improvement in the histological appearance of skeletal muscle. In particular, distribution of type I fibers returned to normal, and type IIA and IIB fiber diameters improved.

ATP and Phosphorylcreatine Metabolism

Total adenine nucleotide concentrations and energy charge ratio were measured in skeletal muscle of hemodialysis patients (80). As compared to healthy controls, these authors observed lower values (−20%) in adenosine triphosphate (ATP) content and energy charge ratio, which could contribute to their reduced exercise capacity and poor metabolic state. However, more accurate measurements were made in isolated mitochondria obtained by muscle biopsies from hemodialysis patients (81). The results unexpectedly showed a 35% increase in mitochondrial production rate of the ESRD patients before rHu-EPO therapy than in sedentary healthy controls. One year after rHu-EPO treatment, the ATP production rate per kilogram of muscle was decreased to control level in most patients. These results suggest that the enhanced mitochondrial ATP production rate in uremic patients is a metabolic adaptation to decreased oxygen transport and that this state is reversed by long-term rHu-EPO treatment.

Recently, ^{31}P-nuclear magnetic resonance spectroscopy studies (70, 82–84) extended the previous observations made on resting subjects. However, their results are not always similar. As compared to healthy individuals, all investigations reported an identical decrease of phosphorylcreatine (PC), a lower PC/Pi ratio under submaximal and maximal isotonic and dynamic exercises. Meanwhile, there are some discrepancies in intracellular pH values, which are lower than controls in some studies (70, 83, 84), while no changes between groups were recorded in another study (82). A lower muscle cell bioenergetic status and a lower intracellular pH, at a given $\dot{V}O_2$, was found in ESRD patients as compared to controls, even after rHu-EPO treatment (70, 84). A low pH can inhibit cellular enzymes and lower the oxidative muscle capacity. Analysis of submaximal and peak exercise data clearly demonstrates that there were no changes after rHu-EPO treatment. This observation implies that muscle microcirculation and lower intracellular pH might be partially involved in the intrinsic limitation of oxidation in uremic myopathy.

Carbohydrate Metabolism in ESRD

The abnormality of carbohydrate metabolism most commonly demonstrated in uremic patients is a markedly delayed utilization of glucose load under resting conditions (85). Hyperglycemia and impaired glucose tolerance are well-known phenomena even if there is no uniform concept to sustain these observations. Unfortunately, no data are available in the literature on muscle lactate concentration

during exercise in uremic patients. All hypotheses on lactate production have been postulated from blood lactate analyses (see above).

Lipid Metabolism in ESRD

Abnormal fatty acid utilization has been reported in uremic individuals (86, 87). These authors pointed out an incomplete β-oxidation of long-chain fatty acids with a concomitant appearance of short-chain acyl-carnitine in plasma. The mitochondrial transport of free fatty acids depends on the presence of L-carnitine in the cytosol and on the outer surface of the inner-mitochondrial membrane. Skeletal muscle total carnitine content at rest in patients with ESRD has been reported as normal in most studies (87–89), although there is a decreased level of free carnitine as compared to healthy subjects (90). Carnitine supplementation significantly increases plasma and muscle levels of free and acetylcarnitine (91) but its administration is ineffective in altering lipoprotein levels (92) or muscle metabolism (88).

Muscle total carnitine content at rest has been positively correlated with exercise duration on cycle ergometer in patients with ESRD and it has been postulated that low muscle carnitine content may play a role in impaired exercise performance (87). Thus, administration of oral or intravenous carnitine has been used to test this hypothesis. Hiatt and associates (87, 93) and Ahmad and colleagues (94) sustained the hypothesis, while Fagher and associates (88) rejected it. There are, however, major differences in the protocols since different exercises have been applied to these subjects: maximal dynamic strength on an isokinetic ergometer (88) or maximal aerobic capacity on cycle ergometer (87, 94). It seems that carnitine supplementation improves endurance aerobic exercise tolerance by a mechanism that still needs to be defined. Indeed, fatty acid metabolism is not mainly involved in maximal exercise, and nothing up to now is said on the activity of the limiting enzyme carnitine acyltransferase needed for the transfer of the acyl group into the mitochondria.

Muscle Protein and Amino Acid Metabolism in ESRD

There is abundant evidence that loss of renal function leads to a decline in lean body mass, specifically muscle (95). Alterations of plasma and muscle amino acids levels have been described in uremic patients (96). These abnormalities have been attributed to low protein intake, deficiency of amino acid metabolism, and loss of protein and amino acids by the dialytic procedure. Garber analyzed skeletal muscle amino acids in experimental chronic uremia in rats (97, 98). He reported increased alanine and glutamine production and release from skeletal muscle of chronically uremic animals. This increase appears to derive in part from an enhancement of net protein degradation (97) and oxidation

(99). To improve nitrogen balance and nutritional status, Van der Niepen and associates suggested supplementing hemodialysis patients and uremic patients in predialysis state with oral amino acids up to a total daily protein load of 1.2 g/kg body weight (100).

It also appeared that skeletal muscle in chronic uremia acquired insensitivity to the metabolic action of epinephrine or serotonin (98). An important factor that initiates abnormal responses in uremia is metabolic acidosis, which stimulates muscle protein degradation and increases the activity of branched-chain amino acid enzymes (101, 102). Recently, Ikizler and colleagues (103) suggested that the net anabolic processes induced by recombinant human growth hormone could reflect a beneficial shift in amino acid metabolism toward muscle tissue in dialysis patients.

Apparently, no data are yet available on the effect of acute exercise on protein and amino acid metabolism of patients with renal insufficiency.

Steady-State Exercise During Hemodialysis Treatment

The acute effects of mild cycling exercise have been studied during dialysis (8, 75, 104–107). The initial interest in practicing exercise during dialysis was to counteract the decrease of alveolar ventilation observed with acetate dialysis. Indeed, Germain and associates showed that light bicycle exercise (5 minutes at 25 watts) performed 30 minutes after the beginning of hemodialysis reversed the initial decrease in P_{AO_2} (105). Acetate dialysis induced small decreases in pH values; however, light exercise did not worsen this effect, therefore avoiding exercise metabolic acidosis (106). It is hoped that acetate dialysate is no longer in use. Bicarbonate baths are used instead, so that acidosis and P_{AO_2} decreases do not affect patients.

Moore and colleagues (75) compared exercise (40 watts) "on" and "off" dialysis, and they were unable to show any difference in work capacity, oxygen uptake, or arteriovenous extraction. They concluded that performing the exercise while "on" dialysis did not alter determinants of peak oxygen uptake. The same researchers investigated cardiovascular response to submaximal stationary cycling during different periods of the hemodialysis treatment (108). They found that the cardiovascular exercise response is superimposed on hemodynamic effects of dialysis and is adequately stable during the first 2 hours of treatment. After 2 hours, cardiovascular decompensation may preclude exercise.

Kidney Transplant and Active Life

The number of renal transplants has been increasing steadily in the last decade. The annual number of renal transplants in the United States has been about 9% of the number of patients being dialyzed (109). Clearly, renal transplantation generally offers a more normal lifestyle and full rehabilitation. In a study published in 1985, Evans and associates (110) reported that 79% of transplant patients functioned at nearly normal levels compared with 48% to 59% of those treated with various forms of dialysis. Almost 75% of transplant patients were able to work, compared to 25% to 59% of the dialysis patients.

Successful renal transplantation is recognized by disappearance of toxic uremic effects. However, cardiovascular disease is a major cause of morbidity and mortality among renal transplant patients (111). Moreover, Goffin and colleagues reported that within 6 months after renal transplantation, 10% of patients develop a syndrome of transient, severe musculoskeletal pain in the lower limbs, typically in the knees and ankles (112). Kosch and associates reported altered bone structure expressed by low bone stiffness values measured by quantitative ultrasound in kidney transplant patients (113). Osteogenic agents (e.g., cyclosporine and steroids) could cause the epiphyseal impaction, and these authors suggested that additional factors such as excessive physical exercise should be limited, even avoided, in transplanted patients. However, no data are available to suggest that moderate, low-impact activities cause epiphyseal impaction in patients after transplantation. In fact, injury rates in participants in the U.S. Transplant Games show very low rates of injury during high-level competition (114). It is highly probable that progressive exercise implemented following transplantation will result in increased muscle and bone strength, which has the potential to prevent problematic bone trauma during activity.

Working Capacity

Painter and colleagues have investigated exercise tolerance to treadmill test (35). They showed that renal transplant patients had a higher peak $\dot{V}_{O_2}$ than dialyzed patients. Clyne and associates and Painter and colleagues also showed that, 3 to 6 months posttransplantation, the maximal working capacity increased by 18% to 27% (60, 61). Table 22.2 summarizes these results, as well as personal unpublished data.

The improvement of peak $\dot{V}_{O_2}$ does not lead transplant patients to normalized working capacity as compared to healthy subjects. However, transplant recipients who participate in high-level training are able to exceed normal values of peak $\dot{V}_{O_2}$ (115).

The correction of anemia (60) and reduction of toxic uremia (35, 61) could be involved in the improvement of working capacity in kidney recipients. The lower values of maximal load could also be attributed to a decreased skeletal muscle oxidative capacity (-40%) after kidney transplantation as compared to healthy moderately trained subjects (62).

Renal Functions

From the beginning, the GFR of the transplanted kidney is usually within the range of 40 to 80 ml/min/1.73 m^2 (109).

The toxicity of cyclosporine on renal structure and function is well documented. It is been pointed out that increased urinary protein concentrations contribute to the progressive nature of renal disease (116), kidney recipients included (117). The determination of specific plasma protein excretion revealed that glomerular (118) and tubular (119) transplant disease exists in almost all apparently well-functioning long-term grafts.

Clyne (120) reported a significant but moderate ($r = 0.37$, $P < 0.005$) correlation between a low GFR (0.3–32 ml/min) and maximal exercise capacity of 59 uremic patients, but did not reevaluate this correlation after kidney transplantation (GFR 45 ± 19 ml/min, mean $\pm$ SD). In a recent work, Poortmans and colleagues analyzed blood lactate and protein excretion rate of kidney transplant patients after maximal exhaustive cycling exercise (24) (Figure 22.3). They observed that total protein and albumin excretion rate remained within the normal physiological range, despite a high blood lactate level, while healthy controls had a typical postexercise proteinuria at maximal exercise. This clearly pointed out the primacy of absolute load instead of relative load on protein handling by the kidney. Given the relationship during exercise between plasma noradrenaline level and albumin excretion (13) in healthy individuals after maximal exercise, one may argue that the low figure observed with kidney recipients could be related to the kidney denervation, which thus reduces the hypothetical induction of catecholamines in the genesis of increased glomerular membrane permeability. Indeed, plasma renin activity is higher than normal in kidney transplant recipients (121). This could be due to a stimulating effect on plasma renin activity by the immunosuppressive drug cyclosporine. The increase in plasma renin activity normally seen during exercise is abolished in the kidney transplant patient due to the denervation of the kidney. However, Di Bona (122) assumed that renal denervation is not permanent, and Gazdar and Dammin (123) noted that regeneration of renal nerves begins as early as 28 days after transplantation in humans.

Exercise Training

Rehabilitation in patients with renal diseases, ESRD, and kidney transplants is an increasingly important concept, as emphasized at a symposium of the American Society of Nephrology (124). The debilitating symptoms of anemia profoundly affect the patient's quality of life; however, this can be partly improved by treatment with rHu-EPO, mode of dialysis, and **exercise therapy** (125, 126).

The Effects of Exercise Training on Kidney Disease Progression

Exercise training apparently does not cause disease progression in humans. Boyce and colleagues showed no

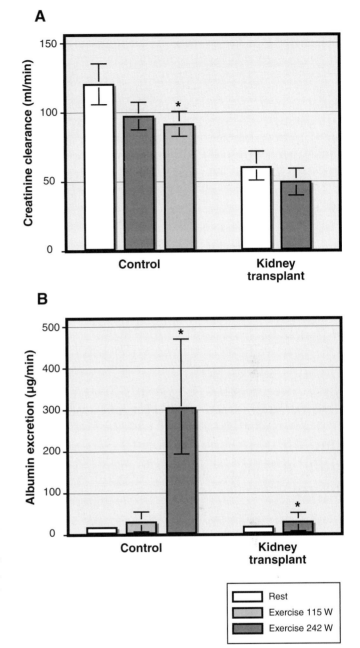

FIGURE 22.3. Glomerular filtration rate (A) and albumin excretion rate (B) in kidney transplant recipients and healthy controls at rest and at maximal exercise on cycle ergometer. The kidney transplant patients reached a power output of 115 watts while the healthy controls attained 242 watts. The upper limit of albumin excretion under resting condition in a healthy population should be under 20 μl/min.

* $P = 0.05$ between exercise and rest.

changes in GFR over a period of 4 months of exercise training in 16 patients with chronic renal insufficiency (127). More data exist for animal models.

Heifets and associates have induced impaired kidney function in rats by subtotal nephrectomy (128). One group of animals was trained by regular exercise for a period of 2 months while another group remained sedentary. GFR was higher and proteinuria was reduced in trained animals as compared with sedentary animals. The degree of glomerulosclerosis was much less prominent in trained rats. This observation suggests that regular exercise has beneficial effects on slowing the progression of renal disease. Other studies on animal models appear to reach the same conclusion. Mice with various degrees of renal mass reduction may augment GFR by physical training (20 minutes daily in a rotating cylinder, for 30 days) (129). However, this positive effect is dependent upon the amount of remaining functional renal tissue. Osato and colleagues also reported that swimming exercise training (2 hours daily, 6 days a week, 20 weeks) can prevent progressive renal dysfunction in nephritic rats induced by injection of Adriamycin, a potent drug for chronic progressive focal glomerulosclerosis (130). Eventually, Darnley and associates conducted a study on rats carrying a dominant mutation for PKD, an accepted model for human PKD (10). The rats were exercised on treadmill (30 minutes daily, 3 days a week, 6 weeks). The results support the safety of moderate exercise in PKD rats.

However, there has been one study showing that strenuous exercise superimposed on active immune complex-mediated glomerulonephritis resulted in worsening of abnormal glomerular function (131). It is difficult to say whether this unique study remains an anecdotal incidence of regular bovine serum albumin injection in rabbits.

Diabetes, Kidney Reactions, and Exercise Training Program

Information is lacking about the potential beneficial effects of training on kidney functions during exercise training. Poortmans and colleagues investigated the renal handling of plasma proteins in a young diabetic population during repeated exercises (participants 11–18 years of age, with diabetes for an average of 13 years) (132). These adolescents participated in a 15-day sport camp, with 6 hours daily of various physical activities (Figure 22.4).

With exercise training, both albumin and β_2-microglobulin excretion rates were reduced by half for the same load of exercise. In other words, the training session attenuated the glomerular membrane changes and tubular impairment in the active population. Whether this effect is beneficial for the diabetic adolescents remains an open question.

ESRD and Exercise Training Program

The importance of exercise training in the rehabilitation of patients with ESRD has been emphasized by the reviews of Painter (58) and Clyne (9), reinforcing previous investigations (83, 104, 133, 134). It is common knowledge that, in healthy subjects, an endurance-training program improves most physiological functions from the lungs and heart to

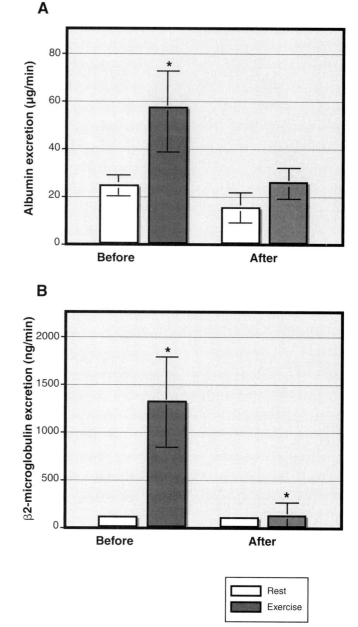

Figure 22.4. Albumin (A) and β_2-microglobulin (B) excretion rates at rest and at the end of exercise before and after exercise training in adolescents with insulin-dependent diabetes mellitus.
* $P = 0.05$ between exercise and rest.

the inside of mitochondria. Because anemia and muscle metabolism are impaired in patients with ESRD, investigators proposed regular exercise as part of the process of rehabilitating these patients to a better level of adaptation to their illness.

Fitts and associates investigated predialysis and dialysis patients who were engaged in strengthening and stretching exercises for 30 minutes per day, 5 days a week for 26 weeks, either at home or at a physical therapy gymnasium near the dialysis center (135). Kouidi and colleagues investigated the effects of exercise training on muscle atrophy in 7 hemodialysis patients (136). Before training, all patients showed muscular atrophy and reduced muscle strength and nerve conduction velocity. A rehabilitation program (cycle ergometer, treadmill, low-weight resistance exercises) of 90-minute sessions, 3 times per week during 6 months improved leg muscle strength by about 45%, while peak $\dot{V}_{O_2}$ increased by 48%. The authors also found a 51% increase in the proportion of type II fibers and a 42% decrease in the proportion of type I fibers in the vastus lateralis after the 6-month aerobic training program. Thus, the rehabilitation program improved muscle atrophy markedly and had beneficial effects on overall work performance. Rehabilitation programs should begin prior to dialysis to achieve the greatest and most lasting benefits.

Predialysis uremic patients improved their aerobic exercise capacity by 11% following 3 months of submaximal exercise (45 minutes per session at 60%–70 % of peak $\dot{V}_{O_2}$) with 3 sessions per week (134). Since total hemoglobin, blood volume, blood pressure, and echocardiographic variables remained unchanged during the observation period, the author concluded that predialysis uremic patients showed an essentially improved muscular function.

Indirect evidence of beneficial effects of endurance training on muscle has been reported in an animal model (137). Rats were made uremic by right nephrectomy and 50% left renal infarction by ligation of some terminal branches of the renal artery. The associated renal failure was characterized by enhanced catabolism of muscle protein. The rats were then subjected to a swimming program for 2 hours daily, 5 days per week for 1 month. In epitrochlearis muscle obtained from exercised uremic rats, net protein degradation was 25% less compared with muscle obtained from sedentary uremic rats, with no modifications in protein synthesis. Moreover, the endurance effect was also sustained by an 82% increase in mitochondrial citrate synthase activity. Thus, exercise training reduced the enhanced muscle protein degradation in moderate renal insufficiency.

Endurance exercise training reduces resting blood pressure in some hemodialysis patients (104, 133, 138). The hemodialysis patients have an average peak $\dot{V}_{O_2}$ that is 50% below that of healthy nonuremic age- and sex-matched subjects (89, 139). Various authors have reported improvement in the aerobic capacity of hemodialyzed patients (35, 89, 138, 140, 141). A mean increase of 17% to 32% has been reported according to the duration of the training period (3–6 months). Nevertheless, even after 12 to 18 months of an exercise-training program, the mean level of maximal aerobic capacity of the trained hemodialysis patient is still almost 35% below that of a normal population.

Goldberg and associates have also reported beneficial effects of endurance training on blood carbohydrate and lipid profiles (138, 142). After 9 months of training sessions of 70% to 80% of peak $\dot{V}_{O_2}$, during sessions lasting 45 to 60 minutes, 3 times a week, hemodialyzed patients improved

the abnormal glucose metabolism and insulin resistance usually observed in dialysis patients. As compared to controls, exercise training increased glucose disappearance rates by 42% to 48%, lowered insulin resistance by reducing basal insulin levels by 18% to 20%, and improved insulin receptor-binding affinity to mononuclear cells by 25% to 71% (138, 142). Fasting plasma triglyceride levels were reduced by 23% to 33%, and high-density lipoprotein cholesterol concentrations were increased by 16% to 21%. These changes might have potential positive effects on several factors that contribute to the development of atherosclerosis in this population.

A few teams have investigated the effect of exercise training on muscle metabolism of ESRD patients. A 3-month period of endurance training on a cycle ergometer to 70% of peak heart rate increased by 44% the succinate dehydrogenase and phosphofructokinase activities in the rectus femoris muscle of hemodialysis patients; however, neither change was correlated with change in peak $\dot{V}_{O_2}$ (75). Type I and II fiber areas were unaffected by training.

Stationary cycling during hemodialysis treatment has been used as an alternative to exercise training (8, 104, 143). Patients were exercised during the second and third hour of hemodialysis treatment for a total of 30 to 45 minutes using heart rates at 65% of peak $\dot{V}_{O_2}$. Peak $\dot{V}_{O_2}$ increased 10% after 3 months of training and 23% after 6 months of training. Successful implementation of an exercise-training program during dialysis depends on cooperation and caring for the patient's well being, as well as on the personal decision of the patient. For example, Painter reported on a total of 358 patients receiving dialysis treatment in her Satellite Dialysis Centers; 171 performed exercise tests for pre-exercise screening (144). A total of 113 patients started the exercise program; during the 11-month trial, 52 patients discontinued the exercise for different reasons (disinterest, home exercise, renal transplantation, cardiac and diabetes complications, deceased). Thus, 54% of the initial exercise population (17% of the total population) fully participated and benefited from the positive effects of the exercise training. Recent investigations of long-term exercise training on rats with induced chronic renal failure (145) and on predialysis patients (127) were unable to demonstrate any detrimental effects on renal function, but did show beneficial improvement in aerobic capacity of the animals and patients.

Recent reports on hemodialysis patients have shown that self-reported physical functioning in these patients is low (146, 147). The authors demonstrated that reduced physical activity and evidence of poor nutritional status lead to higher mortality (146). Moreover, the beneficial impact of regular exercise training seems to be more profound in the lowest functioning patients (148). It has been suggested that some of the benefit observed in physically trained patients following correction of the anemia with rHu-EPO is due to an improvement in voluntary skeletal muscle function (38).

Transplant Patients and Exercise Training Programs

There are only limited data from the literature, despite more than 10 years of World Transplant Games in which transplant recipients have exhibited extraordinary performance in high-level competition. In the average patient older than 60 years of age, Nyberg and colleagues did not observe any improvement in physical performance (grip strength, stepping up on a chair, rising from sitting on a floor, standing on toes) 1 year after successful kidney transplantation (63). In their view, the corticosteroids are likely to have contributed to the patients' weakness. The study by Miller and associates involved 10 patients (mean age 32 years) who, after undergoing renal transplantation, began an exercise program (141). The modes of physical activity used were walking on a treadmill and bicycling between 40% and 60% of peak $\dot{V}O_2$ for 25 to 40 minutes, 3 sessions per week, in addition to walking on their own. This program was sustained for 38 days. Peak $\dot{V}O_2$ increased from 18 ml/kg/min at entry into the exercise program to 34 ml/kg/min at the end. Two years after completion of the supervised program, peak $\dot{V}O_2$ remained at the same level (34 ml/kg/min). However, this improvement obtained after 5 to 6 weeks of training appears astounding.

In the study by Kempeneers and associates, a 24-week exercise-training program was implemented for 16 renal transplant recipients (mean age 33 years) (62). The training routine consisted of 60-minute sessions of supervised exercises (calisthenics, walking, jogging, aerobics, and ball games) 3 times per week at a maximal allowed exercising heart rate of 80% of maximal heart rate measured during a treadmill exercise test. The subjects increased their peak $\dot{V}O_2$ from 29 to 38 ml/kg/min, but the latter value still represented 78% of a healthy control population of similar mass, although the subjects were younger (mean age is 24 years). The isokinetic muscle power also showed an average increase of 25% for the quadriceps and 56% for the hamstrings. Muscle biopsies (vastus lateralis) of 6 subjects showed a lower oxidative capacity (64%) as compared to healthy, moderately trained subjects (100%). Yet, even after training, the exercise capacity of renal transplant recipients remained lower than that of untrained control subjects.

Conclusions and Practical Considerations

Participation in an active life is certainly a major goal for all those who are suffering from any metabolic disturbance. People with renal pathology, patients with diabetes, and organ transplant recipients are concerned with the reaction of their kidneys when exercising regularly. Is it safe, or not, to participate in rehabilitation programs?

Besides the cardiovascular and respiratory benefits of regular exercise, the present contribution emphasized that submaximal exercise does not impair renal functions to any extent (diabetes, organ transplant). However, beforehand, it would be safer to monitor kidney reactions to exercise in laboratory and/or field conditions to avoid any anecdotal incidence.

By definition, ESRD patients are people with disabilities. The debilitating symptoms of anemia have a profound effect on the patient's quality of life. Weakness, dyspnea, headache, and fatigue can be reduced by implementing rHu-EPO therapy, which can largely correct the anemia. Levin assessed the quality-of-life studies and showed that rHu-EPO therapy improved patients' sense of well being, sexual function, sleep habits, social activity, exercise capacity, and appetite in 30% to 90% hemodialysis patients (125). The beneficial effects of rHu-EPO on exercise tolerance and myocardial function have been clearly demonstrated and the hormone treatment has been found to improve markedly the subjective symptoms in hemodialysis patients (126). Aerobic exercise training in healthy individuals has been shown to facilitate muscle oxygen uptake and utilization. So does exercise in ESRD patients, and there is evidence that exercise training in conjunction with rHu-EPO therapy may affect exercise capacity. In an anecdotal note, Painter reported that 2 patients on dialysis who participated in the 1991 California Transplant Games finished first and second in the race, with a peak $\dot{V}O_2$ approaching levels observed in well-trained transplant recipients (58). According to Painter (58) and Clyne (9), each patient with chronic failure should also receive an appropriate dose of exercise training, according to their needs and ability, enabling them to fight against fatigue, to strengthen muscle power, and to enjoy life more fully. One of the ironies of present-day medical care is the lack of efforts to improve the rehabilitation of patients with ERSD who are treated by dialysis and transplantation. The benefits of optimal dialysis and maximum opportunity for rehabilitation could be significant, the costs being not entirely offset by the savings (149). It is high time for every self-respecting nephrology unit to incorporate a physiotherapist in the team and make physical training an integral part of the treatment of ESRD (9).

Successful incorporation of an exercise program by the patient depends on the support received from the nephrologist and the dialysis care staff. Some information to initiate an exercise rehabilitation program for dialysis patients may be found in specific publications (58, 150, 151, 152). Painter has proposed 4 stages to achieve this goal in the dialysis unit (58): (1) incorporate exercise in the patient care plan (ask what the patient does for regular exercise); (2) make automatic referrals for physical therapy (decide how to increase strength and endurance); (3) develop contacts with community programs for referral of patients for participation (exercise at home or in a community program); and (4) develop an intercenter program (dialysis units, stationary exercise instruments).

When is it appropriate for hemodialysis patients to train? Exercise training should be done whenever the patient feels best, which is typically on nondialysis days. Prior to dialysis, patients may be fluid overloaded, thus limiting the amount of exercise tolerated. Exercise immediately after dialysis may be difficult for many patients due to posttreatment fatigue. Moreover, because fluid is lost during treatment, blood pressure is maintained through vasoconstriction. The vasodilatory challenge of exercise at that time may result in hypotension. However, some patients may be able to tolerate exercise either before or after treatment, and should not be discouraged from exercising.

Until now, there has been no longitudinal study that indicates whether endurance exercise training and a more active lifestyle would prolong the survival of uremic patients and kidney transplant patients. However, one may recognize that quality of life is enhanced. It is certainly better to add life to years instead of the reverse, but to reach this level active encouragement by physicians is required, both to the patients and to the staff involved. Let us hope that such a change will lead to greater independence and improved rehabilitation results.

REFERENCES

1. Epstein M. Effects of aging on the kidney. Fed Proc 1979;38:168–172.
2. Macias Nunez JFM, Cameron JS. Renal function and disease in the elderly. London: Butterworth; 1987:548.
3. Miescher E, Fortney SM. Responses to dehydration and rehydration during heat exposure in young and older men. Am J Physiol 1989;257:R1050–R1057.
4. Phillips PA, Rolls BJ, Ledingham JG, et al. Reduced thirst after water deprivation in healthy elderly men. N Engl J Med 1984;311:753–759.
5. Zappe DH, Bell GW, Swartzentruber H, Wideman RF, Kenney WL. Age and regulation of fluid and electrolyte balance during repeated exercise sessions. Am J Physiol 1996;69:R71–R79.
6. Hricik DE, Chung-Park M, Sedor JR. Glomerulonephritis. N Engl J Med 1998;339:888–899.
7. Keane WF. Proteinuria: its clinical importance and role in progressive renal disease. Am J Kidney Dis 2000;35(suppl 1):S97–S105.
8. Painter PL. Exercise in end-stage renal disease. Exerc Sport Sci Rev 1988;16:305–339.
9. Clyne N. Physical working capacity in uremic patients. Scand J Urol Nephrol 1996;30:247–252.
10. Darnley MJ, DiMarco NM, Aukema HM. Safety of chronic exercise in a rat model of kidney disease. Med Sci Sports Exerc 2000;32:576–580.
11. Wilson PD, Falkenstein D. The pathology of human renal cystic disease. Curr Top Pathol 1995;88:1–50.
12. Taverner D, Craig K, Mackay I. Effects of exercise on renal function in patients with moderate impairment of renal function compared to normal men. Nephron 1991;57:288–292.
13. Poortmans JR, Vanderstraeten J. Kidney function during exercise in healthy and diseased humans. Sports Med 1994;18:419–437.
14. Mogensen CE, Vittinghus E, Solling K. Urinary albumin excretion during exercise in juvenile diabetes. A provocative test for early abnormalities. Scand J Clin Lab Invest 1975;35:295–300.
15. Jefferson IG, Greene SA, Smith MA, Smith RF, Griffin NKG, Baum JD. Urine albumin to creatinine ratio-response to exercise in diabetes. Arch Dis Childhood 1985;60:305–310.
16. Poortmans JR, Dorchy H, Toussaint D. Urinary excretion of total protein, albumin and β_2-microglobulin during rest and exercise in diabetic adolescents with and without retinopathy. Diabetes Care 1982;5:617–623.
17. Johansson B-L, Berg U, Bohlin A-B, Lefvert A-K, Freyschuss U. Exercise-induced changes in renal function and their relation to plasma noradrenaline in insulin-dependent diabetic children and adolescents. Clin Sci 1987;72:611–620.
18. Bertoluci MC, Friedman G, Schaan BD, Ribeiro JP, Schmid H. Intensity-related exercise albuminuria in insulin dependent diabetic patients. Diabetes Res Clin Pract 1993;19:217–225.
19. Groop L, Stenman S, Groop PH, Mäkipernaa A, Teppo AM. The effect of exercise on urinary excretion of different size proteins in patients with insulin-dependent diabetes mellitus. Scand J Clin Lab Invest 1990;50:525–532.
20. Ala-Houhala I. Effects of exercise on glomerular passage of macromolecules in patients with diabetic nephropathy and in healthy subjects. Scand J Clin Lab Invest 1990;50:27–33.
21. Hoogenberg K, Dullaart RPF. Abnormal plasma noradrenaline response and exercise induced albuminuria in type 1 (insulin-dependent) diabetes mellitus. Scand J Clin Lab Invest 1992;52:803–811.
22. Niset G, Poortmans JR, Leclercq R. Metabolic implications during a 20-km run after heart transplantation. Int J Sports Med 1985;6:340–343.
23. Haywood GA, Counihan PJ, Sneddon JF, Jennison SH, Bashir Y, McKenna WJ. Increased renal and forearm vasoconstriction in response to exercise after heart transplantation. Br Heart J 1993;70:247–251.
24. Poortmans JR, Hermans L, Vandervliet A, Niset G, Godefroid C. Renal responses to exercise in heart and kidney transplant patients. Transpl Int 1997;10:323–327.
25. McLachlan M. Anatomic, structural and vascular changes in the aging kidney. In: Macias Nunez JF, Cameron JS, eds. Renal Function and Disease in the Elderly. London: Butterworth; 1987:3–26.
26. Blachley JD, Knochel JP. The biochemistry of uremia. In: Brenner BM, Stein JH, eds. Contemporary Issues in Nephrology: Chronic Renal Failure. New York: Churchill Livingstone; 1981:28–45.
27. Wayand D, Baum H, Schätzle G, Schaärf J, Neumeier D. Cardiac troponin T and I in end-stage renal failure. Clin Chem 2000;46:1345–1350.
28. Clyne N, Jogestrand T, Lins L-E, Pehrsson SK, Ekelund L-G. Factors limiting working capacity in predialytic uremic patients. Acta Med Scand 1987;222:183–190.
29. Clyne N, Jogenstrand T, Lins LE, Pehrsson SK. Progressive decline in renal function induces a gradual decrease in total hemoglobin and exercise capacity. Nephron 1994;67:322–326.
30. Mayer G, Thum J, Graf H. Anaemia and reduced exercise capacity in patients on chronic haemodialysis. Clin Sci 1989;1989:265–268.
31. Zabetakis PM, Gleim GW, Pasternack FL, Saraniti A, Nicholas JA, Michelis MF. Long-duration submaximal exercise conditioning in hemodialysis patients. Clin Nephrol 1982;18:17–22.
32. Barnea N, Drory Y, Iaina C, et al. Exercise tolerance in patients on chronic hemodialysis. Isr J Med Sci 1980;16:17–21.
33. Lundin AP, Stein RA, Frank F, et al. Cardiovascular status in long-term hemodialysis patients: an exercise and echocardiography study. Nephron 1981;28:234–238.
34. Metra M, Cannella G, La Canna G, et al. Improvement in exercise capacity after correction of anemia in patients with end-stage renal disease. Am J Cardiol 1991;68:1060–1066.
35. Painter P, Messer-Rehak, Hansen P, Zimmerman SW, Glass NR. Exercise capacity in hemodialysis, CAPD and renal transplant patients. Nephron 1986;42:47–51.
36. Clyne N, Jogestrand T. Effect of erythropoietin treatment on physical exercise capacity and on renal function in predialytic uremic patients. Nephron 1992;60:390–396.
37. Fahal IH, Bell GM, Edwards RHT. Physiological abnormalities of skeletal muscle in dialysis patients. Nephrol Dial Transplant 1997;12:119–127.
38. Davenport A. The effect of treatment with recombinant human erythropoietin on skeletal muscle function in patients with end-stage renal failure treated with regular hospital hemodialysis. Am J Kidney Dis 1993;22:685–690.

39. Robertson HT, Haley NR, Guthrie M, Cardenas D, Eschbach JW, Adamson JW. Recombinant erythropoietin improves exercise capacity in anemic hemodialysis patients. Am J Kidney Dis 1990;15:325–332.

40. Diesel W, Noakes TD, Swanepoel C, Lambert M. Isokinetic muscle strength predicts maximum exercise tolerance in renal patients on chronic hemodialysis. Am J Kidney Dis 1990;16:109–114.

41. Winearls CG, Oliver DO, Pippard MJ, Reid C, Downing MR, Cotes PM. Effects of human erythropoietin derived from recombinant DNA on the anaemia of patients maintained by chronic haemolysis. Lancet 1986;II:1175–1178.

42. Eschbach JW, Egrie JC, Downing MR, Browne JK, Adamson JW. Correction of the anemia of end-stage renal disease with recombinant human erythropoietin. N Engl J Med 1987;316:73–78.

43. Montini G, Zacchello G, Baraldi E, et al. Benefits and risks of anemia correction with recombinant human erythropoietin in children maintained by hemodialysis. J Pediatr 1990;117:556–560.

44. Jacquot C, Berthelot JM, Chiappini-Judith D, et al. Correction de l'anémie des hémodialysés chroniques par l'érythropoïétine recombinante humaine: résultats à long terme sur quinze malades. Néphrologie 1990;11:11–16.

45. Mayer G, Thum J, Cada EM, Stummvoll HK, Graf H. Working capacity is increased following recombinant human erythropoietin treatment. Kidney Int 1988;34:525–528.

46. Frenken LAM, Verberckmoes R, Michielsen P, Koene RAP. Efficacy and tolerance of treatment with recombinant-human erythropoietin in chronic renal failure (predialysis) patients. Nephrol Dial Transplant 1989;4:782–786.

47. Lim VS, DeGowin RL, Zavala D, et al. Recombinant human erythropoietin treatment in pre-dialysis patients. Ann Intern Med 1989;110:108–114.

48. Davenport A, Will EJ, Khanna SK, Davison AM. Blood lactate is reduced following successful treatment of anaemia in hemodialysis patients with recombinant human erythropoietin both at rest and after maximal exertion. Am J Nephrol 1992;12:357–362.

49. Horina JH, Schwaberger G, Brussee H, Sauseng-Fellegger G, Holzer H, Krejs GJ. Increased red cell 2,3-diphosphoglycerate levels in haemodialysis patients treated with erythropoietin. Nephrol Dial Transplant 1993;8:1219–1222.

50. Juric M, Rupcic V, Topuzovic N, et al. Haemodynamic changes and exercise tolerance in dialysis patients treated with erythropoietin. Nephrol Dial Transplant 1995;10:1398–1404.

51. Grunze M, Kohlmann M, Mulligan M, Grüner I, Koeppel M, Bommer J. Mechanisms of improved physical performance of chronic hemodialysis patients after erythropoietin treatment. Am J Nephrol 1990;10(suppl 2):15–23.

52. Lewis NP, Macdougall IC, Willis N, Coles GA, Williams JD, Henderson AH. Effects of the correction of renal anaemia by erythropoietin on physiological changes during exercise. Eur J Clin Invest 1993;23:423–427.

53. Macdougall IC, Cochlin DL, Fox KAA. Long-term cardiorespiratory effects of amelioration of renal anaemia by erythropoietin. Lancet 1990;335:489–493.

54. McMahon LP, Johns JA, McKenzie A, Austin M, Fowler R, Dawborn JK. Haemodynamic changes and physical performance at comparative levels of haemoglobin after treatment with recombinant erythropoietin. Nephrol Dial Transplant 1992;7:1199–1206.

55. Wizemann V, Kaufmann J, Kramer W. Effect of erythropoietin on ischemia tolerance in anemic hemodialysis patients with confirmed coronary artery disease. Nephron 1992;62:161–165.

56. Braumann KM, Nonnast-Daniel B, Böning D, Böcker A, Frei U. Improved physical performance after renal anemia with recombinant human erythropoietin. Nephron 1991;58:129–134.

57. Laupacis A. Association between recombinant human erythropoietin and quality of life and exercise capacity of patients receiving haemodyalisis. BMJ 1990;300:573–578.

58. Painter P. The importance of exercise training in rehabilitation of patients with end-stage renal disease. Am J Kidney Dis 1994;24(suppl 1):S2–S9.

59. Painter PL, Moore GEM. The impact of rHu erythropoietin on exercise capacity in hemodialysis patients. Adv Ren Replace Ther 1994;1:55–65.

60. Clyne N, Jogestrand T, Lins LE, Pehrsson SK. Factors influencing physical working capacity in renal transplant. Scand J Urol Nephrol 1989;23:145–150.

61. Painter P, Hanson P, Messer-Rehak D, Zimmerman SW, Glass NR. Exercise tolerance changes following renal transplantation. Am J Kidney Dis 1987;10:452–456.

62. Kempeneers G, Noakes TD, van Zyl-Smit R, et al. Skeletal muscle limits the exercise tolerance of renal transplant recipients: effects of an exercise training program. Am J Kidney Dis 1990;16:57–65.

63. Nyberg G, Hallste G, Norden G, Hadimeri H, Wrammer L. Physical performance does not improve in elderly patients following successful kidney transplantation. Nephrol Dial Transplant 1995;10:86–90.

64. Parrish AE, Ostapenko E. The effect of minimal exercise on blood lactate in azotemic subjects. Clin Nephrol 1981;16:35–39.

65. Kettner A, Goldberg A, Hagberg J, Delmez J, Harter H. Cardiovascular and metabolic responses to submaximal exercise in hemodialysis patients. Kidney Int 1984;26:66–71.

66. Latos DL, Strimel D, Drews MH, Allison TG. Acid-base and electrolyte changes following maximal and submaximal exercise in hemodialysis patients. Am J Kidney Dis 1987;10:439–445.

67. Lundin AP, Stein RA, Brown CD, et al. Fatigue, acid-base and electrolyte changes with exhaustive treadmill exercise in hemodialysis patients. Nephron 1987;46:57–62.

68. Lewis NP, Macdougall IC, Coles GA, Williams JD, Fox KAA. Increased exercise capacity and reversal of exercise induced myocardial ischaemia in haemodialysis patients treated with recombinant human erythropoietin. Br Heart J 1989;61:436.

69. Meierhenrich R, Jedicke H, Voigt A, Lange H. The effect of erythropoietin on lactate, pyruvate and excess lactate under physical exercise in dialysis patients. Clin Nephrol 1996;45:90–96.

70. Marrades RM, Alonso J, Roca J, et al. Cellular bioenergetics after erythropoietin therapy in chronic renal failure. J Clin Invest 1996;97:2101–2110.

71. Bradley JR, Anderson JR, Evans DB, Cowley AJ. Impaired nutritive skeletal muscle blood flow in patients with chronic renal failure. Clin Sci 1990;79:239–245.

72. Marrades RM, Roca J, Campistol JM, et al. Effects of erythropoietin on muscle O_2 transport during exercise in patients with chronic renal failure. J Clin Invest 1996;97:2092–2100.

73. Brautbar N. Skeletal myopathy in uremia: abnormal energy metabolism. Kidney Int 1983;24(suppl 16):S81–S86.

74. Floyd M, Ayyar DR, Barwick DD, Hudgson P, Weightman D. Myopathy in chronic renal failure. Q J Med 1974;172:509–524.

75. Moore GE, Parsons DB, Stray-Gundersen J, Painter P, Brinker KR, Mitchell JH. Uremic myopathy limits aerobic capacity in hemodialysis patients. Am J Kidney Dis 1993;22:277–287.

76. Clyne N, Esbjörnsson M, Jansson E, Jogestrand T, Lins L-E, Pehrsson SK. Effects of renal failure on skeletal muscle. Nephron 1993;63:395–399.

77. Diesel W, Emms M, Knight BK, et al. Morphologic features of the myopathy associated with chronic renal failure. Am J Kidney Dis 1993;22:677–684.

78. Nakao T, Fujiwara S, Isoda K, Miyahara T. Impaired lactate production by skeletal muscle with anaerobic exercise in patients with chronic renal failure. Nephron 1982;31:111–115.

79. Bergström J, Hultman E. Glycogen content of skeletal muscle in patients with renal failure. Acta Med Scand 1969;186:177–181.

80. Cleminson WG, Manchester KL, Diesel WJ, Margolius LP. Adenosine nucleotide concentrations and energy charge in muscle of chronic haemodialysis patients. Nephron 1992;60:232–234.

81. Barany P, Wibom R, Hultman E, Bergström J. ATP production in isolated muscle mitochondria from haemodialysis patients: effects of

correction of anaemia with erythropoietin. Clin Sci 1991;81:645–653.

82. Moore GE, Bertocci LA, Painter PL. ^{31}P-magnetic resonance spectroscopy assessment of subnormal oxidative metabolism in skeletal muscle of renal failure patients. J Clin Invest 1993;91:420–424.

83. Park JS, Kim SB, Park SK, Lim TH, Lee DK, Hong CD. Effect of recombinant human erythropoietin on muscle energy metabolism in patients with end-stage renal disease: a ^{31}P-nuclear magnetic resonance spectroscopy study. Am J Kidney Dis 1993;21:612–618.

84. Durozard D, Pimmel P, Baretto S, et al. ^{31}P NMR spectroscopy investigation of muscle metabolism in hemodialysis patients. Kidney Int 1993;43:885–892.

85. Fröhlich J, Schollmeyer P, Gerok W. Carbohydrate metabolism in renal failure. Am J Clin Nutr 1978;31:1541–1546.

86. Ricanati ES, Tserng K-Y, Hoppel CL. Abnormal fatty acid utilization during prolonged fasting in chronic uremia. Kidney Int 1987;32 (suppl. 22):S145–S148.

87. Hiatt WR, Koziol BJ, Shapiro JI, Brass EP. Carnitine metabolism during exercise in patients on chronic hemodialysis. Kidney Int 1992;41:1613–1619.

88. Fagher B, Cederblad G, Erikkson M, et al. L-carnitine and haemodialysis: double blind study on muscle function and metabolism and peripheral nerve function. Scand J Clin Lab Invest 1985;45:169–178.

89. Lennon DLF, Shrago E, Madden M, Nagle F, Hansen P, Zimmerman S. Carnitine status, plasma profiles, and exercise capacity in dialysis patients: effects of a submaximal exercise program. Metabolism 1986;35:728–735.

90. Savica V, Bellinghieri G, Di Stefano C, et al. Plasma and muscle carnitine levels in haemodialysis patients with morphological-ultrastructural examination of muscle cramps. Nephron 1983;35: 232–236.

91. Bellinghieri G, Savica V, Mallamace A, et al. Correlation between increased serum and tissue L-carnitine levels and improved muscle symptoms in hemodialyzed patients. Am J Clin Nutr 1983;38:523–531.

92. Nilsson-Ehle P, Cederblad G, Fagher B, Monti M, Thysell H. Plasma lipoproteins, liver function and glucose metabolism in haemodialysis patients: lack of effect of L-carnitine supplementation. Scand J Clin Lab Invest 1985;45:179–184.

93. Brass EP, Hiatt WR. Carnitine metabolism during exercise. Life Sci 1994;54:1383–1393.

94. Ahmad S, Robertson HT, Golper TA, et al. Multicenter trial of L-carnitine in maintenance hemodialysis patients. II. Clinical and biochemical effects. Kidney Int 1990;38:912–918.

95. Holliday MA, Chantler C. Metabolic and nutritional factors in children with renal insufficiency. Kidney Int 1978;14:306–312.

96. Bergström J, Alvestrand A, Fürst P. Plasma and muscle free amino acids in maintenance hemodialysis patients without protein malnutrition. Kidney Int 1990;38:108–114.

97. Garber AJ. Skeletal muscle protein and amino acid metabolism in experimental chronic uremia in the rat. J Clin Invest 1978;62(3): 623–632.

98. Garber AJ. The regulation of skeletal muscle alanine and glutamine formation and release in experimental chronic uremia in the rat. J Clin Invest 1978;62(3):633–641.

99. Odetti P, Garibaldi S, Gurreri G, et al. Protein oxidation in hemodialysis and kidney transplantation. Metabolism 1996;45: 1319–1322.

100. Van der Niepen P, Allein S, Verbeelen D. Muscle metabolism in uremia and the effect of amino acid supplementation. Nephron 1998;79:387–398.

101. Mitch WE, Jurkovitz C, England BK. Mechanisms that cause protein and amino acid catabolism in uremia. Am J Kidney Dis 1993;21:91–95.

102. Mochizuki T. The effect of metabolic acidosis on amino and keto acid metabolism in chronic renal failure. Jpn J Nephrol 1991;33:213–224.

103. Ikizler TA, Wingard RL, Flakoll PJ, Schulman G, Parker RA, Hakim RM. Effects of recombinant human growth hormone on plasma and dialysate amino acid profiles in continuous ambulatory peritoneal dialysis patients. Kidney Int 1996;50:229–234.

104. Painter PL, Nelson-Worel JN, Hill MM, et al. Effects of exercise training during hemodialysis. Nephron 1986;43:87–92.

105. Germain MJ, Burke EJ, Braden GL, Fitzgibbons JP. Amelioration of hemodialysis-induced fall in PaO$_2$ with exercise. Am J Nephrol 1985;5:351–354.

106. Burke EJ, Germain MJ, Braden GL, Fitzgibbons JP. Mild steady-state exercise during hemodialysis treatment. Phys Sports Med 1984;12:153–157.

107. Moore GE, Brinker KR, Stray-Gundersen J, Mitchell JH. Determinants of $\dot{V}O_2$ peak in patients with end-stage renal disease: on and off dialysis. Med Sci Sports Exerc 1992;25:18–23.

108. Moore GE, Painter PL, Brinker KR, Stray-Gundersen J, Mitchell JH. Cardiovascular response to submaximal stationary cycling during hemodialysis. Am J Kidney Dis 1998;31:631–637.

109. Braun WE. Long-term complications of renal transplantation. Kidney Int 1990;37:1363–1378.

110. Evans RW, Manninen DL, Garrison LP Jr, et al. The quality of life of patients with end-stage renal disease. N Engl J Med 1985;312: 553–559.

111. Kuzuhara K, Dobashi Y, Aikawa M, et al. Evaluation of cardiac function of renal transplants using stress and rest cardiac pool gated scintigraphy and myocardial scintigraphy with [99]mTc-MIBI. Transplant Proc 1996;28:1618–1620.

112. Goffin E, Vande Berg B, Pirson Y, Malghem J, Maldague B, van Ypersele de Strihou C. Epiphyseal impaction as a cause of severe osteoarticular pain of lower limbs after renal transplantation. Kidney Int 1993;44:98–106.

113. Kosch M, Hausberg M, Link T, et al. Measurement of skeletal status after renal transplantation by quantitative ultrasound. Clin Nephrol 2000;54:15–21.

114. Green GA, Moore GEM. Exercise and organ transplantation. J Back Musculoskelet Rehabil 1998;10:3–11.

115. Painter PL, Luetkemeier MJ, Moore GEM, et al. Health related fitness and quality of life in organ transplant recipients. Transplantation 1997;64:1795–1800.

116. Bruzzi I, Benigni A, Remuzzi G. Role of increased glomerular protein traffic in the progression of renal failure. Kidney Int 1997;52(suppl 62):S29–S31.

117. Rosenkranz AR, Mayer G. Proteinuria in the transplanted patient. Nephrol Dial Transplant 2000;15:1290–1292.

118. Hemmingsen L, Jensen H, Skaarup P. The urinary excretion of ten plasma proteins in long-term renal transplant patients. Acta Med Scand 1976;199:311–316.

119. Manuel Y, Poli S, Bernhardt JP, Revillard JP, Claudey D, Traeger J. Proteinuria in human renal allografts. Helv Med Acta 1969;35:3–19.

120. Clyne N. Effects of renal failure on the heart and on exercise performance. In: Dept Medicine. Stockholm, Sweden: Karolinska Hospital; 1991:45.

121. Kjaer M, Beyer N, Secher NH. Exercise and organ transplantation. Scand J Med Sci Sports 1999;9:1–14.

122. Di Bona GF. Renal innervation and denervation: lessons from renal transplantation reconsidered. Artif Organs 1987;11:457–462.

123. Gadzar AF, Dammin GF. Neural degeneration and regeneration in human renal transplants. N Engl J Med 1970;283:222–224.

124. Sadler JH. Renal rehabilitation and health care reform: strategies for a changing era [guest editor's introduction]. Am J Kidney Dis 1994;24(suppl 1):S21.

125. Levin NW. Quality of life and hematocrit level. Am J Kidney Dis 1992;20(suppl 1):16–20.

126. Lundin AP. Quality of life: subjective and objective improvements with recombinant human erythropoietin therapy. Semin Nephrol 1994;9(suppl 1):22–29.

127. Boyce ML, Robergs RA, Avasthi PS, et al. Exercise training by in-

dividuals with predialysis renal failure: cardiorespiratory endurance, hypertension, and renal function. Am J Kidney Dis 1997;30:180–192.

128. Heifets M, Davis TA, Tegtmeyer E. Exercise training ameliorates progressive renal disease in rats with subtotal nephrectomy. Kidney Int 1987;32:815–820.

129. Averbukh Z, Marcus E, Berman S, et al. Effect of exercise training on glomerular filtration rate of mice with various degrees of renal mass reduction. Am J Nephrol 1992;12:174–178.

130. Osato S, Onoyama K, Okuda S, Sanai T, Hori K, Fujishima M. Effect of swimming exercise on the progress of renal dysfunction in rats with focal glomerulosclerosis. Nephron 1990;55:306–311.

131. Cornacoff JB, Hebert LA, Sharma HM, Bay WH, Young DC. Adverse effect of exercise on immune complex-mediated glomerulonephritis. Nephron 1985;40:292–296.

132. Poortmans JR, Waterlot B, Dorchy H. Training effect on postexercise microproteinuria in type I diabetic adolescents. Pediatr Adolesc Endocrinol 1988;17:166–172.

133. Hagberg JM, Goldberg AP, Ehsani AA, Heath GW, Delmez JA, Harter HR. Exercise training improves hypertension in hemodialysis patients. Am J Nephrol 1983;3:209–212.

134. Clyne N, Ekblom J, Jogenstrand T, Lins L-E, Pehrsson SK. Effects of exercise training in predialytic uremic patients. Nephron 1991;59:84–89.

135. Fitts SS, Guthrie MR, Blagg CR. Exercise coaching and rehabilitation counseling improve quality of life for predialysis and dialysis patients. Nephron 1999;82:115–121.

136. Kouidi E, Albani M, Natsis K, et al. The effects of exercise training on muscle atrophy in haemodialysis patients. Nephrol Dial Transplant 1998;13:685–699.

137. Davis TA, Karl IE, Tegtmeyer ED, Osborne DF, Klahr S, Harter HR. Muscle protein turnover: effects of exercise training and renal insufficiency. Am J Physiol 1985;248:E337–E345.

138. Goldberg AP, Geltman EM, Hagberg JM, et al. Therapeutic benefits of exercise training for hemodialysis patients. Kidney Int 1983;24(suppl 16):S303–S309.

139. Goldberg AP. A potential role for exercise training in modulating risk factors in uremia. Am J Nephrol 1984;4:132–133.

140. Ross DL, Grabeau GM, Smith S, Seymour M, Knierim N, Pitetti KH. Efficacy of exercise for end-stage renal disease patients immediately following high-efficiency hemodialysis: a pilot study. Am J Nephrol 1989;9:376–383.

141. Miller TD, Squires RW, Gerald TG, Ilstrup DM, Frohnert PP, Sterioff S. Graded exercise testing and training after renal transplantation: a preliminary study. Mayo Clin Proc 1987;62:773–777.

142. Goldberg AP, Geltman EM, Gavin IJR, et al. Exercise training reduces coronary risk and effectively rehabilitates hemodialysis patients. Nephron 1986;42:311–316.

143. Sams B, Thompson J, Stray-Gundersen J. Three months of cycling while on hemodialysis improves work capacity by improving peripheral extraction in chronic renal failure patients. Med Sci Sports Exerc 1996;28:S55.

144. Painter P. Exercise training during hemodialysis: rates of participation. Dial Transplant 1988;17:165–168.

145. Bergamaschi CT, Boim MA, Moura LA, Piçarro IC, Schor N. Effects of long-term training on the progression of chronic renal failure in rats. Med Sci Sports Exerc 1997;29:169–174.

146. Johansen KL, Chertow GM, Ng AV, et al. Physical activity levels in patients on hemodialysis and healthy sedentary controls. Kidney Int 2000;57:2564–2570.

147. Painter P, Carlson L, Carey S, Paul SM, Myll J. Physical functioning and health-related quality-of-life changes with exercise training in hemodialysis patients. Am J Kidney Dis 2000;35:482–492.

148. Painter P, Carlson L, Carey S, Paul SM, Myll J. Low-functioning hemodialysis patients improve with exercise training. Am J Kidney Dis 2000;36:600–608.

149. Blagg CR. The socioeconomic impact of rehabilitation. Am J Kidney Dis 1994;24(suppl 1):S17–S21.

150. Stugart P, Weiss J. Exercise, rehabilitation, and the dialysis patient: one unit's positive experiences. Dial Transplant 1999;28:134–157.

151. Oberley ET, Sadler JH, Alt PS. Renal rehabilitation: obstacles, progress, and prospects for the future. Am J Kidney Dis 2000;35(suppl 1):S141–S147.

152. Tawney KW, Tawney PJW, Hladik G, et al. The life readiness program: a physical rehabilitation program for patients on hemodialysis. Am J Kidney Dis 2000;36:581–591.

153. Pedersen EB, Danielsen H, Nielsen AH, et al. Effect of exercise on plasma concentrations of arginine vasopressin, angiotensin II and aldosterone in hypertensive and normotensive renal transplant recipients. Scand J Clin Lab Invest 1986;46:151–157.

154. Poortmans JR, Niset G, Godefroid C, Lamotte M. Responses to exercise and limiting factors in hemodialysis and renal transplant patients. In: Rieu M, ed. Physical Work Capacity in Organ Transplantation. Basel: Karger; 1998:113–133.

CHAPTER 23

Menstrual Dysfunction

Ifigenia Giannopoulou, Jill Kanaley

Overview

The acceptance of women's sports into the Olympic Games of 1912 resulted in a dramatic increase in women's participation in athletics (1). Currently millions of women worldwide participate in sports, either recreationally or competitively. In the United States, female sports participation has escalated since 1982 with the inception of Title IX. This ruling allowed more women to participate in sports, and increased the level of competition. Through sports participation, women have achieved not only health benefits, but also psychological and social benefits. However, paralleling the increased participation of women in sports are over-training effects, which have adverse ramifications for the reproductive system. More specifically, higher incidences of reproductive health problems (e.g., **amenorrhea, anovulation, delayed menarche, shortened luteal phase**) have been reported in women involved in intense exercise training (2–4). Among the general female population, 1% to 5% report some reproductive dysfunction, while in elite level female athletes the reported incidence of reproductive dysfunction is as high as 40% to 50% (5–8) (Box 23.1).

The most common forms of reproductive dysfunction are delayed menarche, luteal phase deficiency, anovulation, oligomenorrhea, and amenorrhea (9). Since the recognition of these reproductive problems in female athletes in the 1970s, several different physiological mechanisms have been proposed; many of these theories have been rejected, and many are still being considered (4, 10–15). The underlying mechanism of these reproductive problems has been proposed to be a disturbance on the **hypothalamic-pituitary-ovarian axis** and/or the **hypothalamic-pituitary-adrenal axis**. Further, it is not known whether this reproductive dysfunction is a negative effect of intense exercise training, or whether it is an adaptive effect of the female body to intense exercise stress in order to achieve and sustain high performances.

The primary concern in trained athletes is the potential health consequences of **menstrual dysfunction**. The earliest effect observed is menstrual dysfunction and anovulation (6), often associated with disordered eating. However,

if these conditions persist, reductions in bone mineral density (BMD), or osteopenia, have been observed. In the long term, reproductive dysfunction can also lead to **osteoporosis** (16, 17). This cluster of health problems—eating disorders, amenorrhea, and osteoporosis—is referred to as the **female triad**. Research is currently trying to identify the specific mechanism of this disorder in an attempt to provide adequate treatment for these women to prevent long-term ramifications.

This chapter defines athletic menstrual dysfunction, presents the possible mechanisms of reproductive dysfunction, and discusses the health consequences and treatments available.

Characterization of Menstrual Dysfunction

The reproductive system involves the integrated and coordinated activity of the hypothalamic-pituitary-ovarian axis. The secretion rate and hence the plasma concentrations of estrogens (E_2), **progesterone** (P), and gonadotropins vary considerably according to menstrual phase. Prior to discussing menstrual disturbances, an understanding of normal **menstrual cycle** functioning is essential. Normal follicular development is dependent upon both **follicle-stimulating hormone** (FSH) and **luteinizing hormone** (LH) release from the anterior pituitary gland (Figure 23.1). Re-

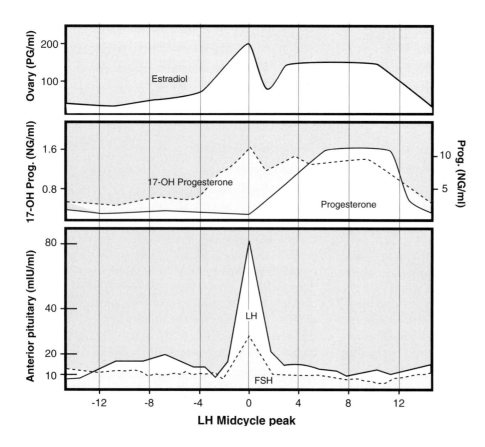

FIGURE 23.1. Changes in the circulatory hormone levels during the menstrual cycle (based on a 28-day cycle). From Turner CD, Bagnara JT. General Endocrinology, 6th ed. Philadelphia: WB Saunders, 1976.

lease of FSH and LH is under the control of gonadotropin-releasing hormone (GnRH) originating in the hypothalamus. FSH and LH stimulate the development of a single follicle, which synthesizes large amounts of estrogens, particularly **17β-estradiol**, thus increasing E_2 levels. The low levels of E_2 in the early follicular phase inhibit LH release; however, late in the follicular phase high concentrations of E_2 induce a surge of LH, which leads to ovulation (18). During the luteal phase, high levels of P and E_2 are secreted by the corpus luteum, suppressing gonadotropin production. After approximately 12 days, E_2 and P levels begin to decrease, stimulating menses and gonadotropin release. Normal menstrual functioning is dependent upon negative feedback of the menstrual cycle.

Definitions of amenorrhea that have been used in the literature are the absence of menstruation for 3, 4, or 6 months per year; less than 3 menstrual periods per year; or no more than 1 menstrual period in the last 10 months (6, 19). Currently, the International Olympic Committee defines athletic amenorrhea as "1 menstrual period or less per year," to reduce the degree of inconsistency between research studies and their outcomes (8, 20). However, theirs is the most stringent definition; most researchers use the absence of 3 to 6 consecutive menstrual cycles (21), since missing this many menstrual cycles may result in health complications (Box 23.2).

Athletic amenorrhea is usually classified as a secondary amenorrhea. Primary amenorrhea refers to the condition where menarche has not occurred by age 16, or the absence of sexual development by age 14. Primary amenorrhea is frequently associated with an underlying defect in the reproductive system or may be due to anorexia nervosa. Secondary amenorrhea occurs in females who previously had menstrual cycles with some regularity, but now have an absence of at least 3 to 6 consecutive cycles (20, 21). Athletic amenorrhea refers only to those women who have secondary amenorrhea and whose onset of amenorrhea is associated with intense athletic training. If an athlete initiates a high level of training at a young age (e.g., gymnasts, figure skaters), this can potentially result in primary amenorrhea. It should be noted that many factors can cause secondary amenorrhea without any athletic training (Table 23.1). The athlete's background, health history, nutritional status, and exercise regimen must be considered carefully to appropriately identify the reproductive dysfunction.

TABLE 23.1. SOME OF THE POSSIBLE CAUSES OF AMENORRHEA

Hypothalamic Defect

Absence of GnRH
Constitutional delay
Psychological or physical stress
Anorexia nervosa
Hyperprolactinemia

Pituitary Defect

Inability to make gonadotropins
Tumors (prolactinomas)
Granulomatous disease

Ovarian Defect

Turner's syndrome
Polycystic ovary syndrome
Autoimmune disease
Idiopathic premature ovarian failure

Uterine Defect

Granulomatous disease

The most common type of athletic amenorrhea is chronic anovulation (19). The rhythm of the reproductive system is disrupted so that ovulation does not occur, but the ovarian follicles continue to function. The reproductive disruptions are not necessarily manifested only as anovulation. Although a biphasic cycle may be seen, the hormonal pattern may be that of a shortened or inadequate luteal phase. Most variation seen in the menstrual cycle usually occurs in the follicular phase, with the length of the luteal phase remaining relatively constant (12–14 days). Bonen and associates (22) showed a shortened luteal phase in teenage swimmers. Bonen and Keizer (23) also reported that in marathon runners 33% of the menstrual cycles appeared normal, but a shortened luteal phase of only 6 days was found. Shangold and colleagues (24) have reported a negative relationship between mileage run during the follicular phase and length of luteal phase. Therefore, excessive training may cause an obvious disruption of the cycle such as anovulation, or may cause changes from the normal rhythm (e.g., shortened luteal phase (luteal phase less than 14 days) or **oligomenorrhea** (less than 10 menstrual cycles/year), which remains hidden to the individual until a hormonal profile is made.

Methodological Problems of Research on Exercise-Induced Menstrual Dysfunction

Research conducted on women has increased dramatically in the last 25 years, coinciding with the increased participation in sports. Despite these research efforts, the exact

---

BOX 23.2. Menstrual Dysfunction

- Amenorrhea: 1 menstrual cycle/year or less
- Reproductive endocrine function similar to women over 50
- Irregular menstrual patterns: luteal insufficiency, shortened luteal phase
- Anovulation

physiological mechanisms of athletic amenorrhea and the factors that cause it still have not been elucidated. One of the major reasons for this lack of knowledge is the methodological difference in the research studies. Listed below are some of the factors that confound the research on menstrual dysfunction.

1. *Multiple definitions of athletic amenorrhea.*

   As mentioned earlier, multiple definitions of athletic amenorrhea have been used to classify female athletes as amenorrheic. This has led to a wide variation in the reported percentages of the incidence of athletic amenorrhea for both the female recreational and athletic populations. Most researchers define athletic amenorrhea as 3 to 6 menstrual periods missed consecutively (21).

2. *Determination of ovulation.*

   Establishing whether ovulation has occurred is critical to the determination of the specific reproductive dysfunction and its severity. It is necessary to establish whether the cycle is anovulatory or not. The most accurate method of establishing ovulation is ultrasound. Ultrasound is valid and reliable, and can establish if there is follicular development. Because ultrasound requires special equipment and is associated with a high cost, this method has not been used widely in research studies. Further, the measurement of hormone concentrations, in particular E_2, P, LH, or FSH, provides strong evidence of ovulation. Ideally a blood sample should be obtained daily for hormone analysis, but the cost of the hormone assay prohibits this in many research studies. Obtaining only one hormone concentration on a given day can be somewhat misleading because the range of normal hormonal values is quite large, making it difficult to precisely establish menstrual phase. For convenience, many research groups try to establish ovulation by measuring early morning **basal body temperature** (BBT). With ovulation there should be a slight increase in BBT (increases of 0.3° or 0.5°F), but this increase can be very subtle and difficult to detect. For this reason measurement of BBT, although inexpensive and convenient, may be prone to error.

   Another method that has been used is the urine assay for urinary estrogen and progesterone metabolites. This method can detect whether the menstrual cycle is ovulatory or anovulatory (25). This method is advantageous because it provides minimal disturbance to the training schedule and is noninvasive, requiring urine collection on day 1 of the menstrual cycle and then every second day.

3. *Confounding variables that influence reproductive function.*

   The most well studied variables recognized to impact menstrual function are as follows:
   • Low percent body fat

• Anorexia nervosa/eating disorders
• Diet and energy availability
• Exercise intensity

These specific variables will be discussed in detail later in the chapter.

Exercise Training and Menstrual Dysfunction

Since the early 1930s, numerous researchers have observed the absence of menstrual cycles in highly exercise trained females (6, 26). Initially, amenorrhea was associated only with endurance-trained female athletes, such as long-distance runners (2–4, 27), or athletes in sports where having a very low body fat is advantageous (e.g., ballet dancers, gymnasts) (28, 29). Many amenorrheic athletes have presented with bulimia, anorexia, or disordered eating patterns. Currently, a wider variety of athletes appear to suffer from reproductive dysfunction. Studies have shown that martial arts athletes, swimmers, weight lifters, track and field athletes, volleyball, basketball and handball players, javelin athletes, and tennis players demonstrate some incidence of irregular menstrual cycles (6). Moreover, these reproductive dysfunctions are not only found in competitive athletes, but also in recreational athletes (Box 23.3).

Exercise Training and Delayed Menarche

Numerous reports indicate that a high percentage of young female athletes initiating intense exercise training before puberty may have a delayed onset of menstruation (28, 30–32). Delayed **menarche** has been primarily observed in young female athletes such as gymnasts, ballet dancers, and runners. In these sports a small body size (ideally, low body fat and high muscle mass) is believed to provide an advantage for performance. The "normal" age of menarche is approximately 12.2 years, and studies on athletes have reported a mean age of menarche of 13.6 years in track athletes, 14.2 years in volleyball players, and 14 years in ballet dancers (33). In many of these sports young athletes

---

BOX 23.3. Eating Disorders

Of 42 college gymnasts studied:
• 62% reported disordered eating
• 26% reported vomiting
• 24% reported diet pill use
• 24% fasted
• 12% used diuretics
• 7% used laxatives

are encouraged to severely restrict their eating, while at the same time train at extremely high intensity levels and for prolonged periods of time daily. As a result, delayed menarche is a very common occurrence.

There are many research studies on the adverse effects of intense exercise on the onset of menarche (30, 32), but the validity of the results and conclusions of these studies have received severe criticism. Due to the cross-sectional nature of these studies, some researchers argue that it is very difficult to differentiate the independent effects of exercise from other confounding effects such as diet, genetics, percent body fat, and biological age (34). Moreover, it has been proposed that females who are genetically predisposed to have a delayed menarche may be more likely to participate in specific sports where a competitive advantage is gained from the delayed pubertal development (5). Although delayed menarche is associated with exercise training, evidence is lacking to support the claim that there is a causative relationship between delayed menarche and exercise training.

Exercise Training and Short Luteal Phase and Anovulation

Many studies on recreational and competitive female athletes have also indicated reproductive dysfunction in the form of a shortened luteal phase, anovulation, or oligomenorrhea (2–4, 15, 18, 22, 35). Intense exercise training has been suggested to result in a shortened luteal phase of less than 7 days, accompanied by reduced levels of serum LH, FSH, and E_2 concentrations. It is unclear, however, whether these cycles are anovulatory cycles. Ronkainen and colleagues (36) have shown differences in menstrual disorders dependent upon the volume of training the athlete is participating in, and whether training began before or after menarche (Figure 23.2). Due to the large variation in cycle duration and luteal phase duration, these athletes need to be carefully monitored. Many athletes may be oligomenorrheic, and frequently these cycles are anovulatory and remain undetected (6). This is often the case with women athletes who are not trying to get pregnant or whose altered cycles are not tested to establish if they are ovulatory. Thus, anovulatory cycles may be underreported in athletic women.

Reproductive function has also been studied during high-volume training to establish if vulnerability of luteal function is limited to either the follicular or luteal phase (37). Nine untrained women were studied over 19 menstrual cycles to establish if short-term high-intensity exercise in either the follicular or luteal phase would cause menstrual disruption. The follicular group started exercising in the late luteal phase (just prior to menses) and exercised until ovulation was completed, while the luteal group started exercising just as progesterone levels would begin to rise until menses. Subjects exercised twice daily, 5 days per week at 84% to 96% of maximum heart rate. They exercised 3.2 km/bout during the first week and increased by 1.2

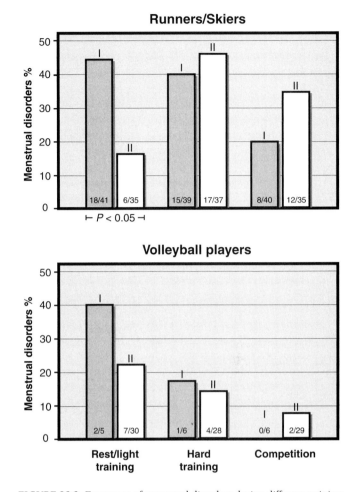

FIGURE 23.2. Frequency of menstrual disorders during different training periods of runners and skiers and volleyball players. Numbers at the bottom of each column indicate the number of women with menstrual disorders in all women evaluated. I = beginning of training before menarche; II = beginning of training after menarche. Adapted from Ronkainen H, Pakarinen A, Kauppila A (36).

km/week. Following 3 months of training the menstrual cycle length was still stable, but in the 5 women who exercised in their follicular phase, 3 of the 9 menstrual cycles examined (33%) had disturbed luteal phases as compared to controls. In the women who exercised in the luteal phase, 50% (or 5 of the 10 cycles examined) had luteal abnormalities. There was no difference between the follicular and luteal phase groups in the proportion of women having luteal problems. Williams and colleagues (37) demonstrated that development of luteal disturbances coincided with the sudden onset of strenuous training. Others have reported similar findings (Figure 23.3, Box 23.4).

Exercise and Menstrual Dysfunction

Numerous research studies have indicated that high levels of exercise-induced amenorrhea occur in a large percentage of female athletes. Compared to sedentary controls, a large

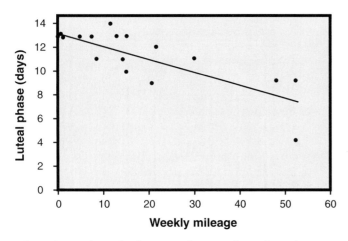

FIGURE 23.3. Relationship between mileage run during first 7 days of the follicular phase and length of luteal phase in 18 cycles. ($y = 13.3 - 01.11x$; $r = -0.81$, $P < 0.001$). Adapted from Shangold M (24)

percentage of female athletes exhibit amenorrhea, with the incidence ranging from 5% to 20% in the general population but from 1% to 50% in the athletic population (6, 28, 38–42). This high variation is attributable to the definition of amenorrhea employed, as well as the athletic population studied (6).

Studies conducted since 1932 on a wide variety of sports indicate that intense exercise training or high volume of training can lead to loss of menstruation or amenorrhea. Soon after the initiation of high-intensity training, female athletes have been found to exhibit signs of reproductive dysfunction (27, 43), which in the long term lead to menstrual irregularities and potentially amenorrhea. These disturbances are related both to the intensity of training as well as the volume of training, but no cause-and-effect relationship has been established (6, 15, 44, 45).

Mechanisms of Athletic Menstrual Dysfunction

Alterations in the hormonal milieu have been associated with menstrual dysfunction. As stated earlier in this chapter, the reproductive system is modulated by the hypothalamic-pituitary-ovarian axis. Normally LH is released in discrete pulses, which are necessary for the ovaries to detect the LH signal. Disruptions in LH release from the pituitary have been observed in amenorrheic women (Figure 23.4) (35). The disruption of both amplitude and frequency of the LH pulse may be the result of an interaction between the hypothalamic-pituitary-ovarian axis and the hypothalamic-pituitary-adrenal axis under chronic stressful conditions (9, 35). In addition to changes in LH pulsatility, low E_2, P, and FSH levels have been reported (35, 46–49). Mechanisms such as hyperprolactinemia, hypercortisolemia, or low serum iron levels have been proposed but have not re-

---

BOX 23.4. Menstrual Function and Strenuous Training

In humans, it is difficult to document changes in menstrual function with training as they occur; therefore, most research is cross-sectional in nature. Recently, Williams and colleagues (62) reported on exercise training-induced amenorrhea in monkeys. They examined individual susceptibility of reproductive function and the progression of changes in reproductive function with training. Sixteen female monkeys were run trained until they were capable of running 12.3 km/day. In response to this strenuous training, body weight did not change, but the time it took to induce amenorrhea varied widely among the animals (7–24 months [mean = 14.3 months]). The changes in reproductive function occurred abruptly, with menstrual dysfunction occurring only 1 to 2 cycles before amenorrhea occurred. Plasma reproductive hormone levels declined significantly; follicular phase length increased; and luteal phase progesterone secretion decreased. There was a high level of interindividual variability in development of reproductive dysfunction, but the transition to exercise-induced amenorrhea was abrupt, occurring within a couple of menstrual cycles. The earliest significant change observed was a decrease in late luteal phase FSH level, which is important in the recruitment of follicle development in each cycle. Time to menstrual dysfunction was not associated with initial body weight, training distance, or food intake.

In another study, Williams and colleagues (111) tested the hypothesis that low energy availability, and not other factors associated with exercise, induced the development of exercise-related reproductive disruptions. They studied the role of low energy availability on the development and reversal of exercise-induced amenorrhea. Using 8 female monkeys in a protocol similar to the one described previously (62), amenorrhea was induced by gradually increasing their daily running to 12.3 km/day over a period of 7 to 24 months. Food intake remained constant during exercise training; however, 4 of the 8 monkeys were given supplemental calories. All 4 monkeys receiving supplemental calories increased reproductive hormone levels and reestablished ovulatory cycles, with recovery time ranging from 12 to 57 days from initiation of supplemental feeding. Rapidity of recovery was directly related to the amount of energy consumed during supplemental feeding. The suppression of reproductive function was primarily due to the energy cost associated with exercise, rather than resulting from other exercise-associated factors (e.g., psychological or physical stress). The reversal and development of amenorrhea were tightly correlated with circulating levels of T_3. Levels of T_3 were significantly decreased in association with the onset of amenorrhea.

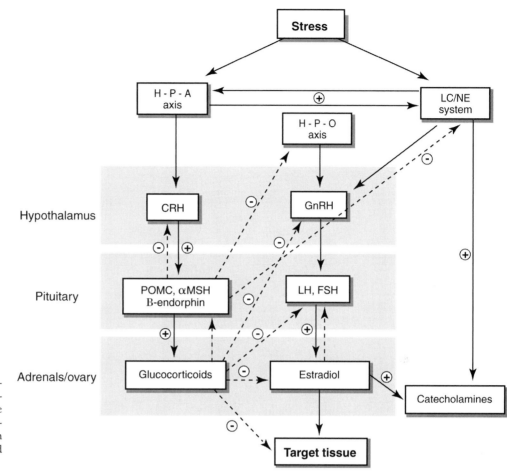

FIGURE 23.4. Interaction of the reproductive system with the hypothalamic-pituitary-adrenal axis and the locus ceruleus-norepinephrine system (LC/NE). Adapted from Chrousos GP, Torpy DJ, Gold PW (9).

ceived strong support. As early as 1932, researchers believed that hormonal variations associated with the menstrual cycle were crucial to physical performance, such that physical efficiency was highest in the intermenstrual phase and lowest during the menstrual phase (26). Exercise-induced changes in hormone levels were posited as one of the underlying causes for athletic menstrual cycle irregularity. Selye (50) was the first to propose a "general adaptation syndrome" as a possible association between the disruptions in menstrual cycle functioning and exercise stress. Selye postulated that a modified reproductive function was one of the nonspecific reactions of an organism adapting to changes in its external or internal environment. The adaptation of the body to stress involves the hypothalamic-pituitary-adrenal axis, together with the arousal and autonomic nervous system (9). In the hypothalamic-pituitary-adrenal axis, the principal modulator is the peptide corticotrophin-releasing hormone (CRH) from the hypothalamus. CRH, together with the nonpeptide arginine-vasopressin, causes the release of adrenocorticotropin hormone (ACTH) from the pituitary, which stimulates the release of glucocorticoids (cortisol) from the adrenal cortex. Under stressful conditions the locus ceruleus-norepinephrine system (central arousal system) also stimulates the hypothalamic CRH

and arginine-vasopressin neurons and contributes to the above-mentioned stressful reaction, resulting in the release of cortisol (9) (Figure 23.5).

It has been proposed that exercise stress chronically elevates cortisol levels in female athletes. This in turn may inhibit or suppress the secretion of **gonadotropin-releasing hormone** (GnRH) from the hypothalamus (9). Inadequate GnRH will result in the suppression of LH and FSH secretion, which in turn will cause inadequate estradiol and progesterone release. Further, at a higher hypothalamic level it has been shown that elevated CRH and CRH-induced β-endorphin release also inhibit GnRH release, causing the physiological suppression of the hypothalamic-pituitary-ovarian axis (see Figure 23.5). Similarly, E_2 has been found to exert a positive effect on to the hypothalamic-pituitary-adrenal axis by stimulating CRH release, and inhibits the re-uptake and catabolism of catecholamines by the central arousal system (9). Thus, stressful conditions (e.g., intense exercise) inhibit the female reproductive system by the suppression of the hypothalamic-pituitary-adrenal system.

Catecholamines have also been proposed to induce reproductive dysfunction. Periodic marked elevations in norepinephrine levels due to intense exercise have been shown

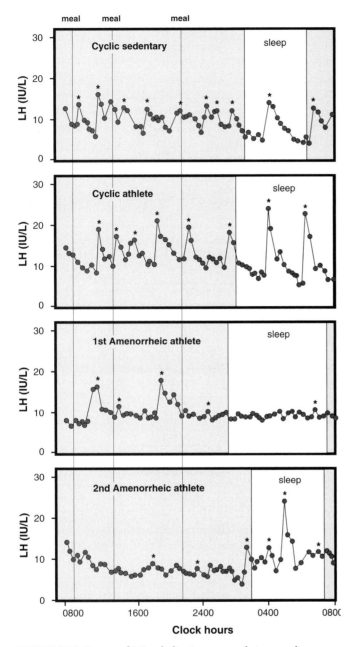

FIGURE 23.5. Pattern of LH pulsality in eumenorrheic controls, eumenorrheic athletes, and 2 amenorrheic athletes. Plasma LH concentrations were measured every 20 minutes. Adapted from Loucks A, Mortola J, Girton L (35).

to interfere with the pulsatile release of LH, and in turn lead to reproductive disturbances (51). For this reason athletic amenorrhea is also called "stress-induced or functional hypothalamic amenorrhea" (9).

It has been speculated that inhibition of the gonadotropins may also be due to elevated levels of prolactin and β-endorphins (52). It is posited that prolactin and β-endorphins interfere with the production or release of GnRH such that it cannot act upon the pituitary to induce release of gonadotropins. The mechanism of action of pro-

lactin and β-endorphins is still unknown, but these levels have repeatedly been shown to increase with exercise and are susceptible to exercise intensity, duration, and frequency.

In addition to the aforementioned physiological mechanisms, a recently postulated theory involves the hormone leptin. Leptin is a relatively newly discovered hormone that is secreted by the adipose tissue and regulates the size of adipose tissue stores (48, 53). Under normal conditions, leptin is known to suppress the hypothalamic-pituitary-adrenal axis by inhibiting CRH and cortisol secretion. Leptin is also known to potentiate the activity of GnRH. Amenorrheic athletes have been found to have low leptin levels and an absence of the typical diurnal pattern of leptin levels (54, 55). With low leptin levels, the inhibition of the hypothalamic-pituitary-adrenal axis is removed. As a result, CRH and cortisol levels are elevated and may cause adverse effects on the hypothalamic-pituitary-ovarian axis (9, 56, 57). More research is needed to clarify the role of leptin in the female reproductive system.

Etiologic Factors of Athletic Menstrual Dysfunction

Despite the recognition that reproductive dysfunction is a stress-related response, the specific "stress" factors that cause it are still not known. Numerous factors have been identified, but many have been criticized and rejected, while others still seem to play an important role in the etiology of athletic amenorrhea. Four of the most commonly discussed factors are highlighted in this section.

Body Composition

Several factors have been associated with athletic amenorrhea and may contribute to reproductive system disruptions by altering the hormonal milieu. Body composition is one of the factors closely associated with amenorrhea. Amenorrheic runners frequently are noted to have a lower body weight to height ratio, a greater weight loss since the onset of training, and a lower percent body fat compared to **eumenorrheic** runners (18, 27, 42). Frisch and colleagues proposed that a critical percent of body fat (>18% body fat) was necessary to sustain reproductive function. Supporting this hypothesis was the observation that many amenorrheic athletes had lower percent body fat than eumenorrheic athletes (e.g., ballet dancers, marathon runners, gymnasts) (11, 12, 31, 58) and this lower body weight was comprised of smaller amounts of both fat mass and lean mass (11). The low body weight was suggested to contribute to menstrual disturbances. The mechanism by which body composition influenced amenorrhea was speculated to be via inappropriate steroid feedback on the hypothalamic-pituitary-ovarian axis. In addition, adipose tissue is a site of androgen-to-estrogen conversion (19). It was believed that low body fat will modify the estrogen levels, resulting in inadequate feedback to the hypothalamus; however, it is still controversial as to whether this estrogen conversion is great enough in premenstrual women to be of significance.

It is now recognized that many women are very lean and still reproductively stable, while other athletes with higher percent body fat suffer from amenorrhea. Numerous studies have reported amenorrheic and eumenorrheic runners to have similar percent fat and height to weight ratios (27, 59, 60). For example, female shot putters and javelin throwers have been found to have a high incidence of athletic amenorrhea, even higher than other leaner athletes (6, 61). Carlsberg and colleagues (11) have suggested that a "threshold" for weight or body fat in a menstruating athlete may apply only to an individual and not to a population of athletes. Contradictions in the results regarding body fat and menstrual dysfunction may arise because various methods of determining body fat have been employed. Some investigators use only height and weight to estimate percent fat (12); others use skinfolds or a more accurate method like hydrostatic weighing (27, 42, 60). Further, many of the statistics reported on height, weight, and percent body fat comparing amenorrheic and eumenorrheic women are based on surveys. Poor recall and erroneous recording by the athletes may contribute to the discrepancies, and could bias the data.

More recently, it has been reported that low energy availability, rather than low body fat, results in amenorrhea (53, 62). This may be occurring in these athletes and is discussed in more depth later in the chapter. Thus, not only very lean athletes but also more normal or even "well-constituted" athletes can suffer from reproductive dysfunctions (6). This phenomenon challenges the theory that low body fat is a causative factor in athletic amenorrhea.

Exercise Training Volume and Intensity

Athletic amenorrhea has also been positively correlated with the training regimen. In runners, a relationship between the incidence of amenorrhea and training distances has been reported, with a greater incidence associated with increased training mileage. However, no relationship was found to exist in swimmers or cyclists (63). Sanborn and colleagues (63) observed a 43% incidence of amenorrhea with training mileage greater than 70 miles/week. Lutter and Cushman (40) noted an incidence of 17% with training distances of 50 miles/week.

Bullen and colleagues (44) studied a group of regularly menstruating untrained women over a period of physical inactivity versus a period of physical activity. After the inactive period, subjects were put on an 8-week high-volume running program consisting of training 2 times per day, 5 days per week, starting at 6.5 km/day and progressing to 16 km/day by the end of the study. In addition, subjects had to complete 3.5 h/day of swimming or cycling training. At the end of 8 weeks, approximately 25% of the participants had developed a shortened luteal phase and about 50% of the women had become anovulatory. The irregularities were resolved a few months later, after the volume of physical activity was reduced. Other studies that investigated the effects of exercise volume on reproductive function have found similar results (24, 40, 64, 65).

Exercise duration may play a key role in menstrual dysfunction because exercise stimulates hormonal release, and the longer the duration of exercise, the longer the hormone levels remain elevated. Exercise has been shown to decrease the metabolic clearance of E_2; however, the time duration of the decreased E_2 is still unknown (66). The mechanisms whereby training practices alter the menstrual cycle are speculated to be due to either changes in basal hormone concentrations or the cumulative effect of repeated transitory hormonal responses to acute exercise (19).

In addition to increasing exercise volume, the intensity of exercise is also a crucial etiologic factor to female reproductive problems. Hormonal responses are often dependent upon threshold intensity; hence higher intensity exercise would tend to cause greater modification of the hormonal milieu (19). Keizer and colleagues (45) studied the effects of short-term, high-intensity exercise on reproductive function. Two days of very intense and fatiguing exercise (4–5 hours per day of field hockey or handball) resulted in diminished LH pulse frequency and a smaller pulse amplitude ($P < 0.01$). In a subsequent study, women trained with either high-intensity aerobic or anaerobic exercise for the first 5 days of their menstrual cycle, and then with low-intensity exercise for days 8 to 28 of their cycle (45). The menstrual cycle of the subjects became significantly longer after the high-intensity anaerobic training as compared to the control cycle ($P < 0.05$). It was observed that during an acute bout of exercise the LH response to GnRH stimulation was reduced with both high-intensity training modes. Data from Keizer and associates (45) suggested a direct suppressive effect of acute exercise on the pituitary. Changes in LH pulsatility characteristics did not seem to be related to changes in training intensity, provided the training volume was kept constant, yet menstrual cycle length was changed.

Exercise training above the anaerobic threshold seems to result in more reproductive problems in female runners compared to exercise training below the anaerobic threshold (49). One year of training, either above or below the lactate threshold, resulted in a slight decrease in LH pulse number and an increase in the LH peak amplitude and nadir, but only in the above-lactate threshold group. In this group, there was a trend for a decrease in luteal phase length but not in total cycle length. This 1-year training study did not find any cases of amenorrhea or oligomenorrhea (<10 menstrual cycles per year). The lack of menstrual disturbances may be due to this cohort of women being more gynecologically mature (age = 30 years) (49) compared to studies using younger athletes, who seem more susceptible to menstrual disruption (22, 44). This study supported the hypothesis that a threshold of exercise intensity exists and it must be exceeded to induce menstrual cycle disruptions (49).

Finally, the psychological stress accompanying training and intense competition is also hypothesized to be a cause of amenorrhea. Studies have presented conflicting results on how athletes perceive the stress of training. In one study, amenorrheic middle-distance runners and long-distance runners showed no differences in level of stress (42). Galle and associates (67) evaluated psychological stress in amenorrheic and eumenorrheic runners, and only found significantly higher scores for obsessive-compulsive behavior in both groups, but these were not outside the norm.

Energy Intake

Energy intake, and in particular low caloric consumption, has been associated with athletic menstrual dysfunction. Dietary differences between amenorrheic and eumenorrheic athletes have been observed in numerous investigations (68–71). There is agreement in the literature that amenorrheic runners consume a lower number of calories compared to eumenorrheic athletes (68, 69, 71). Clark and colleagues (69) reported that amenorrheic runners perceive that they need fewer calories, which corresponds to a lower caloric intake. Lower protein intake has also been observed in amenorrheic women (42, 71). Other studies have shown that 82% of amenorrheic runners were found to have a 12% lower protein intake than the Recommended Daily Allowances, as compared to 35% of cyclic runners (71). Deuster and colleagues (70) reported that dietary fat intake was also lower in amenorrheic (66 g/day) than eumenorrheic (97 g/day) runners. Similarly, Bruemmer and Drinkwater (68) reported that amenorrheic women consumed significantly less fat ($P < .05$) than eumenorrheic women, with intakes of 51 g and 68 g, respectively. The dietary habits and intakes of macronutrients or micronutrients were not significantly different between these groups; however, Deuster and colleagues (70) noted that amenorrheic women consumed large amounts of vitamin A, low amounts of zinc, and high quantities of crude fiber. More recently, a 1-year prospective study of recreational runners found no differences in the mean energy intake or macronutrient intake, but did observe that the amenorrheic and oligomenorrheic runners had increased fiber intake and approximately a two-fold increase in fluid intake (72).

A few investigators have associated the endocrine status with dietary habits of runners in an attempt to isolate some causes of amenorrhea (73). Pirka and colleagues (73) studied 9 women with normal menstrual cycles. These women dieted for 6 weeks and lost 6 to 8 kg of body weight. During the 6 weeks, low LH and E_2 levels were observed and 6 of the 9 subjects showed no hormonal indications of ovulation. Similarly, Nelson and colleagues (71) found amenorrheic athletes to be hypoestrogenic and to have a 25% lower total energy consumption. Low calcium intakes were reported but could not be associated with low bone mineral status in athletes. How the associated endocrine status and dietary differences interact is still subject to considerable speculation, but it has been postulated that the metabolic consequences of dieting may interfere with gonadal steroid production, causing reproductive disturbances (73). Also, it has been suggested that a diet inadequate in calories lacks the necessary precursors for hormone synthesis, hence causing reproductive disturbances (74).

The possibility has been considered that runners may become metabolically more efficient in an attempt to conserve energy, thus allowing them to have low caloric intakes (75). One study recruited 7 amenorrheic runners, 10 eumenorrheic runners, and 10 sedentary women, and examined their resting and postprandial metabolic rates, dietary intake, and hormonal levels. Resting metabolic rate was significantly lower in amenorrheic runners (4667 ± 184 kJ/d) compared to eumenorrheic runners and sedentary controls (5559 ± 239 and 6116 ± 184 kJ/d, respectively, $P < 0.01$), suggesting that there is an adaptive response in amenorrheic women to conserve energy (75). A similar study did not find significant differences between amenorrheic, eumenorrheic, and untrained women for dietary intake and resting metabolic rate, but the investigators indicated that there may have been underreporting or restriction of dietary intake with these women (76). Further, they noted that 6 of the 8 amenorrheic women had an eating disorder, either anorexia and/or bulimia. In conclusion, a high association appears to exist between low energy intake and athletic amenorrhea, but more research is needed to identify the mechanism behind this association.

Low Energy Availability

Expanding on the above concept of energy restriction and reproductive problems, Loucks and colleagues (14, 46, 47, 77, 78) have conducted numerous elegant studies examining the effects of low energy availability on menstrual dysfunction. These authors have shown low thyroid hormone (T_3) levels, a sign of energy deficiency, in amenorrheic athletes compared to eumenorrheic athletes. The low-T_3 condition, which has been found to coexist with an increase of reverse T_3 levels (rT_3), has been named "low-T_3 syndrome" and appears to occur selectively in amenorrheic athletes and not regularly menstruating athletes (78). These studies have manipulated energy availability, either through exercise-induced energy expenditure or low dietary intake, and have shown that low energy availability can induce low-T_3 syndrome in healthy exercising women (77–79). In one study (77), 27 young, healthy, regularly menstruating women were randomly assigned to 4 days of aerobic exercise using 30 kcal/kg lean body mass per day. They were randomized to receive no, one-quarter, one-half, or complete dietary compensation for this exercise energy utilization. Low T_3 syndrome was prevented when dietary intake replenished one half of the energy cost, but a diet of one quarter of the energy cost was not sufficient to prevent this syndrome. It was concluded that energy availability, and not the exercise stress itself, is the critical factor for the induction of low-T_3 syndrome in regularly menstruating women (77).

More recently, Loucks and colleagues (14) tested the hypothesis that the GnRH pulse generator is disrupted by inadequate dietary intake. These authors combined 4 days of intense exercise with either energy balance or low energy availability. The intense exercise had no disruptive effect on LH pulsatility, other than impacting the energy cost on energy availability. Furthermore, exercise LH pulsatility is disturbed less by exercise energy expenditure, than with an equivalent amount of dietary energy restriction. Restricted energy availability disrupted both LH pulse frequency and amplitude (Figure 23.6). Thus, the impact of exercise occurs primarily by its effect on energy availability. It is not the exercise that disturbs LH pulsatility, but the exercise-induced low energy availability (14). Unlike other mammals, extremely high energy availability greater than the energy balance cannot restore the LH pulsatility in 24 hours in humans (47).

Current research demonstrates that energy availability, and not exercise stress per se, plays an etiologic role in re-

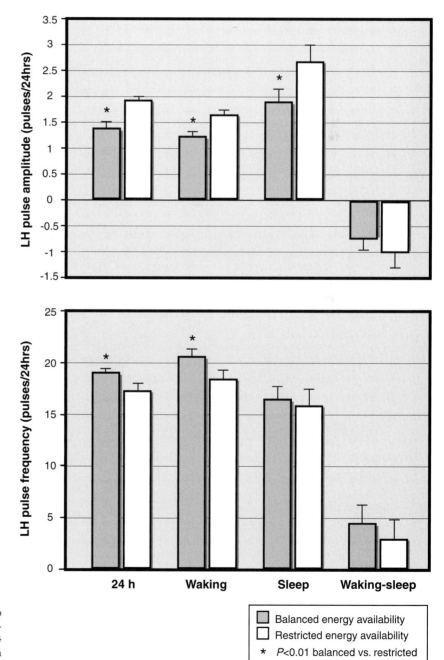

FIGURE 23.6. Effects of energy availability and sleep on LH pulse frequency and pulse amplitude in exercising women. Mean ± SE; units = number of pulses/24 h. Adapted from data from Loucks A, Verdun M, Heath E (14).

■ Balanced energy availability
□ Restricted energy availability
* $P<0.01$ balanced vs. restricted

productive disturbances such as athletic amenorrhea, as well as thyroid disturbances in physically active women (14). These observations agree with the earlier untested hypothesis by Warren (80) that reproductive disorders in physically active women are caused by the so-called "energy drain," and not by the sole effect of exercise stress. The physiological mechanism behind the "energy availability hypothesis" is still not complete. According to Loucks and colleagues (14), the GnRH pulse generator is disrupted by a still unidentified signal from the low energy availability induced by dietary restriction or exercise. Insufficient dietary intake causing the low energy availability effect is proposed to be linked to low glucose availability to the brain that can cause disturbances in reproductive and thyroid function. Leptin receptors have been found on the hypothalamic neurons (81), and alterations in leptin levels with low energy availability may control the GnRH pulse generator. Despite extensive research supporting this hypothesis, more research is needed to identify the signal that links the low energy availability to the reproductive disruptions, and to further establish this hypothesis.

In summary, exercise training, by either increasing the volume or intensity of exercise, as well as excessive dietary restriction, can lead to reproductive problems and eventually result in amenorrhea and other female reproductive dysfunctions. Two hypotheses have been developed to explain this phenomenon. The "exercise stress" hypothesis refers to the sole effect of chronic exercise that activates the hypothalamic-pituitary-adrenal axis and in turn disrupts the GnRH pulse generator and suppresses LH pulsatility. The second hypothesis focuses on low energy availability and refers to the effects of exercise and/or diet on energy availability. Energy intake and energy output needs to be matched, otherwise reproductive disturbances may ensue. Whether these reproductive disturbances are due to increased "energy drain" or to an increased stress response in the female athletes is still unclear (5). More research is certainly needed to test both hypotheses and establish one correct theory of the etiology of reproductive disturbances in female athletes.

Effects of Acute Exercise on the Hormonal Responses

Acute exercise has also been shown to impact hormone levels. As early as 1978, Jurkowski and colleagues found that after a session of light, moderate, or heavy exercise, hormonal changes were observed during both the luteal and follicular phases of the menstrual cycle. Plasma E_2 levels were increased in both phases of the menstrual cycle, but the increase in E_2 during the follicular phase was only significant at exhaustion. No change in plasma LH occurred at any phase, while FSH increased with exercise in the follicular phase. During 90 minutes of submaximal exercise at 60% $\dot{V}O_2$max, Kanaley and colleagues (82) demonstrated

that the greatest E_2 response to exercise occurred in the late follicular phase. Amenorrheic athletes had a significantly lower response in any phase of the menstrual cycle than the eumenorrheic athletes (Figure 23.7). Differences in the absolute resting levels of E_2 with menstrual phase did not in-

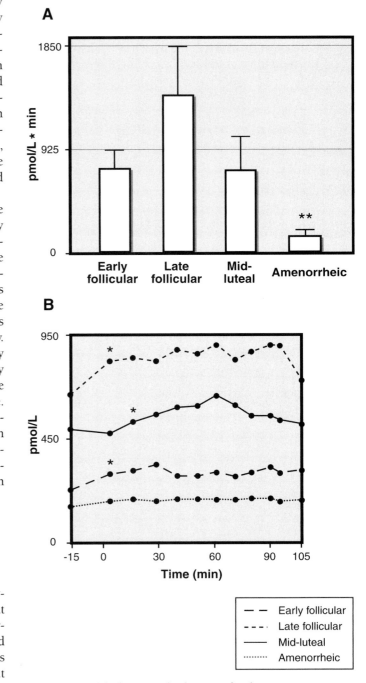

FIGURE 23.7. (A) The area under the curve of E_2 during exercise in amenorrheic and eumenorrheic athletes in each menstrual phase. (B) The pattern of response during exercise in both amenorrheic and eumenorrheic athletes. *First significant increase from rest, $P < 0.05$, **$P < 0.01$ from all phases of the eumenorrheic athletes. Adapted from Kanaley J, Boileau R, Bahr J, Misner, JE, Nelson R (82).

fluence the temporal pattern of the response to the exercise stimulus. Exercise-induced progesterone responses followed a different pattern. The pattern of release was altered in the mid-luteal phase and the net increase (integrated area under the curve above baseline) was greater than in the early follicular and late follicular phases. Discrepancies in the literature (82–86) on the exercise-induced E_2 and progesterone responses are reported and most likely are due to differences in the phase of the cycle tested and the method of data analysis. For example, Kanaley and colleagues (82) demonstrated that examining only the pattern of E_2 response to exercise would have been misleading, as the net increase of the hormone response illustrated other subtle differences in the hormone response. Although the temporal pattern of E_2 release was not different between amenorrheic and eumenorrheic women, the net increase in E_2 levels was higher in the eumenorrheic than in the amenorrheic athletes.

Acute exercise has been found to produce changes in the stress hormones of female athletes. Significant differences in the catecholamine levels of sedentary and athletic women with normal and abnormal menses have been observed (51). During a maximal exercise stress test, amenorrheic and oligomenorrheic runners displayed a significantly higher percent change in norepinephrine values. However, during constant load exercise (60% $\dot{V}O_{2max}$ for 30 min), no differences between groups were observed in norepinephrine or epinephrine levels, nor were differences observed during a subsequent 15-minute bout at 80% $\dot{V}O_{2max}$. These authors speculated that marked elevations in norepinephrine levels during maximal exercise might interfere with pulsatile LH release. Studies of the effects of exercise on other stress hormones have reported similar results. Prolactin, β-endorphin, melatonin, growth hormone, cortisol, and other stress hormones (66, 82, 86–91) have been found to increase with acute exercise and have been proposed to potentially affect the reproductive disturbances observed in female athletes with long-term exercise. Recently it was shown that amenorrheic athletes have an increase in the half-life of GH and the number of secretory bursts, as well as a decrease in the mass of GH secreted per burst (92). These data demonstrate that the amenorrheic state, beyond the exercise, alters the neuroendocrine control of GH output in amenorrheic athletes.

Cortisol levels have also been demonstrated to increase during prolonged exercise. Ding and colleagues (93) have found basal cortisol levels to be higher in amenorrheic than eumenorrheic runners. Others have reported that resting cortisol concentrations are greater in the amenorrheic athletes ($P < 0.01$), and the net increment in cortisol levels during exercise were distinctly higher ($P < 0.01$) in these athletes than in eumenorrheic athletes at any phase of the menstrual cycle (Figure 23.8) (90). In fact, throughout the exercise period, the metabolic clearance rate of cortisol increased in the eumenorrheic athletes, resulting in an overall net decline in cortisol by the end of exercise, while the

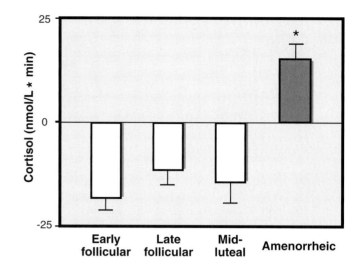

FIGURE 23.8. Integrated area under curve above baseline in eumenorrheic and amenorrheic athletes. *$P < 0.05$ between groups. Adapted from Kanaley J, Boileau R, Bahr J, Misner, JE, Nelson R (90).

amenorrheic athletes completed the exercise bout with a net increase in cortisol levels (90). In animals, exogenous glucocorticoids have been shown to interfere with LH release, hence high cortisol levels may be a marker for altered interactions between the hypothalamic-pituitary-adrenal and hypothalamic-pituitary-ovarian axes (9).

Effects of Menstrual Dysfunction on Athletic Performance

The effects of amenorrhea on athletic performance are controversial. Some authors have reported a reduced performance (94) during the luteal phase of the menstrual cycle of normal cycling women; others have proposed the possibility that amenorrheic athletes might have an advantage and improved performance (10, 95). During the luteal phase, maximum ventilation has been shown to occur at lower exercise intensities compared to the nonluteal phase performance, suggesting a reduced athletic performance (94). These authors concluded that the luteal phase of the cycle is associated with elevated aerobic demands at lower intensities of exercise, which can reduce performance (94). Elevated lactate levels during the luteal phase in comparison to the follicular phase have also been reported, suggesting more anaerobic metabolism (27, 96).

In contrast, many studies have found no differences in athletic performance between the luteal and follicular phase of the menstrual cycle in the following variables: heart rate, respiration, $\dot{V}O_2$, cardiac output, thermoregulation, and lactate levels, implying that performance is not affected by menstrual phase (7, 13, 97, 98). A few studies have indicated an improved performance during the luteal phase (10, 95). This improved performance, which has also been demonstrated in animal studies, is attributable to the hypothesized positive effects of estrogen on fuel metabolism, as well as the protective effect of estrogen on muscle injuries (6).

Health Consequences of Athletic Menstrual Dysfunction

Athletic amenorrhea is considered one part of the female triad that starts with short-term health consequences, which can develop into long-term ramifications. The female triad consists of an interaction of eating disorders, amenorrhea, and osteoporosis. Currently, it is suspected that **disordered eating** or low energy availability interferes with the hypothalamic-pituitary axis, and as a consequence menstrual disruption occurs that can precipitate amenorrhea. Short-term anovulation/amenorrhea only hinders the ability to conceive (20), which appears to be reversible by reducing the exercise training intensity so that the menstrual cycle resumes (6, 15, 74). During periods of low levels of exercise training or vacations, the reproductive function of female amenorrheic athletes has been found to normalize hormonal levels and the menstrual cycle resumes. For many elite athletes, however, there is no low-intensity training period, thus prolonged amenorrhea can cause substantial long-term health damage.

One of the primary concerns with the absence of the menstrual cycle for prolonged periods of time is the low levels of circulating estrogens that may lead to osteopenia (59, 99, 100). Forty eight percent of skeletal mass is attained during adolescence and accumulation of bone continues into our thirties (48); however, bone mass accretion may be compromised in late maturing girls and low bone mineral density (BMD) is constently reported in athletes with hypoestrogen amenorrhea (48). If an athlete has missed more than 6 consecutive menstrual periods, there is an increased risk of premature bone loss (20). Lower BMD of the total body, lumbar spine, pelvis, femoral neck, trochanter, and humerus has been observed in female runners with amenorrhea than in eumenorrheic runners or in female soccer players (100) (Figure 23.9). Most studies suggest that bone loss in amenorrheic athletes is limited to specific sites, specifically to areas of high trabecular bone content. Trabecular bone is more sensitive to hypoestrogenemia than cortical bone because of its higher turnover rate. However, cortical bone changes may appear after 5 to 6 years of estrogen deprivation (101). Pettersson and colleagues (100) have shown that this bone loss can occur in the axial as well as in the appendicular skeleton, and physical weight-bearing activity alone does not override the side effects of reduced estrogen levels.

Accumulating evidence suggests that metabolic factors associated with nutritional deprivation may be important in regulating bone activity. An acute or chronic energy deficit elicits metabolic aberrations. Recently leptin receptors have been found in bone (102), thus depression of leptin levels

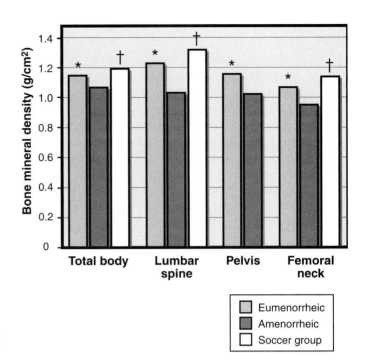

FIGURE 23.9. Bone mineral density measurements in amenorrheic (n = 10) and eumenorrheic (n = 10) runners and soccer players. *Eumenorrheic > amenorrheic ($P < 0.05$); †soccer players > amenorrheic ($P < 0.01$). Adapted from data from Pettersson R, Stalnacke B, Ahlenius G, Henriksson-Larsen K, Lorentzon R (100).

and suppression of the diurnal leptin rhythm associated with low energy inake may mediate not only reproductive function but also bone accretion (48, 54).

Experts in the field have questioned the reversibility of the bone loss. Small gains (6%) in vertebral BMD have been reported in the first year following the resumption of menstrual function (99, 103, 104). A follow-up study of these athletes indicated that this gain ceased and that vertebral BMD was well below average in these women 4 years later (105). In a study of 29 athletes over 8 years, vertebral BMD was significantly lower in the amenorrheic group compared to regularly menstruating women. The oligomenorrheic group had intermediate values that did not differ significantly from the amenorrheic or eumenorrheic athletes. They demonstrated that despite several years of normal menstrual function or the use of oral contraceptives, the vertebral BMD was low in the oligomenorrheic/amenorrheic group. Thus, early prevention is necessary (103).

The resumption of normal menstrual function does appear to help the athlete to regain some of the lost bone mass but does not completely offset what was lost (20, 99). In a 1-year study, the resumption of menstrual function led to only a 1.5% improvement in spinal BMD (106) and the addition of calcium supplementation has not been shown to have any significant effect on BMD (106) (Figure 23.10). Additionally, a direct correlation has been found between the incidence of stress fractures and the number of missed

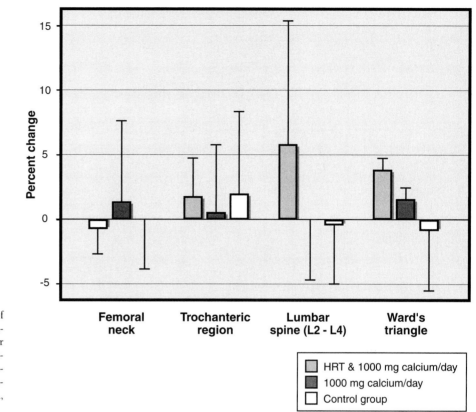

FIGURE 23.10. Percent change per year of bone mineral density in athletes with menstrual irregularity comparing before and after treatment. HRT group, 903 months of treatment; calcium group, 11.2 months of treatment; control group, 11.7 months of no treatment. Adapted from Gibson JH, Mitchell A, Reeve J, Harries MG (106).

menstrual periods in several studies (107, 108). Those women with menstrual dysfunction have been found to have longer interruptions in their training schedules due to musculoskeletal injuries than those with regular cycles (34 days of interruption versus 9 days in 1 year) (109).

Increased risk of cardiovascular disease is another possible consequence of prolonged athletic amenorrhea (5). It is well known that the reduced estrogen levels with menopause are highly associated with a substantially increased risk of cardiovascular disease due to a poor lipid profile and in particular low-density lipoprotein-cholesterol concentration (LDL-C). Compared to eumenorrheic women, amenorrheic women have been shown to possess elevated levels of both LDL-C (2.81 $\pm$ 0.09 versus 3.16 $\pm$ 0.15 mmol/l, respectively, $P < 0.04$) and total cholesterol (4.84 $\pm$ 0.12 versus 5.47 $\pm$ 0.17 mmol/L, respectively, $P < 0.003$) (110). There seem to be cardioprotective elevations in high-density lipoprotein-cholesterol (HDL-C) 1 and 2, which result in the LDL-C/HDL-C ratio being similar between these groups of athletes. Athletic amenorrhea has also been associated with premature cardiovascular disease. One study found that 21 year-old amenorrheic runners had vascular integrity similar to that of women 30 years older (21). These women had a decreased capacity for dilation of the brachial artery, and this was similar to the vasodilation seen in postmenopausal women (21). If more evidence accumulates suggesting that premature cardiovascular disease is occurring in these women, this cluster of interrelated

health problems may actually form a quartet: eating disorders, amenorrhea, osteoporosis, and cardiovascular disease.

Treatment of Athletic Menstrual Dysfunction

In preparing a treatment plan for amenorrheic athletes, a physician must take into consideration the complex and multidimensional nature of these reproductive disorders. Numerous issues need to be addressed in addition to the hormonal changes. For example, nutritional status, eating disorders, exercise training program, and hormone levels need to be examined. Although low or inappropriate hormone levels can be dealt with by using hormone supplements, this does not get to the actual cause of the problem. Treatment needs to deal first with the short-term problems, yet recognizing the long-term complications (e.g., osteoporosis) is essential. Treatment also must include education and modification of both nutrition and the exercise-training program. Careful analysis needs to focus not only on the absolute caloric intake of the athlete but also on whether the energy intake meets the daily energy demands. Ideally, a reproductive endocrinologist with experience with athletic menstrual dysfunction should conduct a complete evaluation. This is critical because much of the recent data (62, 111) suggest that increasing energy intake may restore normal menstrual function. The exercise-training program needs to be evaluated to determine the energy expenditure, and to establish if it matches the energy intake. Adjustments in both energy intake and expenditure may be needed (Box 23.5).

Hormone replacement therapy (HRT) similar to menopausal therapy or oral contraceptive pills should be considered to correct the loss of hormonal release; however, higher doses than are used for the postmenopausal women may be needed (112). Daily calcium supplementation, as well as vitamin D supplementation, may be required to reduce the risk of low bone density problems, and also to ensure safe participation in sports with a reduced risk of bone fractures. No adverse effects have been reported on the prescription of HRT or oral contraceptives in the health and performance of the female athletes, but no research has been conducted on this population (4). Further, it is important to measure bone density in these athletes, whether they have had bone fractures or not. In conclusion, the specific mechanisms for this disorder are not completely understood, and treatment must incorporate nutritional, exercise, and behavioral changes. The aim of the therapy should be to balance energy intake and output so that the athlete is not in a condition of low energy availability. This most likely will require the athlete to decrease exercise volume and to improve dietary intake. Overall, the treatment needs a 3-pronged approach of pharmacotherapy, psychological counseling, and lifestyle changes (113).

Conclusions

Athletic amenorrhea is a growing phenomenon in female athletes all over the world. It is a serious reproductive problem characterized by menstrual cycle disruption, anovulation, and eventually amenorrhea. Low estrogen and progesterone levels, a shortened luteal phase, anovulation, and other reproductive problems result from this overtraining, and in particular this "energy drain" or low energy availability.

Despite the serious consequences and the number of research studies conducted, the physiological mechanism of amenorrhea is still not clear. Two hypotheses of the mechanism responsible for athletic amenorrhea have been put forth. Low energy availability due to exercise and/or dietary restriction is currently hypothesized to cause disruption to the hypothalamic-pituitary-ovarian axis. This paradigm includes a suppression of GnRH secretion from the hypothalamus, decreased pituitary release of LH and FSH levels, and eventually attenuated estrogen and progesterone concentrations. The stress response hypothesis ties changes in the hypothalamic-pituitary-adrenal axis to changes in the hypothalamic-pituitary-ovarian axis. The increased levels of CRH and cortisol present in the amenorrheic athlete due to the increased physiological and psychological stress may interact with the hypothalamic-pituitary-ovarian axis. Furthermore, leptin also appears to contribute to athletic amenorrhea, but the potential mechanism needs to be elucidated.

Amenorrhea or menstrual dysfunction is a serious health problem present in many female athletes. Prolonged menstrual dysfunction can have serious health consequences, such as **infertility**, loss of BMD, and increased risk of cardiovascular disease, and may result in osteoporosis. It is agreed that some of these complications may be partially reversible as long as treatment is provided. To acquire new knowledge about this complex and multidimensional health problem, new methodologically stable and consistent research is certainly needed.

BOX 23.5.   Treatment

- Prevention and early identification
- Education of athletes, coaches, parents, athletic trainers, physicians, health educators
- Consultants: psychologists and nutritionists
- Counseling if needed for eating disorders
- Hormonal intervention: oral contraceptives or hormone replacement therapy
- Nutritional intervention: adequate caloric intake to meet energy expenditure. Increase caloric intake: 1200–1500 mg/day
- Bone scan

What We Know
About Menstrual Dysfunction and Exercise

1 With intense physical training, menstrual dysfunction can occur; this may include anovulation, amenorrhea, shortened or inadequate luteal phase, and oligomenorrhea.

2 The most common type of athletic amenorrhea is chronic anovulation. The reproductive system's rhythm is disrupted so that ovulation does not occur, but the ovaries continue to function.

3 The mean age of menarche is 12.2 years, and intense training before this age may lead to delayed menarche.

4 Menstrual dysfunction has been associated with a high volume of training, low percent body fat, eating disorders, and energy availability.

5 Numerous physiological mechanisms have been suggested as the body adapts to this chronic stress.

6 Chronic hormonal changes seen with training are disturbances in LH pulsatility, elevated CRH levels, marked elevation in catecholamines, elevated prolactin and β-endorphin levels, and low leptin levels.

7 Some studies have shown that an amenorrheic athlete has lower percent body fat than eumenorrheic athletes, but there are also numerous studies that do not support this. No strong association can be made between low percent body fat and amenorrhea.

8 Amenorrheic athletes usually consume a lower energy intake, with some studies showing lower percent protein intake and lower dietary fat.

9 Lower energy availability is now a widely supported hypothesis for athletic amenorrhea. This results in lower glucose availability to the brain that causes disruption of the GnRH pulse generator, in reproduction and thyroid function.

10 The short-term consequences of amenorrhea are anovulation and infertility. The long-term consequences are possibly a lower total body bone density, as well lower regional differences in bone density between amenorrheic and eumenorrheic women. In the short term this is recognized as osteopenia, but in the long term may cause osteoporosis. Premature cardiovascular disease is also a possible long-term consequence.

11 Resumption of the menses in the young athlete may restore some of the bone mineral content lost during the amenorrheic period, but will not recover all of the lost bone.

Women with menstrual dysfunction for a prolonged period of time are susceptible to stress fractures in their lower limbs. These stress fractures are often associated with pain and discomfort at the level of the stress fracture, resulting in a decrease in performance despite maintenance of a high training volume.

What We Would Like To Know About Menstrual Dysfunction and Exercise

1 Is the incidence of amenorrhea really increasing, or is it a phenomenon related to better awareness and/or better diagnosis?

2 Is the bone loss completely reversible? Does reversibility depend upon the age that amenorrhea occurs (pubertal versus postpubertal)?

3 How does the energy availability induce this reproductive disturbance? Is this an adaptive response?

4 Does the low energy availability truly hinder athletic performance?

5 Does early, intense exercise training affect the accrual of peak bone mass?

6 Is hormone replacement therapy effective in restoring bone density similar to a normal cycle?

7 Do men have a similar syndrome due to overtraining that may also have long-term consequences?

Summary

The female reproductive system is highly sensitive to chronic physiological stress. As a result of this chronic stress, reproductive abnormalities may occur, including delayed menarche, shortened luteal phase and oligomenorrhea, and primary and secondary amenorrhea. These reproductive problems typically occur in women engaged in sports that emphasize low weight (e.g., ballet, long-distance running, gymnastics, figure skating), but can also occur in women in any sport that involves intense athletic training. Many of these women have eating disorders of some type in their efforts to minimize their body weight. This reproductive dysfunction is characterized by hypoestrogenism resulting from disruption of the hypothalamic-pituitary-ovarian axis, and may also result in hypercortisolism. Originally, a low percent body fat was speculated to cause the reproductive disturbances; however, recent evidence suggests that low energy availability occurs in these women, whose energy expenditure exceeds dietary energy intake, and may cause the disruption to this axis. The reproductive abnormalities observed usually originate in the hypothalamus and are expressed by disturbances of the gonadotropin-releasing hormone (GnRH) pulse generator. The energy drain may be a primary factor affecting GnRH pulsatility, but the specific mechanism triggering the reproductive dysfunction may vary across athletic disciplines.

Many eumenorrheic athletes may actually be suffering from hidden menstrual irregularities; their evaluation involves serial measurement of hormone levels. Absence of the menstrual cycle is the only overt sign of reproductive disturbances. The clinical consequence of this disruption includes infertility in the short term; long-term effects may be osteopenia or even osteoporosis, and possibly cardiovascular disease. Hypoestrogenemia in pubertal athletes may result in these women failing to attain peak bone mass or may demonstrate bone loss (osteopenia). This bone loss may be irreversible and may lead to osteoporosis. This cluster of disorders—eating disorders, amenorrhea, and osteoporosis—must be treated with a 3-pronged approach that considers and addresses each problem. For optimal results, a team of physicians, nutritionists, endocrinologists, and exercise specialists should be involved in the treatment of this complex disorder.

DISCUSSION QUESTIONS

1 Why is an appropriate diet important for normal reproductive function?

2 Menstrual dysfunction includes anovulation, shortened luteal phase, and missed cycles. Do all of these dysfunctions have similar short-term and long-term consequences?

3 What are the recommendations for care of these individuals?

4 Does amenorrhea affect trabecular and calcaneus bone similarly?

5 Are there any injuries associated with amenorrhea?

CASE STUDY

Patient Information

Eleni is a 21-year-old distance runner at a Division I university. Since her freshman year in college, she has done extensive training both in-season and out-of-season. Despite maintaining her workouts in the off-season to maintain her personal best times, the coaches are concerned with her fitness. She is not running her best times and has been plagued with injuries. The athletic trainers are continually treating her, but she has complaints about her shins and feet. It is beginning to impair her running performance. The coaches are concerned if she will be able to remain healthy during the race season. Discussion of her problems with the team's head athletic trainer has led to an appointment with the team physician.

Assessments

Despite Eleni training hard and being in excellent shape, she is constantly working with the athletic trainers about her shin splints or "aching feet." During her exam with the team physician, it was revealed that she had only 2 menstrual cycles during the summer and none during the previous academic year. An x-ray revealed a stress fracture in her left foot. In addition, although she had an apparently healthy diet, it did not seem balanced and she was referred to a nutritionist. Her diet was composed of 60% carbohydrates, 20% fat, and 20% protein, and the caloric intake was approximately 2200 kcal/day. The nutritionist estimated that she was burning 3000 to 3500 kcal/day with training.

Her hormone panel revealed that her estrogen levels were low but not out of the normal range (25 pg/ml—follicular phase), cortisol levels were high (4 to 27 μg/dl), and there were no signs of hyperprolactinemia.

Questions

1. What factors must you consider when evaluating Eleni's training regimen?
2. What factors must you consider when looking at Eleni's estrogen levels?
3. If Eleni were eating 2200 kcal/day, why would her caloric intake be of concern?
4. What recommendations do you think would be given by the team physician?

REFERENCES

1. Orley J. Sports-related problems in reproductive function. Ann NY Acad Sci 1997;816:285–294.

2. Prior J, Cameron K, Yuen B. Menstrual cycles changes with marathon training: anovulation and short luteal phase. Can J Appl Sport Sci 1982;177:173–177.

3. Prior J, Ho Yuen B, Clement P. Reversible luteal phase changes and infertility associated with marathon training. Lancet II 1982;8292:269–270.

4. Shangold M. Sports and menstrual function. Phys Sportsmed 1980;8(8):66–70.

5. Chen E, Brzyski R. Exercise and reproductive dysfunction. J Fertil Steril 1999;71:1–8.

6. De Crèe C. Sex steroid metabolism and menstrual irregularities in the exercising female: a review. Sports Med 1998;25:369–406.

7. De Souza M, Maguire M, Rubin K. Effects of menstrual phase and amenorrhea on exercise performance in runners. Med Sci Sports Exerc 1990;22:575–580.

8. Marshall L. Clinical evaluation of amenorrhea in active and athletic women. Clin Sports Med 1994;13:371–387.

9. Chrousos GP, Torpy DJ, Gold PW. Interactions between the hypothalamic-pituitary-adrenal axis and the female reproductive system: clinical implications. Ann Intern Med 1998;129:229–240.

10. Baker E. Menstrual dysfunction and hormonal status in athletic women: a review. Fertil Steril 1981;36:691–696.

11. Carlsberg K, Burkman M, Peake G. Body composition of oligo/amenorrheic athletes. Med Sci Sports Exerc 1983;15(3):215–217.

12. Frisch R, MacArthur J. Menstrual cycles: fatness as a determinant of minimum weight for height necessary for the maintenance or onset of menstruation. Science 1974;185:949–951.

13. Jurkowski J, Jones N, Walker W. Ovarian hormonal responses to exercise. J Appl Physiol 1978;44:109–114.

14. Loucks A, Verdun M, Heath E. Low energy availability, not the stress of exercise, alters LH pulsatility in exercising women. J Appl Physiol 1998;84:37–46.

15. Prior J. Endocrine conditioning with endurance training, a preliminary review. Can J Appl Sport Sci 1982;7:157.

16. Harber V, Webber C, Sutton J. The effect of amenorrhea on bone calcaneal bone density and total bone turnover in runners. Int J Sports Med 1991;12:505–508.

17. Heinrich G, Going S, Pamentier R. Bone mineral content of cyclically menstruating female resistance and endurance trained athletes. Med Sci Sports Exerc 1990;22:558–563.

18. Shangold M. Menstrual irregularity in athletes: basic principles, evaluation and treatment. Can J Appl Sport Sci 1982;7:66–70.

19. Loucks A, Horvath S. Athletic amenorrhea: a review. Med Sci Sports Exerc 1985;17:56–72.

20. Fagan K. Pharmacologic management of athletic amenorrhea. Sports Pharmacol 1998;17:327–341.

21. Ill-Effects of female athlete triad may go beyond osteoporosis. The Back Letter 2001;16(8):94.

22. Bonen A, Belcastro A, Ling W. Profiles of selected hormones during menstrual cycle of teenage athletes. J Appl Physiol 1981;50:545–551.

23. Bonen A, Keizer H. Athletic menstrual cycle irregularity: endocrine response to exercise and training. Phys Sportsmed 1984;12:78–94.

24. Shangold M. Exercise and the adult female: hormonal and endocrine effects. In: Wilmore J, Keogh J, eds. Exercise and Sport Science Reviews. New York: Academic Press; 1979:53–79.

25. Morris FL, Wark JD. An effective, economic way of monitoring menstrual cycle hormones in at risk female athletes. Med Sci Sports Exerc 2001;33:9–14.

26. Scott G, Tuttle W. The periodic fluctuation in physical efficiency during the menstrual cycle. Res Q 1932;3:137–144.

27. Baker E, Mathur R, Kirk R. Female runners and secondary amenorrhea: correlation with age, parity, mileage, and plasma hormonal and sex hormone binding globulin concentrations. Fertil Steril 1981;36:183–187.

28. Frisch R, Wyshak G, Vincent L. Delayed menarche and amenorrhea in ballet dancers. N Engl J Med 1980;303:17–19.

29. Warren M, Jeweewicz R, Dyrenfurth I, Ans R, Khalaf S, Vande Wiele R. The significance of weight loss in the evaluation of pituitary response to LH-RH in women with secondary amenorrhea. J Clin Endocrinol Metab 1975;40:601–611.

30. Brisson G, Dulac S, Peronnet F. The onset of menarche: a late event in pubertal progression to be affected by physical training. Can J Appl Sport Sci 1982;7:61–67.

31. Frisch R, Gotz-Welbergen A, MacArthur J. Delayed menarche and amenorrhea of college athletes in relation to age of onset of training. JAMA 1981;246:1559–1563.

32. Mesaki N, Sasaki J, Shoji M. Hormonal changes during continuous exercise in athletic women. Acta Obstet Gynaec Jpn 1984;39:63–69.

33. Malina R, Spirduso W, Tate C, Baylor A. Age at menarche and selected menstrual characteristics in athletes at different competitive levels and in different sports. Med Sci Sports Exerc 1978;10:218–222.

34. Stager J, Wigglesworth J, Hatter L. Interpreting the relationship between age of menarche and prepubertal training. Med Sci Sports Exerc 1990;22:54–58.

35. Loucks A, Mortola J, Girton L. Alterations in the hypothalamic-pituitary-ovarian and the hypothalamic-pituitary-adrenal axes in athletic women. J Clin Endocrinol Metab 1989;68(2):402–411.

36. Ronkainen H, Pakarinen A, Kauppila A. Pubertal and menstrual disorders of female runners, skiers and volleyball players. Gynecol Obstet Invest 1984;18:183–189.

37. Williams N, Bullen B, McArthur J, Skrinar G, Turnbull B. Effects of short-term strenuous endurance exercise upon corpus luteum function. Med Sci Sports Exerc 1999;31:949–958.

38. Bonen A. Exercise-induced menstrual cycle changes: a functional temporary adaptation to metabolic stress. Sports Med 1994;17:373–392.

39. Glass A, Deuster P, Kyle S. Amenorrhea in Olympic marathon runners. Fertil Steril 1987;48:740–745.

40. Lutter J, Cushman S. Menstrual patterns in female runners. Phys Sportsmed 1982;10:60–72.

41. Mann G. Menstrual effects of athletic training. Endocrinol Metab 1989;68:402–411.

42. Schwartz B, Cumming D, Riordan E. Exercise-induced amenorrhea: a distinct identity. Am J Obstet Gynecol 1981;141:662–670.

43. Speroff L, Redwine D. Exercise and menstrual dysfunction. Phys Sportsmed 1980;8:41–52.

44. Bullen B, Skrinar G, Beitins I. Induction of menstrual cycle disorders by strenuous exercise in untrained women. N Engl J Med 1985;312:1349–1353.

45. Keizer H, Platen P, Menheere P. The hypothalamic/pituitary axis under exercise stress: the effects of aerobic and anaerobic training. In: Rogol A, Laron A, eds. Hormones and Sport. Vol. 55. Serono Symposium Publications; 1989:101–115.

46. Loucks A, Heath E. Dietary restriction reduces LH pulse frequency during waking hours and increases LH pulse amplitude during sleep in young menstruating women. J Clin Endocrinol Metab 1994;78:910–915.

47. Loucks A, Verdun M. Slow restoration of LH pulsatility by refeeding in energetically disrupted women. Am J Physiol 1998;275:R1218–R1226.

48. Warren MP, Perlroth NE. The effects of intense exercise on the female reproductive system. J Endocrinol 2001;170:3–11.

49. Rogol A, Weltman A, Weltman J, Evans W, Vendhuis J. Durability of the reproductive axis in eumenorrheic women during one year of endurance training. J Appl Physiol 1992;72:1571–1580.

50. Selye. The effects of adaptation to various damaging agents on the female sex organs in the rat. Endokrinologie 1939;25:615–624.

51. Chin N, Chang F, Dodds W, Kim M, Malarkey W. Acute effects of exercise on plasma catecholamines in sedentary and athletic women

with normal and abnormal menses. Am J Obstet Gynecol 1987;157:938–944.

52. Carr B, Bullen B, Skrinar G, et al. Physical conditioning facilitates the exercise-induced secretion of beta-endorphins and beta-lipotropin in women. New Engl J Med 1981;305:560–562.

53. Hilton LK, Loucks AB. Low energy availability, not exercise stress, suppresses the diurnal rhythm of leptin in healthy young women. Am J Physiol Endocrinol Metab 2000;278:E43–E49.

54. Laughlin GA, Yenn SSC. Hypoleptinemia in women athletes: absence of a diurnal rhythm with amenorrhea. J Clin Endocrinol Metab 1997;82:318–321.

55. Thong FSL, McLean C, Graham TE. Plasma leptin in female athletes: relationship with body fat, reproductive, nutritional and endocrine factors. J Appl Physiol 2000;88:2037–2044.

56. Ahima R, Prabakaran D, Mantzoros C, et al. Role of leptin in the neuroendocrine response to fasting. Nature 1996;382:250–252.

57. Boden G, Chen X, Mozzoli M, Ryan I. Effects of fasting on serum leptin in normal human subjects. J Clin Endocrinol Metab 1996;81:3419–3423.

58. Frisch R, Revelle R, Cook S. Components of weight at menarche and the initiation of the adolescent growth spurts in girls: estimated total water, lean body weight and fat. Hum Biol 1973;45:449–483.

59. Drinkwater BL, Nilson K, Chesnut CH 3rd, Bremner WJ, Shainholtz S, Southworth MB. Bone mineral content of amenorrheic and eumenorrheic athletes. N Engl J Med 1984;311:277–281.

60. Loucks A, Horvath S. Exercise-induced stress responses of amenorrheic and eumenorrheic runners. J Clin Endocrinol Metab 1984;59:1109–1120.

61. Higher R. Athletic amenorrhea: an update on aetiology, complications and management. Sports Med 1989;7:82–108.

62. Williams NI, Caston-Balderrama AL, Helmreich DL, Parfitt DB, Nosbisch C, Cameron JL. Longitudinal changes in reproductive hormones and menstrual cyclicity in cynomolgus monkeys during strenuous exercise training: abrupt transition to exercise-induced amenorrhea. Endocrinol 2001;142:2381–2389.

63. Sanborn C, Martin B, Wagner W. Is athletic amenorrhea specific to runners? Am J Obstet Gynecol 1982;143:859–861.

64. Gray P, Dale E. Variables associated with secondary amenorrhea. J Sports Sci 1983;1:55–67.

65. Tomten S, Hostmark A, Stromme S. Exercise intensity: an important factor in the etiology of menstrual dysfunction? Scand J Med Sci Sports 1996;6:329–336.

66. Keizer H, van Soest O, Beckers E. Exercise-induced changes in estradiol metabolism and their possible physiological meaning. Med Sport 1981;14:141–147.

67. Galle P, Freeman E, Galle M, Huggins G, Sondheimer S. Physiologic and psychologic profiles in a survey of women runners. Fertil Steril 1983;39:633–639.

68. Bruemmer B, Drinkwater B. Nutrient intake in amenorrheic and eumenorrheic athletes. Med Sci Sports Exerc 1987;19(suppl):S37.

69. Clark N, Nelson M, Evans W. Elite women runners: association between menstrual status, dietary practices and eating disorders [abstract]. Med Sci Sport Exerc 1987;19(suppl):S37.

70. Deuster P, Kyle S, Moser P. Nutritional survey of highly trained women runners. Fertil Steril 1986;46:636–643.

71. Nelson M, Fisher E, Catsos P, Meredith C, Turksoy R, Evans W. Diet and bone status in amenorrheic runners. Am J Clin Nutr 1986;43:910–916.

72. Rosetta L, da Silva Fraga EC, Mascie-Taylor CGN. Relationship between self-reported food and fluid intake and menstrual disturbance in female recreational runners. Ann Hum Biol 2001;28:444–454.

73. Pirka L, Schweiger U, Lemmel W, Kreig J, Berger M. The influence of dieting on the menstrual cycle of healthy young women. J Clin Endocrinol Metab 1985;60:1174–1179.

74. Sanborn C, Albrecht B, Wagner W Jr. Athletic amenorrhea: lack of association with body fat. Med Sci Sports Exerc 1987;19:207–212.

75. Myerson M, Gutin B, Warren MP, et al. Resting metabolic rate and energy balance in amenorrheic and eumenorrheic runners. Med Sci Sports Exerc 1991;23:15–22.

76. Wilmore J, Wambsgans K, Brenner M. Is there energy conservation in amenorrheic compared with eumenorrheic distance runners? J Appl Physiol 1982;72:15–22.

77. Loucks A, Callister R. Induction and prevention of low T3 syndrome in exercising women. Am J Physiol 1993;264:R924–R930.

78. Loucks A, Heath E. Induction of low T3 syndrome in exercising women occurs at a threshold of energy availability. Am J Physiol 1994;266:R817–R823.

79. Loucks A, Laughlin G, Mortola J, Girton L, Nelson J, Yen S. Hypothalamic-pituitary-thyroidal function in eumenorrheic and amenorrheic athletes. J Clin Endocrinol Metab 1992;75:514–518.

80. Warren M. The effects of exercise on pubertal progression and reproductive function in girls. J Clin Endocrinol Metab 1980;51:1150–1157.

81. Cheung CC, Thornton JE, Kuijper JL, Weigle DS, Clifton DK, Steiner RA. Leptin is a metabolic gate for the onset of puberty in the female rate. Endocrinol 1997;138:855–858.

82. Kanaley J, Boileau R, Bahr J, Misner, JE, Nelson R. Substrate oxidation and GH response to exercise are independent of menstrual phase and status. Med Sci Sports Exerc 1992;24:873–880.

83. Bunt J, Bahr J, Bemben D. Comparison of estradiol and testosterone levels during the immediately following prolonged exercise in moderately active and trained males and females. Endocr Res 1987;13:157–172.

84. Bunt J. Metabolic actions of estradiol: significance for acute and chronic response. Med Sci Sports Exerc 1990;22:286–290.

85. Mesaki N, Sasaki J, Shoji M. Hormonal changes during incremental exercise in athletic women. Acta Obstet Gynaec Jpn 1986;38:45–52.

86. Mesaki N, Motobu M, Sasaki J. Hypothalamic-pituitary function in female athletes. Jpn J Fertil Steril 1988;33:291–296.

87. Baker E, Mathur R, Kirk R. Plasma gonadotropins, prolactin and steroid hormone concentration in female runners immediately after a long distance run. Fertil Steril 1982;38:38–41.

88. Brisson G, Volle M, DeCaruifel D. Exercise disassociation of the blood prolactin response in young women according to sports habits. Horm Metab Res 1980;12:201–205.

89. Chang F, Dodds W, Sullivan M. The acute effects of exercise on prolactin and growth hormone secretion: comparison between sedentary women and women runners with normal and abnormal menstrual cycles. J Clin Endocrinol Metab 1986;62:551–556.

90. Kanaley J, Boileau R, Bahr J, Misner J, Nelson R. Cortisol levels during prolonged exercise: the influence of menstrual phase and menstrual status. Int J Sports Med 1992;13:100–105.

91. Mesaki N, Sasaki J, Nabeshima Y. Exercise decreases the pulsatile secretion of luteinizing hormone. Jpn J Fertil Steril 1992;37:16–21.

92. Waters DL, Qualls CR, Dorin R, Veldhuis JD, Baumgartner RN. Increased pulsatility, process irregularity, and nocturnal trough concentrations of growth hormone in amenorrheic compared to eumenorrheic athletes. J Clin Endocrinol Metab 2001;86:1013–1019.

93. Ding J, Sheckter C, Drinkwater B, Soules M, Bremmer W. High serum cortisol levels in exercise-associated amenorrhea. Ann Intern Med 1988;108:132–135.

94. Schoene R, Pierson D, Lakshminaragavan S. Effect of medroxyprogesterone acetate on respiratory drives and occlusion pressure. Bull Eur Physiopathol Respir 1980;16:645–653.

95. Nicklas B, Hackney A, Sharp R. The menstrual cycle and exercise: performance, muscle glycogen and substrate responses. Int J Sports Med 1987;10:264–269.

96. Lavoie JM, Dionne N, Helie R. Menstrual cycle phase disassociation of blood glucose homeostasis during exercise. J Appl Physiol 1987;62:1084–1089.

97. Bemden D, Salm P, Salm A. Ventilatory and blood lactate responses to maximal treadmill exercise during the menstrual cycle. J Sports Med Phys Fitness 1995;35:257–262.

98. De Bruyn-Prevost P, Masset C, Sturbois X. Physiological response from 18–25 years of women to aerobic and anaerobic physical fitness tests at different periods during the menstrual cycle. J Sports Med Phys Fitness 1984;24:144–148.

99. Drinkwater B, Nilson K, Ott S, Chesnut C. Bone mineral density after resumption of menses in amenorrheic athletes. JAMA 1986;256:380–382.

100. Pettersson R, Stalnacke B, Ahlenius G, Henriksson-Larsen K, Lorentzon R. Low bone mass density at multiple skeletal sites, including the appendicular skeleton in amenorrheic runners. Calcif Tissue Int 1999;64:117–125.

101. Myerson M, Gutin B, Warren MP, Wang J, Litchman S, Pierson RN. Total body bone density in amenorrheic runners. Obstet Gynecol 1992;79:973–978.

102. Bradley SJ, Taylor MJ, Rover JF, et al. Assessment of brain function in adolescent anorexia nervosa before and after weight gain. J Clin Exp Neuropsychol 1997;19:20–33.

103. Keen AD, Drinkwater BL. Irreversible bone loss in former amenorrheic athletes. Osteoporos Int 1997;7:311–315.

104. Lindberg JS, Powell MR, Hunt MM, Ducey DE, Wade CE. Increased vertebral bone mineral in response to reduced exercise in amenorrheic runners. West J Med 1987;146:39–42.

105. Drinkwater BL, Bruemner B, Chestnut CH. Menstrual history as a determinant of current bone density in young athletes. JAMA 1990;263:545–548.

106. Gibson JH, Mitchell A, Reeve J, Harries MG. Treatment of reduced bone mineral density in athletic amenorrhea: a pilot study. Osteoporos Int 1999;10:284–289.

107. Myburgh K, Hutchins J, Fataar A, Hough S, Noakes T. Low bone density is an etiologic factor for stress fractures in athletes. Ann Intern Med 1990;113:754–759.

108. Warren M, Brooks-Gunn J, Hamilton Lea. Scoliosis and fractures in young ballet dancers. N Engl J Med 1986;314:1348–1353.

109. Henriksson GB, Schnell C, Hirschberg AL. Women endurance runners with menstrual dysfunction have prolonged interruption of training due to injury. Gynecol Obstet Invest 2000;49:41–46.

110. Friday K, Drinkwater B, Bruemmer B, Chestnut III C, Chait A. Elevated plasma low-density lipoprotein and high-density lipoprotein cholesterol levels in amenorrheic athletes: effects of endogenous hormone status and nutrient intake. J Clin Endocrinol Metab 1993:1605–1609.

111. Williams NI, Parfitt DB, Caston-Balderrama A, Cameron JL. Evidence for a causal role of low energy availability in the induction of menstrual cycle disturbances during strenuous exercise training. J Clin Endocrinol Metab 2001;86:5184–5193.

112. Warren M. Health issues for women athletes: exercise-induced amenorrhea. J Clin Endocrinol Metab 1999;84:1892–1896.

113. Kleposki RW. The female athlete triad: a terrible trio. Implications for primary care. J Am Acad Nurse Pract 2002;14:26–31.

SUGGESTED READINGS

1. Arena B, Maffulli N, Maffulli F, Morleo MA. Reproductive hormones and menstrual changes with exercise in female athletes. Sports Med 1995;19(4):278–287.

2. Beim G, Stone DA. Issues in the female athlete. Sports Med 1995;26(3):443–451.

3. DeCree C. Sex steroid metabolism and menstrual irregularities in the exercising female: a review. Sports Med 1998;25(6):369–406.

4. Chen EC, Brzyski RG. Exercise and reproductive dysfunction. J Fertil Steril 1999;71(1):1–8.

5. Chrousos GP, Torpy DJ, Philip W. Gold. Interactions between the hypothalamic-pituitary-adrenal axis and the female reproductive system: clinical implications. Ann Intern Med 1998;129:229–240.

6. Loucks AB, Verun M, Heath EM. Low energy availability, not the stress of exercise, alters LH pulsatility in exercising women. J Appl Physiol 1998;84(1):37–46.

7. Williams NI, Helmreich DL, Parfitt DB, Caston-Balderrama A, Cameron JL. Evidence for a causal role of low energy availability in the induction of menstrual cycle disturbances during strenuous exercise training. J Clin Endocrinol Metab 2001;86:5184–5193.

8. Yen SSC. Effects of lifestyle and body composition on the ovary. Endocrinol Metab Clin North Am 1998;27:915–926.

Pediatric Obesity

Linda M. LeMura

Overview

Pediatric **obesity** has increased to epidemic proportions in the United States, with 20% to 30% of children and adolescents now classified as clinically obese, an increase of over 20% in the past decade (1). The environmental conditions and the typical lifestyle of technologically developed countries, particularly the reduction of **physical activity**, have contributed to the development of this epidemic. Fortunately, the numbers of affected children and the resulting concerns expressed by the medical community have sparked increasing research on the etiology, diagnosis, treatment, and prevention of pediatric obesity. However, a complete understanding of the root causes and proper treatment of this major public health problem remains elusive.

It is imperative that the evaluation of obesity occurs early in childhood, for several reasons. First, obesity tends to "track" throughout life; its presence at any age increases the risk of persistence in adulthood. Second, it is necessary to rule out endocrine or genetic causes of obesity (e.g., hypothyroidism or Turner's syndrome). Third, an early diagnosis is the best hope for preventing the numerous disease progressions that can occur in adulthood as a consequence of obesity (2). Specifically, obesity is associated with significant **morbidity**, including cardiovascular disease, hypertension, **hyperlipidemia**, **type 2 diabetes**, **hyperuricemia**, respiratory disorders, orthopaedic problems, and some forms of cancer (particularly colon and breast cancer) (3). Furthermore, the negative impact of obesity on a child's self-esteem may have significant implications for happiness and success in later life.

The most recent data obtained from the National Health and Nutrition Examination Survey (NHANES III) provides large-scale epidemiologic evidence that pediatric obesity is increasing at an alarming rate across all racial and ethnic groups (4). The definition of pediatric obesity and severe obesity varies by source, and no single definition has been generally accepted; suggested criteria are summarized in Table 24.1 Regardless of the definition used, the trends for pediatric obesity are not encouraging (5).

Pathophysiology of Pediatric Obesity

In the simplest terms, a person gains weight when energy input (caloric intake) exceeds energy output, thereby creating a positive energy balance. Interestingly, investigators have reported that obese children do not necessarily consume significantly more calories than their thin counterparts; rather, it is their energy expenditure that is often deficient (6). Energy output is composed of the **basal metabolic rate** (the minimal level of energy required to sustain the body's vital functions in the waking state), the **thermal effect of food** (the energy-requiring processes of digesting, absorbing, and assimilating food nutrients), and physical activity. Of these 3 output factors, physical activity is the least affected by genetic influences, and therefore the most susceptible to alteration. Since 3,500 **kilocalories**

| BOX 24.1. **Relevant Statistics** |

Did You Know?

- Obese children *under* 3 years of age (without obese parents) are at low risk for obesity in adulthood. But among older children, obesity is an increasingly important predictor of adult obesity (regardless of whether both parents are obese) (8).
- Parental obesity *more than doubles* the risk of adult obesity among both obese and nonobese children less than 10 years of age (8).
- After a child reaches age 6, the probability that obesity persists exceeds 50% (8).
- The probability that obese adolescents will become obese adults is 70% to 80% (9).
- Roughly 25% to 35% of the cases of pediatric obesity occur in families of *normal weight parents* (10).
- Recent studies combining measurements of individuals' BMI with information obtained from parents and siblings indicate that the genetic contribution to obesity ranges from 25% to 40% (10).

(kcal), equal to14,700 kilojoules (kJ), is equivalent to 1 pound (lb) or 2.2 kilograms (kg), an excess of only 100 kcal (420 kJ) per day can result in a weight gain of 10 lb in a single year. (The international standard for expressing energy is the kilojoule; to convert kilocalories to kilojoules, multiply the kilocalorie value by 4.2.) Obviously, even a small imbalance between energy input and output can potentially result in a serious weight gain over time. Recent research confirms that most obese children demonstrate slow, consistent weight gain during childhood (7). The relative risk of and the genetic contribution to obesity are summarized in Table 24.2.

It is a gross simplification to state that excess body fat can be explained entirely by energy input versus energy output; in fact, it is a complex, multifactorial problem (Box 24.1) (8, 9). Obesity emerges from the interaction of molecular, cellular, physiological, metabolic, social, and behavioral influences. For example, it is well established that obesity runs in families. However, the **familial aggre-**

TABLE 24.1. DEFINITIONS OF OBESITY AND SEVERE OBESITY

Index	Obesity	Severe Obesity	Relevant Information
1. 0 weight for height	>120 percent	>140 percent	Weight is 20% or more above the 0 weight for children of this height
2. Weight for Height	>85 percentile	>95 percentile	See available reference charts; but do do not consider body fat vs. lean mass
3. Triceps Skin fold	>85 percentile	>95 percentile	Direct measurement of subcutaneous fat
4. Body Mass Index (BMI) (kg/m^2)	>85 percentile	>95 percentile	Percentiles are age and gender specific
5. Ponderal Index (PI) (kg/m^3)	>85 percentile	>95 percentile	Percentiles are age and gender specific

0 = mean
Adapted with permission from Williams CL, Campanaro LA, Squillace M, Bollella M (5).

gation (characteristics affecting more members of the same family than can be accounted for by chance) cannot be fully accounted for by shared environmental conditions, and is actually more consistent with the notion that affected relatives share specific genetic characteristics. This has been demonstrated in studies of twins reared together and apart, adoptees and their biologic and adoptive parents, and large cohorts of nuclear families (10).

The genes and **mutations** responsible for the individual's susceptibility to a persistently positive energy balance and consequent enhanced fat storage have not yet been identified, but the number of genetic markers is increasing steadily. Whatever the influences of the identified genes, they may be attenuated or exacerbated by nongenetic factors. Specifically, body fat is altered during one's lifetime by numerous genetically controlled environmental interactions. These interactions vary among individuals because of changing environments or lifestyles. Factors that influence gene-environment interactions include a high-fat diet, a low level of habitual physical activity, a low resting metabolic rate for a given body mass and body composition, a high **respiratory quotient** in the resting state (i.e., a tendency to oxidize more carbohydrates than lipids under standardized conditions), high insulin sensitivity, and perhaps many others. In addition, the fat distribution pattern is an inherited characteristic governed by the regional activity of the rate-limiting enzyme lipoprotein lipase (LPL). This enzyme facilitates triglyceride storage by the fat cell or adipocyte (11). Any variation in LPL will contribute to differences in fat distribution, as well as changes in fat patterns that occur during pregnancy and in middle age.

All of the contributory causes of pediatric obesity must be explored, because the nature of its origin will dictate treatment. Only a relatively small percentage (approximately 10%) of obesity is associated with a hormonal or genetic defect; the most common **endogenous** causes of pediatric obesity are summarized in Table 24.2. An endogenous cause for obesity can usually be verified or eliminated in most children after obtaining a detailed family history and a physical examination. Additionally, psychological problems and medication patterns should be reviewed to determine potential causes.

Differentiating **exogenous** pediatric obesity (which accounts for 90% of cases) from the less common endocrine and genetic causes requires recognition of the key features of both conditions (12) (Figure 24.1). For example, children with genetic forms of obesity typically are shorter than average (less than the 5th percentile for height) and may have a low intelligence quotient (IQ). Other physical defects (e.g., skeletal abnormalities) may be noticed upon physical examination, and family members are unlikely to be obese. In contrast, children with exogenous obesity generally have a normal IQ, tend to be tall (greater than the 50th percentile), and have physical examinations that are normal. (13).

TABLE 24.2. ENDOGENOUS CAUSES OF CHILDHOOD OBESITY

Hormonal Causes	Diagnostic Evidence
1. Hypothyroidism	↑ TSH, ↓ thyroxine (T_4) levels
2. Hypercortisolism (Cushing's syndrome)	Abnormal dexamethasone suppression test; ↑ 24-hour free urinary cortisol level
3. Primary hyperinsulinism	↑ plasma insulin
4. Pseudohypoparathyroidism	Hypocalcemia, hyperphosphatemia; ↑ PTH levels
5. Acquired hypothalamic	Presence of hypothalamic tumor; infection; trauma; vascular lesion

Genetic Syndromes	Characteristics
1. Prader-Willi	Obesity, insatiable appetite, mental retardation, hypogonadism, strabismus
2. Laurence-Moon/Bardet-Biedl	Obesity, mental retardation, hypogonadism, spastic paraplegia
3. Alstrom	Obesity, deafness, diabetes mellitus
4. Börjeson-Forssman-Lehman	Obesity, mental retardation, hypogonadism, hypometabolism, epilepsy
5. Cohen	Truncal obesity, mental retardation, hypogonadism
6. Turner's	Short stature, cardiac abnormalities, webbed neck, undifferentiated gonads
7. Familial lipodystrophy	Muscular hypertrophy, acromegalic appearance, insulin resistance, hypertriglyceridemia, mental retardation
8. Beckwith-Wiedemann	Gigantism, exomphalos, visceromegaly
9. Sotos'	Cerebral gigantism, physical overgrowth, hypotonia, delayed motor and cognitive development
10. Weaver	Infant overgrowth syndrome, accelerated skeletal maturation
11. Ruvalcaba	Mental retardation, microcephaly, skeletal abnormalities, hypogonadism

Gene Associations

Leptin
Beta$_3$ adrenergic receptor

TSH = thyroid-stimulating hormone; PTH = parathyroid hormone
Adapted from Moran R (7).

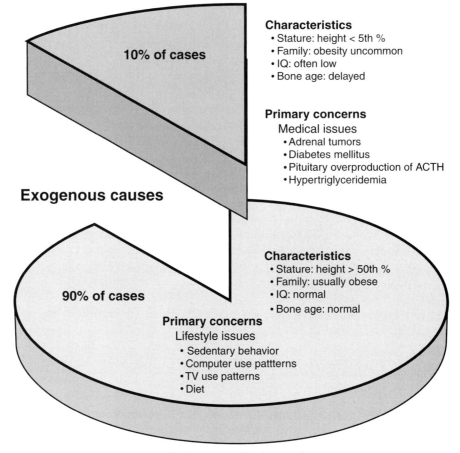

Characteristics
- Stature: height < 5th %
- Family: obesity uncommon
- IQ: often low
- Bone age: delayed

Primary concerns
Medical issues
- Adrenal tumors
- Diabetes mellitus
- Pituitary overproduction of ACTH
- Hypertriglyceridemia

10% of cases

Exogenous causes

90% of cases

Characteristics
- Stature: height > 50th %
- Family: usually obese
- IQ: normal
- Bone age: normal

Primary concerns
Lifestyle issues
- Sedentary behavior
- Computer use pattterns
- TV use patterns
- Diet

FIGURE 24.1. The diagnosis of pediatric obesity.

Measurement of Body Composition

Several criterion laboratory methods are available for evaluating body composition in children. Typically, either fat mass (FM) or fat-free mass (FFM) is measured, and the other value is then calculated by subtraction from total body weight. Although **hydrodensitometry** (underwater weighing) is considered the reference method for the determination of body fat in adults, its suitability for use in young children has been questioned (13, 14). An alternative for analyzing pediatric body composition is **dual x-ray absorptiometry** (DEXA). This technique is increasingly popular for the measurements of FM, FFM, and body fat percentage in children because it uses a low radiation dose, requires minimal subject cooperation, and has demonstrated high reliability (15). However, the cost is a major limitation. Other established methods include **magnetic resonance imaging** (MRI) and **total body potassium concentration** (TBP). Although all of these methods are available for the determination of pediatric body composition for basic and clinical research, measurements are often needed in field settings (i.e., physicians' offices and large-scale epidemiologic studies). Available field-measurement

techniques include skinfold thickness and **bioelectric impedance analysis** (BIA). However, although these methods provide a reasonable estimate of body composition in the field setting, they do compromise some accuracy when compared to the criterion laboratory methods (16).

Currently, the most commonly used measure of fatness among adults is the **body mass index** (BMI), expressed in kilograms (kg) per square meter (kg/m_2). The advantages of using the BMI are numerous:

- It is completely safe for the subject;
- The measurement is inexpensive and easy to calculate in the clinical setting;
- It correlates with subcutaneous fat and FM; and
- It yields statistical properties well suited for pediatric screening (17, 18).

A recent investigation comparing the use of BMI and DEXA in children validated BMI as a measure of adiposity (18). The results of the study confirmed that a strong correlation exists between BMI and fatness in both girls and boys. In addition, the BMI may serve as a surrogate marker of fatness in epidemiologic studies. Children with progressive obesity who cross into higher percentiles of the BMI run a significant risk of obesity in adulthood (10, 18); it would therefore be clinically useful to follow a child's BMI, in addition to height and weight, over time. These data would identify potential problems and highlight the need for intervention. Table 24.3 provides age-specific, normative data for BMI in U.S. children.

The Maximal Exercise Test

Evaluation of the obese child may include a maximal exercise test. This test has an important role in the management of therapeutic exercise prescribed for intervention. The objectives of the exercise test include development of an appropriate exercise prescription, and in some cases, disease diagnosis. A critical outcome of the maximal exercise test is the establishment of effective, accurate exercise intensity for the obese child; essential to this objective is the measurement of the **peak aerobic capacity** ($\dot{V}O_2$peak). The $\dot{V}O_2$peak is selected, rather than the frequently used $\dot{V}O_{2max}$ (the criterion measure for a "true maximal" aerobic capacity in adults), because the plateau effect is atypical in children (19). Other assessments that may prove useful include the following:

- Medical history,
- Nutritional assessment,
- Patterns of eating, and
- Body composition assessment.

Pretest Considerations

Pretest preparation requires special care and attention for the obese child. It is important to instill confidence in children in general; however, the need to assure the obese child that he or she can successfully complete the test is particularly acute. The typical pretest "jitters" will be magnified in obese children who often do not experience success in exercise-related activities. In addition, the normal preparation that occurs with the maximal exercise test may be embarrassing to some children who fear revealing any part of their bodies. Every effort must be made to make the child feel as confident and comfortable as possible.

Other important pretest considerations regard technical issues. For example, special care must be taken to ensure that the proper cuff size is used to measure blood pressure (BP). A cuff that is too small may result in falsely elevated readings (7). Proper electrode placement for electrocardiograph (ECG) monitoring is also important. Placing the leg ECG electrodes near the right and left inferior rib margins, between the midclavicular and anterior axillary line (rather than at a lower position), can significantly reduce signal artifact (20).

Evaluation of Peak Aerobic Capacity: Which Protocol Is Best?

The data generated from maximal exercise tests provide important information about cardiovascular function. The measure commonly reported for this value is the absolute $\dot{V}O_2$peak (L/min), but difficulty arises in normalizing absolute $\dot{V}O_2$peak for growth during the pediatric years. Typically, this is achieved by obtaining the relative measure of $\dot{V}O_2$peak to body weight (ml/kg/min). However, relative $\dot{V}O_2$peak is also an indicator of the body's ability to move excess body fat in a weight-bearing activity, such as treadmill exercise. Thus, if the value of $\dot{V}O_2$peak derived from an exercise test is used to assess cardiovascular function, relative $\dot{V}O_2$peak falsely elevates values for slender individuals and depresses values for those who are obese. In short, absolute $\dot{V}O_2$peak is the preferable measure of cardiovascular function, whereas relative $\dot{V}O_2$peak provides an index of performance capabilities (21).

From a therapeutic standpoint, the distinctions between relative and absolute measures of $\dot{V}O_2$peak are important because the program for improving cardiopulmonary fitness (**exercise training**) is different from that for reducing body fat (diet and increased physical activity). In other words, using poor running performance (i.e., if a treadmill test is chosen) as the basis for an interpretation of poor cardiorespiratory fitness in an obese child may be misleading, because the problem may be poor running economy as a result of over-fatness (22).

This leads to questions regarding the nature of which apparatus (cycle ergometer versus treadmill) and testing protocols are most appropriate for obese children. There is no single best protocol or apparatus that will meet the needs of all clinicians and researchers. Furthermore, arguments can be made regarding the advantages and disadvantages of various ergometers, the use of the treadmill, and choice of protocols. It is well established that treadmill exercise places greater physiological stress on the cardiovascular system in comparison to cycle exercise. Maximal or peak oxygen con-

TABLE 24.3. BODY MASS INDEX (BMI) BY AGE AND GENDER FOR SELECTED PERCENTILES

Age (y)	50th M	50th F	85th M	85th F	95th M	95th F
6	15.4	15.2	16.8	17.1	18.2	18.5
7	15.6	15.4	17.1	17.6	18.9	19.6
8	16.0	15.9	18.1	18.6	20.2	21.1
9	16.2	16.3	19.0	19.5	22.4	22.9
10	16.5	16.9	19.2	20.6	21.8	23.6
11	17.2	17.5	20.9	21.7	24.2	24.8
12	17.8	18.6	21.4	22.6	24.1	26.2
13	18.7	19.4	22.6	23.4	26.6	26.8
14	19.6	20.2	23.2	24.1	26.7	26.5
15	20.4	20.7	24.0	24.7	27.8	29.4
16	20.8	20.9	24.0	24.9	26.9	29.6
17	21.5	21.0	24.9	24.3	28.5	29.3

Adapted from Rowland TW (16).

sumption values derived from treadmill protocols (e.g., Bruce and modified Balke) are approximately 10% higher on the treadmill than on the cycle, a difference that has been documented in both adults (23) and children (24). This discrepancy in $\dot{V}O_{2max}$ values is explained by the fact that cycling involves less muscle mass than running, and that a significant increase in local muscle fatigue limits maximal performance during cycling. In addition, cycle exercise results in significantly higher **respiratory exchange ratio** (RER) and lactate levels, both indicators of anaerobic work.

However, studies have reported that healthy children are more comfortable on the cycle ergometer than the treadmill (21,24). In addition, many children are reluctant to adjust to treadmill belt motion. Preference for the cycle ergometer is especially apparent when the subject's stability and anxiety are concerns. Given the limited influence of body weight during cycle exercise, obese children are best tested with cycle protocols. One disadvantage of cycle ergometry is that very young, poorly fit, and obese subjects may have difficulty sustaining the proper pedal rate for the duration of the test. With mechanically braked cycle ergometers, the work rate depends upon the subject pedaling at a constant rate. The pace can be better controlled by using an electronically braked bike. The optimal cycle protocol provides for uniform submaximal stages that are of sufficient duration to obtain steady-state data and physiologic measurements, yet short enough to avoid boredom. The load increments need to be appropriate for body size. A good example is the McMaster protocol (21), with 2-minute stages and loads related to body height (Table 24.4) (25, 26)

Although children indicate a clear preference for cycle ergometry, either the ergometer or the treadmill may be used successfully to test obese children (21). The decision regarding the optimum test apparatus and protocol should consider the subject's fitness level, age, and comfort level with testing procedures, and the physiologic measurements desired. Researchers and clinicians should attempt to satisfy as many of the pediatric exercise testing guidelines as possible (Box 24.2).

TABLE 24.4. THE McMASTER PROTOCOL

Rate (rpm)	Body Measure	Initial Load	Increment	Stage Duration
50	**Height (cm)**	**Watts (W)**	**W**	**Minutes**
	<120	12.5	12.5	2
	120–140	12.5	12.5	2
	140–160	25	25	2
	>160	25	50 (male) 25 (female)	2

Note: Optimal testing conditions include: crank arm length of 13 cm in 6-year-olds and 15 cm in 8- to 10-year-olds; pedal rate = 50 rpm; saddle height should be adjusted to create a knee angle of 160° when the leg is extended (25, 26).

BOX 24.2. Summary of Test Protocol Guidelines

1. The exercise test should not be too long. Boredom, decreased motivation, and an insufficient effort are associated with long tests. On the other hand, a short, overly intense test may be unsafe for children with cardiovascular disease. The ideal test duration is 8 to 12 minutes.

2. The exercise test should be uniform in terms of submaximal stages and work increment. Treadmill protocols should not include overly steep steps and excessively high speeds. If the child feels compelled to hold the handrails, the test is most likely inappropriate.

3. The exercise test protocol should allow for the determination of various physiologic measurements (e.g., blood pressure and cardiac output).

4. The exercise test should evaluate cardiovascular function rather than local muscular fatigue.

5. The exercise test should be safe and adaptable to all children regardless of age, fitness, and body composition.

Adapted from Rowland, TW. Pediatric Exercise Testing. Champaign, Ill: Human Kinetics Press, 1993 (21).

Exercise Responses

The research literature on maximal exercise responses in the obese child reveals agreement on some metabolic variables, but inconsistent results on some physiologic and hemodynamic variables; research is wholly lacking on some variables. Table 24.5 summarizes what we know about maximal exercise responses in the obese versus nonobese child (27–37). Based upon the available data, obese children (i.e., 85th percentile for BMI) do not usually generate significantly different physiologic responses than their lean counterparts (20). Whether this holds true for the severely obese child (≥95th percentile for BMI) requires further investigation. The comments included in the table reflect the interpretation of existing data by researchers and clinicians.

Exercise Training Options

If the physiologic and metabolic responses of the maximal exercise test are within normal ranges, and if a physical examination excludes endogenous causes of obesity, the next logical step is to establish reasonable and attainable goals for the child. The amount of weight that should be lost can be determined by data derived from body composition assessment, or through the use of the BMI. Although it is possible to lose body fat by reducing caloric intake, there are numerous compelling reasons to combine caloric reduction with increased energy expenditure through enhanced physical activity. Examples include enhanced self-esteem, increased aerobic fitness, and a reduction in risk factors for cardiovascular disease (10). In fact, the most successful fat

TABLE 24.5. EXPECTED MAXIMAL RESPONSES IN THE OBESE VERSUS NONOBESE CHILD

Variable (Reference Numbers)	Obese Child (O)	Nonobese Child (NO)	Comments
Heart rate (HR) (27, 28)	HR: 200 bpm on TM HR: 195 bpm on CE; HR ↑ vs. NO	HR: 200 bpm on TM HR: 195 bpm on CE	Data remain conflicting
Systolic blood pressure (SBP) (29, 30)	+ correlation with body fat and BSA; no differences with NO	Normal responses: (SBP rarely exceeds 200 mm Hg)	Data remain conflicting
Diastolic pressure (DBP) (20)	?	?	"Difficult to measure and interpret"
Cardiac output (Q) (20, 31)	No differences with NO; Q is ↑ in O	Normal responses	Comparative studies needed
Electrocardiograph responses (20, 32)	*Paucity of data	Normal responses	Data remain inconclusive
V̇o₂ peak ml/kg/min vs. L/min (10, 28, 33)	TM test: ml/kg/min ↓ vs. NO, but in L/min, no difference	CE test: ml/kg/min ↑ vs. NO, but in L/min, no difference	Data are in good agreement
Ventilatory anaerobic threshold (VAT) (20, 22, 27)	VAT occurs at ↓ V̇o₂ peak ml/kg/min vs. NO	VAT occurs at ↑ V̇o₂ peak ml/kg/min vs. O	Data in good agreement, but more research required

↑ = increase; ↓ = decrease; + = positive; *indicates the use of normal pediatric testing guidelines in the obese child, i.e., ST segment depression (J-point depression ≥2 mm and an ST depression >1 mm with a flat or down-sloping ST segment at 60 msec) and test termination guidelines (ST segment depression or elevation >3 mm; significant arrhythmia precipitated by the exercise test.

TM = treadmill; CE = cycle ergometer; BSA = body surface area.

reduction programs are those that include diet and exercise combined with behavior modification (5, 7, 10).

Currently, no data are available that provide the optimal dose of physical activity for the obese child. However, researchers suggest a program of gradually increased activity over a prolonged period. Overwhelming the child with unattainable goals (attempting to accomplish too much, too soon) may cause the child to become discouraged and lose the resolve to continue the program, and even result in orthopaedic distress. The general guidelines for an exercise prescription must consider the appropriate type, intensity, frequency, and duration of exercise. The well-considered exercise prescription optimizes energy expenditure, yet minimizes the potential for injury.

Finally, motivational aspects are paramount in developing an exercise program for obese children; they often lack confidence in their ability and may feel inhibited when asked to exercise in front of others. Thus, an additional goal of the exercise program should be to strengthen self-confidence. This requires tailoring the program to the child's capabilities; to encourage adherence, it is equally essential that the activities are enjoyable. Reasonable examples of exercise prescription options are provided in Box 24.3.

Exercise is the single most flexible component of the energy balance equation. A 35-kg child whose energy expenditure is 2 kcal/day (8.4 kJ/day) can increase it by approximately 10% to 15% through 40 to 50 minutes of aerobic activities. This increase can result in 1 kg of fat loss in 1 month. Ideally, exercise is chosen that entails a high energy output, emphasizing the quantity of exercise rather than intensity. When designing an exercise prescription for the obese child, it is important to remember special considera-

BOX 24.3. Exercise Prescription Options

Mode
- Non-weight-bearing activities are preferable (swimming, water aerobics, cycling)
- Walking
- Resistance exercise (free weights, resistance machines) to increase FFM. (Emphasis should be placed on high repetitions.)
- Cross-training: Alternating the type of activities (e.g., aerobic exercise and resistance exercise). The combination not only stresses different organ and energy systems, it is an effective method to reduce boredom

Frequency
- Preferably daily, or a minimum of 5 times per week

Duration
- 10 minutes, several times per day (exercise must fit into the child's lifestyle), with a goal directed toward:
- 20 minutes twice per day, or
- 45 minutes per day

Intensity
- 50–60% of V̇o₂peak or HR peak

Special Considerations
- Gradual progression of intensity and duration
- Low-impact or non-weight-bearing activities are preferred
- Encourage exercise in thermoneutral environments
- Wear loose-fitting clothing
- Encourage an adequate warm up and cool down

tions (i.e., age, body mass); do not merely adopt adult exercise programs.

Dietary Intervention and Behavior Modification

It is vital that dietary programs used in weight management for obese children include the requirements necessary for optimal growth and health maintenance. Assessment of the child's and family's diet will assist in the development of an appropriate dietary prescription, as well as the need for nutrition education. A nutrition specialist may recommend the use of a food diary (recorded by the child or parents) that will provide a quantitative assessment of caloric intake when analyzed by a variety of software programs.

However, a thorough assessment should also include a qualitative analysis that answers the following questions (5, 7):

- Where is food eaten?
- What time of day?
- Who is present when eating?
- Does the family eat together?
- Who prepares the meals?
- Does the family appear to eat a high-fat diet?
- How often does the family eat out (particularly at fast-food restaurants)?
- Does the child pack lunch or buy it at school?
- How many fruits and vegetables does the child eat daily?
- What are the typical snacks?
- Are more calories consumed on snacks versus meals?

Eating pattern data such as these are integral to the development of a behavior modification program. Stimulus control, for example, is a frequently successful strategy that involves limiting the amount of high-calorie foods in the home (7). Every effort must be made to avoid situations where overeating might occur, such as in front of the television or while doing homework. The child should eat meals at the designated time and in the designated area. Finally, parents should respect the child's sense of satiety and should not force him or her to clean the plate before leaving the table.

The ideal pace for weight loss is approximately 1 kg (2.2 pounds) per week. The 14,700 kJ (3500 kcal) that must be eliminated to accomplish this goal should be achieved through a combination of decreased caloric intake (diet) and increased caloric expenditure (exercise). The rationale for this combination is directly related to the metabolic consequences of dieting. In essence, reducing caloric intake may result in a loss of lean body mass; this in turn decreases the BMR, and a depressed BMR makes it harder to lose weight (7, 10, 15). In some cases, it may be appropriate to increase protein intake slightly during caloric restriction to avoid a negative protein balance and the consequent loss of

lean body mass. But by increasing physical activity, BMR is increased and FFM is increased or at least preserved. Furthermore, exercise may cause the BMR to remain elevated for a long period after the cessation of activity, providing an additional mechanism for caloric expenditure.

Implementing the dietary component of the weight reduction program requires knowledge of portion size and permissible food exchanges; these are explained in detail in the Exchange Lists for Weight Management (34). It is essential that parents receive specific recommendations regarding daily caloric intake that follow the guidelines for the percentages of protein, fat, and carbohydrate. A comprehensive nutrition education program should emphasize the following (5):

- A healthy balanced diet is essential for children over 2 years of age;
- Fat calories should not exceed 30% of the total caloric intake;
- Protein should constitute 20% of the diet;
- The remainder of the caloric intake should come from carbohydrates;
- Low caloric density is preferable (i.e., 1 gram of fat produces 37.7 kJ (9 kcal), but 1 gram of carbohydrate and protein each produce only 16.8 kJ (4 kcal).

One effective dietary strategy is the inclusion of dietary fiber, which displaces fat and (as a consequence) reduces caloric density. Fiber promotes a feeling of satiety, slows down digestion, and delays gastric emptying (5, 7). The recommended daily allowance of fiber is equivalent to the child's age, plus an additional 5 to 10 grams per day. A list of high-fiber foods is easily obtainable from a nutrition specialist or pediatrician.

Alternative Therapy: Medications

Currently, there are no anorectic (causing lack of appetite) medications approved by the U.S. Food and Drug Administration for use in children. Surgical procedures such as the gastric bypass have not been sufficiently researched to advise their use as a potential weight loss option in obese children.

Mechanisms of Weight Loss: The Role of Energy Expenditure

Although a reduction in physical activity and increased time spent in sedentary activities (e.g., television and computer games) are implicated as causal factors in childhood weight gain, the etiology of obesity remains elusive. Intuitively, we expect to explain the mechanism of obesity (in part) through energy expenditure; however, data on the regulation of energy expenditure in children are lacking.

It is known that **total energy expenditure** (TEE) consists of 3 components: BMR; the **thermic effect of food** (TEF), or internal work; and the energy expended in physical activity, or external work (35, 36). Internal work is determined by the energy necessary for maintenance of body functions and varies with body composition. The amount of between-subject variation in BMR has been calculated as ranging from 60% to 80% (37). It is also likely that differences in FFM (i.e., primarily the amount of skeletal muscle) and genetic factors directly affect the BMR. Because FFM is metabolically active in comparison to fat, there exists a strong positive correlation between FFM and BMR. It is now well established that changes in body composition will alter BMR. Specifically, weight loss in the absence of physical activity reduces BMR, and the reduction is directly proportional to the amount of lost FFM. In contrast, weight gain increases BMR, and the increase is directly proportional to the amount of FFM gained. For this reason, resistance training consisting of high repetitions with light weights (which may preserve or increase FFM) may be an effective training option for older children and adolescents (38).

The TEE is defined as the total amount of physical activity or external work performed by the body. Various techniques (direct or indirect) for measuring TEE in children have been described in the literature. For example, a direct evaluation of physical activity is the study of simple movements. This method would provide an index of movement rather than an estimation of energy expenditure. Other methods include recording physiological variables (e.g., heart rate [HR]) and using physiological markers (which are more complex and expensive), such as direct or indirect calorimetry and oxygen consumption. Kinematic analysis is very valuable, but also is limited by the expense. **Accelerometry** has been validated in the pediatric literature; however, the evidence to date suggests that **triaxial accelerometers**, which measure three-dimensional movement, provide a better estimate of physical activity or energy expenditure than a **single-plane accelerometer**, which measures vertical movement only (39). Accelerometry has been used as an effective measurement tool in epidemiologic research. Questionnaires have emerged as a common measurement tool because they are simple, less expensive, and require little analytical equipment. More recently, the determination of the caloric cost of physical activity in both laboratory and field studies has been made possible with the application of the **doubly labeled water** technique. It is currently the "gold standard" for assessing energy expenditure, and is used as the criterion for validating more practical approaches (36, 37).

The quantity of physical activity may certainly vary greatly between children; however, it also varies within the same child over time in response to changes in chronic exercise patterns, or in response to changes in spontaneous daily movements. Some of the variation in TEE can be explained by fitness and body weight, but the largest source of variation in energy requirements remains the total quantity of physical activity. In fact, one of the few studies on this topic reported that FFM, BMR, and HR (which are directly

related to physical activity) explained 86% of the interindividual variation in TEE in children (35). To enhance fat loss, one must force the establishment of new energy requirements by changing the factors associated with energy expenditure and nutrient balance. Physical activity is the best way to effect these changes.

It has been documented that healthy, nonobese children generate low TEE values primarily because they engage in low amounts of physical activity. In other words, although children may appear to be physically active, they do not engage in high-intensity exercise for sufficiently long periods of time to significantly alter TEE. In fact, the energy cost of playing is less than a slow walk for equivalent time periods (40). In one of the rare comparative analyses of TEE and patterns of physical activity in obese and nonobese children, it was revealed that obese children actually had a higher TEE than nonobese children despite being excessively sedentary (41). This was explained (in part) by the hypothesis that 50% of excess weight in obese children is actually FFM needed to support excess weight. This paradox was further explained by the higher energy cost to perform weight-bearing activities and a higher absolute BMR in obese children (42).

Of course it must be noted that the dietary composition alters the efficiency of how the body converts and stores excess fat. Roughly 3% of the calories in ingested fat are required to convert the calories into body fat. In contrast, 25% of the calories in carbohydrate are oxidized in the fat conversion process. It is biochemically far easier to synthesize body fat from dietary lipids than from equivalent carbohydrate calories (43). Therefore, in the event of caloric excess, additional carbohydrate would result in a smaller deposition of body fat.

Finally, the net effect of physical activity on the oxidation rates of carbohydrate, protein, and fat in obese children is unclear. Although there are substantial data about RER during exercise, few data are available on the effects of varying the intensity, duration, and types of exercise on 24-hour substrate oxidation in children. For example, while carbohydrate oxidation may be the primary energy substrate during weight training (resulting in an elevated RER), it is possible that fat oxidation may increase well after the activity (thereby lowering RER). This may be a consequence of the more effective use of available carbohydrate for the restoration of glycogen stores (42). This information could directly impact the exercise prescription developed for an obese child.

Physiologic Adaptations and Mechanisms After Training

It has been proposed that the spontaneous daily habits of children control peak or maximal aerobic capacity and subsequently the risk for cardiovascular disease; thus, additional exercise training would have little or no effect on improving these variables (44). But, as previously mentioned, the short duration of sustained heart rates during daily physical activity fails to produce a significant relationship between patterns of physical activity and $\dot{V}O_2$peak, and its associated determinants (i.e., **cardiac output** and the **arteriovenous oxygen difference**). The most recent research investigating the relationship between physical activity and $\dot{V}O_2$peak clearly revealed that chronic exercise training, not daily physical activity, promotes the adaptations normally experienced by endurance-trained individuals (24, 37).

Few data are available to explain the mechanisms responsible for adaptive changes after exercise in the obese child. It is known that aerobic training induces nonspecific changes in the obese child, such as an increase in peak aerobic capacity ($\dot{V}O_2$peak), a decrease in resting and submaximal heart rate, and in submaximal **minute ventilation** ($\dot{V}_E$) (21, 24). But changes in body fat after short-term training (2–3 months) are typically small and often do not persist after the conclusion of the training period. The impact of longer exercise programs on obese children remains unclear. It is well known, however, that regular training has an anabolic effect on muscle protein metabolism, thereby increasing FFM. This anabolic effect is essential for children because growth requires a positive nitrogen balance (5).

Exercise training also induces several important biochemical changes in obese children, particularly in regard to plasma insulin concentration, which is usually increased in obesity. Regular exercise causes a decrease in plasma insulin concentration, an increase in receptor sensitivity to insulin, and improved glucose tolerance (45). There is also evidence to suggest that alterations in the lipoprotein-lipid profile in obese children are possible as a consequence of exercise training. For example, a decrease in serum triglycerides (TG), an increase in high-density lipoprotein (HDL), and a decrease in low-density lipoprotein (LDL) have been reported (46). Other studies, however, have reported inconsistent or no changes in lipoprotein fractions and subfractions (47–49). Additional research is needed to determine the dose of exercise required to elicit favorable changes, as well as the long-term effects on the lipid-lipoprotein after exercise intervention programs have ended.

With regard to hemodynamic changes, exercise training has been demonstrated to decrease both systolic and diastolic blood pressure by as much as 11 to 16 mm Hg in obese children. When exercise training was performed in conjunction with dietary and behavior modification, the reduction in blood pressure was even greater (50). Another study reported that a 1-year exercise program resulted in an increase in **left ventricular end-diastolic dimension** as a consequence of volume overload hypertrophy. Upon additional study of their data, it was revealed that there was no increase in left ventricular wall thickness (51). Hence the investigators postulated that the increase in end-diastolic dimension occurred because of increased diastolic filling, resulting from exercise-induced **bradycardia**. The effects of exercise training that are specific to the obese child are summarized in Table 24.6 (45).

TABLE 24.6. TRAINING ADAPTATIONS IN THE OBESE CHILD

Parameter	Effects of Physical Training
Body Composition	
Body weight	nc/ ↓
% body fat	↓
Fat-free mass	↑
Appetite	?
Biochemical Changes	
Plasma insulin	↓
Sensitivity to insulin	↑
Glucose tolerance	↑
Free fatty acid mobilization	↑
Low-density lipoprotein	↓
Serum triglycerides	↓
Total cholesterol	nc/ ↓
High-density lipoprotein	↑
Hemodynamic Changes	
Systolic and diastolic blood pressure	↓
Energy Expenditure	
Resting (basal metabolic rate)	Reverses reduction by diet/ ↑
Energy expenditure after exercise	Remains ↑

↓ = decrease; ↑ = increase; nc = no change; ? = still unclear
Adapted from Bar-Or O (45).

The Molecular Basis for Obesity

The frenetic pace of research directed toward the identification of physiologic mechanisms that underlie disease has resulted in a better understanding of the effects and causes of obesity. For example, the molecular mechanism that links obesity and diabetes has been elusive. Recently, researchers have discovered a hormone secreted by fat cells that counteracts insulin (52). The hormone, dubbed resistin (for resistance to insulin), caused poor glucose regulation in mice; but a combination of antidiabetic drugs and antibodies neutralized resistin. The end result was an insulin-stimulated glucose uptake by adipocytes, demonstrating the potential of resistin to form at least part of the link between obesity and diabetes in humans. Two exciting lines of research inquiry on the molecular basis of exercise and obesity are summarized in Box 24.4 (53, 54).

Another recent study with important clinical ramifications has revealed a significant relationship between asthma and obesity, although it remains unclear which condition is the cause and which condition is the effect (55). The researchers speculated that asthma could promote obesity because children with asthma often have a sedentary lifestyle, which encourages obesity. Conversely, obesity could contribute to asthma by reducing the extent to which bronchial muscle is stretched, thereby causing air passages to narrow. The results of this research revealed a need for more study to clarify the nature of this relationship.

1. Research on the molecular basis of exercise adaptations can elucidate the influence of energy expenditure and energy intake on the cellular mechanisms that regulate fat metabolism. For example, a recent exciting study revealed that exercise training makes adipocytes more sensitive to epinephrine, a hormone that induces lipolysis (which shrinks fat cells) (53). Another hormone, adenosine A1, "forces" the cells to retain fat. Fortunately, exercise-trained adipocytes have fewer receptor sites that can bind the hormone, but, unfortunately, overeating blunts adipocytes' ability to ignore adenosine A$_1$. This "hold-on" message results in a drastic reduction in lipolysis. The end result is that fat cells remain fat. These data were derived from research on exercise-trained, restricted-fed and full-fed miniature swine. In effect, excess energy intake or overindulgence attenuates the positive effects of exercise training. These data will augment our understanding of the molecular control of lipolysis with and without exercise, and during controlled and uncontrolled energy intake in children and adults.

2. In addition to having a role in energy storage, adipocytes also secrete substances such as **leptin** that might lead to insulin resistance or other complications of obesity. Leptin is best known as the adipocyte hormone whose absence causes profound obesity in rodents and humans, but it also has potent effects on insulin's action. In rodents, for example, an inherited deficiency in leptin causes both severe insulin resistance and obesity. Researchers have determined that returning leptin to these rodents reverses insulin resistance, but by mechanisms that are independent of effects on food intake and body weight (54). This reversal in insulin resistance may result from leptin working within the brain as well as directly on target issues. In contrast to rodents, in which leptin deficiency causes obesity, levels of leptin are higher than normal in most obese people. So additional research is currently directed toward understanding how alterations in leptin might affect insulin resistance.

Although the relationship between cardiovascular disease and obesity in adults has been thoroughly substantiated through empirical study, a recent investigation demonstrated the potential of obesity in childhood for predicting heart disease in adult life. Researchers determined that obese children as young as 8 years of age have an ominous bloodstream inflammation that is linked to cardiovascular disease (56). The study found that overweight and obese children were 3 to 5 times more likely than normal weight children to have elevated levels of C-reactive protein (CRP) and white blood cell counts, both of which suggest the presence of an inflammation. The researchers postulated that elevated CRP emerges in response to plaque buildup in the arteries by releasing disease-fighting cells (the CRP and white cells), which ultimately results in a bloodstream inflammation designed to attack the plaque.

The emergence of data describing or measuring the factors involved with obesity will continue to proliferate at an exponential rate. In the meantime, it is well established that obese children are often physiologically and emotionally different from their normal weight peers. Therefore, successful intervention includes the recognition that programs should be specific to each child's level of obesity and special needs. The multifactorial nature of obesity necessitates a multidisciplinary team consisting of a pediatrician, nutrition specialist, exercise specialist, behaviorist, and parents is optimal. Some of the issues that clinicians, researchers, and parents should monitor are listed in Box 24.5 (5, 7, 12):

For Clinicians

- Skin Disorders (especially if deep skinfolds are present): Obese children are prone to heat rash, **intertrigo**, **monilial dermatitis**, and **acanthosis nigricans**. Acne should be treated, if present, to help improve self-esteem.
- Orthopaedic Problems: Because they carry more weight, obese children are prone to increased tibial torsion, bowed legs, and symptoms of stress in the joints and lower extremities.
- Psychiatric Problems: Obese children often suffer from depression, negative self-esteem and self-image, and withdrawal.
- Motivational Problems: Obese children are often caught in a vicious cycle of low motivation causing increased weight gain, and vice-versa.
- Type 2 diabetes: The prevalence of this obesity-related diabetes has surged and now accounts for more than 2000 cases. Testing should occur every 2 years beginning in children at age 10 who are more than 20% overweight and have a family history of type 2 diabetes.

For Parents:

- Establish regular family activities such as walks, games, or other outdoor activities.
- Limit television viewing and computer activities not related to homework.
- Respect the child's appetite. Don't force children to "clear the plate."
- Do not buy high-calorie foods and avoid packaged, prepared foods.
- Do not use food as a reward or for comfort.
- Include fiber in the child's diet.
- Provide a healthy, balanced diet with 30% or fewer calories from fat.
- Encourage fruits and vegetables as snacks.
- Encourage and reward physical activity.
- Do not offer sweets or high-calorie desserts in exchange for a completed meal.

What We Know
About Pediatric Obesity

1 Current dietary patterns promote overweight and obesity. The intake of fats among children is above currently recommended levels, and only about 30% of youth meet the goals of daily intake of fruits, meats, grains, and dairy.

2 Current patterns of physical activity promote overweight and obesity. Levels of physical activity are inversely related to levels of overweight and obesity in children and adolescents.

3 For many children, obesity starts in the preschool years. Although many adults acquire their obesity during adolescence or adult life, those children who develop severe lifelong obesity often acquire it very early in life.

4 Prevention is better than treatment. It must be acknowledged that treating obesity is difficult at best. In pediatrics, the promise of new pharmacological approaches must be tempered, because their risk and cost-effectiveness are sure to be understood later for children than for adults. In addition, there is reason to worry that for some children, the social experience of being obese can be damaging itself. Although it will always be necessary to treat some children for obesity, prevention should be the focus.

5 In addition to reducing body fat, physical training has an anabolic effect on muscle protein metabolism, resulting in an increase in fat-free mass (FFM). This is in contrast to the effect of a low- or very-low-calorie diet (i.e., 750 kcal [3,150 kJ] or less per day), which may induce a loss of FFM.

6 Physical training causes a decrease in plasma insulin concentration, an increase in receptor sensitivity to insulin, and improved glucose tolerance.

7 The plasma lipid profile is frequently abnormal in pediatric obesity. Obese children tend to have abnormally high levels of serum triglycerides (TG), very-low-density lipoprotein (VLDL) and low-density lipoprotein (LDL), and low levels of high-density lipoprotein (HDL).

8 Resting arterial blood pressure is often high in obese children. Aerobic exercise may induce a decrease in both systolic and diastolic pressures of such patients.

9 The delayed onset of menarche confers various health benefits, one of which is the reduction in fat deposition during and after puberty.

What We Would Like to Know
About Pediatric Obesity

1 Why are some children more likely to develop obesity than others? Research indicates that Hispanic, African American, and Native American children are more prone to develop obesity than other groups. Additionally, why have low-income children been identified as a high-risk group?

2 Does intense physical exercise in children result in a suppression of appetite? If so, what is the mechanism to explain reduction in appetite?

3 What impact does regular physical exercise have on counteracting the reduction in basal metabolic rate that occurs with caloric restriction?

4 What are the benefits of physical activity in relation to regular physical training? Can physical activity be an effective method to reduce the incidence of pediatric obesity? If so, how?

5 Why is pediatric obesity more prevalent among young girls as opposed to boys?

6 Does pediatric obesity result primarily from **adipocyte hypertrophy**, **hyperplasia**, or a combination of both?

7 Do adipocytes reach a biologic limit, so that the adipocyte number determines the extent of obesity?

8 If the adipocyte number becomes stable before adulthood, is weight gain thereafter related to adipocyte hypertrophy?

Summary

The epidemic of obesity is inextricably linked to inactivity. Physical activity plays a critical role in both prevention and treatment of pediatric obesity. Increased physical activity is also a vital component of weight loss strategies. In addition, physical activity confers a variety of health benefits, including favorably altering body composition, increasing metabolism, and psychological well being.

Because the prevalence of pediatric obesity is high and still growing, it is important to understand who is at risk and for what reasons, so that preventive measures can be implemented. Unfortunately, it is still not possible to determine which children will be obese as adults, which will be affected by the conditions commonly associated with obesity in adulthood, or when these conditions will develop. This is due in part to the limited controlled data on physical activity in pediatric obesity treatment (57). However, it is known that obesity is heterogeneous; several factors have the potential to cause a positive energy balance over long periods.

Based upon the available basic and epidemiologic research, it is well established that physical activity is a critical adjunctive therapy for pediatric obesity. Additional research is needed to explain the mechanisms involved in weight gain and loss, and the proper dose-response relationship between exercise and fat loss. An even more important research extension is the benefit of regular physical activity on the prevention of pediatric obesity.

DISCUSSION QUESTIONS

1 What are the current attitudes and behaviors among parents and children in various demographic groups related to eating, exercise, and obesity in children?

2 How do current family structures—including extended and single-parent families, families with 2 or no working parents, and isolated nuclear families—affect eating and exercise patterns? How can beneficial effects be encouraged and deleterious ones reduced?

3 How do community patterns of activity in many areas of life affect the behaviors and attitudes of families and children related to eating exercise and overweight?

4 How do the electronic and other aspects of our broader cultural environment affect food choices of families and children, and how can any deleterious effects be reduced?

CASE STUDY

Patient Information

Casey is a 10-year-old girl who is severely obese. Her parents have attempted to assist in her weight loss efforts since she was 8 years old. They have encouraged her to diet and exercise, but it seems with every successive diet, Casey gains additional weight. She has vowed never to attempt a weight-loss program again. Casey refuses to engage in any physical activities in her school (at recess and in physical education class) and has become increasingly withdrawn. Her favorite pastime is "surfing the Internet." She eats very little at mealtime, and prefers to snack between meals while doing her homework or while at the computer. In frustration, her parents brought her to a wellness clinic at the local hospital and indicated that they were in desperate need of counseling.

Assessments

A preliminary examination by a pediatrician indicated Casey was mildly hypertensive, and had an elevated lipid profile. Her height was 136.5 cm, weight was 45.3 kg, and body fat percentage as measured by skinfold analysis was 33.2%. Casey's BMI was determined to be at the 95th percentile for her age and gender. A maximal exercise test reveals good cardiopulmonary function (a good *absolute* $\dot{V}O_{2max}$) but a low *relative* $\dot{V}O_{2max}$, and an elevated blood pressure response to increasing exercise intensity. She was evaluated by a psychologist and was found to be mildly depressed. Her pediatrician recommended a 16-week program of exercise and nutritional counseling. She is not on any medications.

The American Diabetes Association recommends testing every 2 years starting at age 10 for children who are greater than 20% overweight and have risk factors such as a family history of type 2 diabetes or African, Native American, or Hispanic ancestry. Casey should have a baseline test for diabetes that accompanies the lipid profile analysis. Furthermore, Casey and her parents should provide a family history that may offer valuable information regarding her risk for type 2 diabetes.

Questions

1. What factors must you take into consideration before you develop an exercise program for Casey?

2. Develop a program of exercise. Describe the intensity, frequency, duration, and mode of exercise that would be safe and appropriate. How long should the program last?

3. What other health care professionals might be engaged in assisting Casey to make substantive lifestyle changes? Why?

4. How would you evaluate Casey's progress at the conclusion of your program? Would follow-up be advised? Why? How often?

REFERENCES

1. Troiano RP, Flegal KM, Kuczmarski SM, Campbell SM, Johnson JC. Overweight prevalence and trends for children and adolescents. Arch Pediatr Adolesc Med 1995;149:1085–1091.

2. Pratt M, Macera CA, Blanton C. Levels of physical activity and inactivity in children and adults in the United States: current evidence and research issues. Med Sci Sports Exerc 1999;31(11):S526–S533.

3. Grundy SM, Backburn G, Higgins M, Lauer R, Perri MG, Ryan D. Physical activity in the prevention and treatment of obesity and its co-morbidities. Med Sci Sports Exerc 1999;31(11):S502–S508.

4. Flegal KM, Carroll MD, Kuczmarski RJ, Johnson CL. Overweight and obesity in the United States: prevalence and trends, 1960–1994. Int J Obes 1998;22:39–47.

5. Williams CL, Campanaro LA, Squillace M, Bollella M. Management of childhood obesity in pediatric practice. Ann NY Acad Sci 1997;817:225–240.

6. DeLany PD. Role of energy expenditure in the development of pediatric obesity. Am J Clin Nutr 1998;68(suppl):950S–955S.

7. Moran R. Evaluation and treatment of childhood obesity. Am Fam Physician 1999;59(4):861–868.

8. Whitaker RC, Wright JA, Pepe MS, Seidel KD, Dietz WH. Predicting obesity in young adulthood from childhood and parental obesity. New Engl J Med 1997;337(13):869–873.

9. Epstein L, Wing R, Valoski A. Childhood obesity. Pediatr Clin North Am 1985;32:363–379.

10. Bar-Or O, Foreyt J, Boutchard C, et al. Physical activity, genetic, and nutritional considerations, in childhood weight management. Med Sci Sports Exerc 1998;31(11):2–10.

11. Durstine JL, Haskell WL. Effects of exercise training on plasma lipids and lipoproteins. Effects of exercise training on plasma lipids and lipoproteins. Exerc Sports Sci Rev 1994;22:477–497.

12. Williams CL, Bollella M, Carter BJ. Treatment of childhood obesity in pediatric practice. Ann NY Acad Sci 1999;207–219.

13. Weil WB. Obesity in children. Pediatr Rev 1981;3:180–189.

14. Boileau A, Lohman TG, Slaughter MH, Horswill CA, Stillman RJ. Problems associated with determining body composition in maturing youngsters. In: Brown EW, Branta CF, eds. Competitive Sports for Children and Youth. Champaign, Ill: Human Kinetics Press; 1988:3–16.

15. Owens S, Gutin B, Allison J, et al. Effect of physical training on total and visceral fat in obese children. Med Sci Sports Exerc 1999;31(1):143–148.

16. Rowland TW. Developmental Exercise Physiology. Champaign, Ill: Human Kinetics Press; 1996.

17. Rosner B, Prineas R, Loggie J, Daniels SR. Percentiles for body mass index in US children 5 to 17 years of age. J Pediatr 1998;132:211–222.

18. Pietrobelli A, Faith M, Allison DB, Gallagher D, Chiumello G, Heymsfield S. Body mass index as a measure of adiposity among children and adolescents: a validation study. J Pediatr 1998;132:204–210.

19. Rowland TW. Does peak $\dot{V}_{O_2}$ reflect $\dot{V}_{O_{2max}}$ in children? Evidence from supramaximal testing. Med Sci Sports Exerc 1993;25:689–693.

20. Owens S, Gutin B. Exercise testing of the child with obesity. Pediatr Cardiol 1999;20:79–83.

21. Rowland TW. Aerobic exercise testing protocols. In: Rowland TW, ed. Pediatric Laboratory Exercise Testing: Clinical Guidelines. Champaign, Ill: Human Kinetics Press; 1993:19–41.

22. Sallis JF. Epidemiology of physical activity and fitness in children and adolescents. Crit Rev Food Sci Nutr 1993;33:403–408.

23. Åstrand PO. Definitions, testing procedures, accuracy, and reproducibility. Acta Paediatr Scand 1971;217:9–12.

24. LeMura LM, von Duvillard SP, Carlonas R, Andreacci J. Can exercise training improve maximal aerobic power ($\dot{V}_{O_{2max}}$) in children: a meta-analytic review. J Exer Physiol 1999; 2(3):1–17.

25. Klimt F, Voight ED. Investigations on the standardization of ergometry in children. Acta Paediatr Scand 1971;217:35–36.

26. Bar-Or O. Pediatric Sports Medicine for the Practitioner. New York, NY: Springer-Verlag; 1983:315–338.

27. Maffeis C, Schena F, Zaffanello M. Maximal aerobic power during running and cycling in obese and non-obese children. Acta Paediatr 1994;83:113–116.

28. Zanconato S, Baraldi E, Santuz P. Gas exchange during exercise in obese children. Eur J Pediatr 1989;148:614–617.

29. Elliot DL, Goldberg L, Kuehl KS, Hanna C. Metabolic evaluation of obese and nonobese siblings. J Pediatr 1989;114:957–962.

30. Gutin B, Islam S, Treiber F, Smith C, Manos T. Fasting insulin concentration is related to cardiovascular reactivity in children. Pediatrics 1995;96:1123–1125.

31. Davies CTM, Godfrey S, Light M, Sargeant AJ, Zeidifard E. Cardiopulmonary responses to exercise in obese girls and young women. J Appl Physiol 1975;38:373–376.

32. Klein AA. Pediatric exercise testing. Pediatr Ann 1987;16:546–558.

33. Washington RL, Bricker TJ, Alpert BS. Guidelines for testing in the pediatric age group. Circulation 1994;90:2166–2179.

34. American Dietetic Association and American Diabetes Association. Exchange Lists for Weight Management. Rev ed. Chicago, Ill, and Alexandria, VA: Authors; 1995.

35. Goran M, Carpenter W, Poehlman E. Total energy expenditure in 4-to-6-yr-old children. Am J Physiol 1993;264:E706–711.

36. Goran M, Carpenter W, McGloin A, Johnson R, Hardin JM, Weinsier R. Energy expenditure in children of lean and obese parents. Am J Physiol 1995;268:E917–E924.

37. DeLany JP. Role of energy expenditure in the development of pediatric obesity. Am J Clin Nutr 1998;68(suppl):950S–955S.

38. Payne GV, Morrow JR, Johnson L, Dalton SN. Resistance training in children and youth: a meta-analysis. Res Quarterly Exer Sport 1997;68:80–88.

39. Montoye HJ Kemper HCG, Saris WH, Washburn RA. Measuring Physical Activity and Energy Expenditure. Champaign, Ill: Human Kinetics Press; 1996.

40. Sothern MS, Hunter S, Suskind RM, et al. Motivating the obese child to move: the role of structured exercise in pediatric weight management. Southern Med J 1999;92:577–584.

41. Maffeis C, Zaffanello M, Pinelli L, Schutz Y. Total energy expenditure and patterns of activity in 8–10-year-old obese and nonobese children. J Pediatr Gastroenterol Nutr 1996;23:256–261.

42. Hill JO, Melby C, Johnson SL, Peters JC. Physical activity and energy requirements. Am J Clin Nutr 1995;62 (suppl):1059S–1066S.

43. Sims EAH, Danforth E. Expenditure and storage of energy in man (perspective). J Clin Invest 1987;80:1019–1024.44.

44. Rowland TW. Effect of prolonged inactivity on aerobic fitness of children. J Sports Med Phys Fitness 1994;34:147–155.

45. Bar-Or O. Physical activity and physical training in childhood obesity. J Sports Med Phys Fitness 1993;33:323329.

46. Sasaki J, Shindo M, Tanaka H, Ando M, Arakawa K. A long-term aerobic exercise program decreases obesity index and increases high-density lipoprotein cholesterol concentration in obese children. Int J Obesity 1987;11:339–345.

47. Bar-Or O. Physical conditioning in children in children with cardiorespiratory disease. Exerc Sports Sci Rev 1990;18:243–261.

48. Depres JP, Bouchard C, Malina RM. Physical activity and coronary heart disease risk factors during childhood and adolescence. Exerc Sport Sci Rev 1990;18:243–26.

49. Rowland TW, Martel L, Vanderburgh P, Manos T, Charkoudian N. The influence of short-term aerobic training on blood lipids in healthy 10–12-year-old children. Int J Sports Med 1996;17:487–492.

50. Rocchini AP, Katch V, Anderson J. Blood pressure in obese adolescents: effect of weight loss. Pediatrics 1998;82:16–23.

51. Hayashi T, Fujino M, Shindo M, Hiroki T, Arakawi K. Echocardiographic and electrocardiographic measures in obese children after an exercise program. Int J Obesity 1987;11:465–472.

52. Steppan CM, Bailey ST, Bhat S, et al. The hormone resistin links obesity to diabetes. Nature 2001;409:307–312.

53. Carey GB. Cellular adaptations in fat tissue of exercise-trained miniature swine: role of excess energy intake. J Appl Physiol 2000;88:881–887.

54. Oksana G, Marcus-Samuels C, Leon LR, Vinson C, Reitman L. Hormones: leptin and diabetes in lipoatrophic mice. Nature 2000; 403(6772):850.

55. Figueroa-Munoz J, Chinn S, Rona RJ. Association between obesity and asthma in 4–11-year-old children in the UK. Thorax 2001;56: 133–137.

56. Visser M, Bouter LM, McQuillan GM, Wener MH, Harris TB. Low-grade systemic inflammation in overweight children. Pediatrics 2001; 107(1):e13–20.

57. LeMura LM, Maziekas MT. Factors that alter body fat, body mass, and fat-free mass in pediatric obesity. Med Sci Sports Exer 2002;34(3): 487–496.

SUGGESTED READINGS

American College of Sports Medicine Roundtable. Physical activity in the prevention and treatment of obesity and its comorbidities. Med Sci Sports Exer 1999;31:(11), November: Special Supplement.

Rowland TW, ed. Pediatric Laboratory Exercise Testing: Clinical Guidelines. Champaign, Ill: Human Kinetics Press; 1993.

IMMUNOLOGICAL AND HEMATOLOGICAL DISEASES AND DISORDERS

CHAPTER 25

Cancer

*Kerry S. Courneya, John R. Mackey, Ryan E. Rhodes**

Overview

Normal body cells grow, divide, and die in a tightly regulated fashion. Imbalances in cellular regulation may result in a mass called a tumor or neoplasm (i.e., "new and abnormal growth"). Benign tumors grow and enlarge only at the site where they began. Malignant or cancerous tumors, on the other hand, have the potential to compress, invade, and destroy the normal tissues that surround them. Moreover, they are able to spread (i.e., metastasize) throughout the body via the bloodstream or lymph system and form "colony" tumors at a new site where they continue their destructive behavior. The term cancer is used to describe over 100 diseases that can occur in virtually any body tissue or organ. Most cancers, however, fall into four major classifications, based on the type of cell from which they arise: **carcinoma, leukemia, lymphoma,** and **sarcoma.**

Carcinomas are cancers that develop from epithelial cells that line the surface of the body, glands, and internal organs. They account for 80% to 90% of all cancers and include prostate, colon, lung, cervical, and breast cancer (see Chapter 26). Cancers also can arise from the cells of the blood (i.e., leukemias), the immune system (i.e., lym-

*Kerry S. Courneya is supported by an Investigator Award from the Canadian Institutes of Health Research and a Research Team Grant from the National Cancer Institute of Canada (NCIC) with funds from the Canadian Cancer Society (CCS) and the CCS/NCIC Sociobehavioral Cancer Research Network. John R. Mackey's research program is supported by the NCIC and the Alberta Cancer Board. Ryan E. Rhodes is supported by a graduate studentship from the Alberta Heritage Foundation for Medical Research.

phomas), and connective tissues such as bones, tendons, cartilage, fat, and muscle (i.e., sarcomas).

Epidemiology

Over 1 million Americans are diagnosed with invasive cancers other than breast each year (1). Prostate, colorectal, and lung cancer are the three most common cancers besides breast (Box 25.1). These cancers result in more than 500,000 deaths each year in the United States (1). The probability of developing most cancers increases dramatically with age, making cancer a disease that affects primarily older persons. There are, however, some cancers that affect mostly younger people, including Hodgkin disease, non-Hodgkin lymphoma, leukemia, and testicular cancer (see Box 25.1).

Fortunately, early detection and improved treatments for many cancers has resulted in increased survival rates over the last few decades (1). The current **5-year relative survival rate** (adjusted for normal life expectancy) is estimated to be about 60%, although this figure varies considerably depending on the type of cancer and extent of the disease at diagnosis. Because of increased incidence rates and improved survival rates, millions of Americans are alive today who have been through the cancer experience (1). Consequently, fitness professionals may expect to serve a large and increasing number of cancer survivors.

Etiology and Risk Factors

Although the causes and risk factors for human cancer are diverse, ranging from genetics to behavior to the environment, lifestyle factors appear to be paramount. The Harvard Report on Cancer Prevention (2) concluded that nearly two thirds of cancer mortality in the United States can be linked to tobacco use, poor diet, and lack of exercise. Only 5% to 10% of most types of cancer are due to defects in single genes that run in families, and only a similarly small percentage are due to occupational and environmental exposures.

Physical inactivity as a risk factor for cancer has received significant recent research attention based on a number of plausible biologic mechanisms. More than 130 studies on the topic are currently available (3). The strongest evidence for a protective effect of physical activity comes from research on colon cancer, where there is an estimated 50% risk reduction for the most active compared to the least active people. Colditz et al. (4) estimate that if everyone in the United States increased their amount of physical activity by 3 hours of walking per week, there would be 17% fewer cases of colon cancer. "Evidence also is available to suggest that physical activity may have a protective effect against breast (see Chapter 26), prostate, endometrial, and lung cancer, although definitive conclusions cannot be made at this time (3). Evidence for a relation between exercise and other cancers (e.g., pancreas, ovarian, testicular, stomach) currently is too sparse to make even tentative conclusions. Many organizations recommend 30 to 45 minutes of exercise of at least moderate intensity on most days of the week as a method of reducing cancer risk (5).

Screening, Diagnosis, and Staging

A key to improving survival rates from cancer is early detection of the disease. **Screening** is the process of identifying disease in people who are asymptomatic. The major advantage of screening is that it can identify abnormalities that may be cancer at an early stage before physical signs and symptoms develop. Screening tests are available for many of the most common types of cancer, including breast (see Chapter 26), colorectal, prostate, and uterine cervix. Unfortunately, there are no effective screening tests for lung cancer at this time. Screening tests for prostate cancer include the digital rectal examination (DRE) and prostate-specific antigen (PSA) tests. Prostate-specific antigen is a substance produced only by the prostate. It is measured by a blood test, with PSA values below 4.0 ng/mL considered normal, values between 4.0 ng/mL and 10.0 ng/mL considered borderline, and values over 10.0 ng/mL

BOX 25.1. Estimated New Cases and Deaths for Cancers Other Than Breast, United States, 2000

	Estimated New Cases			Estimated New Deaths		
Site	Total	Male	Female	Total	Male	Female
All cancers Other than breast	1,035,900	618,300	417,600	511,000	283,700	27,300
Prostate	180,400	180,400	—	31,900	31,900	—
Lung	164,100	89,500	74,600	156,900	89,300	67,600
Colorectal	130,200	63,600	66,600	56,300	27,800	28,500

Note: Excludes basal and squamous cell skin cancers and in situ carcinomas except urinary bladder.

Adapted from the American Cancer Society. Cancer Facts & Figures 2000. Atlanta, GA: American Cancer Society,

considered high and suggestive of prostate cancer. Testing the PSA level is considered a more definitive screening tool for prostate cancer than DRE. Screening tests for colorectal cancer includes DRE, fecal occult blood test, flexible sigmoidoscopy, double contrast barium enema, and colonoscopy. The most definitive test for colorectal cancer is a colonoscopy, which involves visualizing the internal surface of the rectum and large bowel using a flexible fiberoptic tube.

The effects of exercise on the accuracy of screening and diagnostic tests for cancer are largely unknown. One study (6) found a threefold increase in PSA concentration in serum after a 15-minute session of cycle ergometer exercise. Consequently, the authors suggested that extensive exercise should be avoided before PSA blood sampling for prostate cancer screening. Moreover, the study also found that the amount of PSA liberated by exercise was a better measure of prostate volume than PSA measured at rest. This finding led the authors to suggest that measuring PSA change from rest to postexercise may improve assay specificity while maintaining its sensitivity, making PSA an even more important and useful marker for prostate carcinoma. However, a similar study found no effects of acute exercise on PSA using treadmill exercise (7), and no other research has examined the effects of acute or chronic exercise on the results of other cancer screening and diagnostic tests.

Screening tests cannot diagnose cancer. A diagnosis of cancer requires analysis of a tissue sample taken by biopsy. By examining cells under the microscope, a trained pathologist can almost always distinguish malignant cells from their benign (i.e., nonmalignant) counterparts. The pathologist looks for cells that are dividing often, are invading normal surrounding tissue, or have unusual cellular features such as large and disorganized nuclei. In some cases, it is possible to determine that suspicious cells are malignant by identifying cancer-related genetic mutations using the techniques of molecular biology.

After the initial diagnosis, it is important to learn the extent to which the disease has spread or progressed (i.e., stage) to assess the patient's prognosis and guide the choice of therapy. **Cancer stage** is determined by patient history, physical examination, laboratory testing, or diagnostic imaging (e.g., chest radiography, computed tomography, or magnetic resonance imaging). A number of different systems currently are used to classify tumors, but the most common is the Tumor (T), Node (N), **Metastasis** (M) system (8). The **TNM system** stages cancer based on the size of the primary tumor and extent of local invasion (T), the involvement of regional lymph nodes (N), and the presence or absence of distant metastases (M). Once the T, N, and M have been determined a "stage" of I (least advanced) through IV (most advanced) is assigned. In general, regionally confined cancers are stages I and II, locally advanced cancers are stage III, and cancers with overt distant metastases are stage IV.

Surgical and Medical Treatments

Cancer treatments may be used to cure cancer, to prolong life when a cure is not possible, or to improve quality of life (e.g., symptom relief). The three primary cancer treatment modalities are surgery, **radiation therapy**, and **systemic therapy** (i.e., drugs). Surgery is the oldest and most commonly used modality in cancer therapy. Cancer surgeries include operations to remove high-risk tissues to prevent the development of cancers, biopsies of abnormal tissue to establish the diagnosis of cancer, excision of tumors with curative intent, insertion of central venous catheters to support chemotherapy infusions, reconstruction after definitive surgery, and palliative or symptom relief for incurable disease (e.g., surgery to relieve bowel obstruction). About 60% of cancer survivors have surgical removal of their tumor. Some operations attempt to remove all gross and microscopic tumor in a single operation. These operations commonly involve excision of the tumor and draining regional lymph nodes as a single specimen. Other, more conservative, operations minimize the volume of tissue removed and preserve organ function. In general, conservative surgeries require additional nonsurgical treatment with radiation therapy or systemic therapy to eradicate residual cancer cells. Some common operations to remove cancers other than breast are described in Table 25.1.

Radiation therapy is the treatment of cancer using ionizing radiation. It is considered a locoregional treatment with the goal being to irradiate the known tumor volume while sparing adjacent radiation-sensitive tissues. Over 50% of all cancer survivors may undergo radiation therapy at some point during the treatment process. Of these, about one third are treated with curative intent (of which about half are cured) and about two thirds with palliative intent. Several types of radiation are used, but most radiation therapy treatments are external beams of high-energy photons produced by linear accelerators or from the decay of cobalt-60. These photons penetrate into tissue and produce ionized (electrically charged) particles that damage DNA. This DNA damage usually inhibits cell replication and often leads to cell death. Radiation therapy is delivered in repeated small doses (i.e., fractions) over an extended period of time to kill cancer cells without undue damage to normal cells. Treatment typically is given each day, Monday through Friday, for between 5 and 8 weeks. For example, a patient with prostate cancer may receive a total dose of 70 grays (Gy) "fractionated" into two Gy every weekday for 7 weeks. A full course of external beam radiation therapy can range from 8 weeks of low-fraction therapy administered each weekday given with curative intent to higher-dose treatments lasting only several days, for instance as palliative treatment for a painful bone metastasis. Although malignant cells typically are more radiosensitive than normal cells, normal tissue toxicity does occur and is entirely dependent on what part of the body is irradiated (Table 25.2).

TABLE 25.1. COMMON OPERATIONS AND THEIR SEQUELAE FOR CANCERS OTHER THAN BREAST

Operation	Description	Sequelae
Pulmonary lobectomy	Removal of one lobe of one lung	Reduced lung capacity and function, dyspnea, deconditioning
Pneumonectomy	Removal of one entire lung	Reduced lung capacity and function, dyspnea, deconditioning
Radical neck dissection	Removal of cervical lymphatics	Reduced neck range of motion and muscle strength, occasional cranial nerve XI palsy
Pelvic lymph node dissection	Removal of groin or retroperitoneal nodes	Lymphedema
Radical prostatectomy	Removal of prostate, seminal vesicles, and ampullae of vasa deferentia	Urinary incontinence, erectile dysfunction; deconditioning
Abdominoperineal resection	Removal of rectum and draining lymphatics	Patient may require ostomy; deconditioning
Hemicolectomy	Removal of involved colon and draining lymphatics	Patient occasionally requires ostomy; deconditioning, diarrhea
Limb amputation	Removal of tumor with margin of normal tissue	Occasional chronic pain syndromes, deconditioning
Limb-sparing surgery	Removal of tumor and reattachment of distal limb	Postoperative casting leads to decreased joint range of motion and muscle atrophy, occasional chronic pain syndromes, deconditioning

Adapted from Courneya KS, Mackey JR, Quinney HA. Neoplasms. In Myers J (Ed). ACSM's Resource Manual for Clinical Exercise Physiology for Special Populations. Baltimore: Lippincott Williams & Wilkins, in press.

Systemic therapy (i.e., drugs) is prescribed for many advanced solid tumors if cancer cells are suspected of metastasizing beyond the primary site and regional lymph nodes. Moreover, systemic therapy is the mainstay of curative treatment for leukemia and lymphoma, where cancer cells, by definition, are not regionally confined. The three major types of systemic therapy are **chemotherapy**, **endocrine therapy**, and **biologic therapy** (Table 25.3).

Chemotherapy exploits biologic differences between normal and malignant cells to preferentially kill malignant cells. Over 80 drugs currently are approved for the treatment of cancer, most of which have been selected to be toxic to rapidly proliferating cells. Over half of all cancer survivors may receive chemotherapy at some point during the treat-

TABLE 25.2. COMMON ADVERSE EFFECTS OF RADIATION THERAPY

Radiation Site	Common Adverse Effects
Skin	Redness, pain, dryness, peeling, sloughing, reduced elasticity
Brain	Nausea and vomiting, fatigue, memory loss
Pharynx	Mouth ulceration
Salivary gland	Xerostomia (dry mouth)
Thorax	Some degree of irreversible lung fibrosis, heart *may* receive radiation, causing pericardial inflammation or fibrosis; premature atherosclerosis; cardiomyopathy
Abdomen	Vomiting, diarrhea
Pelvis	Diarrhea, pelvic pain, bladder scarring, occasionally incontinence and sexual dysfunction
Joints	Connective tissue and joint capsule fibrosis; possible decreased range of motion

Adapted from Courneya KS, Mackey JR, Quinney HA. Neoplasms. In Myers J (Ed). ACSM's Resource Manual for Clinical Exercise Physiology for Special Populations. Baltimore: Lippincott Williams & Wilkins, in press.

ment process, with about one quarter of those being cured. Chemotherapy usually is administered intravenously or orally and is given in repeated courses or cycles 2 to 4 weeks apart. In general, curative chemotherapy requires combinations of several chemotherapy drugs typically given over several treatment cycles spanning 3 to 6 months. Adult cancers that can be cured by chemotherapy include acute leukemias, Hodgkin disease, some lymphomas, and testicular cancers. Because the goal of treatment is cure, most cancer survivors are willing to accept the multiple side effects of chemotherapy. If these particular cancers recur after standard chemotherapy, treatment with high-dose chemotherapy (requiring **bone marrow transplantation** or **peripheral blood stem cell transplantation** to restore the blood-forming system) can provide long-term survival.

Endocrine or hormone therapy is used to treat hormone-dependent cancers. About 20% of cancers in males and about 40% in females arise in hormone sensitive organs (e.g., prostate, breast, and uterus). The hormonal environment of the body can directly stimulate the growth of established cancers. Depriving an established prostate, breast, or uterine tumor of its sustaining hormones can halt growth and may even induce regression. For example, men with advanced prostate cancer derive substantial benefit from depletion of testosterone. Hormonal treatments usually are administered continuously or intermittently for many years and can have significant side effects. Glucocorticoid hormonal therapy is cytotoxic to some leukemic and lymphoma cells, and may be used at high doses for these cancers. Additionally, glucocorticoids commonly are given to prevent and treat chemotherapy-induced nausea, to treat brain metastases and spinal cord compression, to reduce cancer-related pain, and to treat and prevent allergic reactions from chemotherapy drugs. Unfortunately, use of these agents causes muscle loss, proximal muscle weakness, fat

TABLE 25.3. CLASSES OF SYSTEMIC THERAPY FOR CANCER AND THEIR COMMON ADVERSE EFFECTS

Class	Examples	Common Adverse Effects
Chemotherapies		
Antimetabolite chemotherapy (intravenous)	Methotrexate, fluorouracil, gemcitabine	Fatigue, anorexia, nausea, anemia, neutropenia, thrombocytopenia
Antitubulin chemotherapy (intravenous)	Taxol, Taxotere, vinorelbine, vincristine	Fatigue, muscle pain, sensory and motor peripheral neuropathy, ataxia, anemia, neutropenia, thrombocytopenia
Alkylator chemotherapy	Cyclophosphamide, chlorambucil	Fatigue, anorexia, nausea, anemia, neutropenia, thrombocytopenia
Anthracycline chemotherapy (intravenous)	Doxorubicin (Adriamycin), mitoxantrone	Fatigue, cardiotoxicity (cardiac failure in <5% of patients), nausea, vomiting, anemia, neutropenia, thrombocytopenia
Platinum salt chemotherapy (intravenous)	Cisplatin, carboplatin	Fatigue, nausea, sensory and motor peripheral neuropathy, anemia neutropenia, thrombocytopenia
High-dose chemotherapy with bone marrow/stem cell transplantation	Combinations of 2 to 4 chemotherapy drugs in maximally tolerated doses	Loss of muscle mass, deconditioning, nausea, vomiting, neuropathy, anemia, neutropenia, thrombocytopenia, infection
Endocrine Therapies		
Glucocorticoid hormonal therapy (oral)	Dexamethasone (Decadron), prednisone	Fat redistribution (truncal and facial obesity); proximal muscle weakness, osteoporosis, edema, infection
Antiestrogen hormonal therapy (oral)	Tamoxifen	Weight gain, fatigue, hot flashes
Antiandrogen hormonal therapy (oral)	Flutamide	Weight gain, fatigue, loss of muscle mass, hot flashes, osteoporosis
Luteinizing hormone-releasing hormone agonists (subcutaneous injection)	Goserelin, buserelin	Weight gain, fatigue, hot flashes, osteoporosis
Biologic Therapies		
Antibody therapy (IV injection)	Herceptin, Rituxan	Fevers or allergic reactions on first injection. Herceptin can increase risk of cardiotoxicity from anthracycline chemotherapy
Interferons	IFN-α	Chills, fever, headache, fatigue, neutropenia
Interleukins	IL-2	Chills, fever, fatigue, nausea, low blood pressure
Tyrosine kinase Inhibitors (oral)	Iressa	Skin rash
	STI-571	Anemia, neutropenia, thrombocytopenia

accumulation in the trunk and face, osteoporosis, and an increased susceptibility to infection.

It has only been in the past few years that cancer researchers have begun to understand the molecular changes that convert a normal cell into a cancerous cell. This knowledge has led to a new class of systemic treatments for cancer called biologic therapy. These drugs differ from standard chemotherapy or endocrine therapy, and attempt to target the specific molecular changes found in cancer. For example, antibody injections can help control certain breast cancers and lymphomas by interacting with target proteins that are found on cancer cells but absent in normal tissues. Another new class of drugs, the tyrosine kinase inhibitors, target the abnormal intracellular signaling pathways that drive some cancers to grow and resist the effects of chemotherapy and radiation. Other biologic therapies influence the body's own defense mechanisms to act against cancer cells. The interferons and interleukins work in this fashion, but produce side effects similar to a flu-like illness. The number of bio-

logic therapies is likely to increase very rapidly, and this class of drugs is expected to further revolutionize cancer therapy and provide treatments that are more effective and better tolerated.

Combinations of the main cancer treatment modalities (surgery, radiation therapy, and systemic therapy) are being used increasingly often to treat cancer. The timing and order of the treatments varies depending on the cancer and its stage. When the primary treatment is given first, all subsequent therapy is referred to as **adjuvant therapy**. For example, after resection of a colon cancer, some patients may receive adjuvant chemotherapy. Alternatively, some cancers are best treated by deferring the primary treatment until **neoadjuvant therapy** is given first. Occasionally, two modalities of cancer treatment can be given simultaneously. For example, the concurrent use of chemotherapy and radiation is referred to as chemoradiotherapy. The major advantages of combined modality treatment are as follows: (1) cancer cells remaining after locoregional therapy may still be treated by systemic therapy (i.e., adjuvant therapy); (2) tumor shrinkage by radiation therapy or systemic therapy (i.e., neoadjuvant therapy) can allow a more conservative surgery and thereby preserve organ function; and (3) tumors may respond more dramatically to combined therapy. Combined modality therapy is now the standard of care for most high-risk or locally advanced cancers.

Impact of Cancer and its Treatments on Quality of Life

Not surprisingly, cancer and its treatments often result in significant reductions in quality of life. The physical and functional effects include cytopenias (**anemia**, **neutropenia**, and **thrombocytopenia**), **asthenia**, **ataxia**, **cachexia**, reduced cardiovascular and pulmonary function, muscle weakness and atrophy, **dyspnea**, weight change, difficulty sleeping, fatigue, nausea, vomiting, and pain (9–13). Moreover, cancer and its treatments also result in significant declines in exercise levels (14–17). It is not clear, therefore, how much of the decline in physical function is due to the cancer itself, the associated medical treatments, or the inactivity secondary to the disease and treatments. In any case, these declines in physical functioning may, in part, also underlie some of the psychologic and emotional sequelae of the cancer experience, which include depression, anxiety, stress, body image concerns, decreased self esteem, and loss of a sense of control (18, 19). Although most physical and psychosocial side effects tend to peak during treatment and dissipate quickly thereafter, chronic or late-appearing effects may develop months or even years after treatment (18).

Acute and Chronic Responses to Exercise in Cancer Survivors

Interestingly, the majority of studies on exercise during and after cancer treatments have focused exclusively on breast cancer (see Chapter 26) (20). In this chapter, we review studies that included persons diagnosed with any cancer other than breast. A literature search was conducted in February 2001 using the CD-ROM databases CancerLit, CINAHL, HERACLES, MEDLINE, PsycINFO, and SPORT Discus. Key words that related to cancer (cancer, oncology, tumor, neoplasm, carcinoma), the postdiagnosis time period (rehabilitation, therapy, adjuvant therapy, treatment, intervention, palliation), and exercise (exercise, physical activity, physical therapy, sport, weight training) were combined and searched. Relevant articles were then hand-searched for further pertinent references. To be included in the review, a study had to be published in a peer-reviewed journal and examine aerobic or resistance exercise training. Studies restricted solely to movement therapy or stretching and flexibility exercises for range of motion were excluded.

Moreover, studies that did not separate the effects of exercise from a multiple intervention package (e.g., exercise combined with diet, social support, counseling) also were excluded. The search located 18 studies, nine of which examined exercise during cancer treatment (Table 25.4) and nine of which examined exercise after cancer treatment (Table 25.5).

Exercise During Treatments for Cancers Other Than Breast

Nine studies have examined the effects of exercise during treatments for cancers other than breast (17, 21–28). Four of the studies examined a mixed group of cancer survivors (e.g., breast, testicular, non-Hodgkin lymphoma, multiple myeloma) immediately after high-dose chemotherapy and bone marrow or peripheral blood stem cell transplantation; two studies examined leukemia survivors immediately after high-dose chemotherapy and bone marrow transplantation; and one study each examined adolescents with mixed cancers (e.g., leukemia) on mixed chemotherapies, adults with mixed cancers (e.g., Hodgkin and non-Hodgkin lymphoma) on mixed treatments, and postsurgical stomach cancer survivors. Two of the studies used descriptive designs and seven used experimental designs. One of the descriptive designs was a prospective study of 78 consecutive cancer survivors admitted for chemotherapy and bone marrow transplantation. That study found that maximal performance on a treadmill correlated negatively with fatigue even after controlling for age and sex. The second descriptive study also used a prospective design to study 25 consecutive mixed cancer survivors who had just completed high-dose chemotherapy and bone marrow transplantation. This study found that self-reported cycling ergometry and walking correlated positively with various indicators for quality of life.

Of the seven experimental studies performed during cancer treatment, five studies used randomized controlled trial (RCT) designs with usual-care controls, and two studies used pre–post tests with no controls. The sample sizes ranged from 5 to 70 participants with a mean of 30. Supervised exercise programs were reported in six of the studies; the other study reported a home-based exercise program. Following traditional exercise prescription guidelines, six of the studies tested an aerobic exercise intervention (three cycling, two walking, and one mixed aerobic exercise), whereas one intervention focused upon resistive exercise. The length of the exercise programs ranged from 2 to 16 weeks. The studies examined a wide range of biopsychosocial outcomes including functional capacity, body composition, natural killer cell cytotoxic activity, mood states (e.g., anxiety and depression), symptoms (e.g., nausea, fatigue, pain) and general quality of life. All seven of the experimental studies showed significant beneficial effects of exercise during cancer treatment in multiple domains of functioning despite some small sample sizes (see Table 25.4).

Exercise After Treatments for Cancers Other Than Breast

Nine studies have examined exercise after treatments for cancers other than breast (14, 16, 29–35). Three studies examined mixed cancer survivors (e.g., breast, non-Hodgkin lymphoma, leukemia, prostate), two studies each examined colorectal cancer survivors and mixed childhood/adolescent cancer survivors (e.g., Hodgkin disease, lymphoma, leukemia), and one study each examined prostate cancer survivors and head and neck cancer survivors. Four of these studies used descriptive designs and five used experimental designs. The four descriptive studies surveyed cancer survivors several months to many years postdiagnosis who had completed one or more treatments (e.g., surgery, radiation therapy, or chemotherapy). Three of these studies used cross-sectional/retrospective designs, whereas only one used a prospective design. All studies used self-reported measures of exercise. Sample sizes ranged from 53 to 420 participants, with a mean of 159. The descriptive studies focused exclusively on psychosocial outcomes such as fatigue, satisfaction with life, depression, self-concept, psychological impact of cancer, and quality of life. All of these studies found significant associations between exercise and these various psychosocial outcomes (Table 25.5).

Of the five experimental studies on exercise after cancer treatments, two studies used pre–post tests with matched controls and three used pre–post tests with no controls. The sample sizes ranged from 6 to 32 (mean, 19). All studies reported supervised exercise interventions. One study used a walking program, three studies used a mixed aerobic and resistive program, and one study used an unspecified aerobic program. Four of the five studies followed traditional exercise prescription guidelines in terms of frequency, intensity, and duration. Length of the programs ranged from 5 to 52 weeks. The studies examined biopsychosocial outcomes including functional capacity, body composition, hemoglobin levels, and general quality of life. All five studies showed beneficial effects of exercise, with three reaching statistical significance (see Table 25.5).

Overall, despite methodological limitations, the 18 studies on exercise and cancers other than breast have demonstrated that exercise has beneficial effects on a wide variety of biopsychosocial outcomes, both during and after treatment. In fact, all studies showed beneficial changes or trends in at least one biopsychosocial outcome. Although much more research is needed, it appears that exercise will be a useful therapy for persons diagnosed with cancers other than breast. Whether postdiagnosis exercise may influence tumor growth, disease progression, recurrence, or survival is still an open question. Consequently, at this time fitness professionals should promote exercise in cancer survivors for its quality-of-life benefits and not as a means of fighting the cancer or improving survival.

Special Precautions When Exercise Testing Cancer Survivors

Exercise testing after a cancer diagnosis may serve several clinical purposes, including the following: (1) quantifying the physical condition of a person prior to a given treatment; (2) quantifying the short- and long-term functional effects of the disease and its treatments; (3) identifying comorbid conditions that may preclude exercise (e.g., cardiovascular disease); (4) developing or modifying an exercise prescription; and (5) determining the functional benefits of the prescribed exercise program. Because cancer and its treatments may affect all aspects of physical functioning in cancer survivors (e.g., cardiorespiratory endurance, muscular strength and endurance, flexibility, anthropometry and body composition, gait and balance), a comprehensive fitness test assessing all such parameters is warranted. If possible, exercise testing should be performed before treatment, during treatment (if treatment lasts longer than 3 months), immediately after treatment, and 3 to 6 months posttreatment. Not surprisingly, exercise testing in cancer survivors requires special precautions and considerations (Table 25.6) in addition to those recommended for healthy, asymptomatic middle-aged and older adults (36). These special precautions arise from the significant morbidity experienced by cancer survivors during and after treatments.

Before beginning exercise testing, it is important to have cancer survivors complete a cancer history questionnaire in addition to other exercise and medical history questionnaires that may be indicated (e.g., Revised PAR-Q). The cancer history questionnaire should collect information on important diagnostic and treatment variables such as time since diagnosis, type and stage of disease, type of surgery and adjuvant therapy, and known or suspected side effects of treatments (e.g., ataxia, cardiomyopathy, pulmonary complications, or orthopaedic conditions). It may be necessary to consult the patient's oncology team to get complete and accurate information. A sample cancer history questionnaire is provided in Figure 25.1.

In principle, the exercise tests should stress the patient to at least the level that will be experienced during the exercise program so that any symptoms that might be experienced are identified under the more controlled environment of an exercise test. Moreover, it is desirable to stress the patient as close to maximum capacity as is safely possible to provide better diagnostic information about cardiorespiratory function and to serve as a more accurate and reliable basis for exercise prescription. Notwithstanding the special precautions and considerations highlighted in Table 25.6, most otherwise healthy cancer survivors can safely perform symptom-limited maximal testing.

The decision concerning what types of exercise tests to use depends on the limitations imposed by each specific cancer/treatment combination. These are too numerous to

TABLE 25.4. SUMMARY OF STUDIES EXAMINING EXERCISE DURING TREATMENTS FOR CANCERS OTHER THAN BREAST

Study	Sample/Treatment	Design	Exercise Intervention/ Measures	Outcomes/Measures	Results
Descriptive					
Dimeo et al., 1997 (23)	78 consecutive cancer patients admitted for chemotherapy and bone marrow transplantation: 34 breast cancer, 11 testicular cancer, 3 sarcoma, 1 lung, 2 myeloma, 6 Hodgkin disease, 21 non-Hodgkin lymphoma	Prospective	Maximal performance assessed by treadmill test	Profile mood states and Symptom Checklist–90-Revised	Performance significantly correlated with and distress fatigue in a negative direction.
Courneya et al., 2000 (17)	25 cancer patients who had just completed chemotherapy and bone marrow transplantation: 8 breast, 7 multiple myeloma, 7 non-Hodgkin lymphoma, 2 Hodgkin disease, 1 other	Prospective	Self-reported cycle ergometry and walking during hospital stay	Functional assessment of Cancer Therapy Fatigue Scale and QOL	Cycling duration per day correlated significantly with fatigue at discharge ($r = -.27$, $P < .05$). Exercise during hospital stay correlated with QOL.
Experimental					
Cunningham et al., 1986 (21)	26 leukemia patients who had just completed high dose chemotherapy and total body irradiation followed by an allogeneic bone marrow transplant	Randomized controlled trial with two exercise arms (3/wk vs. 5/wk) and usual care controls	Supervised 5 weeks of resistive exercise for either 3 or 5 days/wk for 30 min	Body composition, creatine excretion, and 3-methyl-histidine excretion	Experimental groups maintained creatine excretion level whereas control group decreased
Decker et al., 1989 (22)	12 patients with acute leukemia who underwent bone marrow transplants	Pre–post test	Home-based exercise program for 30 min, 3/week, at 85% of HR_{max} starting 1 week before bone marrow transplant and lasting 4 months	Functional capacity, and depresson	Decreased maximal aerobic capacity and 20 lb. weight loss from pretransplant to 4 mos posttransplant. Patients found exercise program worthwhile
Dimeo et al., 1997b	70 mixed cancer patients undergoing autologous peripheral blood stem cell transplant: 46 breast, 13 germ cell, 5 sarcoma, 4 lung, 1 adreno-carcinoma, 1 neuroblastoma	Randomized controlled trial with usual care controls	Supervised biking using a bed ergometer 7/week for 30 min at 70% intensity from time of high dose chemotherapy until discharge	Physical performance, hematologic indexes, symptoms, and length of hospital stay	Experimental group showed increases in functional capacity at program end; decreased neutropenia, thrombopenia; platelet transfusions; severity of pain and diarrhea; and hospital stay

Dimeo et al., 1998 (25)	Patients with solid tumors / 5 cancer patients who reported fatigue: 1 medulloblastoma, 1 non-Hodgkin lymphoma, 1 Hodgkin disease, 1 disseminated non-small cell bronchial carcinoma, 1 breast carcinoma; 3 were on treatment	Pre-post test	Daily supervised treadmill walking for 6 weeks, 15–30 min at 80% HR_{max}	Treadmill stress test until exhaustion and clinical observation of fatigue	Significant increase in maximal physical performance and clear decrease in fatigue
Dimeo et al., 1999 (26)	59 cancer patients who had just completed high-dose chemotherapy and bone marrow transplantation: 31 breast, 6 seminola, 2 sarcoma, 4 lung carcinoma, 7 Hodgkin disease, 9 non-Hodgkin lymphoma)	Randomized controlled trial with usual care controls	Daily supervised recumbent biking during hospitalization (about 2 weeks) for 30 min at 50% HR reserve	Profile of mood states and the symptom checklist –90 revised	Exercise group showed decrease in psychological distress; controls showed increase in fatigue and decrease in vigor
Shore & Shepard, 1999 (28)	3 children aged 13–14 successfully treated for acute lymphoblastic leukemia and other types of neoplasms and 11 healthy controls	Pre-post test with healthy controls	Supervised 12 weeks of aerobic exercise 3/week for 30 min at 7–85% of the child's HR_{max}	Mood state, body composition, physical fitness, and immune measures	Low maximum oxygen intake, excess body fat, and high anxiety all reduced with exercise training. Immune responses were impaired during acute exercise but changes were insufficient to cause concern for health
Na et al., 2000 (27)	35 stomach cancer patients who had undergone curative surgery	Randomized controlled trial with usual care controls	From postoperative day 2, moderated exercise using arm and bicycle ergometers performed 2/day, 5/week, for 14 days at 60% of HR_{max}	Mean sequential change of natural killer cell cytotoxic activity (NKCA)	Mean sequential change of NKCA demonstrated a significant increase in the exercise group over controls at day 14

HR; heart rate; HR_{max}, maximum heart rate; NKCA, natural killer cell cytotoxic activity; QOL, quality of life.

Kerry S. Courneya is supported by an Investigator Award from the Canadian Institutes of Health Research and a Research Team Grant from the National Cancer Institute of Canada (NCIC) with funds from the Canadian Cancer Society (CCS) and the CCS/NCIC Sociobehavioral Cancer Research Network. John R. Mackey's research program is supported by the NCIC and the Alberta Cancer Board. Ryan E. Rhodes is supported by a graduate studentship from the Alberta Heritage Foundation for Medical Research

TABLE 25.5. SUMMARY OF STUDIES EXAMINING EXERCISE DURING TREATMENTS FOR CANCERS OTHER THAN BREAST

Study	Sample/Treatment	Design	Exercise Intervention/Measures	Outcomes/Measures	Results
Descriptive					
Courneya & Friedenreich 1997 (14)	110 colorectal cancer survivors from provincial cancer registry	Retrospective	Self-reported exercise prediagnosis during treatment and posttreatment	Functional assessment of Cancer Therapy Fatigue Scale and Satisfaction with Life Scale	Survivors who permanently relapsed from pretreatment to posttreatment reported lowest quality of life
Courneya et al., 1999 (16)	53 postsurgical colorectal cancer patients	Prospective	Self-reported exercise over 4 months	Physical, functional, emotional, social quality of life, and fatigue	Increase in frequency of light exercise from pre- to postsurgery correlated with quality of life satisfaction
Keats et al., (32) 1999 (32)	53 adolescent cancer survivors (17 Hodgkin disease or lymphoma, 12 leukemia, 8 central nervous system; 85% had completed treatment)	Retrospective	Self-reported exercise, pre-diagnosis, during and after treatment	Depression and multiple self-concept indices	Patients active at all three points had best psychological status
McBride et al., 2000 (33)	420 prostate cancer survivors (10–74 mos postdiagnosis) who had completed various treatments	Cross-sectional	Self-reported exercise frequency, duration, length of time, and intentions using stage of change measure	Psychological impact of cancer (impact of events scale)	Those who reported exercising regularly had significantly lower impact scores than those who were not exercising
Experimental					
Seifert et al., 1992 (34)	6 head and neck cancer survivors in Germany who had undergone surgery and radiation and un-specified number of controls	Pre-post test with nonrandomized controls	Supervised group exercise program for 1 year 1/week for 60 min posttreatment	Physical capacity, flexibility, muscle endurance, and quality of life	Trends in favor of experimental group but no significant differences due to small number
Sharkey et al., 1993 (35)	10 childhood cancer survivors (5 leukemia, 2 Ewing tumor, 1 each—rhabdomyosarcoma, neuroblastoma, Wilms tumor) who completed at least 1 year chemotherapy	Pre-post test	Supervised exercise program for 12 weeks, 2/week 60–80% of HR_{max} 30 minutes post-treatment. Home-based exercise 1/week added for last 6 weeks	Physical functioning, body composition, and pulmonary function	Exercise resulted in significant increase in total exercise time and trend toward increased peak oxygen update and ventilatory threshold
Dimeo et al., 1997 (29)	32 cancer patients (17 breast car-cinoma, 12 non-Hodgkin lymphoma, 1 nonsmall cell lung carcinoma, 1 sarcoma, 1 seminola) who under-went high-dose chemotherapy and autologous peripheral blood stem cell transplantation	Pre-post test with non-randomized controls	Treadmill walking 5/week for 6 weeks, 15–30 min at 80% HR_{max} using interval training	Clinical observation, treadmill test, hemoglobin levels	Hemoglobin level was significantly decreased in exercise group. Physical performance was signifi-cantly greater at discharge in the exercise group, but 25% of controls, reported fatigue with usual daily activities
Durak & Lilly et al., 1998 (30)	20 cancer survivors (17 carcinoma, 1 lymphoma, 2 leukemia) who had just completed adjuvant therapy (M = 14 months postdiagnosis)	Pre-post test	Supervised aerobic and weight training 2/week at own RPE for 10 weeks	Physical performance, quality of life	Significant increase in muscle strength, endurance, quality of life
Durak et al., 1999 (31)	25 prostate and leukemia cancer survivors (84% had completed treatment	Pre-post test	Supervised aerobic and weight training 2/week at own RPE for up to 20 weeks	Time of machines, muscle strength, quality of life	Increased overall strength by 38–52%, increased time on machines by 24–30%, increased quality of life, but only for leukemia patients

HR_{max}, maximum heart rate; RPE, rate of perceived exertion; M, males.

TABLE 25.6. SPECIAL PRECAUTIONS WHEN EXERCISE TESTING CANCER SURVIVORS

Complication	Precaution
Complete blood count	
Hemoglobin level < 8.0 g/dL	Avoid tests that require significant oxygen transport (e.g., maximal aerobic tests).
Absolute neutrophil count ≤ 0.5 × 10 * 9/L	Ensure proper sterilization of equipment and avoid maximal tests
Platelet count < 50 × * 9/L	Avoid tests that increase risk of bleeding (e.g., high-impact exercises).
Fever > 38°C	May indicate systemic infection and should be investigated. Avoid exercise testing.
Ataxia/dizziness/peripheral sensory neuropathy	Avoid tests that require significant balance and coordination (e.g., treadmill, free weights).
Severe cachexia (loss of > 35% of premorbid weight)	Loss of muscle mass usually limits exercise to mild intensity depending on the degree of cachexia. Avoid exercise testing altogether.
Mouth sores/ulcerations	Avoid mouthpieces for aerobic tests. Use face masks.
Dyspnea	Avoid maximal tests.
Bone pain	Avoid tests that increase risk of fracture (e.g., high impact/stress tests such as treadmill and 1 RM).
Severe nausea/vomiting	Avoid maximal tests.
Extreme fatigue/weakness	Begin tests at lower power output, use smaller incremental increases, avoid maximal tests.
Surgical wounds/tenderness	Select a test that avoids pressure/trauma to the surgical site.
Poor functional status	Avoid exercise testing altogether if Karnofsky Performance Status score ≤ 60%.

Modified from Courneya KS, Mackey JR, Jones LW. Coping with cancer: Can exercise help? Phys Sportsmed 2000;28(5):49–73.

list and discuss individually; some simple examples, however, will provide the general idea. Cancer survivors who have recently undergone rectal or prostate surgery may prefer a treadmill test to a cycle ergometer test for assessing functional capacity. Similarly, cancer survivors presenting with specific limitations in range of movement in the upper extremities following surgery or radiation therapy (e.g., head and neck) probably will not be able to perform tests involving upper body movements (e.g., arm ergometer tests, bench press). Moreover, cancer survivors who have neurologic complications affecting coordination or balance (i.e., ataxia) will require stable testing modes such as a recumbent cycle ergometer as opposed to less stable tests such as treadmill or step tests. Finally, some cancer survivors will experience severe sickness and fatigue at certain times during chemotherapy or radiation therapy treatments and are unlikely tolerate maximal testing. For these patients, submaximal tests should be used with lower initial power outputs and smaller incremental increases.

Body composition tests also may have to be modified. More specifically, skinfold tests may need to be modified based on the surgical or radiation sites, and existing equations may not be accurate for cancer survivors. Moreover, hydrostatic weighing is contraindicated for cancer survivors who are neutropenic or myelosuppressed because of increased risk of infection. Modifications also may be necessary for muscular fitness and flexibility tests. The bottom line for fitness professionals is that creativity will be needed to develop a testing protocol that is comprehensive yet personalized for a given cancer survivor.

Exercise Programming Options for Cancer Survivors

Specific exercise prescription guidelines for cancer survivors are challenging because cancer is not a uniform disease with limited treatment options that elicit predictable responses. Rather, cancer is more than 100 different diseases with myriad treatment protocols that produce a unique constellation of side effects for each individual. Consequently, the appropriate exercise prescription will vary depending on the type of cancer (e.g., prostate, colon, lung), the treatment protocol (e.g., surgical procedure, specific drugs), individual responses to treatment (e.g., level of fatigue, nausea, pain, cachexia, ataxia), baseline fitness, and participant preferences. To date, the only cancer/treatment combination outside of breast cancer that has received even modest research attention is mixed cancer survivors treated with high-dose chemotherapy and bone marrow or peripheral blood stem cell transplant. Even for this cancer/treatment combination, however, we do not know the optimal type, frequency, duration, intensity, or progression of exercise because all studies have compared single exercise prescriptions to a "no exercise" condition. Clearly, determining the optimal exercise prescription for each cancer/treatment combination is a large challenge awaiting future research. Nevertheless, some general guidelines can be drawn from the exercise and cancer literature (13, 37–39), the literature on older adults with other chronic diseases (40), as well as a recent survey on exercise programming preferences of cancer survivors (41). A general summary of these guidelines is provided in Box 25.2.

Cancer history questionnaire

- Date of cancer diagnosis (day/month/year): _____

- Type of cancer (e.g., breast, colon): _____

- Stage of cancer at diagnosis (i.e., I, II, III, IV): _____

- Did/will treatment include surgery?　　Y　　N　　(circle)
  - If yes:　Type of surgery? _____
  - 　　　　Date of surgery (day/month/year): _____
  - 　　　　Limitations imposed by surgery: _____

- Did/will treatment include radiation therapy?　　Y　　N　　(circle)
  - If yes:　Beginning and end dates (day/month/year) _____
  - 　　　　Treament schedule: _____
  - 　　　　Sites of the body irradiated: _____
  - 　　　　Acute/chronic side effects: _____

- Did/will treatment include include radiation therapy?　　Y　　N　　(circle)
  - If yes:　Beginning and end dates (day/month/year) _____
  - 　　　　Treatment schedule: _____
  - 　　　　Sites of the body irradiated: _____
  - 　　　　Acute/chronic side effects: _____

- Please describe anything else relevant about your cancer diagnosis or treatment: _____

_____
_____
_____
_____
_____
_____
_____
_____

FIGURE 25.1. Sample cancer history questionnaire. Adapted with permission from Courneya KS, Mackey JR, Quinney HA. Neoplasms. In Myers J (ed). ACSM's Resource Manual for Clinical Exercise Physiology for Special Populations. Baltimore: Lippincott, Williams & Wilkins, in press.

Exercise goals for cancer survivors will vary depending on the treatment trajectory. It may be useful to begin an exercise program before treatment to build physical conditioning as much as possible. During treatment, exercise goals likely will emphasize exercising regularly, preventing functional decline, and managing specific symptoms and side effects. Immediately after treatment, the goals may shift to rehabilitation of specific problems. Finally, after recovery from the acute effects of cancer treatments, goals may become more long-term, including the optimization of general health and the prevention of specific diseases for which cancer survivors are at higher risk (e.g., osteoporosis, second cancers, cardiovascular disease).

Most of the studies on cancer survivors and exercise have tested walking or cycle ergometer interventions. Walking has been prescribed for home-based programs and is the form of exercise preferred by over 80% of cancer survivors (41). Prescription of walking takes advantage of this natural choice and also has direct implications for activities of daily living.

Most studies prescribing cycle ergometry have been laboratory-based and the most likely reason for prescribing this type of exercise is the availability of the equipment and the particular cancer survivors studied (i.e., breast). The advantages of cycle ergometry include that it is done in a sitting position with leg exercises that minimize the effects of ataxia (i.e., coordination and balance problems) and limitations in upper extremity movement. Some cancer survivors, however, may not be able to perform cycle ergometry (e.g., following rectal or prostate surgery) and only 4% of cancer survivors actually prefer this mode of exercise (41).

The key point when prescribing activity mode in cancer survivors is to take into account any acute or chronic physical impairments that may have resulted from medical treatment. At this time there is no evidence that one type of aerobic exercise is superior to another for the general rehabilitation of cancer survivors. As with all older populations with chronic disease, safety must be the primary issue (40, 42). Swimming should be avoided by those survivors with nephrostomy tubes, non-indwelling central venous access catheters, and urinary bladder catheters. Swimming is not contraindicated for survivors with continent urinary diversions, uterotomies, or colostomies, but survivors should wait 8 weeks postsurgery and avoid open-ended pouch appliances. High-impact exercises or contact sports should be avoided in cancer survivors or palliative care patients with primary or metastatic bone cancer. From a clinical perspective, it is probably safest to prescribe walking. Although ev-

---

BOX 25.2. General Aerobic Exercise Recommendations for Otherwise Healthy Cancer Survivors

Parameter	Guideline/Comment
Mode	Most exercises involving large muscle groups are appropriate, but walking and cycling are especially recommended. The key is to modify exercise mode based on acute and chronic treatment effects from surgery, chemotherapy, or radiation therapy and patient preferences.
Frequency	At least 3 to 5 times per week, but daily exercise may be optimal for deconditioned cancer patients beginning with exercise of lighter intensity or shorter duration. The key is to exercise regularly while allowing for missed days due to treatment toxicities.
Intensity	Moderate intensity depending on current fitness level and severity of side effects from treatments. Guidelines are as follows: 50% to 75% $\dot{V}O_{2max}$ or HRreserve, 60% to 80% HR_{max}, or 11 to 14 RPE. $HR_{reserve}$ is the best guideline if HR_{max} is estimated rather than measured.[a]
Duration	At least 20 to 30 continuous minutes, but this goal may have to be achieved through multiple intermittent shorter bouts (e.g., 5–10 minutes) with rest intervals in deconditioned patients or those experiencing severe side effects of treatment.
Progression	Initial progression should be in frequency and duration, and only when these goals are met should intensity be increased. Progression should be slower and more gradual for deconditioned patients or those experiencing severe side effects of treatment. Progression may not always be linear; rather, it may be cyclical with periods of regression.

[a]$HR_{reserve}$ = maximal heart rate (HR_{max}) minus standing resting heart rate (HR_{rest}). Multiply $HR_{reserve}$ by 0.60 and 0.80. Add each of these values to HR_{rest} to obtain the target heart rate range. HR_{max} can be estimated as $220 - age$ (years).

RPE, rating of perceived exertion.

Adapted from Courneya KS, Mackey JR, Jones LW. Coping with cancer: Can exercise help? Phys Sportsmed 2000; 28(5):49–73.

idence for the efficacy of weight training is only beginning to emerge, the optimal rehabilitation program for older persons with chronic diseases, including cancer, probably will combine aerobic and weight training (40).

The volume of exercise (i.e., frequency, intensity, and duration) prescribed for cancer survivors has closely followed the guidelines set out by the American College of Sport Medicine (36). Most studies have prescribed moderate intensity exercise performed 3 to 5 days per week for 20 to 30 minutes per session. This prescription appears appropriate for most cancer survivors (13, 38, 39, 43) but may need to be modified based on fitness level and morbidity resulting from medical treatments. Many cancer survivors will not be able or willing to exercise at certain times during treatment because of severe side effects such as fatigue, nausea, pain, and diarrhea. However, because the type and severity of side effects are different for each cancer patient, it is essential to build flexibility into the exercise prescription. This flexibility allows cancer survivors to modify the frequency, intensity, or duration of their exercise depending on how well they are tolerating treatment.

High-intensity exercise probably should be avoided during and after cancer treatment because of the potential immunosuppressive effects (44). Fortunately, most cancer survivors prefer low- to moderate-intensity exercise, so high-intensity exercise is not difficult to avoid (41). It is likely that many cancer survivors will not be able to tolerate 30 minutes of continuous exercise at the start of their treatments, especially if they were previously sedentary. Some researchers have used intermittent or interval training (i.e., alternating short sessions of exercise and rest) for survivors during chemotherapy treatment (39, 45) or immediately following bone marrow transplantation (23, 24) as a way of accumulating the 30 minutes. This approach is recommended for older, deconditioned persons with chronic diseases (40, 42) and also may be optimal for cancer survivors who have been sedentary or who are receiving palliative care (13, 43).

In terms of the physical and social context of exercise, a recent survey has provided valuable information on the preferences of cancer survivors (41). For example, 44% of cancer survivors prefer to exercise alone, 27% prefer to exercise with other cancer survivors, and 11% prefer to exercise with others who are not cancer survivors (19% had no preference). Clearly, there is a market for exercise classes specifically designed for cancer survivors. Forty percent of cancer survivors prefer to exercise at home, 19% at a cancer center, 16% outdoors, and 13% at a community center (12% had no preference). These findings suggest that home-based exercise programs also will be popular for many cancer survivors, presumably many of those who prefer to exercise alone. Finally, 48% of cancer survivors prefer to exercise in the morning compared to 23% in the afternoon and only 5% in the evening (24% had no preference). Offering evening exercise programs for cancer survivors may not meet the need of this population.

It is important to recognize that cancer survivors exercise as much for psychological health as for physiological health (16, 46, 47). Consequently, it is important to take psychological benefits into account when prescribing exercise for cancer survivors. As a general guideline, fitness professionals should prescribe exercise that addresses at least several of the following goals: is enjoyable, builds confidence, facilitates perceptions of control, develops new skills, incorporates social interaction, and takes place in an environment that engages the mind and spirit. In a previous publication we have discussed dragon boat racing as the quintessential example of an exercise that may optimize psychological health (20).

Finally, although exercise generally is a safe therapeutic modality for cancer survivors, certain precautions in addition to those related to age must be taken to avoid unnecessary risks. One of the most important things to watch for is the possible presence of metastatic bone disease, which occurs at some point in about 50% of all cancer survivors. Although bone metastases most commonly occur in the vertebra, pelvis, femur, and skull, the most common site of major fracture is the hip. Survivors at particular risk of hip fracture have hip pain that is worse on activity, lytic lesions in the peritrochanteric area of the femur, and metastases that measure more than half the diameter of the bone on plain films. Such survivors should be referred to their treating physician for radiation therapy to the hip or prophylactic surgery, and should avoid contact sports or high-impact exercise. Other important precautions are listed and described in Table 25.7.

Exercise Motivation in Cancer Survivors

The effectiveness of physical exercise as a quality-of-life intervention for cancer survivors depends to a large extent on the motivation and adherence of participants. Exercise adherence is a major challenge in the general population and probably is even more difficult during and after cancer treatments. As mentioned earlier, there is a significant decline in the volume of physical exercise performed by cancer survivors during treatments that has not been recovered even years after treatments are completed (14, 15, 32). Nevertheless, 84% of cancer survivors are interested in receiving exercise counseling at some point during their cancer experience (41). Of these, 39% would prefer to receive that exercise counseling before treatment, 19% during treatment, and 22% immediately after treatment (41).

Fortunately, research has started to examine the major incentives and barriers to exercise in cancer survivors (16, 17, 46–50). Although some general conclusions can be made, the specific incentives and barriers are likely to vary depending on the type of cancer, extent of disease, type of medical treatments, existence of other comorbid condi-

TABLE 25.7.   SPECIAL PRECAUTIONS WHEN PRESCRIBING EXERCISE TESTING TO CANCER SURVIVORS

Complication	Precaution
Complete blood count	
Hemoglobulin level <8.0 g/dL	Avoid activities that require significant oxygen transport (i.e., high intensity).
Absolute neutrophil count ≤0.5 × 10*9/L	Avoid activities that may increase risk of bacterial infection (e.g., swimming)
Platelet count <50 × *9/L	Avoid activities that increase risk of bleeding (e.g., contact sports or high-impact exercises).
Fever >38°C and >40°C	May indicate systemic infection and should be investigated. If neutropenic, avoid exercise altogether. If not neutropenic, avoid high-intensity exercise if fever > 38°C and all exercise if fever > 40°C
Ataxia/dizziness/peripheral sensory neuropathy	Avoid activities that require significant balance and coordination (e.g., treadmill).
Severe cachexia (loss of >35% of premorbid weight)	Loss of muscle mass usually limits exercise to mild intensity, depending on the degree of cachexia.
Dyspnea	Investigate etiology; exercise to tolerance.
Bone metasteses/pain	Avoid activities that increase risk of fracture at the location of bone pain/metastases (e.g., contact sports or high-impact exercises).
Severe nausea	Investigate etiology; exercise to tolerance.
Extreme fatigue/muscle weakness	Exercise to tolerance
Severe lymphedema	Avoid exercises with the affected limb.
Dehydration	Ensure adequate hydration.

Modified from Courneya KS, Mackey JR, Jones LW. Coping with cancer: Can exercise help? Phys Sportsmed 2000;28(5):49–73.

tions, timing of the exercise, and other personal factors (16, 46, 47). Box 25.3 lists some of the common incentives and barriers to exercise during cancer treatments. Not surprisingly, some of the incentives and barriers are unique to the cancer experience, whereas others are common to the general population. The key point for fitness professionals is that cancer survivors will present with unique incentives and barriers to exercise that need to be understood and addressed. Creative exercise programming and adherence strategies will be required for this population, which may be facilitated by an understanding of cancer survivors' exercise preferences (41).

Summary

Over 1 million Americans will be diagnosed with cancers other than breast in the year 2000. Treatments for these cancers are intensive and cause significant morbidity that results in acute and chronic reductions in quality of life. Preliminary evidence from 18 studies suggests that exercise may be a beneficial therapeutic modality for a wide variety of cancer survivors. Exercise testing and prescription in this population must take into account the diverse morbidities caused by the disease and treatments. Guidelines for exercise prescription include moderate-intensity exercise performed three to five times per week for 30 to 60 minutes in an environment that optimizes psychosocial health. Finally, facilitating exercise adherence among cancer survivors will require a good understanding of the unique incentives and barriers in this population and their preferences for exercise counseling and programming.

BOX 25.3. Common Exercise Incentives and Barriers for Cancer Survivors

Incentives
Maintain a normal lifestyle
Recover from surgery and treatment
Gain control over cancer and life
Cope with the stress of cancer and treatment
Get mind off cancer and treatment
Feel better and improve well-being
General health benefits
Social aspects
Enjoy weather/outdoors

Barriers
Bad weather
Fatigue/tiredness
Concurrent medical condition
Lack of time/too busy
Nausea
Diarrhea
Family responsibilities
Pain/soreness
Lack of support for exercise
Lack of counseling for exercise

DISCUSSION QUESTIONS

1 What is the role of lifestyle in reducing the risk of cancer?

2 What special precautions should be taken when exercise testing or prescribing exercise for cancer survivors?

3 What are some examples of creative programing options that may optimize exercise adherence in cancer patients?

What We Know
About Exercise After Cancers Other Than Breast:

1 The number of persons being diagnosed with and surviving cancer will continue to increase.

2 Exercise levels are significantly reduced during cancer treatments, and they are not recovered even years after treatment is completed.

3 Exercise appears safe and feasible for most cancer survivors.

4 Exercise probably improves physical function and quality of life both during and after cancer treatments.

5 Exercise testing and programming require modifications based on the diverse morbidities resulting from each cancer/treatment combination.

What We Would Like to Know
About Exercise After Cancers Other Than Breast:

1 What is the safety, feasibility, and efficacy of exercise for persons diagnosed with cancers other than breast (e.g., prostate, colorectal, lung, endometrial)?

2 What is the safety, feasibility, and efficacy of exercise during treatments other than dose-intensive chemotherapy with stem cell support (e.g., external beam radiation therapy, brachytherapy, conventional chemotherapies, hormonal therapies, biologic therapies)?

3 What is the safety, feasibility, and efficacy of exercise for cancer survivors with advanced disease receiving palliative care?

4 What is the optimal time course for initiating exercise after a cancer diagnosis (e.g., before treatment, during treatment, immediately after treatment, 3 to 6 months posttreatment)?

5 What is the optimal mode (e.g., aerobic versus resistance), frequency, duration, intensity, progression, and context (e.g., home-based versus supervised) of exercise for optimizing quality of life after a cancer diagnosis?

6 Who is most likely to benefit from an exercise intervention after a cancer diagnosis, based on such factors as disease stage, previous exercise levels, or patient's personality?

7 How does exercise compare to other interventions (e.g., psychotherapy, group support, diet, medical interventions) known to benefit quality of life in cancer survivors? Are the effects of exercise redundant or complementary to these interventions?

8 What are the effects of exercise on tumor growth, disease progression, recurrence, and survival after a cancer diagnosis? And what are the effects of exercise on intermediate markers of survival in cancer survivors (e.g., immune system functioning, endocrine system functioning, obesity, dose-intensity received)?

9 What are the major determinants of exercise after a cancer diagnosis (e.g., demographic, medical, social cognitive, environmental)?

10 What interventions will be most effective in promoting exercise after a cancer diagnosis (e.g., persuasive communications, environmental supports, physician recommendation, behavior modification strategies)?

CASE STUDY

Patient Information

Shirley is a 48-year-old woman who has been diagnosed with colon cancer. She completed surgery 9 months ago and chemotherapy 3 months ago. She states that she had always considered adopting a more physically active lifestyle but never moved beyond this contemplation. After treatment, she had continued to think about exercising but had not yet started an exercise program. Shirley had trouble with fatigue from the cancer treatment. Further, she has had complications of diarrhea and pain that have since thwarted her intentions to be physically active. However, after listening to our recruitment seminar about the possible advantages of moderate exercise after cancer treatment, Shirley decided that participation in the study might provide the motivation she needed to begin an exercise program.

Although postoperative pain and diarrhea are not uncommon after colon cancer surgery and chemotherapy, they probably should have dissipated by this stage of Shirley's recovery process. It would be prudent to recommend that she undergo a medical evaluation to determine the cause of her continuing symptoms prior to undergoing fitness testing and programming.

Assessments

A baseline fitness test evaluating body composition, strength, flexibility, and cardiovascular fitness indicated that Shirley was in moderately poor physical condition. Her body mass index and sum of skinfold (biceps, triceps, subscapular, suprailiac, medial calf) were 27 and 93 mm, respectively, placing her in approximately the 30th percentile of the population for her age and sex. However, her results for grip strength and flexibility were within the excellent range for age and sex, with 76 kg and 40 cm, respectively. Finally, using a modified Bruce protocol on the treadmill (2 miles an hour at 0% grade), Shirley reached 70% of her predicted maximum heart rate in 154 seconds, suggesting moderately poor cardiovascular fitness. Following this assessment, a 10-week exercise program was prescribed.

Questions

1. What factors must you take into consideration before you develop an exercise program for Shirley?

2. Develop a program of exercise for this patient. Describe the intensity, frequency, duration, and mode of exercise that would be safe and appropriate.

3. How would you be able to evaluate Shirley's progress at the conclusion of your program? Would follow-up be advised? Why? How often?

REFERENCES

1. American Cancer Society. Cancer Facts and Figures 2000. Atlanta, GA: American Cancer Society, 2000.

2. Harvard Center for Cancer Prevention. Harvard report on cancer prevention. Volume 1: causes of human cancer. Cancer Causes Control 1996; 7(Suppl 1):S3–S59.

3. Friedenreich CM. Physical activity and cancer prevention: from observational to intervention research. Cancer Epidemiol Biomarkers Prev 2001;10:287–301.

4. Colditz GA, Cannusico CC, Frazier AL. Physical activity and reduced risk of colon cancer: Implications for prevention. Cancer Causes & Control 1997;8:649–667.

5. Marrett L, Theis B, Ashbury F. Workshop report: Physical activity and cancer prevention. Chronic Diseases in Canada 2000; 21:143–149.

6. Oremek GM, Seiffert UB. Physical activity releases prostate-specific antigen (PSA) from the prostate gland into blood and increases serum PSA concentrations. Clin Chem 1996;42:691–695.

7. Leventhal E, Rozanski T, Morey A, Rholl V. The effects of exercise and activity on serum prostate specific antigen levels. J Urol 1993;150:893–894.

8. American Joint Committee on Cancer. AJCC Cancer Staging Manual. Philadelphia: Lippincott-Raven Publishers, 1998.

9. Ferrell BR. The impact of pain on quality of life: a decade of research. Nurs Clin North Am 1995;30:609–624.

10. Jenny ME, Faragher EB, Morris-Jones PH, Woodcock A. Lung function and exercise capacity in survivors of childhood leukemia. Med Pediatr Oncol 1995;24:222–230.

11. Morrow GR, Dobkin PL. Anticipatory nausea and vomiting in cancer patients undergoing chemotherapy treatment: Prevalence, etiology, and behavioral interventions. Clin Psychol Rev 1988; 8:5517–5556.

12. Pelletier C, Lapointe L, LeBlanc P. Effects of lung resection on pulmonary function and exercise capacity. Thorax 1990;45:497–502.

13. Winningham ML. Exercise and cancer. In Goldberg L, Elliot DL, eds. Exercise for Prevention and Treatment of Illness. Philadelphia: FA Davis, 1994:301–305.

14. Courneya KS, Friedenreich CM. Relationship between exercise across the cancer experience and current quality of life in colorectal cancer survivors. J Alternative Comp Med 1997;3:215–226.

15. Courneya KS, Friedenreich CM. Relationship between exercise during treatment and current quality of life among survivors of breast cancer. J Psychosocial Oncol 1997; 15:35–57.

16. Courneya KS, Friedenreich CM, Arthur K, Bobick TM. Understanding exercise motivation in colorectal cancer patients: A prospective study using the theory of planned behavior. Rehab Psychol 1999;44:68–84.

17. Courneya KS, Keats MR, Turner AR. Social cognitive determinants of hospital-based exercise in cancer patients following high dose chemotherapy and bone marrow transplantation. International J Behav Med 2000;7:189–203.

18. Spiegel D. Psychosocial aspects of breast cancer treatments. Semin Oncol 1997;24:S136–S147.

19. Zabora J, Brintzenhofeszoc K, Curbow B, et al: The prevalence of psychological distress by cancer site. Psycho-Oncol 2001;10:19–28.

20. Courneya K, Mackey JR, McKenzie DC. Exercise for breast cancer survivors: research evidence and clinical guidelines. Physician Sport Med (in press).

21. Cunningham BA, Morris G, Cheney CL. Effects of resistive exercise on skeletal muscle in marrow transplant recipients receiving total parental nutrition. J Parenter Enteral Nutr 1986;10:558–563.
22. Decker W, Turner-McGlade J, Fehir K. Psychosocial aspects and the physiological effects of a cardiopulmonary exercise program in patients undergoing bone marrow transplantation (BMT) for acute Leukemia (AL). Transplant Proc 1989; 21:3068–3069.
23. Dimeo F, Stieglitz RD, Novelli-Fischer U, et al. Correlation between physical performance and fatigue in cancer patients. Ann Oncol 1997; 8:1251–1255.
24. Dimeo FC, Tilmann MHM, Bertz H, et al. Aerobic exercise in the rehabilitation of cancer patients after high dose chemotherapy and autologous peripheral stem cell transplantation. Cancer 1997; 79:1717–1722.
25. Dimeo F, Rumberger BG, Keul J. Aerobic exercise as therapy for cancer fatigue. Med Sci Sports Exerc 1998;30:475–478.
26. Dimeo FC, Stieglitz RD, Fischer-Novelli U, et al. Effects of physical activity on the fatigue and psychologic status of cancer patients during chemotherapy. Cancer 1999; 85:2273–2277.
27. Na Y, Kim M, Kim Y, et al. Exercise therapy effect on natural killer cell cytotoxic activity in stomach cancer patients after curative surgery. Arch Phys Med Rehabil 2000; 81:777–779.
28. Shore S, Shephard R. Immune responses to exercise in children treated for cancer. J Sports Med Phys Fitness 1999;39:240–243.
29. Dimeo F, Fetscher S, Lange W, et al. Effects of aerobic exercise on the physical performance and incidence of treatment-related complications after high-dose chemotherapy. Blood 1997;90:3390–3394.
30. Durak EP, Lilliy PC. The application of an exercise and wellness program for cancer patients: A preliminary outcomes report. J Strength Condition Res 1998;12:3–6.
31. Durak EP, Lilly PC, Hackworth JL. Physical and psychosocial responses to exercise in cancer patients: A two year follow-up survey with prostate, leukemia and general carcinoma. Journal of Exercise Physiology on line (JEPonline) 1999; 2. Available at www.css.edu/users/tboone2/asep/june1.htm.
32. Keats MR, Courneya KS, Danileson S, Whitsett SF. Leisure-time physical activity and psychosocial well-being in adolescents after cancer diagnosis. J Pediatr Oncol Nurs 1999;16:180–188.
33. McBride CM, Clipp E, Peterson BL, et al. Psychological impact of diagnosis and risk reduction among cancer survivors. Psycho-Oncol 2000;9:418–427.
34. Seifert E, Ewert S, Werle J. Bewegungs—und sporttherapie fur patienten mit kopf-hals-tumoren. Rehabilitation 1992;31:33–37.
35. Sharkey AM, Carey AB, Heise CT, Barber G. Cardiac rehabilitation after cancer therapy in children and young adults. Am J Cardiol 1993;71:1488–1490.
36. American College of Sports Medicine. Position stand on the recommended quantity and quality of exercise for developing and maintaining cardiorespiratory and muscular fitness, and flexibility in healthy adults. Med Sci Sports Exerc 1998;30:975–991.
37. Hicks J. Exercise for cancer patients. In: Basmajian J, Wolf S, eds. Therapeutic Exercise. Baltimore: Williams & Wilkins, 1990.
38. Mock V. The benefits of exercise in women with breast cancer. In: Dow K, ed. Contemporary Issues in Breast Cancer. Sudbury, MA: Jones & Bartlett, 1996.
39. Winningham ML, MacVicar MG, Burke C. Exercise for cancer patients: guidelines and precautions. Physician Sports Med1986; 14:125–134.
40. Petrella RJ. Exercise for older adults with chronic disease. Physician Sports Med 1999;27:79–102.
41. Jones LW, Courneya KS. Exercise counseling and programming preferences of cancer survivors. Cancer Pract 2002;10(4):208–215.
42. American College of Sports Medicine. Position stand on exercise and physical for older adults. Med Sci Sports Exerc 1998;30:992–1008.
43. Winningham ML. Walking program for people with cancer: getting started. Cancer Nurs 1991;14:270–276.
44. Shephard RJ, Shek PN. Exercise, immunity, and susceptibility to infection: A J-shaped relationship? Physician Sports Med 1999; 27:47–71.
45. Mock V, Burke MB, Sheehan P, et al. A nursing rehabilitation program for women with breast cancer receiving adjuvant chemotherapy. Oncol Nurs Forum 1994;21:899–907.
46. Courneya KS, Friedenreich CM. Determinants of exercise during colorectal cancer treatment: An application of the theory of planned behavior. Oncol Nurs Forum 1997;24:1715–1732.
47. Courneya KS, Friedenreich CM. Utility of the theory of planned behavior for understanding exercise following breast cancer treatment. Psychooncology 1999;8:112–122.
48. Cooper H. The role of physical activity in the recovery from breast cancer. Melpomene Journal 1995;14:18–20.
49. Leddy SK. Incentives and barriers to exercise in women with a history of breast cancer. Oncol Nurs Forum 1997;24:885–890.
50. Nelson JP. Perceived health, self-esteem, health habits, and perceived benefits and barriers to exercise in women who have had and who have not experienced stage I breast cancer. Oncol Nurs Forum 1991;18:1191–1211.

CHAPTER 26

Breast Cancer

Ann Ward, Jackie Kuta, Lisa Sanborn, Cathy Burt

Overview

Breast cancer is the most common **cancer** among women and the second leading cause of cancer death in women (1, 2). One out of every eight women in the United States will develop breast cancer at some point in her life. The incidence of breast cancer increases with age, with women older than 50 accounting for over 75% of all breast cancer diagnoses. Women under the age of 40 years account for only 5% of breast cancer cases. Men also can get breast cancer. However, for every man who is diagnosed, over 100 women are found to have breast cancer. Early-stage breast cancer has an excellent prognosis, with a 5-year survival rate of over 90% (1). Currently more than two million women in North America are survivors of breast cancer. For this growing group of women, the emphasis of **complementary therapy** is on diminishing the effects of treatment and improving quality of life.

Cancer treatment varies widely depending on the type and stage of cancer and the age and medical history of the patient. Treatment may include surgery (**lumpectomy** or **mastectomy**), **chemotherapy**, **radiation therapy**, and **hormonal therapy**, or—very commonly—combinations of these therapies. All of these treatments have side effects. Common side effects include anxiety, depression, lowered self-concept, difficulty sleeping, fatigue, nausea, weight gain, and limited range of motion and **lymphedema** of the arm on the affected side (3). Women with breast cancer also experience diminished self-concept and self-image (4). These side effects can decrease independence and affect quality of life. During cancer treatment many women become fearful of overexertion and are uncertain of what they can do. Physicians also are not sure how much exercise to recommend and often instruct breast cancer patients to go home and rest. Consequently, many women decrease their level of physical activity, which leads to reductions in functional capacity (5, 6).

With increases in survival and growing recognition of the importance of quality of life, the focus of complementary treatments is shifting to managing symptoms and promoting and restoring optimal function. Exercise training is emerging as one complementary treatment that can help meet these goals. Exercise can address many of the physiologic and psychologic needs of the cancer patient.

This chapter presents background on the pathophysiology of breast cancer and surgical and adjuvant treatments, followed by guidelines for exercise screening and prescription. The focus is on the unique issues that women with breast cancer encounter with exercise.

Pathophysiology of Breast Cancer

The breasts are made up of sections or lobes. Each lobe contains many lobules (glands that make milk), which are linked to the nipple by ducts. Fatty, connective, and lymphatic tissue surrounds the lobules and ducts. The lymphatic vessels in the breast lead to lymph nodes under the arm called *axillary nodes*. Cancer is characterized by uncontrolled growth and spread of cells; breast cancer can start in the ducts or lobules. Most types of tumors that form in the breast are **benign**, but other tumors are cancerous. Cancer tumors that have not spread beyond the area where they began are defined with the term *in situ*.

Breast cancer is staged from 0 to IV based on how far the cancer has spread (Table 26.1). The **stage** determines the

treatment and outlook for recovery (2). In general, the lower the number, the less the cancer has spread. Stage 0 is sometimes called noninvasive carcinoma or carcinoma in situ and is the earliest stage of breast cancer. **Lobular carcinoma in situ (LCIS)** refers to abnormal cells in the lining of a lobule. These abnormal cells seldom become **invasive cancer**. **Ductal carcinoma in situ (DCIS)** refers to abnormal cells in the lining of a duct. The abnormal cells have not spread beyond the duct to invade the surrounding breast tissue. Women with DCIS are at increased risk of developing invasive breast cancer, however.

Stages I and II are early stages of breast cancer in which the cancer has spread beyond the lobe or duct and invaded nearby tissue. Stage I means that the tumor is no larger than about 2 cm in diameter and cancer cells have not spread beyond the breast. Stage II means one of the following: either the tumor in the breast is less than 2 cm in diameter and the cancer has spread to the axillary lymph nodes; or the tumor is between 2 and 5 cm in diameter, with or without spread to the axillary lymph nodes; or the tumor is larger than 5 cm but has not spread to the axillary lymph nodes.

Stage III also is called *locally advanced* cancer. In this stage, the tumor in the breast is large (>5 cm across) and the cancer has spread to the axillary lymph nodes; or the cancer has spread to other lymph nodes or other tissues near the breast. Stage IV indicates the cancer has metastasized to other organs of the body (e.g., bone, liver, or lung). **Recurrent cancer** refers to cancer that has come back in spite of the initial treatment. Even when a tumor in the breast seems to have been completely removed or destroyed, the disease sometimes returns because undetected cancer cells remained somewhere in the body after treatment. Most recurrences appear within the first 2 or 3 years after treatment, but breast cancer can recur many years later.

Risk Factors for Breast Cancer

The cause of breast cancer is unknown, but several **risk factors** are linked to the disease (1, 2). The biggest risk factors are being a woman and aging. Other risk factors include the following:

- Personal or family history of breast cancer
- History of noncancerous breast tumor
- Recent use of oral contraceptives or postmenopausal estrogens
- Never having children or having first child after age 30
- Chest radiation therapy as a child or young adult
- Consuming two or more alcoholic drinks a day
- Obesity, especially after menopause
- Mutations of the BRCA1 and BRCA2 genes.

Recently, physical inactivity has received attention as a risk factor for breast cancer. A reduced risk of breast cancer has been observed in both pre- and postmenopausal women

TABLE 26.1. BREAST CANCER STAGING

Stage	Definition
Stage 0	In situ
Stage I	Tumor size: ≤2 cm, no evidence of spread to lymph nodes
Stage II	Tumor size: 2–5 cm, no evidence of spread to lymph nodes
	or
	Tumor size ≤2 cm, one or more positive lymph nodes
Stage III	Tumor size >5 cm, usually one or more positive lymph nodes
Stage IV	Tumor size: any size, evidence of cancer spread somewhere else in the body

TABLE 26.2.   SURGICAL INTERVENTIONS FOR BREAST CANCER

Surgical Procedure	Description
Lumpectomy	Removal of a breast lump and the surrounding tissue.
Simple (total) mastectomy	Removal of the entire breast. Does not include removal of the lymph nodes underneath the arm or the muscle tissue beneath the breast.
Modified radical mastectomy	Removal of the entire breast and the lymph nodes underneath the arm.
Radical mastectomy	Removal of the entire breast, the lymph nodes underneath the arm, and the pectoral muscles beneath the breast. This procedure is rarely performed.
Lymph node dissection	Removal of a sampling of lymph nodes in the armpit to determine if the cancer cells have spread beyond the breast. This procedure is performed in conjunction with lumpectomy or mastectomy.
Sentinel node biopsy	Procedure in which a dye or radioactive substance is injected around the breast tumor. The substance flows into the sentinel lymph nodes (the first lymph nodes that cancer is likely to spread to from the primary tumor). The sentinel nodes are removed to check for the presence of tumor cells. This procedure is less invasive than lymph node dissection.
Breast reconstruction	An option for women who have had a mastectomy. It can be done immediately after the removal of the breast or at a later time. An implant or the patient's own tissue can be used.

in several epidemiologic studies (7). Furthermore, several possible mechanisms mediating an association between physical activity and breast cancer have been identified (8).

Surgical Interventions

Almost all women with breast cancer undergo some type of surgery, usually lumpectomy or mastectomy with or without **breast reconstruction** (1,2). The different types of surgery are described in Table 26.2. The primary goal of breast cancer surgery is to remove the cancer from the breast and lymph nodes. Most women with breast cancer also undergo a **lymph node dissection** or **sentinel node biopsy** in conjunction with the lumpectomy or mastectomy.

Lymph node dissection involves removal of lymph tissue located under the arm on the affected side to determine if the cancer has left the breast and to determine the course of treatment. With sentinel node biopsy, only one node is removed (the first node that the cancer would spread to) and examined. If the sentinel node contains cancer, more lymph nodes are removed. If it is free of cancer, further lymph node surgery may not be needed. The advantage of sentinel node biopsy is that it can reduce the incidence of complications associated with more extensive surgery by indicating that further surgery is not required.

Adjuvant Treatments

Adjuvant treatments usually are started after completion of surgery and can include chemotherapy, radiation therapy, hormonal therapy, or a combination of these treatments (2). Chemotherapy and hormonal therapy are **systemic therapies**, whereas radiation is a local treatment to

destroy cancer cells that remain in the chest wall or regional lymph nodes after surgery. Understanding the treatments and their side effects and their impact on exercise is important for prescribing exercise appropriately. General side effects of the adjuvant treatments are listed in Table 26.3.

TABLE 26.3.   SIDE EFFECTS OF ADJUVANT TREATMENTS THAT MIGHT AFFECT EXERCISE PRESCRIPTION

Treatment	Side Effects
Chemotherapy drugs	**Associated with all drugs**
Doxorubicin (Adriamycin)	Fatigue
Cyclophosphamide (Cytoxan)	Nausea, vomiting, diarrhea
Taxanes (Taxol, Paclitaxel)	Decreased appetite
5-fluorouracil	Lower back pain
	Difficulty breathing
	Irregular heartbeat
	Sores and blisters
	Associated with specific drugs
	Cardiac toxicity with long-term use (doxorubicin)
	Joint or muscle pain (cyclophosphamide)
	Peripheral neuropathy (taxanes)
	Bone and muscle aches and pains (taxanes)
	Fainting spells and lightheadedness (taxanes)
Radiation therapy	Fatigue
	Tissue damage, burns
Hormonal therapy	Hot flashes
Tamoxifen	Dry mouth
	Slightly increased risk of thromboembolism

Chemotherapy

Chemotherapy is a systemic treatment for breast cancer that is administered orally, intravenously, or through a port. Chemotherapy is given in cycles, with a period of treatment followed by a recovery period. The total course lasts 3 to 6 months. The side effects of chemotherapy depend on the type of drugs used, the amount given, and the length of treatment and can include loss of hair, nausea, diarrhea, and a drop in white blood cell count (see Table 26.3).

Radiation Therapy

Radiation therapy is a local treatment using high-energy rays such as x-rays to kill or shrink cancer cells. Patients usually receive treatment 5 days per week (Monday through Friday) in an outpatient center for about 6 weeks, beginning about a month after surgery. The main side effects of radiation therapy are swelling and heaviness in the breast, sunburn-like changes in the treated area, and possibly fatigue (see Table 26.3).

Hormonal Therapy

The hormone estrogen promotes the growth of some breast cancers; hormonal therapy prevents cancer cells from getting the hormones they need to grow. Women whose breast cancer tests positive for estrogen or progesterone receptors may respond to hormonal treatment. Such treatment may include the use of drugs such as tamoxifen that change the way hormones work or surgery to remove the ovaries. Patients taking tamoxifen are advised to take it for 5 years. Like chemotherapy, hormonal therapy can affect cancer cells throughout the body. Side effects associated with tamoxifen include hot flashes, dry mouth, and a slightly increased risk of thromboembolism (see Table 26.3).

Lymphedema

Lymphedema, an accumulation of excess lymphatic fluid causing arm swelling, is one of the most common problems associated with lymph node removal (9). The removal of lymph nodes and vessels changes the way lymph fluid flows within the breast and arm area. If the remaining lymph vessels cannot remove enough of the fluid in the breast and underarm area, the excess fluid builds up and causes swelling, or lymphedema. Radiation treatment can affect the flow of lymph fluid in the arm and breast area in the same way, putting the patient at increased risk for lymphedema. Infection and traumatic injury can trigger the onset of lymphedema.

Lymphedema can develop soon after surgery or radiation treatment, or it may not develop until many months or even years later. The swelling can range from mild to severe. It is not fully understood why some patients are more likely to have problems with lymphedema than others. As surgery becomes more conservative (i.e., less tissue is removed) it is hoped that fewer women will be at risk of developing lymphedema. Currently approximately 25% to 30% of women treated for breast cancer develop lymphedema at some point (9). The average onset of lymphedema is 2 to 3 years postdiagnosis.

Women generally are instructed to restrict the use of the affected side and particularly to limit the amount of weight lifted to prevent lymphedema (see Box 26.1) (10). Most of these recommendations are based on conventional wisdom rather than scientific evidence. In fact, we believe appropriate exercises can help women regain their normal range of shoulder and arm movement and actually may help to prevent lymphedema by pumping lymph fluid out of the arm through the undamaged lymph vessels. Patients should be encouraged to keep the arm, shoulder, and chest flexible and loose as well as conditioned and strong. Women should follow a systematic and progressive plan starting with range-of-motion exercise and slowly adding more advanced exercises. Each patient will respond to this exercise in her own way and should be instructed in monitoring for signs of lymphedema. Signs and symptoms of lymphedema include the following (10):

- Feelings of tightness in the extremity
- Rings, watch, or bracelet that feels tight

BOX 26.1. Recommendations for Prevention of Lymphedema

Avoid injury and infection of the affected limb

- Use electric razor for shaving
- Wear gardening and cooking gloves
- Maintain good nail care; do not cut cuticles
- Avoid vaccinations, injections, or having blood drawn from the affected arm
- Wear SPF15 or higher sunscreen when outside or in the sun
- Use insect sprays to help prevent insect bites

Avoid constrictive pressure on the arm

- Wear loose jewelry and clothes with no constricting bands
- Carry handbag on opposite arm
- Do not use blood pressure cuffs on the affected arm
- Avoid carrying heavy objects, moving heavy furniture, or doing other activities that cause excessive force or strain on the affected arm.
- Limit activities that require prolonged use of the arm (pulling, digging, raking).
- Avoid weight gain
- Practice drainage-promoting exercises

- Decreased movement or flexibility in the hand or wrist
- Pain, aching or heaviness of the affected arm
- Redness, fever, swelling, or signs of infection in the affected arm.

Treatment of lymphedema is tailored to the cause. If it is the result of an infection, antibiotics will be prescribed. Other treatment modalities include specific exercises, compression garments, special bandaging techniques, and manual lymphatic drainage. Patients typically are referred to physical therapists for further treatment.

Exercise Testing

Screening and Pretest Considerations

Women with breast cancer should be screened before participating in an exercise program to ensure their safety and to provide appropriate exercise prescriptions. This process should include a thorough medical history, exercise history, and fitness assessment. We also recommend that women have their physicians sign authorization forms before participating in an exercise program or exercise testing.

When working with this population, a common mistake is to focus exclusively on the cancer and the treatment of this disease while overlooking other health concerns that can affect exercise programming. Postmenopausal breast cancer patients often have one or more comorbid conditions (e.g., heart disease, chronic obstructive pulmonary disease, diabetes, hypertension, and arthritis) (11). Keeping this in mind, screening for cardiovascular risk, injury history, arthritis, and other underlying medical conditions is important to develop the best and safest exercise program for an individual participant.

Knowledge of the participant's current treatment regime is essential to designing her program and monitoring her progress. Breast cancer–specific questions include which side is involved, what type of surgical intervention the patient has had, what adjuvant treatments were chosen and when they were received, and whether or not the participant has had any problems with lymphedema. If the cancer has metastasized, it is important to know what organs are affected. Certain sites of metastasis may require modifications to the exercise testing and training program. Contraindications to exercise testing listed in the *ACSM's Guidelines for Exercise Testing and Prescription* should be noted and observed (12). In addition, women with anemia (hemoglobin < 8 g) or fever should be excluded until that condition is resolved. In women with bone metastasis, tests and exercises that increase the risk of fracture must be avoided.

Fitness Assessment

Most women recovering from breast cancer can perform the same fitness assessments as other health and fitness clients

with a few modifications. These assessments include measurements of resting heart rate and blood pressure, body composition, strength, flexibility, and aerobic capacity. In addition, assessment of shoulder range of motion and strength also is helpful for determining if the cancer survivor has any deficits on the affected side and therefore would need specific exercises.

Because of the breast cancer patients' risk of developing lymphedema, it is useful to make circumferential or volumetric measurements periodically, although no criteria for diagnosing lymphedema have been established. Water displacement measurement 15 cm above the epicondyle has been suggested as the best objective criterion (9). An increased displacement of 200 ml included 96.4% of patients with subjective lymphedema in one study.

When using arm circumferences for evaluation, Harris and Niesen-Vertommen (13) recommend comparing at four consistent landmarks: across the midpalm of the hand; at the wrist (just distal to the ulnar styloid process); 5 cm distal to the lateral epicondyle; and 5 cm proximal to the lateral epicondyle. A clinically significant difference in arm circumference is defined as a difference of more than 2.5 cm between the ipsilateral and contralateral upper extremities.

Evaluation of Peak Aerobic Capacity

We use a submaximal test to estimate peak aerobic capacity. The submaximal test can be performed using a treadmill, bicycle ergometer, or walking track. The single-stage submaximal treadmill test and the 1-mile walk test are simple protocols that provide accurate estimates of aerobic capacity and work well in this population (14, 15). The 6- or 12-minute walk tests may be more appropriate in extremely debilitated women as an assessment of functional ability.

Maximal or peak aerobic capacity testing is possible in women recovering from breast cancer. However, some participants may still be undergoing treatment; requiring them to perform a maximal test may be challenging, therefore, and, in some cases, contraindicated. In addition, this level of testing is time-consuming and expensive. Appropriate exercise prescriptions can be developed by an experienced exercise professional using data obtained from a submaximal performance. Participants who are at higher risk based on their personal medical history or risk factors for cardiovascular disease should be referred to their primary care physician for an appropriate work-up and clearance for exercise, which may include a diagnostic exercise test.

If maximal testing is chosen, several options are available. A protocol such as the Modified Balke Protocol, which uses a constant walking speed of 2.5% increases in elevation, works well. With this protocol, peak oxygen capacity can be either measured or estimated from the final completed stage using ACSM metabolic equations.

Program Design and Exercise Prescription

Most women with breast cancer can start exercising once they have recovered from surgery. The goal for women undergoing treatment is to maintain strength, endurance, and functional ability and minimize side effects of treatment. After treatment has ended, the goal may shift to improving the woman's functional ability and fitness. Home programs are safe and feasible, but we have found that many breast cancer survivors enjoy exercising in a group. Fitness levels may vary according to age and past experience with exercise. For women undergoing adjuvant treatment, the type of treatment may affect how they feel day to day and the amount of energy they want (or are able) to expend. It is important to be sensitive to the needs of each individual patient and to set reasonable and realistic goals for each woman.

Exercise Prescription and Format

The exercise session should include a warm-up phase, aerobic activity, and a cool-down phase. No research is available on the optimal exercise dose, but the ACSM guidelines for exercise can be followed, with a few modifications (12):

Mode: Aerobic, flexibility, and resistance exercise
Frequency: 3 to 7 days/week (depending on intensity and duration)
Intensity: 40% to 80% $\dot{V}O_{2max}$ or heart rate reserve
Duration: 20 to 40 minutes of aerobic activity

The recommended format for an exercise session is as follows:

1. *Warm-up/stretching for flexibility (10–15 minutes).* The warm-up should include activities that use large muscle groups, such as walking, biking, and swimming. The activity should be performed in a slow and deliberate manner. This activity is followed by a stretching routine that involves the whole body but with a strong emphasis on the upper body (shoulder and back) to facilitate return to presurgery range of motion.
2. *Aerobic activity (20–40 minutes).* A variety of modalities are appropriate for this population. These include walking, jogging, biking, rowing, swimming, and use of stationary equipment. The intensity and duration of aerobic training depends on the woman's current health status and exercise capacity. If the participant has not been exercising, she should be encouraged to start slowly at 50% to 60% of aerobic capacity for 10 to 20 minutes, gradually working up to 75% to 80% of aerobic capacity for 30 to 40 minutes, as tolerated. Specific workloads and programs are recommended on an individual basis. Recommendations for exercise for women undergoing treatment are different from those for women who have completed treatment. While undergoing treatment, participants often will have to vary their workouts on a day-to-day basis because fatigue and other side effects will affect their ability to exercise. Women who have recovered from treatment can follow exercise prescriptions and progress similar to those for clients who do not have cancer.
3. *Cool-down (10–15 minutes).* The cool-down includes slow aerobic movements for a few minutes, additional stretching, and strengthening activities. Resistance bands and tubes, free weights, Physioballs, and calisthenics are appropriate, depending on the individual's ability. The progression of exercises should be gradual—beginning with no resistance and progressing to limb/body weight for resistance, easy resistance bands, challenging resistance bands, free weights, and possibly the use of resistance machines. For upper-body exercise, it is necessary to monitor each step in this progression to ensure that the involved arm is ready and capable of this level of resistance. Participants often will have different needs and abilities on one side of the body than on the other. In this case, the use of different resistance on each side is appropriate and should be encouraged.

Precautions and Modifications to the Exercise Program

Each type of breast cancer intervention requires some special consideration when the patient is exercising. Many different types of drugs or combinations of drugs are used for chemotherapy, but they share some common side effects. General side effects of chemotherapy include extreme fatigue and nausea. Health care professionals generally recommend that women not exercise for 24 to 48 hours following chemotherapy. However, some women can exercise the day after chemotherapy and report that the exercise helps them recover from the treatment faster. Because women are at increased risk for dehydration during chemotherapy treatment, they should be encouraged to drink plenty of fluids before, during, and after exercise. Due to the nausea that may accompany chemotherapy, many women lose their appetite and therefore skip meals. Women should be encouraged to eat in the hours before exercising. Women who have recently had a port implanted or are being treated for a port infection should not exercise in a pool. Day-to-day fluctuations in ability to perform exercise should be expected, and participants should be informed that this is common. On days that a woman is not feeling well or has a high level of fatigue, she should be encouraged to continue exercise but at a lower intensity and duration. Women often report feeling better and less fatigued after exercise. A very fine line exists between remaining active and overdoing.

General side effects of radiation therapy include fatigue and burns to the local area. It may be necessary to adjust exercise programs, because burns may be irritated by clothing that moves over the skin surface in response to body motion. Fatigue usually is worse toward the end of treatment, but individuals respond differently. In many cases the workload needs to be reduced, and it may be necessary to modify or discontinue exercises that include arm motion until the burns heal. Pool use should be discontinued until the burns have healed completely. Participants should be encouraged to use the ointments that they are given by their health care providers and to be optimistic that their energy level will return. Tissue damage continues after treatment ends, so exercise program modifications must be maintained for a week or two after the last treatment is administered.

Hormonal therapy is the simplest of the breast cancer treatments. Tamoxifen is the most common drug prescribed for this treatment. Tamoxifen has several side effects including, but not limited to, weight gain, joint pain, dry mouth, and hot flashes. Exercise may counter some of these side effects. When joint pain is an issue, exercise may be useful—symptoms often can be alleviated by keeping the joint active. Participants should be encouraged to try a variety of modes of exercise. Patients with joint pain often enjoy water activities as an option.

When participants present with symptoms of lymphedema, the exercise prescription must be reviewed and often altered. If the symptoms are mild, the first adjustments to try are gentle stretching and a decrease in resistance exercise in the involved side. These adjustments often allow for a safe return to activity. If the symptoms are severe, upper body exercise should be discontinued. In either case, pool activities are strongly encouraged. Specific adjustments made on stationary equipment include not gripping the side railings on treadmills and stepping machines, allowing the involved arm to "ride along" (not actively pushing or pulling) on equipment such as cross trainers and the Schwinn AirDyne bicycle and limiting the use of rowing machines. With aerobic equipment, arm placement and use are key in preventing further swelling. The arm should not be allowed to hang at the side or clenched on equipment. These actions impair circulation of the lymph fluid out of the arm. Proper motion in the arm will aid in the circulation of the fluid. In mild cases upper body ergometers (UBE) may be used to aid in the circulation of lymph fluid. When lymphedema is present, the resistance program must be adapted. In cases of severe swelling, resistance training on the involved side should be discontinued until the swelling decreases. In milder cases, resistance training can be maintained, but resistance on the involved side should be decreased (Table 26.4).

Special Issues

Several concerns are unique to women with breast cancer. These issues are focused primarily on a new body aware-

TABLE 26.4. EXERCISE MODIFICATIONS RELATED TO SIDE EFFECTS OF TREATMENT

Side Effect	Exercise Modifications
Fatigue	Decrease workload by decreasing intensity and duration.
Radiation burns	Modify or discontinue exercises that include arm motion until burns heal. Pool use should be discontinued.
Blisters	Decrease weight-bearing activities such as walking and jogging. Pool use should be discontinued.
Peripheral neuropathy	Be concerned with balance issues. Patient may want to use a cane or walking poles to enhance balance (4).
Lymphedema	*Mild symptoms:* Gentle stretching and a decrease in resistance in the involved side. *Severe symptoms:* Discontinue resistance activities on the involved side until swelling decreases. *Aerobic equipment:* Do not grip handrails or arm levers. Allow the arm to "ride along" without actively pushing or pulling.

ness postsurgery and during treatment and recovery. For some women, body image is an issue when changing and dressing in more public areas (e.g., locker rooms and shower rooms). For others, who have lost their hair as a result of treatment, the question is what to wear on their head while exercising (e.g., wig, scarf or nothing at all). Others must deal with **prostheses** or burns from radiation therapy. These issues may deter women from joining a health/fitness facility to get good, sound advice. Therefore, exercise professionals are responsible for addressing these issues and developing a comfortable environment where women feel free to participate and get the assistance they may need. The exercise professional plays an instrumental role in making the women feel comfortable and secure.

A comfortable environment starts with a staff that understands and is sensitive to the issues of breast cancer survivors. The next step is evaluating the physical environment—for example, is the locker room designed to provide participants with privacy when changing or showering? The final area for consideration is the mix of clientele. For some participants, the more diverse the clientele in the facility the easier it is for them to feel comfortable. However, some participants are so driven to return to exercise or to start a program that the environment will not be a consideration.

Another issue is headwear. Women undergoing chemotherapy usually lose their hair, and most choose to wear wigs. Because wigs limit heat loss, they can become very hot and uncomfortable while exercising. Scarves and light hats are more comfortable. These options allow for heat to escape while providing some head cover in air-conditioned environments. Some women are comfortable wearing nothing on their heads while exercising, even in public places.

Swimwear and pool exercise provide another potentially challenging area for women surviving and undergoing treatment for breast cancer. Many women who undergo mastectomies choose not to have reconstructive surgery. Some choose to wear prostheses. Because prostheses are buoyant, maintaining the correct position of the prosthetic breast while in the pool can be difficult. Fortunately, swimsuits that are designed to secure the prosthesis in place are available.

A prosthetic breast also can be uncomfortable when exercising. Because the prosthesis is not part of the body, it does not always move with the body while exercising. The exercise professional should reassure women that wearing a prosthesis while exercising is not necessary and help them feel comfortable if they choose to go without.

All of these issues may seem minor, but they are very important to survivors of breast cancer. Exercise professionals need to be resourceful and encouraging in this process of helping women incorporate exercise into their lifestyle (Box 26.2).

Physiologic and Psychological Adaptations Associated With Exercise

Only a few studies have evaluated the effects of exercise on women with breast cancer. Most of these studies focused on the impact of exercise on treatment side effects and quality of life (Tables 26.5 and 26.6). Extensive reviews on the effects of exercise training on women with breast cancer also are available (3, 16, 17).

Several observational studies have compared women with breast cancer who exercise with those who do not. Demark-Wahnefried and coworkers measured physical activity in women with breast cancer before and during chemotherapy and found that levels of physical activity decreased during treatment (5). The retrospective survey by Courneya and Friedenreich (4) showed that women decreased their level of physical activity from prediagnosis to active treatment and then increased physical activity posttreatment. Whereas moderate intensity exercise returned to prediagnosis levels, strenuous and total activity remained depressed up to 2 years postdiagnosis. However, women who exercised while receiving treatment demonstrated a higher quality of life and overall satisfaction with life. Demark-Wahnefried and coworkers (18) found that weight gain during chemotherapy was associated with a reduction in physical activity rather than an increased energy intake. Other cross-sectional studies indicate that women who exercise after being diagnosed with breast cancer score higher on quality-of-life scales, have fewer barriers to exercise, have higher self-esteem, and report less confusion, more social support and more vigor (19–21).

Most of the exercise intervention studies have included women with cancer in stages I through III. In most, aerobic exercise conducted 3 days per week for 20 to 30 minutes at 60% to 85% maximum heart rate was compared to control groups who did not exercise. All but two of the studies were 12 weeks or less in duration, and until the recent study by Segal and coworkers, the sample sizes have been very small (22, 23). Some of the studies included only women posttreatment (24, 25). Others were designed to evaluate the effects of exercise on symptoms associated with ongoing chemotherapy or radiation therapy (18, 26–34).

The results of studies conducted in women posttreatment indicate that aerobic exercise training is associated with improvements in functional capacity and mood, and decreased anxiety and depression (24, 25). Nieman and coworkers randomized 16 women (3 years postdiagnosis) to either an aerobic and resistance training program or no exercise (24). After 8 weeks, the subjects in the exercise group demonstrated modest improvements in aerobic capacity and strength, but there was no significant effect on natural killer cells compared to the nonexercise group.

Aerobic training studies involving women undergoing treatment also have found positive results. In these studies, aerobic exercise has been associated with increased aerobic capacity or functional ability, improved strength, improved body composition, less nausea, improvement in scores on the Symptom Checklist-90-R, decreased symptoms of fatigue, fewer sleep problems, improved body image, improvements in internal locus of control, and improved quality of life (23, 27–34).

BOX 26.2. Tips for the Exercise Professional

Client Concerns	Tips for Professionals
Comfortable environment	Private changing areas
	Clientele mix: other clinical populations in the facility may make some participants more comfortable.
Headwear	For women who lose their hair, wigs, scarves, and light hats are options. Wigs are hot and do not allow for proper heat loss when exercising. Scarves and light hats work well in air-conditioned environments. Wearing nothing on their heads should always be an option.
Prosthesis	Can be uncomfortable when exercising. Does not always move with the body when exercising. Encourage women to exercise without it if becomes uncomfortable. The prosthesis can be challenging in the pool because it is buoyant. Swimsuits are available that are designed to secure the prosthesis in place.

TABLE 26.5. OBSERVATIONAL STUDIES OF EXERCISE AND BREAST CANCER

Study	Research Design	Subjects and Methods	Results
Young-McCaughan and Sexton, 1991 (19)	Retrospective cohort study	71 patients diagnosed with Stage I–IV breast cancer (23 receiving treatment) Age: 60 (range, 29–84) Exercise, 42; no exercise, 29 One-time mailing of questionnaires 7 months to 7 years postdiagnosis (85.9% within 2 years of diagnosis)	Patients who exercised reported higher QOL, fewer barriers to exercise
Nelson, 1991 (20)	Retrospective case-control study	54 patients with Stage I breast cancer who had completed treatment Exercise, 40; no exercise, 14 Control group consisted of 54 patients: exercise, 46; no exercise, 8	Exercise associated with self-esteem $r = .34$; patients who exercised perceived greater exercise benefits and fewer barriers
Courneya and Friedenreich, 1997 (4)	Retrospective survey	167 patients with Stage I–IV breast cancer within 2 years of diagnosis, who had completed treatment (87% of patients were Stage I–II) Age: 53 ± 9 years Self-administered questionnaire that assessed exercise behavior prediagnosis, during active treatment, and posttreatment, as well as quality of life	Levels of exercise declined from prediagnosis to active treatment, then increased from active treatment to posttreatment. Exercise during treatment was associated with a higher quality of life.
Demark-Wahnefried et al., 1997 (5)	Observational	20 premenopausal women with Stage I or II breast cancer enrolled prior to chemotherapy. Assessments were made of resting energy expenditure, energy intake, physical activity, and body composition before, during, and after chemotherapy.	Levels of physical activity and energy intake decreased during chemotherapy compared to baseline. Resting energy expenditure decreased during treatment, but rebounded at completion.
Pinto et al.,1998 (21)	Cross-sectional descriptive	71 patients, 248 ± 105 days postdiagnosis Age: 57 ± 13 Control group: n = 14, vigorous exercise 3 d/wk, 20 min/day or moderate exercise 5 d/wk, 30 min/day Breast cancer group: n = 37, vigorous or moderate exercise irregularly IG: n = 20, no exercise	Exercise groups report less confusion, more social support and vigor.
Demark-Wahnefried et al., 2001 (18)	Observational	53 premenopausal women receiving chemotherapy (n = 36) or localized treatment (n = 17). Assessments of body composition, resting energy expenditure, dietary intake and physical activity.	Weight gain during chemotherapy was associated with decreased physical activity, not with increased energy intake.

In the largest clinical trial published to date, self-directed home exercise and supervised exercise were compared in women with stages I and II breast cancer receiving adjuvant therapy (chemotherapy, radiation therapy, or hormonal therapy) to evaluate the effect of structured exercise on physical function and other dimensions of health-related quality of life (22). The women in both groups walked 5 days per week at 50% to 60% predicted maximal oxygen uptake for 6 months. In this study, self-directed exercise was found to be an effective way to improve physical function. No significant differences were observed among the groups for changes in quality of life scores. Supervised exercise improved aerobic capacity and reduced body weight compared to usual care only in participants not receiving chemotherapy.

Kolden and coworkers have conducted one of the most comprehensive studies on exercise in women being treated for breast cancer (23). Forty women aged 45 to 76 years

with breast cancer of stages I through III enrolled in a supervised exercise program 3 days per week for 16 weeks. Assessments were made of body composition, flexibility, strength, aerobic capacity, and multiple dimensions of quality of life (mood/distress, well-being, and functioning). The women experienced significant improvements in strength, flexibility, aerobic capacity, and quality of life (measured as increased positive affect, decreased distress, enhanced well-being, and improved functioning).

Schwartz and coworkers investigated the effects of exercise on daily fatigue in women with breast cancer receiving chemotherapy (34). Seventy-two women newly diagnosed with breast cancer enrolled in a home-based, moderate-intensity exercise program. Subjects maintained daily records of fatigue and exercise duration, frequency, and intensity. Fatigue was significantly reduced on exercise days. The reduction in intensity of fatigue was related to exercise duration. The effect of exercise on fatigue was greatest on the

TABLE 26.6. EXERCISE INTERVENTION STUDIES IN WOMEN WITH BREAST CANCER

Study	Research Design	Subjects	Interventions	Results
Winningham, 1983 (26)	Quasi-experimental	8 women with Stage II breast cancer receiving chemotherapy Exercise, 4 patients Control group, 4 patients H: 4 healthy women	Cycle ergometer 10 to 12 wks 3 d/wk, 30 min, 60% to 85% HR_{max}	Increased functional capacity and internal locus of control
MacVicar and Winningham, 1986 (27)	Quasi-experimental	10 women with Stage II breast cancer receiving chemotherapy Exercise, 6 patients Control group, 4 patients H = 6 healthy women	Cycle ergometer 10 to 12 wks 3 d/wk, 30 min, 60% to 85% HR_{max}	Increased functional capacity and improved mood
Winningham and MacVicar, 1988 (28)[8]	Randomized controlled trial	42 women with Stage II–IV breast cancer receiving chemotherapy Exercise: 16 patients, age 46 ± 12 P = 14, age 48 ± 11 Control group: 12 patients, age 45 ± 9	Cycle, 60% to 85% HR_{max}, 3 d/wk, for 10 wks P = flex and stretch, 3 d/wk, for 10 wks C = normal daily activities	Exercise group showed improvements in Symptom Checklist-90-R and decreased nausea
Winningham et al., 1989 (29)	Randomized controlled trial	24 women with Stage II breast cancer receiving chemotherapy Exercise: 12 patients, age 45 ± 10 Control group: 12 patients, age 45 ± 10	Cycle 20 to 30 min, 3 d/wk, 60% to 85% HR_{max}, for 10 wks	Both groups gained weight Exercise group lost fat and gained lean body mass Control group gained fat and lost lean body mass
MacVicar et al., 1989 (30)	Randomized controlled trial	45 women with Stage II breast cancer receiving chemotherapy Exercise: 18 patients, age 45 ± 10 P = 11, age 46 ± 10 Control group: 16 patients, age 44 ± 9	E: Cycle 3 d/wk, 30 min, 60% to 85% HR_{max}, for 10 wks P: flex and stretch 3 d/wk, for 10 wks C: normal daily activities	Improved functional capacity in Exercise group versus P and Control group
Mock et al., 1994 (31)	Randomized controlled trial	14 women with Stage I and II breast cancer, some receiving treatment Exercise: 9 patients Control group: 5 patients	Walking 10 to 45 min, 4-5 d/wk, for 4-6 mos	Increased 12-min walk distance Improved body image, decreased fatigue, nausea, depression
Nieman et al., 1995 (24)	Randomized controlled trial	12 women ± 1 year post-diagnosis and treatment Exercise: 6 patients, age 61 ± 4 Control group: 6 patients, age 51 ± 5	60 min supervised weight training and aerobic activity, 75% HR_{max}, 3 d/wk, 8 wks, 30 min track walking and 2 sets 12 reps	E decreased submax HR increased leg strength No change in NKCA
Mock et al., 1997 (32)	Pre-post experimental design	46 women with Stage I–II breast cancer receiving radiation therapy Exercise: 23 patients, age 48 ± 5 Control group: 23 patients, age 50 ± 8	E = home-based walking (6 wks) C = usual care (6 wks)	E increased physical functioning and decreased rating of fatigue, anxiety and sleep difficulties
Segar et al., 1998 (25)	Crossover randomized	24 women, 41.8 mos postsurgery Exercise: 10 patients, age 47 ± 7 E + BM = 10, age 52 ± 8 Control group: 10 patients, age 49 ± 8	E = 30 min, 4 d/wk, = 60% HR_{max}, 10 wks E+BM = same exercise, rewarded daily C = maintain sedentary lifestyle	E groups showed less depression and state and trait anxiety No change in self-esteem
Schwartz, 1999 (33)	Pre-post test	27 women with Stage I–IV breast cancer enrolled prior to the start of chemotherapy, average age 47 (range, 35–57)	Home-based exercise program, monitored by the Caltrac accelerometer and exercise logs for 8 wks	Exercise improved QOL, functional ability, and fatigue. Improvements in QOL mediated by decreased fatigue.
Segal et al., 2001 (22)	Randomized controlled trial	123 women with Stage I–II breast cancer receiving treatment SD = self-directed exercise SE = supervised exercise C = usual care	Walking 5 d/wk at 50% to 60% aerobic capacity for 6 mos	Both self-directed and supervised exercise resulted in increased physical functioning.

(continued)

TABLE 26.6. EXERCISE INTERVENTION STUDIES IN WOMEN WITH BREAST CANCER (*continued*)

Study	Research Design	Subjects	Interventions	Results
Schwartz et al., 2001 (34)	Pre-post test	72 women with Stage I–III breast cancer enrolled prior to start of chemotherapy, age 27 to 69.	8-week home-based program monitored by Caltrac accelerometers and exercise logs; daily assessment of fatigue	Exercise decreased level of fatigue; intensity of fatigue decreased with duration of exercise.
Kolden et al., 2002 (23)	Pre-post test	40 women with Stage I–III breast cancer, age 45-76 enrolled within 12 mos of diagnosis; most concurrently undergoing adjuvant therapy	Supervised aerobic exercise 30 to 40 min 3 d/wk at 70% heart rate reserve, strength, and flexibility for 16 weeks	Increased strength, flexibility, aerobic capacity, and QOL (increased positive affect, decreased distress, enhanced well-being, and improved functioning)

C, control group; E, exercise group; H, healthy comparisons; HR_{max}, maximum heart rate; P, placebo; QOL, quality of life; BM, behavior modification.

day of exercise and did not necessarily carry over to subsequent days. These data suggest daily low- to moderate-intensity exercise may reduce fatigue in women with breast cancer undergoing chemotherapy.

The results of these studies indicate that exercise training is feasible and safe for women undergoing treatment for primary breast cancer and women who have completed treatment. Exercise can address a wide range of quality of life outcomes among women recovering from breast cancer treatment. Improvements occur in functional capacity, body composition, side effects of treatment, mood, self-image, and quality of life. Future research is needed to examine mechanisms of action and long-term health benefits.

4 Women can exercise while undergoing adjuvant therapy. The exercise dose may vary day to day depending on the severity of side effects.

5 Exercise training is associated with many benefits. Women improve their functional capacity, flexibility, and strength as expected for the intensity, duration, and frequency prescribed. Side effects of treatment such as fatigue, nausea, anxiety, depression, and weight gain are attenuated, and overall quality of life is improved.

6 Women feel better and enjoy participating!

What We Know
About Breast Cancer and Exercise

1 Women decrease their level of physical activity when cancer is diagnosed. The decreased physical activity is associated with decreased functional capacity and increased body fatness.

2 Cancer treatment is associated with many side effects, including fatigue, nausea, anxiety, depression, and weight gain. Exercise can attenuate many of these side effects.

3 Exercise training is feasible and safe. Treatment for breast cancer is not an obstacle to prescribing exercise. Other underlying medical conditions are more challenging to the prescription. If progression is gradual, aerobic and resistance exercise should not trigger lymphedema, and, in fact, they may help prevent lymphedema.

What We Would Like to Know
About Breast Cancer and Exercise

1 What is the optimal type and dose (frequency, intensity, and duration) of exercise training for women recovering from breast cancer? Are the recommendations the same for women undergoing different types of treatment (i.e., different combinations of chemotherapy or radiation therapy)?

2 Why do some women gain fat while undergoing chemotherapy? Can regular exercise minimize or prevent the fat gain?

3 How does exercise training compare with other complementary treatments in the management of side effects?

4 What are the mechanisms for the reduction in side effects with exercise training?

5 Does exercise training provide protection against breast cancer recurrence and improve survival? If so, what are the mechanisms? Evidence supports the role of exercise in primary prevention of cancer, including plausible mechanisms. Does exercise play a role in secondary prevention through the same or other mechanisms?

6 What causes lymphedema? Why do some women develop lymphedema whereas other women do not? Why is the risk lifelong? What is the explanation for lymphedema that develops decades after treatment? Is early-onset lymphedema the same as lymphedema developed years later? What are the best methods for preventing lymphedema? What is the role of resistance exercise in causing or preventing lymphedema?

7 Do women return to the levels of exercise they engaged in before the diagnosis of breast cancer? Do functional capacity, strength, and shoulder range of motion return to prediagnosis levels?

8 Very little information is available on exercise for women with metastatic breast cancer. Is exercise safe and feasible for them? Can exercise help maintain physical functioning and quality of life and help in the management of treatment side effects?

Summary

More than two million women in North America are breast cancer survivors. Exercise training is emerging as a complementary treatment for women with breast cancer. A growing body of research supports the safety and efficacy of exercise both during and following the treatment of breast cancer. Most breast cancer survivors can perform fitness assessments and undergo exercise training with few modifications. The main precaution is to avoid activities that might trigger or exacerbate lymphedema. For individuals who were active before cancer diagnosis, cancer rehabilitation programs should emphasize the importance of continuing to exercise during active treatment. Women who were inactive before diagnosis should start low- to moderate-intensity exercise programs after recovery from surgery. Exercise training is associated with many benefits, including improved aerobic capacity, strength, flexibility, and multiple dimensions of quality of life. Women who exercise while undergoing treatment also experience an improvement in side effects associated with treatment.

DISCUSSION QUESTIONS

1 Should all women recovering from breast cancer undergo fitness assessments before initiating an exercise program? What modifications should be made to the fitness assessments? What additional assessments should be included?

2 What are the pros and cons of performing maximal aerobic and strength testing in women undergoing treatment for breast cancer?

3 Describe specific exercise precautions and modifications for each type of breast cancer intervention.

4 What are some specific measures a health or fitness facility can incorporate to make women recovering from breast cancer feel more comfortable?

5 What are the benefits of regular exercise for women recovering from breast cancer?

CASE STUDY 1

Patient Information

Lisa is a 48-year-old woman diagnosed with Stage II breast cancer in her left breast. Initial intervention included a lumpectomy of the 1-cm tumor and lymph node dissection in which it was determined she had 17 out of 20 positive nodes. Lisa began a series of chemotherapy treatments every 3 weeks for a total of eight treatments. The first four treatments consisted of a combination of adriamycin and Cytoxan (AC), and the fifth through eighth treatments were with Taxol. She experienced fatigue and mild nausea with these drugs. Lisa started an exercise program during the final AC treatments. During the subsequent Taxol treatments, Lisa experienced body aches, fatigue, and mild neuropathy of the feet and fingertips. Chemotherapy was followed by 6 weeks of radiation therapy. The radiation resulted in skin burns from her sternum to the midaxillary line.

Assessments

During the initial assessment the following information was gathered: Lisa has Tourette syndrome and reports that she smoked as a teenager. Lisa had been physically active prior to her diagnosis. She walked on a regular basis and enjoyed golf. The results of Lisa's initial fitness assessment are as follows:

Height: 68.5 inches
Weight: 137.5 pounds
Resting heart rate: 87 bpm
Resting blood pressure: 94/60 mm Hg
Sit-n-reach score: 15 inches
Estimated percentage of body fat: 25.6%
Estimated aerobic capacity: 39.8 ml/kg/min (11.4 METs)
Estimated maximal bench press: 44 pounds
Estimated maximal leg press: 132 pounds.

Questions

1. What factors must you take into consideration before developing an exercise program for Lisa?

2. What additional information might be relevant to your decision-making?

3. Develop an appropriate exercise program for Lisa. Describe the frequency, intensity, duration, and mode(s) of exercise that would be safe and effective.

4. Would you expect to be able to progress Lisa through her program in a systematic fashion?

CASE STUDY 2

Patient Information

Cathy is a 54-year-old woman diagnosed with right-sided stage III breast cancer. The surgical intervention was a lumpectomy of a 3- to 4-cm tumor and a lymph node dissection with 2 positive nodes out of 19. Cathy participated in a clinical trial of chemotherapy, which included a total of 12 treatments (four with adriamycin, four with Taxol, and four with Cytoxan). During her adriamycin treatments, Cathy experienced nausea, fatigue, and blistering in the mouth, throat, and on the soles of her feet. In addition to these side effects, during her second cycle of chemotherapy (Taxol), Cathy developed peripheral neuropathy, extreme body aches, and joint pain. These symptoms and side effects continued through her final cycle of chemotherapy (Cytoxan).

Assessments

During the initial fitness evaluation Cathy shared that she has not been active in years, although she has been doing some arm exercises postsurgery. Her medical history includes allergies to sulfa drugs and tetanus shots. She reports that she had elevated lipid values (borderline) a couple of years ago, but no intervention was initiated. These values have not been checked since that time. The results of Cathy's initial fitness assessment are as follows:

Height : 63.75 inches
Weight: 240.5 pounds
Resting heart rate: 90 bpm
Resting blood pressure: 104/70 mm Hg
Sit-n-reach score: 14 inches
Estimated percentage of body fat: 43.9%

Estimated aerobic capacity: 31.2 ml/kg/min (8.9 METs)
Estimated maximum bench press: 44 pounds
Estimated max leg press: 132 pounds.<\ul>
Cathy's plan is to use the fitness facility where she and her family have a membership.

Clinical trials are prospective trials that study a new treatment by having one group of subjects receive the new treatment while another group (the control group) does not get the treatment. The control group usually receives standard treatment. These research studies usually are randomized so that there is no possibility that subjects will be chosen with any bias toward their current situation.

Questions

1. What modes of exercise should Cathy avoid during her adriamycin treatments?

2. During Cathy's second cycle of chemotherapy (Taxol) she developed peripheral neuropathy. What is peripheral neuropathy and what exercise modifications should be considered?

REFERENCES

1. American Cancer Society. Breast Cancer Facts & Figures 2001-2002. Available at *http://www.cancer.org.*
2. National Cancer Institute. What you need to know about breast cancer. Available at *http://cancer.gov/cancer_information/cancer_type/breast/.*
3. Mock V. The benefits of exercise in women with breast cancer. In: Dow KH, ed. Contemporary Issues in Breast Cancer. Boston: Jones and Bartlett Publishers, 1996:99–106.
4. Courneya KS, Friedenreich CM. Relationship between exercise during treatment and current quality of life among survivors of breast cancer. J Psychosocial Oncol 1997;15:35–56.
5. Demark-Wahnefried W, Hars V, Conaway MR, et al. Reduced rates of metabolism and decreased physical activity in breast cancer patients receiving adjuvant chemotherapy. Am J Clin Nutr 1997;65:1495–1501.
6. Schwartz A. Patterns of exercise and fatigue in physically active cancer survivors. Oncol Nurs Forum 1998;25:485–491.
7. Gammon MD, John EM, Britton JA. Recreational and occupational physical activities and risk of breast cancer. J Natl Cancer Inst 1998;90:100–117.
8. Hoffman-Goetz L, Apter D, Demark-Wahnefried W, et al. Possible mechanisms mediating an association between physical activity and breast cancer. Cancer 1998;83:621–628.
9. National Cancer Institute. Lymphedema (PDQ). *http://cancernet.nci.nih.gov.*
10. American Cancer Society. Lymphedema. Available at *http://www.cancer.org.*
11. Satariano WA. Comorbidity and functional status in older women with breast cancer: implications for screening, treatment and prognosis. J Gerontol 1992;47:24–31.
12. American College of Sports Medicine. ACSM's Guidelines for Exercise Testing and Prescription. 6th Ed. Philadelphia: Lippincott Williams & Wilkins, 2000.
13. Harris SR, Niesen-Vertommen SL. Challenging the myth of exercise-induced lymphedema following breast cancer: a series of case reports. J Surg Oncol 2000;74:95–99.
14. Ebbeling C, Ward A, Puleo E, et al. Development of a single-stage submaximal treadmill walking test. Med Sci Sports Exerc 1991;23:966–973.
15. Kline GM, Porcari JP, Hintermeister R, et al. Estimation of $\dot{V}O_{2max}$ from a one-mile track walk, gender, age, and body weight. Med Sci Sports Exerc 1987;19:253–259.
16. Friedenreich CM, Courneya KS. Exercise as rehabilitation for cancer patients. Clin J Sport Med 1996;6:237–244.
17. Pinto BM, Maruyama NC. Exercise in the rehabilitation of breast cancer survivors. Psycho-Oncology 1999; 8:191-206.
18. Demark-Wahnefried W, Peterson BL, Winer EP, et al. Changes in weight, body composition, and factors influencing energy balance among premenopausal breast cancer patients receiving adjuvant chemotherapy. J Clin Oncol 2001; 19:2381-2389.
19. Young-McCaughan S, Sexton DL. A retrospective investigation of the relationship between aerobic exercise and quality of life in women with breast cancer. Oncol Nurs Forum 1991; 18:751-7.
20. Nelson JP. Perceived health, self-esteem, health habits, and perceived benefits and barriers to exercise in women who have and have not experienced Stage I breast cancer. Oncol Nurs Forum 1991; 18:1191-7.
21. Pinto BM, Maruyama NC, Engelbretson TO, Thebarge RW. Participation in exercise, mood, and coping in survivors of early stage breast cancer. J Psychosocial Oncol 1998;16:45–58.
22. Segal R, Evans W, Johnson D, et al. Structured exercise improves physical functioning in women with stages I and II breast cancer: results of a randomized controlled trial. J Clin Oncol 2001;19:657–665.
23. Kolden GG, Strauman TJ, Ward A, et al. A pilot study of group exercise training (GET) for women with primary breast cancer: Feasibility and health benefits. Psychooncology 2002;10:1–10.
24. Nieman DC, Cook VD, Henson DA, et al. Moderate exercise training and natural killer cell cytoxic activity in breast cancer patients. Int J Sports Med 1995;16:334–337.
25. Segar ML, Katch VL, Roth RS, et al. The effect of aerobic exercise on self-esteem and depressive and anxiety symptoms among breast cancer survivors. Oncol Nurs Forum 1998;25:107–113.
26. Winningham ML. Effects of a bicycle ergometry program on functional capacity and feelings of control in women with breast cancer [Dissertation]. Columbus, OH: Ohio State University, 1983.
27. MacVicar MG, Winningham ML. Promoting the functional capacity of cancer patients. Cancer Bull 1986;38:235–239.
28. Winningham ML, MacVicar MG. The effects of aerobic exercise on patient reports of nausea. Oncol Nurs Forum 1988;15:447–450.
29. Winningham ML, MacVicar MG, Bondoc M, et al. Effects of aerobic exercise on body weight and composition in patients with breast cancer on adjuvant chemotherapy. Oncol Nurs Forum 1989;16:683–689.
30. MacVicar MG, Winningham ML, Nickel JL. Effects of aerobic interval training on cancer patients' functional capacity. Nurs Res 1989;38:348–351.
31. Mock V, Burke MB, Sheehan P, et al. A nursing rehabilitation program

for women with breast cancer receiving adjuvant chemotherapy. Oncol Nurs Forum 1994;21:899–907.

32. Mock V, Dow KH, Meares CJ, et al. Effects of exercise on fatigue, physical functioning and emotional distress during radiation therapy for breast cancer. Oncol Nurs Forum 1997;24:991–1000.

33. Schwartz AL. Fatigue mediates the effects of exercise on quality of life. QOL Res 1999;8:529–538.

34. Schwartz AL, Mori M, Gao R, et al. Exercise reduces daily fatigue in women with breast cancer receiving chemotherapy. Med Sci Sports Exerc 2001;33:718–723.

SUGGESTED READINGS AND RESOURCES

Love SM, Lindsey K. Dr. Susan Love's Breast Book. 3rd Ed. Perseus Publishing, 2000.

The Susan G. Komen Foundation. http://www.komen.org/bci/.

CancerNet. http://cancernet.nci.nih.gov

National Cancer Institute. http://cancer.gov

National Cancer Institute Information Service. http://www.cancer.gov/cancerinfo/

National Alliance of Breast Cancer Organizations. http://www.nabco.org

National Lymphedema Network. http://www.lymphnet.org

Y-Me National Breast Cancer Organization. http://www.y-me.org

Breast Cancer (PDQ) Treatment-Health Professionals. http://cancer.gov/cancerinformation

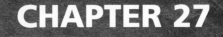
Immune Deficiency

Laurel T. Mackinnon

Overview

The general perception that athletes are susceptible to illness during periods of **intense exercise training** and competition has prompted an interest in whether chronic exercise training suppresses **immune function** in athletes. Epidemiologic evidence and data from short-term studies associate increased risk of **upper respiratory tract infection** (URTI) with endurance training and competition, such as marathon or ultramarathon running. On the other hand, moderate exercise training is not associated with increased risk of illness, and may perhaps provide a small degree of protection against URTI. As will be discussed in this chapter, there is a body of literature suggesting mild chronic suppression of some immune parameters in well-trained athletes. It should be noted, however, that despite evidence for mild **immune suppression** in athletes, they would not be considered clinically immune deficient. That is, athletes do not exhibit severe illnesses associated with clinical im-

mune deficiency. URTI is a relatively mild and short-lived illness, and seems to be the only illness to which athletes seem more susceptible. Nevertheless, the appearance of URTI symptoms at a crucial time in the athlete's training or competition schedule can have adverse effects on performance.

Besides the possible association with URTI, there are other reasons to study the immune system response to intense exercise training in athletes. Both physical and psychological stressors are known modulators of immune function. Physical exercise can provide a useful model to study the immune response to stress, because the stressor (exercise) can be quantified, and repeated exposure to the stressor (exercise training) results in adaptive physiologic responses. In addition, cells of the immune system, in particular neutrophils and macrophages, are involved in inflammatory processes and repair after tissue damage. Some immune cells have been found to localize to sites of injury and inflammation in skeletal muscle damaged by eccentric

421

exercise. Cytokines, soluble mediators of immunity and inflammation produced by some immune cells, also are involved in damage and repair and are released after some types of exercise. Studying the adaptive responses of cells and mediators of the immune system during intense exercise training in athletes may provide a model to understand further the overall regulation of immune function and inflammation, and may have implications for diseases such as chronic fatigue syndrome, arthritis, and immune deficiency diseases.

Experimental Approaches

Approaches to studying the effects of exercise on immune function include both cross-sectional and longitudinal studies. In cross-sectional studies, immune parameters such as illness rate or immune cell number or function may be compared between athletes and matched nonathletes or against clinical reference values. Any differences between groups are inferred to result from exercise training or competition. The disadvantage of such comparisons is that there is a high degree of variability in immune parameters that cannot be discerned from a single measurement. Longitudinal studies may follow a group of athletes over a training season (usually 4 to 8 months), comparing measures of immune function obtained at different times in the season or with samples obtained at the same time from nonathletes. This approach allows a comparison of responses to different levels of training (e.g., moderate versus intense) in the athlete's natural environment. However, it is difficult to control for confounding variables such as competition, psychological stress, diet, travel, and illness, each of which may affect immune function. Sometimes training is intensified for a defined period (usually less than 4 weeks) to study the immune response to **overtraining**. This model does allow more control of variables such as training intensity, but the increases in training volume are generally higher than normal, and some athletes may adapt positively whereas others may show signs of a stress response ("overreaching"). No single approach is without disadvantages, but combining information from all of these approaches provides a more comprehensive view of how the immune system adapts to intense exercise training as experienced by high-performance athletes.

Incidence of Upper Respiratory Tract Infection in Athletes

Symptoms of URTI have been reported to be elevated after endurance competition such as marathon (42 km) or ultramarathon (> 42 km) running. Between 45% and 70% of runners report symptoms of URTI in the 2 weeks after such events (1, 2). Peters and Bateman (1) surveyed 140 South African runners before and after a 56-km ultramarathon.

Compared with age-matched nonathletes living in the same household, runners were more than twice as likely to exhibit symptoms of URTI during the 2 weeks after the race (overall 33% versus 15% in runners and nonrunners, respectively). Moreover, there was a highly significant relation between pace during the race and incidence—that is, the incidence of URTI increased progressively with race pace, with 47% of the fastest runners exhibiting symptoms after the race. Sore throat and nasal symptoms were most often reported, lasting more than 7 days in about half the runners. A subsequent study from the same laboratory also found a higher incidence of URTI in runners after a longer (90 km) race (2).

An epidemiologic study of more than 2000 randomly selected participants in a Los Angeles Marathon showed that runners were nearly six times more likely to exhibit symptoms of URTI during the week after the race compared with runners who entered the race but, at the last minute, chose not to compete for reasons other than illness (3). In contrast, susceptibility to URTI does not appear to be elevated after shorter races, such as half-marathons, 5- to 10-km "fun runs," or middle-distance events (4, 5).

Over the long term, the risk of URTI appears to be related to training volume, at least in runners (1, 6 ,7). For example, Heath and coworkers (6) reported a dose-response relationship between annual training distance and the incidence of URTI symptoms in more than 500 runners. Compared with runners averaging less than 778 km/yr, the odds ratio of URTI was 2 in runners averaging 778 to 1384 km/yr and 3.5 in those averaging more than 1384 km/yr. A high incidence of URTI symptoms may occur during even relatively short periods of intense exercise training. For example, URTI symptoms were noted in more than 40% of the following athletes: swimmers during 4 weeks of intensified training (8); elite hockey players during a 10-day training camp (9); and elite squash players over 10 weeks of intense training (9). In volunteers experimentally infected with a virus that caused symptoms of URTI, moderate exercise training had little effect on the severity and duration of illness (10).

Taken together, these studies suggest that endurance exercise, in particular distance running, is associated with a high incidence of symptoms of URTI. The incidence of URTI symptoms increases for 1 to 2 weeks after major competition, and in a dose-dependent relation to training volume (distance). Moderate or lower volume exercise training does not appear to increase the risk of URTI. These data suggest that intense exercise may alter some aspects of immune function, increasing susceptibility to minor illness such as URTI. The apparent susceptibility to URTI among athletes has prompted a keen interest in whether intense exercise training alters specific aspects of immune function, and if so, whether any of these changes are related to the appearance of illness. It should be noted, however, that virtually all studies on URTI rely on self-reported symptoms, and to date no study has identified any particular infectious agent associated with URTI in athletes. Thus, although symptoms resemble those associated with virally induced URTI, it is not known with certainty that the URTI reported by athletes is actually infectious.

Chronic Training Effects on Selected Immune Parameters

The immune system responds to any challenge in a complex manner, requiring coordinated action by various immune cells and messenger molecules. Any number of stresses, whether physical (e.g., exercise) or psychological (e.g., bereavement), can induce a host of changes in immune function. Because of the complexity of the immune system, it is impossible simultaneously to study all aspects of the immune response to a given event or stressor, such as exercise. Selected immune parameters thus are chosen to give a representative view of particular aspects of immune function. As discussed in the following sections, not all immune parameters respond similarly to the same stimulus; in addition, the extent of change in a particular immune parameter may vary with exercise duration and intensity. Table 27.1 summarizes the responses of selected immune parameters to moderate and intense exercise training in athletes.

Leukocytes (white blood cells) are a heterogenous group of immune cells made up of various subsets with specific functions. Leukocytes circulate among the lymphoid tissues, blood, and lymph, and consist of the following major subsets:

- Polymorphonuclear granulocytes, mainly **neutrophils**, account for about 60% to 70% of circulating leukocytes and are primarily involved in phagocytosis or killing of extracellular pathogens.
- **Lymphocytes** bear cell surface receptors for antigen and make up about 20% to 25% of circulating leukocytes. The two main subsets of lymphocytes are T cells, which initiate much of the immune response and can kill infected cells, and B cells, which produce antibody. Monocytes account for about 10% of circulating leukocytes and are involved in phagocytosis of pathogens and production of soluble mediators of immune function.
- **Natural killer (NK) cells**, about 10% of circulating leukocytes, can kill some tumor and infected cells directly.

Immune Cell Number in Athletes

Resting leukocyte number is generally normal in athletes compared with nonathletes or with clinical norms, and remains relatively unchanged after long periods of exercise training (11–13). A few exceptions have been reported, however. For example, leukocyte count declined progressively after 4 weeks of intensified training, leading to symptoms of overtraining syndrome in middle-distance runners (14). Values at the end of the 4 weeks were near the low end of the clinically normal level (4×10^9/l). Decreases in natural killer (NK) cell number have been noted after short (10–28 days) and long (7 months) periods of intensified training in competitive swimmers (11, 15, 16) and overtrained special services military personnel (17). These changes in NK cell number occurred despite maintenance of normal counts of other immune cells. Thus, although

TABLE 27.1. SUMMARY OF CHRONIC EFFECTS OF EXERCISE TRAINING ON SELECTED IMMUNE PARAMETERS

Immune Parameter	Resting Values In Athletes*	After Moderate Training	After Intense Training
Circulating cell number			
Leukocytes	Normal (11, 12, 29)	No change (12)	No change (11, 12) or decrease (11, 21)
Neutrophils	Normal (11, 22, 29)	No change (12)	No change (12) or increase (22)
Lymphocytes	Normal (11, 22, 29)	No change (12)	No change (11,13)
NK cells	Normal or higher (11, 28, 29, 35)	No change (69)	Decrease (11, 15, 16)
Cell function			
Neutrophil function	Lower (20, 22)	No change (21)	Decrease (21, 22)
NKCA	Normal (28) or higher (29, 30)	No change (34)	Decrease (15)
Lymphocyte activation and proliferation	Normal or higher (11, 29, 35)	No change (29, 36)	Increase (37, 38)
Soluble factors			
Serum Ig level	Low (12)	No change (36)	No change (11, 16)
Serum-specific antibody	Normal (39, 40)	ND	No change in ability to mount specific antibody response (39)
Salivary IgA level	Normal or low (11, 42)	No change (46)	No change (45) or decrease (11)
Plasma glutamine	Normal (14, 48) or low in overtrained athletes (8,49)	ND	No change (8, 14) or decrease (38, 48)

* Resting values are compared with clinical norms or with matched nonathletes.
Ig, immunoglobulin; IgA, immunoglobulin A; NKCA, natural killer cytotoxic activity; ND, no data available.

most studies show normal circulating leukocyte and subset counts in athletes, total leukocyte and NK cell numbers may decline during periods of very intense exercise training. It is unclear whether these changes reflect increased turnover of cells, redistribution of cells out of the circulation to some unknown site or sites within the body, or some other factor. There is evidence of increased leukocyte apoptosis (programmed cell death) acutely after intense exercise (18), but it is unclear whether this contributes to changes in cell number.

Immune Cell Function in Athletes

Despite relatively stable cell counts, there is consistent evidence of alterations in athletes of specific aspects of immune function, including neutrophil function, mucosal immunity, NK cell cytoxicity, and lymphocyte activation; these are discussed separately in this and the following sections. Moderate exercise training seems to have little effect on these variables.

Neutrophil Function

The majority of circulating leukocytes are neutrophils. Neutrophils are essential to the early response to infection by bacteria and fungi, and probably viruses, and also participate in degradation and repair of damaged tissue. Although neutrophil number remains normal, resting and postexercise neutrophil function appears to be reduced during intense exercise training (19). In one of the first studies to note this, trained cyclists exhibited lower neutrophil activation at rest and 6 hours after moderate exercise (60 min cycling) compared with matched nonathletes (20). In another study, neutrophil phagocytic activity was lower at rest and 24 hours after exercise in distance runners assessed during intense compared with moderate training; values during moderate training were not different from those obtained from matched nonathletes (21). In another study on elite swimmers, neutrophil activation declined as training intensity increased over a 12-week training period (22). It appears that a less responsive subset of neutrophil may be recruited to the circulation after a period of intense exercise training (23).

Because neutrophils are involved in inflammatory processes, it has been proposed that this apparent downregulation of neutrophil function reflects the body's attempt to limit inflammation and cellular damage caused by intense daily exercise (19, 24). After intense exercise, neutrophils infiltrate various tissues and organs including the heart, skeletal muscle and nasal mucosa (25–27), where they may release toxic molecules such as reactive oxygen and nitrogen species. Downregulation of neutrophil function may serve to limit inflammatory processes during periods of intense training.

Natural Killer Cell Cytotoxicity

Natural killer cells are a distinct subset of leukocyte capable of recognizing and killing certain tumor and virally infected cells without prior exposure. The cytoxicity of NK cells is important to the body's early defense against viral infection and tumor cell growth. Cross-sectional comparisons of resting natural killer cytotoxic activity (NKCA) find either similar (28) or higher (29, 30) values in endurance athletes compared with nonathletes. In studies showing higher NKCA in athletes, these differences remain after adjustment for any differences in circulating NK cell number. This suggests that basal cytotoxic activity of each NK cell may be higher after endurance training. However, in most studies athletes are rested for 18 to 36 hours before blood sampling, and a long-lasting effect of the previous exercise session cannot be completely discounted (31). The activation state of circulating NK cells, as shown by expression of the activation marker CD69, does not appear to differ between trained and untrained subjects (32). A recent study showed higher resting NKCA during 7 weeks of endurance exercise training in subjects fed a high-carbohydrate compared with a high-fat diet (33). Because endurance athletes often consume a diet higher in carbohydrate than the general public, it is possible that differences in diet may explain the differences in resting NKCA observed in some studies.

Moderate exercise training appears to have little—or, at most, a slight enhancing, effect— on resting NKCA (34). Intense training has been associated with declines in NK cell number, as noted previously, but few studies have addressed the response of NKCA. One study reported a concomitant decline in NKCA and NK cell number over 4 weeks of intensified training in competitive swimmers (15); when NKCA was adjusted for these changes in NK cell number, activity per cell remained unchanged over the 4 weeks. It is unclear whether these declines in NK cell number and NKCA associated with prolonged periods of intense training occur in other types of athletes, and if so, whether these represent simply a redistribution of cells out of the circulation, or increased turnover of cells.

Lymphocyte Activation and Proliferation

Exposure to antigen or other challenges activates lymphocytes to enter the cell cycle, proliferate and differentiate; upon activation, lymphocytes display cell surface markers that can be quantified. Although lymphocyte number remains relatively stable during periods of intense exercise training, lymphocyte activation and proliferation may be altered. For example, compared with nonathletes, resting lymphocytes from runners expressed more cell surface activation markers, such as the low- and high-affinity interleukin-2 (IL-2) receptors (CD 25 and CD 122) (35). Moderate exercise training does not alter lymphocyte activation or proliferation (36). However, intense training may induce activation, as shown by increased expression of CD25 in soldiers after 10 days of intense running training that induced symptoms of overtraining syndrome (37, 38). Other studies, however, have not found increased expression of activation markers in athletes. As mentioned earlier, NK cell expression of the activation marker CD69 is similar in endurance athletes compared with matched nonathletes (32). Expression of the activation marker HLA-DR appears to be similar in distance runners (28) and competitive swimmers (11) compared with nonathletes. Differences in types and levels of athletes and use of various activation markers may explain the discrepancies between studies. The significance of any increase in lymphocyte activation after intense training is unclear. Lymphocyte proliferation tends to remain unchanged or possibly to decrease after periods of intense exercise training (38).

Soluble Factors

An effective immune system requires coordinated activity of soluble mediators, including **immunoglobulin** and antibody (which bind to proteins on pathogens), cytokines (growth factors produced by various cells which stimulate immune cells), and **glutamine** (needed as an energy substrate and for proliferation in lymphocytes).

Immunoglobulin and Antibody

Immunoglobulin (Ig) represents a class of glycoproteins produced by B lymphocytes that appears in serum and other body fluids. Antibody, Ig that binds specifically to antigens (foreign proteins), is important to host defense against infection by its ability to bind to pathogens and to activate other immune cells. Most studies show clinically normal serum Ig levels in athletes and after moderate exercise training (36), although recent reports suggest that low levels may occur during prolonged periods of intense training. For example, serum IgA, IgG and IgM concentrations were in the bottom 10% of clinical norms in elite swimmers assessed during a 7-month season (11). Cell counts were normal and thus could not explain the low Ig levels. Despite these low serum Ig concentrations, the ability to produce specific antibody in response to antigenic challenge is normal in swimmers (39) and triathletes (40).

The mucosal surfaces of the upper respiratory tract (e.g., mouth, nose, and throat) are bathed in mucosal fluids containing Ig primarily of the **IgA** class, and, to a lesser extent, IgM classes. Because of its ability to interfere with viral adherence to mucosal surfaces, mucosal IgA is an important effector of host defense against viruses causing URTI. The apparent high incidence of URTI among athletes has prompted interest in the effects of intense exercise on mucosal IgA levels (41). Low resting salivary IgA concentration has been reported in some elite athletes (42–44). Salivary IgA levels decline during prolonged periods of intense

training (11) and are lower in overtrained than in well-trained swimmers (45). In contrast, moderate exercise training does not alter IgA levels (46). In addition, low salivary IgA concentration early in the season was predictive of URTI later in the season in swimmers; low levels of subclass IgA_2 (but not IgA_1) were associated with URTI (44). To date, salivary IgA is the only immune parameter to be associated with the appearance of URTI (9, 43, 44).

Plasma Glutamine

Glutamine, the most abundant amino acid in the body, is required as an energy substrate and for DNA replication in lymphocytes. After intense exercise, plasma glutamine levels decline for up to 4 hours, and low plasma glutamine concentration has been associated with overtraining (47). It has been suggested that exercise-induced reduction of plasma glutamine may compromise immune function. Plasma glutamine concentration declined progressively after 10 days of intense, twice-daily training, leading to symptoms of overreaching in special forces military personnel (48), and after 8 weeks of intense interval training in runners (38). Lower plasma glutamine concentration has been noted in overreached compared with well-trained swimmers (8). In athletes showing symptoms of overtraining syndrome, plasma and skeletal muscle glutamine concentrations were the only immune parameter that distinguished athletes with symptoms from those without symptoms (49). However, as discussed in the following sections, glutamine supplementation has little effect on the immune system response to intense exercise.

Overtraining, Upper Respiratory Tract Infection, and Immune Function

Overtraining is a process of excessive training with inadequate recovery leading to a state referred to as "overtraining syndrome," which is characterized by poor performance in training and competition, prolonged fatigue, frequent illness, neuroendocrine changes, and alterations in mood state. Despite few empirical studies on URTI and immune function in overtrained athletes, there is a perception that overtraining syndrome is associated with frequent URTIs. In one study of 24 competitive swimmers, training intensity was increased over 4 weeks. Thirty-three percent of the swimmers exhibited symptoms of overreaching (a more transient form of overtraining syndrome), and 42% exhibited symptoms of URTI (8). Surprisingly, fewer of the overreached swimmers (12.5%) exhibited symptoms compared with 56% of the well-trained swimmers. In another study of swimmers, there was no relationship between increased training volume and intensity and URTI symptoms over 8 months (22). In contrast, a study of 25 athletes found that a high proportion of illness was related to athletes exceeding "individual training thresholds," defined as a combination of training volume and monotony (50).

Only a few studies have assessed immune parameters in overtrained athletes (8, 13, 14, 17, 49, 51), and few of these find perturbations of immune parameters associated with the syndrome. As mentioned above, in distance runners 4 weeks of intensified training leading to symptoms of overreaching caused a progressive decline in circulating leukocyte number toward the low end of the clinically normal range; this occurred only with increased training volume, and not training intensity (14). Declines in circulating NK cell number also were reported after 10 days of twice-daily maximal interval training that induced overreaching in soldiers (17). After 4 weeks of intensified training, leukocyte and subset counts were similar in swimmers showing symptoms of overreaching compared with non-overreached swimmers (13), although plasma glutamine concentration was significantly lower in overreached compared with well-trained swimmers (8). The only immune parameter to differentiate overtrained athletes appears to be plasma glutamine concentration (49).

Thus, the few published studies that address this question directly do not support the perceived association among overtraining, immune dysfunction, and frequent URTIs. Rather, it appears that overtraining syndrome, perturbations in immune function, and URTI may result from a common cause—excessive training with inadequate rest and recovery (52). The risk of URTI appears to be high during periods of intense training, regardless of whether athletes exhibit symptoms of overtraining syndrome. Similarly, suppression of immune parameters is associated with prolonged periods of intense exercise training, but not necessarily that which causes overtraining syndrome.

Modifying the Immune Response to Exercise: Can Illness Be Prevented?

As has been discussed, athletes are not clinically immune deficient, and the only illness associated with intense exercise training and competition is an increased risk of URTI symptoms. The risk of URTI and changes in various immune parameters appear to be most closely related to high training volume and intensity (1, 6, 11, 21, 22), suggesting that careful monitoring of these factors may help prevent illness. The same recommendations for monitoring athletes to avoid overtraining syndrome apply to preventing illness in athletes—periodizing training, and ensuring proper nutrition, adequate sleep, rest, and recovery (52–54) (Box 27.1).

Because URTI is thought to occur frequently in athletes, with the potential to disrupt the athlete's ability to train and compete, there is some interest in finding legal (i.e., not banned) means of altering the immune system response to exercise. Many of these involve dietary supplementation.

BOX 27.1. Practical Recommendations for Preventing Illness in Athletes

- Monitor athletes for adaptation or lack of adaptation to training (overtraining syndrome), and modify training accordingly.
- Gradually increase training volume (<10% per week).
- Individualize training for each athlete.
- Include periodized training along with an adequate taper before major competition.
- Program rest and recovery into the training cycle.
- Avoid too frequent competition.
- Ensure adequate dietary intake of total energy, protein, carbohydrate, and fluids.
- Instruct athletes in relaxation and stress management techniques.
- Ensure adequate sleep.
- Limit exposure to potential sources of pathogens (e.g., avoid air travel, large crowds) during and immediately after major competition.
- Vitamin C supplementation *may* have some benefit.

Data from Gleeson M (53); Hooper SL and Mackinnon LT (54); and Peters-Futre EM (55).

Although its effects are controversial, vitamin C is thought to play a role in preventing URTI under some circumstances such as physical stress (55). Moderate doses of vitamin C may be helpful in preventing URTI in athletes. For example, in a double-blind placebo-controlled trial in runners, vitamin C supplementation (600 mg/d for 3 wk) reduced the incidence of URTI symptoms by half during the 2 weeks after an ultramarathon; supplementation had no effect on the occurrence of URTI symptoms in nonathlete control subjects, however (2). It is unclear which mechanisms might be responsible for any protective effect of vitamin C, but they may be related to its antioxidant properties (55).

As discussed earlier, plasma glutamine concentration may decrease during intense exercise, and it is thought that this may impair immune function by limiting availability of this essential substrate for immune cell proliferation. Immunosuppression secondary to trauma such as burns, surgery or chemotherapy, can be partially prevented with glutamine supplementation. One study found that, in runners and rowers, glutamine supplementation during the 2 hours after competition was associated with a lower rate of URTI symptoms in the following week compared with athletes given a placebo (4). Glutamine supplementation appears to have no effect, however, on immune suppression observed after intense exercise. For example, glutamine supplementation to maintain plasma levels had no effect on exercise-induced changes in leukocyte subset numbers, lymphocyte proliferation, NKCA, and lymphokine-activated cytotoxicity (47). A recent report showed no effect of glutamine supplementation on suppression of neutrophil activity after prolonged exercise (56).

To maintain blood glucose levels and attenuate dehydration, thereby delaying fatigue during prolonged exercise, athletes regularly consume carbohydrate supplements, often in the form of sports drinks. Several studies have shown that carbohydrate supplementation using sports drinks during prolonged exercise attenuates some immune responses to exercise (57). For example, compared with placebo, carbohydrate supplementation reduced the increases in circulating leukocyte and subset numbers, neutrophil phagocytic activity and cytokine levels, and attenuated decreases in NKCA and lymphocyte numbers after prolonged exercise such as running, cycling, and rowing (58, 59). During prolonged exercise, carbohydrate supplementation prevents a decline in plasma glucose level and the associated rise in stress hormones such as cortisol and epinephrine. The attenuated immune response implicates neuroendocrine factors, secondary to changes in plasma glucose level, as mediators of much of the immune response to exercise. Saliva flow rate also is maintained by carbohydrate and fluid intake during prolonged exercise (60), which may help maintain salivary IgA secretion rate and thus provide protection from viruses causing URTI. It is unclear at present whether there is any practical benefit for the athlete in modifying the immune cell response to exercise with carbohydrate supplementation.

Psychological stress also has been associated with increased susceptibility to URTI and decreased mucosal IgA levels, and it has been postulated that the high rate of URTI among athletes may reflect the combined effects of psychological and physical stress (31). Athletes cannot avoid the prolonged periods of intense training that are necessary for performance at the elite level. It may be possible, however, to influence URTI risk by altering the level of psychological stress or the way in which athletes respond to that psychological stress. A recent paper showed significant increases in IgA secretion rate after 30 minutes of relaxation (61), suggesting that regular practice of relaxation techniques may have some potential in counteracting decreases in IgA levels in athletes. There is one published report of an attempt to influence IgA levels and URTI susceptibility by exogenous administration of IgA (62). In this study of elite canoeists, therapeutic doses of IgA increased its level in saliva but not in nasal secretions; the incidence of URTI was unaffected but the severity of illness was lessened.

Possible Mechanisms to Explain Apparent Immune Suppression in Athletes

Given the complexity and overlapping functions of different aspects of the immune system, it is unlikely that any suppression of immunity in athletes results from changes in a single immune parameter. The acute response to a single bout of intense exercise may persist for several hours. Many athletes train at least daily, and sometimes twice per day; it is possible, therefore, that chronic suppression of immunity results from the cumulative long-lasting acute effects of each exercise bout. It has been suggested that immune suppression lasting for several hours after a single bout of exercise may act as an "open window" during which the athlete may be susceptible to infection by pathogens encountered during this time (63). In athletes, intense daily exercise training may thus provide multiple extended intervals of susceptibility. In addition, it is possible that chronic suppression may result if a subsequent exercise bout is begun during the open window of the previous bout (i.e., before immune function is fully restored) (31).

Many acute effects of exercise on immune function appear to relate to neuroendocrine changes, in particular release of stress hormones such as cortisol and catecholamines. It is possible that chronic changes also arise from perturbations of neuroendocrine function, such as alterations in hormone released during and after exercise, hormone receptor number or sensitivity (13, 14, 64). Stress hormones are capable of modulating many immune functions, including release of cytokines, neutrophil function, NKCA, leukocyte concentration in blood, and Ig synthesis. For example, salivary IgA secretion is influenced by sympathetic input during psychological stress (65). As mentioned earlier, carbohydrate feeding during exercise attenuates changes in cytokine levels, circulating leukocyte subset numbers, NKCA, neutrophil function, and monocyte phagocytosis by damping the rise in stress hormones such as cortisol, growth hormone, and catecholamines (57). Psychological stress also modulates immune function via neuroendocrine mechanisms, and it is likely that there is a combined effect of physical and psychological stress on immune function in the competitive athlete.

Relation Between Immune Parameters and Upper Respiratory Tract Infection in Athletes

With the exception of salivary IgA, no single immune parameter has been associated with the appearance of URTI in athletes. In elite hockey and squash athletes, athletes who developed URTI demonstrated decreases in IgA concentration after exercise in the 2 days before symptoms appeared (9); in contrast, IgA levels remained unchanged or increased in athletes who did not develop symptoms. In 26 elite swimmers, an inverse relation was observed between salivary IgA level and incidence of URTI (43). Episodes of URTI were predicted by resting concentrations of IgA preseason, IgA levels before training sessions throughout the season, and by the rate of decline in resting IgA concentration over the season. In contrast, other studies have not found an association between IgA concentration and URTI in various athletes such as rowers and swimmers (16, 66). There is no clear explanation for the discrepancies between studies, but they may relate to a number of factors including the following: the relatively small sample size and thus low statistical power in each study; differences and sensitivity of IgA assays, type and level (elite versus non-elite) of athlete; the time in the training season at which samples are obtained; and the way IgA level is expressed (e.g., absolute concentration, concentration relative to protein, or IgA secretion rate).

Although the relation between URTI and specific immune parameters has not been studied extensively, to date no other immune parameter has been directly associated with URTI. For example, despite a reduction in neutrophil function with increasing training intensity over 12 weeks, there was no relation between neutrophil function and URTI in elite swimmers and recreationally active control subjects (22). In another study, plasma glutamine concentration did not differ between competitive swimmers who exhibited symptoms of URTI and those who did not over 4 weeks of intensified training (8). Again in swimmers, NK cell number and serum Ig levels did not correlate with URTI symptoms over 12 weeks of intense training (16). In elite female rowers, a 2-month history of URTI symptoms did not correlate with lymphocyte proliferation, NKCA, plasma cytokine concentrations, or monocyte and granulocyte phagocytic activity (67). Given the complexity and redundancy of the immune system, it is unlikely that changes in a single immune parameter predispose the athlete to risk of URTI during intense training. If there is any effect, it is likely to result from the combined and cumulative effect of small changes in several immune parameters over prolonged periods of time (i.e., months). For example, it has been suggested that lower mucosal IgA levels combined with reduced neutrophil function may inhibit the ability of neutrophils to clear IgA-coated pathogens by phagocytosis (19).

Is the Upper Respiratory Trace Infection Reported in Athletes Really Infectious?

In the research literature, reported symptoms are consistent with URTI of viral origin, and the term *upper respiratory tract infection* is used to describe the "illness." However, to date no infectious agent has been isolated from ill athletes to firmly classify episodes of illness as infectious. Few studies discount athletes with a history of allergic rhinitis, which may present with symptoms similar to URTI. It has been proposed that symptoms of URTI reported after intense exercise may reflect inflammatory rather than infectious processes (68). Neutrophils localize to nasal mucosa after intense exercise (marathon running), and once there may release molecules that may induce inflammation (27). However, competitive performance is significantly impaired in athletes (swimmers) experiencing symptoms of URTI

(41). If symptoms are due simply to local inflammation of the nasal and oral mucosa, it is difficult to explain how this could adversely affect performance.

Alternatively, it has been proposed that viral reactivation secondary to immune suppression may occur acutely after intense exercise or chronically with immune suppression (41). According to this model, exercise-induced disturbances of normal immune function or inflammation could reactivate Epstein-Barr virus (EBV), to which more than 90% of young adults have been exposed and which remains resident in B cells and oropharyngeal epithelial cells after initial infection. This could account for the transitory appearance of symptoms of URTI, which may then disappear as immune competence is restored during recovery after exercise. Further research is needed to document the etiology of symptoms experienced by athletes associated with intense exercise.

What We Know
About Immune Suppression in Athletes

1 Athletes in endurance sports experience a high rate of symptoms of upper respiratory tract infection (URTI) compared with nonathletes. The rate of URTI symptoms is related to training volume (distance) and competition intensity (pace).

2 Upper respiratory tract infection appears to be the only illness to which athletes are more susceptible. Although URTI is a relatively minor illness, its appearance at a crucial time in the athlete's training or competition schedule can have serious effects on performance. Despite the susceptibility to URTI, athletes do not exhibit what would be considered clinical immune deficiency.

3 Although symptoms of URTI are consistent with viral infection, no infectious agent has been identified in athletes, and it is unclear whether such episodes are truly infectious, reflect reactivation of dormant virus(es), or related to some type of inflammatory response.

4 Athletes exhibit signs of mild suppression of some immune parameters, in particular downregulation of neutrophil function, lower salivary IgA and serum immunoglobulin levels, and reduced number of circulating natural killer cells. These changes are associated only with prolonged periods of intense training.

5 Attempts to correlate changes in immune parameters with episodes or risk of URTI generally show no relation, with the exception of salivary IgA concentration, which may predict subsequent appearance of URTI when values are low.

6 Moderate exercise and short periods of intense exercise training are not associated with adverse effects on immune function.

What We Would Like To Know
About Immune Suppression in Athletes

1 Is the upper respiratory tract infection (URTI) observed in athletes really caused by an infectious agent? If so, what is or are the agents? Do these agents vary by geographical location (i.e., are there different agents on different continents)? Or do symptoms of URTI reflect reactivation of dormant viruses, as recently proposed? If so, what is the mechanism by which exercise allows reactivation of the virus?

2 Are small changes in immune parameters related to URTI? If so, what are the responsible mechanisms? Is it any single parameter (e.g., IgA), or is it the combination of changes in several parameters?

3 Is risk of URTI elevated in all athletes or only those in endurance sports? Is there a dose-response relation between the risk of URTI and training volume or intensity? If so, which of these is more important, or is it the combination of the two?

4 How can exercise training be modified to train athletes effectively without increasing the risk of URTI? What other interventions (e.g., relaxation, stress management, dietary supplements) might be helpful?

5 How can we better monitor athletes after viral infection to ensure prompt return to training and competition without risking further (rare, but potentially serious) complications?

6 Does moderate exercise reduce the risk of URTI and other infectious illnesses?

Summary

The incidence of upper respiratory tract symptoms appears to be higher in endurance athletes during periods of intense exercise training and in the recovery period after major competition. The incidence of URTI seems to follow a dose-response relation with training volume, although moderate exercise training does not appear to elevate, and possibly may lower, risk of URTI. Recent evidence suggests that athletes exhibit mild suppression of several immune parameters during periods of intense exercise training. Because URTI symptoms seem to be the only illness to which ath-

letes are susceptible, they are not considered immune deficient. Whereas circulating concentrations of immune cells are clinically normal, there is evidence of modest impairment in a variety of immune parameters such as neutrophil function, natural killer cell number and cytotoxic activity, and serum and mucosal immunoglobulin levels. It is possible that the combined effects of these small changes in these immune parameters may compromise immunity to minor illness, such as URTI, in athletes. Although competitive athletes must train intensely over prolonged periods of time, coaches and athletes may be able to reduce the risk of illness by: monitoring adaptation to training and adjusting training loads accordingly; programming rest and recovery into the training cycle and after competition; and attending to other factors such as relaxation, stress management, adequate sleep and proper nutrition.

DISCUSSION QUESTIONS

1 By what mechanisms do molecules released from activated neutrophils induce inflammation?

2 What mechanisms are thought to underlie the acute changes in leukocyte functions after intense exercise? Are these similar or different for the various cell subsets (e.g., neutrophils, NK cells, lymphocytes)?

3 How could athletes be monitored over the long term to reduce risk of illness during periods of intense training? How could this information be used to adjust training?

4 By what mechanisms might vitamin C be prophylactic against the common cold? Why would vitamin C be effective in athletes but not in nonathletes?

REFERENCES

1. Peters EM, Bateman ED. Ultramarathon running and upper respiratory tract infections. S Afr Med J 1983;64:582–584.
2. Peters EM, Goetzsche JM, Grobbelaar B, Noakes TD. Vitamin C supplementation reduces the incidence of postrace symptoms of upper respiratory tract infection in ultramarathon runners. Am J Clin Nutr 1993;57:170–174.
3. Nieman DC, Johanssen LM, Lee JW, Arabatzis K. Infectious episodes in runners before and after the Los Angeles Marathon. J Sports Med Physical Fitness 1990;30:316–328.
4. Castell LM, Newsholme EA, Poortmans JR. Does glutamine have a role in reducing infections in athletes? Eur J Appl Physiol 1996;73:488–490.
5. Nieman DC, Johanssen LM, Lee JW. Infectious episodes in runners before and after a roadrace. J Sports Med Physical Fitness 1989;29:289–296.
6. Heath GW, Ford ES, Craven TE, et al. Exercise and the incidence of upper respiratory tract infections. Med Sci Sports Exerc 1991;23:152–157.
7. Nieman DC, Berk LS, Simpson-Westerberg M, et al. Effects of long-endurance running on immune system parameters and lymphocyte function in experienced marathoners. Int J Sports Med 1989;10:317–323.

8. Mackinnon LT, Hooper SL. Plasma glutamine concentration and upper respiratory tract infection during overtraining in elite swimmers. Med Sci Sports Exerc 1996;28:285–290.

9. Mackinnon LT, Ginn EM, Seymour GJ. Temporal relationship between decreased salivary IgA and upper respiratory tract infection in elite athletes. Aust J Sci Med Sport 1993;25:94–99.

10. Weidner TG, Cranston T, Schurr T, Kaminsky LA. The effect of exercise training on the severity and duration of a viral upper respiratory illness. Med Sci Sports Exerc 1998;30:1578–1583.

11. Gleeson M, McDonald WA, Cripps AW, et al. The effect on immunity of long-term intensive training in elite swimmers. Clin Exp Immunol 1995;102:210–216.

12. Hooper SL, Mackinnon LT, Howard A, et al. Markers for monitoring overtraining and recovery in elite swimmers. Med Sci Sports Exerc 1995;27:106–112.

13. Mackinnon LT, Hooper SL, Jones, et al. Hormonal, immunological and haematological responses to intensified training in elite swimmers. Med Sci Sports Exerc 1997;29:1637–1645.

14. Lehmann M, Mann H, Gastmann U, et al. Unaccustomed high-mileage vs intensity training-related changes in performance and serum amino acid levels. Int J Sports Med 1996;17:187–192.

15. Gedge VL, Mackinnon LT, Hooper SL. Effects of 4 wk intensified training on natural killer (NK) cells in competitive swimmers [abstract]. Med Sci Sports Exerc 1997;29(suppl):S158.

16. Gleeson M, McDonald WA, Pyne DB, et al. Immune status and respiratory illness for elite swimmers during a 12-week training cycle. Int J Sports Med 2000;21:302–307.

17. Fry RW, Grove JR, Morton AR, et al. Psychological and immunological correlates of acute overtraining. Br J Sports Med 1994;28:241–246.

18. Mars M, Govender S, Weston A, et al. High intensity exercise: a cause of lymphocyte apoptosis? Biochem Biophys Res Communications 1998;249:366–370.

19. Smith JA, Pyne DB. Exercise, training, and neutrophil function. Exercise Immunology Review 1997;3:96–116.

20. Smith JA, Telford RD, Mason IB, Weidemann MJ. Exercise, training and neutrophil microbicidal activity. Int J Sports Med 1990;11:179–187.

21. Hack V, Strobel G, Weiss M, Weicker H. PMN cell counts and phagocytic activity of highly trained athletes depend on training period. J Appl Physiol 1994;77:1731–1735.

22. Pyne DB, Baker MS, Fricker PA, et al. Effects of an intensive 12-wk training program by elite swimmers on neutrophil oxidative activity. Med Sci Sport Exerc 1995;27:536–542.

23. Suzuki K, Naganuma S, Totsuka N, et al. Effects of exhaustive endurance exercise and its one-week daily repetition on neutrophil count and functional status in untrained men. Int J Sports Med 1996;17:205–212.

24. Smith JA. Neutrophils, host defense and inflammation: a double-edged sword. J Leukocyte Biol 1994;56:672–686.

25. Belcastro AN, Arthur GD, Albisser RA, Raj DA. Heart, liver and skeletal muscle myeloperoxidase activity during exercise. J Appl Physiol 1996;80:1331–1335.

26. Fielding RA, Manfredi TJ, Ding W, et al. Acute phase response in exercise III. Neutrophil and IL-1 accumulation in skeletal muscle. Am J Physiol 1993;265:R166–R172.

27. Muns G, Rubinstein I, Singer P. Neutrophil chemotactic activity is increased in nasal secretions of long-distance runners. Int J Sports Med 1996;17:56–59.

28. Nieman DC, Brendle D, Henson DA, et al. Immune function in athletes versus nonathletes. Int J Sports Med 1995;16:329–333.

29. Nieman DC, Buckely KS, Henson DA, et al. Immune function in marathon runners versus sedentary controls. Med Sci Sports Exerc 1995;27:986–992.

30. Pedersen BK, Helge JW, Richter EA, et al. Training and natural immunity: effects of diets rich in fat or carbohydrate. Eur J Appl Physiol 2000;82:98–102.

31. Mackinnon LT. Advances in Exercise Immunology. Champaign, IL: Human Kinetics, 1999.

32. Gedge VL, Mackinnon LT. Natural killer (NK) cell activation at rest and after exercise in trained and untrained subjects [Abstract]. Med Sci Sports Exerc 1998;30(suppl):S174.

33. Pedersen BK, Tvede N, Christensen LD, et al. Natural killer cell activity in peripheral blood of highly trained and untrained persons. Int J Sports Med 1989;10:129–131.

34. Nieman DC, Nehlsen-Cannarelaa SL, Markoff PA, et al. The effects of moderate exercise training on natural killer cells and acute upper respiratory tract infections. Int J Sports Med 1990;11:467–473.

35. Rhind SG, Shek PN, Shinkai S, Shephard RJ. Differential expression of interleukin-2 receptor alpha and beta chains in relation to natural killer cell subsets and aerobic fitness. Int J Sports Med 1994;15:911–918.

36. Mitchell JG, Paquet AM, Pizza FX, et al. The effect of moderate aerobic training on lymphocyte proliferation. Int J Sports Med 1996;1:384–389.

37. Fry RW, Morton AR, Keast D. Biological responses to overload training in endurance sports. Eur J Appl Physiol 1992;64:335–344.

38. Hack V, Weiss C, Friedmann B, et al. Decreased plasma glutamine level and CD4+ T cell number in response to 8 wk of anaerobic training. Am J Physiol 1997;272:E788–E795.

39. Gleeson M, Pyne DB, McDonald WA, et al. Pneumococcal antibody responses in elite swimmers. Clin Exp Immunol 1996;105:238–244.

40. Bruunsgaard H, Hartkopp A, Mohr T, et al. In vivo cell-mediated immunity and vaccination response following prolonged, intense exercise. Med Sci Sports Exerc 1997;29:1176–1181.

41. Gleeson M. Mucosal immune responses and risk of respiratory illness in elite athletes. Exerc Immunol Rev 2000;6:5–42.

42. Tomasi TB, Trudeau FB, Czerwinski D, Erredge S. Immune parameters in athletes before and after strenuous exercise. J Clin Immunol 1982;2:173–178.

43. Gleeson M, McDonald WA, Pyne DB, et al. Salivary IgA levels and infection risk in elite swimmers. Med Sci Sports Exerc 1999;31:67–73.

44. Gleeson M, Hall ST, McDonald WA, et al. Salivary IgA subclasses and infection risk in elite swimmers. Immunol Cell Biol 1999;77:351–355.

45. Mackinnon LT, Hooper S. Mucosal (secretory) immune system responses to exercise of varying intensity and during overtraining. Int J Sports Med 1994;15:S179–S183.

46. McDowell SL, Hughes RA, Hughes RJ, et al. The effect of exercise training on salivary immunoglobulin A and cortisol responses to maximal exercise. Int J Sports Med 1992;13:577–580.

47. Rohde T, Krzywkowski K, Pedersen BK. Glutamine, exercise, and the immune system—is there a link? Exerc Immunol Rev 1998;4:49–63.

48. Keast D, Arstein D, Harper W, et al. Depression of plasma glutamine concentration after exercise stress and its possible influence on the immune system. Med J Aust 1995;162:15–18.

49. Rowbottom DG, Keast D, Goodman, C Morton AR. The haematological, biochemical and immunological profile of athletes suffering from the overtraining syndrome. Eur J Appl Physiol 1995;70:502–509.

50. Foster C. Monitoring training in athletes with reference to overtraining syndrome. Med Sci Sports Exerc 1998;30:1164–1168.

51. Gabriel HHW, Urhausen A, Valet G, et al. Overtraining and immune system: a prospective longitudinal study in endurance athletes. Med Sci Sports Exerc 1998;30:1151–1157.

52. Mackinnon LT. Overtraining effects on immunity and performance in athletes. Immunol Cell Biol 2000;78:502–509.

53. Gleeson M. The scientific basis of practical strategies to maintain immunocompetence in elite athletes. Exerc Immunol Rev 2000;6:75–101.

54. Hooper SL, Mackinnon LT. Monitoring overtraining in athletes: recommendations. Sports Med 1995;20:321–327.

55. Peters-Futre EM. Vitamin C, neutrophil function and upper respiratory tract infection risk in distance runners: the missing link. Exerc Immunol Rev 1997;3:32–52.

56. Walsh NP, Blannin AK, Bishop NC, et al. Effect of oral glutamine supplementation on human neutrophil lipopolysaccharide-stimulated degranulation following prolonged exercise. Int J Sports Nutr Exerc Metab 2000;10:39–50.

57. Nieman DC. Influence of carbohydrate on the immune response to intensive, prolonged exercise. Exercise Immunol Rev 1998;4:64–76.

58. Henson DA, Nieman DC, Nehlsen-Cannarella SL, et al. Influence of carbohydrate on cytokine and phagocytic response to 2 h of rowing. Med Sci Sports Exerc 2000;32:1384–1389.

59. Nieman DC, Nehlsen-Cannarella SL, Fagoaga OR, et al. Effects of mode and carbohydrate on the granulocyte and monocyte response to intensive, prolonged exercise. J Appl Physiol 1998;84:1252–1259.

60. Bishop NC, Blannin AK, Armstrong E, et al. Carbohydrate and fluid intake affect the saliva flow rate and IgA response to cycling. Med Sci Sports Exerc 2000;32:2046–2051.

61. Reid MR, Drummond PD, Mackinnon LT. The effect of moderate aerobic exercise and relaxation on secretory immunoglobulin A. Int J Sports Med 2001;22:132–137.

62. Lindberg K, Berglund B. Effect of treatment with nasal IgA on the incidence of infection disease in world-class canoeists. Int J Sports Med 1996;17:235–238.

63. Pedersen BK, Ullum H. NK cell response to physical activity: possible mechanisms of action. Med Sci Sports Exerc 1994;26:140–146.

64. Schaller K, Mechau D, Scharmann HG, et al. Increased training load and the beta-adrenergic receptor system on human lymphocytes. J Appl Physiol 1999;87:317–324.

65. Ring C, Carroll D, Willemsen G, et al. Secretory immunoglobulin A and cardiovascular activity during mental arithmetic and paced breathing. Psychophysiol 1999;36:602–609.

66. Nehlsen-Cannarella SL, Nieman DC, Fagoaga OR, et al. Saliva immunoglobulins in elite women rowers. Eur J Appl Physiol 2000;81:222–228.

67. Nieman DC, Nehlsen-Cannarella SL, Fagoaga OR, et al. Immune function in female elite rowers and non-athletes. Br J Sports Med 2000;34:181–187.

68. Northoff H, Enkel S, Weinstock C. Exercise, injury and immune function. Exerc Immunol Rev 1995;1:1–25.

69. Tvede N, Steenberg J, Baslund J, et al. Cellular immunity in highly trained elite racing cyclists during periods of training with high and low intensity. Scand J Sci Med Sports 1991;3:163–166.

SUGGESTED READINGS

Gleeson M. Mucosal immune responses and risk of respiratory illness in elite athletes. Exerc Immunol Rev 2000;6:5–42.

Gleeson M. The scientific basis of practical strategies to maintain immunocompetence in elite athletes. Exercise Immunology Review 2000;6:75–101.

Mackinnon LT. Advances in Exercise Immunology. Champaign, IL: Human Kinetics, 1999.

Mackinnon LT. Overtraining effects on immunity and performance in athletes. Immunol Cell Biol 2000;78:502–509.

Nieman DC. Influence of carbohydrate on the immune response to intensive, prolonged exercise. Exercise Immunol Rev 1998;4:64–76.

Rohde T, Krzywkowski K, Pedersen BK. Glutamine, exercise, and the immune system—is there a link? Exercise Immunol Rev 1998;4:49–63.

Smith JA, Pyne DB. Exercise, training, and neutrophil function. Exercise Immunol Rev 1997;3:96–116.

CHAPTER 28

Allergies

Jason Johnson, William W. Briner

Overview

Allergy can occur in many forms in relation to exercise. Although it often is mild or asymptomatic, in some people it can be severe enough to limit physical activity. Exercise-induced asthma is both common and potentially perfor-mance-limiting in athletes, and is addressed in detail in Chapter 13.

Allergy is commonly manifested by **urticaria** and **angioedema**. These conditions, which occur in approximately 20% of the population (1), are characterized by vascular changes and a subsequent edematous rash. A circumscribed, raised, erythematous rash is typical of urticaria, with **edema** involving the superficial portion of the **dermis**. **Wheals**, the classic urticarial lesion, are pruritic, blanching papules that range from several millimeters to several centimeters in diameter (2). Also known as *hives*, they may become confluent into large patches. Typically, these lesions last less than 24 hours, and leave no residual skin changes. There are many potential causes of urticaria, but usually it is idiopathic. A specific cause is identified in only 21% of cases (3). Table 28.1 reviews potential causes of urticaria.

Unlike urticaria, the swelling of angioedema is more severe, with edema extending into the deep dermis or subcuticular layers. It often is less pruritic than urticaria, but it may be painful. The swelling may last up to 72 hours and also may involve the mucous membranes of the gastrointestinal or respiratory tract (2). Pharyngeal edema occasionally may be severe enough to compromise swallowing or breathing, constituting a medical emergency.

Discussions of exercise and allergy center predominantly around the physical urticarias, a subclassification of chronic urticaria. As opposed to the more commonly occurring **idiopathic** forms, these urticarias are unique in that the characteristic wheals are inducible by a physical stimulus. They comprise up to 17% of all chronic urticarias (4). Causative factors include cold, heat, water, pressure, light, and vibration. It is not unusual for individuals to be exposed to these stimuli during athletic activity, and exercise itself may be a provoking factor. Physical urticaria often can be differentiated from other urticarias by the observation of episodic wheals, often limited to areas of skin that came in contact with the inducing stimulus (4). Although the urticaria is widely believed to be secondary to **mast cell** activation and mediator release, the mechanism by which mast cell degranulation is triggered remains unclear. This release of histamine and other **vasoactive** mast cell mediators such as **prostaglandins** and **leukotrienes** subsequently leads to the skin changes and systemic symptoms commonly seen in the physical urticarias.

Although the physical urticarias are not as common as other forms of urticaria, they are the ones most closely related to exercise and the environments in which people train. Therefore, the remainder of this chapter will concentrate on these specific individual forms of urticaria (Table 28.2).

TABLE 28.1. POTENTIAL CAUSES OF URTICARIA AND ANGIOEDEMA

Foods and preservatives	Bites and stings
Medications	Hereditary angioedema
Idiopathic	Skin contacts
Physical allergies	Blood transfusion reaction
Infectious agents	Inhaled substances
Systemic diseases	

TABLE 28.2. PHYSICAL URTICARIAS

Cholinergic urticaria	Solar urticaria
Localized heat urticaria	Symptomatic dermatographism
Exercise-induced anaphylaxis	Aquagenic urticaria
Essential (acquired) cold urticaria	Delayed pressure urticaria/
Familial cold urticaria	angioedema

Pathophysiology of Individual Physical Urticarias

Symptomatic Dermatographism

Dermatographism (dermographism) affects approximately 2% to 5% of the population, making it the most common form of physical allergy (1). Dermatographism ("writing on the skin") is diagnosed by a characteristic reaction after stroking the skin. Initially, the response is a white line secondary to reflex vasoconstriction. This is followed by linear swelling, erythema, and wheal formation. Symptomatic cases may be intensely pruritic. Hot baths, emotion, exercise, and cold exposure can exacerbate the condition (5). Onset is typically rapid, usually in 2 to 5 minutes, with the lesions lasting anywhere from 30 minutes to 3 hours (4). Less commonly, intermediate or late-onset variants can occur, in some cases as long as 6 to 8 hours later. The skin changes of these variants may take 1 to 2 days to resolve (5). Systemic symptoms are notably absent. Fortunately, the majority of cases are asymptomatic, and do not require medical treatment.

The cause of the reaction in dermatographism is unclear. Studies have suggested an **IgE**-mediated reaction in approximately 50% of cases; no associated **antigen** has been found, however (6). Studies also have implicated elevated **histamine** levels, although other vasoactive substances released from cutaneous mast cells likely play a role.

Treatment with the newer non-sedating antihistamines often is adequate in mild cases. For more severe cases, older sedating antihistamines such as Benadryl are more effective. Combining H_2 antagonists with H_1 antagonists seems to add efficacy as well. These medications are discussed at length in the medication section of this chapter.

Cholinergic Urticaria

Heat allergy occurs in both localized and generalized forms. Cholinergic urticaria, the generalized form, is relatively common. It occurs most commonly in teenagers and young adults, and may account for 5% to 7% of all urticarias (4). In this variant, the stimulus for the reaction is an increased core body temperature. This can be due to exercise, anxiety, or **exogenous** heating (such as hot baths) (1). Urticaria is *not* induced in cases of elevated core temperature due to **endogenous pyrogens** (4).

The lesions of cholinergic urticaria typically are small, punctate, very pruritic wheals on a large surrounding erythematous base. Lesions classically start on the neck, upper trunk, and arms, but can spread distally to include the whole body. In some cases, the urticaria becomes confluent and mimics angioedema (6).

It is believed that the **cholinergic nervous system** involved in temperature regulation has a major role in these changes. Acetylcholine release, which is activated in response to the temperature stimulus, ultimately leads to mast cell degranulation (4). Histamine and other mast cell mediator levels are elevated. Subsequently, affected individuals may experience a spectrum of systemic symptoms related to cholinergic or histaminergic stimulation, including headache, dizziness, lacrimation, salivation, **hypotension**, wheezing, and gastrointestinal complaints (4–6).

Several options are available for testing for cholinergic urticaria. In **methacholine** skin testing, a small amount of methacholine is injected intradermally. A localized hive (wheal) surrounded by smaller satellite lesions is diagnostic (6). Unfortunately, the test is definitively positive in only approximately one third of patients. Whereas a positive test, therefore, is helpful, a negative test is nondiagnostic. A more reliable alternative is a heat challenge. Either through exercise or immersion in hot water (40°C to 42°C), an increase in core temperature of more than 0.7°C results in symptoms.

Treatment

Attacks can potentially be aborted, or at least decreased in length and severity, by immediate cooling of the patient. After a severe attack, some individuals have a **refractory period** of decreased susceptibility (4). In some patients, it is possible to induce **tolerance**. By slowly exposing the patient to stimuli of increasing intensity or duration, the response of cholinergic urticaria can potentially be avoided.

Antihistamine medications are useful in the treatment of cholinergic urticaria, which is consistent with the observed increases in blood histamine levels in the condition. Hydroxyzine is the drug of choice and has been shown to be more effective than conventional antihistamines, although the reason for this is unclear. **Anticholinergic** agents have not been shown to be effective (6),

Localized Heat Urticaria

In contrast to the diffuse heat allergy of cholinergic urticaria, in localized heat urticaria the rash occurs only on the part of the skin that comes in contact with a warm stimulus. This type of urticaria occurs in both immediate and delayed forms. The rash itself is similar to that of the diffuse form. The condition is extremely rare; as of 1988 only 16 cases had been reported in the literature (4). Systemic reactions are unlikely.

The pathophysiology of localized heat urticaria is debated, although many believe that mast cell degranulation with release of mediators plays a role. Arguing against this, however, is the fact that passive transfer studies have been negative. In these studies, serum is transferred from affected to unaffected individuals. The induction of a similar reaction in a previously normal individual is considered a positive test, suggesting the disease process involves some serum factor.

The definitive diagnostic test for this condition is the application of a heated cylinder (50°C to 55°C) to the skin for 5 minutes. The appearance of a characteristic rash within a few minutes constitutes a positive test. Unlike the more diffuse form of cholinergic urticaria, exercise and methacholine skin tests do not produce a response.

Treatment

Treatment primarily involves avoidance of topical heat stimuli. As in cholinergic urticaria, tolerance may be induced with graded exposure to increasing stimulus. Attempts to treat with medication, including antihistamines and cromolyn, have been of minimal benefit.

Cold Urticaria

Just as heat can be a causative factor, cold also can trigger urticaria. Approximately 3% to 5% of urticarias can be attributed to the cold (5). There are various types of classifications, but it is most commonly broken down into primary (essential) and familial forms.

Familial cold urticaria is rare, and is inherited as an autosomal dominant trait. After cold air exposure, the individual develops burning, erythematous **macules** or **papules**. Frequently, systemic symptoms such as fever, chills, **myalgia**, **arthralgia**, **leukocytosis**, and headache are associated. This type of urticaria occurs in both an immediate form, where skin lesions occur approximately 30 minutes after cold exposure, and in delayed form, with effects delayed for 9 to 18 hours. It is not a true urticaria—biopsy specimens of skin lesions reveal leukocyte infiltrates as well as the typical edema. Passive transfer, common in the other urticarias, does not occur, and the pathophysiology is unknown. Symptoms typically last 24 to 48 hours. Treatment is primarily prophylactic with cold avoidance. Antihistamines generally have a poor response.

Primary (essential) cold urticaria is an acquired condition. It is brought on by cold, but symptoms typically occur within 2 to 5 minutes upon rewarming. Precipitants include cold air, cold objects on the skin, and cold food or drink. Localized contact usually results in localized swelling, erythema, and **pruritus**. This is particularly problematic if the swelling is of the lips, tongue, or pharynx, which potentially could compromise the airway. With total body exposure, a spectrum of symptoms of **anaphylaxis** can occur (Table 28.2. Anaphylaxis is discussed further later in this chapter.

Diagnosis and Treatment

When the diagnosis is in doubt, the skin changes can often be reproduced by placing an ice cube on the skin for 5 minutes. An alternative is immersing the hand in 10°C water for 5 minutes, again observing for skin changes. It is important to remember that the condition may coexist with cholinergic urticaria, occurring only with exercise in a cold environment.

As in other forms of urticaria, the best treatment is prevention by avoidance of the trigger, in this case cold temperatures. Tolerance may be induced by repeated, graded stimulus, and some cases may resolve spontaneously over a few months to 2 years (4). Whereas antihistamines in general are effective, cyproheptadine (Periactin) is particularly beneficial and is the drug of choice. When cyproheptadine is inadequate or ineffective, doxepin or cromolyn may be helpful.

Solar Urticaria

Solar urticaria is rare, accounting for less than 1% of all urticarias. As implied by the name, it is triggered by exposure to light in the ultraviolet or visible spectrum. Most common in the third or fourth decades of life, it can occur in any age group (6). Within minutes of exposure to light, the reaction typically starts with pruritus followed by erythema and edema in the exposed area only. The rash may start as **morbilliform** erythema, but often progresses to the wheal pattern typical of urticaria. It resolves within 1 to 3 hours, followed by a 12- to 24-hour period of tolerance to light (4). The full spectrum of anaphylactic reactions has been reported when large areas of the body are exposed. Table 28.4 reviews the classification of solar urticaria into six types, based on the causative wavelengths of light and the ability to transfer the disorder passively with serum. Type VI has been shown to be a metabolic disorder in which the photosensitizer is **protoporphyrin IX** (1, 6); the photoallergens have not been identified for the other types. Those that are passively transferred are likely IgE-mediated, and associated

TABLE 28.3. SIGNS AND SYMPTOMS OF ANAPHYLAXIS

Pruritus	Wheezing or bronchiolar constriction
Flushing	Laryngeal or pharyngeal swelling
Nausea	Hypotension
Vomiting	**Tachycardia**
Diarrhea or abdominal cramps	**Syncope**
Urticaria or angioedema	Cardiovascular collapse or shock
Headache	

TABLE 28.4. CLASSIFICATION OF SOLAR URTICARIA

Type	Causative Light Wavelength (nm)	Passively Transferred?
I	280–320	Yes
II	320–400	No
III	400–500	No
IV	400–500	Yes
V	280–500	No
VI	400	No

with mast cell and **eosinophil degranulation**. Histamine levels are elevated.

Diagnosis and Treatment

Diagnosis of solar urticaria is clinical, based on the patient's history and physical examination. The diagnosis can be confirmed with exposure to electromagnetic radiation, using either direct sunlight or artificial devices. Monochromators are useful devices that emit narrow bands of electromagnetic radiation, but they are expensive and are not practical for use by most patients.

Again, the best treatment is avoidance of the sun or inciting wavelengths of light. Covering the skin when outdoors is recommended. Sunscreens are helpful for ultraviolet wavelengths of light, but do little to filter out the visible spectrum of light. Antihistamines, antimalarial medications, and corticosteroids may be beneficial. Tolerance can be induced with long-term, graded exposure to natural or artificial light. Prolonged or permanent remissions do occur spontaneously in 20% to 30% of patients (4).

Delayed Pressure Urticaria and Angioedema

Delayed pressure urticaria, another rare form of physical allergy, is characterized by lesions that develop 4 to 8 hours after sustained pressure on the skin. It accounts for less than 1% of all urticaria. Although it can occur in isolation, it more commonly occurs in association with chronic idiopathic angioedema. Data suggest that food allergy may be a precipitating factor in these patients. Chronic idiopathic angioedema is outside the scope of this chapter.

In delayed pressure urticaria or angioedema, erythema of the skin occurs with painful, burning swelling in the dermis and underlying subcutaneous tissues. It is localized to the area where pressure occurred, and may last for 24 to 48 hours. Although this angioedema is more common, urticaria may coexist or be the predominant skin change. Reactions are common after prolonged walking, sitting, use of hand tools, or wearing tight clothes (1). Watches and belts may be problematic. Systemic symptoms may occur in severe cases, including malaise, fever, arthralgias, and leukocytosis.

Diagnosis and Treatment

History and physical findings, as in all the physical urticarias, are the key to diagnosis. Provocative testing may be helpful however. A 15-pound weight is hung from the shoulder using a 1-inch wide sling for 20 minutes, with inspection for painful skin changes 4 to 6 hours later.

In contrast to some of the other physical allergies, antihistamines generally are ineffective in treating delayed pressure urticaria or angioedema. They may have a role in cases where superficial urticaria is the predominant reaction, however. If angioedema predominates, corticosteroids may be necessary. Nonsteroidal anti-inflammatory drugs (NSAIDs) may be helpful as well.

Aquagenic Urticaria

Aquagenic urticaria is an extremely rare disorder, with only 13 cases reported in the world literature (6). Water, regardless of its temperature or salt content, induces small **hives** similar to those seen in cholinergic urticaria. Lesions occur as soon as 2 minutes after skin exposure, and last up to an hour. The pathophysiology does involve mast cell degranulation and elevated levels of histamine and other mediators. It has been suggested that a water-soluble epidermal antigen may play a role, permeating the skin in the presence of water and activating mast cells (4, 7).

Diagnosis and Treatment

Diagnostically, aquagenic urticaria may mimic cholinergic or cold urticaria. It may be the coldness or heat of the water that actually is inducing the symptoms. Unlike cholinergic urticaria, methacholine skin testing is negative. If the patient's history is suggestive, provocative skin testing may be performed by placing a room temperature compress on the skin for 30 minutes and observing for skin changes.

The mainstays of treatment are antihistamines. Oil-based lotions may be useful by minimizing water contact with the skin.

Vibratory Angioedema

Also quite uncommon, vibratory angioedema occurs in hereditary and acquired forms. The hereditary form follows **autosomal dominant** inheritance. Few cases have been reported in the literature. Afflicted individuals have a reaction within 1 to 5 minutes following inciting stimuli, such as lawn mowing, riding a motorcycle, toweling off, or getting a massage. The severity and duration of the reaction is proportional to the intensity or duration of the stimulus, although symptoms usually resolve within 24 hours. Local changes typical of angioedema predominate, but systemic reactions such as diffuse erythema and headache have been described. Passive transfer attempts have been negative, but histamine release after vibratory challenge has been shown (4).

Diagnosis and Treatment

Vibratory challenge is performed by applying a laboratory vortex or other vibratory stimulus to the skin for 5 minutes. Local skin changes constitute a positive test. The key to treatment is avoidance, although antihistamines are used with variable results. Induction of tolerance has been reported.

Exercise-Induced Anaphylaxis

Exercise-induced anaphylaxis, first reported in 1970 (8, 9), has been recognized with increasing frequency over the last 30 years. More than 1000 cases have been reported, although there has been only one death (10). Of the many forms of physical allergy, it certainly can be the most serious. Although exercise is the major precipitant, food allergies are associated in some cases. Other individuals suffer attacks only postprandially. Approximately one third of affected individuals have a personal history of atopy, or environmental allergy, and about two thirds have a family history of atopy (10, 11). Symptoms may be more likely to occur in women near their menses, and attacks may be more common with the use of aspirin and NSAIDs (10).

Multiple subtypes of exercise-induced anaphylaxis exist. Variant-type exercise-induced anaphylaxis presents similarly to the classic form, with the exception of the urticaria. Accounting for approximately 10% of cases, the lesions of the variant type are 2 to 4 mm in diameter and punctate, similar to those seen in cholinergic urticaria (10, 11). The similarities to cholinergic urticaria stop there, however. There also appears to be a familial form of exercise-induced anaphylaxis. The condition has been reported in two brothers who share an **HLA haplotype** (12). Lastly, a food-dependent form of the condition has been described. Some of these individuals suffer attacks only if they have eaten within a few hours before exercise. Others suffer attacks only in association with specific foods, with wheat, shellfish, and celery being major culprits (13–16). Interestingly, neither the food nor exercise alone is enough to trigger attacks; rather, it is the combination of the two that induces symptoms.

Symptom onset in exercise-induced anaphylaxis occurs anywhere from 5 to 30 minutes into exercise, often starting with a sensation of warmth, flushing, pruritus, and the development of urticaria. Subsequently, angioedema and the full spectrum of anaphylaxis may develop. The urticaria typically is the classic giant-sized wheal, 10 to 15 mm in diameter, as opposed to the punctate lesions seen in cholinergic urticaria (10). Angioedema in the upper airway may lead to obstruction, causing choking and **stridor**. Any of the spectrum of anaphylactic symptoms may occur (Table 28.3). Headache is common, and may persist for up to 72 hours after severe attacks. Hypotension may cause dizziness and can lead to life-threatening vascular collapse. Attacks usually resolve within three hours.

As in other types of physical allergy, degranulation of mast cells has been demonstrated in relation to attacks. Elevated plasma histamine levels also have been found. Therefore, it is thought that mast cell mediators such as histamine, prostaglandins, and leukotrienes play a key role in the onset of symptoms.

Diagnosis and Treatment

Exercise-induced anaphylaxis can be difficult to distinguish from cholinergic urticaria, because both conditions may occur during or soon after exercise. Exercise-induced anaphylaxis is not related to core body temperature, however, and will not occur with passive warming, anxiety, or stress. The urticaria, as mentioned previously, is much larger than the punctate, 1- to 3-mm lesions seen in cholinergic urticaria. Whereas cholinergic urticaria is quite reproducible with rises in body temperature, exercise-induced anaphylaxis occurs inconsistently in response to exercise. The vascular collapse that may be seen in exercise-induced anaphylaxis does not occur in cholinergic urticaria (10).

Provocative testing may be attempted in cases in which the diagnosis is unclear. Because of the potentially serious complications, however, it should be performed only in a controlled setting with resuscitation equipment on hand. While the patient exercises for up to 30 minutes, he or she is monitored closely for the development of urticaria, hypotension, or any of the other myriad symptoms that may occur. A negative test does not rule out the condition, however, because it occurs variably in response to exercise.

Treatment of this condition is symptomatic. Affected individuals must be counseled extensively about avoiding exercise, or stopping immediately at the first sign of symptoms. They should always exercise with a partner. They should also be instructed in the self-administration of subcutaneous epinephrine, which should be given immediately with the development of symptoms. Antihistamines, like most pharmacologic agents, generally have been unsuccessful. Those patients with food-related or postprandial exercise-induced anaphylaxis may be able to continue exercising by avoiding eating anything (or at least eating inciting foods) for 4 to 6 hours prior to exercise. Women may benefit from avoiding exercise near their menses, and aspirin and NSAIDS should be avoided by both men and women on days of exercise.

Atopic Athletes

Symptoms of atopy, or environmental allergy, affect approximately 15% of the population. Many athletes, therefore, are

going to be affected, although exercise per se does not increase the likelihood of symptoms. Symptoms may be more pronounced due to exercise, however. With exercise, minute ventilation dramatically increases, up to 30 times greater than resting ventilation. As a result, exposure to environmental allergens may increase with activity. Treatment starts with avoidance of allergens, including molds and mites indoors and pollens and grasses outdoors. Nonsedating antihistamines are quite helpful, as are corticosteroid nasal inhalers.

Potential Medications

Because most of the proposed pathophysiology of the physical allergies revolves around mast cell degranulation and the release of the mediators histamine, prostaglandins, and leukotrienes, medical management aims to address these issues. Accordingly, antihistamines are the medications most commonly used to combat physical allergies, although corticosteroids, cromolyn, and epinephrine also may be used.

Antihistamines

There are three main types of histamine receptors found on cell membranes throughout the body: H_1-receptors, H_2-receptors, and H_3-receptors. Antihistamines are accordingly broken into classes corresponding to their affinity for receptor type. H_1-receptor antagonists competitively compete with histamine for the H_1-receptor, whereas H_2- and H_3-receptor antagonists compete for the H_2- and H_3-receptors, respectively. Type 2 receptors are most active in the parietal cells of the gastric mucosa, which, when stimulated, help contribute to the release of gastric acid. Type 3 receptors are active within the central nervous system, and their significance has yet to be defined (17). Type 1 receptors, on the other hand, are more notable for their presence throughout the vasculature, the mucus membranes lining the upper respiratory tract, and the brain. When stimulated by histamine, they presumably play a major role in the broad spectrum of allergic response in the physical allergies. Therefore, blocking these receptors with the antihistamine medications, and subsequently preventing the action of histamine, can be very helpful in avoiding or attenuating these allergic responses.

The classic H_1-receptor antagonists are numerous and come from six general classes, the details of which are beyond the scope of this chapter. They are effective, binding to the H_1-receptor in a reversible, concentration-dependent manner. However, they do have an extensive side effect profile, which may limit their usefulness in treating the allergic disorders. Sedation can be so pronounced that these medications are sometimes used specifically for this effect. Table 28.5 reviews the potential side effects of these medications.

This use-limiting sedation led to the development of newer, nonsedating antihistamines. These medications are

TABLE 28.5. POTENTIAL SIDE EFFECTS OF CLASSIC H₁-RECEPTOR ANTAGONISTS

Sedation	Constipation
Dry mouth, nose, throat	Fever
Headache	Urinary retention
Dizziness	Blurred vision
Nausea/vomiting	Tachycardia

long-acting, and tend to act preferentially at the peripheral H₁-receptors rather than in the central nervous system, leading to a lower incidence of sedation. They may also act to inhibit histamine release, although the mechanism for this is not clear. For specifics regarding individual medications within this subclass, the reader is referred to any standard pharmacology text.

In very severe cases of physical allergy, or cases in which H₁-receptor antagonists give a suboptimal result, H₂-receptor antagonists may be **synergistic** with the H₁-receptor antagonists, resulting in better outcomes.

Cromolyn

Cromolyn also may be useful in treating these disorders. Prophylactic use of cromolyn can stabilize mast cell membranes. This inhibits the release of mast cell vasoactive mediators, thus preventing the allergic response cascade. It usually is used as an inhaled medication, but it also is available as a liquid. Side effects usually are minimal, but irritation or drying of the upper respiratory tract, bitter taste, cough, and wheezing can occur.

Corticosteroids

Corticosteroids are potent anti-inflammatory medications that work by inhibiting the formation of arachidonic acid, a precursor to the prostaglandins and leukotrienes. These substances play a role in the inflammatory and allergic response, so corticosteroids can be extremely useful in combating these disorders. They do have numerous potential side effects, however, especially when used on a regular basis. Therefore, the risk-benefit ratio of these medications must be considered carefully before opting for their use.

Nonsteroidal Anti-inflammatory Drugs (NSAIDs)

There are multiple classes of NSAIDS with subtle variations, but all of them act to inhibit the enzyme cyclooxygenase. Inhibition of this enzyme prevents formation of the prostaglandins, potent inflammatory agents that play a role in the allergic response. Paradoxically, some allergy-prone individuals are found to experience a worsening of their allergic symptoms in response to NSAIDs, so their use should be monitored carefully. These agents also have a broad spectrum of potential side effects, including but not limited to peptic ulcer disease, nausea and vomiting, gastrointestinal bleeding, renal damage, liver toxicity, drowsiness, and fluid retention.

Epinephrine

Epinephrine is an **adrenergic neurotransmitter** that has myriad effects on the cardiovascular system. Its use for physical allergy is reserved for life-threatening anaphylaxis only, when a patient has swelling that is threatening the patency of the airway, or is undergoing hypotension or vascular collapse. It functions to strengthen **myocardial** contraction, constrict the peripheral blood vessels to maintain blood pressure, and dilate the airways in the respiratory tract. It can be life-saving in acute situations. Because epinephrine can cause **arrhythmias**, severe hypertension, and stroke in addition to many less serious side effects, however, its use should be reserved for such serious situations.

CASE STUDY

Patient Information

John is a 28-year-old triathlete who presented to his physician complaining of a rash appearing with exercise for the last month. He describes the rash as consisting of many small red spots on his trunk and extremities, typically starting about 10 to 15 minutes into his workout. In several episodes, it has been associated with dizziness and the sensation that he was going to "black out," although he never did. He notes the symptoms have occurred most often with running, although they also have occurred with biking.

Assessment

A thorough physical examination was unremarkable, with the exception of dermatographism. Laboratory analysis was entirely within normal limits. The patient was therefore tested on a cycle ergometer, with full resuscitation equipment on hand. Approximately 10 minutes into the exercise challenge, the patient developed 3- to 4-mm urticarial lesions of the trunk, which rapidly spread to the proximal extremities. The athlete's blood pressure, 116/64 prior to exercise, was 140/70 at the time the challenge was stopped. Two minutes into recovery, he began to feel light-headed, with an associated blood pressure drop to 90/50. This resolved quickly with intravenous administration of fluids, recumbent positioning, and the administration of subcutaneous epinephrine, and did not recur.

Questions

1. What is the diagnosis?
2. In this instance, what testing could help to differentiate cholinergic urticaria from exercise-induced anaphylaxis?
3. The patient did not report symptoms with swimming. Is this relevant?
4. How should this patient be counseled regarding food?

Discussion

John was given and instructed in the use of subcutaneous epinephrine, and also instructed never to exercise without a partner. Multiple antihistamines of the H_1-receptor subtype were tried, with little success. He did find, however, that avoiding eating for several hours before exercise dramatically reduced the number of recurrences. He was subsequently able to return to competition.

What We Know
About Allergy and Exercise

In the physical allergies, the allergic response can be triggered by any number of physical stimuli an athlete may encounter. This leads to urticaria and angioedema that can occur in either localized or generalized form. The physical allergies occur infrequently. They account for about 17% of all chronic urticarias (4), which as a group are still relatively uncommon. Therefore, awareness and understanding of these conditions are crucial to early recognition and treatment.

What We Would Like to Know
About Allergy and Exercise

The urticaria and angioedema of the physical allergies generally is believed to be secondary to mast cell degranulation and release of vasoactive mediators. What is less clear is the mechanism that triggers this mast cell degranulation. Current treatments often are ineffective. Furthermore, the infrequency with which these allergic responses occur makes it difficult to study them effectively. Therefore, much work needs to be done to better understand the pathophysiology behind these conditions. It is hoped that this will lead to more effective treatments, and relief for many frustrated, affected individuals.

Summary

Allergy in its many forms occurs commonly in athletes, and may have profound effects on exercise. Effects may range from the localized and relatively minor skin reaction of dermatographism, to the more severe and potentially life-threatening response of exercise-induced anaphylaxis. Fortunately, the very common forms, such as environmental allergies (atopy) and exercise-induced asthma (see Chapter 13), usually can be well-controlled with medication. The less common physical urticarias are difficult to diagnose, and require a high index of suspicion by the health care practitioner. They may not respond as well to medication, and often force the athlete to avoid the triggering physical stimuli. Continuing research into these conditions should result in better treatments, allowing athletes to train and compete in any physical environment in spite of these physical allergies.

DISCUSSION QUESTIONS

1 Discuss the common symptoms and physical signs of allergy, in particular those relating to the physical allergies. Describe urticaria and angioedema.

2 What physical stimuli have been implicated as causes of physical urticaria? How can these be tested to confirm that the presumed cause is correct?

3 Compare and contrast exercise-induced anaphylaxis with cholinergic urticaria. How does ingested food relate? How can one differentiate the two conditions in symptomatic athletes?

4 Discuss several types of medications used to treat allergy in athletes, particularly in relation to how physical stimuli are thought to trigger symptoms.

REFERENCES

1. Huston DP, Bressler RB. Urticaria and angioedema. Med Clin North Am 1992;76:805–840.
2. Kumar SA, Martin BL. Urticaria and angioedema: diagnostic and treatment considerations. J Am Osteopath Assoc 1999; 99(3 suppl):S1–4.
3. Tharp MD. Chronic urticaria: pathophysiology and treatment approaches. J Allergy Clin Immunol 1996;98:S325–S330.
4. Casale TB, Sampson HA, Hanifin J, et al. Guide to the physical urticarias. J Allergy Clin Immunol 1988;82:758–763.
5. Kantou-Fili K, Borici-Mazi R, Kapp A, et al. Physical urticaria: classification and diagnostic guidelines. An EAACI position paper. Allergy 1997;52:504–513.
6. Kaplan AP. Urticaria and angioedema. In: Middleton E, ed. Allergy: Principles and Practice. St. Louis: Mosby, 1998.
7. Czarnetzki BM, Breethold K, Traupe H. Evidence that water acts as a carrier for an epidermal antigen in aquagenic urticaria. J Am Acad Dermatol 1986;15:623.
8. Castells MC, Horan RF, Sheffer AL. Exercise-induced anaphylaxis. Clin Rev Allergy Immunol 1999;17:413–424.
9. Matthews KP, Pan PM. Postexercise hyperhistaminemia, dermographia, and wheezing. Ann Intern Med 1970; 72:241-49.
10. Briner WW. Physical allergies and exercise: clinical implications for those engaged in sports activities. Sports Medicine 1993;15:365–373.
11. Sheffer AL, Sotter NA, McFadden ER, Austen KF. Exercise-induced anaphylaxis: a distinct form of physical allergy. J Allergy Clin Immunol 1983;71:311–316.
12. Longly S, Panush RS. Familial exercise-induced anaphylaxis. Ann Allergy 1987;58:257–259.
13. Briner WW, Bruno PJ. Case report: 30-year-old female with exercise-induced-anaphylaxis. Med Sci Sports Exerc 1991;23:991–994.
14. Guinnepain M, Eloit C, Raffard M, et al. Exercise-induced anaphylaxis: useful screening of food sensitization. Ann Allergy Asthma Immunol 1996;77:491–496.
15. Palosuo K, Alenius H, Varjonen E, et al. A novel wheat gliadin as a cause of exercise-induced anaphylaxis. J Allergy Clin Immunol 1999;103:912–917.
16. Varjonen E, Vainio E, Kalimo K. Life-threatening, recurrent anaphylaxis caused by allergy to gliadin and exercise. Clin Exp Allergy 1997;27:162–166.
17. Montgomery LC, Deuster PA. Effects of antihistamine medications on exercise performance. Sports Medicine 1993;15:179–195.

CHAPTER 29

Sickle Cell Disease

Kristy F. Woods, Leigh T. Ramsey

SEARCHABLE KEY TERMS

Sickle Cell Disease	Vasoocclusion
Hemoglobinopathy	Hydroxyurea
Sickle Cell Anemia	Rhabdomyolysis
Thalassemia	Exercise Capacity
Globin Chains	Lactate/Lactic Acid
Sickling	Peak $\dot{V}O_2$
Polymerization	Endothelin (ET-1)
Sickle Cell Trait	Nitric Oxide (NO)
Hemolysis	

Overview

More than 600 hemoglobin variants have been identified to date. Sickle cell disease (SCD), the most common hemoglobin disorder worldwide (1), has been well understood on a molecular and genetic level since the early 1950s. Normal human hemoglobin (Hb), Hb A ($\alpha_2\beta_2$), is composed of two α-globin chains, two β-globin chains and four heme molecules that bind oxygen (O_2). In sickle cell disease, the α-globin chains are normal and there is a point mutation in triplet codon six of the β-globin gene (GAG$\rightarrow$GTG). This base exchange, thymine (T) in place of adenine (A), results in a single amino acid substitution at the 6th position of the β-globin chain. A polar, hydrophilic amino acid, glutamic acid, is replaced by the nonpolar, hydrophobic valine (glutamic acid$\rightarrow$valine) producing the abnormal β^s globin (Figure 29.1).

When fully oxygenated, there are few structural distinctions between normal hemoglobin (HbA) and sickle hemoglobin (HbS [$\alpha_2\beta^s_2$]). In the deoxygenated state, however, a conformational change occurs that decreases the solubility of sickle hemoglobin. The HbS molecules form rigid polymers within the red blood cell (erythrocyte) (2). This process of hemoglobin polymerization distorts the normal biconcave disc shape of the erythrocyte. The cell assumes a "sickled" shape, hence the name *sickle cell disease* (Figures 29.2 and 29.3). Upon reoxygenation, the reversibly sickled cell initially resumes the normal erythrocyte shape. As a consequence of repeated configurational changes with reoxygenation and deoxygenation, the cell membrane becomes permanently damaged and the cell irreversibly sickled, and hemolysis occurs (3). The normal erythrocyte lifespan of 120 days is shortened to less than 20 days for sickle erythrocytes, and a chronic hemolytic state exists.

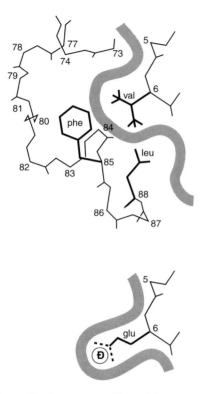

FIGURE 29.1.   Molecular structure of hemoglobin.

The term *sickle cell disease* refers to a group of genetic disorders of hemoglobin production. The four most common forms of SCD in the United States are HbSS (sickle cell anemia [SCA]), HbSC (HbSC disease), and the sickle-β thalassemias (HbSβ$^+$ thalassemia and HbSβ^0 thalassemia). All forms of SCD are characterized by production of HbS, chronic hemolytic anemia, and acute and chronic ischemic tissue damage due to vascular obstruction (vasoocclusion). Individuals with SCA are homozygous for the sickle (β^s) globin gene, whereas individuals with HbSC disease and Hbβ-thalassemia are mixed heterozygous. They inherit both a sickle (β^s) globin gene and the gene for HbC (β^6:glutamic acid→lysine) or thalassemia, respectively. Persons with HbSC disease produce both HbS and HbC. Individuals with sickle thalassemia produce HbS and either a decreased amount (HbSβ$^+$thal) or no (HbSβ^0 thal) normal β-globin chains.

Sickle cell disease is found in Africa, the Middle East, South and Central America, the Caribbean, East India. and the Mediterranean. In the United States, it is most common in those of African ancestry. It is estimated that one out of eight African-Americans are carriers of the gene (AS) known as sickle cell trait. Individuals with sickle cell trait often are unaware of their condition, and it is not considered a form of SCD. Although they do produce some HbS, it usually accounts for less than 30% of their total hemoglobin and rarely results in anemia or medical complications. There are approximately 70,000 Americans with sickle cell disease. The estimated prevalence of SCD in African-Americans is as follows: SCA, 1 case per 375 live births; HbSC disease, 1 case per 835 live births; and HbSβ-thalassemias, 1 per 1667 live births (4).

The clinical hallmark of SCD is the acute vasoocclusive episode, also known as acute painful crisis (Figure 29.4). Painful episodes result from blockage of small blood vessels (vasoocclusion) with resultant hypoxia and ischemic injury to richly innervated cortical bone. In addition, subclinical vasoocclusion can occur to organs throughout the body (the kidneys, liver, lungs, retina, heart, and spleen). Patients with sickle cell disease also are at increased risk for abnormalities of growth and development, infections, cerebrovascular disease, and psychosocial manifestations of chronic illness (5).

Sickle cell disease usually is diagnosed at birth as a result of widespread newborn screening programs that have been implemented across the United States over the past 20 years. Prompt identification of affected individuals, early involvement of families, and pediatric care has resulted in a dramatic decline in childhood mortality from SCD. Many patients are now living well into adulthood—the mean life expectancy currently is about 45 years for those with SCA and about 62 years for those with Hb SC disease (6). However, there is considerable variability in the clinical course between and within genotypes.

Despite new drug therapies and treatment options, SCD remains associated with increased morbidity and functional and psychological dysfunction. On standardized surveys, adults with SCD have poor perceptions of overall health and well-being (7). Psychological and social manifestations of chronic illness are not uncommon in this population (8). People with SCD may become sedentary as a result of sickle cell–related complications such as fatigue, avascular necrosis, leg ulcers, childhood stroke, or chronic sickle lung disease. In addition, because of medical conservatism, some patients may be discouraged from exercising for fear of precipitating acute vasoocclusive episodes. However, a sedentary lifestyle may exacerbate already poor health perceptions and contribute to obesity in adulthood in patients with SCD (9). Long-term management goals should focus on early detection and prevention of complications and improving perceived health status and quality of life. As with other chronic conditions, this includes maximizing physical and psychological functioning. Regular exercise may have a role in preserving or enhancing physical functioning and improving psychological health in this population with chronic disease.

Treatment and Potential Medications

Newborn diagnosis, family education, and early implementation of comprehensive medical care are important aspects of medical management. Daily, oral penicillin, which significantly decreases morbidity and mortality in infants and children with SCD, should be begun at the time of diagno-

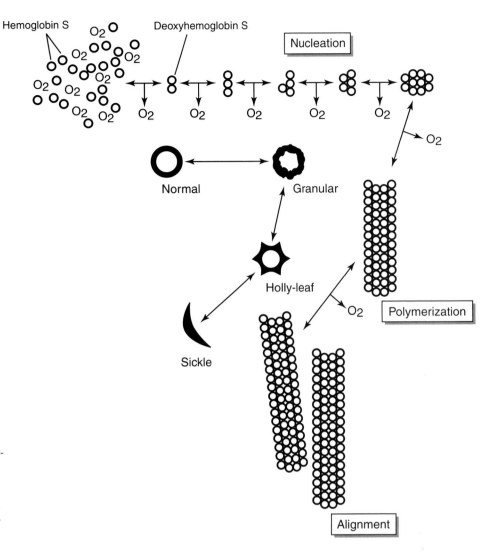

FIGURE 29.2.   Polymerization process of sickle hemoglobin (Hb S). When HbS becomes deoxygenated, the HbS molecules polymerize. The polymers consist of 14-strand fibers that distort the shape of the erythrocyte membrane, changing its normal biconcave disc shape to a number of other shapes such as granular, holly-leaf, and the classic sickle shape. (Reprinted with permission from Bessa EC. Hemoglobin and Hemoglobinopathies in Hematology. Philadelphia: Harwal Publishing, 1992:123–136.)

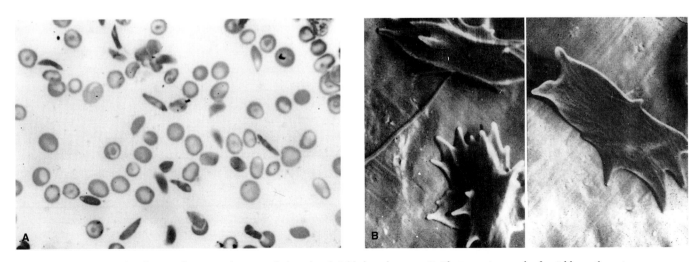

FIGURE 29.3.   **A.** Peripheral smear demonstrating normal-shaped and sickled erythrocytes. **B.** Electron micrograph of a sickle erythrocyte.

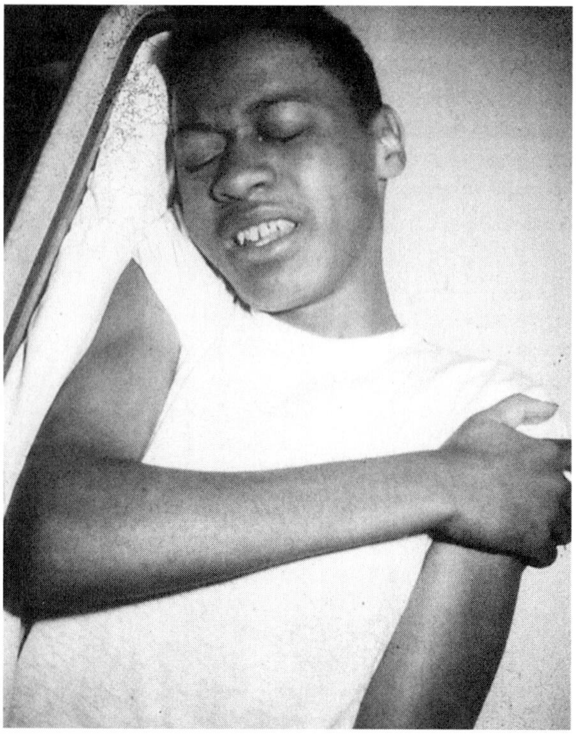

FIGURE 29.4. Patient with sickle cell anemia during an acute vasoocclusive episode (acute pain crisis).

sis (10). Early immunization against *Haemophilus influenzae* and *Streptococcus pneumoniae* is essential for this population. Other immunizations should be done according to the guidelines of the American Academy of Pediatrics or Centers for Disease Control and Prevention, and should include the hepatitis B vaccine, as children with SCD may require blood transfusions (11). In SCD, acute, recurrent painful episodes (acute vasoocclusive episodes) are the most common cause for health care encounters. Specific guidelines for sickle cell pain assessment and appropriate use and monitoring of opioid and nonopioid analgesics are available (12).

As a result of a large, U.S., multicenter clinical trial, the drug hydroxyurea was approved for the treatment of adults with SCD in 1995. The study found that hydroxyurea therapy significantly reduced the frequency of painful episodes, the need for transfusions, and the incidence of acute chest syndrome (13). Preliminary studies in children are encouraging; however, hydroxyurea is not yet approved for children with SCD (14). Hydroxyurea, a ribonucleotide reductase inhibitor, increases the percentage of fetal hemoglobin (HbF;$\alpha_2\gamma_2$) within the red blood cells. Fetal hemoglobin (HbF) normally is present during the gestational period and during adulthood in small amounts (<2%). In SCD, however, normal HbF levels range from 2% to 20%. The presence of HbF inhibits polymerization of sickle hemoglobin (HbS), thus explaining a primary mechanism of action of hydroxyurea (15). Other mechanisms of action may explain the beneficial clinical effects observed before HbF levels increase (16, 17). The long-term effects of hydroxyurea in people with SCD are not completely understood, and investigation is ongoing. Because of potential cytotoxicity, very close monitoring with frequent laboratory assessment is required for patients on hydroxyurea therapy. Other drugs, including arginine butyrate and erythropoietin, also increase HbF production in patients with SCD but have experienced limited success in clinical trials to date.

Red cell transfusions often are used in individuals with SCD and can increase oxygen-carrying capacity, dilute sickle erythrocytes, and suppress erythropoiesis. Transfusion is indicated acutely to correct severe anemia due to sequestration or aplastic crises (due to parvovirus B19 infection). Transfusion also decreases primary and secondary stroke risk for patients with SCD and is beneficial in the treatment of other sickle cell–related complications including acute chest syndrome, priapism, and growth failure. However, transfusion complications, particularly the development of red cell antibodies and iron accumulation, limit usefulness for long-term management. The indications for transfusion, type of transfusion, and the role of chronic transfusion therapy in SCD remain areas of controversy.

Bone marrow transplantation can be curative in SCD. The largest U.S. series, of 22 patients, reported 20 of 22 patients alive and 16 of 22 with stable engraftment at 24 months following transplant (18). This strategy has not been widely used in patients with SCD, however, for a number of reasons. Because SCD is not a fatal disease, the risk of early mortality and long-term complications has resulted in limited patient acceptance. The procedure is costly, and identifying which patients are appropriate for transfusion and suitable matched donors remains challenging. Recently, transcranial Doppler has proven useful in identifying children with SCD who are at increased risk of stroke and cerebrovascular complications and may, therefore, benefit from early transplant. The use of umbilical cord blood as an alternative source of stem cells for transplantation appears promising and may require less stringent tissue matching and improve availability (19). New conditioning regimens that reduce transplant-associated toxicity and the possibility of in utero stem cell therapy also are being investigated (20, 21).

Exercise Response

Adaptations to exercise that occur in patients with SCD include regional hypoxia, lactic acidosis, hypertonicity, and hyperthermia, conditions that promote polymerization of sickle hemoglobin (HbS) in vivo. Justifiable concern exists, therefore, that exercise may promote sickle cell–related medical complications, particularly acute vasoocclusive episodes. In a large, retrospective study of military recruits in basic training, Kark and colleagues reported a 28- to 40-

fold increased risk of exertion-induced sudden death in individuals with sickle cell trait compared to controls (normal hemoglobin; HbA) (22). All recruits were untrained and were performing strenuous exercise in extreme temperatures without access to oral hydration. Rhabdomyolysis (muscle breakdown) often was documented at postmortem examination. Further analysis revealed a correlation between ambient temperature on the day prior to exercise and risk of sudden death (23). A more recent report of Air Force military recruits (1956–1996) found a relative risk for nontraumatic death of 23.53 (CI, 19.55–30.01) when people with sickle cell trait were compared with those without it (24). In addition, a number of isolated cases of exercise-related sudden death have been reported in individuals with sickle cell trait, usually during extreme exertion and high-altitude training (25–29). In these cases, collapse and sudden death were usually associated with rhabdomyolysis, heat stroke, or cardiac arrhythmia (30).

Conversely, there are no known reports of sudden death during exercise in females and few reports of sudden death beyond basic training and preseason sports training in males with sickle cell trait. A study by Martin and colleagues demonstrated that sickling increased significantly during maximal exercise at an altitude of 1270 meters (31). At 4000 meters, sickling increased dramatically, but did not affect overall performance as determined by peak oxygen consumption ($\dot{V}O_2$) and anaerobic threshold. There is no direct evidence that altitude- or exercise-related death in persons with sickle cell trait involves the pathogenesis of microvascular obstruction. Nor is there direct evidence that these deaths are related to the typical life-threatening complications of SCD (29). Although ability to perform intense and prolonged exercise may be decreased, under most circumstances sickle cell trait does not appear to preclude participation in sports activities. Some studies have demonstrated normal to near-normal exercise capacity in individuals with sickle cell trait, and there are several reports of professional athletes with sickle cell trait (32–38).

In summary, sickle cell trait should not be used as a reason to restrict physical activity. Individuals with sickle cell trait should adhere to general guidelines for fluid replacement and acclimatization to hot conditions and altitude during exercise (39). Maximum exercise testing is not contraindicated in this population, but it is not necessary prior to exercise training. Over the past decade, military training has been altered to limit strenuous exercise in extreme conditions among untrained recruits (for example, limiting the duration and intensity of training and allowing access to water). And while the military excludes persons with SCD, it does not exclude those with sickle cell trait.

Individuals with SCA do, however, have a reduced work capacity as evidenced by a low maximal $\dot{V}O_2$ and low muscular exercise tolerance. This may be partially explained by a decreased O_2-carrying capacity due to anemia. Exercise capacity in SCD improves with transfusion, but it also improves with partial exchange transfusion in which the HbA level increases and total hemoglobin is unchanged (40–42). This observation suggests that sickle erythrocytes (or HbS) may directly contribute to low exercise capacity by erythrocyte sickling, decreased deformability, increased blood viscosity or other mechanisms. In addition, children and adults with SCD demonstrate an abnormal ventilatory response to exercise (43, 44). Although this response is due primarily to a large dead space, an increased transit time of blood through the lungs during peak exercise may prevent adequate gas exchange, thus contributing to the reduced exercise capacity. Despite these limitations, the psychological benefits of moderate physical activity may be important in improving perceived health status in patients with SCD, and physical training may improve physical function and overall quality of life in this population.

There have been few clinical studies and no controlled clinical trials addressing the safety of controlled physical training or exercise in persons with SCD. Nor have the long-term effects of physical training in this population been assessed. Regular, moderate exercise as tolerated is recommended during childhood in people with SCD to facilitate physical and psychological growth and development (5). Maximum exercise testing is not required for children prior to regular exercise, but clinical evaluation and monitoring of exercise response by a pediatrician or pediatric hematologist is warranted. There are no exercise recommendations specifically for adults with SCD. The American College of Sports Medicine's (ACSM) general exercise recommendations for adults should be observed, with modifications based on individual functional capacity and status of chronic disease (i.e., number, type and severity of sickle cell-related medical complications). Maximum exercise testing is not contraindicated in adults. In fact, it may provide useful information regarding cardiovascular limitations (e.g., peak $\dot{V}O_2$) and can be used for exercise recommendations. Careful clinical evaluation and monitoring of exercise response by a physician is recommended for adults with SCD.

Exercise Programming Options

Endurance Training Programs

Sickle cell disease has not been studied sufficiently to yield physical training guidelines for aerobic exercise. The general guidelines suggested by the ACSM should be individualized and based on the individual patient's baseline assessment, concomitant medical complications, and physical limitations. Pretraining maximum exercise testing and clearance by a physician are recommended for adults. Exercise programs should take place in a controlled environment and should begin gradually (45). Ability to perform intense or prolonged exercise is limited in this population due to the underlying pathophysiological mechanisms of SCD, discussed in the following sections.

Resistance Training Programs

A preliminary study implementing resistance training in adults with SCD found that although baseline leg strength was average and arm strength was poor, subjects were able to safely perform 8 to 12 repetitions with each of the major muscle groups (Figure 29.5) (45). With 3 to 6 months of resistance training, leg strength increased significantly. Although the data are inconclusive as far as making recommendations for resistance training in this population, ACSM guidelines should be implemented gradually and carefully modified based on individual response and adaptations to training.

Potential Physiologic Adaptations and Associated Mechanisms

General pathophysiologic abnormalities that occur in SCD may affect exercise tolerance and physiologic adaptations to exercise. These abnormalities can be divided into four major categories: anemia; pulmonary limitations; cardiovascular abnormalities; and vascular dysfunction. The associated mechanisms involved and their potential impact on exercise are discussed in the following sections.

Anemia

Chronic anemia in SCD is due to increased red blood cell destruction or hemolysis, which occurs because of cellular membrane damage caused by polymerization of sickle hemoglobin (HbS). The normal lifespan of a red blood cell is 120 days; the lifespan of a red blood cell with sickle hemoglobin (sickle erythrocyte) is less than 20 days. Instead of a normal hemoglobin level of 12 to 16 g/dl, individuals with HbSS, HbSC, and HbSb thalassemia have hemoglobin levels of 6 to 8 g/dl, 10 to 15 g/dl, and 6 to 12 g/dl, respectively.

In anemia, the reduction of circulating erythrocytes decreases oxygen-carrying capacity. To maintain adequate oxygen delivery to the tissue, increased oxygen unloading occurs at given partial pressures of oxygen (pO_2). A shift of the oxygen dissociation curve to the right and increased O_2 unloading also occurs with intracellular polymerization of HbS, increased 2,3-diphosphoglyercol (DPG) concentrations of O_2, and decreased intracellular pH (46) (Figure 29.6). Other compensatory mechanisms for anemia to maintain adequate O_2 delivery and minimize lactic acidosis include increasing cardiac output and respiratory rate.

When oxygen delivery to muscles during exercise is insufficient, anaerobic metabolism occurs and lactic acid accumulates. Compared with healthy individuals, patients who have illness characterized by inadequate oxygen delivery (such as SCA) experience increases in blood lactate concentrations at lower work rates (47, 48). Freund and colleagues reported earlier onset of lactate production in

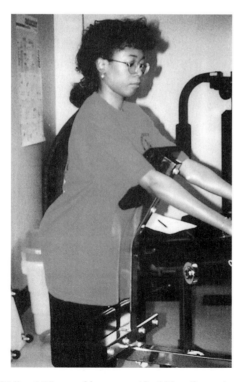

FIGURE 29.5. A 32-year old woman with sickle cell anemia performing supervised resistance-training exercise.

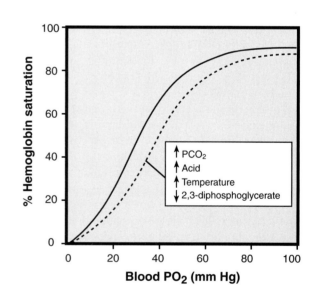

FIGURE 29.6. Oxygen–hemoglobin dissociation curve. The oxy-Hb curve can shift to the right or left. An increase in 2,3-diphosphoglycerol (DPG), temperature, P_{CO_2}, or H^+ ions (decreased pH) will shift the curve to the right. A shift in the curve to the right allows more O_2 to be liberated for a given decrease in PO_2, which allows more O_2 to be freed from hemoglobin. (Reprinted with permission from Sherwood L. Respiratory system. In Fundamentals of Physiology: A Human Perspective. St. Paul: West Publishing Co., 1991:10–25.)

multistage exercise tests and delayed lactate clearance in patients with SCA compared to healthy controls (49) (Figure 29.7). Other studies have demonstrated no difference in lactate exercise and recovery curves between groups when relative work rate and absolute work rate are considered in interpreting the data (50). It is unclear whether the low work rate in SCD is a function of low physical fitness, disease-specific factors, or a combination of these factors.

Pulmonary Limitations

Pulmonary complications are leading causes of morbidity and mortality in patients with SCD (51). Acute complications include bacterial pneumonia, pulmonary edema, and acute chest syndrome. Acute chest syndrome is the most life-threatening of the acute pulmonary complications; its etiology remains incompletely understood. Recent studies suggest that contributing factors may include a combination of vasoocclusion, infection, and embolization of fat from the bone marrow (52). Chronic pulmonary complications include chronic sickle lung disease, pulmonary hypertension, and possibly thrombosis of large pulmonary arteries (53). The incidence of chronic sickle lung disease is unknown—or perhaps underestimated. It is characterized by progressive shortness of breath, exercise intolerance, and hypoxemia and may result from repeated episodes of acute microvascular or infectious events.

The pulmonary vascular bed usually has a large reserve capacity in order to adjust for changes in cardiac output such as those that occur during exercise. In healthy individuals, this includes increased blood flow to the upper regions of the lungs and increased pulmonary ventilation. In persons with SCD, the reserve capacity may be limited due to chronic sickle lung disease or may already be in use because of an anemia-induced compensatory increase in cardiac output and respiratory rate (54, 55). Obstructive and restrictive abnormalities and gas-exchange abnormalities have been documented in adults with SCD. These include decreased forced expiratory volume (FEV_1), forced vital capacity (FVC), and total lung capacity (TLC), increased dead space (V_D), and resting hyperventilation ($pCO_2 < 35$ mm Hg) (56).

Cardiovascular Abnormalities

The compensatory cardiac response to anemia in SCD (an increase in cardiac output) is associated with minimal increase in heart rate but substantial increases in stroke volume due to plasma volume expansion. The increase in plasma volume leads to alterations in cardiac structure and function (57–59). The Cooperative Study of Sickle Cell Disease found elevated dimensions of the right ventricle, left ventricle, and left atrial chamber of the heart and increased interventricular wall thickness (60). It also determined that left ventricular dilatation was inversely related to total he-

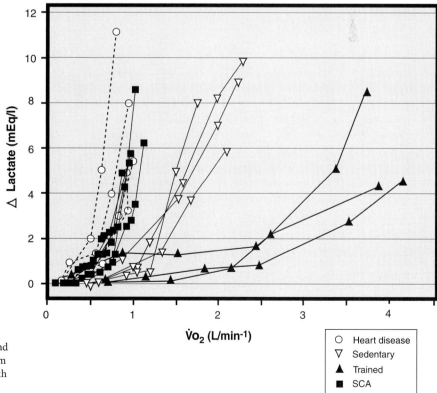

Figure 29.7. Changes in lactate vs. $\dot{V}_{O_2}$. Lactate data are plotted with previously published results of blood lactate measurements in patients with heart disease and in those who were sedentary or trained. (Adapted from Wasserman K, Whipp BJ. Exercise physiology in health and disease. Am Rev Resp Dis 1975;112:219–249.)

moglobin and that left ventricular dimension increased with age. Other potential causes of cardiac abnormality include hypoxia and chronic sickle lung disease (pulmonary artery hypertension), iron overload (deposition in cardiac tissue), arrhythmia, and eventual heart failure.

Early exercise studies suggested an exercise-induced increase in pulmonary arterial pressure and right ventricular work in patients with SCD (57). Studies examining cardiac function in adolescents with SCD found decreased ventricular filling as well as decreased heart rate and blood pressure response during exercise compared to age- and race-matched controls (61–63). In an already compensated heart, the increased metabolic demands of exercise may contribute considerably to limitations in exercise capacity.

Vascular Dysfunction

The exact mechanism of vasoocclusion in SCD remains unclear. Although erythrocyte sickling and increased blood viscosity contribute to the process, other factors also are intimately involved. Sickle erythrocytes have been shown to be more adhesive during steady state than normal erythrocytes (64, 65). Higher levels of tumor necrosis factor alpha (TNFα), interleukin-6 (IL-6), and C-reactive protein (CRP) are found in individuals with SCD compared with controls, suggesting a chronic inflammatory state (66–71). Sickled erythrocytes also affect the vascular endothelium by disrupting local vasoregulatory mechanisms and damaging endothelial cells lining blood vessels (72). In addition, circulating endothelial cells are elevated in patients with SCD, reflecting a state of chronic vascular injury (73).

Maintenance of an appropriate balance between vasodilation and vasoconstriction is important for normal vascular function. Endothelin-1 (ET-1), a potent vasoconstrictor, and nitric oxide (NO),* a vasodilator, are derived from the endothelium and are important determinants of vascular tone. Abnormal control of local vascular tone during steady state conditions and during sickle cell crises has been reported. During steady state, vasodilation is elevated and there is low vascular resistance; during a sickle cell crisis, there is decreased vasodilation and increased

vascular resistance (57). Several studies have demonstrated higher circulating plasma ET-1 concentrations in patients with SCD compared to controls (74–77). This finding may be due to hypoxia, shear stress, or chronic endothelial damage. Nitric oxide (NO) metabolite concentrations also have been shown to be significantly higher in patients with SCD than in controls during steady state, with further increases during acute painful episodes (78, 79). With ischemia, NO is protective by enhancing vasodilatation to increase local blood flow. Nitric oxide also inhibits neutrophil activation, adhesion, accumulation and platelet aggregation and may thereby facilitate passage of sickle erythrocytes (80).

Exercise may upregulate nitric oxide synthase (NOS) gene expression and thus affect NO production, which may partially explain the vascular adaptations seen in aerobic training (81). However, NO is not essential for exercise-related vasodilatation, and some studies point to the role of other vasodilators (82). Likewise, although there are reports of an increase in plasma concentrations of ET-1 with exercise, findings have been inconsistent, and the role of ET-1 in exercise remains ambiguous (83–87). In a recent study examining the effect of exercise on vasoactive mediators in SCD, three consecutive days of exercise did not result in a change in plasma ET-1 concentration in either group. However, the response of NO metabolites to exercise differed between groups. Whereas plasma concentration of NO metabolites increased significantly on the first day in both groups, it increased after exercise on all 3 days only in the SCD group (88). Further analysis of short- and long-term vascular adaptations to exercise in individuals with SCD is indicated.

Summary

Sickle cell disease is the most common hemoglobinopathy in the world and affects approximately 70,000 Americans. Despite advances in early diagnosis, pediatric management, and treatment, the disease still is associated with increased morbidity and early mortality. In the past, many patients avoided exercise for fear of precipitating a sickle cell–related complication or because of medical conservatism (i.e., they were advised by physicians not to exercise). Physiologic adaptations to sickle cell disease may limit exercise capacity. These abnormalities include anemia, pulmonary limitations, cardiovascular abnormalities, and vascular dysfunction. Regular, moderate exercise is recommended during childhood to facilitate physical and psychological growth and development. However, clinical evaluation and monitoring of exercise response by a pediatrician is warranted. Although there are no general exercise guidelines for adults, maximal exercise testing may provide useful information regarding the individual patient's cardiovascular limitations and exercise recommendations.

---

* Nitric oxide (NO), an endothelium-derived relaxing factor, is a potent vasodilator. Because of its short half-life (5–10 seconds), the stable end products of NO catabolism, nitrates and nitrites (NOx), are usually measured.ᵃ NO synthase (NOS) converts L-arginine into NO and L-citrulline. Three forms of NOS have been identified and classified according to where they were isolated: neuronal (nNOS or NOS I), inducible (iNOS or NOS II), and endothelial (eNOS or NOS III). Endothelial-derived NOS is upregulated by exercise, shear stress, hypoxia and ischemia, whereas cytokines upregulate iNOS.

CASE STUDY

Patient Information

A 36-year-old African-American woman with sickle cell anemia (Hb SS) has a past medical history remarkable for infrequent painful episodes and a history of pneumonia (two episodes). She has noted a 10-pound weight gain over the past year and is seeking advice regarding a "safe" exercise regimen. Her laboratory values are as follows:

Hemoglobin: 7.6 g/dl
Hematocrit: 22.8%
Pulse oximetry (room air): 89%

Questions

1. What other assessment would be helpful?
2. Should this patient be referred to a physician?
3. Does this patient need cardiopulmonary exercise testing?

DISCUSSION QUESTIONS

1 What is the primary cause of morbidity in individuals with sickle cell disease?

2 While regular, moderate exercise is recommended for children with sickle cell disease, there are no general guidelines for adults. What are the physiologic differences between sickle cell disease in children and in adults?

3 Are exercise recommendations the same for people with sickle cell disease and those with sickle cell trait? Explain.

4 Identify and discuss four contributing factors to exercise limitations in individuals with sickle cell disease.

Adults with sickle cell disease should be evaluated to determine each one's individual exercise capacity and physiologic limitations before an exercise training program is recommended.

Individuals with sickle cell disease should avoid intense and prolonged exercise; exercise response should be monitored by a physician.

Under conditions of extreme heat and limited access to water, sickle cell trait is associated with increased risk of sudden death.

What we Know
About Sickle Cell Disease and Sickle Cell Trait

1 Sickle cell disease, the most common hemoglobinopathy in the world, is an inherited disorder.

2 Despite advances in diagnosis and treatment, sickle cell disease remains associated with significant morbidity and early mortality.

3 When untrained, individuals with sickle cell trait exercising under conditions of extreme heat and without access to water, have a greater than 20-fold increase in risk of sudden death.

4 Patients with sickle cell disease often are sedentary, and obesity in adults has been documented.

5 No controlled clinical trials have assessed the long-term benefits and risks of exercise in sickle cell disease.

What We Would Like to Know
About Sickle Cell Disease and Sickle Cell Trait

1 What factors determine variability in the clinical course of sickle cell disease among individuals within the same genotype?

2 What are the long-term benefits and risks of controlled exercise in adolescents and adults with sickle cell disease? Do the benefits outweigh the risks?

3 Do chronic complications of sickle cell disease override the potential beneficial physical and psychological benefits of physical activity, particularly in adults?

REFERENCES

1. Schroeder WA, Huisman THJ. The Chromatography of Hemoglobin. New York: Marcel Dekker, 1980.

2. Bessa EC. Hemoglobin and hemoglobinopathies. In: Hematology. Philadelphia: Harwell Publishing, 1992:123–136.

3. McCurdy PR, Sherman AS. Irreversibly sickled cells and red cell survival in sickle cell anemia: a study with both DF32P and 51 CR. Am J Med 1978;64:253–258.

4. Sickle Cell Disease: Screening, Diagnosis, Management, and Counseling in Newborns and Infants. Clinical Practice Guideline No. 6. U. S. Department of Health and Human Services, Public Health Service. Agency for Health Care Policy and Research Publication No. 93-0562, April 1993.

5. Reed CD, Charache S, Lubin B, eds. Management and Therapy of Sickle Cell Disease. 3rd Ed. National Institutes of Health, National Heart, Blood and Lung Institute. No. 95-2117. 1995

6. Platt OS, Brambilla DJ, Rosse WF, et al. Mortality in sickle cell disease: life expectancy and risk factors for early death. N Engl J Med 1994;330:1639–1644.

7. Woods KF, Miller MD, Johnson MH, et al. Functional status and well-being in adults with sickle cell disease. JCOM 1997;4:15–21.

8. Bobo L, Miller ST, Smith WR, et al. Health perceptions and medical care opinions of inner-city adults with sickle cell disease or asthma compared with those of their siblings. So Med J 1989;82:9–12.

9. Woods KF, Ramsey LT, Callahan LA, et al. Body composition and health status in women with sickle cell disease. Ethnicity and Disease 2001;11(1):30–35.

10. Gaston M, Verter J, Woods G, et al. Prophylaxis with oral penicillin in children with sickle cell anemia. N Engl J Med 1986;314;1594–1599.

11. Wethers DL. Sickle cell disease in childhood. Part II: Diagnosis and treatment of major complications and recent advances in treatment. Am Fam Phys 2000;62:1309–1314.

12. Ballas SK, Carlos TM, Dampier C, et al. Guidelines for standards of care of acute painful episodes in patients with sickle cell disease. Philadelphia: Cardeza Foundation for Hematologic Research, Thomas Jefferson University, 2000.

13. Charache S, Terrin M, Moore R, et al. Effect of hydroxyurea on the frequency of painful crises in sickle cell disease. N Engl J Med 1995;322:1317–1322.

14. Kenny TR, Helms RW, O'Branski EE, et al. Safety of hydroxyurea in children with sickle cell anemia: results of the HUG-KIDS study, a Phase I/II trial. Pediatric Hydroxyurea Group. Blood 1999;94:1550–1554.

15. Charache S, Dover GJ, Moore RD, et al. Hydroxyurea: effects on hemoglobin F production in patients with sickle cell anemia. Blood 1992;79:2555–2565.

16. Kim-Shapiro DB, King SB, Bonifant CL, et al. Time resolved absorption study of the reaction of hydroxyurea with sickle cell hemoglobin. Biochim Biophys Acta 1998;1380:64–74.

17. Glover RE, Ivy ED, Orringer EP, et al. Detection of nitrosyl hemoglobin in venous blood in the treatment of sickle cell anemia with hydroxyurea. Mol Pharmacol 1999;55:1006–1010.

18. Walters M, Patience M, Leisenring W, et al. Bone marrow transplantation for sickle cell disease. N Engl J Med 1996;335:369–376.

19. Kelly P, Kurtzberg J, Vichinsky E, et al. Umbilical cord blood stem cell: application for the treatment of patients with hemoglobinopathies. J Pediatr 1997;130:695–703.

20. Hoppe CC, Walters MC. Bone marrow transplantation in sickle cell anemia. Curr Opin Oncol 2001;13(2):85–90.

21. Cowan M, Globus M. In utero hematopoietic stem cell transplant for inherited diseases. Am J Pediatr Hematol Oncol 1994;16:35–42.

22. Kark JA, Posey DM, Schumagher HR, Ruehle CJ. Sickle cell trait as a risk factor for sudden death in physical training. N Engl J Med 1987;317:781–787.

23. Phinney LT, Gardner JW, Kark JA, Wenger CB. Long-term follow-up after exertional heat illness during recruit training. Med Sci Sports Exerc 2001;33:1443–1448.

24. Drehner D, Neuhauser KM, Neuhauser TS, Blackwood GV. Death among US Air Force Basic Trainees, 1956-1996. Mil Med 1999;164:841–847.

25. Kerle KK. Exertional collapse and sudden death associated with sickle cell trait. Mil Med 1996;161:766–767.

26. LeGallais D, Bile A, Mercier J, et al. Exercise-induced death in sickle cell trait: role of aging, training and deconditioning. Med Sci Sports Exerc 1996;28:541–544.

27. Wirthwein DP, Spotswood SD, Barnard JJ, Prahlow JA. Death due to microvascular occlusion in sickle cell trait following exertion. J Forensic Sci 2001;46:399–401.

28. Gardner JW, Kark JA. Fatal rhabdomyolysis presenting as mild heat illness in military training. Mil Med 1994;159:160–163.

29. Kark JA, Ward FT. Exercise and hemoglobin S. Semin Hematol 1994;31:181–225.

30. Browne RJ, Gillespie CA. Sickle cell trait. A risk factor for life-threatening rhabdomyolysis? Phys Sports Med 1993;21:80–88.

31. Martin TM, Weisman IM, Zeballos RJ, Stephenson SR. Exercise and hypoxia increase sickling in venous blood from an exercising limb in individuals with sickle cell trait. Am J Med 1989;87:48–56.

32. Nuss R, Loehr JP, Daberkow E, et al. Cardiopulmonary functioning men with sickle cell trait who reside at moderately high altitude. J Lab Clin Med 1993;122:382–387.

33. Bile A, LeGallais D, Mercier B, et al. Blood lactate concentrations during incremental exercise in subjects with sickle cell trait. Med Sci Sports Exerc 1998;30:649–654.

34. Bitanga E, Rouillon JD. Influence of sickle cell trait heterozygote on energy abilities. Pathol Biol (Paris) 1998;46(1):45–52.

35. Bile A, LeGallais D, Mercier J, et al. Sickle cell trait in Ivory Coast athletic throw and jump champions, 1956-1995. Int J Sports Med 1998;19:215–219.

36. LeGallais D, Perfaut C, Mercier J, et al. Sickle cell trait as a limiting factor for high-level performance in a semi-marathon. Int J Sports Med 1994;15:399–402.

37. Murphy JR. Sickle cell hemoglobin (Hb AS) in black football players. JAMA 1973;25:981–982.

38. Thiriet P, Lobe MM, Gweha I, Gozal D. Prevalence of sickle cell trait in an athletic West African population. Med Sci Sports Exerc 1991;23:389–390.

39. Shaskey DJ, Green GA. Sports haematology. Sports Med 2000;29:27–38.

40. Miller D, Winslow R, Klein H, et al. Improved exercise performance after exchange transfusion in subjects with sickle cell anemia. Blood 1980;56:1127–1131.

41. Charache S, Bleecker ER, Bross DS. Effect of blood transfusion on exercise capacity in patients with sickle cell anemia. Am J Med 1983;74:757–764.

42. Braden DS, Covitz W, Milner PF. Cardiovascular function during rest and exercise in patients with sickle cell anemia and co-existing alpha thalassemia 2. Am J Hematol 1996;52:96–102.

43. Pianosi P, D'Souza J, Esseltine D, et al. Ventilation and gas exchange during exercise in sickle cell anemia. Am Rev Resp Dis 1991;143:226–230.

44. Callahan LA, Woods KF, Mensah GA, et al. Cardiopulmonary responses to exercise in women with sickle cell anemia. Am J Resp Crit Care Med 2002;165:1309–1316.

45. Ramsey LT, Woods KF, Barbeau P, et al. Implementation of a controlled physical training program in women with sickle cell disease. *Am J Hematol,* 2000;66:155–156.

46. Charache S, Grisolia S, Fiedler AJ, Hellegers AE. Effect of 2,3-diphosphoglycerate on oxygen affinity of blood in sickle cell anemia. J Clin Invest 1970;49: 806–812.

47. Wasserman K, Whipp B. Exercise physiology in health and disease. Am Rev Respir Dis 1975;112:219–249.

48. Wasserman K, Hansen JE, Sue DY, et al. Principles of Exercise testing and interpretation. Malvern, PA: Lea and Febiger, 1994.

49. Freund H, Lonsdorfer J, Oyono-Enguelle S, Lonsdorfer A. Lactate ex-

change and removal abilities in sickle cell patients and untrained and trained healthy humans. J Appl Physiol 1992;73:2580–2587.

50. Oyono-Enguelle S, LeGallais D, Lonsdorfer A, et al. Cardiorespiratory and metabolic responses to exercise in HbSC sickle cell patients. Med Sci Sports Exerc 2000;32:725–731.

51. Weil JV, Castro O, Malik AB, et al. Pathogenesis of lung disease in sickle hemoglobinopathies. Am Rev Resp Dis 1993;148:149–156.

52. Vichinski EP, Styles LA, Colangelo LH, et al. Acute chest syndrome in sickle cell disease: clinical presentation and course. Blood 1997;89:1787–1792.

53. Haynes JJ, Manci E, Voelkel N. Pulmonary complications. In: Embury SH, Hebbel RP, Steinberg MH, Mohandas N, eds. Sickle Cell Disease: Basic Principles and Clinical Practice. New York: Raven Press, 1994: 623–631.

54. Varat MA, Adolph RJ, Fowler NO. Cardiovascular effects of anemia. Am Heart J 1972;83:415–426.

55. Lindsay J, Meshel J, Patterson R. The cardiovascular manifestations of sickle cell disease. Arch Intern Med 1974;133:643–651.

56. Ramsey LT. The Implementation of Controlled Physical Training and the Physiological Effects of Exercise in Women With Sickle Cell Disease [dissertation]. Augusta, GA: Medical College of Georgia, 1999:51–54.

57. Sarjeant GR. Sickle Cell Disease. Oxford: Oxford University Press, 1985.

58. Gerry JL, Baird MG, Fortuin NJ. Evaluation of left ventricular function in patients with sickle cell anemia. Am J Med 1976;60:965–972.

59. Arensman FW, Covitz W, Dicks G, et al. Digitized echocardiographic assessment of left ventricular wall motion in children and adolescents with sickle cell anemia. J Cardiovasc Ultrasonogr 1986;5:223–227.

60. Balfour IC, Covitz W, Arensman FW, et al. Left ventricular filling in sickle cell anemia. Am J Cardiol 1988;61:395–399.

61. Covitz W, Espeland M, Gallagher D, et al. The heart in sickle cell anemia. The Cooperative Study of Sickle Cell Disease (CSSCD). Chest 1995;108:1214–1219.

62. Covitz W, Balfour IC, Alpert BS, Arensman FW. The heart as a target organ in sickle cell anemia. J Cardiovasc Ultrasonogr 1986;5:177–181.

63. Covitz W, Eubig C, Balfour IC, et al. Exercise-induced cardiac dysfunction in sickle cell anemia: a radionuclide study. Am J Cardiol 1983;51:570–575.

64. Swerlick RA, Eckman JR, Kumar A, et al. Alpha 4 beta 1-integrin expression on sickle reticulocyte: vascular cell adhesion molecule-1-dependent binding to endothelium. Blood 1993;82:1891–1899.

65. Kasschau MR, Barabino GA, Bridges KR, Golan DE. Adhesion of sickle neutrophils and erythrocytes to fibronectin. Blood 1996;87:771–780.

66. Malave, I, Perdomo Y, Escalona E, et al. Levels of tumor necrosis factor α/Chacectin (TNFα) in sera from patients with sickle cell disease. Acta Haematol 1993;90:172–176.

67. Hedo CC, Aken'ova YA, Okpala IE, et al. Acute phase reactants and severity of homozygous sickle cell disease. J Intern Med 1993;233:467–470.

68. Singhal A, Doherty JF, Raynes JG, et al. Is there an acute-phase response in steady-state sickle cell disease? Lancet 1993;341:651–653.

69. Taylor SC, Shacks SJ, Mitchell RA, Banks A. Serum interleukin-6 levels in the steady state of sickle cell disease. J Interferon Cytokine Res 1995;15:1061–1064.

70. Kuvibidila S, Gardner R, Ode D, et al. Tumor necrosis factor alpha in children with sickle cell disease in stable condition. J Natl Med Assoc 1997;89:609–615.

71. Bourantas KL, Dalekos GN, Makis A, et al. Acute phase proteins and interleukins in steady state sickle cell disease. Eur J Haematol 1998;61:49–54.

72. Weinstein R, Zhou M, Bartlett-Pandite A, Wenc K. Sickle erythrocytes inhibit human endothelial cell DNA synthesis. Blood 1990;76:2146–2152.

73. Solovey A, Lin Y, Browne P, et al. Circulating activated endothelial cells in sickle cell anemia. N Engl J Med 1997;337:1584–1590.

74. Rybicki AC, Benjamin LJ. Increased levels of endothelin-1 in plasma of sickle cell anemia patients. Blood 1998;92:2594–2595.

75. Werdehoff SG, Moore RB, Hoff CJ, et al. Elevated plasma endothelin-1 levels in sickle cell anemia: relationships to oxygen saturation and left ventricular hypertrophy. Am J Hematol 1998;58:195–199.

76. Graido-Gonzalez E, Doherty JC, Bergreen EW, et al. Plasma endothelin-1, cytokine, and prostaglandin E2 levels in sickle cell disease and acute vaso-occlusive sickle crisis. Blood 1998;92:2551–2555.

77. Werdehoff SG, Moore RB, Hoff CJ, et al. Elevated plasma endothelin-1 levels in sickle cell anemia: relationships to oxygen saturation and left ventricular hypertrophy. Am J Hematol 1998;58:195–199.

78. Rees DC, Cervi P, Grimwade D, et al. The metabolites of nitric oxide in sickle-cell disease. Br J Haemotol 1995;91:834–837.

79. Lopez BL, Barnett J, Ballas SK, et al. Nitric oxide metabolite level in acute vasoocclusive sickle cell crisis. Acad Emerg Med 1996;3:1098–1103.

80. Moncada S, Higgs A. The L-arginine-nitric oxide pathway. N Engl J Med 1993;329:2002–2012.

81. Shen W, Zhang X, Zhao G, et al. Nitric oxide production and NO synthase gene expression contribute to vascular regulation during exercise. Med Sci Sports Exerc 1995;27:1125–1134.

82. Green DJ, O'Driscoll G, Blanksby BA, Taylor RR. Control of skeletal muscle blood flow during dynamic exercise: contribution of endothelium-derived nitric oxide. Sports Med 1996;21:119–146.

83. Maeda S, Miyauchi T, Goto K, Matsuda M. Alteration of plasma endothelin-1 by exercise at intensities lower and higher than ventilatory threshold. J Appl Physiol 1994;77:1399–1402.

84. Maeda, S, Miyauchi T, Sakane M, et al. Does endothelin-1 participate in the exercise-induced changes of blood flow distribution of muscles in humans. J Appl Physiol 1997;82:1107–1111.

85. Ahlborg G, Weitzberg E, Lundberg J. Metabolic and vascular effects of circulating endothelin-1 during moderately heavy prolonged exercise. J Appl Physiol 1995;78:2294–2300.

86. Cosenzi A, Sacerdote A, Bocin E, et al. Neither physical exercise nor α1- and β-adrenergic blockade affect plasma endothelin concentrations. Am J Hyperten 1996;9:819–822.

87. Lenz T, Nadansky M, Gossmann J, et al. Exhaustive exercise-induced tissue hypoxia does not change endothelin and big endothelin plasma levels in normal volunteers. Am J Hyperten 1998;11:1028–1031.

88. Barbeau P, Woods KF, Ramsey LT, et al. Consecutive daily bouts of exercise in sickle cell anemia: effect on vasoactive mediators and inflammatory markers, Endothelium 2001;8:147–156.

SUGGESTED READINGS

American College of Sports Medicine. Guidelines for Exercise Testing and Prescribing. 6th Ed. Philadelphia: Lippincott Williams & Wilkins, 2000.

American College of Sports Medicine. ACSM's Exercise Management for Persons with Chronic Diseases and Disabilities. 2nd Ed. Champaign, IL: Human Kinetics, 2003.

Embury SH, Hebbel RP, Steinberg MH, Mohandas N, eds. Sickle Cell Disease: Basic Principles and Clinical Practice. New York: Raven Press, 1994.

Reed CD, Charache S, Lubin B, eds. Management and Therapy of Sickle Cell Disease. 3rd Ed. National Heart, Blood and Lung Institute Publication No. 95-2117. Washington, DC: National Institutes of Health, 1995.

Sickle Cell Disease: Screening, Diagnosis, Management, and Counseling in Newborns and Infants, Clinical Practice Guideline No. 6, US Department of Health and Human Services, Public Health Service, AHCPR Publication No. 93-0562, April 1993.

CHAPTER 30

HIV and AIDS

William W. Stringer

Overview

Infection with human immunodeficiency virus (**HIV**), the cause of the acquired immunodeficiency syndrome (**AIDS**), has reached epidemic levels worldwide. The enormous number of existing (and forecasted) cases and the new therapies available for HIV have made exercise an increasingly important therapeutic modality. Exercise can increase aerobic and functional capacity, improve quality of life, preserve immune function, and perhaps mitigate the effects of current HIV therapies such as highly active anti-retroviral therapy (HAART). In fact, the metabolic and anthropomorphic complications associated with HIV/AIDS and HAART therapy may be a prime target for exercise intervention. This chapter reviews the general biology of the HIV virus, the spectrum of HIV infection (from asymptomatic carriers to overt AIDS), and the role of aerobic and strength exercise in comprehensive HIV therapy. In addition, we review the risk of transmission during sporting events, provide specific recommendations for exercise prescriptions, update the current status of **anabolic therapy**, and discuss the metabolic syndromes associated with HIV infection/therapy. We end by presenting future research directions and a case study in this important, rapidly changing, engaging area of clinical care and research investigation.

HIV

General Biology of the Virus and Mechanisms of Transmission

Human immunodeficiency virus (HIV) is observed in two serotypes (HIV-1 and HIV-2). This chapter will primarily focus on the more common form, HIV-1 (hereafter, HIV). HIV is an RNA retrovirus that transforms its viral RNA into double-stranded DNA which is then incorporated into the host genome. HIV is a very small (100–nm diameter) particle that is transmitted primarily via sexual contact with blood, semen, and vaginal secretions. Once the virus is inside the body, it binds to the CD4 receptor on the surface of affected cells (Figure 30.1)

After binding to the cell surface, the virus fuses with the cell membrane and releases its viral core into the cytoplasm. The HIV virus has a genome of approximately 10 kilobases with three major structural genes (gag, pol, and env). The reverse polymerase creates linear double-stranded DNA, which incorporates into the host genome. Once this DNA is activated, the mRNA is produced and the viral proteins are produced. New viral particles bud off the membrane and subsequently mature (1). Viremia can be quite marked after infection with very high titers of virus on the blood. This can lead to an acute syndrome that resembles any other viral infection (2). During this phase, the virus is widely distributed throughout the body, including the lymphatic system, muscle, heart, lung, and central nervous system. Although the viral levels decrease by 4 to 6 months after the beginning of the infection, the subject remains infectious.

Scope of the Epidemic

As of December 2000, the cumulative number of AIDS cases reported to the CDC was 774,467 (17% were female, 83% male), and the total number of deaths reported with AIDS was 448,060. Most cases were observed in people 25 to 44 years of age. Forty-three percent of all persons with AIDS cases were Caucasian, 38% were African-American, 18% were Hispanic, and 7% were Asian or Pacific Islander. The Centers for Disease Control estimates that 40,000 people per year become infected with the HIV virus in the USA (www.cdc.gov) (3).

Strategies for reducing the disease burden, both in the USA and internationally, currently are underway (4). Infection with HIV has reached epidemic levels on all continents except Antarctica. The Joint United Nations Program on HIV/AIDS estimates that as of December 2000, there were 36.1 million people living with HIV/AIDS worldwide, of whom 34.7 million were adults, 16.4 million were women (47%), and 1.4 million were children under the age of 15. It is estimated that 21.8 million people have died worldwide from AIDS since the epidemic began. The overwhelming majority of people with HIV (approximately 95%) live in the developing world, and the disease increasingly is being spread by heterosexual contact in the underdeveloped world (Figure 30.2).

Effects of HIV on the Immune System

The HIV virus selectively attacks cells with surface CD4 receptors. Although attacks on these cells result in a marked depletion of the CD4⁺ T lymphocytes and a reduction in the ability of the immune system to respond to common infec-

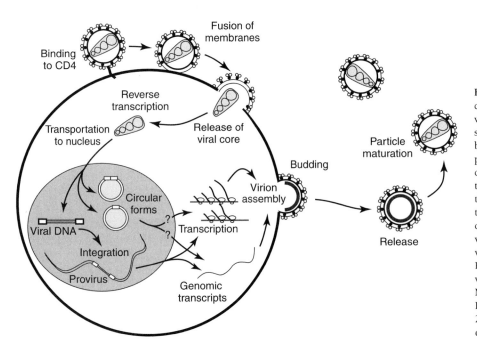

FIGURE 30.1. The life cycle of HIV-1. The life cycle of the virus begins with binding of the virus to CD4 on the cell surface, followed by fusion of the viral envelope with the cell membrane and release of the viral core into the cytoplasm. The process of reverse transcription is completed, and the viral DNA is integrated into the host cell genome to form the provirus. In the presence of appropriate host cell stimulation, viral mRNA transcripts are produced that code for the structural proteins as well as provide a source of genomic transcripts for new viral particles. (Adapted from Streicher HZ, Reitz MSJ, Gallo RC. Human immunodeficiency virus. In: Mandell GL, Bennett JE, Dolin R, eds. Mandell: Principles and Practice of Infectious Diseases. Kent, UK: Churchill Livingstone, 2000:1874–1885 Mandel, Chapter 157, Reference (1).

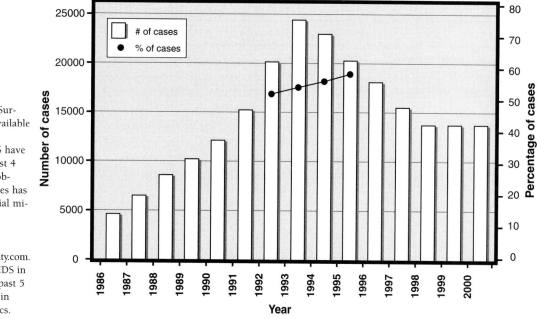

FIGURE 30.2. A. Increasing AIDS/HIV cases in minorities. Adapted from CDC HIV/AIDS Surveillance Data (1986–2000). Available at www.cdc.gov/hiv/graphics/minority.com. As cases of AIDS have decreased in the USA in the past 4 years, the percentage of cases observed in racial/ethnic minorities has increased. B. AIDS cases in racial minorities. Adapted from CDC HIV/AIDS Surveillance Data 1986–2000. Available at www.cdc.gov/hiv/graphics/minority.com. As the percentage of cases of AIDS in Caucasians decreased over the past 5 years, the percentage increased in African-Americans and Hispanics.

tious agents in the environment (opportunistic infections), any cells in the body can be attacked by the HIV virus. The reduction in immune function also leads to an increase in the number and type of malignancies seen in patients with AIDS. Infection with HIV reflects exposure to the virus and incorporation of the viral genome into the host's DNA.

Progression of HIV Infection to AIDS

Progression to AIDS is measured by the progressive damage to the host's immune system, which leaves the host vulnerable to opportunistic infections and malignancies. The average time from initial infection to AIDS among untreated patients is 8 to 10 years (CD4+ cells decrease at a rate of approximately 50 to 75 cells per year); however, this can vary—some people (about 20% of patients) develop AIDS in less than 5 years, whereas others (<5%) remain asymptomatic for more than 10 years (5). As the immune system fails, increased numbers of viral particles circulate in the blood, as measured by HIV **polymerase chain reaction** (PCR). In 1993, the CDC defined AIDS as a CD4 count of less than 200 cells/mm³ (6). The stage of HIV infection can be determined from the CD4 count: more than 500 cells/mm³ represents mild or early disease; 200 to 500 cells/mm³ qualifies as moderate or mid-stage; and less than 200 cells/mm³ indicates advanced or severe infection. Patients with counts below 50 cells/mm³ are considered to have end-stage immunodeficiency.

Therapies for HIV

Therapies for HIV have evolved from a single agent (AZT) in the late 1980s to several categories of agents that are used in combination (as of 2002). The major categories of HIV

drugs are nucleoside analog reverse transcriptase inhibitors (NRTIs); nonnucleoside reverse transcriptase inhibitors (NNRTIs); and protease inhibitors (Table 30.1).

Several Internet sites are very helpful in keeping up with rapidly changing treatments (Table 30.2).

Therapy for HIV should take into account the patient's current clinical status, the stage of HIV, the **CD4+ T cell counts**, and the **viral load**. There is very little controversy about starting HIV medications when the CD4+ count is less than 200 cells/mm³ (or when the patient is symptomatic with an AIDS-defining illness) (Table 30.3) (8). However, the evidence is not convincing that withholding therapy from patients with CD4+ counts higher than 200 cells/mm³ until the count falls below 200 cells/mm³ results in adverse outcomes for the patient. Therefore, due to side effects of the medications, complicated drug therapy regimens, and the risk of virus mutations that may decrease the overall effectiveness of therapy, the decision whether or not to treat asymptomatic patients must be made for each patient individually.

Furthermore, because the number of HIV drugs, drug-related medication complications, and nuances of therapy have become far more intricate, the current recommendation is that HIV care be delivered by an expert in HIV medicine (8).

Monitoring the Effect of Therapy

Several surrogate markers for HIV outcomes have been suggested to monitor the natural history of the HIV infection and to quantify the effects of various interventions, (9–11). CD4+ T cell counts alone, while helpful in understanding the stage of HIV infection, have been shown to an inferior predictor of outcome when compared to plasma viral load

TABLE 30.1. DRUGS LICENSED IN THE UNITED STATES FOR THE TREATMENT OF HIV INFECTION (2000)

Drug	Typical Dosage	Most Common Adverse Effects
Nucleoside Reverse Transcriptase Inhibitors (NRTIs)		
Zidovudine (AZT) (Retrovir)	300 mg PO b.i.d.	Anemia
Didanosine (ddI) (Videx)	400 mg PO qhs	GI upset, pancreatitis
Zalcitabine (ddC) (Hivid)	0.75 mg PO t.i.d.	Neuropathy
Stavudine (d4T) (Zerit)	40 mg PO b.i.d.	Neuropathy, mitochondrial abnormalities
Lamivudine (3TC) (Epivir)	150 mg PO b.i.d.	Rash
Abacavir Sulfate (ABC) (Ziagen)	300 mg PO b.i.d.	Rash, fever
Nonnucleoside Reverse Transcriptase Inhibitors (NNRTIs)		
Nevirapine (Viramune)	200 mg PO b.i.d.	Rash
Delavirdine mesylate (Rescriptor)	400 mg PO t.i.d.	Rash
Efavirenz (Sustiva)	600 mg PO qhs	Altered mental status
Protease Inhibitors (PIs)		
Ritonavir (Norvir)	600 mg PO b.i.d.	GI upset, paresthesias
Indinavir sulfate (Crixivan)	800 mg PO q8h	Nephrolithiasis
Saquinavir (Fortovase)	1,200 mg PO q8h	Nausea
Nelfinavir mesylate (Viracept)	1,250 mg PO b.i.d.	Diarrhea
Amprenavir (Ageneras)	1,200 mg PO b.i.d.	Nausea
Lopinavir/Ritonavir (Kaletra)	400/100 mg (3 capsules) b.i.d.	Diarrhea, nausea

b.i.d., twice a day; PO, orally; qhs, at bedtime; t.i.d., three times a day.
Modified from Wolfe PR. Practical Approaches to HIV Therapy: Recommendation for the year 2000 (7) and the treatment guidelines from the U.S. Department of Health and Human Services, available at http://www.aidsinfo.nih.gov/ (8).

(12). Therefore, within any given range of CD4+ counts, the plasma viral load adds additional information on the patient's risk of progression to an AIDS-defining illness (11, 13–15). The current recommendations are as follows:

- Viral loads should be assessed at the time of diagnosis and every 3 to 4 months thereafter in the untreated patient.
- CD4+ T cell counts should be measured at the time of diagnosis and generally every 3 to 6 months thereafter.
- Viral loads should be assessed between 2 and 8 weeks after initiation of antiretroviral therapy to determine the initial effectiveness of therapy. Most patients should have a large decrease (about 1 $\log_{10}$ reduction) in viral load by this time (8).

Therefore, in assessing the patient's response to an intervention (either clinical or as part of a research protocol), current practice would dictate analysis of both CD4+ cell count and plasma viral load.

TABLE 30.2. WEBSITES OFFERING REGULAR UPDATES ON HIV TREATMENT

Medscape http://hiv.medscape.com/updates/quickguide
JAMA HIV AIDS Information http://www.ama-assn.org/special/hiv
AIDS info, a service of the U.S. Department of Health and Human Services: http://www.aidsinfo.nih.gov/
National Institutes of Health, National Institute of Allergy and Infectious Diseases: Division of Acquired Immunodeficiency Syndrome: http://www.niaid.nih.gov/daids/

Exercise Testing in HIV-Positive Individuals

Cardiopulmonary Exercise Testing

Cardiopulmonary exercise testing (CPET) has several advantages over electrocardiogram (ECG) treadmill testing in HIV-positive individuals because it acquires a wider range of information for analysis (Figure 30.3). The ECG treadmill usually is used in clinical medicine to diagnosis flow-limiting coronary artery disease. Cardiopulmonary exercise testing is used to evaluate exercise tolerance and dyspnea and to discover the specific physiologic mechanisms contributing to exercise limitation as well as for evaluation of coronary artery disease (see Figure 30.3).

Precise information on cardiac, ventilatory, pulmonary vascular, peripheral vascular, and muscle system function can be readily obtained from CPET at rest and during exercise, obviating the need to estimate either metabolic equivalents (**METs**), work rate, or $\dot{V}o_2max$ (Table 30.4). Finally, more subtle indicators of deconditioning, dyspnea, and opportunistic infections can be deduced from information obtained via CPET.

Protecting Current and Future Test Subjects Before Cardiopulmonary Exercise Testing

The CPET protocol is not altered for HIV-positive individuals (16). Both ramp and constant work rate tests are effective protocols for evoking diagnostic cardiopulmonary re-

TABLE 30.3. INDICATIONS FOR INITIATION OF ANTIRETROVIRAL THERAPY IN HIV-INFECTED PATIENTS

Clinical Category	CD4+ T Cell Count	Plasma HIV RNA	Recommendation
Symptomatic (AIDS, severe symptoms)	Any value	Any value	Treat
Asymptomatic, AIDS	CD4+ T cells < 200/mm³	Any value	Treat
Asymptomatic	CD4+cells > 200/mm³ but < 350 mm³	> 55,000 (bDNA or RT-PCR)	Some experts recommend initiating therapy, recognizing that the 3-year risk of developing AIDS in untreated patients is >30%. In the absence of very high levels of plasma HIV RNA, some would defer therapy and monitor the CD4+ T cell count and level of plasma HIV RNA more frequently. Clinical outcomes data after initiation therapy are lacking.
Asymptomatic	CD4+ T Cells > 350/mm³	< 55,000 (bDNA or RT-PCR)	Many experts would defer therapy and observe, recognizing that the 3-year risk of developing AIDS in untreated patients is < 15%.

From Fauci AS, Bartlett JG, Goosby EP, et al. Guidelines for the use of antiretroviral agents in HIV-infected adults and adolescents. http://www.hivatis.org 2002;1:1–111. Data from Table 30.6, p 37 (8).

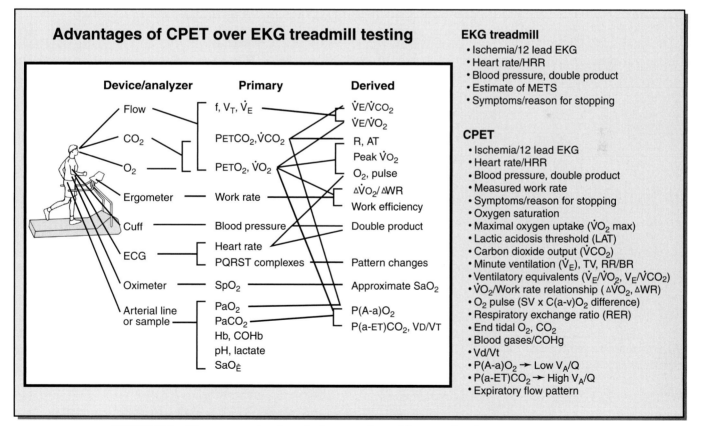

FIGURE 30.3. The amount and quality of information obtained from a cardiopulmonary exercise test (CPET) relative to electrocardiogram (ECG) treadmill testing is enormous. The ECG treadmill is used primarily to diagnose flow-limiting coronary artery disease. The CPET provides additional information to assess the cardiac, ventilatory, pulmonary vascular, peripheral vascular, and muscle systems. HRR, heart rate reserve; V_d/V_t, ratio of dead space to tidal volume.

TABLE 30.4. CARDIOPULMONARY PARAMETERS AND THEIR CLINICAL USE DURING EXERCISE TESTING

Exercise Parameter	Measurement	Usual Range	Significance of Low Values	Significance of High Value
Cardiovascular				
Oxygen uptake	$\dot{V}O_2$ (L/min) = cardiac output $\times$ C(a-v) O_2 difference	Predicted based on age, gender, height, weight, type of protocol (treadmill vs. bike).	Consider anemia, heart or lung disease, pulmonary or peripheral vascular disease, ischemia, mitochondrial dysfunction, or poor effort	Training effect
Anaerobic threshold	AT (L/min)	> 40% of $\dot{V}O_{2max}$	Consider anemia, heart or lung disease, pulmonary or peripheral vascular disease, ischemia, mitochondrial dysfunction	Training effect
Heart rate, heart rate reserve	HR (bpm), HRR	50–200, (for a maximal test)	Maximal effort, cardiovascular limitation	Poor effort, beta-blocker, peripheral arterial disease, sick sinus syndrome, lung disease, skeletal muscle weakness
Oxygen pulse	O_2 Pulse (ml/dl) = stroke volume $\times$ C(a-v) O_2 difference	Normal about 15 ml/dl at peak exercise	Low stroke volume, low a-v oxygen extraction, anemia	Training
Hematocrit	Hct (g/dl)	13–15 g/dl (male > female)	Anemia	Polycythemia, erythropoietin therapy, androgen therapy
Ventilatory				
Minute ventilation	V_E (L/min) = Alveolar ventilation (V_A) + dead space ventilation (V_D)	6–200 L/min	Chronic obstructive lung disease (COPD), muscle weakness, poor effort	Increased ventilatory requirements at a given work level, increased dead space ventilation (increased V_D/V_T), training, anxiety, hyperventilation
Ventilatory equivalents	$V_E/\dot{V}O_2$, $V_E/\dot{V}CO_2$ (unitless)	$V_E/\dot{V}O_2$ = 22 to 27 $V_E/\dot{V}CO_2$ = 26 to 30	Efficient gas exchange, high arterial PCO_2	Increased ventilatory requirements at a given work level, increased dead space ventilation (increased V_D/V_T), anxiety, hyperventilation
Oxygen saturation	O_2 Sat (%)	94–100%	Arterial desaturation, hypoxemia	NA
End-tidal CO_2 and O_2	ETO_2 mm Hg $ETCO_2$ mm Hg	ETO_2 = 90–120 $ETCO_2$ = 35–45	$ETO_2 \rightarrow$ hypoventilation, decreased FIO_2, altitude $ETCO_2$ = hyperventilation, anxiety, chronic metabolic acidosis	$ETO_2 \rightarrow$ Hyperventilation, increased FIO_2 $ETCO_2$ = hyperventilation, anxiety, chronic metabolic acidosis
Breathing reserve	BR (L/min)	> 11 L/min	Primary lung disease, cardio-vascular disease	Training

sponses, and the data generated can be used for a spectrum of indications, from diagnosing subtle pulmonary vascular disease (e.g. opportunistic pulmonary infections in an HIV-positive individual) to generating an exercise prescription for a deconditioned subject who wants to initiate an exercise training program. However, much greater attention must be given to protecting current and future test subjects.

The risks of disease transmission (e.g., tuberculosis), and even HIV transmission (from saliva or blood) in the laboratory must be considered. Although theoretically there may be risk of HIV disease transmission from contact with tears, sweat, and urine, the primary vehicles for spread of the virus appear to be blood, tissue, or sexual contact (17). These risks vary with CD4+ count and plasma viral loads; however, universal precautions should be observed at all times in the laboratory. During the initial interview, the subject should be questioned regarding cough, fever, chills, weight loss, or other symptoms that might indicate an acute (or subacute) infectious illness. If any of these symptoms are present, the exercise test should be postponed until the symptoms have been clinically evaluated, and a chest x-ray should be obtained to exclude active disease such as tuberculosis or Pneumocystis pneumonia (PCP).

During Cardiopulmonary Exercise Testing

During the CPET, attention should be devoted to decreasing the risk of infectious disease transmission to other subjects. These measures should include use of disposable mouthpieces and flow meters during exercise testing, strict adherence to proper blood-drawing technique with safety needles, and proper use and disposal of all biological specimens. It is important for the exercise personnel (preferably a physician during the initial exercise testing) to be attentive and monitor several cardiopulmonary markers before and during the exercise test. These include heart rate (12-lead ECG at start and every 2 minutes during exercise), oxygen uptake, **anaerobic threshold**, minute **ventilation**, **ventilatory equivalents**, respiratory exchange ratio (**RER**), end-tidal CO_2 and O_2, and work rate during the exercise test. The subject should be questioned during the test regarding any symptoms (e.g., chest pain, dyspnea, leg pain, palpitations, severe fatigue) prior to exercise, at 1- to 2-minute intervals during exercise, and after completion of the test.

After Cardiopulmonary Exercise Testing

After exercise the subject should be monitored closely during the early recovery period while on the bike or treadmill (the first 3 minutes of recovery) with gas exchange and ECG. The subject should continue to move his or her legs slowly to prevent venous pooling. After 3 minutes, the subject should sit in a chair (or gurney if needed) and recover completely before being discharged from the laboratory. Once the mouthpiece is out, the subject should be questioned closely regarding symptoms during exercise and any

factors that limited exercise (e.g. legs, lungs, chest pain). The subject should not leave the laboratory until any exercise-related symptoms have resolved. Once the CPET is over, the exercise data can be organized into a 9-panel plot as well as the tabular data (Figure 30.4) and scrutinized in detail for more subtle exercise parameter changes.

Mechanisms of Exercise Limitation in Patients With HIV

Several mechanisms of aerobic exercise limitation can be present in HIV-positive individuals. In this section we review the various broad categories (e.g., cardiovascular, ventilatory, pulmonary vascular, peripheral vascular, muscle, anemia, deconditioning) that may present limitations and determine what types of mechanisms are supported by the exercise literature in HIV-positive individuals.

Cardiopulmonary exercise testing is performed routinely for diagnostic, therapeutic, and research purposes in HIV-positive individuals. A uniform and systematic output of the enormous amount of data obtained during exercise testing is important to prevent missing or misinterpreting diagnostic information. A nine-panel output montage (see Figure 30.4) is helpful to rigorously evaluate the results of progressively increasing work rate (usually cycle ergometer) CPET testing (16).

The exercise responses in the normal subject shown in Figure 30.4 (non–HIV-positive subject with normal oxygen uptake, **lactic acidosis threshold**, ventilatory mechanics, gas exchange, and peripheral oxygen delivery) is compared in the following sections with the responses observed in HIV-positive individuals to identify the important clinical implications of CPET tests results (see also Table 30.4).

Cardiovascular Variables

Figure 30.4 represents the response to progressively increasing work ("ramp") cycle ergometer exercise in a normal subject. **The maximal oxygen uptake** ($\dot{V}O_{2max}$) and work rate are consistent with predicted values (16) (see Figure 30.4, panel 3). Oxygen uptake is an important cardiac variable because it is related to cardiac output (C.O.) and arteriovenous oxygen content ($C_{(a-v)}O_2$) by the following equation:

Equation 30.1:
$$\dot{V}O_2 = C.O. \times C_{(a-v)}O_2$$
where C.O. = heart rate (HR) × stroke volume (SV)
Content (C) = oxygen saturation × concentration of hemoglobin (Hg) × 1.34

Therefore, progressive increases in $\dot{V}O_2$ during exercise reflect the product of changes in cardiac output and arterial mixed venous oxygen content difference. In fact, it has been

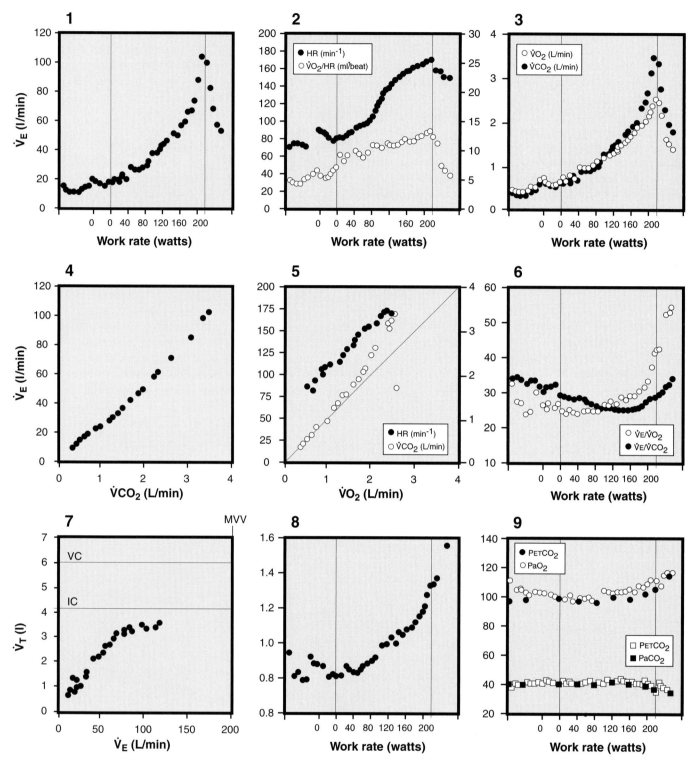

FIGURE 30.4. Cardiopulmonary exercise testing data from a normal subject. *Panel 1:* Ventilation ($\dot{V}_E$) as a function of work rate. *Panel 2:* Heart rate (HR) and O_2 pulse ($\dot{V}O_2$/HR) as a function of work rate. *Panel 3:* Oxygen uptake ($\dot{V}O_2$) and carbon dioxide output ($\dot{V}CO_2$) as a function of work rate. *Panel 4:* $\dot{V}_E$ as a function of $\dot{V}CO_2$. *Panel 5:* $\dot{V}CO_2$ and HR as a function of $\dot{V}O_2$. *Panel 6:* Ventilatory equivalents for oxygen ($\dot{V}_E$/$\dot{V}O_2$) and carbon dioxide ($\dot{V}CO_2$) as a function of work rate. *Panel 7:* Tidal volume (V_T) as a function of $\dot{V}_E$. *Panel 8:* R ($\dot{V}CO_2$/$\dot{V}O_2$) as a function of work rate. *Panel 9:* End-tidal partial pressure values for oxygen ($P_{ET}O_2$) and carbon dioxide ($P_{ET}CO_2$) (both open symbols), and arterial PO_2 and PCO_2 as a function of work intensity (both closed symbols). All panels display the physiologic variables during rest, unloaded cycling, exercise, and early recovery. (Panel 5 does not display recovery data.) (Reprinted with permission from Wasserman K, Hansen JE, Sue DY, et al. Principles of Exercise Testing and Interpretation: Pathophysiology and Clinical Applications. Baltimore: Lippincott Williams & Wilkins, 1999.)

shown that the A-V oxygen content in subjects with heart failure and normal subjects is quite similar, allowing estimation of cardiac output during exercise in these groups (18). Finally in panel 3, the slope of the relationship of oxygen uptake to work rate ($\dot{V}o_2$/WR) is normal (approximately 10 mL/min/watt, *solid line*).

The lactic acidosis threshold (LAT), another important cardiovascular variable during exercise, is defined as the oxygen uptake where net lactate accumulation occurs. The lactic acid produced as work rate increases is immediately buffered by bicarbonate (HCO$_3$-), creating excess CO_2— that is, above and beyond the aerobic production of CO_2—during exercise. Therefore plotting $\dot{V}CO_2$ as a function of $\dot{V}o_2$ on equally sized and scaled axes (Figure 30.4, panel 5) and noting where $\dot{V}CO_2$ begins to increase out of proportion to $\dot{V}o_2$ (the "V slope" method [19]) allows rapid identification of the LAT. The LAT value in this particular case is approximately 1.2 L/min, and is normal. Ventilatory equivalents for oxygen ($\dot{V}_E/\dot{V}o_2$) and ($\dot{V}_E/\dot{V}CO_2$) (Figure 30.4, panel 6) reflect the amount of ventilation required to exchange 1 liter of oxygen (or carbon dioxide) and thus reflect the efficiency of pulmonary gas exchange. These values have a U-shaped appearance during exercise, and generally fall to 28 (or below) at the LAT in healthy subjects. A second method of obtaining the gas exchange anaerobic threshold involves determining the WR at which the ventilatory equivalent for oxygen ($\dot{V}_E/\dot{V}o_2$) begins to increase (Figure 30.4, panel 6) while the ventilatory equivalent for carbon dioxide ($\dot{V}_E/\dot{V}CO_2$) remains stable. End-tidal oxygen (P_{ETo_2}) and carbon dioxide (P_{ETco_2}) are displayed in Figure 30.4, panel 9. The gas exchange anaerobic threshold can be confirmed subsequently by observing an increase in P_{ETo_2} and subsequent decrease in P_{ETco_2} as a function of work rate in Figure 30.4, panel 9. The $\dot{V}o_2$ at this work rate is an independent confirmation of the LAT obtained from the V-slope method shown in Figure 30.4, panel 6.

The final cardiovascular variables, heart rate (HR) and O_2 pulse, are displayed in Figure 30.4, panels 2 and 5. The exercise heart rate response is an important noninvasive marker of exercise training ranges, which is useful for the exercise training prescription. The oxygen pulse (oxygen uptake divided by heart rate, or $\dot{V}o_2$/HR in mL of oxygen per beat) estimates the amount of oxygen in each stroke volume. Dividing both sides of Equation 30.1 by heart rate:

Equation 30.2:

$$\frac{\dot{V}o_2/HR = [C.O. \times C_{(a-v)}O_2]/HR}{\text{since CO/HR = SV}}$$

Equation 30.3:

$$\text{Oxygen pulse } (\dot{V}o_2/\,HR) = SV \times C_{(a-v)}O_2$$

Therefore, we can evaluate the product of stroke volume (SV) and arterial–mixed venous oxygen content difference continuously during exercise by assessing the oxygen pulse.

Ventilation Variables

Figure 30.4, panel 1 displays the minute ventilation ($\dot{V}_E$) as a function of work rate. The relation of ventilation to **carbon dioxide output** ($\dot{V}CO_2$) is displayed in Figure 30.4, panel 4. The slope of this relation changes (steepens) at the respiratory compensation point (approximately 2.3 L/min) representing the point at which $\dot{V}_E$ responds to the H$^+$ ion stimulus (lactic acid) of carotid body.

The ratio $\dot{V}CO_2/\,\dot{V}o_2$, or the **respiratory exchange ratio** (RER) is graphed as a function of work rate in panel 8. This value is approximately 0.8 in resting subjects and increases to well above 1.0 at the end of a maximal exercise test. This is another marker that can be used to determine if the LAT has been reached; however, the LAT occurs prior to reaching an R value of 1.0 (the additional CO_2 output needed to drive the R value up is supplied by bicarbonate buffering of lactic acid). As mentioned above in the cardiac section, the ventilatory equivalents for oxygen ($\dot{V}_E/\dot{V}o_2$) and ($\dot{V}_E/\dot{V}CO_2$) (panel 6) reflect the amount of ventilation required to exchange 1 liter of oxygen (or CO_2). They can be envisioned as an efficiency marker for pulmonary gas exchange, and elevations in these values (>28 at the LAT) can indicate subtle abnormalities (high ventilation-to-perfusion ratio units reflecting increases in dead space ventilation, V_d/V_t) as can be seen with early pulmonary infections in HIV. Caution is advised, however, because hyperventilation due to anxiety (e.g., lack of familiarity with the laboratory environment) also can elevate the ventilatory equivalents and R. One indication of hyperventilation is a very low end-tidal PCO_2 at rest or during exercise with an elevated R value.

The final respiratory variables are tidal volume (V_T) and respiratory rate (RR) as a function of the increased minute ventilation. These variables demonstrate the mechanical characteristics of the respiratory pump during exercise. This plot can be used to discover ventilatory limitations to exercise stemming from an obstructive defect (e.g., low breathing reserve and normal—or slightly reduced—V_T with a low RR) or a restrictive ventilatory defect (e.g., V_T approaches the inspiratory capacity [IC], low V_T with increased RR). In addition, resting pulmonary function testing done before exercise testing can identify abnormalities of respiratory mechanics as well as a reduced gas transfer (diffusing capacity for carbon monoxide [DLCO]).

Moving from the normal CPET, we can now describe the responses that may be obtained during CPET testing in HIV-positive individuals. Several mechanisms may be responsible for the exercise limitation observed in HIV-positive individuals, including cardiac, ventilatory, pulmonary vascular, anemia, peripheral muscle, deconditioning, carboxyhemoglobin (smoking), decreased motivation, and combination defects. The manifestations of these abnormalities on the 9-panel plot for CPET testing are described in the following sections.

Cardiac Limitation in HIV

Several studies have observed a reduction in LAT and $\dot{V}O_{2max}$ during CPET in HIV-positive individuals (20–23) (Table 30.5). Johnson (20) studied 32 subjects who were HIV-positive and compared them to other active military duty service members. He found a small, but not statistically significant, decrease in $\dot{V}O_{2max}$ (2.61 ± 0.58 vs 2.84 ± 0.58 l/min), and a statistically significantly lower LAT (1.44 ± 0.40 l/min or 49.2 ± 13.0% of $\dot{V}O_{2max}$ vs 1.83 ± 0.34 l/min or 61.9 ± 9.1% of $\dot{V}O_{2max}$). Despite the fact that these were active duty service members, nine of the 32 (28%) subjects in the HIV-positive group had a LAT below 43% of their predicted $\dot{V}O_{2max}$. In this group, the measured $\dot{V}O_{2max}$ was only 69.9% ± 11.2% of predicted. Pothoff (22) also reported reductions in $\dot{V}O_{2max}$ (averaging 65% of predicted) and LAT (ranging from 34% to 42% of predicted $\dot{V}O_{2max}$). Stringer (23) reported a reduction in $\dot{V}O_{2max}$ (averaging 85% of predicted) with LAT (averaging 54% of predicted $\dot{V}O_{2max}$). Perna (21) reported a reduction in $\dot{V}O_{2max}$ averaging 85% of predicted. Smith (28) found a low normal baseline $\dot{V}O_{2max}$ (34.9 ml/kg/min) that did not increase at the end of the training intervention (although treadmill time did increase 11%). These studies suggest that a cardiac limitation may have been present; however, studies of vigorous aerobic training in HIV-positive individuals (21, 23, 25) over 6- to 12-week periods, involving bicycle or treadmill exercise (work rate ranges of 60% to 80% $\dot{V}O_{2max}$) with training sessions lasting about 1 hour, three times per week (see Table 30.5) have shown that the $\dot{V}O_{2max}$ and LAT can be restored to normal values. This suggests that the majority of the initial exercise limitations are related to deconditioning. All of these studies were completed prior to aggressive antiretroviral therapy with HAART, however. In conclusion, although a cardiovascular limitation to exercise appears to be present in untrained subjects, an **aerobic exercise training** program can return the cardiovascular variables to normal ranges within 6 to 12 weeks.

Ventilatory Limitation in Patients With HIV

What manifestations should we expect on the CPET test if the patient has a ventilatory limitation to exercise? Certain infectious diseases that might occur more often in HIV-positive individuals, e.g. early Pneumocystis pneumonia, could result in a restrictive ventilatory defect (rapid respiratory rate [RR] at peak exercise [>50], and a V_T that approaches the IC). Also, resting pulmonary function tests might show mild restriction with a decreased gas transfer. Pothoff (22) and Johnson (20) performed pulmonary function tests before exercise testing in their HIV-positive subjects. They found no systematic abnormality in the resting pulmonary function tests (FEV$_1$ and FVC were 95% to 100% of predicted), but Pothoff did observe a slight reduction in gas transfer (KCO) (69.1% ± 14.5 vs. 88.9% ± 14.7 of predicted).

This patient with severe interstitial lung disease displays a very rapid respiratory rate at end exercise, and the V_T approaches the IC. The tidal volume is reduced, and the end-exercise $\dot{V}_E$ is near the maximal voluntary ventilation (MVV) measured prior to exercise (Figure 30.5).

Johnson and coworkers (20) observed no restrictive ventilatory pattern during exercise in HIV-positive individuals. They found that although the peak exercise ventilation was statistically significantly lower in the HIV-positive individuals (101 ± 28 vs. 117 ± 24 L/min), the respiratory rates at peak exercise were identical (38.7 ± 6.6 vs. 40.9 ± 7.7 l/min). There was no specific evidence for a restrictive ventilatory pattern in HIV-positive individuals. In addition, no evidence of desaturation on pulse oximeter was observed. In both of these groups of HIV-positive patients, the immune status and asymptomatic nature (i.e., no acute respiratory symptoms) would make it less likely that changes would be observed on CPET. However, the CPET remains an important screening test for subtle ventilatory changes, which may suggest early stages of infectious diseases.

Pulmonary Vascular Limitation in HIV

Evidence of pulmonary vascular disease can be inferred on CPET when changes consistent with a cardiovascular limitation (e.g., reduced $\dot{V}O_2$/WR, O_2 pulse, LAT, and $\dot{V}O_{2max}$) are coupled with elevated ventilatory equivalents for carbon dioxide ($\dot{V}_E$/$\dot{V}CO_2$) at the LAT. The elevated $\dot{V}_E$/$\dot{V}CO_2$ suggests abnormalities of ventilation/perfusion matching (V_A/Q). As shown in Figure 30.6, the $\dot{V}_E$/$\dot{V}CO_2$ is elevated at rest and throughout exercise.

Coupled with the cardiovascular abnormalities noted above, this finding would be very suggestive of pulmonary vascular disease. One important variable to examine is the end-tidal values for carbon dioxide ($P_{ET}CO_2$) during the early phases of exercise, because reduction in this value would indicate either acute (R > 1) or chronic (R < normal) hyperventilation.

If the $P_{ET}CO_2$ is abnormal at rest (reduced) then the measured ventilatory equivalents may be artificially elevated by hyperventilation. This situation, then, does not necessarily indicate a primary abnormality of ventilation/perfusion matching (V_A/Q). However, an elevated ventilatory equivalent in the face of normal $P_{ET}CO_2$ values, generally suggests an abnormality of V_d/V_t such as can be seen in early pulmonary disease. If the question still persists regarding the presence of abnormal ventilation/perfusion matching (V_A/Q), an arterial blood gas obtained during exercise (and a calculation of V_d/V_t) is the most effective way to rule out hyperventilation vs. early pulmonary vascular disease. Finally, Stringer and coworkers (23) evaluated the ventilatory equivalents in 34 asymptomatic HIV-positive patients and found no evidence for elevated $\dot{V}_E$/$\dot{V}CO_2$ (unpublished data).

TABLE 30.5. STUDIES OF AEROBIC EXERCISE IN HIV-POSITIVE INDIVIDUALS

Study	No. Subjects/ Gender Distribution/ Ethnicity (When Reported)	HIV Stage/ HIV Therapy	Type of Exercise	Baseline $\dot{V}O_{2max}$/LAT Drop-Out Rate	Smoking and Anemia	Training Duration	Immunology Outcome/ Weight Change	Quality of Life Outcome
Johnson et al., 1990 (20)	32 subjects 32 male, 0 female	Walter Reed Class I–V (1 Patient on Zidovudine)	Cycle ergometry	$\dot{V}O_{2max} \downarrow$ (~70% of predicted), LAT ↓ (~32% of $\dot{V}O_{2max}$)	19 (59.3%) subjects were smokers; 2 subjects (6%) were anemic	No training intervention	NA	NA
Rigsby et al., 1992 (24)	19 subjects 19 male, 0 female	Mean Walter Reed Class III Mean CD4+ 335 ± 166	Cycle ergometry/ flexibility activities/ strength training	No gas exchange Drop-out rate: 68%	NA	12 weeks 11% decrease in heart rate with training; strength improved	Mean CD4+ from 335 ± 166 to 393 ± 221	NA
MacArthur et al., 1993 (25)	25 subjects 24 male, 1 female	Mean CD4+ (6 who completed study) 209 ± 115	Treadmill	$\dot{V}O_{2max} \downarrow$ (~80% of predicted) Drop-out rate: 76%	No data presented	24 weeks of low- and high-intensity training 24% increase in $\dot{V}O_{2max}$ O_2 pulse increased 20%, both essentially normal at the end of the study	No change in CD4+ counts pre- or post-exercise training	Improved anxiety and depression scores with training
Pothoff et al., 1994 (22)	20 subjects 18 female, 2 male ⊗	Group I (WR IV-V) Group II H/O PCP (~one half of subjects on Zidovudine)	Cycle ergometry	$\dot{V}O_{2max} \downarrow$ ~65% of predicted), LAT → (~30% of $\dot{V}O_{2max}$)	Number of smokers not listed Groups I, II, and III were anemic: 13.5 ± 1.3, 12.4 ± 1.5, and 12.6 ± 2.1, respectively	No training intervention	NA	NA
Stringer et al., 1998 (23)	26 subjects 24 male, 2 female 29% Hispanic, 20% African-American	CD4 counts: Mean 266 ± 128 HIV PCR: range 11,706 to 56,101 copies/ml All subjects on zidovudine or zidovudine plus didanosine	Cycle ergometry	$\dot{V}O_{2max} \downarrow$ (~85% of predicted), LAT → (~54% of $\dot{V}O_{2max}$) Drop-out rate 23%	27% smokers No anemia noted	6 weeks moderate and heavy-intensity training vs. non-exercising control Training improved LAT (both groups) and $\dot{V}O_{2max}$ (heavy group).	No change in CD4 or HIV PCR. Improvement in skin test reactivity (Candida), small weight increase (about 1 kg)	Significant improvement in quality-of-life markers relative to non-exercising HIV-positive control group
Perna et al., 1999 (21)	28 subjects 18 male, 10 female 17% Hispanic, 47% African-American	CD4 counts: mean 472 ± 150 No protease inhibitors	Cycle ergometry Weight Increase	$\dot{V}O_{2max} \downarrow$ (~62% of predicted), no LAT reported Drop-out rate: ~33%	9 (32%) smokers No anemia noted.	12 weeks heavy-intensity training (60% to 80% $\dot{V}O_{2max}$) $\dot{V}O_{2max}$ increased 14%	CD4 count up 13%. No HIV PCR	NA
Terry et al., 1999 (26)	21 subjects 14 male, 7 female 100% Hispanic	CD4 counts: mean 592 ± 245 No protease inhibitors	Walking treadmill	No gas exchange Drop-out rate: ~23%	No data on smoking presented Subjects were mildly anemic (hemoglobin of 8.1 to 8.3 ± 1.2)	12 weeks moderate and high-intensity training	CD4 counts up 13% No HIV PCR Weight up 1.4 kg, body fat down 2%	NA

(continued)

TABLE 30.5. STUDIES OF AEROBIC EXERCISE IN HIV-POSITIVE INDIVIDUALS

Study	No. Subjects/ Gender Distribution/ Ethnicity (When Reported)	HIV Stage/ HIV Therapy	Type of Exercise	Baseline $\dot{V}o_{2max}$/LAT Drop-Out Rate	Smoking and Anemia	Training Duration	Immunology Outcome/ Weight Change	Quality of Life Outcome
Roubenoff et al., 1999 (27)	25 subjects 21 male, 4 female 26% African-American, 60% Caucasian, 4% Native American, 0% Hispanic)	CD4 counts: mean 335 (range, 10–744) Viral loads: mean 410,000 ± 70,000 18 were taking zido-vudine, either alone, or in combination with lamivudine, or lamivudine with or without stavudine. Twelve were on pro-tease inhibitors. Two were on no antiretro-viral therapy.	15 minutes of 60-cm (vertical distance) step aerobic	No gas exchange Drop-out rate: ~ 23%	Subjects were mildly anemic (hemoglobin of 13.8 ±1.4)	NA	No change in viral load for 168 hours after the acute exercise bout	NA
Smith et al., 2001(28)	60 subjects 52 male, 8 female 26% of subjects were African-American or Hispanic—more in intervention group (n = 10) than control (n = 3)	CD4 counts: mean 328 ± 69 HIV PCR ~ 5,011 to 7,943 copies/ml[-1] Most subjects on two or fewer antiretroviral medications. Seven subjects in each group (29% of those en-rolled) were on pro-tease inhibitor therapy.	Walking—treadmill or track	Baseline $\dot{V}o_{2max}$ was ~ normal (34.9 ml/kg/min (experimental group) and 31.0 (control group) Drop-out rate: ~ 18%	29/48 or 60% No data on anemia presented.	12 weeks of 20-minute warm up (walking or jogging) followed by 30 minutes of high-intensity aerobic exer-cise training (60% to 80% of $\dot{V}o_{2max}$). No statistically significant change in $\dot{V}o_{2max}$ although treadmill time increased 1 minute (11% increase, 9.2 to 10.2 minutes).	CD4 counts: no change. HIV PCR: no change. Experimental subjects lost 1.5 kg, controls lost 0.5 kg. Triceps skinfold, sum of central skinfolds, and circumference of the abdomen all decreased.	No change in rating of perceived exertion.

[⊕ Walter Reed Classification: WRI, no signs or symptoms, CD4 count ≥ 400 mmm[-3]; WRII, adenopathy present, CD4 ≥ 400 mmm[-3]; WRIII, normal delayed hypersensitivity, CD4 ≥ 400 mmm[-3]; WRIV, partial cutaneous anergy, CD4 < 400 mmm[-3]; WRV, complete cutaneous anergy or oral thrush present, CD4 < 400 mmm[-3]; WRVI, opportunistic infection present. NA; not assessed.

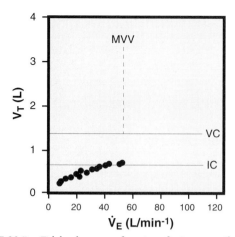

FIGURE 30.5. Tidal volume as a function of minute ventilation in a patient with restrictive (interstitial) lung disease. The V_T rapidly reaches the inspiratory capacity (IC), and further increases in minute ventilation are achieved by increases in respiratory rate (> 50 at end exercise). (Reprinted with permission from Wasserman K, Hansen JE, Sue DY, et al. Principles of Exercise Testing and Interpretation: Pathophysiology and Clinical Applications. Baltimore: Lippincott Williams & Wilkins, 1999.)

Anemia in HIV

Anemia reduces the oxygen-carrying capacity of the blood and, therefore, reduces the size of the arteriovenous content difference (equation 2 and 3). This results in reduced maximal oxygen uptake, earlier lactic acidosis threshold, and a reduced maximum oxygen pulse. Heart rate and minute ventilation (above the LAT) are generally elevated for any given work intensity; however, the gas exchange variables

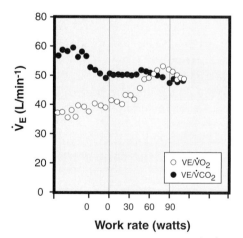

FIGURE 30.6. Ventilatory equivalents for oxygen ($\dot{V}_E/\dot{V}O_2$) and carbon dioxide ($\dot{V}_E/\dot{V}CO_2$) during exercise in the same patient shown in Figure 30.5. (Reprinted with permission from Wasserman K, Hansen JE, Sue DY, et al. Principles of Exercise Testing and Interpretation: Pathophysiology and Clinical Applications. Baltimore: Lippincott Williams & Wilkins, 1999; Case 51A.). Both ventilatory equivalents are elevated at rest >35, and remain elevated during exercise indicating ventilation perfusion inequality (V_A/Q) and wasted ventilation (elevated dead space to tidal volume ratio (V_D/V_T). End-tidal CO_2 values were not elevated. Coupled with a low $>\dot{V}O_2/WR$, O_2 pulse, LAT, and $\dot{V}O_{2max}$, it is most likely related to pulmonary vascular disease.

below the LAT (ventilatory equivalents, end-tidal oxygen and carbon dioxide, and V_d/V_t) are all normal.

The most striking study regarding anemia in the HIV-positive group was that reported by Pothoff and coworkers (22), where the HIV-positive group had a hemoglobin of 13.5 ± 1.3 g/dl, compared to 15.3 ± 0.8 g/dl in the control group. This difference alone could account for a 12% reduction in maximal oxygen uptake, a low oxygen pulse, and earlier lactic acidosis thresholds in the HIV-positive individuals. Johnson and coworkers (20) found that five of the nine subjects with markedly reduced lactic acidosis thresholds were anemic (hematocrit $< 45\%$). A more recent study by Roubenoff and coworkers (27) again revealed moderate anemia (hemoglobin was 13.8 ± 1.4 g/dl). Because anemia may be a primary manifestation of HIV infection, or a side effect of current antiretroviral and prophylactic therapy, anemia must remain an important consideration in the exercise limitation observed in this patient population.

Carboxyhemoglobin (Smoking) in HIV

Carboxyhemoglobin elevations reduce the oxygen-carrying capacity of the blood (each 1% increase in carboxyhemoglobin level reduces the oxygen carrying capacity by 1%), thus the size of the arterial–venous content difference in equations 2 and 3. In addition, and perhaps as important for oxygen delivery to the tissue, when bound to hemoglobin carbon monoxide shifts the oxyhemoglobin dissociation curve to the left. This decreases the amount of oxygen unloaded at any given PO_2 in the tissue capillaries. Both of these effects reduce the maximal oxygen uptake and lactic acidosis threshold (29), and increase the ventilation and heart rate for any given exercise intensity (above the LAT). Indeed, 59% of the HIV-positive individuals in the study by Johnson and coworkers (20) were current smokers, and eight of the nine subjects (88%) with the most markedly reduced LATs were smokers. The studies by Stringer and coworkers (23) and Perna and coworkers (21) involved 27% and 32% smokers, respectively, and the study by Smith and coworkers (28) included 60% smokers! Because smoking is a potentially modifiable form of exercise limitation, separate from other HIV mechanisms, smoking cessation should be strongly encouraged in this group. Research studies should be performed without smoking for more than12 hours, or carboxyhemoglobin values should be obtained.

Peripheral Muscle Abnormalities in HIV

Abnormalities of cytoplasmic (e.g., glucose metabolism, redox state, tricarboxylic acid cycle) or mitochondrial (e.g., oxidative phosphorylation) function related to HIV infection or HIV therapy (e.g., HAART) would be expected to affect high-energy phosphate (ATP) production in the exercising muscle cell. Several agents have been shown to induce a mitochondrial myopathy and adversely affect cellular bioenergetics, including the nucleoside reverse transcriptase inhibitors (NRTIs), such as zidovudine (30–32), didanosine, zidovudine, fialuridine (33), stavudine, and zalcitabine. Abnormalities associated with NRTI appear to involve differential inhibition of mitochondrial gamma-DNA polymerase, thereby impairing mitochondrial DNA replication and reducing mitochondrial DNA (mDNA) content. This results in a reduction in mitochondrial synthesis of the proteins involved in oxidative phosphorylation and reduced ability to generate ATP.

Despite this argument, the majority of the patients studied with CPET testing after aerobic exercise training reveal very little residual abnormality of work capacity, $\Delta\dot{V}$ O_2/Δwork rate, RER, or maximal oxygen uptake. If a significant abnormality of muscle cell or mitochondria existed with these medications, persistent deficits in these variables would be observed, however, the majority of these studies were performed prior to the widespread use of HAART.

Finally, severe resting lactic acidosis can be induced by HIV or T-cell-mediated inflammatory myopathies (34), regardless of the stage or control of the HIV infection (31).

Deconditioning in HIV

Deconditioning is present in a number of disease processes as well as with physically inactive individuals. This is generally manifested on CPET tests as low LAT, $\dot{V}O_{2max}$, low O_2 pulse, and high heart rates at any given work rate. High lactate values are observed at low exercise intensities, resulting in additional ventilation and the sensation of dyspnea. This might suggest a cardiovascular limitation to exercise; however, additional testing after a 6- to 12–week aerobic exercise training program reveals partial (or complete) resolution of these observed changes (21, 23, 25). Deconditioning also can be confirmed by comparing the current aerobic exercise regimen to 1 year and 5 years previously.

Decreased Motivation in Chronic Diseases

Patients with chronic diseases such as HIV sometimes have decreased motivation to perform regular aerobic exercise. This can be related to illness, musculoskeletal pain, or coexistent depression. This lack of activity results in a vicious cycle of decreased exercise, pain, slow recovery from activity, loss of lean body mass, anxiety about exercise, deconditioning, and reduced gain from aerobic exercise sessions. During testing, if a patient is not sufficiently motivated to perform a maximal effort exercise test, the $\dot{V}O_{2max}$ may be artificially reduced (the LAT, however, which is observed at a submaximal work rate, may still be available and provide useful information).

The CPET manifestations of decreased motivation are large breathing and heart rate reserves, failure to reach LAT, and normal values for cardiac and ventilatory variables just before exercise cessation. Proper coaching of the patient with vigorous encouragement during the CPET test may appreciably improve patient effort.

Combination Defects in HIV

Any combination of the previously mentioned defects may result in exercise limitation on CPET testing. This makes the methodical review of all the cardiac, ventilatory, peripheral vascular, pulmonary vascular, and motivational variables during the exercise test even more important. For instance, in the study by Johnson and coworkers (20) the nine patients with the lowest LAT values were those who had either anemia, carboxyhemoglobin (current smokers), or deconditioning (no regular aerobic training program), all of which might have contributed to exercise limitation. Finally, the various medications used for HIV treatment (HAART therapy) may have variable effects on exercise tolerance and motivation.

Exercise in HIV-Positive Individuals

Review of Prior Studies of HIV and Exercise

A number of studies have examined the effects on HIV-positive individuals of exercise and aerobic or strength (progressive resistance) training. Some of the desirable effects of these types of exercise training include the following:

- Improved aerobic capacity and functional status
- Increased strength
- Reduction in fat mass
- Improved immune function/indices
- Maintenance of (or improvement) in lean body mass or weight
- Improved mood (reduced depressive symptoms)
- Improvement in the overall quality of life.

Methods to Assess the Effectiveness of an Exercise Training Program

To determine the effectiveness of an aerobic, strength, or combined exercise program, as well as determine the beneficial effects of interventions such as aerobic exercise training, strength training, nutritional and medical therapy (e.g. HAART), or adjuvant therapies, several specialized tests are available for clinical and research purposes. These tests supplement the history and physical examination (e.g., questions and examination focused on weight loss or gain, changes in body habitus and image, dietary habits, drug regimen/schedule, functional capacity, regular exercise activity, anthropomorphic evaluation, fasting lipid abnormalities) and assist with documentation and quantification of the current physiologic, anatomic, and nutritional status. These tests include the following:

- **Dual energy x-ray absorptiometry** (DEXA) scanning (35–40) is used to evaluate changes in body composition (e.g., muscle, fat, bone) using the differential absorption of two different electron energy sources by tissues of different density .
- **Bioelectrical impedance** (BIA) (39, 41) is used to assess fat-free mass (FFM) and fat mass (i.e., it is a two-compartment model). The test measures electrical conductivity through ionic charged liquid media. When validated against established measures of body composition, differential equations can be generated to estimate body cell mass or FFM, indirect measures of muscle and other components of lean tissue. Fat is derived by subtracting FFM from total weight, but BIA has not been validated to assess changes in body fat in persons with HIV.
- **Computed tomography (CT)** or **magnetic resonance imaging (MRI)** scanning (35, 39, 42) (although expensive are perhaps the most anatomically precise of the readily available clinical methods to determine body composition, allowing quantification of fat, muscle, and bone as well as the amount of visceral and regional fat accumulation (or loss).
- Anthropomorphics is used to assess various body measurements, including weight, skinfold thickness, girth, and other measurements of various areas of the body (e.g. thigh, arm, chest, abdomen).
- Cardiopulmonary exercise testing (CPET) (16, 20–23, 25, 26, 28) (see Table 30.5) is an integrative physiologic test that measures oxygen uptake, lactic acidosis threshold, ventilation, heart rate, cardiac effects (via 12-lead ECG), and oxygen saturation continuously during exercise. It can be used to evaluate exercise limitation in HIV-positive individuals (44), as well as document the effects of an aerobic exercise training program, medical intervention, or other adjunctive therapy on the entire individual from the respiratory and cardiovascular system to the muscle mitochondria.
- **Strength testing** (Table 30.6) (35, 38, 39, 42) evaluation can be an effort-dependent (maximal voluntary muscle strength) or effort-independent test (amount of electromyographic signal at a specific work intensity). It is used as an objective evaluation of the effects of a **progressive resistance training** program.

These tests can be used individually or in combination to document the current status of the HIV-positive individual and his or her response to medical and adjuvant therapies.

Aerobic Exercise and Training in HIV-Positive Patients

Studies dating back into the early years of the HIV epidemic have evaluated whether the patient can achieve benefits with aerobic exercise training. Nine studies (20–28) contribute significant information to the HIV aerobic exercise literature (see Table 30.5). The characteristics of patients entered into these studies were quite variable. Although all were HIV-positive, they varied dramatically in their immune dysfunction, ranging from asymptomatic to recovering from an AIDS-defining diagnosis (although most participants in the trials listed did not have AIDS, or an AIDS-defining diagnosis). Weight loss greater than 10% of body mass was uncommon. The ethnic and gender makeup of these studies has gradually changed, reflecting the change in demographics of the epidemic in industrialized countries, from the earlier studies which included primarily homosexual Caucasian men to the more recent studies with greater diversity in ethnic background, gender, and mechanism of transmission (e.g., heterosexual, intravenous drug use). Even with these changes, most of the patients examined were still men (considerably more women are included in later studies). The entry CD4+ T cell counts of the HIV-positive individuals also were quite variable, ranging from 209 ± 115 to 592 ± 245. Finally, markers of aerobic function (e.g., maximal oxygen uptake [$\dot{V}O_{2max}$], anaerobic threshold [AT]) (where measured) were slightly decreased at study entry—the $\dot{V}O_{2max}$ averaged between 66% (20) and 85% (23) of predicted, and the LAT was on average 54% of $\dot{V}O_{2max}$ (24), suggesting a mild cardiovascular limitation or deconditioning (44).

The primary aerobic exercise intervention was cycle ergometry. However, two studies used the treadmill (25, 26), one study had no exercise intervention (20), and one study only followed subjects for 168 hours (7 days) after exposure to heavy exercise to evaluate the acute effect of heavy exercise on viral load (27). The usual aerobic exercise protocol duration in most of these studies was between 6 and 12 weeks, although the study with the highest dropout rate (76%) lasted 24 weeks (25). Dropout rates in the other studies averaged 30%, with dropout rates in three studies as low as 185 to 23% (23, 26, 28). Some of these studies used a mixture of stretching and aerobic exercise; one added strength training as well (24). (See also the section Strength Training and Table 30.6). Exercise sessions usually lasted for 1 hour, were supervised, and were conducted three times per week.

Three studies attempted to determine the effect of aerobic exercise at two different exercise intensities (25). The subjects in these groups received either moderate- (exercise intensity below the LAT) or high (exercise intensity above the anaerobic threshold) intensity exercise (23, 26) and the observed changes in aerobic parameters, immune indices, and quality of life/depression scores were recorded. All three of these studies found more marked im-

TABLE 30.6. STUDIES OF STRENGTH AND RESISTIVE EXERCISE TRAINING IN HIV-POSITIVE INDIVIDUALS

Study	No. Subjects/ Gender Distribution/ Ethnicity (When Reported)	HIV Stage/ HIV Therapy/ Androgenic Therapy	Type of Strength Exercise Training/ % Compliance	Baseline Strength Measurements (Arm/Leg), Anthropometrics Weight	Smoking and Anemia	Training Duration, Mechanism of Assessment, and Training Results	Immunology Outcome/Weight Change
Spence et al., 1990 (43)	24 subjects 24 male, 0 female 12 control and 12 intervention. No data on ethnicity. Drop-out rate: 0%	Outpatients who were S/P PCP (at least 2 weeks), therefore, presume CD4+ counts < 200 All on zidovudine therapy No androgenic therapy	Supervised progressive resistance exercise (PRE) ~100% compliance	OmniTron computerized hydraulic resistance testing machine measuring torque, maximum power, and total work. Body weight, girth (arm and thigh), and skinfold thickness at 6 weeks.	No data	PRE three times per week for 6 weeks. Prior to PRE, subjects performed stretching exercises and a 5 minute warm-up on a leg-crank ergometer at low power output. Both leg and arm torque (force), maximum power, and total work increased (10–56% increase, mean 26%). The sum of skinfolds (mm) increased 8%, and girth (cm) increased 4.3%.	Weight increased 2.4% (1.7 kg)
Roubenoff et al., 1999 (38)	14 subjects 14 male, 0 female 20% African-American Drop-out rate: 28%	CD4+ counts: mean 339 (range 75–622) Outpatients: 9 of 10 on antiretroviral therapy (Indinavir (2), Saquinavir plus Ritonavir (3), Nelfinavir (4)) No androgenic therapy	Largely (2 of 3 sessions) unsupervised health club setting 77% compliance with training.	One repetition max (1 RM) strength testing. Percentage of body fat and lean body mass measured by DEXA scanning (initial and at 16 weeks). Total cholesterol and triclyceride levels determined pre- and post-intervention.	No data	Three times per week for 16 weeks: 20 min aerobic exercise (treadmill or stationary bike) followed by 1 hour high-intensity resistance training (legs, back, arms). On 1 RM strength testing, the group improved on both leg and arm strength: 5% to 19% increase (mean 14%).	Weight increased 1.9% (1.1 kg). Overall body fat decreased 1.9% (20.4 to 18.3%), and trunk fat decreased (54.1 to 52.2%) of total body fat.
Strawford et al., 1999 (45)	24 subjects 24 male, 0 female 100% Caucasian Drop-out rate: 8.3%	CD4+ counts: mean, 234 to 337 Viral loads ranged from 7,943 to 79,432 copies /ml Outpatients: 76% on antiretroviral therapy (54% on HAART). All with 10% weight loss. Androgenic therapy: all received testosterone 100 mg/week and then received either placebo or oxandrolone tablets 20 mg/day.	Supervised passive resistance exercise and aerobic conditioning. No data on compliance.	1 RM strength testing established baseline and followed up postexercise training. Percentage of body fat and lean body mass measured by DEXA (initial and at 8 weeks). Total cholesterol, HDL, and nitrogen balance, were also determined pre- and post-intervention.	No data	Three times per week (1 hour) for 8 weeks: mixture of upper and lower body exercise. The intervention (supraphysiologic doses of oxandrolone) relative to placebo increased arm and leg strength by over 100% compared to nontraining. All subjects increased nitrogen retention.	Weight increased ~ 3% (2.5 kg on oxandrolone). Total cholesterol did not change; HDL decreased in response to oxandrolone therapy compared to placebo.

Study	Subjects	Patient characteristics	Intervention	Outcome measures		Training protocol	Results
Grinspoon et al, 200 (46)	54 subjects 54 male, 0 female 100% Caucasian Drop-out rate: 13%	CD4+ counts: Mean, 313 to 430. Viral loads ranged from 38,810 to 50,011 copies /ml. Outpatients: 76% on antiretroviral therapy (72% on HAART) All with >10% weight loss. Androgenic therapy: testosterone 200 mg/week	Supervised passive resistance exercise and aerobic conditioning. No data on compliance with training.	1 RM strength testing established baseline and followed up post-exercise training. Percent body fat and lean body mass measured by DEXA (initial and at 12 weeks). Total cholesterol, LDL, HDL, triglyceride, were also determined pre- and post-intervention.	No data	Three times per week for 12 weeks: 20 min of aerobic activity followed by 15-min cool-down period and then 2 sets of 8 repetitions per set. Increased to 3 sets by week 7. Mixture of upper and lower body exercise. The intervention (exercise) increased arm and leg cross-sectional area by over 100% compared to non-training subjects. The testosterone intervention relative to placebo increased arm and leg mass by approximately the same amount as training. There was no statistically significant increase of testosterone and exercise over either therapy alone by 23% to 28% and leg strength by 11% to 38% on 1 RM.	Weight increased about 3% (2.6 kg on testosterone without PRE). Overall lean body mass increased (4.2 kg on testosterone). Total cholesterol did not change, but LDL decreased in response to testosterone therapy compared to placebo.
Yarasheski, 2000 (40)	18 subjects 18 male, 0 female 100% Caucasian Drop-out rate: 28%	CD4+ counts: mean range 152 to 840. Viral loads ranged from 1,700 to 93,000 copies/ml (11 with viral load < 400). Outpatients: all on antiretroviral therapy (16 HAART, 2 PI-naïve). No androgenic therapy	Supervised free weights. No data on compliance with training	One repetition max (1 RM) strength testing. Percent body fat and lean body mass measured by DEXA (initial and at 16 weeks). Total cholesterol, LDL, HDL, triglyceride, insulin levels, C-peptide levels, proinsulin, and glucagon levels were also determined pre- and post-intervention.	No data	Four times per week for 16 weeks: 1.5 hour of a weight-lifting program consisting of 3 upper body and 4 lower body exercises. Initial sessions were low-intensity (50% to 65% of maximum strength) and high-repetition (10+ lifts/exercise). A personal trainer monitored the subjects' progress, and by the end of the study (week 16) the exercise intensity was 75% to 85% of final maximum voluntary muscle strength at low repetition (5–8 lifts/exercise). The intervention group increased upper body strength by 23% to 28% and leg strength by 11% to 38% on 1 RM. All of these observed improvements were smaller than in HIV-negative subjects from a prior study (those ranged from 14% to 63%).	Weight increased 1.9% (1.4 kg). Overall lean body mass increased, but fat mass did not change. Total cholesterol, LDL, HDL, insulin levels, C-peptide levels, proinsulin, and glucagon did not change, but triglyceride levels decreased (300 → 200 mg/dl).

(continued)

TABLE 30.6. STUDIES OF STRENGTH AND RESISTIVE EXERCISE TRAINING IN HIV-POSITIVE INDIVIDUALS (continued)

Study	No. Subjects/ Gender Distribution/ Ethnicity (When Reported)	HIV Stage/ HIV Therapy/ Androgenic Therapy	Type of Strength Exercise Training/ % Compliance	Baseline Strength Measurements (Arm/Leg), Anthropometrics Weight	Smoking and Anemia	Training Duration, Mechanism of Assessment, and Training Results	Immunology Outcome/Weight Change
Bhasin et al., 2000 (35)	61 subjects 61 male, 0 female Ethnicity mixed Drop-out rate: 20%	Involuntary weight loss of at least 5% in the past 6 months with a low testosterone level (<12.9 nmol/l). CD4+ counts: mean range 279 to 357. No data on viral loads. Outpatients: 82% to 100% on antiretroviral therapy, 40% to 60% on protease inhibitors. Testosterone enanthate 100 mg/week intramuscularly	Resistance exercise No data on compliance with training.	One repetition max (1 RM) strength testing. Changes in thigh muscle volume measured by MRI, and FFM by DEXA. Body weight, and health-related QOL were also determined pre- and post-intervention.	No data	Three times per week for 16 weeks (upper and lower body): For the first 4 weeks, the exercise regimen consisted of a high-volume (3 sets of 12–15 repetitions), low-intensity (60% of maximal 1 RM) resistance exercise. Weeks 5 to 10 involved 90% of 1 RM on heavy days, 80% of 1 RM on medium days, and 70% of 1 RM on light days. For weeks 11 to 16, the loads were increased by 7% for upper body and 12% for lower body work. There were four groups (1 control, 1 testosterone, 1 exercise, and 1 exercise plus testosterone). The control group did not change from baseline, the testosterone group increased strength by 16%, the exercise group increased strength by 27%, and the testosterone plus exercise group increased by 21% (leg press). Therefore, both testosterone and resistance exercise increased strength, but there was no additive effect of testosterone and exercise demonstrated.	Weight increased 2.3% to 3.7% (1.7 to 2.9 kg). Fat-free mass increased for testosterone, exercise, and exercise plus testosterone.
Sattler et al., 1999 (39)	30 subjects 30 male, 0 female 53% Hispanics, 33% Caucasians, 13% African-American Drop-out rate: 10%	Stable weight CD4+ counts: mean range of 216 to 228 cells/mm³ Undetectable viral loads in 11 on Indinavir, 2 on saquinavir, 3 on ritonavir, and 2 on nelfinavir, and 6 on saquinavir plus second protease drug. Nandrolone decanoate: first week 200 mg IM, 2nd week 400 mg IM, and weeks 3 to 12, 600 mg/week IM	Progressive resistive training (PRT) with free weights No data on compliance . with training	One repetition max (1 RM) strength testing. Changes in thigh muscle volume measured by MRI, and FFM by DEXA. Body weight, bioelectrical impedance analysis (BIA) were determined pre- and post-intervention	No anemia	Three times per week for 12 weeks (upper and lower body): After 1 warm-up set of 5 to 8 repetitions at 50% of the 1 RM max, subjects performed 3 sets of 8 repetitions at 80% of the 1 RM with the final set performed to failure. There were two groups: 1 nandrolone (n = 15) and nandrolone + progressive resistance training. Strength increased in both upper and lower body exercises (10%–31% with nandrolone, and 14%–53% with nandrolone and PRT.	Weight increased 4.3% to 5.6% (3.2–4.0 kg). Fat-free mass increased more for the progressive resistance training than the nandrolone alone group. BIA went up in both groups, and cross-sectional area by MRI went up in thigh, quads, and hamstrings.

Agin et al., 2001 (47)	30 subjects 0 male, 30 female 73% African-American, 6% Caucasian, 20% Hispanic Drop-out rate: 23%	Stable weight CD4+ counts: mean range, 215–335 cells/mm³ 44,449 to 100,343 viral copies/ml No androgenic therapy (did give whey protein)	Progressive resistive training (PRT)—free weights No data on compliance with training. No control group, but each group had a 6-week control period.	One repetition max (1 RM) strength testing. Changes in skeletal muscle and fat mass measured by total body MRI, body cell mass by total body potassium measurements, fat-free mass by DXA and MRI were determined pre/post intervention.	No data	Three times per week for 14 weeks (7 major muscle groups): subjects performed three sets of 10 exercises at 8 to 10 repetitions per ACSM guidelines. Week 1 was set at 50% of the baseline 1 RM. Thereafter, weight loads were approximately 75% 1 RM. There were three groups: protein supplementation (PRO), passive resistance (PRE), and combined (PRO + PRE). Strength increased in both PRE and PRO + PRE groups relative to PRO (40% to 96%).	Weight increased 4.4% (3.6 kg) in the PRO group, with little change in the PRE or PRO + PRE groups. Body cell mass increased in both PRE and PRO + PRE groups, and PRE increased skeletal muscle as well. Fat-free mass by DXA increased 1.4 to 1.6 kg in all three groups. QOL went up in the PRE group and worsened in the PRO group.
Roubenoff et al., 2001 (48)	25 subjects 20 male, 5 female 64% Caucasian, 36% African-American Drop-out rate: 23%	6 with AIDS wasting, 19 without. CD4+ counts: Mean range of 181 to 368 cells/mm³ 10,191 to 16,999 viral copies/ml No androgenic therapy	Progressive resistive training (PRT) with free weights No data on compliance with training. No control group, but each group had a 6-week control period.	One repetition max (1 RM) strength testing. Changes in lean body mass, bone mineral content, and fat mass were estimated using DEXA pre- and post-intervention.	No data	Three times per week for 8 weeks (upper and lower body major muscle groups): Week 1 was set at 50% of RM of their first session, week 2 at 60%, and remaining sessions (unsupervised) at 75 to 80%. Subjects performed three sets of eight repetitions on each machine. PRE increased strength (44% nonwasted and 60% wasted) and lean body mass (LBM).	Lean body mass increased 2.3% in the nonwasted and 5.3% in the wasted subjects.

provements in aerobic parameters with heavy than with moderate exercise. The observed reduction in LAT and $\dot{V}O_{2max}$ at study entry probably represented deconditioning rather than a true cardiovascular abnormality (44). Immune indices (CD4$^+$ T cell counts) were unaffected by whether the exercise training was of moderate or heavy intensity; one study (23), however, demonstrated statistically significant improvements in the size of skin tests to *Candida* antigen for moderate exercise. Viral loads were measured in three studies (23, 27, 28) and were not significantly affected by aerobic exercise training. No opportunistic infections were observed for the combined 224 participants in the exercise training studies.

In aggregate, these studies strongly support the contention that moderate to heavy aerobic exercise training (three times per week for 1 hour) is safe, both short- and long-term, in HIV-positive individuals. They also document that significant improvements in aerobic parameters can be achieved that are proportional to exercise intensity. Aerobic exercise training had no observed deleterious effects on immune indices (very little change was observed in CD4$^+$ T cell counts or viral load), and moderate-intensity exercise may actually improve skin test reactivity to *Candida* spp. These study findings support the recommendation of aerobic exercise training in HIV-positive individuals to increase aerobic performance and leave little doubt that aerobic exercise training can be recommended with confidence in HIV-positive individuals (49). Finally, several of the studies document that anxiety, depression, and quality of life scores certainly do not worsen, and may indeed improve with exercise training.

Advantages of Low- vs. High-Intensity Exercise

In reviewing all of the studies in Table 30.5 regarding aerobic exercise training at moderate or high intensity, there does not appear to be any negative effect on immune function from exercise training at either intensity. One training study (23) did show that skin test reactivity was better at moderate rather than heavy exercise training intensities; however, CD4$^+$ T cell counts and viral loads were not changed in this or other studies in Table 30.5. Roubenoff and coworkers (27) looked at the acute changes in CD4$^+$ T cells and viral loads in the 168 hours (7 days) after a bout of acute (heavy or intensive) exercise and found no statistically significant changes in these values. Finally, heavy (60% to 80% of $\dot{V}O_{2max}$) exercise training provoked a statistically significant improvement in both global parameters of exercise performance (a 23% increase in LAT and 13% increase in $\dot{V}O_{2max}$) relative to moderate exercise (below the LAT). [LAT improved (13% increase), but not $\dot{V}O_{2max}$ (2% decrease)] or the non-exercising group [LAT (4% decrease), $\dot{V}O_{2max}$ (7% decrease)], the *maximal*

aerobic benefits of aerobic exercise training are obtained with heavy exercise.

Strength Training

Table 30.6 summarizes the studies currently available on strength and progressive resistive exercise (PRE) training in HIV-positive individuals. Although the PRE protocols varied, most consisted of three 1-hour sessions per week. One repetition max (1 RM) values were determined at the start of the program, and the first few sessions were performed at 50%, advancing to 75% of 1 RM by the second week. Subsequent training was three sets of 8 to 12 repetitions per session at 75% of 1 RM. With this type of protocol, PRE has been shown to improve strength (10–60%, with higher percentages in wasted individuals) and lean body weight (1% to 4%). Interestingly, when androgenic therapy (e.g., testosterone, nandrolone, oxandrolone) is added to PRE, there are not significant improvements in strength over PRE alone, although weight and fat free mass did increase (35, 39) (see Table 30.6). The combination of strength and aerobic exercise training has not been studied in large trials, there is only limited data (24). From these studies, it appears that upper body strength is best predicted by lean body mass (measured using DEXA, MR imaging, or CT scanning), and lower body strength and performance on the 6-minute walk test were best predicted by lower extremity cross-sectional area (42). Therefore, the central and peripheral benefits of aerobic exercise training may be additive to the gains in upper body and lower body strength (and lean body mass) achieved with progressive resistance training.

Exercise Training Recommendations in HIV-Positive Individuals

There is convincing evidence from existing studies (see Table 30.5) that aerobic exercise training is safe and effective in promoting aerobic fitness, without documented detrimental effects on immune function. Most studies have been based on 6 to 12 weeks of regular cycle or treadmill exercise. The intensity has been either moderate (below the LAT) or heavy (60% to 80% of $\dot{V}O_{2max}$), with training sessions scheduled on average three times per week and lasting 1 hour each (49).

The beneficial effects of strength or PRE training also have been documented in the literature (see Table 30.6). The effects of aerobic exercise training are less dramatic and less well studied than those of strength or progressive resistance training on lean body mass. Although it seems likely that these therapies (i.e., aerobic and strength training) may be combined for optimal outcomes in HIV-positive individuals, a large trial has not yet been completed in this area.

Generating an Exercise Prescription

Exercise prescriptions for HIV-positive individuals should be generated following ACSM guidelines (50), recognizing that a large percentage of these individuals will be deconditioned and may require a more gradual and graded return to activity. Any patient over 40 years of age should have a CPET to evaluate his or her fitness for resuming exercise and to exclude flow-limiting coronary artery disease. Direct measurement of $\dot{V}O_{2max}$, LAT, heart rate, and work rate during the initial exercise test allows precise calculation of an appropriate exercise prescription. This information can then be converted to intensity—either treadmill (speed and incline) or cycle ergometer work rates (watts), with an appropriate duration (time). Finally, although a combined exercise program involving both aerobic and strength training features would appear to be desirable, the data are not adequate to make that a definitive recommendation at this time.

Anabolic Therapy Strategies in HIV-Positive Individuals

Therapies other than aerobic or strength training aimed at improving muscle mass have focused on testosterone, oxandrolone, growth hormone (GH), and insulin-like grown factor-1 (42, 45, 51–56). These studies have studied primarily patients with AIDS-associated wasting syndrome, defined as low body mass index (BMI), e.g., less than 20 kg/m², or recent weight loss of more than 10% from baseline weight). Although these studies have not applied exercise uniformly as an adjuvant to hormonal therapy, the results support administration of testosterone to both men and women suffering from HIV-associated wasting (see Table 30.6). The current recommendation is to use GH only for patients with severe AIDS-associated wasting, and other strategies (including androgens, nutritional augmentation, and intensification of HAART therapy, and exercise training (both strength and aerobic) for patients with normal or even increased body mass indexes (BMI) (57). This recommendation is related to the cost, toxicity, and variable benefit of GH to patients with normal BMIs.

More recently, GH has been used as a lipolytic agent in HIV-infected patients with lipodystrophy (58); however, GH can affect glucose metabolism adversely (i.e., it may be diabetogenic) and increase insulin resistance (especially at higher doses), so the long-term use of GH in HIV-positive individuals on HAART therapy remains controversial. Growth hormone does appear to stabilize or increase lean body mass; however, it appears to increase resting energy expenditure and lipid oxidation while decreasing protein oxidation. These effects may represent a detrimental redistribution of body energy stores (59).

Metabolic Syndromes Associated With HIV Infection and HAART Therapy

AIDS Wasting Syndrome and Sarcopenia

Several distinct syndromes are observed with HIV infection and current therapy (HAART) (60), including the loss of body mass secondary to decreased intake (reduction in calories, starvation) and reduced appetite (8, 61). AIDS wasting syndrome (AWS) is established when there is loss of greater than 10% of body weight and is case-defining for AIDS in up to 18% of HIV-positive subjects. Loss of weight due to inadequate intake of dietary calories usually occurs during serious secondary infections when appetite is impaired (62). Diarrhea and malabsorption also are common contributing factors to the AIDS wasting syndrome. Another syndrome observed with HIV infection is cachexia due to ongoing inflammation, which results in loss of lean body mass despite adequate or even increased caloric intake. This type of loss of lean body mass (especially muscle) is associated with active retroviral replication and opportunistic infections, and should therefore be mitigated by appropriate antiretroviral therapy. Muscle myopathy with muscle pain, tenderness, sarcopenia, and elevated muscle enzymes also can occur occasionally even with optimally controlled HIV infection (i.e., high CD4+ T cell counts and low HIV viral loads).

Lipodystrophies

Metabolic dysregulation (e.g., lipohypertrophy, lipoatrophy, glucose intolerance, overt diabetes mellitus, and hyperlipidemia) is very common in patients being treated with HAART therapy. The changes in fat storage and lipid metabolism and distribution probably are related to changes in adipose cell function, and have a prevalence of 2% to 84% (63). The deposition of fat known as lipohypertrophy may be observed in 1% to 56% of patients (63). Initial reports of this syndrome noted that a "buffalo hump" had formed in several males despite a lack of evidence of abnormal adrenal cortical function (e.g., Cushing syndrome) (64). Subsequent studies, however, have revealed deposition of tissue in the breasts, upper torso, and neck in both men and women. In men, lipohypertrophy with central obesity may represent an acceleration of the normal aging process, which usually results in increased waist-to-hip ratio (WHR). A significant problem is the lack of a gold standard for diagnosis based on these changes. Loss of body fat (lipoatrophy) may occur with loss of adipose tissue in the face, arms, or legs, with a prevalence of 1% to 24% (63). Moreover, lipohypertrophy and lipoatrophy may occur in the same patient.

Hyperlipidemia

Although changes in fat deposition are troublesome and usually progressive, the most important changes may be at the biochemical level (36). Carr and coworkers studied 113 HIV-positive patients receiving protease inhibitor (PI) therapy. They studied the morphologic changes just described, along with the biochemical changes in lipid, glucose, uric acid, and insulin levels. They found that increases in serum lipids—total cholesterol (TC), low-density lipoprotein cholesterol (LDL), and triglycerides (TG)—with reductions in high-density lipoprotein cholesterol (HDL) were common in subjects receiving PI therapy. The elevation in blood sugar observed with PI therapy was similar to the changes observed with type 2 diabetes mellitus: high blood sugars, high insulin levels, and insulin receptor resistance (36). Associated risk factors often seen in type 2 diabetes, including hypertension and hyperuricemia, also may be observed in these HIV-positive individuals. Control of HIV infection was excellent in this study, as evidenced by increases in CD4+ T cell counts and undetectable levels of HIV PCR RNA, suggesting that the changes in lipids were not related to poor control of HIV. Furthermore, HIV infection and PI treatment were associated with elevations in both triglycerides and cholesterol, similar to the changes observed with diabetes mellitus in non–HIV-positive individuals (59).

Syndrome X and Glucose Intolerance

In 1999 Carr and coworkers (36) found overt diabetes mellitus (defined as fasting blood glucose greater than 7.0 mmol/L [> 126 mg/dl] or a 2-hour post–glucose-tolerance test blood glucose greater than 11.1 mmol/L [>200 mg/dl]) in 7% of the subjects treated with PIs, and impaired glucose tolerance (defined as fasting blood glucose of 6.1 to 7.0 mmol/L [110–126 mg/dl] or a 2-hour post–glucose-tolerance test blood glucose of 7.8–11.1 mmol/L [140–200 mg/dl]) in a further 16%. Subjects not being treated with PIs did not have overt diabetes or glucose intolerance.

Most subjects with HAART-induced diabetes were asymptomatic and required an oral glucose tolerance test for diagnosis. In addition, the degree of insulin resistance was significantly associated with the degree of lipodystrophy: no, mild, moderate, and severe lipodystrophy were associated with increasing insulin resistance levels: 1.73, 2.25, 2.60, 3.86 mIU/mmol/L^{-2}, respectively. Table 30.7) presents the case definition proposed by Carr and coworkers (36) for PI-related lipid and glucose metabolism changes.

Therapy for the lipid and glucose changes associated with HAART therapy is focused on standard glucose control agents (e.g., sulfonamides, metformin, acarbose, repaglinide, and rosiglitazone) and cholesterol and triglyceride lipid-lowering agents (e.g., pravastatin, atorvastatin, gemfibrozil, and fenofibrate) (61).

Mitochondrial Toxicity and Lactic Acidosis

Lactic acidosis and hepatic steatosis are rare, but important, complications of antiretroviral therapy (65). Certain medications used in the treatment of HIV, especially the class of nucleoside analog reverse transcriptase inhibitors (NRTIs) (30, 66), can affect the ability of the muscle and liver cells to generate adenosine triphosphate (ATP). Medications used in treatment of HIV have the capacity to affect the ability of the cytosol (e.g., glucose metabolism, tricarboxylic acid cycle) or, more likely, mitochondria (e.g., oxidative phosphorylation) to produce energy, resulting in lactic acidosis. This disruption appears to result from a disturbance in the metabolic machinery (type B lactic acidosis) and is not associated with lack of oxygen (67). A mitochondrial myopathy has been described with long-term zidovudine therapy (31, 34). Other newer NRTI HIV medications, however, including didanosine (68), staduvine, and zalcitabine, also have been associated with this syndrome (32, 33, 69). The oxidative phosphorylation enzymes present in the mitochondria are produced from a combination of nuclear (nDNA) and mitochondrial (mtDNA) DNA (except

TABLE 30.7. CASE DEFINITION FOR PROTEASE INHIBITOR–RELATED LIPID AND GLUCOSE METABOLISM CHANGES

Physical Features	Metabolic Features	Exclusion Criteria
Clinical evidence (physical examination or patient's report) of one or more of the following since the start of PI therapy • Fat wasting of the face, arms, legs, or buttocks (possibly with prominence of leg and arm veins) • Fat accumulation in the abdomen or over the dorsocervical spine	One or more of the following since start of PI therapy • Fasting hyperlipidemia (cholesterol ≥ 212 mg/dl or triglyceride ≥ 200 mg/dL) • Fasting C-peptide > 200 pmol/l • Impaired fasting glucose (110–126 mg/dL) or diabetes mellitus (≥ 200 mg/dl) on 2-h blood glucose by oral glucose tolerance test	Patients should not have any of the following with 3 months of assessment: • AIDS-defining event or other severe clinical illness • Anabolic steroids, glucocorticosteroids, or immune modulators

From Carr et al (36).

complex II in DNA) (30). A leading hypothesis regarding HAART-induced mitochondrial toxicity, therefore, is impairment of the mtDNA polymerase-γ function, resulting in difficulty with mitochondrial DNA synthesis (70) and reduced oxidative phosphorylation function. The presentation of HAART-associated mitochondrial disorders is remarkably similar that of the inherited disorders of mitochondrial function (71–73). As with the inherited disorders, although defects in oxidative function are uniformly present in the cells, the clinical manifestations of a single biochemical defect are protean. Patients with mitochondrial disorders may present with exercise intolerance, diabetes, neuropathy, cardiomyopathy, fatigue, hearing loss, and pancreatitis (74, 75)—strikingly similar to the spectrum of side effects of HAART (30, 76, 77). Finally, just like the inherited disorders of mitochondrial function, although the defect is clearly systemic, the clinical presentation may be limited to a single organ system (30, 78).

Recognition of the clinical syndrome of hepatic steatosis and lactic acidosis may be difficult, because the symptoms usually are mild and nonspecific (e.g., nausea, vomiting, fatigue, or muscle or abdominal pain) and have a subacute presentation (e.g., symptoms present for weeks to months), and elevations of hepatic enzymes (e.g., AST, ALT) are not uniformly present. Even muscle markers of inflammation or dysfunction (e.g., creatine kinase, aldolase) may not be elevated in the clinical setting of a myopathy. The electrolytes or arterial blood gases may indicate a severe metabolic acidosis (lactic acidosis), and a serum lactate level should be obtained to document the diagnosis (>2.5 mEq/l without recent strenuous activity or other medication known to cause lactic acidosis). Liver biopsy or abdominal CT scanning may document hepatic fat deposition. Withdrawal of all medications with cautious reinstitution of HIV medications when the metabolic abnormalities have resolved (avoiding the suspected NRTI) may be effective.

Osteopenia and Osteoporosis

Finally, osteopenia and osteoporosis have been observed in female patients who have AIDS wasting syndrome. Potential contributors to osteopenia or osteoporosis in this group are reduced lean body mass (primarily muscle mass), reduction in anabolic hormones (e.g., estrogen and androgens), and medication effects (e.g., from HAART therapy) (79). Additional research is needed to determine the optimal treatment strategy.

Future Research Directions

Because many of the studies reported in this chapter were performed before HAART therapy was widely used, and the baseline viral loads (23, 27, 28, 38) were much higher than

would be desirable with currently available therapy, future research must focus on the effect of exercise in HIV-positive subjects already receiving optimal retroviral therapy (HAART). Aerobic and strength training are likely to become increasingly important in mitigating or preventing the metabolic syndromes associated with HIV infection and HAART therapy. Additional studies that combine strength and aerobic exercise training will be important to assist in generation of a rational, focused, and complete exercise prescription for this patient population.

As the extreme heterogeneity of mitochondrial toxicity related to the reverse transcriptase inhibitors becomes more widely appreciated (30), and the typical therapies for mitochondrial dysfunction are used routinely (78) (including aerobic exercise training), cardiopulmonary exercise testing (CPET) is likely to emerge as an excellent choice to assess mitochondrial function or energy synthesis impairment (assessing oxygen flow from the mouth to the mitochondria).

As HIV-positive people are living longer, we must focus our investigations on the long-term health benefits observed with sedentary and non–HIV-positive adults (80). One specific area to investigate is whether the benefits (81, 82) with regard to lipid metabolism, insulin sensitivity, weight control, and long-term coronary artery disease risk carry over to the HIV-positive population. Also, aerobic exercise may be useful for mitigating or even preventing the metabolic syndromes observed with HAART therapy (e.g., lipodystrophy, mitochondrial toxicity, glucose intolerance, or osteopenia), and studies in this area are proceeding.

Finally, additional research into vaccines (83) and other creative therapeutic strategies (e.g., the use of exercise to generate anti-HIV (anti-VIP) antibodies that might be protective for both HIV-positive and HIV-negative individuals) (84) will be important fields for further investigation.

Risk of HIV Transmission During Sporting Events

In 1995, a joint statement of the American Medical Society for Sports Medicine (AMSSM) and the American Academy of Sports Medicine (AASM) (14) addressed the issues regarding blood-borne pathogen transmission among athletes during sporting events. The statement noted: "HIV is usually transmitted through sexual contact, parenteral exposure to blood and blood components, contamination of infected blood into open wounds or mucous membranes, or perinatally from mother to fetus or infant." Because no large epidemiologic studies are available at this time and anecdotal cases have lacked sufficient documentation to be considered reliable, the risk during sports competition appears to be low, but not zero. In 1992, the National Football League estimated that the risk of HIV transmission on the field is 1 per 1 million games (34). In 1997, Feller (53) reached similar conclusions regarding the very small risk of HIV transmission during athletic events. Finally, the American Academy of Pediatrics in a consensus statement released in 1999 (17) states that "...athletes with HIV infection be permitted to participate in all competitive sports" and that "Gloves should be readily available in the event an injury occurs with bleeding that requires intervention. Disinfection of soiled surfaces with a freshly prepared 1:10 dilution of household bleach is recommended."

The joint statement from the AMSSM and AASM also states that widespread mandatory HIV testing probably is not warranted for competitive sports at this time. Voluntary testing, however, should be suggested, with counseling for those with multiple sexual partners, intravenous drug abuse, sexually transmitted diseases, blood transfusions prior to 1985, or other HIV risk factors.

What We Know
About HIV and Exercise

1 Cardiopulmonary exercise testing has a number of advantages over conventional treadmill testing in HIV-positive individuals, including risk stratification, identifying subtle pulmonary infectious complications, designing an exercise prescription, and documenting improvement with exercise training. Aerobic and strength exercise training is safe and effective in HIV-positive individuals.

2 Most patients who are HIV-positive have deconditioning as a prominent or sole mechanism of exercise limitation.

3 High-intensity aerobic exercise training appears to generate maximal improvements in conditioning, without detrimental effects on the immune system of HIV-positive individuals.

4 Anabolic strategies for HIV-positive individuals (e.g., testosterone, oxandrolone, growth hormone) in addition to exercise training should be reserved for those with significant wasting (BMI < 20 kg/m^2 or $> 10\%$ recent weight loss from baseline weight).

5 Several metabolic syndromes have been associated with highly active antiretroviral therapy (HAART), including insulin resistance, hyperlipidemia, redistribution of body fat, and mitochondrial toxicity with lactic acidosis.

6 The risk of HIV transmission during competitive sporting events is very low, but not zero.

What We Would Like to Know
About HIV and Exercise

1 Most of the studies reviewed in this chapter were performed before highly active antiretroviral therapy (HAART) was widely utilized. The effects and value of aerobic and strength exercise training should be documented in a large study involving patients who are on optimal HAART therapy.

2 Aerobic and strength exercise training may be very important for mitigating many of the metabolic syndromes associated with HIV infection and HAART therapy. These important questions remain unanswered in the current literature.

3 Will combining the two modalities of strength and aerobic exercise training improve short- and long-term outcomes in HIV-positive individuals?

4 Is cardiopulmonary exercise testing (CPET) the optimal, non-invasive examination to identify and follow mitochondrial toxicity in HAART- treated patients?

5 Because HIV-positive individuals live longer with newer therapy, will the long-term benefits of regular exercise be similar to those for non–HIV-positive adults?

6 Will vaccine development or other creative therapeutic strategies for HIV prevention be potentiated or mitigated by regular aerobic exercise?

Summary

This chapter has reviewed the general biology of HIV as well as current HIV therapies and modalities of therapeutic monitoring. The specifics of cardiopulmonary exercise testing are discussed in relation to HIV-positive individuals. The potential mechanisms of exercise limitation are identified, as are the results of current aerobic and strength exercise training studies in the literature. Recommendations for exercise training and anabolic therapy strategies for HIV-positive individuals are presented, and the metabolic syndromes associated with HIV infection and HAART therapy, as well as the possible use of exercise training to mitigate these syndromes, are discussed. Finally, the risk of transmission of HIV during competitive sporting events is reviewed.

DISCUSSION QUESTIONS

1 Name three advantages of cardiopulmonary exercise testing relative to conventional treadmill exercise testing in the HIV-positive population.

2 Name five potential mechanisms of exercise limitation in the HIV-positive population.

3 Name several anatomic or physiologic tests that can be used to assess changes in body composition in HIV-positive individuals. Discuss their relative advantages and disadvantages.

4 Design a specific exercise program (aerobic and strength training) for the patient described in the case study. ($\dot{V}O_2$max 28 ml/min, HR at the AT 124, Age 41.) Describe in detail the length and duration of sessions, specific treadmill and bicycle settings, the overall goals of training, and so forth.

CASE STUDY

Patient Information

A 41-year-old man has been HIV-positive for 39 months. He desires a nonpharmacologic method to improve his exercise tolerance, mood, strength and muscle mass, and immune system function. He also desires to lose some weight. His CD4$^+$ T cell count is 300 and his viral load is undetectable on current highly active antiretroviral therapy (HAART).

Assessments

On physical examination, his weight is 83 kg, and his body mass index (BMI) is 27. His waist-to-hip ratio (WHR) is 0.97.

A number of the HAART medications can adversely affect glucose tolerance, insulin sensitivity, and lipid profiles. Although he is young and does not have a history of diabetes in his family, this patient's fasting blood sugar and lipid panel (total cholesterol, LDL, HDL, and triglycerides) should be checked during his evaluation (85).

Questions

1. What are the risks and benefits of aerobic or strength training exercise in this patient?

2. What testing should be done before this patient begins an exercise training program to ensure safety and exclude occult cardiopulmonary diseases?

3. What exercise program would you recommend for this patient?

REFERENCES

1. Streicher HZ, Reitz MSJ, Gallo RC. Human immunodeficiency virus. In: Mandell GL, Bennett JE, Dolin R, eds. Mandell: Principles and Practice of Infectious Diseases. Kent, UK: Churchill Livingstone, 2000:1874–1885.

2. Kahn JO, Walker BD. Acute human immunodeficiency virus type I infection. N Engl J Med 1998; 339:33–39.

3. Centers for Disease Control and Prevention, Division of HIV/AIDS Prevention: http://www.cdc.gov/hiv/pubs/facts.htm.

4. Dayton JM, Merson MH. Global dimensions of the AIDS epidemic: Implications for prevention and care. Infect Dis Clin North Am 2000;14:808.

5. Vergis EN. Natural history of HIV-1 infection. Infect Dis Clin North Am 2000;14:809–825.

6. Castro KG, Ward JW, Slutsker JW, et al. 1993 revised classification system for HIV infection and expanded surveillance case definition for AIDS among adolescents and adults. MMWR 1992;41:961–962.

7. Wolfe PR. Practical approaches to HIV therapy: recommendations for the year 2000. Postgraduate Medicine 2000;107:127–136.

8. Fauci AS, Bartlett JG, Goosby EP. et al. Guidelines for the use of anti-retroviral agents in HIV-infected adults and adolescents. http://www.aidsinfo.nih.gov/ 2002;1:1–111.

9. Choi S, Lagakos SW, Schooley RT, et al. CD4+ lymphocytes are an incomplete surrogate marker for clinical progression in persons with asymptomatic HIV infection taking zidovudine. Ann Intern Med 1993;118:674–680.

10. Fei DTW, Paxton H, Chen AB. Difficulties in precise quantitation of CD4$^+$ T lymphocytes for clinical trials: a review. Biologicals 1993;21:221–231.

11. Mellors JW, Munoz A, Giorgi JV, et al. Plasma viral load and CD4+ lymphocytes as prognostic markers of HIV-1 infection. Ann Intern Med 1997;126:946–954.

12. Mulder J, McKinney N, Christopherson C, et al. Rapid and simple PCR assay for quantitation of human immunodeficiency virus type 1 RNA in plasma: application to acute retroviral infection. J Clin Microbiol 1994;32:292–300.

13. Lee TH, Sheppard HW, Reis M, et al. Circulating HIV-1 infected cell burden from seroconversion to AIDS: importance of postseroconversion viral load on disease course. J AIDS 1994;7:381–388.

14. Mellors JW, Rinaldo CR, Gupta P, et al. Prognosis in HIV infection predicted by the quantity of virus in plasma. Science 1996;272:1167–1170.

15. O'Brien WA, Hartigan PM, Martin D, et al. Changes in plasma HIV-1 RNA and CD4+ lymphocyte counts and the risk of progression to AIDS. Veterans Affairs Cooperative Study Group on AIDS. N Engl J Med 1996;334:426–431.

16. Wasserman K, Hansen JE, Sue DY, et al. Principles of Exercise Testing and Interpretation: Pathophysiology and Clinical Applications. Baltimore: Lippincott Williams & Wilkins, 1999.

17. American Academy of Pediatrics. Issues related to human immunodeficiency virus transmission in schools, child care, medical settings, the home, and community. Pediatrics 1999;104:318–324.

18. Stringer WW, Hansen JE, Wasserman K. Cardiac output estimated noninvasively from oxygen uptake during exercise. J Appl Physiol 1997;82:908–912.

19. Beaver WL, Wasserman K, Whipp BJ. A new method for detecting the anaerobic threshold by gas exchange. J Appl Physiol 1986;60:2020–2027.

20. Johnson J, Anders G, Blanton H, et al. Exercise dysfunction in patients seropositive for the human immunodeficiency virus-1. Am Rev Respir Dis 1990;141:618–622.

21. Perna FM, LaPerriere A, Klimas NG, et al. Cardiopulmonary and CD4 changes in response to exercise training in early symptomatic HIV infection. Med Sci Sports Medicine 1999;31:973–979.

22. Pothoff G, Wasserman K, Ostmann H. Impairment of exercise capacity in various groups of HIV-infected patients. Respiration 1994;61:80–85.

23. Stringer WW, Berezovskaya M, O'Brien WA, et al. The effect of exercise training on aerobic fitness, immune indices, and quality of life in HIV⁺ patients. Med Sci Sports Exerc 1998;30:11–16.

24. Rigsby LW, Dishman RK, Jackson AW, et al. Effects of exercise training on men seropositive for the human immunodeficiency virus-1. Med Sci Sports Exerc 1992;24:6–12.

25. MacArthur RD, Levine SD, Berk TJ. Supervised exercise training improves cardiopulmonary fitness in HIV-infected persons. Med Sci Sports Exerc 1993;25:684–688.

26. Terry L, Sprinz E, Ribeiro JP. Moderate and high intensity exercise training in HIV-1 seropositive individuals: a randomized trail. Int J Sports Med 1999;20:142–146.

27. Roubenoff R, Skolnik PR, Shevitz A, et al. Effect of a single bout of acute exercise on plasma human immunodeficiency virus RNA levels. J Appl Physiol 1999;86:1197–1201.

28. Smith BA, Neidig J, Nickel J, et al. Aerobic exercise: effects on parameters related to fatigue, dyspnea, weight and body composition in HIV-infected adults. AIDS 2001;15:693–701.

29. Koike A, Weiler-Ravell D, McKenzie DK, et al. Evidence that the metabolic acidosis threshold is the anaerobic threshold. J Appl Physiol 1990;68:2521–2526.

30. Brinkman K, ter Hofstede HJ, Burger DM, et al. Adverse effects of reverse transcriptase inhibitors: Mitochondrial toxicity as common pathway. AIDS 1998;12:1735–1744.

31. Dalakas MC, Illa I, Pezeshkpour MD, et al. Mitochondrial myopathy caused by long term zidovudine therapy. N Engl J Med 1990;322:1098–1105.

32. Roy PM, Gouello JP, Pennison-Besnier I, et al. Severe lactic acidosis induced by nucleoside analogues in an HIV-infected man. Ann Emerg Med 1999;34:282–284.

33. Honkoop P, Scholte HR, de Man RA, et al. Mitochondrial injury: lessons from the fialuridine trial. Drug Safety 1997;17:1–7.

34. Mhiri C, Baudrimont M, Bonne G, et al. Zidovudine myopathy: a distinctive disorder associated with mitochondrial dysfunction. Ann Neurol 1991;29:606–614.

35. Bhasin S, Storer TW, Javanbakht M, et al. Testosterone replacement and resistance exercise in HIV-infected men with weight loss and low testosterone levels. JAMA 2000;283:763–770.

36. Carr A, Samaras K, Thorisdottir A, et al. Diagnosis, prediction, and natural course of HIV-1 protease-inhibitor-associated lipodystrophy, hyperlipidaemia, and diabetes mellitus: a cohort study. Lancet 1999;353:2093–2099.

37. Hadigan C, Miller K, Corcoran C, et al. Fasting hyperinsulinemia and changes in regional body composition in HIV-infected women. J Clin Endocrinol Metab 1999;84:1932–1937.

38. Roubenoff R, Weiss L, McDermott A, et al. A pilot study of exercise training to reduce trunk fat in adults with HIV-associated fat redistribution. AIDS 1999;13:1373–1375.

39. Sattler FR, Jaque SV, Schroeder ET, et al. Effects of pharmacological doses of nandrolone decanoate and progressive resistance training in immunodeficient patients infected with HIV. J Clin Endocrinol Metab 1999;84:1268–1276.

40. Yarasheski KE, Tebas P, Stanerson B, et al. Resistant exercise training reduces hypertriglyceridemia in HIV infected men treated with antiviral therapy. J Appl Physiol 2000;90:133–138.

41. Kotler DP, Burastero S, Want J, et al. Prediction of body cell mass and total body water using bioimpedance analysis: effects of race, gender, and disease. Am J Clin Nutr 1996;64(3 Suppl):489S–497S.

42. Grinspoon S, Corcoran C, Rosenthal D, et al. Quantitative assessment of cross-sectional muscle area, functional status, and muscle strength in men with the acquired immunodeficiency syndrome wasting syndrome. J Clin Endocrinol Metab 1999;84:201–206.

43. Spence DW, Galantino MLA, Mossberg KA, et al. Progressive resistance exercise: effect on muscle function and anthropometry of a selected AIDS population. Arch Phys Med Rehabil 1990;71:644–648.

44. Stringer WW. Mechanisms of exercise limitation in HIV⁺ individuals. Med Sci Sports Exerc 2000;32:S412–S421.

45. Strawford A, Barbieri T, Van Loan M, et al. Resistance exercise and supraphysiologic androgen therapy in eugonadal men with HIV-related weight loss: a randomized controlled trial. JAMA 1999;281:1282–1290.

46. Grinspoon S, Corcoran C, Parlman K, et al. Effects of testosterone and progressive resistance training in eugonadal men with AIDS wasting. Ann Intern Med 2000;133:348–355.

47. Agin D, Gallagher D, Wang J, et al. Effects of whey protein and resistance exercise on body cell mass, muscle strength, and quality of life in women with HIV. AIDS 2001;15:2431–2440.

48. Roubenoff R, Wilson IB. Effects of resistance training on self-reported physical conditioning in HIV infection. Med Sci Sports Exerc 2001;33:1811–1817.

49. Nixon S, O'Brien K, Glazier RH, Wilkins AL. Aerobic exercise interventions for people with HIV/AIDS. Cochrane Database Syst Rev 2001;(1):CD001796. Review. Update in: Cochrane Database Syst Rev. 2002;(2):CD001796.

50. Mahler DA. ACSM's Guidelines for Exercise Testing and Prescription. Baltimore, MD: Williams & Wilkins, 1995.

51. Ellis KJ, Lee PD, Pivarnik JM, et al. Changes in body composition of human immunodeficiency virus-infected males receiving insulin-like growth factor I and growth hormone. J Clin Endocrinol Metab 1996;81:3033–3038.

52. Grinspoon S, Corcoran C, Askari H, et al. Effects of androgen administration in men with AIDS wasting syndrome. A randomized, double-blind, placebo-controlled trial. Ann Intern Med 1998;129:18–26.

53. Miller K, Corcoran C, Armstrong C, et al. Transdermal testosterone administration in women with acquired immunodeficiency syndrome wasting: a pilot study. J Clin Endocrinol Metab 1998;83:2717–2725.

54. Mulligan K, Tai VW, Schambelan M. Effects of chronic growth hormone treatment on energy intake and resting energy metabolism in patients with human immunodeficiency virus-associated wasting—a clinical research center study. J Clin Endocrinol Metab 1998;83:1542–1547.

55. Schambelan M, Mulligan K, Grunfeld C, et al. Recombinant human growth hormone in patients with HIV-associated wasting. A randomized, placebo-controlled trial. Serostim Study Group. Ann Intern Med 1996;125:873–882.

56. Wagner G, Rabkin J, Rabkin R. Exercise as a mediator of psychological and nutritional effects of testosterone therapy in HIV+ men. Med Sci Sports Exerc 1998;30:811–817.

57. Grinspoon S. Editorial: The rational use of growth hormone in HIV-infected patients. J Clin Endocrinol Metab 2001;86:3478–3479.

58. Wenke C, Gerrior J, Kantaros J, et al. Recombinant human growth hormone improves the fat redistribution syndrome (lipodystrophy) in patients with HIV. AIDS 1999;13:2099–2103.

59. Meigs JB, Nathan DM, Wilson PWF, et al. Metabolic risk factors worsen continuously across the spectrum of nondiabetic glucose tolerance. The Framingham Offspring Study. Ann Intern Med 1998;128:524–533.

60. Stringer WW, Sattler FR. Metabolic syndromes associated with HIV infection and therapy. Phys Sports Med 2001;29(12):19–26.

61. Stenzel MS, Carpenter CC. The management of the clinical complications of antiretroviral therapy. Infect Dis Clin North Am 2000;14:851–878.

62. Grunfeld C, Feingold KR. The role of the cytokines, interferon alpha and tumor necrosis factor in the hypertriglyceridemia and wasting of AIDS. J Nutr 1992;122(2 Suppl):749–753.

63. Safrin S, Grunfeld C. Fat distribution and metabolic changes in patients with HIV infection. AIDS 1999;13:2493–2505.

64. Lo JC, Mulligan K, Tai VW, et al. "Buffalo hump" in men with HIV-1 infection. Lancet 1998;351:867–870.

65. Olano JP, Borucki MJ, Wen JW, et al. Massive hepatic steatosis and lactic acidosis in a patient with AIDS who was receiving zidovudine. Clin Infect Dis 1995;21:973–976.

66. Lewis W, Dalakas MC. Mitochondrial toxicity of antiviral drugs. Nat Med 1995;1:417–422.

67. Aggarwal A, al Talib K, Alabrash M. Type B lactic acidosis in an AIDS patient treated with zidovudine. Mol Med J 1996;45:929–931.

68. Bissuel F, Bruneel FHF, Habersetzer F, et al. Fulminant hepatitis with severe lactate acidosis in HIV-infected patients on didanosine therapy. J Intern Med 1994;235:367–371.

69. Miller KD, Cameron M, Wood LV, et al. Lactic acidosis and hepatic steatosis associated with the use of stavudine: Report of four cases. Ann Intern Med 2000;133:192–196.

70. Tsai CH, Doong SL, Johns DG, et al. Effect of anti-HIV 2'-beta-fluoro-2',3'-dideoxynucleoside analogs on the cellular content of mitochondrial DNA and on lactate production. Biochem Pharmacol 1994;48:1477–1481.

71. Brook MH. Metabolic muscle diseases. In: Brooke MH, ed. A clinician's view of neuromuscular diseases. Baltimore: Williams & Wilkins, 1989:243–331.

72. Dandurand RJ, Matthews PM, Arnold DL, et al. Mitochondrial disease: pulmonary function, exercise performance, and blood lactate levels. Chest 1995;108:182–189.

73. Elliot DL, Buist NR, Goldberg L, et al. Metabolic myopathies: evaluation by graded exercise testing. Medicine 1989;68:163–172.

74. Andreu AL, Hanna MG, Reichmann H, et al. Exercise intolerance due to mutations in the cytochrome b gene of mitochondrial DNA. N Engl J Med 1999;341:1037–1044.

75. Walker UA. Clinical manifestations of mitochondrial toxicity. J HIV Ther 2001;6(1):17–21.

76. Brinkman K. Evidence for mitochondrial toxicity: Lactic acidosis as proof of concept. J HIV Ther 2001;6(1):13–16.

77. Rustin P. Mitochondrial dysfunction in HIV infection: An overview of pathogenesis. J HIV Ther 2001;6(1):4–12.

78. Walker UA, Byrne E. The therapy of respiratory chain encephalomyopathy: a critical review of the past and current perspective. Acta Neurol Scand 1995;92:273–280.

79. Huang JS, Wilkie SJ, Sullivan MP, et al. Reduced bone density in androgen-deficient women with acquired immune deficiency syndrome wasting. J Clin Endocrinol Metab 2001;86:3533–3539.

80. Blair A, Kohl H, Paffenbarger R, et al. Physical fitness and all-cause mortality: a prospective study of healthy men and women. JAMA 1989;262:2395–2401.

81. Fletcher GF, Ballady G, Blair SN, et al. Statement on Exercise: Benefits and Recommendations for Physical Activity Programs for all Americans: A statement for health professionals by the Committee on Exercise and Cardiac Rehabilitation of the Council on Clinical Cardiology, American Heart Association. Circulation 1996;94:857–862.

82. Pate RR, Pratt M, Blair SN, et al. Physical activity and public health: A recommendation from the Centers for Disease Control and Prevention and the American College of Sports Medicine. JAMA 1995;273:402–407.

83. Levy JA. What can be achieved with an HIV vaccine? Lancet 2001;357:223–224.

84. Veljkovic V, Metlas R, Jevtovic D, et al. The role of passive immunization in HIV+ patients: A Case Report. Chest 2001;120:662–666.

85. NCEP Expert Panel. Executive summary of the Third Report of the National Cholesterol Education Program (NCEP) Expert Panel on Detection, Evaluation, and Treatment of High Blood Cholesterol in Adults (Adult Treatment Panel III). The National Heart, Lung, and Blood Institute (NHLBI)-National Institutes of Health 2001. Available at *http://www.nhlbi.nih.gov/guidelines/cholesterol/atp_iii.htm.*

SUGGESTED READINGS

Brinkman K, ter Hofstede HJ, Burger DM, et al. Adverse effects of reverse transcriptase inhibitors: mitochondrial toxicity as common pathway. AIDS 1998;12:1735–1744.

Fauci AS, Bartlett JG, Goosby EP, et al. Guidelines for the Use of Anti-retroviral Agents in HIV-Infected Adults and Adolescents. http://www hivatis org 2001;1:1–111.

Mahler DA. ACSM's Guidelines for Exercise Testing and Prescription. Baltimore, MD: Williams & Wilkins, 1995.

Stenzel MS, Carpenter CC. The management of the clinical complications of antiretroviral therapy. Infect Dis Clin North Am 2000;14:851–878.

Vegis EN. Natural history of HIV-1 infection. Infect Dis Clin North Am 2000;14:809–825.

Wasserman K, Hansen JE, Sue DY, et al. Principles of Exercise Testing and Interpretation: Pathophysiology and Clinical Applications. Baltimore: Lippincott Williams & Wilkins, 1999.

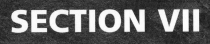

ORTHOPEDIC DISEASES AND DISORDERS

CHAPTER 31

Osteoporosis

Ronald T. Smith, Diane M. Cullen

Overview

Bone health may be defined as the ability to avoid fracture, whereas **osteoporosis** is a disease of skeletal fragility characterized by fractures resulting from low levels of trauma. Osteoporotic fractures occur when bone mass and structure become too weak to support forces created during activities of daily living. They can occur in any bone, but are most common in the hip, vertebrae, and forearm as well as the humerus and bones of the foot (Figure 31.1). Osteoporosis is commonly perceived as a woman's disease, with the lifetime risk of fracture 40% in women (1). However, bone fragility is not limited to women. The lifetime risk of fracture is estimated to be 13% in men (2). The prevalence of male femoral neck osteoporosis averages 27% after age 80

(1). Independent of age, risk factors for both sexes include a genetic history of fracture or height loss with age, low bone mass, low gonadal hormones (**amenorrhea**, menopause), steroid use, hormonal imbalance (thyroid, parathyroid, insulin), poor nutrition (calcium deficiency, eating disorders), disuse and overuse, and alcohol and cigarette use.

One of the most important components of bone health is the peak bone mass achieved at the end of growth. It is estimated that 90% of adult bone mass is acquired by the end of puberty (3, 4), with the remainder of peak bone mass accumulating through the twenties (5–7). Children with bone density lower than age- and gender-matched controls have a higher risk of fracture (8, 9). In older adults peak bone mass has also been associated directly with fragility frac-

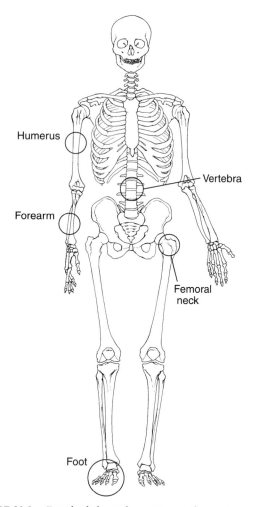

FIGURE 31.1.   Female skeleton demonstrating the most common sites of fracture. Osteoporotic fractures in the vertebrae can occur at any level. They result in loss of height and may cause a dowager's hump. Fractures in the distal forearm are referred to as Colles fractures; fractures at the femoral neck or greater trochanter are referred to as hip fractures.

tures (10–13). For every standard deviation that bone mass is below normal bone mass, the relative risk of fracture in postmenopausal women increases by as much as 2.6 times (14). Although genetics play a major role in determining potential peak bone mass, bone accrual depends upon lifestyle factors such as calcium intake and exercise. Many scientists now view osteoporosis as a disease of pediatric origin, because bone gain during growth is crucial for lifelong bone health.

Osteoporosis can be diagnosed by clinical measures of bone mass, but the morbidity of the disease is not noticeable until fractures occur. Falls are a common cause of hip or wrist fractures. These falls can be related to poor balance, muscle weakness, poor vision, side effects of drugs, tripping on rugs or other objects, or slipping on ice. Hip fractures occur most commonly with falls to the side, whereas forearm or Colles fractures usually occur with a forward fall when the person tries to catch herself or himself with the

hands. The most devastating osteoporotic fracture is of the hip or femoral neck, with a 12–20% mortality rate within 1 year after fracture; 50% of the victims never regain independent mobility (15, 16). Bed rest following fracture can be harmful especially for the frail elderly, in whom strength losses can prevent return to independent living or susceptibility to infection (e.g., pneumonia) can be fatal. Vertebral fractures result in a permanent compression of the vertebra; they can occur with falls or with simple motions such as twisting, but commonly occur while lifting a weight in front of the body (e.g., bag of groceries, grandchild, or garage door). Vertebral fractures may be the most insidious osteoporotic fracture. The compression can occur in stages until the bone is almost pancake-like; progressive compression will eventually involve multiple vertebrae. These fractures can be painful, requiring bed rest and medication, or "silent" and unrecognized. The accumulation of multiple vertebral fractures results in height loss, shortening of the trunk, and in later stages a dowager hump. In the most severe cases, the vertebral column may compress to such an extent that the ribs rest on the hipbones. The obvious problems with these physical deformities include pain, limited range of motion, and inability to find clothes that fit properly. However, severe problems result when the deformations compress the digestive organs and respiratory system, limiting the ability to eat and breathe.

Review of Physiology and Pathophysiology

Bone metabolism has a complex physiology geared toward maintaining serum calcium levels for homeostasis and bone strength for movement. There are 3 primary bone cells: **osteoblasts**, which form new bone; **osteocytes**, which maintain bone; and **osteoclasts**, which remove bone. The activities of these cells are synchronized through intracellular communication to maintain bone balance. The major bone cell activity during growth is modeling. This involves new bone formation to increase bone size, and removal of less structurally important bone to reshape the immature bone to the adult shape. An example would be the growth in outside diameter of cortical bone while the marrow cavity expands. Although the osteoblast and osteoclast work on different surfaces during modeling, their combined activities create a mechanically sound structure. In adult bone, the major cellular activity is remodeling or bone turnover. With remodeling, osteoclasts are activated to remove bone, which is immediately replaced by the osteoblasts. When the osteoclast/osteoblast activities are perfectly coupled, then no net bone loss or gain occurs with remodeling. This system works well for replacing old or damaged bone or for releasing calcium into the serum. With aging, hormonal deficiency, or disuse, the quantity of osteoblast bone formation is less than the quantity of osteoclast resorption, and remodeling results in net bone loss.

Bone Mass Regulation

Our body size and bone size are genetically determined, but mechanical forces and hormonal stimuli modulate our genetic potential. The skeleton serves 2 major roles. The first and most important is calcium storage for homeostasis. The skeleton contains 99% of all calcium found in the body. Serum calcium homeostasis is critical for all life functions and serum levels rarely vary outside the normal value of 10 mg/dl $\pm$ 1. When dietary calcium is insufficient to maintain serum levels, then **parathyroid** hormone (PTH) levels increase to stimulate osteoclast bone resorption, increase renal retention of calcium, and increase intestinal absorption of calcium. Endogenous PTH acts systemically on all bones as a stimulus to resorb bone and release calcium into the serum. If serum calcium levels begin to rise, then calcitonin is released from the thyroid gland to suppress osteoclast bone resorption. In concert, PTH and **calcitonin** act systemically to maintain serum calcium homeostasis.

The second role of the skeleton is to provide structural support for the body. The bones act as levers during muscle contraction and withstand forces many times that of body weight during locomotion. It is crucial that bones have adequate strength to resist bending and ultimately resist fracture during mechanical loading. Bone size and structure are regulated locally at the cellular level within bone to assure adequate strength for daily activities. As with muscle, bones that are loaded or involved with heavy exercise hypertrophy, and bones that are in disuse atrophy. The method of mechanical regulation is not well understood, but it appears that when a bone bends due to loading then bone cells such as the osteocytes and osteoblasts detect stretch, fluid flow, and/or electrical currents (17). These cells transduce the mechanical signal into a cellular response that initiates the adaptive response. The bone adapts to loading by increasing bone formation and mass in areas of greatest strain and reducing mass in areas of least strain. This mechanical regulation results in a very efficient bone shape providing the greatest strength with the least amount of mass or weight.

The **mechanostat** is a term coined by Frost (18–20) to describe the integration of local mechanical regulation and systemic regulation of bone mass. Systemic factors such as hormones and pharmacological agents alter cellular activity throughout the body. Factors that tend to cause bone loss may decrease the sensitivity of the bone cells, whereas factors that increase bone mass may increase the sensitivity of the cells to mechanical loads. When the systemic and local stimuli are integrated, the net result is bone gain in areas of greatest load and bone loss in areas of least load. This results in the most efficient distribution of bone for the prevention of fractures. The local versus systemic struggle is best demonstrated in amenorrheic runners in whom bone mass in the legs is less than in **eumenorrheic** runners but greater than in sedentary controls, whereas bone mass in the upper body is below normal. Repetitive loading on the legs during strenuous training maintains bone in those sites, but the less loaded bones (e.g., ribs or arms) are more susceptible to the systemic effects of estrogen deficiency. It is not unusual for these runners to fracture ribs during low-trauma activities, much like an osteoporotic patient.

Bone Strains

When force is applied to bone, the bone bends such that the shape is distorted momentarily. This distortion seems to initiate the bone response to exercise. The momentary change in length relative to normal length is measured as strain and can reach up to a 0.3% change in length or 3000 $\mu\epsilon$ at maximal loading (21). Strain is a relative measure of bending: the larger the bone, the larger the force required to create the same strain. For example, trotting causes about 2500 $\mu\epsilon$ in the radius of the horse, pig, and dog despite differences in body weight and speed. In each case the bone structure has adapted to the animal's size, so that across species there tends to be a "normal" or common strain range at maximal forces (21, 22). In humans, strains approach 2000 $\mu\epsilon$ with strenuous downhill zigzag running (23). Healthy bones have a large safety margin between normal maximal strains and damage. In mechanical testing, bone begins to show damage around 6,800 $\mu\epsilon$ and completely fracture around 15,700 $\mu\epsilon$ (24). Therefore, in healthy bone, damage would begin at strains twofold to threefold higher than normal peak strains and fracture would occur at strains fivefold higher than normal peak strains. This safety margin decreases with age or disease until, in an osteoporotic person, bones fracture with normal daily loads.

Compared to larger bones, small, thin bones have less resistance to bending and therefore experience greater strains for a given load. The strength of the bone or its ability to resist fracture depends upon the bone quantity or bone mineral content (BMC), bone quality, and bone structure. Given an equal quantity and quality of bone, the greater the cortical diameter and greater the number, thickness, and connectivity of **trabecular** struts, the stronger the bone. Osteoporotic bone is not brittle and does not necessarily have different bone quality than normal bone, but it does have poor bone quantity and structure. With aging and osteoporosis, cortical wall thickness decreases due to expansion of the marrow cavity, and trabecular bone struts decrease in number and connectivity. This bone loss is seen as decreased bone mineral content within the same bone area, resulting in decreased bone mineral density. Loss of bone mass and structure results in decreased bone strength, such that normal loads cause excessive bone bending or strain and fracture. The cumulative effect of loss of bone structure is shown in Figure 31.2.

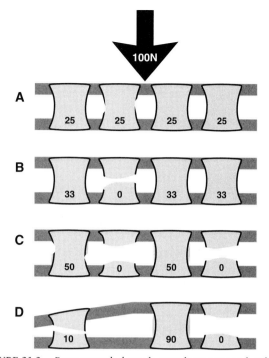

FIGURE 31.2. Bone strength depends upon bone mass and architectural structure. The 4 vertebrae here show how trabecular struts support weight, distributing it among the supports. (A) The 100-Newton weight is evenly distributed among 4 struts, but 1 strut is weakened during bone reabsorption and may show greater strain. (B) When that strut breaks, then the remaining struts must distribute the load. Some trabeculae will adjust by increasing mass to resist bending, but others will continue remodeling and may fracture with the added load. (C) Old broken struts that are no longer loaded will be reabsorbed. Although the structure participating in load bearing is decreased greatly, bone mass and density are decreased only slightly compared with that shown in A. (D) When loads become too great, the vertebrae compress. This can occur in the anterior region or along the length of the bone, and can occur in stages until multiple vertebrae are compressed.

Stress Fractures

Osteoporotic fractures are not limited to the elderly. Many athletes suffer from bone fragility, referred to as stress fractures. These fractures are a subset of overuse injuries that are commonly seen in athletes and military recruits during periods of intense physical training. As with other patients, the incidence of stress fracture in young adult athletes and military recruits has been associated with lower than average bone density and bone size (25–29). When strains are great enough or continue for sufficient numbers of cycles, they result in fatigue damage with loss of bone strength (30). The cumulative effects of repetitive loads are such that even small loads repeated a sufficient number of times will cause fatigue damage (31) and stress fracture. The skeleton is robust and normally increases formation to increase size and resistance to bending while it repairs microdamage quickly by remodeling or removing and replacing damaged bone (20, 30). When loads occur over a period of weeks or months, the balance between injury rate and repair rate determines the ac-

cumulation of damage. Injury rate depends upon the initial bone strength, relative increase in loads, number of load cycles, and rate of adaptive growth. The repair rate depends upon metabolic conditions at both systemic and tissue levels.

Bone Response to Changes in Mechanical Loading

Exercise creates mechanical loads or force on bone as muscles contract or as the body lands, takes off, or contacts objects. These forces cause momentary and slight bending of the bone, or strain. When mechanical loads create excessive strains, bone mass increases and shape changes until what was once an overload is within a "normal" range. Conversely, when training discontinues or disuse occurs and bone loads or strains fall below normal, bone mass decreases until strains return to a "normal" range. Bone cell formation is activated by high strains, and bone loss occurs in the absences of strains.

Cellular Response to Mechanical Loading

Mechanical loads regulate bone size through transient changes in cell activity. Increased mechanical loading transforms quiescent and even resorbing surfaces into bone-forming surfaces (32–35). Once adaptation is complete and the structure is sufficient to meet the new strength demands, then cell activity returns to nonexercise levels and the new structure is maintained. A permanent acceleration of bone formation would overcompensate for a discrete load change, so as bone strength changes, the stimulus for formation decreases. The pattern should resemble muscle training, where muscle mass and strength plateau at each training level until the training level is increased.

Adaptation to increased loads is seen with exercise training (35–42), external loading (43–46), and osteotomy (47–49). The early bone changes associated with mechanical loading include increased mRNA expression, osteoblast number, and bone formation within 5 days after loading (32, 33, 44, 50, 51).

Some studies have shown indirectly the waning of bone formation with long-term loading (41, 46). With repeated loading in artificial loading devices, formation may be consistently elevated between 2 and 6 weeks with increased mineralizing surface, mineral apposition rate, and bone formation rate (44, 52–55). From weeks 12 to 18 of loading, the formation rate declines to age-matched sedentary levels (43, 54). Baseline labels show that the majority of bone is added within the first 6 weeks and maintained through 12 and 18 weeks of loading (54). This discrete gain in bone mass with a discrete increase in load is consistent with Frost's theory of skeletal adaptation to mechanical usage (SATMU), which suggests that bone modeling occurs to accommodate new forces (56).

Inactivity and Weightlessness

Disuse does not create the normal mechanical load signals in bone that act to maintain bone balance and results in an increase in bone resorption with insufficient bone formation. Complete localized disuse **osteopenia** is clearly documented in the lower limbs of paraplegic individuals; immediately after spinal cord injury, bone loss is rapid, averaging 1% to 2% per month for the femur and twice that for the tibia (57–59).

Long-term bed rest and space flight are dramatic forms of bone disuse and appear to share similar characteristics. Temporary bed rest results in bone loss averaging 1% per week (60–62). However, space flight removes all normal gravitational loads from bone and creates more extreme disuse than bed rest. This weightless environment results in a marked decline in bone mass (63, 64). With unloading or disuse, the rate of bone loss is proportional to the relative changes in loading. This is supported by the greater percentage of bone loss from weight-bearing bones and little or no loss in non-weight-bearing bones such as the upper limbs (64). In the calcaneus bone loss can be as high as 1.8% per week and ranges from 0.13% to 0.27% per week in the tibia, femur, and spine. As with bed rest, greater bone loss occurs in the lower than in the upper limb bones during space flight (64, 65).

Bone loss can be prevented partially with intermittent exercise. However, even with a strenuous exercise program, bone mineral loss averages 1% per month in space flight (63, 65). Although muscle and bone loss during space flight and subsequent gain after flight parallel each other, bone recovery after disuse may take 2 to 3 times longer (60). Studies have shown that even after 6 months, young men have not regained initial bone mass (62). Recovery time to replace bone mineral is dependent on the length of time in disuse and the bone compartment sustaining the loss (63, 64), and may take several years. This incomplete recovery of bone mass is especially seen in the trabecular compartment (64). When individual trabecula or struts break and no longer bear loads, then they are removed and are rarely replaced. A challenge to the research community is to devise methods for simulating normal skeletal loads in microgravity to prevent irreversible bone losses during space flight. Although it appears that with exercise countermeasures, the rate of muscle loss during flight reaches a plateau, there is no support for the same phenomenon in bone (63). This continued loss of bone at 1% to 2% per month would present serious challenges for extended space flight, extended work on the International Space Station, or the estimated 3-year Mars trip.

Implications

The common recommendation for bed rest for the relief of back pain after fracture may induce additional bone loss and muscle atrophy and can lead to increased risk of subsequent fracture. Bone loss of the hip and lumbar spine with bed rest may be more detrimental for older, sedentary individuals with osteoporotic vertebral fractures than for younger, healthy individuals. In addition, the elderly are less likely to resume an active lifestyle sufficient to stimulate recovery of loss of bone mass. After hip fracture, there is often a prolonged period of bed rest or non-weight bearing. Not only is this deleterious for bone mass, but it can have disastrous consequences for the patient's independence. As many as 20% of those with a hip fracture live less than a year after fracture due to secondary illnesses such as pneumonia, and another 50% never regain mobility due to loss of physical abilities (15, 16). Many of the frail elderly are living near maximal exercise capacity, and any loss of strength or coordination can sentence them permanently to a wheelchair.

Bone Measurements (Table 31.1)

There are several methods for estimating bone mass and size. These devices are capable of measuring whole body as well as regional sites and are the same devices used to determine body composition. The normal distribution curves and standard deviations for peak bone mass are based upon a large sample of young premenopausal women and men. Recently, the World Health Organization (WHO) defined osteoporosis based on bone mass measurements relative to this young normal population. In addition to being defined by low-trauma fracture, osteoporosis is now diagnosed as bone density at a Z score below −2.5 or 2.5 standard deviations below normal (1). Bone density from −1 to −2.5 standard deviations below normal in the absence of fractures is termed osteopenia. The most common method for assessing bone mass or density is by dual energy x-ray absorptiometry (DEXA) (Figure 31.3). This is a noninvasive, low-radiation device that calculates bone mineral content and bone area for common sites such as the lumbar spine, femoral neck, forearm, and whole body. The dual beam or energy technology allows separation of body mass from the whole body scans into 3 compartments of bone, fat, and lean tissue. A more precise method of measuring bone density is quantitative computed tomography (QCT). The DEXA devices report density in grams of mineral per area of

TABLE 31.1. BONE DENSITY MEASUREMENTS AND OSTEOPOROSIS CLASSIFICATION

Classification	Standard deviation from mean
Healthy Young Normal	0
Osteopenia	−1 to −2.5
Osteoporosis	<−2.5

Based on WHO.

Adapted from Kanis JA, Melton J, Christiansen C, Johnston CC, Khaltaev N (1).

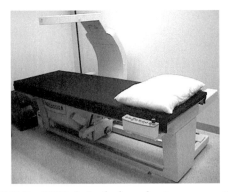

FIGURE 31.3. DEXA device for bone density measures. With the subject lying supine, the device is programmed to measure whole body, lumbar spine, hip, or forearm. The device measures radiation that passes through body regions and can estimate bone mineral content, lean body mass, and body fat mass. It is often used in body composition studies.

bone, using only bone width and assuming consistent bone shapes, while CT measures the full cross-sectional area. CT has a much higher radiation dose and cost, but provides measures of trabecular and cortical bone separately from the same region and is useful for research studies. It is sensitive to differences in mass distribution and can compute moments of inertia, and therefore is more predictive of bone strength. CT has the added benefit of measuring muscle cross-sectional area in the same region as the bone measurements. The other common bone measurement devices use ultrasound to record the speed of sound and signal attenuation through bone. They provide data on the combined bone density, structure, and quality. Ultrasound values of the calcaneus and forearm have similar predictive value to DEXA measures of the arm for fracture. Although commonly used as screening tests, the results are only suggestive of osteoporotic risk when applied to individuals.

Diseases That Cause Osteoporosis

The Female Triad: Disordered Eating, Amenorrhea, and Osteoporosis

Stress fractures in female athletes, especially track and field participants and performance dancers, are a result of several risk factors including low BMD, menstrual irregularities, nutrition intake, and history of stress fracture. The term *female triad* emphasizes health issues of active women and the consequences of excessive physical activity with inadequate nutrition. Poor nutrient intake or inadequate caloric intake can have serious health consequences. In the extreme, anorexia and bulimia can result in permanent disability or even death. As the body adapts to inadequate diet, bone calcium is depleted to maintain serum calcium homeostasis and often the ovaries shut down, resulting in the loss of menses (amenorrhea). Amenorrhea, like menopause, is an outward sign that the body is estrogen deficient, and estrogen is essential for maintaining bone mass in adult women. Hip BMD has been negatively correlated with amenorrhea of 3 months or longer (66). The impact of these health issues is amplified when they occur during growth, when these girls and women should be realizing large increases in bone density but unfortunately are experiencing substantial bone loss. Conditions that reduce peak bone mass have a lifetime impact on risk for osteoporosis. Treatments for eating disorders include dietary counseling and usually medical interventions. Amenorrhea is sometimes reversed by improved dietary habits to ensure adequate caloric intake for current exercise levels, cutting back on training if overtraining is an issue, and/or hormone replacement therapy to increase bone density (16).

The prevalence of eating disorders in young women has been estimated at 3% (67) and reported as high as 35% in female college athletes (68). Bulimia has been reported to affect 1% to 10% of adolescent girls and college women (69). The loss of bone in anorexia nervosa is a result of greater resorption than formation. Bone loss in eating-disordered individuals is in the range of 50% to 70% reduction in BMD (70, 71). This bone loss leads to osteopenia, secondary osteoporosis, and increased fracture risk (67, 72).

Drugs With Adverse Effects on Bone

Glucocorticoids and corticosteroids are important therapy for inflammatory disorders and are often used in the treatment of allergies and asthma, as anticonvulsant therapy, and for immunosuppression with transplants. However, the adverse effects of these drugs on bone can be substantial. Bone loss can be as high as 50% at selected sites after 6 months of treatment, and this loss has been associated with a 30% to 40% increase in fracture incidence (73). Patients on long-term corticosteroid treatment have a 50% increased risk of hip fractures and 30% to 35% higher risk of vertebral fracture (74, 75).

The mechanisms for action of steroids on bone involve several organ systems. The direct effect on bone cells is impaired function of osteoblasts and osteoclasts, with decreased tissue repair. Parathyroid activity on bone is enhanced, renal calcium excretion is increased, and intestinal absorption of calcium decreased. In addition, the anabolic action of sex steroids is impaired (76).

Anticonvulsant/antiepileptic drug therapy was first associated with osteomalacia/osteoporosis in the late 1960s. The Study of Osteoporotic Fractures (77) and work by Stephen (78) has identified long-term anticonvulsant drugs as an independent factor in osteoporosis. The effect of these drugs is associated with duration of drug use and the number of different drugs used (79). Depending on the type of drug used, the reduction of BMD has been shown to approach 12% in men and 15% to 16% in women (80). Of the patients studied by Sato, 23% had BMD values suggestive of osteoporosis and an additional 15% had BMD values that were classified as osteomalacia (80). Biochemical markers in this study indicated an increase in bone resorption may have been a primary cause of the lower BMD (80). Anticonvulsant drugs have also been shown to reduce new bone formation in addition to altering calcium and vitamin D homeostasis (81). Although new drugs improve the treatment of this condition, they also increase the risk for low bone density for individuals receiving long-term anticonvulsant treatment (82).

Addictive Chemicals

Caffeine intake, usually in coffee, has been associated with low bone mass. Coffee intake of 4 cups per day has been associated with 5% lower than normal total body bone calcium and doubled the hip fracture risk (83). A possible explanation is that caffeine drinks often replace high-calcium beverages, such as milk, reducing daily calcium intake below required levels. When intake was adjusted for level of calcium, there was also a decrease in the efficiency of calcium absorption (84). The effect of caffeine may be decreased or eliminated by meeting the daily calcium requirement (83). Excessive intake of alcohol has been shown to increase the risk of osteoporosis (85–88). The amount of intake and length of time over which the alcohol consumption occurs exacerbates the bone loss. However, moderate amounts of alcohol have been associated with a reduced risk of osteoporosis (87). The amount of alcohol deemed moderate is somewhat variable; in general, moderate consumption is 1 to 2 beers, 1 to 2 mixed drinks, or 1 to 2 glasses of wine per day, but not more than a total of 4 to 5 drinks per week.

The effect of alcohol on bone is difficult to determine because of a lack of longitudinal studies, differing amounts of alcohol intake, frequency of alcohol consumption, number of years of consumption, and inaccuracies in self-reports. In animals, alcohol has been shown to reduce bone formation (87) and decrease proliferation of cultured osteoblastic cells (89). The potential mechanisms of action of alcohol on bone are varied and may involve disturbances to one or more of the following (87): calcium-regulating hormones; vitamin D metabolism (especially associated with liver disease); mineral homeostasis of calcium, magnesium, and zinc; decreased mechanical loading; poor nutrition; malabsorption as a result of chronic pancreatitis; cigarette smoking; and aluminum contamination from antacids.

Incidence of Osteoporosis

The World Health Organization (WHO) has established an operational definition of osteoporosis as a bone density at 2.5 standard deviations below the mean (90). In the United States the incidence of osteoporosis has been reported at 13% to 18% for women and 3% to 6% for men (91). When the WHO criteria were applied to Canadian women and men over 50 years of age, the incidence of osteoporosis in the lumbar spine of women was 12.1% and in the femoral neck 7.9%. Prevalence was less in the men, 2.9% in the lumbar spine and 4.8% in the femoral neck. Combined prevalence of osteoporosis in women was 15.8%, whereas in men it was 6.6% (92). The incidence of osteoporosis has been reported in Australia (93) for women as 28% at the hip and 21% at the spine, and men were 10% and 7% at the hip and spine, respectively. In Swedish populations the estimated prevalence in postmenopausal women is 21.1%, and in men of a similar age, 6.3% (94). Around the world, it is generally accepted that the incidence of osteoporosis is higher in women than in men of the same ethnic group.

Risk of hip fracture in men is approximately one third that of women and is associated with greater bone mass in men. This is similar in several different cultures. However, the lifelong risk of osteoporotic fracture has been increasing in men (95–96). Although in some cases there are explanatory factors for low bone mass, no etiology has been found in approximately 50% of osteoporotic men.

The average rate of osteoporosis in Mexican women 50 years and older is 16% (97), which is less than that of Caucasians in other countries. This is consistent with National Health and Nutrition Examination Survey (NHANES) III data suggesting that Mexican American women have as much as 4% greater bone mineral density than non-Hispanic whites (98). This translates to an estimated 300,000 to 400,000 Mexican Americans with osteopenia compared to 10 to 15 million non-Hispanic whites using the WHO standard. The estimated incidence for osteoporosis using the same standard is 100,000 Mexican Americans compared to 5 to 6 million non-Hispanic whites (98).

African American populations, both women and men, have had a lower incidence of osteoporotic fracture than that found in White populations. Black women have a 1.3 to 2.4 lower incidence than non-Hispanic white women (98). When comparing different femoral regions of non-Hispanic Whites with non-Hispanic Blacks, the osteoporosis prevalence is higher in the non-Hispanic Whites by 1.5 to 2.8 times, depending on the femur site (91). This lower rate may be a result of greater peak bone mineral density and lower turnover as a result of ethnicity and gender (99).

The incidence of osteoporosis is lower in Asian societies than in Western societies. Although the calcium intake in Asian diets is lower than Western diets, the incidence of fractures is less (100). Some of these differences may be accounted for by differences in body build and lower center of gravity. Asian people tend to have more developed hip muscles, which may be a result of having to repeatedly rise from the floor rather than from a chair. The movement of sitting on the floor and repeatedly rising from that position is thought to improve motor function, agility, and balance, which taken together would contribute to fewer falls and a lower fracture rate (100). Within Asian cultures, higher fracture rates are found in urbanized settings (101), possibly explained by a reduced amount of walking and less physical activity in urbanized compared to rural settings.

Direct Cost of Osteoporosis

More than 25 million Americans are afflicted with osteoporosis (102). The rate of all osteoporotic fractures is over 1.5 million per year, and of this group, 10% to 20% of women with a hip fracture will not survive 1 year (103). The direct cost of treatment of osteoporotic fractures was estimated at between $10 and $15 billion per year (90). Nursing home care for patients with osteoporotic hip fractures is in excess of $4 billion per year (104). These estimates are direct health care costs, and do not include costs for family care, lost independence, and forced changes in lifestyle. At 78 million people, baby boomers between 35 and 53 years of age account for one third of the U.S. population (105). As this group ages, there will be a substantial increase in the numbers of individuals suffering osteoporotic fractures.

Potential Treatments

The first recommendations for the prevention of bone loss are adequate calcium and vitamin D intake combined with exercise. When these actions are not sufficient to maintain or increase bone, then other medical interventions may be necessary.

Importance of Adequate Calcium and Vitamin D Nutrition

Parathyroid hormone (PTH) is the principal hormone regulating plasma calcium ion levels and the primary stimulus to bone remodeling (106). Thus, when plasma calcium levels fall due to insufficient intake or excessive loss of calcium, PTH production is increased in order to stimulate bone resorption and liberate calcium from the skeleton to restore plasma calcium concentration. This homeostatic response is referred to as secondary **hyperparathyroidism**, and can persist for as long as the stress to plasma calcium persists. The bone response to the increased PTH is to increase the activation of bone resorption, thus increasing the remodeling space. This results in an imbalance of bone remodeling in which more bone is lost from the skeleton than is replaced, and skeletal strength is compromised.

Calcium

Although calcium is a necessary building block for bone, it is also required for many body functions including nerve

transmission, blood clotting, and muscle contraction. In terms of bone formation, adequate calcium intake is important to (1) provide adequate calcium for attainment of peak bone mass and for bone adaptation to exercise; (2) maintain bone calcium stores and structural integrity of bone during the aging process; and (3) provide adequate calcium for microfracture repair. Serum calcium homeostasis is essential for life, and when these levels become compromised, calcium is removed from bone. Thus, the strength of the skeleton may be sacrificed to maintain plasma calcium homeostasis. The requirement for calcium varies with gender, age, growth, and hormonal status.

Calcium intakes for women have been historically low, in the range of 600 to 700 mg/day, while the dietary reference intake has been established between 1,000 and 1,200 mg/day for premenopausal women with an upper recommendation of 2,500 mg/day (Table 31.2). The predominant reason for low intake in women, particularly in peak bone-forming years, is poor nutrition education. Concerns about dietary fat content cause some women to avoid dairy products, which are the richest source of dietary calcium. However, many low-fat and fat-free dairy products are available that will help them attain appropriate calcium intake without high caloric intake. In addition, many products have been fortified with calcium to provide additional dietary sources.

Vitamin D

Vitamin D is critically important in the regulation of blood calcium levels and consequently bone calcium. The active form of vitamin D, $1,25(OH)_2D$, regulates the active transport mechanism of calcium absorption from the gut (106). Vitamin D can be obtained by dietary sources or from skin exposure to sunlight. Absent these sources of vitamin D, the individual has a substantial risk of developing bone disease (107). Aside from skeletal benefits, vitamin D also works in the prevention of some cancers, multiple sclerosis, and hypertension (108).

Cutaneous synthesis of vitamin D from exposure to sunlight can make a substantial contribution to vitamin D sta-

TABLE 31.2. CALCIUM (MG/DAY) DIETARY REFERENCE INTAKES

Age	Females		Males	
	DRI	**Upper Limits**	**DRI**	**Upper Limits**
9–13	1,300	2,500	1,300	2,500
14–18	1,300	2,500	1,300	2,500
19–30	1,000	2,500	1,000	2,500
31–50	1,000	2,500	1,000	2,500
51–70	1,200	2,500	1,200	2,500
>70	1,200	2,500	1,200	2,500

DRI = dietary reference intake

tus. However, many people have limited opportunity for exposure to sunlight. This is especially true for latchkey children and adolescents spending increasing amounts of time on computers and the Internet, video games, and television. The increased use of sunscreen to protect against skin cancer may drastically reduce available vitamin D from sunlight during peak bone-forming years. Adults are working longer hours indoors, reducing exposure to daily sunlight. The elderly have reduced exposure to sunlight because of inclement weather and difficulty with mobility that adversely affects activities of daily living. This leads to a significant risk for developing vitamin D deficiency and resulting bone problems (109).

Sunlight is a major source of vitamin D in the summer. The Institute of Medicine (IOM) report acknowledged that cutaneous synthesis of vitamin D is markedly diminished or absent in the winter months in latitudes greater than 40 degrees north or 40 degrees south. In the United States the 40th parallel runs through New Jersey, Illinois, and northern California. When sun exposure is blocked completely, vitamin D levels decrease rapidly. The main dietary source of vitamin D in the United States is vitamin-D fortified milk. Unfortunately, many young women avoid milk due to concerns about fat content or because they prefer carbonated beverages. When necessary, vitamin D supplements are available. Although supplements are convenient, the recommendation is to obtain necessary vitamins from food sources. In addition to the specific vitamin, foods contain other important nutrients that are necessary to good health. Foods also enhance absorption of other nutrients. This enhanced absorption would not occur with supplementation, and excessive supplementation of vitamin D may adversely affect the status of other fat-soluble vitamins (A, E, K).

There is no consensus on optimal vitamin D intake. The IOM (110) recommendation for women between the ages of 19 and 30 years is a minimum of 5 μg per day (200 IU per day) (Table 31.3). However, the report indicated that scant literature was available upon which to base those recommendations. Although this level may prevent osteomalacia, higher levels may be needed to prevent fragility fractures and secondary hyperparathyroidism (108). Serum levels less than 10 ng/ml for vitamin D are considered deficient in terms of osteomalacia; however, evidence is mounting that levels of at least 30 ng/ml may be necessary for bone health (111). Total body sunlight exposure easily provides the equivalent of 2500 μg (10,000 IU) of vitamin D per day in the summer, which suggests that doses much higher than 50 μg (2000 IU) are safe. Evidence is mounting that 5 μg/day of vitamin D per day may be inadequate. Two multivitamins containing 10 μg/day (800 IU/day) might be necessary (107).

Medical Interventions

Pharmaceuticals are available for the treatment of osteoporosis to either prevent the effects of estrogen deprivation, slow or stop bone loss, or more recently to increase bone mass. These drugs are effective while taken but have limited long-term effects after withdrawal. Often they are used to delay bone loss at menopause or to stop loss in those with the highest risk of fracture.

Estrogen has been the longest available drug for prevention of postmenopausal bone loss, and can be taken either as estrogen alone or in combination with progesterone. In the 3 years around menopause, women can lose up to 10% of total bone mass due to estrogen deficiency (112). Similarly, ovariectomy and amenorrhea result in rapid bone loss. Estrogen acts to suppress the osteoclasts so that when estrogen is absent, bone remodeling is accelerated with inadequate new bone formation. Estrogen actually can cause a small increase in bone mass and has shown effectiveness in the elderly when given at low doses (113). Serious adverse effects that may be associated with estrogen or estrogen and progesterone include risk of uterine, breast, or ovarian cancers, as well as increased risk of blood clots and strokes.

Alternatives to estrogen have been developed with decreased cancer risk. These are specific estrogen-receptor modulators (SERMs) (77, 114). They are designed to target bone cells, but not other estrogen-sensitive tissue. One, in particular, actually decreases the risk of breast cancer. However, as of now, these drugs are not as effective as estrogen for maintaining bone and may actually increase hot flashes.

Bisphosphonates are a popular class of pharmaceuticals developed to treat osteoporosis. These drugs prevent bone resorption, prevent further bone loss, and actually cause about an 8% gain in bone mass (114). However, there are strict rules for taking bisphosphonates; if taken incorrectly, there can be a risk of stomach/esophageal complications. Their long-term effects have not been determined; therefore bisphosphonates are normally not prescribed for young adults on a long-term basis. Other treatments to prevent bone loss include the hormone calcitonin and soy products as a natural food substitute. However, there is no consistent evidence for effects of these compounds on bone.

TABLE 31.3. VITAMIN D (μg/DAY) DIETARY REFERENCE INTAKES

Age	Females		Males	
	DRI	Upper Limits	DRI	Upper Limits
9–13	5	–	5	–
14–18	5	–	5	–
19–30	5	50	5	50
31–50	5	50	5	50
51–70	5	50	5	50
>70	5	50	5	50

1 μg = 40 IU of vitamin D; DRI = dietary reference intake

Agents that increase bone mass include low-dose fluoride combined with calcium and parathyroid hormone (PTH). Initial trials with fluoride showed large gains in bone mass, but when fluoride was incorporated into the bone mineral structure, bone strength decreased and fracture risk increased despite an increase in bone mass (115). The new low-dose fluoride treatments with high calcium intake do not seem to have the same problem (116). PTH is an anabolic bone agent that can increase bone mass as much as (117). PTH is delivered as an injection; when treatment is stopped bone mass returns to original levels unless some other treatment is used to preserve the bone.

A relatively new treatment for osteoporosis is surgical repair of the vertebrae (118). Both kyphoplasty and vertebroplasty restore strength to the vertebrae by filling it with a plastic that quickly solidifies. This method is the only one available to restore function, but must be performed within a few months of injury before the fracture has time to heal.

Hip Fracture Prevention

A relatively new treatment for the prevention of hip fractures is the hip pad (119). These pads, which are embedded in form-fitting undergarments and are unobtrusive, have been very successful in preventing hip fractures from falls. They cover the greater trochanter and disperse the force when a patient falls to the side. Compliance is the major problem with use of the pads, because the person must wear them 24 hours a day, 7 days a week, so that every time they fall, they have the pads on. Because hip fractures are associated with the greatest morbidity and mortality, the pads are a very smart choice for osteoporotic patients. The challenge is to convince the patient that the change in lifestyle is necessary and not too cumbersome.

Impact on Ameliorating Symptoms

The symptoms of osteoporosis are primarily pain associated with recent fractures and physical limitations. Although some vertebral fractures are "silent" or pain free, others result in considerable back pain that can last for several weeks. Although bed rest relieves pressure on fractured regions, extensive bed rest can result in additional bone loss and physical weakness. The surgical interventions, such as kyphoplasty, that restore vertebral height often relieve pain and restore function.

Vertebral osteoporosis results in loss of height, spinal curvature, and even a dowager's hump. In the later stages the vertebral column shortens so much that the ribs actually rest upon the hips. This limits range of motion, lung capacity, and stomach volume. Physical therapy and exercise prescriptions can help relieve muscle strain, build strength, and increase range of motion, but must be done with care to prevent further fractures.

Hot flashes are a common and disruptive symptom of menopause. Although not directly associated with bone loss, they occur as estrogen levels decrease and while bone loss is most rapid. Estrogen replacement therapy prevents bone loss and can ameliorate hot flashes. The SERMs often do not affect hot flashes and sometimes actually can increase their incidence.

Impact on the Exercise Response

The interaction of pharmaceuticals and exercise are not well understood. Frost's mechanostat theory suggests that drugs and hormones interact with exercise to alter bone sensitivity and magnify or diminish the response to exercise. This has not been well demonstrated in animals and is untested in humans. However, calcium and vitamin D are essential for maximal bone response to mechanical loading or exercise. These are the building blocks and without sufficient nutrients bone gain will be limited (5).

The Exercise Response

Potential Exercise Benefits

The goals of an exercise program in the prevention of osteoporosis are to (1) maintain or increase bone mass and strength, (2) prevent falls, and (3) maintain or improve the ability to perform activities of daily living. The ability to increase bone mass through exercise is limited by an individual's fitness level and ability to carry on a strenuous exercise program. In terms of bone mass, the gains usually occur within the first year and are less than 5% (36, 120–122). However, exercise can be an effective means of maintaining bone mass with age. This is especially true if a person can reverse sedentary lifestyle habits. Men and women average 5% bone loss per decade with aging (123), but it is not known whether this rate is due to aging, disease, or disuse.

The real benefit of exercise for the elderly person with osteoporosis may not be bone strength, but fitness. Hip and wrist fractures are directly associated with falls, and factors that increase the risk of falls include muscle weakness, functional limitations, a history of falls, environmental hazards, psychoactive medication, and alcohol. The most effective measures for preventing traumatic fractures may be improving muscle strength, agility, and flexibility, removing environmental hazards, and correcting visual impairments (124–126).

Functional Exercise Benefits

Enhanced range of motion, balance, and agility through exercise provide positive feedback for exercise. They improve the individual's ability to participate in functional activities that further enhance balance, strength, and agility and reduce traumatic fracture risk (127).

Healthy elderly persons who participate in exercise programs can improve their range of motion (128). Range of motion has an important role in osteoporosis prevention by its effect on mobility, activities of daily living, and balance (129, 130). Skeletal deformities, especially in the vertebral column, can limit range of motion and are generally not resolved by exercise. However, exercise can relieve muscle contractures caused by pain and strengthen muscles to help regain some range of motion. Improved shoulder flexibility and range of motion is important for activities requiring overhead movement, such as work in the kitchen or shop, and activities of daily living, such as dressing and personal grooming. Spinal exercises and shoulder girdle exercises have been shown to reduce pain and improve flexibility and function in osteoporotic patients (131).

Agility is the ability to change directions quickly and is important in avoiding falls. Reaction time, movement time, and strength determine whether we are quick enough to grab a support, readjust a foot after it trips, or right ourselves when we lose our balance. Improvements in agility have been shown in exercise programs that include aerobic dance, flexibility exercises, or walking (132). The elderly have shown significant increases in strength and balance with exercise programs that result in improved functional ability and potentially decrease the risk of falls (125, 133–140). Traumatic falls have been estimated to be responsible for 95% of osteoporotic hip fractures; therefore, reducing the risk of falls would reduce the risk of fracture (141).

Is Maximal Exercise Testing Recommended?

Maximal exercise testing may be inappropriate in severely osteoporotic patients due to the potential for injury. In addition, structural and musculoskeletal handicaps may limit the interpretation of maximal aerobic tests. Careful consideration should be given to the purpose of the test, the individual's limitations, the risk of injury, and how the results will be interpreted. In many cases a well-defined, reliable functional test may be more appropriate than a maximal test.

Exercise Programming Options

Exercise Limitations

Exercise for the treatment of osteoporosis needs to be carefully monitored. Because osteoporosis is defined as a high risk of bone fragility fracture, exercises should not expose patients to undue risk. Actions that create high forces relative to bone strength, require rapid movements, or increase the chance of falls would not be recommended. For the severely osteoporotic patient, range of motion and water exercise may be the best approach initially. Physical limitations in lung capacity and range of motion may further limit exercise participation for this group. The primary goal for the patient with severe osteoporosis would be relief of muscular pain and increased ability to perform activities of daily living.

Training Modalities

Exercise for improving or maintaining bone mass in the lower limbs or spine is most effective if it uses weight bearing physical activity such as walking, running, or jumping. Resistance exercises are an effective alternative or are useful for stressing the non-weight-bearing bones. As with muscle, the exercise effects are specific to the bones stressed (125, 142). The specific parameters for stimulation of a bone response are not well defined. In general, if an exercise stresses the muscles in the region, it will probably stress the bones. Although powerful, quick, forceful actions such as those seen in gymnastics will have the most dramatic effects on bone, other activities can have positive effects as well. The primary goal would be to avoid injury, and the secondary goal to create an overload by increasing the loads and number of repetitions.

Training Parameters

The most effective stimulus for bone formation appears to be strain rate (143, 144). Strain is the deformation in bone, and strain rate is how fast that deformation occurs. The force magnitude, frequency of repetitions, and rate of acceleration or deceleration all contribute to strain rate. Sports that incorporate high-power moves such as gymnastics, power lifting, and wrestling are all associated with high bone mass. However, high-strain, powerful activities are not always appropriate and are not easily maintained for years on end. With lower force activities, a greater number of repetitions are required for bone stimulation. However, in very sedentary animals, walking 20 minutes a day was sufficient to stimulate bone formation (37).

There is substantial evidence that resistance training is effective in reversing the effects of osteoporosis while also being a time-efficient and cost-effective preventative measure for increased BMD and muscle strength. Many of the recent bone studies have worked with strength training protocols and attained moderate results for bone gain. The most effective bone exercise studies have relied on muscle strength training protocols and have attained moderate (1–3%) gain in bone mass. However, bone-specific programs have not been identified and may not be much different from guidelines for muscle training. Current research on muscle training suggests that resistance training is effective if it meets the principles of intensity, volume, and frequency (145). Either increasing the weight or increasing the number of repetitions from the previous session can achieve an overload. The most effective strength training programs use a variety of approaches focusing on major muscle groups, and vary the stresses by regularly altering exercises, repetitions, and weights. Strength training has been shown to improve muscle mass, strength, and dynamic balance (120, 125, 146).

Intensity is the percentage of maximum effort required to complete a repetition. Generally, for muscle strength, high force and lower repetitions are most effective (147); this is probably true for bone as well, because strain magnitude is an important variable. Researchers are currently trying to elucidate the appropriate intensity level for resistance training for maximal response. A twice-a-week training program has been shown to produce muscle improvement; although a once-a-week program also shows improvement, these improvements are somewhat less (148). With animal studies, high loads 3 days a week are as effective as 7 days a week (44). Similarly, with high loads, there is no difference in bone response between 36 and 1800 repetitions of force application (46). However, as the loads or forces decrease, the number of repetitions needed for a response increases (55). More recent studies suggest that very low forces can be effective at high frequency (number of repetitions per second) (149). The frequency of training depends upon the relative overloads created during exercise.

For low-intensity exercise, a daily routine would be more effective for bone than a less regular routine. The limiting factor for exercise intensity and frequency is generally muscle and joint strength in healthy individuals. Although symptoms of overuse may be good markers for the average person, in the elderly or the person with osteoporosis, bones may fail with no symptoms detected before fracture. Exercise prescriptions should not include activities that focus stress on the vertebrae and other high-risk bones.

The exercise parameters for bone health are not as well established as they are for muscle training. Especially when working with frail patients, it is important that the training facility have qualified, knowledgeable instructors to assure safety and maximize adherence. Certification from either the American College of Sports Medicine or the National Strength and Conditioning Association is a minimum standard for work with this group. These certified instructors would be capable of designing resistance-training programs. In addition, they would be capable of explaining training principles, demonstrating proper exercise technique, and monitoring and recording progress. These instructors can also provide accurate, scientific-based answers to inquiries.

Potential Physiological Adaptations

The exercise adaptations in bone occur primarily at the local level. The bone response to loading is site specific. Although exercise can induce changes in gonadal hor-

mones, growth hormone, and stress hormones, their effects are thought to either magnify or diminish the local response.

Mechanical Loading and Bone Responses

Mechanical loads create bone bending or strain. They work at the cellular level to alter bone metabolism and thereby adapt bone size, shape, and strength to reduce strains and to prevent fracture (18–20). The magnitude of the bone stimulus depends upon strain magnitude, strain rate, number of cycles, and frequency (46, 150–152). When activity and bone strains are in the normal adapted range, cellular activity is in steady state and bone mass maintained. However, when strains increase to create a mild overload, then local osteoblast formation is stimulated and local bone resorption decreased for a net gain in bone mass (32, 34, 35, 37, 44).

Animal studies have shown that the bone formation response to loading is activated immediately with biochemical and mRNA changes detected within minutes and hours of loading (153). The modeling response is independent of prior osteoclast activation and results in net bone formation. Osteoblasts appear on the surface within 48 hours of loading and bone formation rate is accelerated by day 5 (32, 51). If loads are maintained, maximal bone formation rates are achieved within 3 weeks and may be complete within 12 to 18 weeks (44, 154). Generally the response is relative to strain magnitude and localized to surfaces with the greatest strain (44). The net effect of this modeling response is to quickly increase bone size and mass to reduce strain or deformation.

BMD measures of bone adaptation can be misleading, because maximal strength gains occur with periosteal apposition, which, when combined with normal growth (periosteal formation, endocortical resorption), can result in lower areal BMD, despite greater BMC. A limitation of many published exercise papers is the analysis of BMD without discussion of BMC or areal changes. Measurements that assess changes in bone shape (moment of inertia) as well as bone mass are required to evaluate structural adaptation to loading (i.e., strength changes).

Skeletal Response to Exercise

In humans, physical training can measurably increase bone mineral within weeks. In a 14-week Israeli infantry-training program, bone mineral content at the distal tibia increased 11.1% in the left leg and 5.2% in the right (155). Although that increase was phenomenal, others have shown BMD increases in recruits with 2.2% at the tibia after 15 weeks of training (156); in gymnasts with 2.8% at the spine and 1.6% at the femoral neck after 8 months of training (157); and in men after 16 weeks of strength training with 2% at the spine and 3.8% at the femoral neck (139).

Exercise does not always have a positive effect on bone mass. In some cases where loaded bones show increased bone density, total body bone mass or bone in other regions may be unchanged or lower. Men with increased femoral neck and spine BMD, and elevated formation markers, showed no change in total body BMD (139). This could be because there was a redistribution of calcium from non-loaded to loaded regions or because the gain in bone at the loaded sites was relatively small when compared to total bone mass.

Skeletal Overload and Stress Fracture

When strains on bone during exercise are too great or continue for excessive cycle numbers, then they can create a pathologic overload and bone microdamage. Surface formation rates become maximal, and remodeling is stimulated to remove and replace damaged bone (20, 30, 158, 159). The remodeling period in humans averages 4 months, with 1 month of resorption followed by 3 months of formation (160). Porosity from microdamage repair would peak between weeks 3 and 6 as damage begins to accumulate and before formation is fully activated (30). This time frame corresponds with peak fracture rates during basic training. As fatigue damage increases, bone strength decreases and porosity from remodeling further reduces bone strength. Meanwhile, physical training demands increase, adding additional stresses to the weakened structure. The cumulative effect can range from a periosteal stress reaction to a complete dislocated fracture. To avoid fracture, bone formation must increase at a rapid rate.

Summary

Bone health is defined as the ability to avoid fracture; osteoporosis is a disease of skeletal fragility characterized by low-trauma fractures. Osteoporotic fractures occur when bone mass and structure become too weak to support forces created during activities of daily living. Osteoporosis can be diagnosed by clinical measures of bone mass, but the morbidity of the disease is often not noticeable until fractures occur. Bone metabolism has a complex physiology geared toward maintaining serum calcium levels for homeostasis and bone strength for movement. The 3 primary bone cells are osteoblasts that form new bone, osteocytes that maintain bone, and osteoclasts that remove bone. The activities of these cells are synchronized through intracellular communications to maintain bone balance. Exercise creates mechanical loads, or force, on bone as muscles contract or as the body lands, takes off, or contacts objects. These forces cause momentary and slight bending of the bone, or strain. When mechanical loads create excessive strains, bone mass increases and shape changes until what was

once an overload is within a "normal" range. Conversely, when training discontinues or disuse occurs and bone loads or strains fall below normal, bone mass decreases until strains return to a "normal" range. Bone cell formation is activated by high strains and bone loss occurs in the absence of strains.

What We Know
About Osteoporosis and Exercise

1 Although genetics play a major role in determining potential peak bone mass, bone accrual depends upon lifestyle factors such as calcium intake and exercise. Many scientists now view osteoporosis as a disease of pediatric origin, since bone gain during growth is crucial for lifelong bone health.

2 As with muscle, bones that are loaded or involved with heavy exercise hypertrophy, and bones that are in disuse atrophy. Long-term bed rest and space flight are dramatic forms of bone disuse that appear to share similar characteristics. Temporary bed rest results in bone loss averaging 1% per week (60–62). However, space flight removes all normal gravitational loads from bone and creates more extreme disuse than bed rest.

3 Poor nutrient intake and extreme exercise can have serious health consequences in women. As the body adapts to inadequate diets, bone calcium is depleted to maintain serum calcium homeostasis and often the ovaries shut down, resulting in the loss of menses or amenorrhea. Amenorrhea, like menopause, is an outward sign that the body is estrogen deficient, and estrogen is essential for maintaining bone mass in adult women.

4 Resistance training is effective in reversing the effects of osteoporosis while also being a time-efficient and cost-effective preventative measure for increasing BMD and muscle strength.

What We Would Like to Know
About Osteoporosis and Exercise

1 The method of mechanical regulation is not completely understood, but it appears that when a bone bends due to loading, bone cells such as the osteocytes and osteoblasts detect stretch, fluid flow, and/or electrical currents. It is postulated that these cells transduce the mechanical signal into a cellular response that initiates the adaptive response.

2 The interaction of pharmaceuticals and exercise is not well understood. A potential explanation is that drugs and hormones interact with exercise to alter bone sensitivity and magnify or diminish the response to exercise. This has not been well demonstrated in animals and is untested in humans.

3 Researchers are currently trying to elucidate the appropriate intensity level for resistance training for maximal bone response.

4 With regard to bone responses, the physiologic adaptations to exercise are site specific. Although exercise can induce changes in gonadal, growth, and stress hormones, their effects are thought to either magnify or diminish the local response. These potential adaptations require additional study.

DISCUSSION QUESTIONS

1 What are the most common sites of osteoporotic fractures?

2 Identify the 3 types of bone cells and the function of each.

3 What are the components of the female triad, and how does each influence bone health?

4 What treatment steps should be taken to ensure adequate bone health?

5 Explain the resistance training principles recommended for elderly persons.

REFERENCES

1. Kanis JA, Melton J, Christiansen C, Johnston CC, Khaltaev N. The diagnosis of osteoporosis. J Bone Miner Res 1994;9(8):1137–1141.
2. Melton LJ, Chrischilles EA, Cooper C, Lane AW, Riggs L. Perspective: how many women have osteoporosis. J Bone Miner Res 1992;7:1005–1010.
3. Matkovic V, Jelic T, Wardlaw G, et al. Timing of peak bone mass in caucasian females and its implication for the prevention of osteoporosis: inference from a cross-sectional model. J Clin Invest 1994;93:799–808.
4. Tylavsky F, Bortz A, Hancock R, Anderson J. Familial resemblance of radial bone mass between premenopausal mothers and their college-age daughters. Calcif Tissue Int 1989;45:265–272.
5. Recker RR, Davies KM, Hinders SM, Heaney RP, Stegman MR, Kimmel DB. Bone gain in young adult women. JAMA 1992;268:2403–2408.
6. Rodin A, Murby B, Smith MA, et al. Premenopausal bone loss in the lumbar spine and neck of femur: a study of 225 Caucasian women. Bone1990;11:1–5.
7. Davee A, Rosen C, Adler R. Exercise patterns and trabecular bone density in college women. J Bone Miner Res 1990;2:245–250.
8. Goulding A, Jones LE, Taylor R, Manning PJ, Williams SM. More broken bones: a 4-year double cohort study of young girls with and without distal forearm fractures. J Bone Miner Res 2000;15(10):2011–2018.
9. Goulding A, Cannan R, Williams SM, Gold EJ, Taylor RW, Lewis-Barned N. Bone mineral density in girls with forearm fractures. J Bone Miner Res 1998;13:143–148.
10. NIH Consensus Development Panel on Optimal Calcium Intake. Optimal calcium intake. JAMA 1994;272(24):1942–1948.
11. Ott S. Bone density in adolescents. New Engl J Med 1991;325:1646–1647.
12. Consensus Development Conference. Diagnosis, prophylaxis, and treatment of osteoporosis. 1993:1–10.
13. Adami S. Optimizing peak bone mass: what are the therapeutic possibilities? Osteoporos Int 1994;4(suppl 1):s27–s30.
14. Cummings C, Black D, Nevitt M, et al. Bone density at various sites for prediction of hip fractures. Lancet 1993;341:72–75.
15. Ray NF, Chan JK, Thamer M, Melton LJ. Medical expenditures for the treatment of osteoporotic fractures in the United States in 1995: report from the National Osteoporosis Foundation. J Bone Miner Res 1997;12:24–35.
16. Cummings S, Rubin S, Black D. The future of hip fractures in the United States: numbers, costs, and potential effects of postmenopausal estrogen. Clin Orthop 1990;252:163–166.
17. Lanyon LE. Osteocytes, strain detection, bone modeling and remodeling. Calcif Tissue Int 1993;53:S102–S107.
18. Frost HM. Bone mass and the mechanostat: a proposal. Anat Rec 1987;219:1–9.
19. Frost HM. Why do long-distance runners not have more bone? A vital biomechanical explanation and an estrogen effect. J Bone Miner Res 1997;15:9–16.
20. Burr DB. Bone, exercise, and stress fractures. Exerc Sport Sci Rev 1997;25:171–194.
21. Rubin CT, Lanyon LE. Dynamic strain similarity in vertebrates; an alternative to allometric limb bone scaling. J Theor Biol 1984;107:321–327.
22. Rubin CT, Lanyon LE. Limb mechanics as a function of speed and gait: a study of functional strains in the radius and tibia of horse and dog. J Exp Biol 1982;101:187–211.
23. Burr DB, Milgrom C, Fyhrie D, et al. In vivo measurement of human tibial strains during vigorous activity. Bone 1996;18(5):405–410.
24. Carter DR, Caler WE, Spengler DM, Frankel VH. Fatigue behavior of adult cortical bone: the influence of mean strain and strain range. Acta Orthop Scand 1981;52:481–490.
25. Myburgh KH, Hutchins J, Fataar AB, Hough SF, Noakes TD. Low bone density is an etiologic factor for stress fractures in athletes. Ann Intern Med 1990;113:754–759.
26. Beck TJ, Ruff CB, Shaffer RA, Betsinger K, Trone DW, Brodine SK. Stress fracture in military recruits: gender differences in muscle and bone susceptibility factors. Bone 2000;27(3):437–444.
27. Lauder TD, Dixit S, Pezzin LE, Williams MV, Campbell CS, Davis GD. The relation between stress fractures and bone mineral density: evidence from active-duty Army women. Arch Phys Med Rehabil 2000;81(1):73–79.
28. Winfield AC, Moore J, Bracker M, Johnson CW. Risk factors associated with stress reactions in female Marines. Mil Med 1997;162(10):698–702.
29. Milgrom C, Finestone A, Shlamkovitch N, et al. Youth is a risk factor for stress fracture. A study of 783 infantry recruits. J Bone Joint Surg Br 1994;76(1):20–22.
30. Burr DB, Forwood MR, Fyhrie DP, Martin RB, Schaffler MB, Turner CH. Bone microdamage and skeletal fragility in osteoporotic and stress fractures. J Bone Miner Res 1997;12:6–9.
31. Carter DR, Caler WE, Spengler DM, Frankel VH. Uniaxial fatigue of human cortical bone. The influence of tissue physical characteristics. J Biomech 1981;14:461–470.
32. Boppart MD, Kimmel DB, Yee JA, Cullen DM. Time course of osteoblast appearance after in vivo mechanical loading. Bone 1998;23(5):409–415.
33. Pead MJ, Skerry TM, Lanyon LE. Direct transformation from quiescence to bone formation in the adult periosteum following a single brief period of bone loading. J Bone Miner Res 1988;3:647–655.

34. Hillam RA, Skerry TM. Inhibition of bone resorption and stimulation of formation by mechanical loading of the modeling rat ulna in vivo. J Bone Miner Res 1995;10(5):683–689.

35. Yeh JK, Aloia JF, Chen MM, Tierney JM, Sprintz S. Influence of exercise on cancellous bone of the aged female rat. J Bone Miner Res 1993;8(9):1117–1125.

36. Dalsky GP, Stocke KS, Ehsani AA, Slatopolsky E, Lee WC, Birge SJ. Weight-bearing exercise training and lumbar bone mineral content in postmenopausal women. Ann Intern Med 1988;108:824–828.

37. Raab DM, Crenshaw TD, Kimmel DB, Smith EL. A histomorphometric study of cortical bone activity during increased weight-bearing exercise. J Bone Miner Res 1991;7:741–749.

38. Raab DM, Smith EL, Crenshaw TD, Thomas DP. Bone mechanical properties after exercise training in young and old rats. J Appl Physiol 1990;68:130–134.

39. Steinberg ME, Trueta J. Effects of activity on bone growth and development in the rat. Clin Orthop 1981;156:52–60.

40. Yeh JK, Aloia JF, Tierney JM, Sprintz S. Effect of treadmill exercise on vertebral and tibial bone mineral content and bone mineral density in the aged adult rat: determined by dual energy x-ray absorptiometry. Calcif Tissue Int 1993;52:234–238.

41. Yeh JK, Aloia JF, Chen M. Growth hormone administration potentiates the effect of treadmill exercise on long bone formation but not on the vertebrae in middle-aged rats. Calcif Tissue Int 1994;54:38–43.

42. Forwood MR, Parker AW. Repetitive loading, in vivo, of the tibiae and femora of rats: effects of repeated bouts of treadmill running. Bone Miner 1991;13:35–46.

43. Turner CH, Woltman TA, Belongia DA. Structural changes in rat bone subjected to long-term, in vivo mechanical loading. Bone 1992;13:417–422.

44. Raab-Cullen DM, Akhter MP, Kimmel DB, Recker RR. Bone response to alternate day mechanical loading of the rat tibia. J Bone Miner Res 1994;9:203–211.

45. Chambers TJ, Evans M, Gardner TN, Turner-Smith A, Chow JWM. Induction of bone formation in rat tail vertebrae by mechanical loading. Bone Miner 1993;20:167–178.

46. Rubin CT, Lanyon LE. Regulation of bone formation by applied dynamic loads. J Bone Joint Surg 1984;66-A:397–402.

47. Lanyon LE, Bourn S. The influence of mechanical function on the development and remodeling of the tibia. An experimental study in sheep. J Bone Joint Surg 1979;61A:263–273.

48. Burr DB, Shaffler MB, Yang KH, et al. Skeletal changes in response to altered strain environments: is woven bone a response to elevated strain? Bone 1989;10:223–233.

49. Burr DB, Schaffler MB, Yang KH, et al. The effects of altered strain environment on bone tissue kinetics. Bone 1989;10:215–221.

50. Chow JWM, Wilson AJ, Chambers TJ, Fox SW. Mechanical loading stimulates bone formation by reactivation of bone lining cells in 13-week-old rats. J Bone Miner Res 1998;13:1760–1767.

51. Forwood MR, Owan I, Takano Y, Turner CH. Increased bone formation in rat tibiae after a single short period of dynamic loading in vivo. Am J Physiol 1996;270:E419–23.

52. Hagino H, Raab DM, Kimmel DB, Akhter MP, Recker RR. The effects of ovariectomy on bone response to in vivo external loading. J Bone Miner Res 1993;8:347–357.

53. Raab-Cullen DM, Akhter MP, Kimmel DB, Recker RR. Periosteal bone formation stimulated by externally induced bending strains. J Bone Miner Res 1994;9:1143–1152.

54. Cullen DM, Smith RT, Akhter MP. Time course for bone formation with long term external mechanical loading. J Appl Physiol 2000;88:1943–1948.

55. Cullen DM, Smith RT, Akhter MP. Bone loading response varies with strain magnitude and cycle number. J Appl Physiol 2001;91:1971–1976.

56. Frost HM. Skeletal structural adaptations to mechanical usage (SATMU): 1. Redefining Wolff's law: the bone modeling problem. Anat Rec 1990;226:403–413.

57. Hancock DA, Reed GW, Atkinson PJ, Cook JB, Smith PH. Bone and soft tissue changes in paraplegic patients. Paraplegia 1980;17:267–271.

58. Kiratli BJ. Skeletal Adaptation to Disuse: Longitudinal and Cross-Sectional Study of the Response of the Femur and Spine to Immobilization (Paralysis) [thesis/dissertation]. Madison: University of Wisconsin; 1989.

59. Biering-Sorensen F, Bohr H, Schaadt O. Longitudinal study of bone mineral content in the lumbar spine, the forearm and the lower extremities after spinal cord injury. Eur J Clin Invest 1990;20:330–335.

60. Donaldson CL, Hulley SB, Vogel JM, Hattner RS, Bayers JH, McMillan DE. Effect of prolonged bed rest on bone mineral. Metabolism 1970;19:1071–1084.

61. Hulley SB, Vogel JM, Donaldson CL, Baynor JH, Friedman RJ, Rosen SN. The effect of supplemental oral phosphate on the bone mineral changes during prolonged bed rest. J Clin Invest 1971;50:2506–2518.

62. LeBlanc AD, Schneider VS, Evans HJ, Engelbretson DA, Krebs JM. Bone mineral loss and recovery after 17 weeks of bed rest. J Bone Miner Res 1990;5(8):843–850.

63. LeBlanc A, Schneider V, Shackelford L, et al. Bone mineral and lean tissue loss after long duration space flight. J Bone Miner Res 1996;11:S323.

64. Collet P, Uebelhart D, Vico L, Hartmann G, Roth M, Alexandre C. Effects of 1- and 6-month space flight on bone mass and biochemistry in two humans. Bone 1997;20(6):547–551.

65. LeBlanc A, Shackelford L, Schneider V. Future human bone research in space. Bone 1998;22(5):113S–116S.

66. Rubin J, Fan X, Biskobing DM, Taylor WR, Rubin CT. Osteoclastogenesis is repressed by mechanical strain in an in vitro model. J Orthop Res 1999;17(5):639–645.

67. Escalante-Boleas M, Franco-Vicario R, Bustamante-Murga V, Miguel-de-la-Villa F. Metabolismo oseo y perdida de masa osea en los trastornos de la alimentaction. An Med Interna 2002;19(3):143–150.

68. Nagel DL, Black DR, Leverenz LJ, Coser DC. Evaluation of screening test for female college athletes with eating disorders and disordered eating. J Athletic Training 2000;35(4):431–440.

69. Daluiski A, Rahbar B, Meals RA. Russell's sign. Subtle changes in patients with bulimia nervosa. Clin Orthop 1997;343:107–109.

70. Grinspoon S, Millerl K, Coyle C, et al. Severity of osteopenia in estrogen-deficient women with anorexia nervosa and hypothalamic amenorrhea. J Clin Endocrinol Metab 1999;84(6):2049–2055.

71. Csermely T, Halvax L, Schmidt E, et al. Occurrence of osteopenia among adolescent girls with oligo/amenorrhea. Gynecol Endocrinol 2002;16(2):99–105.

72. Powers PS. Osteoporosis and eating disorders. J Pediatr Adolesc Gynecol 1999;12(2):51–57.

73. Clowes JA, Peel N, Eastell R. Glucocorticoid-induced osteoporosis. Curr Opin Rheumatol 2001;13(4):326–332.

74. Dequeker J. NSAIDs/corticosteroids—primum non nocere. Adv Exp Med Biol 1999;455:319–325.

75. Lane NE. An update on glucocorticoid-induced osteoporosis. Rheum Dis Clin North Am 2001;27(1):235–253.

76. Patschan D, Lodderkemper K, Buttgereit F. Molecular mechanisms of glucocorticoid-induced osteoporosis. Bone 2001;29(6):498–505.

77. Deal CL. Osteoporosis: prevention, diagnosis, and management. Am J Med 1997;102(1A):35S–39S.

78. Stephen LJ, McLellan AR, Harrison JH, et al. Bone density and antiepileptic drugs: a case-controlled study. Seizure 1999;8(6):339–342.

79. Pack AM, Morrell MJ. Adverse effects of antiepileptic drugs on bone structure: epidemiology, mechanisms and therapeutic implications. CNS Drugs 2001;15(8):633–642.

80. Sato Y, Kondo I, Ishida S, et al. Decreased bone mass and increased bone turnover with valproate therapy in adults with epilepsy. Neurology 2001;57(3):445–449.

81. Feldkamp J, Becker A, Witte OW, Scharff D, Scherbaum WA. Long-term anticonvulsant therapy leads to low bone mineral density—evidence for direct drug effects of phenytoin and carbamazepine on human osteoblast-like cells. Exp Clin Endocrinol Diabetes 2000;108(1):37–43.

82. Farhat G, Yamout B, Mikati MA, Demirjian S, Sawaya R, El-Hajj-Fuleihan G. Effect of antiepileptic drugs on bone density in ambulatory patients. Neurology 2002;58(9):1348–1353.

83. Harris SS. Effects of caffeine consumption on hip fracture, bone density, and calcium retention. In: Burckhardt P, Dawson-Hughes B, Heaney RP, eds. Nutritional Aspects of Osteoporosis. New York: Springer-Verlag; 1998:163–171.

84. Barger-Lux MJ, Heaney RP, Packard PP, Lappe JM, Recker RR. Caffeine and the calcium economy revisited. Osteoporosis 1995;5:97–102.

85. Ganry O, Baudoin C, Fardellone P. Effect of alcohol intake on bone mineral density in elderly women: The EPIDOS Study. Am J Epidemiol 2000;151(8):773–780.

86. Boonyaratavej N, Suriyawongpaisal P, Takkinsatien A, Wanvarie S, Rajatanavin R, Apiyasawat P. Physical activity and risk factors for hip fractures in Thai women. Osteoporos Int 2001;12(3):244–248.

87. Turner RT, Kidder LS, Kennedy A, Evans GL, Sibonga JD. Moderate alcohol consumption suppresses bone turnover in adult female rats. J Bone Miner Res 2001;16(3):589–594.

88. Turner CH, Hsieh YF, Muller R, et al. Genetic regulation of cortical and trabecular bone strength and microstructure in inbred strains of mice. J Bone Miner Res 2000;15(6):1126–1131.

89. Farley JR, Fitzsimmons R, Taylor AK, Jorch UM, Lau KH. Direct effects of ethanol on bone resorption and formation in vitro. Arch Biochem Biophys 1985;238(1):305–314.

90. NIH Consensus Statement. Osteoporosis Prevention, Diagnosis, and Therapy. March 27–29, 2000;17(1):1–36.

91. Looker AC, Orwoll ES, Johnston CC, et al. Prevalence of low femoral bone density in older US adults from NHANES III. J Bone Miner Res 1997;12(11):1761–1768.

92. Tenenhouse A, Joseph L, Kreiger N, et al. Estimation of the prevalence of low bone density in Canadian women and men using a population-specific DXA reference standard: the Canadian Multicentre Osteoporosis Study (CaMos). Osteoporos Int 2000;11(10):897–904.

93. Sanders KM, Seeman E, Ugoni AM, et al. Age- and gender-specific rate of fracture in Australia: a population-based study. Osteoporos Int 1999;10(3):240–247.

94. Kanis JA, Johnell O, Oden A, Jonsson B, DeLaet C, Dawson A. Risk of hip fracture according to the World Health Organization criteria for osteopenia and osteoporosis. Bone 2000;27(5):585–590.

95. Kenny A, Taxel P. Osteoporosis in older men. Clin Cornerstone 2000;2(6):45–51.

96. Vanderschueren D, Vandenput L. Androgens and osteoporosis. Andrologia 2000;32:125–130.

97. Murrillo-Uribe A, Deleze-Hinojosa M, Aguirre E, et al. Osteoporosis in Mexican postmenopausal women. Magnitude of the problem. Multicenter study. Ginecol Obstet Mex 1999;May:67227–67233.

98. Looker AC, Johnston CC, Wahner HW, et al. Prevalence of low femoral bone density in older US women from NHANES III. J Bone Miner Res 1995;10(5):796–802.

99. Henry YM, Eastell R. Ethnic and gender differences in bone mineral density and bone turnover in young adults; effect of bone size. Osteoporos Int 2000;11(6):512–517.

100. Fujita T. Osteoporosis in Japan: factors contributing to the low incidence of hip fracture. Adv Nutr Res 1994;9:89–99.

101. Lau EMC, Suriwongpaisal P, Saw SM, Das-De S, Khir A, Sambrook P. The incidence of hip fracture in four Asian countries: the Asian Osteoporosis Study (AOS). Osteoporos Int 2001;12(3):239–243.

102. Ihrke K. Osteoporosis: risk factors, diagnostic methods and treatment options. Internet Journal of Academic Physician Assistants [serial online] 1997;1(1):5 pages. Available at: http://www.ispub.com/journals/ijapa.htm

103. Shoupe D. Androgens and bone: clinical implications for menopausal women. Am J Obstet Gynecol 1999;180(3 Pt 2):S329–S333.

104. Favus M. Reducing hip fracture risk in patients confined to long-term care facilities: a review of clinical data. Ann Long-Term Care 1998;6(10):315–322.

105. Dychtwald K. "Age power": how the new-old will transform medicine in the 21st century. Geriatrics 1999;54(12):22–27.

106. Heaney R, Barger-Lux J. Calcium, bone metabolism, and structural failure. Triangle 1985;24:91–100.

107. Holick MF. Vitamin D requirements for humans of all ages: new increased requirements for women and men 50 years and older. Osteoporos Int 1998;8:24–29.

108. Vieth R. Vitamin D supplementation, 25-hydroxyvitamin D concentrations, and safety. Am J Clin Nutr 1999;69:842–856.

109. Gloth FM, Tobin JD. Vitamin D deficiency in older people. J Am Geriatr Soc 1995;43(7):822–828.

110. Alenfeld F, Wuster C, Funck C, et al. Ultrasound measurements at the proximal phalanges in healthy women and patients with hip fractures. Osteoporos Int 1998;8:393–398.

111. Holick MF. Vitamin D: the underappreciated D-lightful hormone that is important for skeletal and cellular health. Curr Opin Endocrinol Diabetes 2002;9(87):98.

112. Recker RR, Lappe JM, Davies K, Heaney RP. Characterization of perimenopausal bone loss: a prospective study. J Bone Miner Res 2000;15:1965–1973.

113. Recker R, Davies KM, Dowd RM, Heaney RP. The effect of low-dose continuous estrogen and progesterone therapy with calcium and vitamin D on bone in elderly women. Ann Intern Med 1999;130:897–904.

114. Rodan GA, Martin TJ. Therapeutic approaches to bone disease. Science 2000;289:1508–1514.

115. Riggs BL, O'Fallon WM, Lane A, et al. Clinical trial of fluoride therapy in postmenopausal osteoporotic women: extended observations and additional analysis. J Bone Miner Res 1994;9(2):265–275.

116. Pak CY, Sakhaee K, Adams-Huet B, Piziak V, Peterson RD, Poindexter JR. Treatment of postmenopausal osteoporosis with slow-release sodium fluoride. Ann Intern Med 1995;123:401–408.

117. Lane NE, Sanchez S, Modin GW, Genant HK, Pierini E, Arnaud CD. Parathyroid hormone treatment can reverse corticosteroid-induced osteoporosis. Results of a randomized controlled clinical trial. J Clin Invest 1998;102(8):1627–1633.

118. Hardouin P, Fayada P, Leclet H, Chopin D. Kyphoplasty. Joint Bone Spine 2002;69(3):256–261.

119. Kannus P, Parkkari J, Niemi S, et al. Prevention of hip fractures in elderly people with use of a hip protector. N Engl J Med 2000;343:1506–1513.

120. Lohman T, Going S, Pamenter R, et al. Effects of resistance training on regional and total bone mineral density in premenopausal women: a randomized prospective study. J Bone Miner Res 1995;10(7):1015–1024.

121. Bassey EJ, Ramsdale SJ. Weight-bearing exercise and ground reaction forces: a 12-month randomized controlled trial of effects on bone mineral density in healthy postmenopausal women. Bone 1995;16(4):469–476.

122. Bassey EJ, Rothwell MC, Littlewood JJ, Pye DW. Pre- and postmenopausal women have different bone mineral density responses to the same high-impact exercise. Bone Miner 1998;13(12):1805–1813.

123. Heaney RP. Pathophysiology of osteoporosis. Endocrinol Metab Clin North Am 1998;27(2):255–265.

124. Gerber NJ. Prophylaxis of falls and treatment of fractures. Baillieres Clin Rheumatol 1993;7(3):561–571.

125. Nelson ME, Fiatarone MA, Morganti CM, Trice I, Greenberg RA, Evans WJ. Effects of high-intensity strength training on multiple risk factors for osteoporotic fractures: a randomized controlled trial. JAMA 1994;272(24):1909–1914.

126. Butler RN, Davis R, Lewis CB, Nelson ME, Strauss E. Physical fitness: benefits of exercise for the older patient. 2. Geriatrics 1998;53(10):46, 49–52.

127. Merla JL, Spaulding SJ. The balance system: implications for occupational therapy intervention. Phys Occup Ther Geriatr 1997;15(1):21–36.

128. Mazzeo RS, Cavanagh P, Evans WJ, et al. American College of Sports Medicine position stand: exercise and physical activity for older adults. Med Sci Sports Exerc 1998;30(6):992–1008.

129. Vargo MM. Osteoporosis: strategies for prevention and treatment. J Musculoskeletal Medicine 1995;12(5):19–30.

130. Raab DM, Agre JC, McAdam M, Smith EL. Light resistance and stretching exercise in elderly women: effects upon flexibility. Arch Phys Med Rehabil 1988;69:268–272.

131. Pearlmutter LL, Bode BY, Wilkinson WE, Maricic MJ. Shoulder range of motion in patients with osteoporosis. Arthritis Care Res 1995;8(3):194–198.

132. Bravo G, Gauthier P, Roy PM, et al. Comparison of a group- versus a home-based exercise program in osteopenic women. J Aging Physical Activity 1996;4:151–164.

133. Fiatarone MA, O'Neill EF, Ryan ND, et al. Exercise training and nutritional supplementation for physical frailty in very elderly people. N Engl J Med 1994;330(25):1769–1775.

134. Smith EL, Reddan W, Smith PE. Physical activity and calcium modalities for bone mineral increase in aged women. Med Sci Sports Exerc 1981;13:60–64.

135. Vanderhoek KJ, Coupland DC, Parkhouse WS. Effects of 32 weeks of resistance training on strength and balance in older osteopenic/osteoporotic women. Clin Exerc Physiol 2000;2:77–83.

136. Kerschan-Schmidt K, Uher E, Grampp S, et al. A neuromuscular test battery for osteoporotic women: a pilot study. Am J Phys Med Rehabil 2001;80(5):351–357.

137. Buchner DM, Beresford SA, Larson EB, LaCroix AZ, Wagner EH. Effects of physical activity on health status in older adults. II. Intervention studies. Annu Rev Public Health 1992;13469–13488.

138. Butler RN, Davis R, Lewis CB, Nelson ME, Strauss E. Physical fitness: exercise prescription for older adults. 3. Geriatrics 1998;53(11):45–50, 52.

139. Menkes A, Mazel S, Redmond RA, et al. Strength training increases regional bone mineral density and bone remodeling in middle-aged and older men. J Appl Physiol 1993;74:2478–2484.

140. Ryan AS, Treuth MS, Rubin MA, et al. Effects of strength training on bone mineral density: hormonal and bone turnover relationships. American Physiological Society 1994;77:1678–1684.

141. Stevens JA, Olson S. Reducing falls and resulting hip fractures among older women. MMWR Morb Mortal Wkly Rep 2000;49(RR-2):1–12.

142. Tommerup LJ, Raab DM, Crenshaw TD, Smith EL. Does weight bearing exercise affect non-weight bearing bone? J Bone Miner Res 1993;8(9):1053–1058.

143. Rubin C, Turto H, Jerome C, et al. Low magnitude, high frequency mechanical stimulation increases trabecular density of the proximal femur. J Bone Miner Res 1998;23:S179.

144. O'Connor JA, Lanyon LE, MacFie H. The influence of strain rate on adaptive bone remodeling. J Biomech 1982;15:767–781.

145. Fleck SJ, Kraemer WJ. Designing Resistance Training Programs. 2nd ed. Champaign, Ill: Human Kinetics; 1997.

146. Layne JE, Nelson ME. The effects of progressive resistance training on bone density: a review. Med Sci Sports Exerc 1999;31(1):25–30.

147. Kerr D, Morton A, Dick I, Prince R. Exercise effects on bone mass in postmenopausal women are site-specific and load-dependent. J Bone Miner Res 1996;11:218–224.

148. Feigenbaum MS, Pollack ML. Prescription of resistance training for health and disease. Med Sci Sports Exerc 1999;31(1):38–45.

149. Rubin C, Turner AS, Mallinckrodt C, Jerome C, McLeod K, Bain S. Mechanical strain, induced noninvasively in the high-frequency domain, is anabolic to cancellous bone, but not cortical bone. Bone 2002;30(3):445–452.

150. Rubin CT, Lanyon LE. Regulation of bone mass by mechanical strain magnitude. Calcif Tissue Int 1985;37:411–417.

151. McLeod KJ, Rubin CT. Sensitivity of the bone remodeling response to the frequency of applied strain. Transactions of the 38th Annual Meeting Orthopaedic Research Society 1992;17:533.

152. Turner CH, Owan I, Takano Y. Mechanotransduction in bone: the role of strain rate. Am J Physiol 1995;269(3 pt 1):E438–442.

153. Raab-Cullen DM. In vivo bone cell histology and biochemical responses to mechanical loading. In: Maughan RJ, ed. Biochemistry of Exercise IX. Champaign, Ill: Human Kinetics; 1996:543–554.

154. Cullen DM, Iwaniec U, Barger-Lux MJ. Skeletal response to exercise and training. In: Garret W, Kirkendall D, eds. Exercise: Basic and Applied Science. Baltimore, Md: Lippincott Williams & Wilkins; 2000:227–237.

155. Margulies JY, Simkin A, Leichter I, et al. Effect of intense physical activity on the bone-mineral content in the lower limbs of young adults. J Bone Joint Surg 1986;68-A:1090–1093.

156. Casez JP, Fischer S, Stussi E, et al. Bone mass at lumbar spine and tibia in young males—impact of physical fitness, exercise, and anthropometric parameters: a prospective study in a cohort of military recruits. Bone 1995;17:211–219.

157. Taaffe DR, Robinson TL, Snow CM, Marcus R. High-impact exercise promotes bone gain in well-trained female athletes. J Bone Miner Res 1997;12(2):255–260.

158. Bentolila V, Boyce TM, Fyhrie DP, Drumb R, Skerry TM, Schaffler MB. Intracortical remodeling in adult rat long bones after fatigue loading. Bone 1998;23(3):275–281.

159. Verborgt O, Gibson GJ, Schaffler MB. Loss of osteocyte integrity in association with microdamage and bone remodeling after fatigue in vivo. J Bone Miner Res 2000;15(1):60–67.

160. Parfitt AM. The cellular basis of bone remodeling: the quantum concept reexamined in light of recent advances in the cell biology of bone. Calcif Tissue Int 1984;36s:S37–S45.

161. Popovich RM, Gardner JW, Potter R, Knapik JJ, Jones BH. Effect of rest from running on overuse injuries in army basic training. Am J Prev Med 2000;18(suppl 3):147–155.

SUGGESTED READINGS

Gloth FM, Tobin JD. Vitamin D deficiency in older people. J Am Geriatr Soc 1995;43(7): 822–828.

Kanis JA, Melton J, Christiansen C, Johnston CC, Khaltaev N. The diagnosis of osteoporosis. J Bone Miner Res 1994;9(8):1137–1141.

Layne JE, Nelson ME. The effects of progressive resistance training on bone density: a review. Med Sci Sports Exerc 1999;25–30.

Mazzeo RS, Cavanagh P, Evans WJ, et al. American College of Sports Medicine position stand: exercise and physical activity for older adults. Med Sci Sports Exerc 1998;30(6):992–1008.

Rodan GA, Martin TJ. Therapeutic approaches to bone disease. Science 2000;289:1508–1514.

CHAPTER 32

Osteoarthritis and Rheumatoid Arthritis

Laura J. McIntosh, David M. Jenkinson,
Kenneth W. Rundell

Overview: Osteoarthritis

Osteoarthritis (OA) is more than just degeneration of **articular cartilage**; it is a failure of diarthrodial joints. Although degeneration of the cartilage is the most noticeable change, numerous alterations occur in bone structure, synovial fluid, and supporting musculature (1).

Age is the primary risk factor for osteoarthritis (1, 2) occurring in 60% to 70% of people over the age of 65. Women have a twofold increased risk for developing OA in knees, interphalangeal (IP) joints, and thumb metacarpophalangeal joints (4). Men, however, are more likely to have hip involvement (3). Weight and history of repetitive trauma are significant risk factors (4).

The role of exercise in the development of osteoarthritis is currently under investigation. Initial studies showed that regular recreational activity did not affect the probability of developing OA in the hip or knee (5–7). Supporting this concept, a 9-year longitudinal study of older runners (mean age 66) did not find significant radiographic differences in the hip or knee between runners and non-runners (8). However, a Swedish cohort study evaluating a woman's risk of developing hip OA from recreational and occupational activity (6) concluded that heavy participation in sports (>800 hours total) before the age of 50 doubled a woman's risk of developing OA. Adding in the risk associated with various occupations (jobs that require knee bending and lifting), some women may face a fourfold risk in developing OA in the hip.

Exercise of a normal joint may not increase the risk of developing degenerative joint disease, although normal joint activity in an abnormal joint does increase OA risk. Any joint abnormality (e.g., ligament disruption or joint laxity) that alters the stress distribution across the cartilage can produce injury with normal use (9). The relationship between exercise and degenerative joint disease is complicated by several factors, including a history of joint injury, genetics of the cartilage, muscle strength, body mass, coordination, training patterns, and choice of sports. Runners (competitive or recreational) seem to be at low risk of OA, but sports that involve more intense impact and torsional loading appear to predispose participants to OA (10).

There seems to be an inverse relationship between the risk of developing OA compared to osteoporosis. In osteoporosis, the thinning of the subchondral matrix due to bone reabsorption by the osteoclasts makes that bone a better shock absorber. The result is decreased load carried by, and less damage to, articular cartilage (4). This insight, when coupled with neuromuscular research on the anterior cruciate ligament (ACL) and female athletes (11, 12), points to the possibility of teaching female athletes to soften the impact to the joints, thereby decreasing the risk of developing OA later in life.

Pathophysiology

Articular cartilage plays diverse roles. Cartilage offers a super-smooth surface that permits one bone to move over another with little friction (4). Cartilage has mechanical properties that offer the ability to withstand compressive and shearing forces, and provide tensile strength or stiffness. This allows even distribution of weight-bearing loads across the joint (13).

Articular cartilage primarily consists of an **extracellular matrix** produced by chondrocytes. About 75% (dry weight) of this matrix consists of **type II collagen fibrils** that provide tissue strength and tensile stiffness. The remaining 25% of the matrix's dry weight is composed of **proteoglycans**—large polymers of aggregating macromolecules called aggregans. Aggregans are responsible for the compressibility of the articular cartilage in load distribution (13). A single aggregan consists of a protein core with glycosaminoglycan chains radiating at 90° angles, giving the appearance of a test-tube brush. The glycosaminoglycan molecules include **chondroitin sulfate** and keratin sulfate chains (4). Individual aggregans are bound together by a single long chain of hyaluronic acid, forming the aggregating proteoglycans of the extracellular matrix. The macromolecule is negatively charged and therefore extremely hydrophilic. The hydrophilic nature of the matrix aids in the ability of the cartilage to deform during load bearing and recover shape when unloaded. The large size of the aggregate proteoglycans makes the macromolecules immobile, fixing it between the type II collagen fibers, creating the matrix. Nonaggregating proteoglycans, biglycan and decorin, are also found in close association with collagen fibers (4).

Matrix composition varies across the thickness of the cartilage. Superficially, the collagen fibers are tightly packed and parallel to the joint surface. The low proteoglycan content of this layer of articular cartilage results in less compressibility and deformation. In the middle layer, collagen fibers are randomly distributed and the proteoglycan content is at its maximum level for the tissue. In the deepest area of articular cartilage, the collagen fibers are larger and bundled and are arrayed perpendicularly to the subchondral bone. The proteoglycan content at this level is low (4, 13).

Turnover of normal extracellular matrix in cartilage is slow but continuous. Metalloproteinases like collagenase1-4, gelatinase, and stromelysin are secreted by chondrocytes and cause degradation of old macromolecules. These proteases, secreted by macrophages, are stimulated by **interleukin-1** (IL-1) and **tumor necrosis factor-α** (TNF-α). Chondrocytes also produce plasminogen, which is a substrate for tissue plasminogen activator. All of these enzymes cause breakdown of collagen and proteoglycans and inhibit proteoglycan synthesis (4).

The degenerative activity of the proteolytic enzymes is regulated by at least 2 inhibitors: **tissue inhibitor of metalloproteinase** and plasminogen activator inhibitor 1. Growth factors like tumor growth factor-B (TGF-B) and insulin-like growth factor-1 (IGF-1) stimulate chondrocyte secretion of proteoglycans as well as inhibiting the catabolic actions of IL-1 (4, 14).

Osteoarthritis develops when normal cartilage and bone are exposed to excessive stresses, or when biomechanically abnormal cartilage or bone is exposed to normal stress. Early in the disease process, thickening of the cartilage occurs (4). Damage to the superficial collagen increases the loading on chondrocytes deeper in the matrix, producing increased production of nonaggregating and aggregating proteoglycans. Immunohistochemistry reveals that structure of the chondroitin sulfate molecules on these up-regulated aggregans is altered (14). An increased concentration of the proteoglycans causes the water content of the extracellular matrix to increase; this process initially helps the joint surface in responding to the superficial damage. As the disease progresses, the reparative ability of the tissue diminishes, the articular cartilage begins to thin and soften, and the integrity of the smooth surface is broken by superficial cracks called **fibrillations**. These fibrillations are associated with a loss of type II collagen fibrils and subsequent loss of the nonaggregating and aggregating proteoglycans (4).

The loss of type II collagen and proteoglycans originates from increased secretion of metalloproteinase. Increased chondrocyte sensitivity to the **cytokines** that activate the metalloproteinase has been demonstrated (e.g., TNF-α, through up-regulation of TNF-α receptors) (14, 15). However, no corresponding up-regulation of the activity to the tissue inhibitor of the metalloproteinase (TIMP) has been observed (15). TIMP is also produced by chondrocytes. Its inability to inhibit the metalloproteinase may be due to the sheer number of proteinases rather than defective action (4).

Nitric oxide synthetase is also up-regulated in OA, most likely because of the stimulating effect of IL-1 and TNF-α. Nitric oxide has been shown to play a role in cell apoptosis and may be involved in the loss of cellularity in osteoarthritic cartilage (14).

In addition to changes in cartilage, OA involves changes in the underlying bone. The cancellous subchondral bone is softer than cortical bone and serves as a **passive shock absorber**. When significant load is placed on the joint, the bone will absorb much of the energy, protecting the cartilage (4). With OA, appositional growth occurs in the subchondral bone, producing the sclerosis seen on x-ray films. Thickening of the cancellous bone reduces its ability to act as a shock absorber; thus more load is placed on the cartilage. This can produce microfractures in the subchondral trabeculae as well as localized osteonecrosis and cyst formation.

Osteophytes formed at the joint margins are a principal bony feature of OA. Osteophytes consist of a cap of articular cartilage and a base of actively remodeling bone. Osteophyte growth seems to be stimulated by transforming growth factor-B (14). Initially, the osteophytes may help stabilize the joint; however, they often grow large enough to interfere with range of motion (9). A second bony feature of OA is the ivory appearance of the eburnated bone. Classically, osteophyte size is evaluated by plain x-ray; however, the rate of bone turnover can be evaluated by measuring the urine level of bone-specific deoxypyridinoline cross-links.

Contracting muscles form an **active shock absorbing system** that shares a portion of the load experienced by a joint. Eccentric contractions of periarticular muscles assist with the greatest loads (e.g., walking, running, jumping) (4). Key to this concept, **quadriceps weakness** has been seen in asymptomatic and early OA (16). Atrophy of the supporting musculature from disease or lack of physical activity reduces the muscle's ability to dissipate energy. The precise cause of periarticular muscle atrophy is unclear. One theory under investigation is that changes in the joint inhibit neural activation of the muscle (17). Other inquiries are focusing on atrophy arising from lack of activation secondary to associated movement pain (18).

The inflammation or **synovitis** associated with OA is usually limited. As in **rheumatoid arthritis**, there seems to be a direct correlation between the amount of joint inflammation, level of hyaluronic acid, and disease progression (40). Accelerated OA progression is associated with persistently elevated levels of serum hyaluronic acid (40). There also seems to be a relationship between the level of hyaluronic acid in the synovial fluid and the amount of **joint space narrowing**. Another marker of joint space narrowing is elevated level of serum cartilage oligomeric protein, secreted by synovial cells and chondrocytes in response to transforming growth factor-B.

OA is an insidious disease. Initially, through compensatory actions described above, the tissue/joint is able to function normally. However, we have not found a way to reverse or halt the degradative process. A great deal of attention has focused on delaying disease progression and alleviating symptoms. Early intervention using appropriate strengthening and muscle-balancing exercise programs may aid in this early treatment of OA.

Clinical Presentation

There is no laboratory test for the diagnosis of OA. The diagnosis is based on the clinical and radiographic evidence. Clinical features include localized pain and inflammation. Initially there is pain with movement that may develop into pain at rest. There is also morning stiffness that resolves approximately 30 minutes after getting out of bed. Nocturnal pain, especially if the knee or hip is involved, may be present.

Physical exam may reveal bony or soft tissue swelling, a mild localized effusion, and/or crepitus. As the disease progresses, there may be loss of motion in the joint(s).

Radiologic Findings

Radiologic findings include osteophytes, **subchondral sclerosing**, and cysts associated with joint space narrowing. There is poor correlation between radiographic changes and the severity of disease. Approximately 80% of people over age 65 will have some evidence of OA changes on x-ray, but only 30% will be symptomatic (9).

Diagnosis

Differential diagnosis of periarticular pain would include bursitis, tendinitis, or periostitis. If systemic symptoms were present, the possibility of lupus, malignancy, polymyalgia rheumatica, rheumatoid arthritis, or gouty arthritis should be considered. Intense swelling, warmth, and erythema should prompt investigation of an infectious or a microcrystalline process.

Treatment

Pharmaceutics

Since no pharmacologic agents are available to slow disease progression in OA, medical therapy focuses primarily on symptom management. There are two mainstays of short-term treatment of knee pain in OA: **acetaminophen** and **nonsteroidal anti-inflammatory agents** (NSAIDs). Nonsteroidal anti-inflammatory agents inhibit the action of cyclooxygenase (COX) in the production of prostaglandins from arachidonic acid. Although prostanoids are integral to the maintenance of gastric mucosal integrity and renal function, prostaglandin E_2 (PGE_2) has been shown to be involved in acute and chronic inflammation (19). Historically, all available NSAIDs have been nonspecific COX-inhibitors and seemed to cause at least some degree of GI mucosal damage. The recent addition to the pharmaceutical armamentarium has been specific COX-2 inhibitors (rofecoxib [Vioxx] or valdecoxib [Bextra]). Initial data suggest COX-2 inhibitors are as effective as nonspecific NSAIDs but without the side effects. To date, long-term safety and efficacy studies are not available (19).

There is concern that NSAIDs may have a negative impact on bone healing. Nonunion of fractures and/or time required for union increases if NSAIDs are used (20). Given that NSAIDs are first-line treatment in OA (and in RA), this finding is significant because of the potential negative impact on the body's ability to combat bony changes in arthritis.

In guidelines for treating osteoarthritis in the hip, Hochberg indicates that many rheumatologists are using acetaminophen (Tylenol) as first-line therapy (21). Studies have shown that high-dose acetaminophen therapy (up to 4000 mg/day) is as effective as NSAIDs in reducing pain and inflammation in patients with OA, without the side effects. NSAIDs should be used when acetaminophen is no longer effective; however, monitor renal function and add prophylactic treatment against GI bleeding or ulceration (e.g., Prilosec or misoprostol). Indomethacin should not be used for long-term therapy because it has been shown to speed up joint destruction in persons with OA in the hip (21). Topical medicines such as capsaicin can be adjuvants to oral therapies (22), and glucocorticoid injections can also be helpful in treating effusions or local inflammation in the knee (21). However, if more than 3 to 4 intra-articular injections are needed, surgical options should be considered. The usefulness of steroid injections into the hip has not been well studied, and there is considerable concern about development of progressive cartilage damage through repeated injections. Moreover, the procedure is technically difficult and is usually done under fluoroscopic guidance.

Surgical Options

A variety of orthopaedic options have been developed for treatment of severe OA. Arthroscopic debridement focuses on removal of intra-articular debris and resection of torn tissue. Abrasion arthroplasty, subchondral drilling, and microfracture methods target significant cartilage deficits. By stimulating a bleeding response, these techniques cause the defect to be filled by secondary fibrocartilaginous scar formation. Unfortunately, this fibrocartilaginous scar is not true hyaline cartilage and its durability is unpredictable (23, 24).

Another surgical option is **osteotomy**, which involves realignment of the joint surface. The procedure creates space between 2 opposing joint surfaces or rotates a cartilage-covered surface within the joint to reduce bone-on-bone contact. The goal of osteotomy is to reduce the load borne by the most damaged part of the joint surface (23). This option tends to be most successful in patients with limited varus angulation (<10°) and stable ligaments. Osteotomies are generally more successful than abrasion arthroplasty. For those with more extreme varus angulation, any degree of valgus angulation or unstable ligaments, **total knee arthro-**

plasty is recommended (25). Joint replacement is also recommended for patients with significant pain despite having a tibial osteotomy. Investigation of return to sports after total knee replacement revealed that more than 77% of persons participating regularly in sports will return to sports after the procedure, especially low-impact sports. Physical activity after total hip replacement increased dramatically, with many patients taking up low-impact activity for the first time. Recommended low-impact activities include swimming, walking, and cycling. High-impact sports like tennis are not recommended (26).

Physical Therapy/Exercise

There is strong evidence that both aerobic and anaerobic exercise provides many benefits for patients with OA. Quadriceps strengthening through an **isokinetic exercise** regimen has been shown to reduce pain (especially with stair climbing) and produce a modest improvement in physical function (16). Aerobic walking and weight training have been shown to greatly reduce postural sway in older adults with OA, thereby improving their balance. Moreover, weight training was shown to be particularly beneficial in situations where test subjects were deprived of sensory cues (27).

Research suggests that people with OA are more likely to lead sedentary lives because of pain and disability stemming from their disease (29). Lack of physical activity places the individual at risk for conditions that are often associated with sedentary lifestyles: high body mass indices, higher systolic blood pressures, high serum glucose levels, and low levels of high-density lipoprotein cholesterol. Besides improving physical function, exercise as a therapy for OA will also reduce the risk of heart disease and diabetes (28).

Cognitive-Behavioral Therapy

Pain coping skills can help reduce the physical and psychological disability as well as the physical pain arising from OA. Training in distraction techniques (e.g., relaxation, imagery), activity pacing, or goal setting and cognitive restructuring are strategies for dealing with negative thinking. These techniques are especially effective when the person is having pain, providing significant short-term improvement in physical and psychological disability (29). Assessment of **cognitive-behavioral therapy** (CBT) 6 months later has demonstrated some decline in pain relief, but improvement in psychological disability and ongoing reduction of physical disability were maintained (29). Adapting CBT to include spouses (e.g., addition of couples' skills: communication and problem-solving skills, behavioral rehearsal, and maintenance training) improved outcome in pain and psychological disability as well as greater self-efficacy and marital adjustment (30).

Nutrition and Diet

Vitamin D

Normal bone metabolism depends on vitamin D. Low levels may impair the ability of bone to respond appropriately to the pathophysiologic changes associated with OA. This inability to respond may increase the probability of disease progression in pre-existing disease. In 1996, investigators from the Framingham Study reported that a relative deficiency of vitamin D (low dietary intake and low serum levels) markedly increased the risk of disease progression. However, there was no increased risk of developing OA in a previously normal knee (31). The specific role of vitamin D in OA is unclear.

Vitamin C

Synthesis of type II collagen requires the presence of vitamin C. It is also an essential player in the synthesis of glycosaminoglycans. A threefold increase in the radiographic progression of OA has been observed in patients with low vitamin C intake (32).

Hyaluronic Acid

Hyaluronic acid (HA), an integral component of the extracellular matrix, was recently approved for use in OA. The goal of injecting HA is to improve elastoviscosity of the synovial fluid and reduce stiffness. Clinical studies have been limited; however, the studies that have been done demonstrate mixed results. Randomized control studies of short-term efficacy have shown no toxicity after a total of four injections (33). Of greater interest was the reduction in number of episodes of knee effusions (33). Articular effusion is considered a marker of disease activity associated with increased joint pain and warmth. There is evidence that suggests a correlation between the number of episodes of effusion and radiological joint space narrowing, suggesting that the incidence of synovial effusion may be predictive of joint space deterioration (33).

Chondroitin Sulfate

Chondroitin sulfate (CS) is an oral therapy believed to stimulate synthesis of proteoglycan and collagen and inhibit their enzymatic degradation. One double blind, randomized, placebo-controlled trial comparing chondroitin sulfate with the NSAID diclofenac sodium showed that the CS group experienced reduction in daily NSAID use, and reported therapeutic benefit that continued up to 3 months after CS stopped. However, therapeutic benefit from NSAIDs ceased immediately after treatment stopped (34).

Glucosamine

In short-term studies done in Europe, glucosamine has been shown to be as effective as NSAIDs in reducing pain and stiffness in OA (35). Although the exact mechanism of action is still unknown, it is believed that glucosamine provides a substrate for the damaged tissue (35). Glucosamine and chondroitin sulfate often are packaged together for a hoped-for additive effect.

Overview: Rheumatoid Arthritis

Unlike OA, rheumatoid arthritis (RA) is a systemic disease that can affect a variety of tissues, including joints, blood vessels, skin, cardiac muscle, and lungs. The primary disease process is a proliferative, invasive synovitis, which causes joint destruction and eventually leads to ankylosis of the involved joint.

Pathophysiology: Genetics and Immune System

One function of the macrophage is to serve as an antigen-presenting cell. In this role, macrophages ingest antigenic proteins, which are then cleaved and presented on special receptor molecules to CD4+ T-helper cells; this initiates a cascade of reactions involved in mounting a cellular immune response. The macrophage receptor, class II major-histocompatibility complex (MCH II) molecules are associated with RA risk (36). People who carry the **HLA-DR4 and/or HLA-DR1 alleles** at a particular locus on the MHC II molecule have increased risk of developing RA. The relative risk of developing RA is increased 2.4- to 3.2-fold in persons carrying the HLA-DR4 allele (37); this association is strongest in Whites. There is also evidence that in addition to predicting incidence, the presence of allele HLA-DR4 allele may predict the severity of the disease. Having two copies of the HLA-DR4 allele seems to present an additive effect of disease severity in terms of joint erosion, extra-articular manifestations, and level of function (38). The HLA-DR4 homozygotes are predominantly male (38).

The primary or initial cause of RA is not known. Abrupt onset of the disease and involvement of specific subcategory antigen presenting molecules suggests that a limited number of antigens, perhaps even a single antigen, triggers an **autoimmune process**. Current investigations are focusing on infectious agents such as bacteria and viruses (parvovirus, mycobacteria, Lyme disease, and mycoplasma); others are exploring autoimmune processes that involve connective-tissue proteins such as collagen and proteoglycans.

The **Epstein-Barr (EB) virus** has been a primary suspect as an infectious trigger of RA for more than 10 years. Eighty percent of patients with RA have circulating anti-Epstein Barr antibodies and have been found to shed more EB virus with throat washings than control subjects (39). EB virus is known to polyclonally activate B-lymphocytes, causing overproduction of immunoglobulins including rheumatoid factor (39). Researchers have also discovered the presence of antibodies that recognize a peptide sequence found within a specific locus on both the EB virus (glycoprotein gp110) and the MCH II HLA-DR4 molecule (39). The current hypothesis is that the presence of this shared isotope may help determine who will develop RA (39).

Elevated titers of anti-type II collagen antibodies are present in the serum of RA patients (39). However, the presence of these autoantibodies does not precede the onset of clinical disease. It is more likely that the cartilage is damaged by the invasive synovitis; the presence of exposed cartilage epitopes triggers an autoimmune response against cartilage, amplifying joint destruction (39).

The earliest changes in RA include neovascularization of the synovial membrane and movement of mononuclear cells, neutrophils, and an oligoclonal subset of memory T-helper cells into the tissue and fluid. This movement is triggered by an increased expression of intercellular adhesion molecule-1 (ICAM-1) by the capillary endothelial cells. Initially, the increased endothelial permeability draws the oligoclonal T-helper cells into the synovial membrane. These **memory T cells** are activated by an unidentified antigen or antigenic immune complex present within the synovium (40). The increased permeability results in synovial thickening (i.e., the start of **pannus** formation). Although T cells play a key role in the development of the synovitis, they are not the predominant cell type found in the synovial membrane or the fluid. Macrophages and **fibroblast-like synoviocytes** are the major cell types found in the synovium, and neutrophils are the primary cells in the synovial fluid (4, 39).

Activation of the cellular immune system within the synovial tissue results in the production of cytokines. Cytokines can be categorized functionally: interleukin IL-2, IL-3, IL-4 and interferon-gamma (IFN-γ) are secreted by T cells and are key players in the activation and proliferation of cellular and humoral immune responses. IL-1, IL-6, TNF-α are synthesized by macrophages and fibroblasts. These cytokines cause cellular proliferation, but more importantly, they stimulate chondrocytes and synoviocytes to release metalloproteinase, causing bone resorption and cartilage destruction; inhibit proteoglycan production; inhibit T cell cytokine production; and increase production of endothelial adhesion molecules, further promoting migration of leukocytes into the synovium (39). Studies show that cytokines originating from lymphocytes are present in lower concentrations than cytokines originating from macrophages; this reflects both cytokine-inhibited T cell activity and the low number of T cells present (39).

The IL-2 secreted by the T-helper cells activates B cells and cytokine production by macrophages. Unlike other T cells, memory T-helper cells do not play a role in the negative feedback loop controlling antibody production. As a result of the lack of T cell inhibition of antibody production, large amounts of immunoglobulin are present in involved joints (40).

Immunoglobulin production by B cells in RA also tends to be oligoclonal. B cells expressing anti-type II collagen and the minor collagen types (V, VI, and IX) have been identified (39). Also, approximately 80% of persons with RA demonstrate autoantibodies (IgM) to the FC portion of autologous IgG molecules. The resulting immunologic complexes are found within the synovial tissue and fluid, promoting synovial inflammation. IgM-IgG complexes are also found deposited in superficial layers of cartilage. Activation of the complement cascade contributes to cartilage destruction (39).

In addition to the chronic inflammation of the synovial tissue, there is also an inflammatory process occurring within the synovial fluid. Here, inflammation is mediated primarily by neutrophils. A number of factors are involved in promoting the migration of neutrophils into the joint space. The cytokines IL-1 and TNF-α promote endothelial cell expression of adhesion molecules specifically for neutrophils (39). Leukotriene B4, activated complement component C5a, and platelet-activating factor are proven chemoattractants found within the synovial fluid (39). Once in the joint space, the neutrophils will ingest immune complexes. This phagocytosis is followed by activation of the NADPH oxidase system and production of reactive oxygen metabolites as well as release of proteinases by means of degranulation within the neutrophil cells (39). Prostaglandins released through the metabolism of arachidonic acid also contribute to joint space inflammation.

As the disease progresses, the synovium becomes hypertrophied and edematous. The synovial lining, normally 1 to 3 cells thick, increases to be 5 to 10 cells thick. This layer consists of mostly macrophages with a smaller number of fibroblastic-like synoviocytes. The major cell types found within the sublining stromal are noninflammatory. The sublining primarily consists of phenotypically immature, highly activated, invasive fibroblastic-like cells and new blood vessels. These fibroblast-like cells behave like transformed cells and are not malignant. These cells will induce production of the proto-oncogenes c-fos and c-jun, the metalloproteinase collagenase, and stromelysin (39); induction of the procolleganase gene and proto-oncogenes is stimulated by IL-1, TNF-α, platelet-derived growth factor, and fibroblast growth factor (4).

Proliferation of the hypertrophic synovium is supported by neovascularization that occurs in response to FGF and TNF-α (4). These activated endothelial cells also secrete metalloproteinases, which facilitate their invasion of the synovial tissue, allowing them to provide nutrients to the proliferating cells.

Joint destruction occurs at several points. The fibroblast-like synoviocytes seem to be primary; they secrete metalloproteinases that destroy both articular cartilage and bone at the edge of the invading synovium. Chondrocytes secrete the same proteinases, causing additional degradation of bone and cartilage (40). The ongoing hypertrophy of the synovium/pannus contributes to reduction of joint space and RA pathology. Eventually, pannus will fill the remaining joint space, causing ankylosis of the joint.

Clinical Presentation

Rheumatoid arthritis has 3 modes of presentation: systemic, pauciarticular, and polyarticular. Each mode of onset carries its own unique characteristics (41).

Systemic onset occurs in only 1% of adults but is seen in 20% of children with RA. It is an acute process that has variable joint manifestations (arthralgia to significant joint swelling). Prominent systemic symptoms are high spiking fever, rheumatoid rash, neutrophilic leukocytosis, generalized lymphedema, hepatosplenomegaly, and possible cardiac involvement (42).

Pauciarticular presentation is most commonly seen in children—as many as 50% of children and only 6% of adults present with swelling of 1 to 4 joints. The knee and digits are most common joints involved. There are no systemic manifestations except for iridocyclitis (43).

Polyarticular onset is seen in 93% of adults and 30% of children. Initial presentation often includes vague complaints of stiffness and aches. These symptoms occur in multiple joints, most commonly the hands, feet, and knees. Systemic symptoms include anorexia, weight loss, fatigue, and numbness or tingling in hands and feet. One striking feature of the initial presentation of polyarticular disease is its bilaterality and symmetry. Findings in one hand mirror findings in the other. The proximal interphalangeal, metatarsophalangeal/metacarpophalangeal, and wrist/ankle joints are most commonly affected (4).

Extra-Articular Manifestations

Sjögren's Syndrome

A secondary form of Sjögren's is associated with RA. Patients develop dry eyes and dry mouth due to autoimmune destruction of their lacrimal and salivary ducts.

Felty's Syndrome

Felty's syndrome is a clinical tetrad of thrombocytopenia, neutropenia, hemolytic anemia, and splenomegaly in the setting of RA.

Subcutaneous Rheumatoid Nodules

Free, subcutaneous nodules arise in regions that are subject to repeated stress: elbows, ulnar aspect of forearm, occiput, and lumbosacral region. The presence of nodules is associated with progressive disease and suggests poor prognosis. Nodules will also appear in heart valves, lung parenchyma, and ocular sclera, although this occurrence is rare.

Radiographic Findings

Early radiographic changes include **juxta-articular osteopenia** and increased radiodensity of surrounding soft tissue, signaling swelling. Later findings are **bony erosion**, loss of cartilage with joint space narrowing, and effusions.

Diagnosis

As in OA, there are no laboratory tests to confirm the diagnosis of rheumatoid arthritis. The most recent guidelines for diagnosing the disease are the American Rheumatism Association criteria from 1987 (Box 32.1). Unfortunately, there is often a delay between onset of symptoms and initiation of treatment, during which joint damage has probably begun.

Development of RA seems to depend on a variety of factors: genetic susceptibility, exposure to an infectious agent, and generation of autoimmune response within the synovium resulting in joint destruction.

Treatment
Pharmaceutics

The goals of treatment of RA include controlling disease activity, managing pain, maintaining function, and maximizing quality of life.

Traditionally, treatment of RA has followed the "**therapeutic pyramid**." Initial therapy begins with fast-acting agents to alleviate symptoms, such as NSAIDs and **glucocorticoids** (44). NSAIDs are the principal pain-relieving agent. Most NSAIDs are well tolerated but can cause adverse side effects (e.g., gastrointestinal bleeding and nephrotoxicity). Glucocorticoids can be given by an intra-articular route, or systemically. Intra-articular injections can be effective in reducing inflammation in a single or limited number of joints. Systemic steroids in an acute disease flare (up to 20 mg) or low-dose therapy in the early stages of the disease (7.5 mg) have been shown to be beneficial (45). In the early disease stage, combining high-dose steroids with a disease-modifying drug can induce remission.

In the therapeutic pyramid, introduction of **slow-acting antirheumatic drugs** (SAARDs)—also known as *symptom-modifying antirheumatic drugs*—is typically delayed until

> **BOX 32.1.   1987 Revised Criteria for Classification of RA**
>
> I. Guidelines for classification
>   a. Four of seven criteria are required to classify a patient as having RA.
>   b. Patients with 2 or more clinical diagnoses are not excluded.
> II. Criteria
>   a. Morning stiffness: Stiffness in and around joints lasting 1 hour before maximal improvement. Present for at least 6 weeks.
>   b. Arthritis of 3 or more joint areas: At least 3 joint areas simultaneously have soft tissue swelling or joint effusions observed by a physician and present for at least 6 weeks. There are 14 possible joint areas: R or L proximal interphalangeal, metacarpophalangeal, wrist, elbow, knee, ankle, and metatarsophalangeal.
>   c. Arthritis of hand joints: arthritis of wrist, metacarpophalangeal, or proximal interphalangeal joints, observed by a physician and present for at least 6 weeks.
>   d. Symmetric arthritis: Simultaneous involvement of the same joint areas on both sides of the body observed by a physician and present for at least 6 weeks.
>   e. Rheumatoid nodules: Physician-observed subcutaneous nodules over bony prominences, extensor surfaces, or juxta-articular regions.
>   f. Serum rheumatoid factor: Lab results indicating presence of abnormal amounts of serum rheumatoid factor—testing method must be positive in less than 5% of normal control subjects.
>   g. Radiographic changes: Typical changes on posteroanterior hand and wrist films, which must include erosions or unequivocal bony decalcification, localized in or adjacent to the involved joints.
>
> *Reproduced with permission granted May 2002.*

after development of joint erosion, as seen radiographically. The rationale behind the slow, step-wise progression of the pyramid is the belief that the most effective antirheumatic drugs were toxic, and that the least toxic (and often least effective) drugs are used first (44). The average time needed to move through the treatment pyramid is 8 years. However, most people with RA experience joint damage and erosion within 2 years of disease onset. Recent evidence suggests that a delay in initiating SAARDs results in irreversible joint damage and loss of function (45, 46). Current disease management includes initiation of SAARD therapy early in the process, before radiographic changes appear.

SAARDs can be thought of as agents used to improve the symptoms and clinical features of synovitis. The mechanisms of action of the SAARDs vary greatly and are poorly understood. Although there is good evidence of short-term benefits from using SAARDs, long-term efficacy is still in question (47); concerns are toxicity and efficacy. Current therapies have not been effective in reducing disease activity to a level where joint damage does not occur. The low efficacy to toxicity ratio explains why 20% of patients take a given SAARD for less than 5 years. However, **methotrexate** has been well tolerated by 50% of patients taking it for more than 5 years (46).

Combination therapies have been very successful in transplant and oncology. In treating RA, synergy may be gained from using 2 less effective drugs together; however, this theory is controversial. The lack of understanding of how SAARDs work makes it difficult to predict which drugs may act synergistically. Moreover, many of the drugs have similar toxicity profiles, raising concern that combination therapies may result in increased toxicity. However, there is some evidence that combination therapies offer improved efficacy, at least in the short term. One 6-month study compared methotrexate or placebo to methotrexate plus **cyclosporine** in patients who had partial response to previous methotrexate treatment (46). Patients receiving the dual therapy showed significant improvement without an associated increase in side effects (46).

The current lack of effective treatments is due to a lack of understanding about the pathogenesis and/or the etiology of RA. A true **disease-controlling drug** would be able to change the clinical course of the disease (i.e., maintain/improve function, decrease rate of joint degeneration, increase life expectancy). New insights into the disease process have identified novel therapeutic targets, which may lead to development of a true disease-controlling agent.

Etanercept (Enbrel), a new rheumatoid drug, binds specifically to TNF-α, blocking the interaction with TNF-α receptors on the cell's surface. Among other things, TNF induces chondrocytes/synoviocytes to secrete a matrix metalloproteinase, stromelysin. In preliminary clinical trials (48), etanercept was significantly better than placebo in reducing the signs of RA disease activity, including number of tender joints, pain, and disability. When etanercept was compared with methotrexate, there was less radiographic change over a 12-month period (49, 50). Although short-term evidence is promising, long-term studies are needed.

Exercise

Traditionally, it was believed that dynamic exercise would exacerbate RA by hastening joint damage, increasing pain, and decreasing function. Until recently, physical rehabilitation has focused on preserving joint mobility and maintaining muscle strength with range of motion and non-weight-bearing, isometric exercises (51). This concept is beginning to change as evidence supporting the use of dynamic exercise in RA grows. In a meta analysis of the small number of randomized studies evaluating the effectiveness of aerobic exercise, Van den Ende showed that exercise performed at an intensity level sufficient to build muscle strength and aerobic capacity is effective in improving strength, aerobic capacity, and joint mobility in the short term (51). These benefits came without increased joint pain or disease activity. The impact on ability to maintain function was less encouraging. However, in these studies functional assessment was focused on the ability to perform activities of daily living, and not on activity level. Neuberger showed that short-term low-impact aerobics could have reduced the level of self-reported fatigue in persons with RA (52). Unfortunately, none of the studies investigated the long-term effect of dynamic exercise on radiographic progression of the disease. Long-term studies of exercise and the effect on ability to maintain or improve function and on radiographic disease progression are necessary.

Although little direct research has been done on how SAARDs affects exercise, there is evidence that some of the SAARDs may have an impact on general cardiovascular function. Methotrexate has been shown to induce ventricular tachycardia, and cyclosporine can have a negative impact on lung function.

Surgical Management

Permanent joint deformities and the associated functional impairment can be corrected surgically. Damage in the wrist, metacarpophalangeal, metatarsophalangeal, rotator cuff, and knee joints can be treated conservatively with surgery. **Synovectomy** (either arthroscopic or open), joint stabilizations or fusions, and joint replacements are possible options. Synovectomy temporarily relieves the pain and swelling associated with RA but does not slow disease progression (25). Total knee and hip replacements are also indicated in patients with advanced secondary RA.

Nutrition and Diet

RA is a catabolic process. A person with RA develops an elevated basal metabolic rate, which often leads to loss of weight and mean body mass. It becomes important to ensure that the body's energy and protein needs are met. It is common for persons with severe disease to become malnourished (53).

Many dietary approaches have been used in an attempt to control RA. Some focus on eliminating "disease-causing toxins" from the body through detoxification or cleansing. Often this includes fasting, which seems to offer immediate symptom relief to some; however, this relief is never long-lived. Others avoid foods that are believed to worsen symptoms. Citrus fruit, chocolate, alcohol, red meats, spices, and carbonated beverages can aggravate symptoms, whereas fish, fresh vegetables, and certain oils improve symptoms. There is evidence that the long-chain omega-3 fatty acids found in fish oils reduce pain and stiffness (53).

What We Know
About Osteoarthritis and Rheumatoid Arthritis

1 The term *arthritis* describes a wide variety of different disease entities, of which osteoarthritis (OA), fibromyalgia syndrome, and rheumatoid arthritis (RA) are the most common. Some other arthritis diseases include juvenile rheumatoid arthritis, systemic lupus erythematous, gout, and ankylosing spondylitis, among others.

2 Arthritis is the leading cause of disability among people age 15 years and older.

3 Nearly 3 of every 5 people with arthritis are younger than 65 years of age.

4 More than 42.7 million Americans have some type of arthritis, or about 1 of every 6 Americans, 27.5 million being over the age of 45. OA affects more than 21 million Americans. RA affects more than 2 million Americans. Fibromyalgia affects more than 3.7 million Americans.

5 OA is the most common type of arthritis and a leading cause of disability in the United States.

6 Virtually everyone over the age of 75 is affected by OA in at least one joint.

7 Women are generally affected by OA at a younger age than men.

8 Direct and indirect costs of RA reached $65 billion in 1992.

9 More than 75% of RA patients are women.

10 Peak onset on RA is between ages 20 and 45.

11 Osteoporosis is common in patients with RA, but is not common in OA patients.

What We Would Like to Know
About Osteoarthritis and Rheumatoid Arthritis

1 Better insight is needed into how to prevent or delay the progression of OA.

2 Why are women generally affected by OA at a younger age than men?

3 Would it be possible to develop biomechanical devices or training methods to prevent the development of OA?

4 Why is RA association strongest among Whites? Is there a genetic basis that predisposes certain individuals to develop RA?

5 Someday, would it be possible to vaccinate to prevent RA?

6 Why does juvenile RA present differently from adult RA?

Summary

Arthritis is an umbrella term that encompasses over 120 different diseases. Literally, it means joint inflammation: swelling, redness, heat, and pain caused by tissue injury or disease in the joint. In the past few decades, we have developed a better understanding of the biomechanical, genetic, and extrinsic influences that govern this group of diseases. Significant advances have been made in the understanding of the basic science behind both rheumatoid arthritis and osteoarthritis. The pharmacological agents developed in the last 10 years, in combination with physical therapy, have dramatically changed the morbidity and mortality of RA. Although some of the pharmacologic agents used in OA have been improved, the overall management has changed little. However, future techniques of genetically engineered cartilage replacement/transplant hold great promise. Today, arthritis is a major health problem, but it is hoped that these advances and those to come will decrease its impact on society.

DISCUSSION QUESTIONS

1 What is the difference between OA and RA?

2 What are the current pharmacologic treatments for RA? For OA?

3 What are the current nonpharmacologic treatments for RA? For OA?

4 What are the age and sex differences between OA and RA?

5 What are the societal costs of OA? Of RA?

6 How would OA/RA be managed surgically?

The authors would like to thank Dr. Melinda Campopiano and Sarah Jenkinson for their help in developing this chapter.

CASE STUDY

Patient Information

Mrs. Whiting is a 65-year-old retired store clerk and an avid gardener. The patient relates increasing right knee pain for approximately 1 year. She states that it is much more pronounced in the last 2 weeks and is accompanied by swelling.

Mrs. Whiting complains of right knee pain, especially after going on a long walk, working in her garden, or carrying something heavy. Her right knee hurts more toward the end of the day, especially if she doesn't rest it. She first began to notice the pain about 12 months ago, 3 months after she fell on it. She did note a previous injury to her right knee while in her 40s, but cannot remember many details. She has joint stiffness in her right knee when she wakes up, and the stiffness usually goes away in about 15 or 20 minutes. The knee also gets stiff when she sits down for an hour or more. Mrs. Whiting relates limitation of motion—sometimes she can't squat down to pick up something heavy. She complains of constant right knee swelling for about 2 weeks. She states that her knee also makes more noise lately when she bends it. The noise is described as "grating or popping." Mrs. Whiting denies back pain, neck pain, sprains, or any other significant medical history, surgery, or medications. She presents today because of its failure to resolve.

Assessments

Mrs. Whiting's physical exam was generally negative except for her musculoskeletal system; no muscular weakness, tenderness, or atrophy. No peripheral edema. No spinal tenderness, abnormal curvature, or obvious deformity. Spinal mobility was within normal limits. Joint inspection was normal except for right knee, which reveals moderate swelling, some tenderness, and barely perceptible erythema. Right knee ROM was moderately limited compared to the left knee. No deformities, subluxation, or masses were noted. Plain x-rays of the right knee showed joint narrowing. Lab studies were performed; CBC, sedimentation rate, and rheumatoid factor were all within normal limits.

At this point, you should be fairly confident that Mrs. Whiting has OA or degenerative joint disease. The history and radiographic findings, together with a negative rheumatoid factor, point to OA. However, it's possible that a patient with this presentation suffers from some other form of arthritis or a syndrome that has a presentation similar to OA. The differential includes:

- Psoriatic arthritis
- Reiter's syndrome
- Arthritis associated with ulcerative colitis
- Ankylosing spondylitis
- Disk syndrome
- Gout
- Infectious arthritis
- Lyme disease
- Polymyalgia rheumatica
- Post-traumatic synovitis
- Pseudogout
- Rheumatoid arthritis
- Sarcoid arthritis

It's also possible that laboratory findings were in error, or that drug effects, inadequate diet, stress, anxiety, trauma, or concomitant illnesses created spurious laboratory results.

Physical therapy will help Mrs. Whiting preserve and improve her muscle strength and ROM. She should also be encouraged to use a cane to reduce the stress on her right knee while she's losing weight

Questions

1. What role does weight reduction play in OA?

2. Can long-term oral steroids be given to patients with OA?

3. What type of exercise should you instruct a patient with OA to use: isometric or isokinetic exercises?

4. What role does diet play in OA?

5. What medication should be tried first?

REFERENCES

1. Ling SM, Bathon JM. Osteoarthritis in older adults. J Am Geriatr Soc 1998;46:216–225.

2. McKinney RH, Ling SM. Osteoarthritis: no cure, but many options for symptom relief. Cleve Clin J Med 2000;67(9):665–671.

3. Deleted.

4. Schumacher HRJ, ed. Primer on the Rheumatic Diseases. 10th ed. Atlanta, Ga: Arthritis Foundation; 1993:8–11, 184–190.

5. Panush RS, et al. Is running associated with degenerative joint disease? JAMA 1986;255(9):1152–1154.

6. Lane NE, Buckwalter JA. Exercise and osteoarthritis. Curr Opin Rheumatol 1999;11:413–416.

7. Puranen J, et al. Running and primary osteoarthritis of the hip. BMJ 1975;1:424–425.

8. Lane NE, et al. The relationship of running to osteoarthritis of the knee and hip and bone mineral density of the lumbar spine: a 9-year longitudinal study. J Rheumatol 1998;26:334–341.

9. Lane NE, et al. Long-distance running, bone density, and osteoarthritis. JAMA 1986;255:1147–1151.

10. Buckwalter JA, Lane NE. Athletics and osteoarthritis. Am J Sports Med 1997;25(6):873–881.

11. Rozzi SL, Lephart SM, Fu FH. Effects of muscular fatigue on knee joint laxity and neuromuscular characteristics of male and female athletes. J Athletic Training Apr/June 1999;34(2):106–114.

12. Cerulli G, Benoit DL, Caraffa A, Ponteggia F. Proprioceptive training and prevention of anterior cruciate ligament injuries in soccer. J Orthop Sports Phys Ther 2001;31(11):655–661.

13. Setton LA, Elliott DM, Mow VC. Altered mechanics of cartilage with osteoarthritis: human osteoarthritis and an experimental model of joint degeneration. Osteoarthritis Cartilage 1999;7:2–14.

14. Poole AR. An introduction to the pathophysiology of osteoarthritis. Front Biosci 1999;4:662–670.

15. Malemud CJ. Fundamental pathways in osteoarthritis: an overview. Front Biosci 1999;4:659–661.

16. Maurer BT, et al. Osteoarthritis of the knee: isokinetic quadriceps exercise versus an educational intervention. Arch Phys Med Rehabil 1999;80:1293–1299.

17. Young A. Current issues in arthrogenous inhibition. Ann Rheum Dis 1993;52:829–834.

18. O'Reilly S, et al. Knee pain, quadriceps weakness and muscle activation in the community. Br J Rheumatol 1996;34(suppl 2):45.

19. McKenna F. COX-2: separating myth from reality. Scand J Rheumatol 1999;28(suppl 109):19–29.

20. Giannoudis PV, et al. Nonunion of the femoral diaphysis: the influence of reaming and non-steroidal anti-inflammatory drugs. J Bone Joint Surg Br 2000;82(5):655–658.

21. Hochberg MC, et al. Guidelines for the medical management of osteoarthritis: Part I. Osteoarthritis of the hip. Arthritis Rheum 1995;38(11):1535–1540.

22. Hochberg MC, et al. Guidelines for the medical management of osteoarthritis: Part II. Osteoarthritis of the knee. Arthritis Rheum 1995;38(11):1541–1546.

23. Rand JA. Role of arthroscopy in osteoarthritis of the knee. Arthroscopy 1991;7(4):358–363.

24. Vangsness CTJ. Complex topics in knee surgery: overview of treatment options for arthritis in the active patient. Clin Sports Med 1999;18(1):1–11.

25. Windsor RE, Insall JN. The knee. In: William N. Kelley, ed. Textbook of Rheumatology. Philadelphia, Pa: WB Saunders; 1997:1739–1758.

26. Bradbury N, et al. Participation in sports after total knee replacement. Am J Sports Med 1998;26(4):530–535.

27. Messier SP, et al. Long-term exercise and its effect on balance in older, osteoarthritic adults: results from the Fitness, Arthritis, and Seniors Trial (FAST). J Am Geriatr Soc 2000;48:131–138.

28. Ettinger WHJ. Physical activity, arthritis, and disability in older people. Clin Geriatr Med 1998;14(3):633–640.

29. Keefe FJ, et al. Pain coping skills training in the management of osteoarthritic knee pain II: follow-up results. Behav Ther 1990;21:435–447.

30. Keefe FJ, Caldwell DS. Cognitive behavioral control of arthritis pain. Adv Rheumatol 1997;81(1):277–290.

31. McAlindon TE, et al. Relation of dietary intake and serum levels of vitamin D to progression of osteoarthritis of the knee among participants in the Framingham Study. Ann Intern Med 1996;125:353–359.

32. Sowers M, Lachance L. Vitamins and arthritis: the roles of vitamins A, C, D, and E. Rheum Dis Clin North Am 1999;25(2):315–332.

33. Dougados M, et al. High molecular weight sodium hyaluronate (hyalectin) in osteoarthritis of the knee: a 1-year placebo-controlled trial. Osteoarthritis Cartilage 1993;1:97–103.

34. Morreale P, et al. Comparison of the antiinflammatory efficacy of chondroitin sulfate and diclofenac sodium in patients with knee osteoarthritis. J Rheumatol 1996;23:1385–1391.

35. Schiedermayer D. Glucosamine sulfate for the treatment of osteoarthritis. Altern Med Alert 1998;1:121–132.

36. Abbas AK, Lichtman AH, Pober JS, eds. Cellular and Molecular Immunology. 2nd ed. Philadelphia, Pa: WB Saunders; 1994:116–135.

37. Wagner U, et al. HLA markers and prediction of clinical course and outcome in rheumatoid arthritis. Arthritis Rheumatism 1997;40(2):341–351.

38. Weyand CM, et al. The influence of HLA-DRB1 genes on disease severity in rheumatoid arthritis. Ann Intern Med 1992;117:801–806.

39. Harris EDJ. Rheumatoid arthritis pathophysiology and implications for therapy. N Engl J Med 1990;322(18):1227–1289.

40. Sewell KL. Pathogenesis of rheumatoid arthritis. Lancet 1993;341:283–286.

41. Calabro JJ, Aldo J, Londino V. Drug therapy in rheumatoid arthritis: based on an understanding of its natural history: Part I. Clin Rheumatol Pract 1985;2(6):244–256.

42. Lems WF, Dijkmans BAC. Rheumatoid arthritis: clinical picture and its variant. In: Firestein GS, Panayi GS, Wolheim F, eds. Rheumatoid Arthritis: New Frontiers in Pathogenesis and Treatment. Oxford Univ Press; 2000:chap 16.

43. O'Gradaigh D, Watts RA, Scott DGI. Extra-articular features of rheumatoid arthritis. In: Firestein GS, Panayi GS, Wolheim F, eds. Rheumatoid Arthritis: New Frontiers in Pathogenesis and Treatment. Oxford Univ Press; 2000:chap 17.

44. Dinant HJ, Dijkmans BAC. New therapeutic targets for rheumatoid arthritis. Pharm World Sci 1999;21(2):49–59.

45. Langenegger T, Michel BA. Drug treatment for rheumatoid arthritis. Clin Orthop 1999;366:22–30.

46. Jain R, Lipsky PE. Treatment of rheumatoid arthritis. Adv Rheumatol 1997;81(1):57–84.

47. VanDenPutte LBA, VanRiel PLCM. Currently used second-line agents: do they control the disease course? Clin Exp Rheumatol 1997;15(suppl 17):S71–S74.

48. Fleischmann RM. Early diagnosis and treatment of rheumatoid arthritis for improved outcomes: focus on etanercept, a new biologic response modifier. Clin Ther 1999;21(9):1429–1442.

49. Bathon JM, et al. A comparison of etanercept and methotrexate in patients with early rheumatoid arthritis. N Engl J Med 2000;343(22):1586–1593.

50. Unknown. Mosby GenRx 2001 [book on CD-ROM]. 11th ed. Harcourt Health Science; 2001.

51. Van Den Ende CHM, et al. Dynamic exercise therapy in rheumatoid arthritis: A systematic review. Br J Rheumatol 1998;37:677–687.

52. Neuberger GB, et al. Effects of exercise on fatigue, aerobic fitness, and disease activity measures in persons with rheumatoid arthritis. Res Nurs Health 1997; 20:195–204.

53. Martin RH. The role of nutrition and diet in rheumatoid arthritis. Proc Nutr Soc 1998;57:231–234.

CHAPTER 33

Back Pain

Ralph S. Bovard, David Rhude

Overview

This chapter reviews the salient features of **low back pain,** examines the relevant literature, and champions the role of exercise in its management. We believe the next millen-nium will see a refocusing of our medical efforts into pre-ventive and proactive health care, as opposed to reactive and treatment-based care. In his Presidential Address to the North American Spine Society in 1990, Haldeman said: "[there] is now a convincing body of research that demonstrates that strengthening exercises together with improvement of cardiovascular fitness and general **functional restoration** can reduce disability and possibly pain in patients with chronic low back pain" (2). In the decade since, research has convincingly demonstrated that an appropriately designed exercise program will not only improve coping and return to function better than traditional passive methods, but can also reduce pain (3–6). This represents what Kuhn called a "paradigm shift" (7) from the previous advocacy of rest, pain avoidance, and passive treatment, to the current recommendation: active motion and individual patient responsibility. In other words, exercise is medicine and is the prescription for low back pain (8).

Scope of the Problem

Low back pain (LBP), a pervasive symptom of little significance in most societies, has become a unique form of disability in ours. Task force groups have found little scientific evidence to justify prolonged passive therapy from the standpoint of either cost or symptom reduction. In contrast, evidence supporting active rehabilitation continues to mount.

Despite incredible medical advances, the solution to "man's most important non-life threatening disease" continues to elude us (9). We don't even know what causes 85% of LBP (3). The likelihood that an adult will suffer a significant episode of LBP at some time is roughly 80% to 85%; in any given year the prevalence approaches 50%, although surveys suggest that only 15% to 20% seek medical care (10). When all musculoskeletal conditions are considered, spinal pain (primarily in the lumbar region) consumes the most resources. It is the leading cause of disability in persons under age 45 and the third leading cause in persons over 45 (11). Recent U.S. Bureau of Labor Statistics demonstrate that LBP injuries occur roughly six times as often as leg, finger, or shoulder injuries; LBP is easily the leading industrial health complaint (12). It is second only to respiratory tract infections as a reason to see a physician (13). There are now about 1 million work-related back injury compensation claims in the United States annually (14). It is estimated that 26% of lost workdays in the United States are attributable to back pain (12). Most individuals (about 75%) are significantly better in 2 to 3 weeks, and 90% to 95% have returned to all normal activities within 2 to 3 months (15); however, at least 60% have a recurrent episode within a year, implying that most sufferers have an underlying (subclinical) back problem with significant risk factors that must be addressed.

Most people experiencing LBP do not seek medical attention. However, Deyo estimates that in a general population seen initially in primary care for lower back complaints, 97% will have mechanical low back or leg pain without underlying malignant, infectious, neoplastic, or inflammatory disease. About 2% of the initial total population

will have systemic or visceral illness (e.g., pelvic organ, renal, or gastrointestinal disease, or aortic aneurysm). The remaining 1% will have other nonmechanical spinal conditions such as neoplasia (0.7%), infection (0.01%), inflammatory arthritis (0.03%), Scheuermann's disease, or Paget's disease (3) (Table 33.1).

Of those with mechanical LBP, the vast majority (≤70%) will have what can be described as nonspecific musculoligamentous lumbar strain/sprain. The remainder in this mechanical LBP group will have symptoms attributable to disc or facet degeneration (10%), **herniated disc** (4%), **spinal stenosis** (3%), osteoporotic compression fracture (4%), **spondylolisthesis** (2%), traumatic fracture (<1%), congenital **kyphosis**/scoliosis (<1%), or **spondylolysis**, **discogenic** pain, or presumed segment instability (3). This seeming lack of diagnostic clarity for most LBP is misleading, because we can usually demonstrate quite convincingly that the pain is not due to any serious malady. Having excluded such problems, the management is usually similar and effective.

Of great concern is the fact that 5% to 10% of individuals with mechanical LBP develop "permanent disability" accounting for 75% to 90% of total costs (16, 17). The average cost (direct and indemnity) per industrial back injury in the United States (involving at least 1 day lost from work, and not including injuries without lost days for which no indemnity is paid) is now over $24,000 (18). Isolated cases have exceeded $900,000 (18).

It has been calculated that the growth rate of reported back pain is now roughly 14 times greater than our population growth rate; and while general disability awards have increased by 347% (as of 1990), awards for back disability increased by 2,680% (16). Estimates have placed the total societal cost of LBP at 50 to 100 billion dollars per annum (16). For perspective, our total health care budget now exceeds 1.5 trillion dollars annually. (See Figure 33.1 and Table 33.2)

Historical Perspectives

Maladies of the back are mentioned in written records throughout history and in literature. The hieroglyphics of the Edwin Smith Papyrus (written circa 1500 BC) refer to "a man having a sprain of the vertebra of his spinal column" (19). Psalm 129:2 reads: "But they have not prevailed against me. The plowers plowed upon my back; and made long furrows" (20). Pain in the lower back was traditionally known as **lumbago** (L., from lumbus, loin), which a modern medical dictionary defines as "backache in the lumbar or lumbosacral region" (21). In 1904, writing in the *British Medical Journal*, Sir William Gowers asked:

What is lumbago? Our conception of its symptoms is sufficiently clear, precise, and perhaps vivid. But our conception of its nature is not at all precise or clear. We think of it as

TABLE 33.1. DIFFERENTIAL DIAGNOSIS OF LOW BACK PAIN

Mechanical Low Back or Leg Pain (97%)	Nonmechanical Spinal Conditions (About 1%)	Visceral Disease (2%)
Lumbar strain, sprain (70%)	Neoplasia (0.7%)	Disease of pelvic organs
Degenerative processes of disks and facets, usually age-related (10%)	Multiple myeloma	Prostatitis
Herniated disk (4%)	Metastatic carcinoma	Endometriosis
Spinal stenosis (3%)	Lymphoma and leukemia	Chronic pelvic inflammatory disease
Osteoporotic compression fracture (4%)	Spinal cord tumors	Renal disease
Spondylolisthesis (2%)	Retroperitoneal tumors	Nephrolithiasis
Traumatic fracture (<1%)	Primary vertebral tumors	Pyelonephritis
Congenital disease (<1%)	Infection (0.01%)	Perinephric abscess
Severe kyphosis	Osteomyelitis	Aortic aneurysm
Severe scoliosis	Septic diskitis	Gastrointestinal disease
Transitional vertebrae	Paraspinous abscess	Pancreatitis
Spondylolysis	Epidural abscess	Cholecystitis
Internal disk disruption or diskogenic low back pain	*Shingles*	Penetrating ulcer
Presumed instability	Inflammatory arthritis (often associated with HLA-B27) (0.3%)	
	Ankylosing spondylitis	
	Psoriatic spondylitis	
	Reiter's syndrome	
	Inflammatory bowel disease	
	Scheuermann's disease (osteochondrosis)	
	Paget's disease of bone	

Figures in parentheses indicate the estimated percentages of patients with these conditions among all adult patients with low back pain in primary care. Diagnoses in italics are often associated with neurogenic leg pain. Percentages may vary substantially according to demographic characteristics or referral patterns in a practice. For example, spinal stenosis and osteoporosis will be more common among geriatric patients, spinal infection among injection-drug users, and so forth.
Adapted from Deyo RA, Weinstein JN (3). (Table 1 and page 365).

muscular rheumatism—and correctly. But if we are asked what muscular rheumatism is, I am afraid the reply which would be given is that "it is rheumatism of the muscles," an answer which, you will admit, does not carry us far (22).

Shakespeare frequently mentions lumbago and **sciatica**, and keenly described the former discomfort as "loads o' gravel in the back" (23). Sufferers of LBP often use stronger and more colorful epithets.

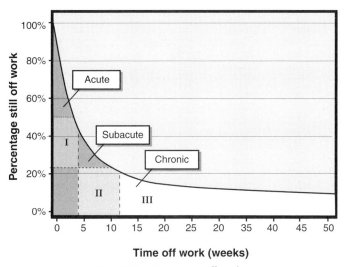

FIGURE 33.1. Percentage off work

Guidelines: From Quebec to Paris

The concepts of prolonged rest and the focus on pain management for the injured back endured for most of the 20th century. In 1986, however, Deyo demonstrated that more than 2 days of rest was neither cost effective nor beneficial to the patient (24). In that same year the Quebec Guidelines were published, offering formalized recommendations based on a careful review of the scientific literature for clinicians managing low back pain (17). In 1994 the U.S. Agency for Health Care Policy and Research (AHCPR) published its algorithms for managing LBP. They endorsed a "shift away from focusing care exclusively on the pain and toward helping patients improve activity tolerance" (10, 11). In 1996 England and New Zealand offered similar recommendations (25).

The Cochran Library reviews have supported early activation in the management of musculoligamentous LBP. A review by Hilde et al. found that the best available evidence from randomized controlled trials (RCTs) suggests that advice to stay active has beneficial effects for patients with acute simple LBP, that activity is not harmful, and that prolonged bed rest has potential harmful effects (26).

In 2000 the Paris International Task Force on Low Back Pain released its collective findings in a comprehensive and updated review of the literature. Representatives of the Quebec, AHCPR, and English groups were members of this

TABLE 33.2. COSTS ASSOCIATED WITH LOW BACK PAIN EVALUATIONS

Study or Procedure	Average Cost/Range
Primary care management (2.3 visits)[a]	$199
Orthopaedic non-operative management (5 visits)[a]	$531
Chiropractic management (10 visits)[a]	$281
Standard x-ray series (AP, lat, sacrum)	$150–200
X-rays (3 views plus obiques)	$200–250
CT scan	$600–800
Magnetic Resonance Imaging study	$1,200–1,500
Electromyelogram	$500–700
Bone scan	$700–100
SPECT scan	$1,300
Physical therapy per session	$75–100/h
Back school program for "failed back" (18-20 sessions)	$2,000
Pool therapy per session	$100–150/h
Epidural steroid injection (each)[b]	$690
Lumbar myelogram	$1,700
Discogram	$2,000
Laminectomy (average worker's compensation case with medical, indemnity, and permanency costs)[b]	$86,000
Spinal fusion (average worker's compensation case with medical, indemnity, and permanency costs)[b]	$168,000
Roman chair for home exercise back extension maintenance	$200–250
Health club membership per year	$400–500
Cigarettes (one pack per day) for one year	$1,200–1,500

[a]Adapted from Shekelle PG, Markovich M, Louie R. Comparing the costs between provider types of episodes of back pain care. Spine 2000;20:221-227. (1982 data)

[b]Adapted from Nelson BW, O'Reilly E, Miller M (5).

task force, and its work is a continuation and elaboration of the previous guidelines (27). The overriding belief of the Paris Task Force is as follows:

It appears that the key to success is physical activity itself— i.e., activity of any form—rather than any specific activity. The Task Force's recommendation that there is scientific evidence in favor of programs combining strength training, stretching, and fitness [italics theirs] is likely to cause a re-thinking of widespread habits and convictions, and there may be some resistance to the implementation of such programs.

Despite all common sense, clinical experience, and solid studies that champion exercise in treating LBP, misconceptions about its lack of effectiveness are still promulgated by groups who cite insufficient proof or lack of randomized clinical evidence (28, 29). However, lack of strict scientific proof does not mean activity and exercise are ineffective (11). We will never do RCTs to prove that tobacco use causes lung cancer, emphysema, and cardiovascular disease, nor will we need to do so, because we know from clinical experience that it does. Controlled, randomized,

blinded investigations into LBP are extremely difficult to perform, which may account for the current lack of statistically significant studies. This should not prevent us from instituting treatment that we know is effective.

Whether acute LBP and chronic LBP are viewed as points on a continuum of dysfunction or as separate entities, the treatment must focus on restoration of function, not treatment of symptoms. According to Herring, the goal of injury rehabilitation has 3 phases: (1) acute phase—rule out serious diagnoses, a brief period of relative or controlled rest, pain reduction, protect the **kinetic chain** from the damaging effects of inactivity, and education; (2) recovery phase—avoid reinjury, promote biologic healing, and restore strength, flexibility, endurance, proprioception, and general fitness; (3) maintenance phase—return to normal function of the injured structure, and develop task-specific skills for the return to activity, risk factor avoidance, and prevention of recurrence (Table 33.3) (30).

Review of Physiology and Pathophysiology

In infancy the human spine is straight, but as the child learns to walk, the spine assumes the natural curves that make ambulation possible. In making this postural adaptation, the child naturally assumes what we call the **power position**, our most stable back position (31). Part of the modern dilemma is that we, who became habitually upright as bipeds, are now habitually sedentary. Prolonged seated postures, especially if slouched, interfere with normal lumbar **lordosis** and result in a functional lumbar kyphosis, shortening of the hamstrings, and weak, unbalanced back muscles. One of the imperative goals of therapy is to regain lumbar lordosis (Figure 33.2).

TABLE 33.3. INJURY REHABILITATION

Phases	Goals
Acute	Accurate diagnosis
	Pain relief
	Relative rest/protect kinetic chain
	Education
Recovery	Promote biologic healing
	Restoration of strength
	Restoration of flexibility
	Restoration of proprioception
	General fitness
Maintenance	Normal function of injured structure
	Development of task specific skills for return to activity

Adapted from Herring SA (30), page 236, Table 22-1.

Herring SA. Sports Medicine Early Care. In: Mayer TG, Mooney V, and Gatchel RJ, eds. Contemporary Conservative Care for Painful Spinal Disorders. Philadelphia. Lea & Febiger, 1991:235-244.

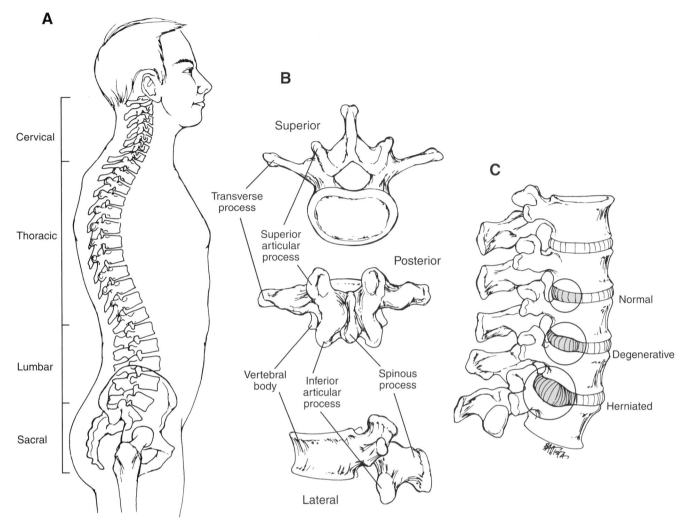

FIGURE 33.2. Lumbar stability by corset of abdominal and paraspinal musculature: (A) vertebrae; (B) components of a vertebra; and (C) normal, degenerative, and herniated disks.

Bipedalism and the Center of Gravity

The human body is subject to the laws of gravity just as any other physical or biomechanical structure. Lifting a weight away from the center of gravity creates an extended lever arm that dramatically increases the compressive forces on the spine. The human body is most energy efficient when it is balanced over this vertical axis, and anything that interferes with this alignment will produce strain and fatigue. The power position, which places the spine in a neutral lordosis position, seems to reduce the risk of injury.

LBP is a common and expected occurrence in pregnancy, and it is readily understood how and why the additional weight and change in center of gravity produces discomfort and alteration in posture. Similarly, an obese individual will require greater reactive forces (thus increasing compressive forces in the spine) to balance an extended mass against the forces of gravity, particularly when bending, lifting, or negotiating stairs. In nonindustrialized societies, people carry

weights on the head or in balanced, tandem loads using a pole across the shoulders; in industrialized societies, we tend to carry to one side or in front with our arms, or with backpacks (some small school children may carry up to one quarter of their body weight), all of which may disrupt the normal spinal alignment (Figure 33.3).

Han showed a positive correlation (after adjusting for confounding factors of aging, smoking, and education) between chronic LBP and disc herniation in women who were overweight and had increased abdominal girth (32). Toda found an association between obesity and LBP in women with a negative straight leg raise (33). Body mass index, which does not differentiate lean from fat mass, was not predictive. It is interesting to note that women tend to develop adiposity "on the outside" whereas men seem to accumulate fat mass more centrally and in retroperitoneal areas. Lee showed that LBP subjects had low muscle strength in both the trunk and lower extremities and that there was a linear correlation between the two (34). Cross-sectional abdominal **computed tomogra-**

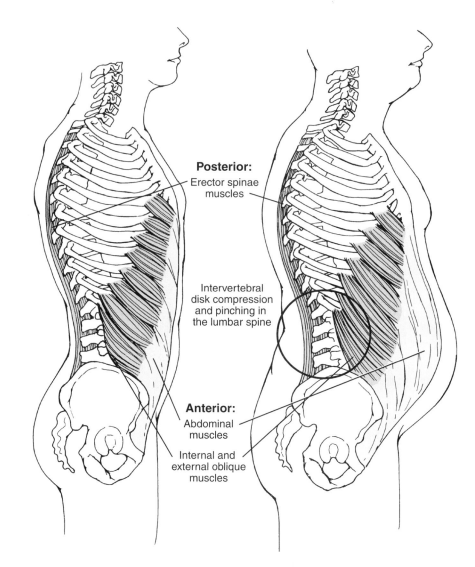

Posterior:
Erector spinae
muscles

Intervertebral
disk compression
and pinching in
the lumbar spine

Anterior:
Abdominal
muscles

Internal and
external oblique
muscles

FIGURE 33.3.   LBP as a result of trunk muscle weakness.

Spinal Anatomy and Biomechanics

Familiarity with the anatomy of the vertebral column is essential. As Hippocrates said, "In the first place, the structure of the spine should be known, for this knowledge is requisite in many diseases" (38). The beauty and marvel of the spine has always been its functional mobility; the Greek term *spondyle* and the Latin *vertebra* both etymologically describe a "turning movement" (39). Ward, a contemporary of Darwin, considered "the vertebral column [as] a remarkable piece of mechanism. Strong enough to support several hundredweight, yet pliant and elastic;...formed, for lightness...yet capable of sustaining...shocks, strains, and con-

phy (CT) scans at the lumbar level help to illustrate how muscle mass and fat distribution may affect the center of gravity and spinal burden. Several studies have documented disuse atrophy of the lumbar extensor muscles, and the role of lumbar extension strengthening programs in reversing such atrophy (18, 35–37) (Figure 33.4).

tortions of considerable violence: this column...performs functions apparently incompatible" (40). The exhortation "Put your back into it, lads" was a tribute to this resolute structure, whereas to be called a "spineless coward" was the nadir of pusillanimity.

The spine serves 3 basic functions: protection, support, and locomotion. It is a protective sheath for the spinal cord and nerve roots and provides a foundation for the ribs and appendicular skeleton, yet allows a great degree of flexibility for postural adaptation and movement. The human has 33 vertebrae (24 are movable): 7 cervical, 12 thoracic, 5 lumbar, 5 fused to form the sacrum, and 4 fused into the coccyx. The spine is a "coupled motion" system consisting of **motion segments** of 2 vertebral bodies and the intervening disc (30). The vertebrae comprise approximately 75% to 80% of the spinal height with approximately 20% to 25% due to the thickness of the **intervertebral disc**. As people age, the disc becomes dehydrated and less elastic, and height is lost (Figure 33.5).

The overall stability of the spinal complex depends upon 3 interrelated systems: (1) inert tissues (bone, ligaments,

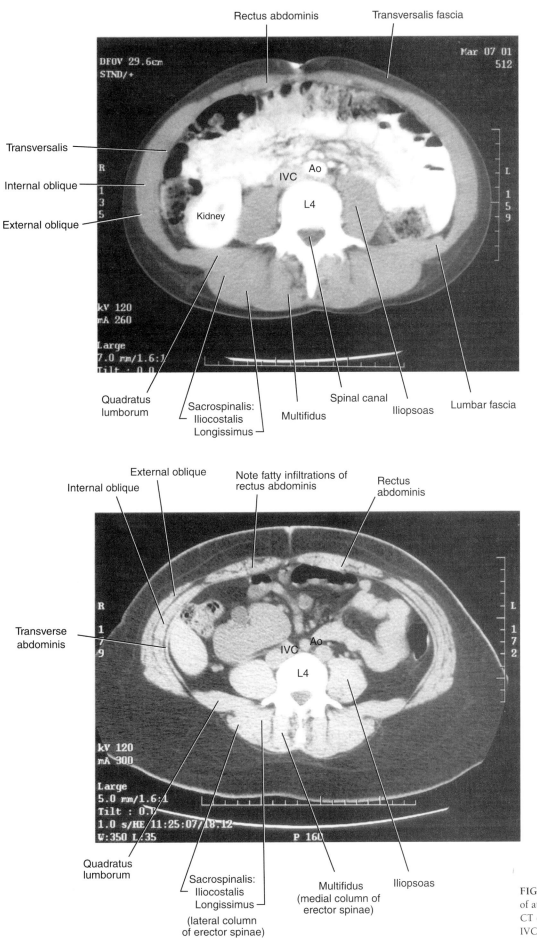

Rectus abdominis

Transversalis fascia

Transversalis

Internal oblique

External oblique

Ao

IVC

L4

Kidney

Quadratus lumborum

Sacrospinalis:
└ Iliocostalis
Longissimus ┘

Multifidus

Spinal canal

Iliopsoas

Lumbar fascia

External oblique

Internal oblique

Note fatty infiltrations of
rectus abdominis

Rectus
abdominis

Transverse
abdominis

Ao

IVC

L4

Quadratus
lumborum

Sacrospinalis:
└ Iliocostalis
Longissimus ┘

(lateral column
of erector spinae)

Multifidus
(medial column of
erector spinae)

Iliopsoas

FIGURE 33.4. (A) Abdominal CT
of athletic female. (B) Abdominal
CT of obese female. (Ao, aorta;
IVC, inferior vena cava)

523

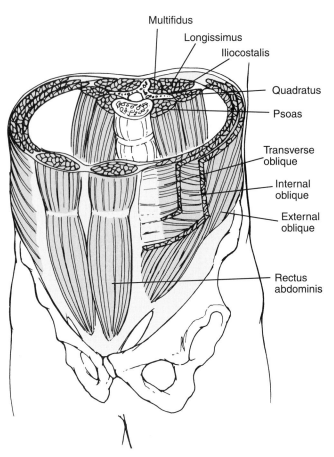

Multifidus
Longissimus
Iliocostalis
Quadratus
Psoas
Transverse oblique
Internal oblique
External oblique
Rectus abdominis

FIGURE 33.5.   Lumbar spinal column with a normal disc, degenerative but asymptomatic level, bulging disc, and protruding disc.

and fascia primarily) provide passive support and stabilization; (2) contractile tissues (muscle-tendon complexes) provide active, dynamic stability; and (3) neural control centers receive sensory feedback from both systems and coordinate output based on both static and dynamic body responses.

The segmental stability of the vertebral couple results from the interlocking of the "articulating triad" of 3 osseous contact surfaces (41). Anteriorly, the intervertebral disc forms a joint with the superior and inferior endplates of the adjacent vertebral bodies. Posteriorly, the 2 articular (zygapophyseal) facets form a true synovial joint where the inferior articular processes, both right and left, of the vertebra above dovetail with the 2 respective superior articular processes of the vertebra below. With flexion, the anterior spine is compressed and the posterior elements open; with extension, the anterior portions of the vertebrae separate while the posterior column elements are compressed, with the spinous processes limiting extension at a certain point. The center of gravity and fulcrum of the motion segment runs through the posterior portion of the vertebral body and disc, but anterior to the spinal cord itself. Dennis has described the 3-column concept of the spine in terms of anterior, middle, and posterior columns (42).

The spine is inherently unstable. With the musculature removed, a cadaver spine will support only 4 or 5 pounds before it collapses (43). To bear substantial weight, the muscles and ligaments must stabilize it. Multiple intervertebral ligaments provide passive stability to the spine. Although usually identified as separate structures, the ligaments of the spine are actually interwoven and functionally form a continuous stocking to provide static support. The major ligaments of the spine are the ligamentum flavum (LF), which forms the rear wall of the spinal canal and joins with the joint capsule of the facet; the anterior longitudinal ligament (ALL); the posterior longitudinal ligament (PLL); and the interspinous ligament (ISL), which thickens posteriorly into the supraspinous ligament (SSL) and the intertransverse ligaments (ITL). Just like ankle or knee ligaments, the ligaments of the spine can be sprained, requiring appropriate healing time, and may be involved in many low back sprain injuries.

The muscles of the back and their tendinous insertions constitute a dynamic set of stabilizers that provide most of the support to the spinal column. The major antero-lateral structures include the quadratus lumborum, iliopsoas, and abdominal muscles; the posterior muscles include the deep intersegmental layer (multifidi, rotatores, and semispinalis), intermediate layer (interspinalis and intertransversarii), and superficial erector spinae layer (spinalis, iliocostalis, and longissimus). The thoracolumbar fascia (TLF) is an essential structure to back stability and functions as a "hydraulic amplifier" by resisting expansion of the erector spinae muscles as they contract, and possibly increasing force generated by the muscles by up to 30% (41, 44, 45). The TLF also contributes to SI joint stability. (See Figure 33.2.)

Viewed écorché (with skin removed), the TLF with its muscular extensions has a notable bias-ply crossover appearance connecting the upper and lower extremities. Like the trunk of a tree, the torso must be adequately buttressed if it is to provide postural support and locomotor activity to the appendicular skeleton. This support is made possible by the synergistic tensions of the gluteus muscles, hamstrings, latissimus dorsi, quadriceps, and other structures described above. The muscles of the back and the appendicular skeleton are connected to the axial spine in this highly integrated and interdependent system. Thus, optimal strengthening of the back requires strengthening of the arms and legs, and vice versa. Kibler and Herring have been vigorous proponents of this kinetic chain approach to rehabilitation (30, 46, 47). Once the value of the kinetic chain mechanism is conceptualized, the need for overall fitness in terms of function and injury prevention is apparent.

There are 24 intervertebral discs; the lumbar spine has 5 discs, with an average thickness of 9 mm. The lumbar discs are thicker anteriorly and thinner posteriorly in concert with the lordosis of the lower spine, which may predispose them to injury posteriorly and the tendency to herniate on either side of the tough PLL. The L4-5 and L5-S1 discs experience the greatest load and hence most commonly herniate, although all may show signs of dehydration and degeneration (48). The annular fibers are anchored to the bony rim of the vertebrae and stabilize the disc between the 2 vertebral segments. The peripheral fibers of the annulus are pain-receptive structures.

The disc itself is a thickened shock absorber of concentric fibrous rings, the **annulus fibrosus**, encircling a gelatinous core called the **nucleus pulposus** (NP). The resiliency of the disc is largely due to the hydraulic forces of the water content of the proteoglycan-rich NP. The intervertebral disc must be able to withstand biomechanical load forces in 6 directions: axial compression, distraction, flexion, extension, multidirectional slide, and rotational shear. The combination of rotation and flexion is most likely to damage the disc. When axially loaded quickly and released, as with a single jump, the disc undergoes elastic deformation and recovery similar to a tennis ball. When loaded over an extended period, such as prolonged sitting, carrying weight, or increased body mass over time, it demonstrates viscoelastic properties and may be compressed and suffer prolonged deformation (41, 48, 49).

In adulthood, the disc is a largely avascular structure, and relies on passive diffusion of fluids (imbibition) through the semipermeable hyaline cartilage interface of the vertebrae above and below to provide nutrients to the AF and central NP. Under normal loading the NP is approximately 80% to 90% water; however, this typically decreases with age (49). An osmotic pressure gradient within the NP normally pulls fluid into the disk. The pressure gradient is enhanced when resting in a recumbent position or during noncompressive horizontal activities (e.g., swimming); nourishment of the disc via osmotic diffusion is reduced by increased or prolonged load on the disc. The thickness of the vertebral disc may be reduced by up to 15% during the day due to the cumulative effects of compressive loading of the vertebral column.

Lack of physical activity and motion reduces blood flow through the vascular channels of the vertebrae, which interferes with metabolic exchange, causes low oxygen concentrations in the disc, and reduces overall disc nutrition, predisposing it to dehydration, microfracture, and fissuring. Smoking substitutes carbon monoxide for oxygen and has been shown to have deleterious effects on nourishment of the intervertebral discs (the largest avascular structures in the body), seen as degenerative change and delayed healing (50–52). In older individuals reduced water content seems to limit the classic flow or extrusion of NP material, and instead radial cracks and delamination of the annulus are seen.

The bony vertebra is about 3 times the thickness of the disk and approximately 6 times as stiff. The trabecular matrix of cancellous bone within the relatively thin shell of cortex is stress moulded according to Wolff's law to resist compressive forces. Because it cannot deform like the more elastic disc, it may fracture even in a young healthy individual under sudden axial overload, particularly with a flexion component. **Osteoporosis** increases the likelihood of

insufficiency fractures of the spine, wrist, and hip in women. Anterior compression fractures in the thoracic vertebrae often produce the kyphotic "dowager's hump" deformity.

The vertebral facets are synovial joints with approximately 2 mL of synovial fluid in each joint capsule. The facet capsule has 3 parts: (1) the articular cartilage, which functions as a connective tissue rim; (2) an adipose tissue pad filled with fat and blood vessels; (3) a 5-mm fibroadipose meniscoid fold that projects from the inner surfaces of the superior and inferior capsules. In the lumbar spine the orientation of the facets allows flexion/extension, but little or no rotation, whereas the facet orientation in the thoracic spine allows rotation and flexion/extension. With increased axial loading compressing the disc, the inferior facets may begin to slip or "creep" abnormally downward to impact the laminae (49). This may damage the joint capsule and result in the classic "degenerative cascade" described by Kirkaldy-Willis (53).

The SI joint is stabilized by several ligaments, particularly the iliolumbar, anterior sacroiliac, sacrospinous, and sacrotuberous ligaments. Both the biceps femoris tendon and the multifidus musculature have attachments to the sacrotuberous ligament and provide additional stabilization to the SI joint. The SI joint motion is called nutation when the sacrum is tilted anteriorly (most commonly in standing), and counternutation when it tilts posteriorly (most often while lying prone). Nutation increases lumbar lordosis, whereas counternutation flattens the back and reduces lordosis. These structures provide "form closure" via a keystone gravitational effect and "force closure" through lateral compression of the iliac wings to the sacrum (54).

Mechanisms of Injury

Our Modern Dilemma: Overload Versus Insufficiency

An early 19th century proverb augurs that "God makes the back to the burden" (55). This may have been true in the past, but given current statistics our backs are not holding up well under the stress of modern existence. It is a common notion, particularly in the work setting, that "back injuries" result from a single episode of excessive lifting. A common explanation is that "I strained my back" or "my back went out" when trying to lift something that was too heavy. Often, however, one was reaching for a relatively light object when the back "went out." Except for falls, traumatic blows, or high-speed injuries, rarely does the back receive its primary insult at the time of perceived injury. It has been shown that in most episodes of axial compression, the vertebral end plates will fail, with collapse of the cancellous or trabecular bone, before the intervertebral disc will rupture. Just as a heart attack that occurs while shoveling snow is less the result of shoveling than the underlying cardiovascular disease, so too LBP is typically more a manifestation of significant underlying debility or insufficiency. The proverbial "straw that broke the camel's back" expresses a basic physiologic wisdom.

Risk Factors

In most cases, the muscle-tendon-bone-ligament-disc complex has undergone gradual insult and weakening over a significant period. This may be due to the effects of many risk factors including poor posture, gradual weight gain, lack of exercise, smoking, poor body mechanics with lifting, or repetitive and/or heavy work demands. All may contribute to poor disc and connective tissue nutrition, increased couple segment motion, and increased fatigability of the back support structures. Sitting, particularly in a slouched position with the head forward, produces intradiscal pressures significantly greater than standing; done for prolonged periods, it is perhaps the most traumatic thing we can do to our backs (56) (Figure 33.6).

Clearly, heavy lifting (especially accelerated lifting), sustained loads over long duration, decreased compressive tol-

erance in the final stages of full flexion, and variations in individual physical capacity increase risk. One seems most prone to injury either when lifting a low load with the major muscles not activated or when an excessive load is attempted. Remember, force equals mass times acceleration (F = MA); lifting slowly reduces forces and vice versa. Although the exact pain generator in most cases of LBP is elusive, we know quite a bit about what can be done empirically to help an individual cope with discomfort and reduce the likelihood that it will chronically interfere with function. It is a mistake to tell a patient they will get better 90% of the time no matter what they do without addressing underlying risks (31).

Numerous behaviors and activities (both vocational and recreational) are associated with an increased risk of LBP, but also can prolong recovery. Individual characteristics often determine how well one copes with such discomfort (57). There is ample documentation of the increased incidence of LBP associated with smoking, depression, job dissatisfaction, lack of exercise, obesity, lifting that requires frequent rotation or twisting, postural habits, sedentary vocation, and repetitive, heavy lifting. Construction workers, baggage handlers, warehouse

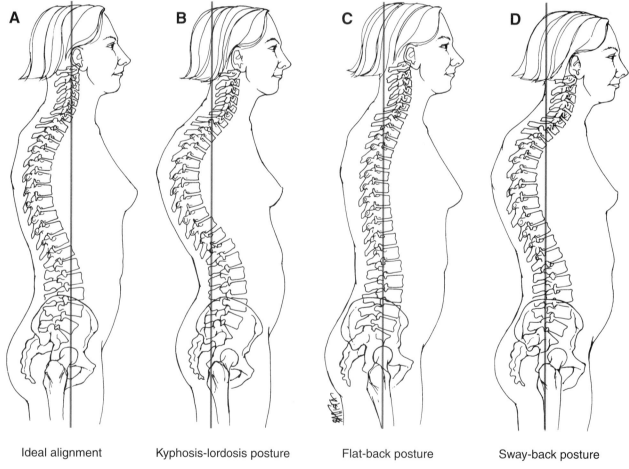

Ideal alignment   Kyphosis-lordosis posture   Flat-back posture   Sway-back posture

FIGURE 33.6.   Four types of postural alignment: (**A**) ideal; (**B**) kyphosis-lordosis; (**C**) flat-back posture; and (**D**) swayback.

workers, fire, police, and ambulance personnel, material handlers, assembly line workers, nurses and nursing assistants, and office workers with desk jobs may be significantly affected. Notably, one of the factors with greatest relative risk in the workplace is depression. Other spine-jarring activities that should be avoided, particularly by individuals under work restriction, include snowmobiling, jet skiing, four-wheeling, and horseback riding. Dr. William Osler said, "It is much more important to know what sort of patient has a disease than what sort of a disease a patient has" (58).

Classification

Nonsurgical LBP goes by many names: lumbago, mechanical low back pain, musculoligamentous low back pain, idiopathic low back pain, nondiscogenic back pain, and paralumbar strain are commonly used. The multiple ICD-9 codes for pain in the lower back region reflect these diagnostic vagaries. Hadler suggests the need to differentiate systemic from regional back pain (59). Because most LBP episodes are soft tissue or musculoligamentous in nature, no readily identifiable mechanical abnormality will be found despite extensive imaging studies. Nachemson suggested only 10% to 20% of patients with lumbosacral pain could be given an exact pathomechanical diagnosis (60). Pragmatically, rehabilitation specialists and therapists are finding that the management protocols are similar, regardless of the etiology (and whether treatment is problem or diagnosis focused).

Attempts to classify LBP by diagnostic category for guideline recommendations often meet with frustration. The Quebec group listed 13 diagnostic categories (17). The Paris Group uses 4 categories: (1) LBP with no radiation; (2) LBP radiating no further than the knee; (3) LBP radiating beyond the knee, with no neurologic signs; and (4) LBP radiating to a precise and entire leg dermatome (27). Under this approach patients are grouped by symptoms, rather than by a specific pathophysiologic diagnosis. Waddell suggests that we avoid the often-misused term "sciatica," and simply make the distinction between "referred leg pain" (which typically does not extend more distal than the knee) and classic nerve root irritation (with dermatomal motor, sensory, or reflex changes) (14).

In addition, LBP is traditionally differentiated by duration of symptoms: acute (0–4 weeks), subacute (4–12 weeks), and chronic (beyond 12 weeks). Other sources define acute LBP as 1 to 2 weeks' duration and chronic LBP as beyond 8 weeks. Clearly, the nomenclature designating a transition from acuity to chronicity is subject to discussion. Yet our current knowledge of soft tissue healing timelines and recovery suggests a Gaussian distribution model with a median of at least 50% of patients recovered at 6 weeks and 95% (2 standard deviations) healing at 3 months after injury. A classification based only on overt symptom duration may fail to recognize underlying pathology, which underscores the need to address comorbid risk factors in all cases.

Ergonomics and Workplace Concerns

The National Institute for Occupational Safety and Health (NIOSH), in a large study of more than 9,000 employees, found no evidence that back belts reduce back injury or back pain "for retail workers who lift or move merchandise" (61). NIOSH last updated its "Applications Manual for the Revised NIOSH Lifting Equation" on January 1, 1994, in a 73-page document accessible through the Centers for Disease Control and Prevention (CDCP) and NIOSH Web site (62). The lifting index (LI) and the recommended weight limit (RWL) are calculated based on a multiplicative model that factors 6 task variables. Although these theoretical models can be useful in some industries, they are not of immediate use to the nursing assistant who must suddenly support an unsteady or falling patient.

Many caregivers now endorse the concept of the "industrial athlete," and believe the workplace should adopt an aggressive sports medicine model of prevention and rehabilitation, which should be applied to both sedentary and heavy labor employees. A desk-bound individual who is 50 or even 25 pounds overweight may actually be placing a greater strain on the back on a daily basis than a warehouse laborer. Given that employees spend 75% of their time away from the workplace and 60% of all compensable injuries actually occur away from the job, injury prevention needs to change its focus from the workplace to the worker (63). With torso and core-body strengthening the worker is better able to withstand the daily stresses placed on the spine both at and away from work. And because a major risk factor for LBP is a previous back injury, prevention to avoid the initial episode makes sense. Companies that have offered fitness programs to their employees have shown consistent cost-benefit, decreased absenteeism, improvements in morale and productivity, and a reduction of injury rates (64–68).

Diagnostic Evaluation

Patient History

A careful history is essential to the evaluation of an individual with low back pain. A thorough history explores issues such as date and mechanism of injury, previous injury, occupation, recreational and other habits, symptoms (including any daily variation, and radicular and constitutional symptoms), nature and distribution of the pain, risk factors, tobacco and ethanol use, previous surgeries, medical problems, family history, allergies, medication use, and complementary treatments. A visual analogue scale (VAS), **Oswestry Low Back Pain Questionnaire**, Roland, or other

TABLE 33.4. COMMON SPINAL CONDITIONS BY AGE GROUP

Age Group	Common Conditions
Younger than 10 years	Intervertebral diskitis, myelomeningocele, osteoblastoma, leukemia, congenital kyphosis, and scoliosis
Teens	Spondylolisthesis, kyphosis (Scheuermann's disease)
Twenties	Disk injuries (central disk protrusion, disk sprain), spondylolisthesis, spinal fracture
Thirties	Cervical and lumbar disk herniation or degeneration
Forties	Cervical and lumbar disk herniation or degeneration spondylolisthesis with radicular pain
Fifties	Disk degeneration, herniated disk, metastatic tumors
Sixties and older	Spinal stenosis, disk degeneration, herniated disk, spinal instability, metastatic tumors

Adapted from Snider RK, ed. Essentials of Musculoskeletal Care. Rosemont, Ill: American Academy of Orthopaedic Surgeons; 1997:493.

similar test, and a depression scale (such as MMPI) are helpful to assess pain and measure changes in functional status (Table 33.4).

Clinical Examination

A thorough clinical examination includes vital signs; comment on general body habitus and overall appearance; inspection of the back for asymmetry, atrophy, or other spinal or muscular abnormalities; leg length assessment; gait; range of motion of the lumbar spine (forward flexion, extension, axial rotation, and lateral flexion) and hips; palpation to localize any bony, muscular, or other soft tissue tenderness; straight leg raise (SLR); hamstring tightness and other lower extremity abnormality; a complete neurologic evaluation of tendon reflexes; evidence of **radiculopathy**; dermatomal changes of motor strength or sensation to pin prick and light touch; and ability to change position and balance. The patient should be examined standing, seated, supine, and prone. Separating lumbar motion and pelvic motion may also be done by inclinometer. It is important to conceptualize lumbo-pelvic motion and recognize that hip flexion (110 degrees) can easily conceal or compensate for a stiff lumbar spine (normal range 72 degrees). Other specific tests may include Lasegue's sciatic nerve test, Stork, flexion in abduction and external rotation (FABER) or Patrick's tests, slump test, and dural tension tests (69). **Waddell signs** are a series of 7 tests designed to help distinguish behavioral (nonorganic) responses from true organic/physical injury (14, 70). These tests assess nonanatomic and superficial tenderness, simulated spinal rotation and axial loading, straight leg raise while dis-

tracted, and regional weakness or sensory disturbance. They may be performed quickly during the physical examination. Waddell emphasizes the need for dispassionate clinical observation rather than judgmental assessment.

Imaging

Radiologic imaging should be used as a confirmatory tool rather than a screening device. In most instances, imaging studies done to evaluate routine musculoligamentous LBP lack specificity (i.e., there are a high number of false-positive findings). If trauma to the back has occurred or other red-flag indications are present, radiographs (or the appropriate study) should be obtained at the initial visit; otherwise, the patient is better served by minimizing the radiation and cost, and spending the time on education and prevention counseling. Labeling of imaging findings as "degenerative joint disease," "arthritis," "protruding disc," and so forth often misleads the patient into thinking the condition is more serious than it really is; "normal wear and tear" and "simple" back pain descriptors cause less apprehension. (We tell patients by analogy that even the best car tires will show wear and tear after miles of use, yet function perfectly well and we trust our lives to them.) However, imaging studies may be indicated for the patient with persistent LBP for more than 6 weeks, despite appropriate management. In certain situations, specialized modalities may be indicated: CT scanning for bony abnormalities; **magnetic resonance imaging** (MRI) for disc and nerve root abnormalities; **bone scan** for suspected stress fractures or pathologic bone changes; single photon emission computed tomography (SPECT) to differentiate disc infections from degenerative vertebral endplate processes; discograms; and myelography (71) (Figures 33.3 and 33.8).

Kirkaldy-Willis and others have demonstrated that the anterior (discovertebral) and posterior (facet) structures show progressive degeneration with age (53). Changes in the synovium and joint capsule, annular ligament tears, ligamentous, muscular, and fascial wear are inevitable for all of us. Yet these progressive changes, as documented in several landmark imaging studies, generally lack specific correlation with back pain symptoms. If abnormalities are discovered with imaging, it must be remembered that more than 50% of asymptomatic persons under age 50, and close to 100% of asymptomatic persons over age 60, will have signs of degenerative joint disease, bulging discs, or other structural changes, yet have no complaint of pain. This has been documented on plain radiographs by Nachemson et al. (56), on computed tomography by Weisel (72), and on MRI by Boden et al (73) and Jensen et al (74). Boden showed that among asymptomatic persons 40 to 59 years old, 59% had degenerative changes, 54% had a bulging disc, and 22% had a herniated disc, whereas among an asymptomatic population older than age 60 the percentages were 93%, 79%, and 36%, respectively (73). Jensen found bulging and her-

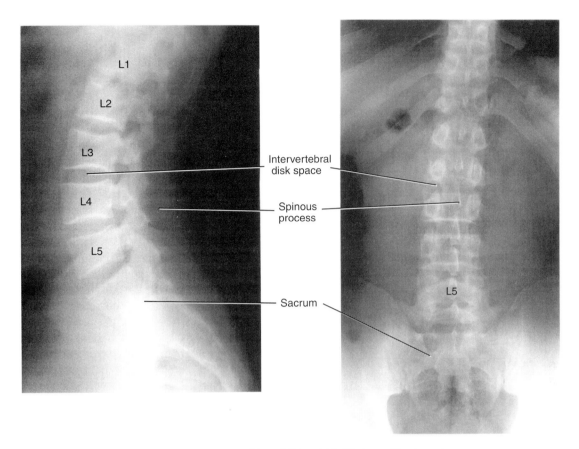

FIGURE 33.7.   Normal lateral (A) and AP (B) views of lumbar spine.

niated discs in asymptomatic patients at rates of 52% and 28%, respectively (74).

The layman's term "slipped disc" is a misnomer, because the intervertebral disc does not actually slide from between the 2 vertebrae. In reading an MRI, radiologists will usually describe a disc as bulging, protruding, extruded, or sequestered. A bulging disc, often the wall of the annulus fibrosus (AF), may indent the thecal sac midline; however, depending on the level, if it does not compress the cord or a nerve root, it often produces no symptoms. Protrusion of disc material, usually nucleus pulposus (NP), if lateral, can narrow the foramina or encroach/impinge on a nerve root and produce characteristic radicular symptoms. Extruded or sequestered fragments of either NP or AF can produce findings similar to a protruded disc, but are less likely to resorb; persistent symptoms may need to be treated surgically to remove the mass effect (Table 33.5).

Differential Diagnosis: Red Flags and Yellow Flags

It is obviously crucial to exclude the possibility of other potentially serious spinal or systemic disorders before reaching a working diagnosis of generic musculoligamentous LBP. The differential diagnosis should include spinal steno-

sis, **cauda equina syndrome**, vascular disease such as abdominal aortic aneurysm, spondylolysis, spondylolisthesis, disc infection or vertebral osteomyelitis (especially due to intravenous drug use or immune compromised status), primary or metastatic tumor (especially breast, prostate, thyroid, lung, and kidney), rheumatologic disease and arthritides, osteoporotic insufficiency fracture, and renal, or gynecologic disease. Fortunately, many of these maladies can be suspected or diagnosed with a thorough medical history and clinical examination (10). "**Red flags**" that should alert the examiner are listed in Table 33.5. Although it is not within the scope of this chapter to discuss them at length, these conditions require specialized medical referral and in most situations more elaborate diagnostic or procedural intervention.

Nonorganic (psychosomatic, social, legal, workers' compensation) issues must be considered in the evaluation of LBP, particularly chronic pain (41). Waddell's nonorganic signs, discussed previously, are often associated with psychosocial issues (14, 70). The New Zealand task force has labeled these concerns "**yellow flags**" to distinguish them from medical "red flags" (75). Litigation and workers' compensation are negative predictors for timely return to function. The longer a patient is off work because of LBP, the greater the risk of ongoing or chronic LBP, and the less the chance of ever returning to work (76). Samuel Butler, the

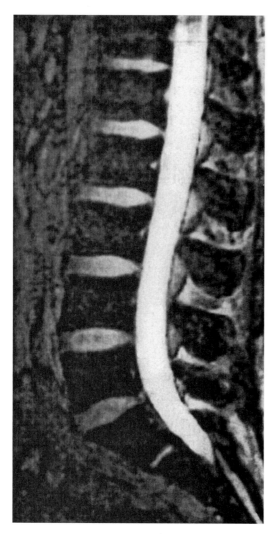

FIGURE 33.8.   Normal MRI of lumbar spine, sagittal view.

English novelist, once said, "I reckon being ill is one of the greatest pleasures of life, provided one is not too ill and is not obliged to work till one is better" (58). Intentional abuse of the system is not widespread, but should be considered when history, exam, and clinical progress are inconsistent.

Prevalence in Sport

The incidence of idiopathic back pain in athletes generally parallels that of the general population, though it may be increased in certain sports. The incidence of chronic or disabling conditions is extremely low, and there is no increase in the incidence of disc pathology associated with participation in recreational sport. Low back soreness or strain may occur with many sporting activities; however, the core body strength/conditioning and increased motivation associated with these activities usually results in a fairly rapid return to activity and competition. Consequently, it is rare for an athlete to become debilitated or be forced to retire from sport due to chronic back pain. The importance of trainers and coaching to ensure proper technique and avoid muscle imbalance injury should not be overlooked (77). In the athlete under 20 years of age with persistent LBP symptoms (particularly in gymnastics, throwing, and hitting sports with forced hyperextension activity), **pars interarticularis** injuries are most common.

Michelli and Wood compared adolescent sports medicine patients (age 12–18) and adult orthopaedic patients (21–77 years), both with LBP, and found the incidence of spondylolysis to be 47% and 5%, respectively; overall, 62% of the adolescent back complaints were felt to be due to posterior element derangements (78). Female gymnasts, presumably due to repeated biomechanical hyperextension microtrauma,

TABLE 33.5.   "RED FLAGS" THAT SUGGEST A NONMUSCULOSKELETAL ETIOLOGY FOR LOW BACK PAIN

Symptoms: Back pain with...	Diagnostic concern
Progressive sensory/motor changes in dermatomal distribution	Herniated disc
Changes in bowel or bladder function; saddle anesthesia; decreased rectal tone.	Cauda equina/spinal stenosis
Pulsatile abdominal mass	Abdominal aortic aneurysm
Fever; history of IV drug use	Osteomyelitis of vertebra
Cough and night sweats; immunocompromised	Tuberculosis
Age < 20 years; athlete	Spondylolysis/spondylolisthesis
Age > 50 years	Cancer/metastases
Female of middle age	Gynecologic or breast cancer
Gastrointestinal symptoms	Visceral disorders
Female > 60	Osteoporosis/compression fracture
Pain following trauma or fall	Fracture
Generalized discomfort with/without symmetric appendicular symptoms, and/or family history of arthridities	Immune spondyloarthropathies
Night pain unrelieved by rest	Tumor/cancer
Low back pain with urinary symptoms	Urolithiasis or pyelonephritis
Pain in gluteal region	Piriformis or other myofascial syndrome
Stocking/glove numbness or global pain	Nonorganic/psychosocial symptoms
Pain increased with walking and relieved by standing	Vascular claudication

Diagnostic concerns should be further evaluated with additional x-ray views, bone scan, ultrasound, CT scan, MRI, fluoroscopic biopsy, and/or subspecialty consultation as appropriate.

have been shown in particular to have a high risk for spine abnormalities. In one study using MRI scans, 9% of pre-elite, 43% of elite, and 63% of Olympic-level female gymnasts had spine "abnormalities" versus 15.8% of swimmers of comparable level (79). Another study showed an incidence of frank spondylolysis of 11% in gymnasts, probably due to neural arch fatigue fracture (80). Spondylolysis and spondylolisthesis is also common in football (especially blocking linemen), weight lifting (30–37%), diving, dance, and throwing sports (e.g., javelin, baseball, tennis, and cricket bowling). Using high-speed photography, the range of motion of the lumbar spine in pole-vaulting has been recorded to go from 40 degrees of extension to 130 degrees of flexion in 0.65 seconds (81). Golfers, perhaps due to the unique rotational motion of the torso, have one of the highest rates of reported back pain of all pro athletes (77% of PGA golfers had injuries in a 1-year period, with 42% being lumbosacral); 38% of professional tennis players have missed tournaments due to LBP (81). In the general population, spondylolysis occurs in roughly 6% of adults (81, 82).

The Enigma of Pain Generators: Mechanical, Chemical, and Biopsychosocial Factors

The issue of pain perception lies at the crux of regional low back discomfort. The gate control theory suggested mechanisms of pain modulation to link the mind-body dichotomy. Clearly, LBP may result from diverse mechanical, chemical, or complex biopsychosocial factors (83, 84). Many individuals with significant bony abnormalities have no pain; others with no evident pathology of the spinal complex have disabling symptoms. A depressed patient (who may not even realize that they are depressed) may perceive ordinary aches and pains as incapacitating. The traditional disease model of illness assumed that pain equaled tissue injury and that treating the pain would result in a cure. Clearly, however, pain does not necessarily equal injury or disability.

Except for the avascular center of the disc itself, the spine is interlaced with pain fibers. The sinovertebral nerve is the major sensory nerve supplying structures of the lumbosacral region. Nociceptive receptors are sensitive to stretch, inflammation, and perhaps disuse. Traditionally, radicular symptoms were thought to be due to mechanical injury, usually with a disc fragment exerting pressure or impinging on a nerve root, with resulting ischemia of the vasa vasorum. Research by Kawakami has shown that the nerve root may respond to chemical irritation from inflammatory substances including phospholipase A_2 (chemically similar to cobra venom), cytokines, substance P, TNF-α, PGE_2, and free radical nitric oxide synthase (85). These mediators may be released from macrophages in response to inflammatory changes secondary to an extrusion of NP. This notion of a chemical radiculitis—that it may be the "disc juice," rather than the NP itself, eliciting radicular pain—explains some of the acute nerve root symptoms experienced in the absence of a demonstrable mechanical lesion, but does not explain why people function differently with pain on a daily basis.

Therapy and rehabilitation have traditionally focused on symptom relief. "Iatrogenic" factors (caused by the caregiver) may ensue from the overprescription of rest and admonitions that "if it hurts, don't do it" and "let pain be your guide," which in LBP may result in disability through exercise avoidance and general **deconditioning**. Complex mechanisms of anticipatory pain behaviors may also develop in response to back discomfort, which are no less real physiologically than the Pavlovian response of salivation in anticipation of a meal. The perception of disability often combines with the anticipation of pain to further interfere with a patient's recovery (57, 83). Fordyce noted that behavior response mechanisms and injury education need to be vigorously addressed to overcome these barriers, and showed a nearly linear inverse relationship between activity levels and pain perception (86). Those who were least active had the highest pain levels, whereas subjects who performed increasingly greater amounts of exercise had a corresponding reduction in pain levels.

Musculoligamentous and soft tissue injuries typically show a normal healing curve to resolution (generally within 12 weeks), when range of motion and strengthening is initiated, despite discomfort, early in the course to ensure that the patient regains mobility and independence in timely fashion. We are aggressive with visible musculoskeletal injury; yet seem afraid to start active functional rehabilitation in LBP patients with no evident pathology other than pain. Waddell, in his timely work *The Back Pain Revolution*, says: "My whole argument is that back pain should settle unless physical dysfunction and illness behavior block recovery. The basic management strategy should be to overcome dysfunction and illness behavior, to restore normal function and behavior, and so permit the pain to settle" (14). Cognitive goals need to reinforce wellness, decrease the fear of pain, and increase self-reliance. Our failure to consistently achieve this aim is not for lack of knowledge, but rather failure to implement what we know.

Pharmaceutical Management

Impact on Ameliorating Symptoms

Medicinal treatment for LBP includes salicylates, **nonsteroidal anti-inflammatory drugs** (NSAIDs), narcotics, corticosteroids (oral and epidural), cartilage rejuvenators, ethanol, and over-the-counter herbals. A typical discharge prescription for the acute sufferer seen initially in urgent care or the emergency room may include an anti-inflammatory, a muscle relaxant, and/or a narcotic for pain control. The benefit of these medications in ameliorating symptoms is highly variable, and depends on the underlying nature of the LBP and the characteristics of the patient. Most individuals will gain enough relief to begin return to function in several days; others may require or demand stronger medication (e.g., intramuscular narcotics). Most physicians try to wean the patient off narcotics and antispasmodics within a few days, but chronic sufferers often feel that these medications provide their only relief. Excessive use of NSAIDS is an underappreciated problem; even the new **COX-2 inhibitors** may cause GI bleeding and renal complications. Corticosteroids (and to a lesser degree, NSAIDs) may delay histologic healing. Although the analgesic properties of NSAIDs may be of benefit, their cavalier long-term use should be questioned (87, 88) (Table 33.6).

Epidural corticosteroid injections remain controversial in the treatment of LBP. They are rarely used acutely, but their application in subacute and chronic LBP is widespread. Though invasive, and generally performed by an anesthesiologist or pain specialist, they offer a treatment option in management that frequently yields positive results. Nelemans et al. reviewed 40 papers, of which 21 met criteria for inclusion in the Cochran Library assessment of injection therapy for subacute and chronic low back pain (89). **Epidural anesthesia** means injection, typically of an anesthetic and a soluble corticosteroid, into the epidural space where the fluid diffuses across the dura into the subarachnoid space to act on nerve roots. The drug also diffuses into

the paravertebral area through the intervertebral foramina. **Local injection therapy** may include trigger point injections, iliolumbar injections, acupuncture, or intradiscal injections. They concluded that, at present, facet, epidural, and local injections lack statistically significant results; however, due to the low rate of side effects and a tendency toward positive results, the authors felt that there was not compelling data to argue for abandoning injection treatment. Variable effects were noted in the use of short-acting anesthetics like procaine or lignocaine (lidocaine) versus long-acting bupivacaine or etidocaine without definite long-term benefit of one over another. Issues of short-term versus long-term pain relief need to be further researched.

Impact on Exercise Response

Narcotics medications have a well-defined depressive effect on the central nervous system, and the performance of activities requiring fine motor skills will be significantly altered. Similarly, muscle relaxants will cause a reduction in the muscle twitch response based on neuromuscular inhibition. NSAIDs, although often used at work and by athletes in competition, do have potentially deleterious effects on the kidneys in a dehydrated state and are known for their gastrointestinal irritation via cyclooxygenase system-mediated inhibition. The new COX-2 inhibitors have a

TABLE 33.6. MEDICATIONS FOR TREATING LOW BACK PAIN

Generic	Brand	Dose	Class	Side Effects
Aspirin	Many	650 mg q 4-6 h	Analgesia	Gastrointestinal
Ibuprofen	Motrin, Advil	200–800 mg po q 6–8 h	NSAID	Gastrointestinal/renal
Naproxen	Naprosyn	250–500 mg po bid	NSAID	Gastrointestinal/renal
Etodolac	Lodine	200–400 mg po bid-qid	NSAID	Gastrointestinal/renal
Piroxicam	Feldane	20 mg po qd	NSAID	Gastrointestinal/renal
Diclofenac	Voltaren	50–75 mg po bid-tid	NSAID	Gastrointestinal/renal
Oxaprozin	DayPro	1200 mg qd	NSAID	Gastrointestinal/renal
Celecoxib	Celebrex	200 mg po qd	NSAID	Gastrointestinal/renal
Rofecoxib	Vioxx	25–50 mg qd	NSAID	Gastrointestinal/renal
Diclofenac/mistoprostol	Arthrotec	1 tab po bid-qid	NSAID/buffer	Gastrointestinal/renal
Ketorolac	Toradol	30–60 mg IM	NSAID	Gastrointestinal/renal
Acetaminophen	Tylenol	1–2 tabs po q 4–6 h	Analgesic	Hepatic
Tramadol	Ultram	50–100 mg po qd to qid	Analgesic	Renal/hepatic/seizures
Cyclobenzaprine	Flexeril	10 mg po qd-tid	Muscle relaxant	Sedation
Chlorzoxazone	Parafon Forte	500 mg po qid	Muscle relaxant	Gastrointestinal/renal
Carisoprodel	Soma	300 mg po qid	Muscle relaxant	Sedation
Methocarbamol	Robaxin	750 mg po qid	Muscle relaxant	Sedation
Metaxalone	Skelaxin	800 mg po tid-qid	Muscle relaxant	Sedation
Orphenadrine citrate	Norflex	100 mg po bid	Muscle relaxant	Sedation
Tylenol with codeine		1–2 tabs po q 3–4 h prn pain	Analgesic and Narcotic	Sedation, constipation, addiction
Hydrocodone	Vicodin	1 tab po q 6–8 h	Narcotic	Sedation, nausea, addiction
Oxycodone	Percocet/Tylox	1 tab po q 6–8 h	Narcotic	Sedation, nausea, addiction
Corticosteroids	Medrol dose	tapering	Steroid	Emotional lability, avascular necrosis, immune suppress
Morphine	MS Contin	30 mg po q 8–12 h	Narcotic	Respiratory depression/addiction
Meperidine	Demerol	50–100 mg IM	Narcotic	Respiratory depression/addiction
Herbal therapy	Various	Variable	Herbal	Variable to none

lent total body (kinetic chain)-conditioning program. (One of the authors [RB] has found that a Vasa trainer swim bench has the advantage of incorporating flexibility, strength, and endurance training with the benefits of back extension, traction, and strengthening of the latissimus dorsi groups and thoracolumbar fascia.)

Physiological Adaptations and Associated Mechanisms

Adaptation refers to the body's response to the physiologic challenge of exercise and physical training. The cells, tissues, and organs of the body, and the neuromuscular system in particular, show a significant degree of plasticity and adaptability to physical stimuli and demands. The specificity and regularity of exercise determines the systematic adaptations that occur. Short-duration, high-intensity exercise and endurance exercise are important components in preventing fatigue. Acute and chronic physiologic adaptations are well studied and are discussed in depth elsewhere in this text.

Central Mechanisms

Reduced strength with decreased use has been shown to be greater than by muscle atrophy alone, and central nervous system (CNS) drive is recognized as an essential component in the feedback mechanism of neuromotor recruitment. When an individual exercises, they strengthen the musculoskeletal system, increase flexibility, and affect cardiovascular parameters, and impact the central nervous system in diverse ways. With training adaptation, neural drive, synchronization of motor units, and activation of the contractile apparatus are all increased.

Numerous health benefits accrue from exercise (see other chapters for elaboration) in addition to strengthening the back (111, 116). Habitual exercise reduces the incidence of hyperlipidemia, hypertension, obesity, type 2 diabetes, osteoporosis, depression, and colon cancer, and is beneficial to immune system, endocrine, and metabolic function in general. Not the least of the values of exercise is the production of pain-mediating enkephalins/endorphins, which may improve mood, decrease anxiety and depression, increase pain tolerance, and induce better sleep (8, 11, 117). Health benefits appear to be largely proportional to the amount of activity; by exceeding minimum thresholds of activity, autonomy and independence are maximized. The "dose-response" relationship between physical activity and health benefit has relevance to back pain as well (111).

Peripheral Mechanisms

Training increases the size (cross-sectional area) and strength of ligaments, muscles, tendons, and bone density.

It increases aerobic enzyme activity and improves energy substrates as well as the ability to recruit a greater percentage of type I and II motor units. In tissues normally unaccustomed to exercise, microscopic "damage" to the contractile portion of the muscle bundle may occur, causing both acute and/or delayed-onset muscle soreness (DOMS) (88). It is likely that many deconditioned individuals discontinue an exercise program due to these early symptoms. When musculotendinous strain or ligament sprain injuries occur, a period of localized pain typically may last 24 to 72 hours. Weakness and reduction in range of motion may last for a week or more. When individuals avoid further challenge to the muscles, a cycle of deconditioning begins. Lumbar extensor muscles demonstrate selective atrophy of type II fast-twitch muscle fibers due to inactivity (disuse) in patients with back pain and in asymptomatic sedentary controls (36, 118). Characteristically, however, if these tissues are stressed with successive bouts of exercise, there is adaptive hypertrophy of muscle fiber size, increased capillary and mitochondrial density, and progressive strengthening along with gradually decreased discomfort. An "overload" strengthening program in an otherwise healthy adult may increase general muscle strength by 20% to 40% in 2 to 4 months (11). In the lumbar spine, the strength will often increase by 100% or more (108) (Figure 33.10).

TABLE 33.9. TESTS FOR ASSESSMENT OF STRENGTH AND FLEXIBILITY

Test[a]	Satisfactory Response
1. Lumbar Flexion	Lumbar spine flattens to neutral during sitting toe touch
2. Lumbar Extension	Ability to achieve test position with smooth lumbar curve
3. Lumbar Rotation	Ability to achieve test position
4. Hamstring Flexibility	Ability to achieve test position with 80–110° hip flexion
5. Hip Flexor Flexibility	Ability to achieve test position with knee (on side of extended hip) flexed to 80°
6. Hip Joint Flexion Flexibility	Ability to achieve test position with hip (on side of flexed hip) flexed to 125°
7. Squat to Stand Strength and Flexibility	Ability to achieve test position and repeat correctly 10 times
8. Shoulder Girdle Strength and Flexibility	Ability to achieve and maintain test position (stick 9" off floor) for 30 seconds
9. Back and Hip Extension Strength	Ability to maintain test position for 60 seconds
10. Abdominal Strength	Ability to maintain test position for 10 seconds (repeat with right and left twist)
11. Abdominal Strength	Ability to maintain test position for 10 seconds
12. Anterior Thigh Strength	Ability to maintain test position for 60 seconds

[a]See Figure 33.10 **(A-L)** for tests.

Adapted from Saunders HD, Saunders R (31), page 377.

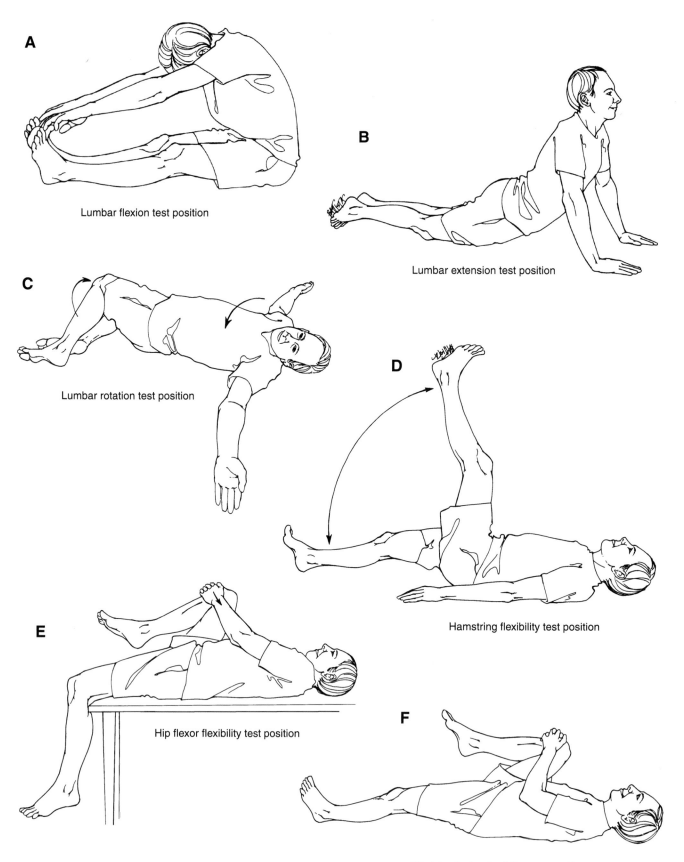

A Lumbar flexion test position

B Lumbar extension test position

C Lumbar rotation test position

D Hamstring flexibility test position

E Hip flexor flexibility test position

F Hip joint flexion flexibility test position

FIGURE 33.10. Tests for assessment of strength and flexibility (A–L).

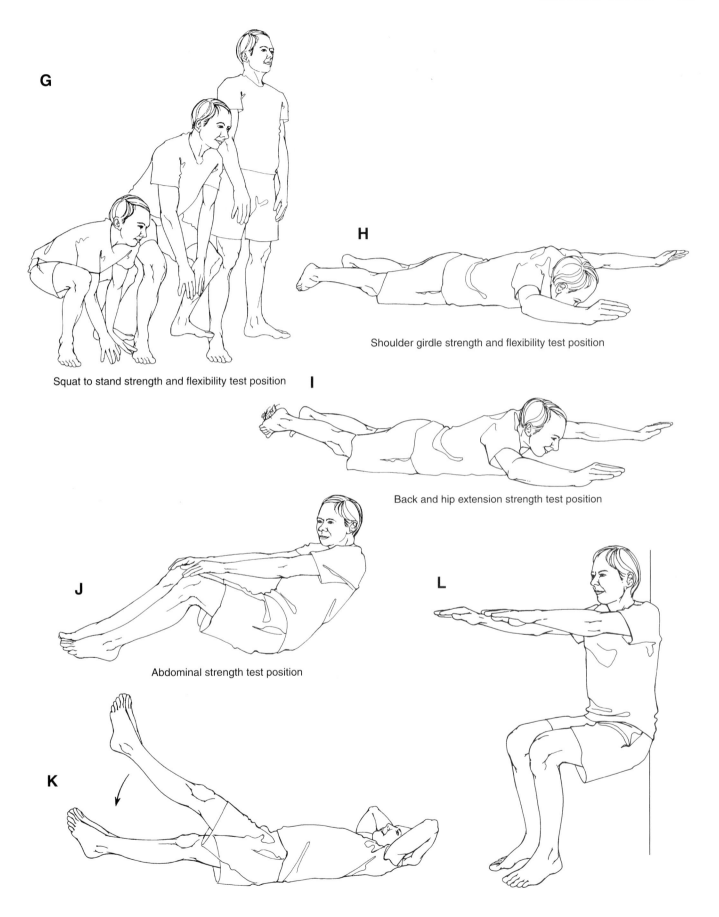

G

Squat to stand strength and flexibility test position

H

Shoulder girdle strength and flexibility test position

I

Back and hip extension strength test position

J

Abdominal strength test position

K

L

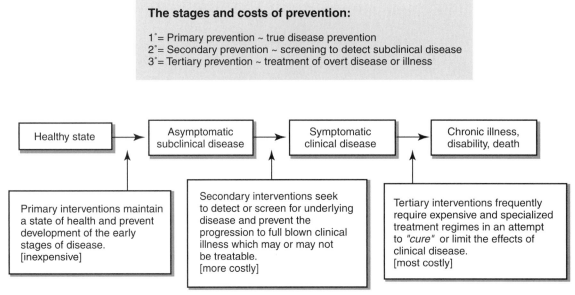

The stages and costs of prevention:

1° = Primary prevention ~ true disease prevention
2° = Secondary prevention ~ screening to detect subclinical disease
3° = Tertiary prevention ~ treatment of overt disease or illness

| Healthy state | → | Asymptomatic subclinical disease | → | Symptomatic clinical disease | → | Chronic illness, disability, death |

Primary interventions maintain a state of health and prevent development of the early stages of disease. [inexpensive]

Secondary interventions seek to detect or screen for underlying disease and prevent the progression to full blown clinical illness which may or may not be treatable. [more costly]

Tertiary interventions frequently require expensive and specialized treatment regimes in an attempt to *"cure"* or limit the effects of clinical disease. [most costly]

FIGURE 33.11. The stages and costs of prevention.

This adaptation to work demand is seen in both sport and vocational activities. Two variables that significantly increase a muscle's susceptibility to strain are weakness and fatigue. Muscle injury typically occurs at the musculotendinous junction. The more energy a muscle can absorb and the less its fatigability, the greater its resistance to injury. Once injured, however, it is important to allow appropriate healing time before return to full activity, or the risk of reinjury is increased.

Prevention

Epidemiologists use the terms *primary*, *secondary*, and *tertiary prevention* to refer, respectively, to (1) interventions to prevent the initial stages of disease; (2) screening to detect subclinical disease; and (3) curative or treatment-based care for full-blown clinical disease. Clearly, primary prevention is the preferred option because it saves the cost and consequences of illness. The annual health care budget in the United States is now more than 1.5 trillion dollars, largely because we have replaced true illness and infectious disease with the "new morbidities" of lifestyle, nearly all of which are risk factors for LBP. A consensus is emerging among caregivers that most LBP is less a medical illness than a fitness problem; less due to work site demands or changes in recreational activity than to our contemporary lifestyle. Numerous studies now suggest that the incidence of LBP can be decreased, the duration of symptoms reduced, and the risk of recurrence significantly lessened by behavior modifications that try to eliminate known risk factors and increase general physical fitness. As a society in general, and as caregivers in particular, we should not be content to practice tertiary medicine, waiting for the disease process to advance to

the stage of chronic illness requiring expensive curative management. Instead, we must begin to refocus our resources on primary prevention methods (Figure 33.11).

What We Know **About Back Pain**

1 Low back pain is a common occurrence that in most cases is a result of lifestyle choices rather than a single event. It is rarely due to serious disease. For most people, reduction of any or all of the risk behaviors (smoking, obesity, deconditioning, depression, job dissatisfaction, ongoing litigation, sedentary lifestyles that encourage poor posture, faulty body mechanics, and heavy, repetitive lifting) will increase functional coping and reduce severity, duration, and recurrence of symptoms.

2 Bed rest and immobility are largely contraindicated. Return to function should take priority over pain avoidance behaviors (in the absence of "red flags"). Early motion and return to activities should be strongly encouraged. Swimming, walking, and low-impact, gliding activities are recommended.

3 Virtually all persons will develop "degenerative" changes (both disc and bony) in the spine as they age; the changes may be evident on imaging studies. In most instances, little or no correlation exists between these changes and the presence or absence of back pain symptoms.

4 Disc nutrition depends on passive diffusion and relies on contact between the avascular disc and blood vessels at the periphery of the annulus fibrosus. The permeability of the bone-disc interface is fragile and can be compromised by the risk factors described above.

5 Treatment for chronic LBP with or without radicular symptoms seems best achieved by an aggressive and quantifiable back extensor strengthening program in concert with aerobic and flexibility work. Depending on the baseline degree of deconditioning, improvement may take 3 to 6 months; the exercise prescription for maintenance and prevention of reinjury is lifelong.

6 The back is not an isolated structure. It is part of the kinetic chain and relies on the support of its many muscle and ligament groups to help it provide support, protection, and movement to the torso and body. For this reason, strength of the arms and legs, general aerobic fitness, flexibility, and endurance to prevent fatigue are important factors in the healthy back.

7 Even if disc herniation has occurred, as many as 75% to 80% of patients can avoid surgery and return to normal function, including recreational activity and vigorous labor. Careful collaboration among the physician, therapist, surgeon, and patient is necessary. Disc material is usually resorbed through macrophagocytosis over time; discs seem to heal without scarring if range of motion and nourishment are preserved.

8 Corporate groups who encourage workers to exercise or have fitness facilities on site show reduced rates of LBP, general indicators of health, and absenteeism; they show increased employee satisfaction, marginal increases in production, and a positive return on investment.

What We Would Like to Know About Back Pain

1 Why is disc and segmental degeneration inevitable? Why do some people with severe degenerative changes have no pain, whereas others with minimal changes have severe pain?

2 How can we unravel and better explain the nature of pain perception? Can our current pain and functional ability scales be modified to better reflect the underlying nature of the patient's malady? Further definition of nociceptive pain generators in the spine is needed. What role do substance "P" and other neuromediators that influence chemical radiculitis play?

3 How do we help reduce perceived barriers to physical activity? How do we help people cross what Covey calls the "gap between stimulus and response"? How can we best increase the patient's confidence in the ability to self-manage pain and maintain activity?

4 Continued research is needed into the nature of applied loads as they affect the shear, rotational, and compressive/tensile stresses on the spine.

5 What is an adequate trial of "conservative management"? Are there quantifiable ways to determine if a patient has failed therapeutic options?

6 What are the best "outcome" measures or tests: patient satisfaction, return to work and function, and/or pain control/elimination?

7 How do we discriminate between the relative contributions of occupational and nonwork physical loads in the development of musculoskeletal symptoms, particularly with respect to "cumulative" strain disorders?

8 Motion and exercise have beneficial effects (with an identifiable dose-response curve); however, at what point, in terms of frequency, duration, magnitude, or rate, do load stressors exceed the biomechanical limits of tissue leading to pathologic damage? How do we discriminate between true extrinsic force overload (workplace hazard) versus biological insufficiency (human deconditioning) on an individual basis? How do we distinguish between association and causation?

Summary

"The future challenge, if costs are to be controlled, appears to lie squarely with prevention and optimum management of disability, rather than perpetrating a myth that low back pain is a serious health disorder" (16).

Low back pain in our society is significantly affected by lifestyle and can frequently be managed by reducing risk factors. Despite the common belief that LBP is the result of an isolated injury, it may be our best true example of a cumulative injury disorder. Whether this malady is more a consequence of disuse than true illness remains a semantic and philosophical issue. Significant disagreement exists in the medical community, as well as in political, business, and labor circles, with regard to the distinction between causation and association in "repetitive" musculoskeletal injury (119, 120). The current costs, both in terms of human suffering and spiraling health care dollars, are unnecessarily high. Our management of back pain in particular, and musculoskeletal disorders in general, needs to address not only environmental hazards, but patient risk factors as well. As Pogo said, "We have met the enemy, and he is us" (121).

Perhaps the greatest service that we can provide back pain patients is education and a prescription to take ownership of their back problem. People are conditioned to believe that the greater the pain, the more serious the injury. In many human conditions this is true; however, for LBP, the pain is often out of proportion to the seriousness of the condition (i.e., "terrible" pain and unable to walk, but still a benign condition). Not knowing this, people go to the doctor who medicalizes a benign condition and makes the problem worse by giving bad advice or ordering imaging with false-positive findings. The patient needs reassurance that the condition is rarely "serious," and that with participatory support they can almost always overcome their symptoms and return to normal function. Patients need to understand the difference between passive modalities, which do little to speed recovery (and may be detrimental by encouraging dependent behaviors), and those which foster active participation and self-healing. Bronowski reminds us that the "real content of evolution (biological as well as cultural) is the elaboration of new behavior" (122). Medically, we are faced with "new morbidities" resulting from lifestyle rather than from chance illness or misfortune, and issues of prevention in altering behavior may be more effective than any pill or treatment. Recovery needs to focus on return to function rather than pain avoidance, otherwise a downward spiral of deconditioning and dysfunction frequently occurs (123).

Some have suggested that we "demedicalize" LBP and accept it as one of the eventualities of life (124). Low back pain may be the evolutionary fate of 2-legged, tech-

nologically advanced beings, but it remains important to provide assessment, rule out bad things (which almost always can be done by history and exam without expensive testing), and guide/educate the patient to recovery. Clearly, individuals who have active lifestyles and few or no risk factors will cope better with activities of daily living and work responsibilities, have LBP of lesser duration, and are less likely to have chronicity or disability. The crux is to translate this knowledge into improved health status for our patients and a reduction of society's health care costs. A lifelong exercise program (incorporating aerobic fitness, strengthening, and flexibility), whether pursued independently, in schools, with a health club, or as part of a worksite wellness program, seems to offer the best promise of preventing debilitating back pain and many other health conditions. The demands of accountability exist in every business and profession. Experience-based treatment of LBP is a legitimate expression of that need.

The goal of this chapter has been to serve as a reminder that primary prevention, in the form of exercise, remains the most effective and responsible way to approach the dilemma of LBP. The benefits are many and the side effects, in contrast to medicinal or surgical remedies, are few to none. There is no magic pill or treatment for routine back pain that is stronger than human resolve. It is ironic that our "new wisdom" with respect to the prevention and treatment of LBP should essentially be a return to the principles of physical activity advocated by Hippocrates centuries ago when he wrote: "If we could give every individual the right amount of nourishment and exercise, not too little and not too much, we would have found the safest way to health" (1).

CASE STUDY 1

Patient Information

A 42-year-old female office manager presents with localized low back pain and no radicular symptoms; sleep is unaffected. She is overweight, smokes a pack of cigarettes daily, and does no exercise other than walking from her car to the office. She wants time off work to rest at home. No other complaints.

Assessment

Her exam is unremarkable except for localized low back discomfort with activity; negative straight leg raise. The rest of the exam is unremarkable.

Questions

1. Are x-rays necessary?
2. Should she be referred to physical therapy immediately?
3. What is her long-term prognosis?

CASE STUDY 2

Patient Information

A 57-year-old male foundry worker presents with sudden onset of low back pain while trying to lift a 100-pound casting which he has lifted "for years" without problem. He complains of numbness on the lateral aspect and sole of the right foot and some unusual numbness in the groin. His right leg feels "weak." He is otherwise healthy.

Assessment

There is an absent Achilles reflex with weak plantar flexion of the foot on the right; Achilles reflex is 1+ (normal = 2+) on the left. He can barely stand without support. He has "saddle anesthesia" in the groin region and decreased rectal tone. He has decreased sensation and discrimination of pinprick and light touch in the S1 dermatome on the right.

 Acute onset of symptoms with focal neurologic signs including rectal tone changes.

Questions

Which imaging studies would you pursue? Would you consult a specialist at this point, or treat his pain with narcotic pain medication? What is the differential diagnosis?

CASE STUDY 3

Patient Information

A highly competitive 16-year-old female volleyball player complained of gradual onset of pain in her lower back aggravated by serving and spiking activity. She denied any direct trauma or history of LBP. She is left-hand dominant. State tournament play starts in 2 weeks.

Assessments

Mild pain with palpation over the spine midline and left paralumbar musculature at the L4-L5 level. Symptoms are aggravated with left leg only hyperextension "stork test" (placing increased stress on the left posterior elements); less uncomfortable with right leg unipodal test. Her straight leg raise was equivocal on the left. Exam is otherwise normal.

 Adolescent with focal back pain in sport with significant hyperextension forces.

Questions

Would you do any tests, give her pain medications, and/or recommend rest and/or play as tolerated?

Acknowledgments

Special thanks to Brian Nelson, MD, Joseph Wegner, MD, MPH, and Richard Timming, MD.

REFERENCES

1. Birrer RB, ed. Sports Medicine for the Primary Care Physician. New York: CRC Press, 1994.
2. Haldeman S. Presidential Address, North American Spine Society. Failure of the pathology model to predict back pain. Spine 1990;15:718.
3. Deyo RA, Weinstein JN. Low back pain. N Engl J Med 2001;344(5):363–370.
4. Fordyce WE, McMahon R, Rainwater G, et al. Pain complaint-exercise performance relationship in chronic pain. Pain 1981;10:311–321.
5. Nelson BW, O'Reilly E, Miller M. The clinical effects of intensive, specific exercise on chronic low back pain: a controlled study of 895 consecutive patients with 1-year follow up. Orthopaedics 1995;18:971–981.

6. Rainville J, Sobel J, Hartigan C, Monlux G, Bean J. Decreasing disability in chronic back pain through aggressive spine rehabilitation. J Rehabil Res Dev 1997;34(4):383–393.

7. Kuhn TS. The Structure of Scientific Revolutions. Chicago, Ill: Univ. of Chicago Press; 1970.

8. Elrick H. Exercise is medicine. Physician Sports Med 1996;24(2):72–79.

9. White AA III, Gordon SL. American Academy of Orthopaedic Surgeons: Idiopathic Low Back Pain. St Louis, Mo: CV Mosby, 1982.

10. Bigos S, Bowyer O, Braen G, et al. Acute Low Back Problems in Adults. Clinical Practice Guideline, Quick Reference Guide Number 14. Rockville, Md: US Department of Health and Human Services, Public Health Service, Agency for Health Care Policy and Research; 1994. AHCPR Pub. No. 95-0643.

11. Casazza BA, Young JL, Herring SA. The role of exercise in the prevention and management of acute low back pain. Occup Med 1998;13(1):47–60.

12. Courtney TK, Webster BS. Disabling occupational morbidity in the United States. J Occup Environ Med 1999;41(1):60–69.

13. Hart GL, Deyo RA, Cherkin DC. Physician office visits for low back pain: frequency, clinical evaluation and treatment patterns from a national survey. Spine 1995;20:11–19.

14. Waddell G. The Back Pain Revolution. Edinburgh: Churchill Livingstone; 1998.

15. Carpenter DM, Nelson BW. Low back strengthening for the prevention and treatment of low back pain. Med Sci Sports Exerc 1999;31(1):18–24.

16. Frymoyer JW, Cats-Baril WL. An overview of the incidences and costs of low back pain. Orthop Clin North Am 1991;22(2):263–271.

17. Spitzer WO. Scientific approach to the assessment and management of activity-related spinal disorder. A monograph for clinicians. Report of the Quebec Task Force on Spinal Disorders. Spine 1987;12(suppl 7):S1–S59.

18. Nelson BW, Carpenter DW, Dreisinger TE, Mitchell M, Kelly CE, Wegner JA. Can spinal surgery be prevented by aggressive strengthening exercises? A prospective study of cervical and lumbar patients. Arch Phys Med Rehabil 1999;80:20–25.

19. Frymoyer JW, ed. The Adult Spine: Principles and Practice. 2nd ed. Philadelphia, Pa: Lippincott Williams & Wilkins; 1997.

20. The Holy Bible. Revised standard version. New York, NY: Thomas Nelson; 1952.

21. Blakiston's Gould Medical Dictionary. New York, NY: McGraw-Hill; 1979:782.

22. Gowers WR. Lumbago: its lessons and analogues. BMJ 1904;16:117–121.

23. Shakespeare. Troilus and Cressida 5.1, 16–21.

24. Deyo RA, Diehl AK, Rosenthal M. How many days of bed rest for acute low back pain? N Engl J Med 1986;315:1064.

25. Waddell G, Feder G, McIntosh A, Lewis M, Hutchinson A. Low Back Pain Evidence Review. London: Royal College of General Practitioners; 1996.

26. Hilde G, Hagen KB, Jamtvedt G, Winnem M. Advice to stay active as a single treatment for low back pain and sciatica (Cochrane Review). In: The Cochrane Library, Issue 4, 2002. Oxford: Update Software.

27. Abenhaim L, Rossignol M, Valat JP, et al. The role of activity in the therapeutic management of back pain: report of the International Paris Task Force on Back Pain. Spine 2000;25(4):1S–33S.

28. Tulder M van, Malmivaara A, Esmail R, Koes B. Exercise therapy for low back pain. Spine 2000;25(21):2784–2796.

29. Tulder MW van, Malmivaara A, Esmail R, Koes BW. Exercise therapy for low back pain. (Cochrane Review). In: The Cochrane Library, Issue 4, 2002. Oxford: Update Software.

30. Herring SA. Sports medicine early care. In: Mayer TG, Mooney V, Gatchel RJ, eds. Contemporary Conservative Care for Painful Spinal Disorders. Philadelphia, Pa: Lea & Febiger; 1991:235–244.

31. Saunders HD, Saunders R. Evaluation, Treatment, and Prevention of Musculoskeletal Disorders. Vol 1: Spine. 3rd ed. Chaska, Minn: Saunders Group; 1995.

32. Han TS, Schouten JSAG, Lean MEJ, Seidell JC. The prevalence of low back pain and associations with body fatness, fat distribution and height. Int J Obes 1997;21:600–607.

33. Toda Y, Segal N, Toda T, Morimoto T, Ogawa R. Lean body mass and body fat distribution in participants with chronic low back pain. Arch Intern Med 2000;27(160):3265–3269.

34. Lee JH, Ooi Y, Nakamura K. Measurement of muscle strength of the trunk and the lower extremities in subjects with history of low back pain. Spine 1995;20(18):1994–1996.

35. Mooney V, Kron M, Rummerfield P, Holmes B. The effect of workplace based strengthening on low back injury rates: a case study in the mining industry. J Occup Rehabil 1995;5(3):157–167.

36. Parkkola R, Kormano M. Lumbar disc and back muscle degeneration on MRI: correlation to age and body mass. J Spinal Disord 1992;5:86–92.

37. Parkkola R, Rytokoski U, Kormano M. Magnetic resonance imaging of the disks and trunk muscles in patients with chronic low back pain and healthy control subjects. Spine 1993;18:830–836.

38. Buckwalter JA. The fine structure of human intervertebral disc. In: White AA, Gordon SL, eds. AAOS Symposium on Idiopathic Low Back Pain. St Louis, Mo: CV Mosby; 1982:108–143.

39. O'Malley CD, Saunders JB de CM. Leonardo da Vinci on the human body. New York, NY: Wing Books; 1982:43.

40. Jayson MIV, ed. The Lumbar Spine and Back Pain. 2nd ed. London: Pitman Publishing; 1985.

41. Norris CM. Back Stability. Champaign, Ill: Human Kinetics; 2000.

42. Greenspan A. Orthopaedic Radiology: A Practical Approach. 3rd ed. Philadelphia, Pa: Lippincott Williams & Wilkins; 2000.

43. Panjabi MM, Abumi K, Duranceau J, Oxland T. Spinal stability and intersegmental muscle forces: a biomechanical model. Spine 1989;14:194–200.

44. Bogduk N, Twomey LT. Clinical Anatomy of the Lumbar Spine. Melbourne: 1987.

45. Vleeming A, Pool-Goudzwaard AL, Stoeckart R, Wingerden JP, Snijders CJ. The posterior layer of the thoracolumbar fascia: its function in load transfer from spine to legs. Spine 1995;20:753–758.

46. Kibler WB. Clinical aspects of muscle injury. Med Sci Sports Exerc 1990;22(4):450.

47. Kibler WB, Chandler TJ, Pace BK. Principles of rehabilitation after chronic tendon injuries. Clin Sports Med 1992;11(3):661–671.

48. Nordin M, Andersson GBJ, Pope MH. Musculoskeletal Disorders in the Workplace. St. Louis, Mo: Mosby; 1997.

49. Watkins J. Structure and Function of the Musculoskeletal System. Champaign, Ill: Human Kinetics; 1999.

50. Deyo RA. Low-back pain. Scientific American 1998;August:48–53.

51. Battie MC, VidemanT, Gill K, et al. Smoking and lumbar intervertebral disk degeneration: an MRI study of identical twins. Spine 1991;16:1015–1021.

52. Leboeuf-Yde DC, Kyvik KO, Bruun NH. Low back pain and lifestyle. Part I: smoking. Information from a population-based sample of 29,424 twins. Spine 1998;23(20):2207–2213.

53. Kirkaldy-Willis WH. Pathology and pathogenesis of low back pain. In: Kirkaldy-Willis WH, Burton CV, eds. Managing Low Back Pain. 3rd ed. New York, NY: Churchill Livingstone; 1992:49–79.

54. Vleeming A, Mooney V, Dorman T, Snijders C, eds. The Integrated Function of the Lumbar Spine and Sacroiliac Joint. Parts I and II. Rotterdam: ECO, 1995.

55. Oxford Dictionary of Quotations. 5th ed. Knowles E, ed. Oxford Univ. Press; 1999:601–614.

56. Nachemson AL. Newest knowledge of low back pain. A critical look. Clin Orthop1992;279:8–20.

57. Kendall NAS. Psychosocial approaches to the prevention of chronic pain: the low back paradigm. Balliere's Clinical Rheumatology. 1999;13(3):545–554.

58. Fitzhenry RI, ed. The Harper Book of Quotations. 3rd ed. New York, NY: Harper Collins; 1993:287

59. Hadler NM, Carey TS. Low back pain: an intermittent and remittent predicament of life. Ann Rheum Dis 1998;57:1–2.

60. Nachemson A. Advances in low-back pain. Clin Orthop 1985;200:266.
61. Coping with back pain. JAMA 2000;284(21):2826.
62. Waters TR, Putz-Anderson V, Gary A. Centers for Disease Control and Prevention 1994;1–73.
63. Accident Facts. National Safety Council, 1997.
64. Beadle CE. Addressing health care and health care costs at their roots. Prev Med 1996;25:66–67.
65. McCunney RJ, Anstadt G, Burton WN. The competitive advantage of a healthy work force: opportunities for occupational medicine. J Occup Environ Med 1997;39(7):611–613.
66. Mooney V, Saal JA, Saal JS. Evaluation and treatment of low back pain. Clinical Symposia (Ciba) 1996;48(4):1–32.
67. Papenfuss RL. Work site health promotion and disease prevention. Occup Health 1994;21(2):387–398.
68. Shephard RJ. Corporate wellness. Current Comment from the ACSM. April 1999.
69. Cipriano JJ. Photographic Manual of Regional Orthopaedic and Neurological Tests. 3rd ed. Baltimore, Md: Williams & Wilkins, 1997:173–260.
70. Waddell G, McCulloch JA, Kummel E, Venner RM. Nonorganic physical signs in low back pain. Spine 1980;5(2):117–125.
71. Jarvik JG, Deyo RA. Diagnostic evaluation of low back pain with emphasis on imaging. Ann Intern Med 2002;137(7):586–597.
72. Weisel S. A study of computer-assisted tomography: the incidence of positive CAT scans in an asymptomatic group of patients. Spine 1984;9(6):
73. Boden SD, Davis DO, Dina TS, Patronas NJ, Wiesel SW. Abnormal magnetic-resonance scans of the lumbar spine in asymptomatic subjects. J Bone Joint Surg Am 1990;72(3):403–408.
74. Jensen MC, Brant-Zawadzki MN, Obuchowski N. Magnetic resonance imaging of the lumbar spine in people without back pain. N Engl J Med 1994;331:69–73.
75. Kendall NAS, Linton SJ, Main CJ. Guide to Assessing Psychosocial Yellow Flags in Acute Low Back Pain: Risk Factors for Long-term Disability and Work Loss. Wellington: Accident Rehabilitation and Compensation Insurance Corporation of New Zealand and the National Health Committee; 1997.
76. Biering-Sorensen F, Bendix AF. Working off low back pain. Lancet 2000;355:1929–1930.
77. Montgomery S, Haak M. Management of lumbar injuries in athletes. Sports Med 1999;27(2):135–141.
78. Micheli LJ, Wood R. Back pain in young athletes. Significant differences from adults in causes and patterns. Arch Pediatr Adolesc Med 1995;149(1):15–18.
79. Goldstein JD, Berger PE, Windler GE, Jackson DW. Spine injuries in gymnasts and swimmers. An epidemiologic investigation. Am J Sports Med 1991;19(5):463–468.
80. Jackson DW, Mannarino F. Lumbar spine injuries in athletes. In: Scott WN, Nisonson B, Nicholas JA, eds. Principles of Sports Medicine. Baltimore, Md: Williams & Wilkins; 1984:212–225.
81. Watkins RG, Dillin WM. Lumbar spine injuries. In: Fu FH, Stone DA. Sports Injuries. Baltimore, Md: Williams & Wilkins, 1994:877–893.
82. Lonstein JE. Spondylolisthesis in children. Spine 1999;24(24):2640–2648.
83. Trafimow D, Trafimow JH. Predicting back pain sufferer's intentions to exercise. J Psychol 1998;132(6):581–592.
84. Sizer PS, Phelps V, Matthijs O. Pain generators of the lumbar spine. Pain Practice 2001;1(3):255–273.
85. Kawakami M. Clin Orthop 1998;351:241–251.
86. Fordyce WE. Psychological factors in the failed back. Int Disabil Studies 1988;10(1):29–31.
87. Almenkinders LC. Anti-inflammatory treatment of acute and chronic soft-tissue sports injuries. Medscape Pharmacotherapy 2000. Available at: http://www.medscape.com/medscape/pharmacology/journal/2000/v02.n0.../mp7267.alme.htm. Accessed March 5, 2001.
88. Kirkendall DT, Garrett WE. Muscle strain injuries: research findings and clinical applicability. Medscape Orthopaedics Sports Medicine 1999;3(2). Available at: http://orthopaedics.medscape.com/medscape/OrthoSports Med/journa.../pnt-mos3028.kirk.htm. Accessed March 5, 2001.
89. Nelemans PJ, Bie RA de, Vet HCW de, Sturmans F. Injection therapy for subacute and chronic benign low back pain (Cochran Review). In: The Cochrane Library, Issue 4, 2002. Oxford: Update Software.
90. Robertson JT. The rape of the spine. Surg Neurol 1993;39:435–472.
91. Saal JA, Saal JS. Nonoperative treatment of herniated lumbar intervertebral disc with radiculopathy. Spine 1989;14(4):431–437.
92. Saal JA, Saal JS, Herzog RJ. The natural history of lumbar intervertebral disk extrusions treated nonoperatively. Spine 1990;15:683–686.
93. Saal JA. Natural history and nonoperative treatment of lumbar disc herniation. Spine 196;21(24S):2S–9S.
94. Kumori H, Shinomiya K, Nakai O, Yamaura I, Takeda S. The natural history of herniated nucleus pulposus with radiculopathy. Spine 1996;21(2):225–229.
95. Maigne JY, Rime B, Deligne B. Computerized tomographic follow-up study of forty-eight cases of nonoperatively treated lumbar intervertebral disc herniation. Spine 1992;17(9):1071–1074.
96. McKenzie RA. Treat Your Own Back.
97. Cherkin DC, Deyo RA, Wheeler K, Ciol MA. Physician verification in diagnostic testing for LBP. Who you see is what you get. Arthritis Rheum 1994;37(1):15–22.
98. Malanga GA, Nadler SF. Nonoperative treatment of low back pain. Mayo Clin Proc 1999;74:1135–1148.
99. Greenman PE. Principles of Manual Medicine. New York, NY: Lippincott Williams & Wilkins; 1996:39.
100. Konlian C. Aquatic therapy: making a wave in the treatment of low back injuries. Orthop Nurs 1999;Jan/Feb:11–19.
101. Saal JA. Dynamic muscular stabilization in the nonoperative treatment of lumbar pain syndromes. Orthop Rev 1990;19(8):691–700.
102. Jull GA, Richardson CA. Rehabilitation of active stabilization of the lumbar spine. In: Physical Therapy of the Low Back. Edinburgh: Churchill Livingstone; 1994.
103. Nelson BW. A rational approach to the treatment of low back pain. J Musculoskel Med 1993;May:67–82.
104. Carpenter DM, Pollock ML, Graves JE, Leggett SH, Foster D. Effect of 12 and 20 weeks of resistance training on lumbar extension torque production. Phys Ther 1991;71(8):580–588.
105. Foster D, Avillar M, Pollock M, et al. Adaptations in strength and cross-sectional area of the lumbar extensor muscles following resistance training. Med Sci Sports Exerc 1993;25(5):S47.
106. Graves JE, Webb D, Pollock ML, et al. Pelvic stabilization during resistance training: Its effect on the development of lumbar extension strength. Arch Phys Med Rehabil 1994;75:210–215.
107. Pollock ML, Garzarella L, Graves JE, et al. Effects of isolated lumbar extension resistance training on bone mineral density of the elderly. Med Sci Sports Exerc 1992;24(5):S66.
108. Pollock ML, Leggett SH, Graves JE, Jones A, Cirulli J, Fulton MN. Effect of resistance training on lumbar extension strength. Am J Sports Med 1989;17:624–629.
109. Risch SV, Norvell N, Pollock ML, et al. Lumbar strengthening in chronic low back pain patients: physiologic and psychological benefits. Spine 1993;18(2):232–238.
110. Manniche C, Lundbergg E, Christensen I, Bentzen L, Hesselsoe G. Intensive dynamic back exercises for chronic low back pain: a clinical trial. Pain 1991;47:53–63.
111. American College of Sports Medicine. The recommended quantity and quality of exercise for developing and maintaining cardiorespiratory and muscular fitness, and flexibility in healthy adults. Med Sci Sports Exerc 1998;30(6):975–991.
112. Foster DN, Fulton MN. Back pain and the exercise prescription. Clin Sports Med 1991;10:197–209.
113. McGill SM. Low back exercises: evidence for improving exercise regimens. Phys Ther 1998;78(7):754–765.

114. Nordin M, Campello M. Exercises and the modalities: when, what and why? Neurol Clin North Am: Low Back Pain 1999;17(1):75–89.
115. Nordin M, Campello M, Weiser S. Exercises for the patient with low back pain: when and how. Bull Hosp Jt Dis 1996;55(3):142–146.
116. Pate RR, Pratt M, Blair SN, et al. Physical activity and public health: a recommendation from the Centers for Disease Control and Prevention and the American College of Sports Medicine. JAMA 1995;273(5):402–407.
117. Strauss E, Durand E, Blaustein A. Keeping in shape: exercise fundamental for the midlife patient. Geriatrics 1997;52(11):62–79.
118. Kalimo H, Rantanen J, Viljanen T, Einola S. Lumbar muscles: structure and function. Ann Med 1989;21:353–359.
119. Amadio PC, Frymoyer J. Repetitive stress injury [separate but consecutive letters to editor with combined response]. J Bone Joint Surg Am 2001;83(1):136–141.
120. Szabo RM, King KJ. Repetitive stress injury: diagnosis or self-fulfilling prophecy? J Bone Joint Surg Am 2000;82(9):1314–1322.
121. Kelly W. Pogo. New York, NY: Simon & Schuster; 1953.
122. Bronowski J. The Ascent of Man. Boston, Mass: Little, Brown; 1973:41.
123. Waddell G. A new clinical model for the treatment of low-back pain. Spine 1987;12:632–644.
124. Carey TS, Garrett JM, Jackman A, Hadler N. Recurrence and care seeking after acute back pain: results of a long-term follow-up study. Med Care 1999;37(2):157–164.

SUGGESTED READINGS

Bigos SJ. Perils, pitfalls, and accomplishments of guidelines for treatment of back problems. Neurol Clin North Am 1999;17(1):179–192.
Bloomfield J, Fricker PA, Fitch KD. Science and Medicine in Sport. 2nd ed. Victoria, Australia: Blackwell Science Pty Ltd; 1995.
Borenstein DG. Low back pain. In: Barker LR, Burton JR, Zieve PD, eds. Principles of Ambulatory Medicine. 5th ed. Baltimore, Md: Williams & Wilkins; 1999:913–927.
Brown RL, Fleming MF, Patterson JJ. Chronic opioid analgesic therapy for chronic low back pain. J Am Board Fam Pract 1996;9(3):191–204.
Cady LE, Bischoff DP, O'Connell ER, Thomas PC, Allan JH. Strength and fitness and subsequent back injuries in firefighters. J Occup Med 1979;21 (4):269–272
Carragee EJ, Paragioudakis SJ, Khurana S. Lumbar high-intensity zone and discography in subjects without low back problems. Spine 2000;25(23):2987–2992.
Cedraschi C, Nordin M, Nachemson AL, Vischer TL. Health care providers should use a common language in relation to low back pain patients. Baillieres Clin Rheumatol 1998;122(1):1–15.
D'Orazio BP. Low Back Pain Handbook. Wooburn, Mass: Butterworth-Heinemann; 1999.
Frank JW, Kerr MS, Brooker A-S, et al. Disability resulting from occupational low back pain. Spine 1996;21:2908–2929.
Hadler NM. Occupational Musculoskeletal Disorders. 2nd ed. Philadelphia, Pa: Lippincott Williams & Wilkins, 1999.
Hides JA, Stokes MJ, Saide M, Jull GA, Cooper DH. Evidence of lumbar multifidus muscle wasting ipsilateral to symptoms in patients with acute/subacute low back pain. Spine 1994;19(2):165–172.
Frymoyer JW, Phillips RB, Newberg AH, MacPherson BV. A comparative analysis of the interpretations of lumbar spinal radiographs by chiropractors and medical doctors. Spine 1986;11(10):1020–1023.
Ito T, Yamanda M, Ikuta F, Fukuda T, et al. Histologic evidence of absorption of sequestration-type herniated disc. Spine 1996;21(2):230–234.
Kendall FP, McCreary EK, Provance PG. Muscles: Testing and Function. 4th ed. Baltimore, Md: Williams & Wilkins, 1993.
Kopec JA, Esdaile JM. Functional Disability Scales for Back Pain. Spine 1995;20(17):1943–1949.
Koury JM. Aquatic Therapy Programming: Guidelines for Orthopaedic Rehabilitation. Champaign, Ill: Human Kinetics, 1996.

Lahad A, Malter A, Berg AO, Deyo RA. The effectiveness of four interventions for the prevention of low back pain. JAMA 1994;272(16):1286–1291.
Liebenson C. Rehabilitation of the Spine. Baltimore, Md: Williams & Wilkins; 1996.
Linton SJ, Hellsing AL, Andersson D. A controlled study of the effects of an early intervention on acute musculoskeletal pain problems. Pain 1993;54(3):353–359.
Malmivaara A, Hakkinen U, Timo A, et al. The treatment of acute low back pain: bed rest, exercises, or ordinary activity? N Engl J Med 1995;332(6):351–355.
Mannion AF, Muntener M, Taimela S, et al. A randomized clinical trial of three active therapies for chronic low back pain. Spine 1999;24:2435–2448.
McKenzie RA. The Lumbar Spine. Waikanae, NZ: Spinal Publication; 1984.
McNab I. Backache. Baltimore, Md; Williams & Wilkins; 1977.
Mink JH, Deutsch AL. MRI of the Musculoskeletal System: A Teaching File. New York, NY: Raven; 1990:117–191.
O'Sullivan PB, Twomey LT, Allison GT. Altered abdominal muscle recruitment in patients with chronic back pain following a specific exercise intervention. J Orthop Sports Phys Ther 1998;27:114–124.
Panjabi MM. The stabilizing system of the spine. Part 1. Function, dysfunction, adaptation, and enhancement. J Spinal Disord 1992;5:383–89.
Poussaint AF. Psychological and psychiatric factors in the low back pain patient. In: White AA, Gordon SL, eds. AAOS Symposium on Idiopathic Low Back Pain. St Louis, Mo: CV Mosby; 1982:39–45.
Read MT. Single photon emission computed tomography (SPECT) scanning for adolescent back pain. A sine qua non? Br J Sports Med 1994;28(1):56–57.
Reider B. The Orthopaedic Physical Examination. Philadelphia, Pa: WB Saunders; 1997.
Rosen NB, Hoffberg HJ. Conservative management of low back pain. Phys Med Rehabil Clin North Am 1998;9(2):435–472.
Saal JA. The pathophysiology of painful lumbar disorder. Spine 1995;20:180–183.
Schellhas KP, et al. Lumbar disc high intensity zone: correlation of magnetic resonance imaging and discography. Spine 1996;21:79–86.
Seidenwurm D, Litt AW. The natural history of lumbar spine disease. Radiology 1995;195:323–324.
Snider RK, ed. Essentials of Musculoskeletal Care. Rosemont, Ill: American Academy of Orthopaedic Surgeons; 1997:490–546.
Steinberg GG, Akins CM, Baran DT. Orthopaedics in Primary Care. 3rd ed. Baltimore, Md: Lippincott Williams & Wilkins; 1999:139–170.
Sundararajan V, Konrad TR, Garrett JM, Carey TS. Patterns and determinants of multiple provider use in patients with acute low back pain. J Gen Intern Med 1998;13:528–533.
Swindler DR, Wood CD. An Atlas of Primate Gross Anatomy. Malabar, Fla: Robert E Krieger; 1982.
Takahashi H, Soguro T, Okazima Y, Motegi M, Okada Y, Kakiuchi T. Inflammatory cytokines in the herniated disc of the lumbar spine. Spine 1996;21(2):218–224.
Tollinson CD, Kriegel ML. Interdisciplinary Rehabilitation of Low Back Pain. Baltimore, Md: Williams & Wilkins; 1989.
Twomey LT, Taylor JR. Physical Therapy of the Low Back. New York, NY: Churchill Livingstone; 1987.
Ward FO. Outlines of Human Osteology. London: Henry Renshaw; 1838:23. [In Jayson, 2nd ed.)
Weiner BK, McCulloch JA. Taking the mystery out of low back pain. J Musculoskeletal Med 2000;August:450–466.
Winkel D, Aufdemkampe G, Matthijs O, Meijer OG, Phelps V. Diagnosis and Treatment of the Spine. Gaithersburg, Md: Aspen; 1996.
Witt, Inge, et al. A comparative analysis of x-ray findings of the lumbar spine in patients with and without lumbar pain. Spine 1984;9(3):
Young JL, Press JM, Herring SA. The disc at risk in athletes: perspectives on operative and nonoperative care. Med Sci Sports Exerc 1997;29(7):S222–S232.

EXERCISE AND AGING

Aging

Roy J. Shephard

Late Middle Age
Lean Tissue Mass
Life Expectancy
Life Span
Longevity
Maximal Heart Rate
Maximal Aerobic Power
Medical Examination
Middle Age
Middle Old
Military Personnel
Mood-State
Mortality Rate
Movement Time
Muscle Force
Muscle Strength
Natural Killer Cell
Naughton Test
Obesity
Osteoarthritis
Osteoporosis
Peak Aerobic Power
Peak Heart Rate
Peak Muscle Force
Peripheral Vascular Disease
Physical Activity
Physical Condition
Posture
Premature Death
Proprioception

Prostaglandins
Public Safety Officers
Quality-Adjusted Life Expectancy
Quality of Life
Reaction Speed
Reaction Time
Resistance Exercise
Resting Metabolism
Retirement
Scintigraphy
Sit-and-Reach Test
Sleep
Smoking
Sphygmomanometer
Stabilometer
Stork Stand
Stress Testing
Stroke Volume
Sympathetic Activity
Tomography
Training
Type 2 Diabetes Mellitus
Type 2 Muscle Fibers
Very Old
Vitamins
Warm-up
Weight-Bearing
Young Adults
Young Old

Overview

Aging is associated with a progressive decline in most biological functions, somewhat more obvious in sedentary than in athletic individuals. Decreases in **peak aerobic power, muscle force** and endurance, **flexibility**, and **balance** progressively limit an elderly person's ability to undertake the **activities of daily living**, with a corresponding deterioration in **quality of life**. Regular physical activity is thus particularly important for the senior citizen. Increased physical activity has little, if any, effect on **longevity** in this age group; however, functional disturbances can be at least partially reversed. Increased functional capacity extends the period of independent living and enhances **quality-adjusted life expectancy**. Detailed **medical examination, exercise testing**, and **exercise prescription** may be desirable for the person who wishes to engage in high-level Masters' competition, but the interpretation of data is difficult, because many test results show features that would be regarded as abnormal in a younger person. A modest increase in physical activity (e.g., gentle walking) is safe, and even if it does not extend average **life expectancy**, it will increase the individual's quality-adjusted life expectancy. Changes in habitual activity patterns are best recommended in simple terms, without creating the potential barriers of detailed medical clearance, **stress testing**, and an elaborate exercise prescription.

The primary focus of this chapter is old age. Investigators commonly distinguish the **young old** (those with little overt loss of function, typically age 65 to 75 years), the **middle-old** (those with some physical limitations in daily activities, typically age 75 to 85 years), and the **very old** or **frail elderly** (typically over 85 years of age, often severely incapacitated and confined to institutions). Popular wisdom long suggested that old age and retirement offered an opportunity to slow down and take a "well-earned rest." Recent population surveys from the United States and elsewhere have shown that the proportion of men and women who take no leisure-time physical activity increases progressively with age. As many as 38% of men and 50% of women older than 75 years are totally inactive (1). Health professionals have sometimes contributed to this trend by expressing alarm at routine exercise test findings, and by overemphasizing the need for the elderly to be cautious when exercising. However, evidence is accumulating that regular moderate physical activity, whether supervised or unsupervised, will prolong survival even in very old age (2). More important, regular physical activity enhances **functional capacity**, reducing the likelihood of becoming dependent and increasing the individual's quality-adjusted life expectancy (3).

We will first look briefly at the extent of functional loss with aging, and the potential to reverse this change by an appropriate program of preventive or therapeutic exercise. We will then look at the influence of an active lifestyle on longevity, **health** and quality-adjusted life expectancy. Finally, we will discuss advice for the senior citizen about exercise testing and exercise prescription.

Functional Losses With Aging and the Potential for Their Reversal

Age-related patterns of functional loss differ between sedentary individuals and athletes who have maintained a rigorous **training** program. Particularly in the sedentary population, the response to training is substantial, even if the individual is very old.

Functional Losses in Sedentary Individuals

In theory, the best way to determine the extent of **functional loss** with aging would be to carry out a longitudinal experiment over a period of 30 to 50 years. However, in practice it is difficult to follow a substantial group of adults for such a long time. Those who volunteer for such a study are not typical members of the community, and the initial bias in subject selection is exacerbated by subsequent "drop-outs." Further, involvement in the program may itself modify habitual physical activity and other lifestyle as-

> **BOX 34.1. Functional Losses With Aging of Sedentary Adult**
>
> - Peak aerobic power: 5 mL/kg/min per decade in sedentary person
> - Peak muscle force and lean tissue: 25% loss from age 40–65 years, accelerating thereafter
> - Flexibility: 7% loss per decade
> - Progressive decrease in bone calcium and deterioration of bone matrix
> - All changes smaller in physically active individuals

pects. The great majority of reports are thus based on the age-related changes that are seen in cross-sectional data. Conclusions about the rate of functional loss (Box 34.1) have reasonable validity through the age of 65 years; however, in older age groups it is important to remember that data are obtained only on those survivors of the original cohort who have remained in sufficiently good health to agree to continue testing. We will comment briefly on age-related decreases in peak aerobic power.

Peak Aerobic Power

Peak aerobic power decreases steadily between the ages of 25 and 65 years. The loss in peak oxygen transport per decade (5–6 ml/kg/min) corresponds to 10% or more of the initial value. Findings are less well established for older individuals, because chronic diseases that also reduce peak aerobic power affect a high proportion of most elderly samples. However, recent data suggest that in those who continue to live independently, the peak oxygen intake declines exponentially to the threshold needed for independent living, a value of about 15 ml/kg/min (4).

A part of the age-related functional loss reflects changes in the **cardiovascular system**. Cardiovascular changes include:

- A decrease in **maximal heart rate** from about 195 beats/min at age 25 to an average of 165 beats/min at age 65;
- Decreased **compliance** of the heart wall (and thus less effective diastolic filling);
- Decreased response of the ventricular muscle to the **catecholamines** secreted during exercise (and thus less complete emptying of the heart during systole); and
- An increase in the afterload against which the heart must contract (due to more rigid arteries, an increase in systemic **blood pressure**, and weaker skeletal muscles).

The **stroke volume** is thus less well sustained in the elderly than in young adults, particularly as the individual approaches peak effort. One widely cited study (5, 6) suggested that the elderly person could compensate for the decrease in maximal heart rate by an increase of end-diastolic volume and thus of peak stroke volume. However, the group studied was not typical of the general population. In addition to willingness to participate in an extended study, the subjects had been cleared of all suspicion of ischemic heart disease by a combination of **electrocardiogram (ECG)** and **scintigraphy**. Moreover, their supposedly peak heart rates were relatively low, and one may hypothesize that if a true peak effort were to have been elicited, these subjects, also, would have shown a decrease rather than an increase in peak stroke volume with aging.

Other factors that often contribute to the age-related decrease of peak oxygen transport include detraining (due to a progressive reduction in habitual physical activity), and an accumulation of **body fat** (if peak oxygen intake is expressed relative to body mass). One large cross-sectional study attributed as much as 50% of the age-related variance in peak aerobic power to lower levels of habitual physical activity and greater **obesity** among older members of the sample (7).

Peak Muscle Force

In general, peak muscle force is well sustained through the age of 35 to 40 years. Thereafter, loss of strength accelerates. The rate of functional deterioration varies from one muscle group to another, but the cumulative effect is commonly a loss of about 25% of the initial strength by age 65 years. During the retirement years, this loss continues and even accelerates (8). An associated loss of **lean tissue mass** occurs, with a selective atrophy of the **type 2** (fast-twitch) **muscle fibers**. The peak muscle force is further compromised by a decreased synchronization of motor unit firing in older adults.

Deterioration in Other Body Systems

The progressive development of cross-bridges between individual filaments of **collagen** causes decreased flexibility in older adults. Often, **osteoarthritis** of the joints exacerbates decreased flexibility. A loss of function is readily demonstrated in middle age by such methods as the "**sit-and-reach test**" (9), but changes are not large enough to affect the performance of most everyday activities until at least age 70 years.

Increased postural sway when standing still demonstrates a deterioration of balance in older adults. Poor balance, slower righting reflexes, less powerful muscles, and impairment of the special senses make the elderly more susceptible to **falls** while exercising (10).

Progressive loss of bone **calcium** and deterioration of the skeletal organic matrix increase vulnerability to fracture from falls and sudden muscular contractions. At any given age, **bone density** is lower in women than in men, and women are correspondingly more susceptible to fractures (11).

Functional Losses in Active Individuals

Technical Problems of Assessment

There are widely divergent reports on the rate of functional loss in individuals who train regularly. Some early longitudinal data found a more rapid aging of peak aerobic power in athletes than in sedentary persons, presumably because the extent of training decreased as the athletes became older. Other longitudinal observations on small samples of active subjects have shown almost no functional loss over periods of 20 years or more. In such samples, one may presume that the **physical condition** of the subjects at recruitment was no more than moderate. Progressive improvement of physical condition over the course of the study thus counteracted the inherent effect of aging (12, 13). In other words, observers were comparing unfit young men with the same individuals who had become fit 20 to 30 years later.

Decreases in Peak Aerobic Power

In some large cross-sectional studies of groups such as Masters' athletes, the training volume has been well maintained in older cohorts. Such observations have suggested that the age-related rate of loss of peak aerobic power ranges from 2.8 to 4.2 mL/kg/min per decade (14). This is appreciably less than the rate of loss of 5 to 6 mL/kg/min anticipated in sedentary individuals; however, it is in keeping with the hypothesis that half the loss seen in sedentary subjects is due to a decrease in habitual physical activity and an accumulation of body fat, and is not inherent in the aging process (7). It also agrees with the findings from one small training study in which 15 men were followed for 33 years, beginning at an average age of 45 years. Throughout this period, they trained at 77% to 84% of the heart rate reserve, 3 to 4 times per week. Much as in sedentary subjects, their peak heart rates decreased by 25 beats/min, but the decrease in peak oxygen transport was 5.8% to 6.8% rather than the 10% per decade seen in sedentary individuals.

Decreases in Lean Tissue Mass

Lean body mass is well conserved in Masters' athletes through age 70 years (14), but a loss occurs subsequently, even if vigorous training is maintained. A similar pattern of change has been observed in the 33-year longitudinal study of active individuals (FW Kasch, personal communication, June 2, 2000). The probable explanation is an age-related decrease in secretion of **androgens**.

Enhancement of Physical Function by Training

 Training counteracts many of the functional effects of aging. Effects can be as large as a 10- to 20-year decrease in **biological age***.*

Peak Aerobic Power

The peak aerobic power of an elderly population responds well to an appropriately graded and progressive training program. In percentage terms, gains in peak aerobic power can be as large (15%–20%) as in young adults; however, because of low initial readings, absolute response declines with age (15). The importance of the training-induced change is highlighted when compared with the anticipated rate of aging in a sedentary person. An increase in peak aerobic power of 5 mL/kg/min is equivalent to a 10-year reduction in biological age.

Peak Muscle Force

Training-induced gains of peak muscle force are impressive. Fiatarone and coworkers (16) found a 113% increase of muscle strength in a small group of institutionalized nonagenarians who undertook high-intensity **resistance exercises**. Initially, much of the increase in performance was attributed to better coordinated contractions; however, as the study continued, **tomography** demonstrated a substantial increase of lean tissue mass in the muscles that had been exercised. Other investigators found a 29% increase in the cross-sectional area of type 2b fibers in the thigh muscles when elderly subjects undertook 50 weeks of weighted stair-climbing; control subjects showed a 22% decrease of fiber area over the same period (17).

Flexibility

Cross-sectional comparisons have shown a positive association between habitual physical activity and the flexibility of the hip and spine. A 2-year program of aerobic, strength, and flexibility exercises yielded an 11% increase in flexibility, as assessed by hamstring length (18), and a 9% improvement of sit-and-reach score was seen when 57- to 77-year-old women undertook a 12-week program of stretching, walking, and dancing (19). This last study also yielded a 12% improvement in balance. Not all investigators have found a significant improvement in balance with training. Nevertheless, a combination of increased **reaction speed**, stronger muscles, enhanced **proprioception** in the joints, and better control of blood pressure seems likely to decrease the risk of falls for active seniors (20); one report suggested that involvement in a simple walking program was enough to reduce the likelihood of a fall by 15% to 20% (21).

Influence of Physical Activity Upon Longevity

Substantial subject numbers are needed to calculate survival curves, and practical considerations generally preclude the random assignment of participants to exercise and control programs for such a purpose. The usual approach is thus a cross-sectional comparison of survival between active and inactive individuals. The effectiveness of regular physical activity in extending life span depends on success in maintaining an active lifestyle, and benefits apparently vary inversely with the age when activity is begun.

Young and Middle-Aged Adults

For the present purpose, we may classify those age 20 to 35 years as **young adults**, those 35 to 45 as in early **middle age**, and those 45 to 65 as in late **middle age**. Studies found that individuals who were athletes while at university had no advantage of survival compared to control groups during late middle and old age (22). There are two probable reasons for this negative outcome. Athletes were likely to have been selected for their university sports team in part because they had a muscular body build (a characteristic that has a negative impact on longevity), and many failed to continue their chosen sport into middle and old age (23). More recent reports have shown that endurance athletes have a 4- to 6-year advantage of longevity relative to control subjects; however, it is difficult to dissociate this finding from the lean, **ectomorphic** body build and the low prevalence of cigarette **smoking** characteristic of endurance competitors (24, 25). Multivariate analyses have attempted to adjust mortality rates for confounding variables, but the magnitude of confounding is such that the effectiveness of statistical adjustments remains problematic. For instance, high socioeconomic status is associated with a physically active lifestyle, and a comparison of the highest and lowest socioeconomic quintiles across Europe and North America shows that the highest quintile has a survival advantage of 6.3 years in men and 2.8 years in women (26). Similarly, abstinence from cigarette smoking can extend life expectancy by an average of 8 years, and endurance athletes typically are nonsmokers.

A 19- to 23-year followup of Harvard alumni suggested that, after statistical adjustments for important confounding variables, a weekly leisure-time **energy expenditure** of 8 MJ enhanced life expectancy by up to 2 years if the activity was begun at age 35 years (2). However, if adoption of a physically active lifestyle was deferred to age 70 years, the gain in life expectancy was only a few months. The extension of life span seemed somewhat greater if the weekly energy expenditure of 8 MJ was accumulated through sport rather than through low-intensity activity (e.g., walking). In keeping with some (but not all) published reports, one analysis of this data proposed that a threshold **intensity** of effort of 6 METS was required to extend life span (27). However, if there is indeed a threshold intensity of effort for benefit, it seems likely that the threshold will decrease as a person becomes older.

Elderly Adults

Regular physical activity does relatively little to extend **life span** if it is not initiated until the retirement years. A study from eastern Finland suggested that the survival curves for active and inactive individuals converged around age 80 years (28). It thus seems that the main effect of regular physical activity is to avoid **premature death** rather than to prolong the period of frail old age; in other words, an active lifestyle promotes what Fries has termed a "squaring" of the mortality curve (29). One cross-sectional study even suggested that in individuals older than 80 years, vigorous physical activity increased **mortality rate** slightly, although moderate activity continued to yield a small benefit compared to sedentary individuals (30).

Influence of Physical Activity Upon Health (Box 34.2)

In the senior citizen, regular physical activity continues to offer protection against chronic diseases (e.g., **hypertension, cardiac and peripheral vascular disease, and chronic obstructive lung disease**) where benefit has been established in younger persons (31). In old age, however, particular importance attaches to the impact of physical activity upon functional capacity and thus the capacity for independent living. Other benefits include increased **appetite**, stimulation of bowel movements, facilitation of **sleep**, enhanced mood-state, reduction in obesity and the risk of

BOX 34.2. Important Health Benefits of Regular Physical Activity in the Elderly

- Enhanced functional capacity and greater independence
- Improvements of appetite, nutrition, bowel movements, and sleep
- Enhanced mood-state
- Control of obesity and type 2 diabetes mellitus
- Enhanced immune function
- Decreased risk of various cancers
- Amelioration of arthritis
- Decreased risk of osteoporosis
- Enhanced overall quality of life

type 2 **diabetes mellitus**, improved immune function, and decreased risk of various types of **cancer, arthritis,** and **osteoporosis**.

Functional Capacity

Peak Aerobic Power

Enhancement of functional capacity is perhaps the most important reason why the old and very old should increase habitual physical activity. Aerobic activity becomes fatiguing if it demands more than 40% of peak oxygen intake, and the progressive, age-related decline of oxygen transport eventually brings most seniors to the point where they lack the energy needed for ordinary activities of daily living. Walking up a slight incline or carrying a small bag of groceries becomes intolerably fatiguing. By comparing people living in and outside of institutions, Paterson and coworkers (4) inferred that the threshold of **dependency** was a peak aerobic power of about 15 mL/kg/min; no independently living seniors had a peak aerobic power of less than 15 mL/kg/min. Sedentary persons reach this threshold around 80 years of age, but those who remain active may stay above the aerobic threshold for a further 10 to 20 years. Retrospective questioning established that those who were physically active at age 50 were much less likely to be institutionalized as seniors (32). A person who is approaching the independence threshold may undergo a progressive training program, setting back the date of institutionalization by 10 to 20 years.

Peak Muscle Force

Age-related decrease in peak muscle force is often an important factor in loss of independence, particularly in elderly women. Strength becomes inadequate to perform the activities of daily living, including carrying household items, opening containers, lifting the body mass from a chair or a toilet seat, and eventually even getting out of bed without assistance (Figure 34.1). Resistance exercises correct many of these problems, enhancing the speed of rising from a chair, improving gait, and boosting the preferred speed of walking (33).

Flexibility, Balance, and Falls

A progressive decrease in flexibility of the major joints increasingly restricts the possible range of activities for most seniors. Entering a car or climbing stairs to enter a house or a bus becomes difficult. Eventually, it becomes impossible to climb into a bath, or even to dress without assistance. As noted previously, training programs can enhance flexibility by 10%, delaying the time when these changes have a major impact on ability to undertake activities of daily living.

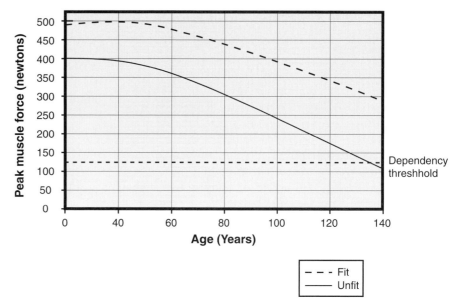

FIGURE 34.1. Impact of fitness on capacity to live independently. Dependency often develops when peak muscle force drops below a critical value (horizontal line). Sedentary individuals with a low level of fitness begin adult life with a lower peak muscle force than their active and physically fit peers. Although both groups lose strength as they age, the peak muscle force of the sedentary group thus drops below the critical threshold much earlier than is the case in those who are fit. Participation in a training program at any age can move the person from the unfit toward the fit aging curve, with a substantial reduction in biological age.

A person who has problems of balance and is susceptible to repeated falls also faces a restricted life. Regular physical activity is helpful in enhancing balance. The stability of blood pressure is increased, reducing the likelihood of hypotensive falls; in the event the person trips over an unperceived obstacle, faster reflexes and stronger muscles enable more rapid righting movements.

Appetite, Bowel Movements, Sleep, and Mood-State

Appetite

Poverty, poor vision, tremor, muscle weakness, stroke, and arthritis can hamper food preparation by the elderly, limiting nutrient intake. Appetite may be limited by unappetizing food, and by deterioration in the senses of taste and smell, poor dentition, difficulty swallowing, or deficient secretion of hydrochloric acid and enzymes in the stomach. Many elderly people are so inactive that they can achieve energy balance by eating little more than the equivalent of their **resting metabolism**. Particularly if they continue to consume 2 to 3 glasses of alcoholic beverages per day, their remaining **food intake** is unlikely to provide sufficient vitamins and micronutrients. In such a situation, increased physical activity plays an important role in stimulating appetite and increasing the intake of vitamins and minerals to a level compatible with nutritional health (34).

Bowel Movements

Many elderly people complain of constipation. Very vigorous physical activity can certainly increase colonic activity. The mechanism is thought to be an exercise-induced secretion of **prostaglandins**. Although claims are sometimes made that more moderate physical activity can also enhance bowel movements, this remains to be proven.

Sleep

Although elderly people take frequent daytime naps, they also tend to complain of difficulty sleeping at night. Exercise early in the day can help to alleviate this problem, in part by increasing the immediate level of **arousal** and reducing daytime napping, and in part by creating a pleasant sense of physical fatigue. It was once held that exercising in the evening was likely to exacerbate sleep problems. This is plausible if the intensity of effort is sufficient to increase arousal, but the gentle walk of most seniors is unlikely to have other than a beneficial effect upon sleep patterns, even if taken relatively late during the day.

Mood-State

Depression and anxiety are common in older people. Causes include poverty, lack of social contacts, chronic illness, and pain. Meta-analyses now suggest that a program of regular physical activity can enhance **mood-state**, particularly in someone who is initially depressed (35). The subjects for some of the investigations included in this meta-analysis were elderly. There are many possible reasons why greater physical activity may reduce depression, ranging from increased experiences and social contacts, through greater neural stimulation and secretion of arousing chemical agents during exercise (various amines and endorphins). Any observed enhancement of mood-state may also reflect incidental consequences of an exercise program, such as increased attention and opportunities for social interaction, rather than the increase in physical activity per se.

Obesity and Type 2 Diabetes Mellitus

Obesity

Obesity reflects a chronic, small (<1%) imbalance between intake and expenditure of food energy. Typically, body fat accumulates over several years because habitual physical activity is reduced without a matching decrease in food intake. It is important to reverse the accumulation of body fat, and not simply to enhance physical appearance: excess body fat reduces peak aerobic power and **peak muscle force** per kilogram of body mass; predisposes to **atherosclerosis**, type 2 diabetes mellitus, and various cancers; and exacerbates existing problems in osteoarthritic joints.

Obesity can be corrected either by decreasing food intake or by augmenting physical activity. However, an increase of physical activity is the preferred option (15, 36), for several reasons:

- Moderate physical activity is pleasant, positive advice, in contrast with the prohibitions implicit in **dieting**.
- Physical activity tends to enhance mood-state, in contrast with the depression induced by dieting.
- Physical activity stimulates metabolism both during and following exercise, thus counteracting the depression of resting metabolism that often neutralizes the effect of dieting alone.
- Moderate physical activity helps to conserve lean tissue mass, whereas with dieting alone, loss of lean tissue may be as great as loss of body fat.

Type 2 Diabetes Mellitus

Cellular resistance to **insulin** develops in many elderly people because of a decrease in the numbers and/or the sensitivity of the insulin receptors, or a failure of the second messenger system that normally initiates intracellular formation of **glycogen** from glucose. Potential etiological factors (37) include the following:

- Increased amounts of **adipose tissue**,
- Decreased amounts of lean tissue,
- Decreased habitual physical activity, and
- Increased **sympathetic** nerve **activity**.

The relationships among decreased physical activity, obesity, and the widespread prevalence of type 2 diabetes mellitus have become particularly obvious in indigenous populations (e.g., Native Americans) as these groups acculturated to a sedentary "western" lifestyle (38). There is now good evidence that regular physical activity reduces the likelihood of developing diabetes (39), and exercise programs are an effective treatment for those who are already showing manifestations of maturity-onset diabetes. In many instances, regular physical activity can correct the need for insulin injections, and in some cases there is no further need to take oral insulin (40).

Immune Function

In young adults, it is widely believed that there is a J-shaped relationship between the volume of physical activity and the immune response: moderate physical activity enhances immune function, but excessive acute or chronic exercise has a depressant effect (41). Maximizing immune function has particular importance for the elderly, because aging is associated with deterioration in **natural killer cell** function. Autoimmune disease and cancers also are more prevalent in the elderly, and chronic pathological changes predispose this age group to **infection** (42). There have been relatively few studies of changes in immune function with exercise in the elderly, but the available information points to both prevention and reversal of some age-related losses by programs of regular, moderate physical activity (43).

Cancer

Cancer is the most frequent cause of death in the elderly. There is growing evidence that a lifetime of regular physical activity reduces the risk of colon cancers. Prolonged physical activity may also offer protection against lung, breast, prostate, and reproductive cancers in women (44). Depending on the tumor site, these findings have many possible explanations. Potential mechanisms include enhanced immune function, reduction of obesity, and accelerated colonic transport (45).

Arthritis

The long-term influence of physical activity upon arthritis remains controversial. Participation in some contact sports appears to increase the risk of developing osteoarthritis (46), but walking and jogging do not seem to be associated with any increased prevalence of this condition (47). Once a joint has been damaged, isometric exercise that strengthens the muscles around the affected joint may be beneficial. Regular physical activity can also help reduce body mass, and thus the load to be supported by the injured joint. Once the acute inflammation has passed, regular physical activity helps maintain mobility and overall cardiorespiratory function in persons with rheumatoid arthritis; weight-supported activities (e.g., cycle ergometry or exercises in a heated pool) are preferred for this purpose (48).

Osteoporosis

Osteoporosis significantly affects both the quality of life and longevity. Elderly people become bed-ridden as a result of osteoporotic fractures, and as many as 20% die of pulmonary emboli or a urinary infection within 12 months of sustaining a hip fracture. Regular **weight-bearing** or resistance exercise is important in both preventing and correcting bone **calcium** loss (11). Adequate intake of calcium and **vitamins** is also necessary to bone health. In the United States, many physicians recommend **estrogen** replacement therapy in postmenopausal women; however, in other countries the value of estrogen for an active and well-nourished older woman is debated relative to the complications that such treatment can cause.

Influence of Physical Activity Upon Quality-Adjusted Life Expectancy

An increase in quality-adjusted life expectancy (Figure 34.2) seems one of the more important reasons to persuade an elderly person to engage in regular physical activity (3). Quality of life may be enhanced by decreased likelihood of acute and chronic disease, improved mood-state, and decreased likelihood of dependency.

Acute and Chronic Disease

Acute Infections

There is evidence that individuals who engage in regular moderate physical activity are less vulnerable to acute infections than those who are sedentary, because regular physical activity enhances immune function (41). However, this factor has only a small impact on quality-adjusted life expectancy. An upper respiratory **infection** may temporarily reduce quality of life by 10% (a decrease of 0.1 units on a scale of the type shown in Fig. 34.2). The average person suffers perhaps two such infections per year, each lasting for about 15 days. It is unlikely that even an optimal dose of physical activity will reduce the period

of infection by more than 25%, or 7.5 days per year. Thus, quality-adjusted life expectancy is likely to be enhanced by (7.5/365 × 0.1), or 0.0021 arbitrary units per year. Given 10 calendar years of survival, the total benefit becomes 0.021 quality-adjusted life years.

Chronic Disease

An analysis by Robine and Ritchie (26) suggested that, in terms of **healthy life expectancy**, circulatory disorders caused an average loss of 4 years, locomotor problems a loss of 5 years, and respiratory problems a loss of 2 years (i.e., total loss of 11 years of healthy life expectancy). Most of these losses were incurred during old age. If we assume that a functional problem in any one of these body systems reduces quality of life by an average of 30%, then the cumulative impact is a loss of 11 (0.3), or 3.3 quality-adjusted life years. For many (although certainly not all) of the relevant conditions, regular physical activity plays both a preventive and a rehabilitative role. Setting the magnitude of the exercise response at a 30% reduction in prevalence of chronic disease, the gain from this consequence of active lifestyle could be as large as 0.99 quality-adjusted life years.

Mood-State

Mood-state is rarely optimal in elderly people. Let us assume that anxiety, depression, and other disorders of affect reduce mood-state from a theoretical ceiling of 100% to an average value of 90% (i.e., a reduction in quality of life from 1.0 to 0.9 in the arbitrary units of Fig. 34.2). There is, then, a cumulative loss of 1 quality-adjusted life year over a 10-year period of survival. One measure of the favorable impact of physical activity upon mood-state (35) is a resulting decrease in demand for medical consultations and hospital

FIGURE 34.2. Impact of fitness on quality of life and quality-adjusted life expectancy. A person who remains vigorously active into old age maintains a high quality of life to near the time of death; indeed, they may die suddenly while engaged in vigorous physical activity. The person who carefully avoids strenuous physical activity in old age may live longer than the active and fit individual, but will have a substantial period of survival with low quality of life, and thus their quality-adjusted life expectancy will be less than that of a fit and active person. As illustrated, quality of life is assessed on an arbitrary scale, ranging from 1.0 (very good quality of life; each calendar year of survival contributes 1 quality-adjusted year of survival) to near zero (very poor; a year of calendar survival has little influence on quality-adjusted years of survival). The fit person maintains a much higher quality-of-life score until about age 80 years, when there is a sudden drop to zero, associated with terminal illness. In the unfit person, poor quality of life persists much longer (in the example, from about 70 years until terminal illness at age 100 years).

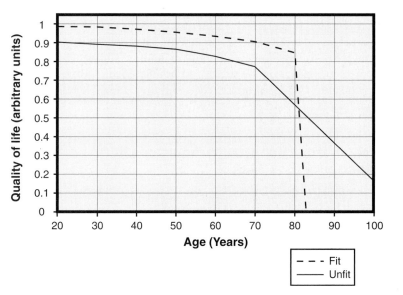

admissions. In middle-aged adults, participation in an exercise program reduced the need for such services by about 25% (49). Given the age-related tendency to depression, benefit may be greater in the elderly than in those who are middle aged. However, on the conservative assumption of a 25% benefit, as in middle age, there would be a cumulative increase in quality-adjusted life expectancy of 0.25 years over 10 calendar years of survival.

Dependency

The causes of institutionalization are varied (50). In some cases, elderly people experience difficulty in ambulation or transfer. Others complain of frequent falls, failure to eat or drink adequately, or incontinence. A decrease in manual dexterity, loss of self-esteem, intellectual deterioration, a sudden stroke or blindness, and loss of support from significant others are all potential crises that precipitate admission to an institution. But often, the underlying problem is that peak aerobic power, **muscle strength**, or flexibility has deteriorated to such an extent that the person can no longer carry out the activities of daily living independently.

Functional dependency is often of relatively slow onset. The impact upon the individual depends on personal coping mechanisms, and the type of environmental aids available. For example, provision of chairs with long legs facilitates standing, and placing electrical outlets at waist height can compensate for impaired flexibility. For many people, there is a progressive change from partial to total dependency over 10 years of survival; we may imagine the quality of life of an elderly person declining gradually from 90% to 50% of its optimal value as dependency develops. Thus, the cumulative effect of the growing dependency is an average loss of 0.2 years per year, or 2 quality-adjusted life years over the decade. In many elderly people, total dependency continues over a final year of life, causing a further loss of 0.4 quality-adjusted life years.

Although regular physical activity is likely to postpone many types of functional deterioration (51 345), perhaps by as much as 10 to 20 years, its impact on other causes of dependency is more limited. The upper limit of the benefit from an exercise program is likely to be a 50% reduction in dependency; the loss is thus decreased from 2.4 to 1.2 quality-adjusted life years.

Overall Impact on Quality-Adjusted Life Expectancy (Box 34.3)

Summing the changes in quality-adjusted life expectancy that are likely to be induced by regular physical activity, we may anticipate a benefit of (0.02 + 0.99 + 0.25 + 1.20), or about 2.5 quality-adjusted life years during the final 10 or 11 years of life. The figure is, as yet, imprecise, and there may be some overlap between the effects that we have at-

---

> **BOX 34.3. Likely Gains in Quality-Adjusted Life Expectancy From an Increase of Physical Activity at Age 65 Years**
>
> - Decrease in impact of acute infections = 0.02 years
> - Decrease in impact of chronic conditions = 0.99 years
> - Enhanced mood-state = 0.25 years
> - Decrease in dependency = 1.20 years
> - Total impact = 2.5 quality-adjusted life years

tributed to the prevention of chronic disease and the maintenance of functional independence. Nevertheless, the anticipated magnitude of benefit is substantially larger than any gain in calendar life expectancy that can be achieved by initiating an exercise program late in life. Moreover, an enhanced quality of life has much greater appeal to most patients than a mere extension of calendar life span. Indeed, the average person will explain the reason that they exercise is that it makes them "feel better."

Clinical Focus: Advising the Senior on Exercise Testing and Exercise Prescription

Given the many benefits that a senior can derive from regular physical activity, it is important that all health professionals who interact with seniors offer appropriate and effective encouragement to an active lifestyle. Information on physical function may also be needed when judging a person's ability to continue in physically demanding employment. What tests should be applied, and what advice should be offered?

Exercise Testing

Information is commonly sought on peak or **maximal aerobic power**, blood pressure, **exercise electrocardiogram**, muscle strength, body fat content, flexibility, balance, and reaction speeds. In the very old, it is also useful to assess ability to undertake activities of daily living, using such measures as the Continuous Scale Physical Functional Performance Test (51). Given a relatively small number of subjects, adequate equipment, and sufficient personnel, tests are best carried out in the laboratory.

Peak Aerobic Power

Peak aerobic power can be estimated by a treadmill or cycle ergometer test, carried to subjective exhaustion under the supervision of a physician. It is best to measure oxygen consumption directly, but if values are predicted from the treadmill stage that is reached (as in the **Naughton test**), it is important to ensure that the subject does not support body weight by using the handrail. Because of interindividual differences in motivation to maximal effort, day-to-day variations in physical condition, the effects of any intercurrent illness, and technical errors, about one test in 40 will underestimate a person's true aerobic power by as much as 10 mL/kg/min, equivalent to a 20-year error in determination of biological age. Further, the test results only indicate the person's ability to carry out the form of exercise that was used in testing; abilities may differ substantially, for example, between walking and cycle ergometry. If simple submaximal predictions of aerobic power are derived from cycle ergometer, step, shuttle run, or 6-minute walk tests, errors in assessment of physical status become even larger. This underlines the difficulty in using either laboratory or field test data for purposes of exercise prescription and work evaluation.

Blood Pressure

Resting blood pressure is usually determined by means of a standard clinical **sphygmomanometer** cuff, although portable battery-operated devices for the measurement of blood pressure are also now available. It is important to allow adequate preliminary seated rest, to deflate the cuff slowly, and to avoid rounding blood pressure readings to numbers ending with a five or a zero. The systolic reading is indicated by the pressure at which pulsation (the Korotkov sounds) is first heard under the sphygmomanometer cuff, and the diastolic reading corresponds to the fifth phase (the pressure at which the pulsating sounds disappear). The exercise systolic reading can be measured in similar fashion, but it is difficult to determine the diastolic reading during exercise.

Exercise Electrocardiogram

Because of baseline abnormalities, the exercise electrocardiogram (ECG) is often difficult to interpret in older people. A horizontal or down sloping depression of the ST segment of the ECG in excess of 1 mm (0.1 mV) during near-maximal effort implies a statistical increase in the risk of a heart attack, but unfortunately this is a **false-positive** response in many people. ST segmental depression is more likely to be a true-positive finding if the person shows other **cardiac risk factors** (e.g., history of cigarette smoking, high resting blood pressure, or blood lipid abnormalities).

Muscle Strength

Muscle strength can be assessed using **isotonic** or **isometric** tests, or less directly through the determination of lean tissue mass (total body mass minus fat mass). Possible field assessments of muscle strength include the number of sit-ups or modified push-ups that can be performed in a minute, and the speed of rising from a chair. One problem with most tests of muscle strength is that scores are specific to the muscle group tested. Leg strength contributes to the restoration of balance and the prevention of falls. Grip, shoulder, and arm strength are important to the performance of activities of daily living, and trunk lifting may be important in some occupations. However, strength measurements show a relatively weak correlation with the ability to perform either daily or occupational tasks, accounting for only about 25% of interindividual differences in the performance of such activities.

Body Fat

Body fat is determined by underwater weighing; however, this procedure is often difficult in the elderly, because of problems in using a mouthpiece underwater. Body fat can be determined more simply by applying standard Lange or Harpenden calipers to a double fold of skin and subcutaneous tissue at selected sites (e.g., triceps, subscapular, and suprailiac skinfolds). The skinfold figure represents superficial body fatness, but it does not measure intra-abdominal fat (which is more important in cardiovascular risk). In elderly people, the skin is thinner than in young adults, and often has only a loose attachment to underlying tissue. It is thus important to ensure that subcutaneous tissue is included in the measured skinfold. Age-specific readings should be used to convert the data to body density and thus an estimated percentage of body fat, since bone demineralization reduces the average density of the lean tissues.

Flexibility

Flexibility can be examined in the laboratory, using a **goniometer**, and an overall field assessment can be made by means of the sit-and-reach test. As with muscle strength, flexibility is specific to the joint that is tested, particularly in older people who are affected by local arthritic conditions.

Balance and Reaction Speed

Balance and reaction speed are critical to the prevention of falls. Overall balance can be assessed from the extent of body sway, shown by the forces generated when standing on a **force plate**. A **stabilometer** provides a simple overall assessment of the time a person can stand astride a balanced beam and keep it from hitting the ground. For field surveys, it is also possible to time the interval a person can remain on one foot with the eyes closed (the "**stork stand**" test).

The speed of reaction is commonly assessed from the time needed to make an electrical contact in response to a colored light or a noise. It comprises both the true **reaction time** (delays in the processing of information by the brain) and the **movement time** needed to execute a response at a given joint. Because of differences in the length of nerve pathways and the efficiency of various muscle groups, determinations must be made for movements of interest (e.g., the time to apply the foot brake in a car simulator).

Exercise Prescription

Traditional Approach

The traditional approach to exercise prescription in the older adult has been a full medical examination followed by laboratory testing that includes an exercise stress test with ECG and direct measurement or prediction of peak or maximal aerobic power. Detailed exercise testing leads, in turn, to detailed exercise prescription. Typically, the prescription indicates an appropriate intensity, frequency, and duration of exercise sessions, and often recommends specific forms of exercise, including resistance training (52 344, 53).

If vigorous exercise is planned, at least 5 minutes should be allocated to gentle stretching and a progressive **warm-up** to minimize the risk of musculoskeletal injuries. Similarly, a bout of vigorous exercise should be followed by a 5- to 10-minute **cool-down** (e.g., slow walking) to reduce the likelihood of a sudden drop in blood pressure and resulting cardiac problems postexercise. Muscular contractions should be slow and controlled. In elderly people with advanced osteoporosis, overly vigorous contractions can cause bone fractures. Sustained contractions with a closed glottis should also be avoided, because such activity can cause an undesirably large rise in blood pressure. Often, older people tolerate extreme environmental conditions poorly, and exercise should move indoors during very hot or very cold weather, or if outdoor surfaces become ice covered. If there is a history of frequent falls, or **posture** is unstable, exercise in a seated position is advisable. Low-impact, weight-supported activity such as pool exercise is a preferred option if there is a history of back problems or arthritis in weight-supporting joints.

A detailed exercise prescription is desirable if a senior citizen expresses interest in preparing for a competitive Masters' marathon run or other athletic event (54 342). However, most seniors wish to do no more than begin some light gardening or gentle walking, and in this contributor's view it is inappropriate to constrain enthusiasm for such health-giving activity by an excess of preliminary tests and regulations. Further, many of those carrying out fitness testing are more familiar with the performance of young athletes than with the responses of an 80-year-old patient. Thus, they may be concerned by a mild elevation of blood pressure, or what appears to be a small abnormality of the exercise ECG. Too often, it seems that North American physicians are prepared to treat an ECG anomaly rather than respond to any symptoms the patient may develop. So, in practicing defensive medicine, the result of an exercise stress test may be that an 80-year-old exercise candidate is advised to be "very careful," and sometimes the planned increase in physical activity is totally prohibited.

Vigorous, unaccustomed exercise can sometimes hasten the death of such an individual compared to the alternative of living "very carefully." Similarly, an excessive rate of progression of conditioning, or vigorous exercise sessions with an inadequate warm-up, may cause tiresome musculoskeletal **injuries**. Nevertheless, most seniors exercise prudently, and would prefer to enjoy their final years, possibly dying of a sudden **heart attack** on the golf course rather than sitting around a nursing home awaiting death from cancer or some other unpleasant disease. Thus, the traditional approach of detailed, test-based restrictions on exercise seems inappropriate for those who plan only a moderate increase in daily physical activity.

Nontraditional Approach

In advising seniors who wish to begin moderate exercise and physical activity, a few simple principles should be observed. Rather than proposing a complex exercise prescription that may be difficult to understand, the best plan is to review current activities and suggest how a little more exercise may be undertaken in the next 2 weeks. The program should include aerobic exercise, stimulation of the major muscles, and increased movement at each of the major joints. If the suggestions are followed without causing symptoms other than a pleasant tiredness a few hours after exercise, activity may be increased progressively in subsequent weeks until the fitness objectives of the exercise specialist and the patient have been satisfied.

Warning signs of an excessively vigorous approach may include an increase of resting heart rate, persistent fatigue, and swelling of the ankles. But the advisor should recognize that most old people do not overexercise, and that the likely long-term effect of regular moderate physical activity is an extension rather than a shortening of calendar life span, with an even larger increase in quality-adjusted life expectancy. The advisor's role is thus to encourage rather than to restrict movement. The very old may not always remember to attend organized exercise sessions, and thus much of the required physical activity should be built into a program of **active living**: walking to the store for a newspaper, or to the cafeteria for lunch, as well as gardening and other activities around the home. Good shoes with adequate heel support should be worn, and any exercise area should be well lighted and free of objects that may cause tripping or collisions. Other general precautions are as suggested for a traditional exercise prescription.

Occupational Assessment

Some organizations have specified physiological standards that must be met for an older person to retain employment. For example, it has been suggested that **public safety officers** (e.g., police and firefighters) need a peak oxygen transport of 3 L/min to carry out their duties effectively. Similarly, **airline pilots** must show that they are free of ST depression on an exercise ECG, and **military personnel** must meet specific criteria of isotonic lifting ability. However, it is difficult to enforce these standards in court, in part because adjudicators have found difficulty in relating physiological test scores to job demands, and in part because of errors inherent in the measurements. In some instances, retention of personnel has thus been based on reaching minimum test scores in **job simulations** (e.g., a timed obstacle pursuit for police officers). Others have used averaged physiological data to establish fixed retirement ages; however, this approach is unsatisfactory because it fails to account for wide differences in biological age and functional ability at the normal **retirement** age.

What We Know
About Exercise for the Older Adult

1 Regular physical activity is a powerful method of counteracting the decline in peak aerobic power, muscle strength, and flexibility that otherwise progressively limits the independence of the elderly person.

2 An effective exercise program can decrease the biological age of an older adult by as much as 10 to 20 years, with major gains in quality-adjusted life expectancy.

3 Moderate physical activity is a pleasant and safe form of treatment for most seniors, with positive effects on many aspects of health.

4 In general, older adults can and should be encouraged to make moderate increases in their habitual physical activity without excessive preliminary testing and detailed exercise prescription.

What We Would Like to Know
About Exercise for the Older Adult

1 Improved methods of assessing the quality of life are needed for adults of all ages.

2 Accurate assessment of the magnitude of the gains in function and quality of life that result from various patterns and intensities of exercise would be helpful in advising seniors on an optimal lifestyle.

3 It would be helpful to know the extent to which very vigorous physical activity may shorten the life span of the very old.

4 Given that a high proportion of seniors are currently totally sedentary, there is an urgent need for information about ways in which health professionals can encourage older people to adopt a more active lifestyle.

Summary

Most biological functions decline progressively with age. This change is somewhat more obvious in sedentary than in athletic individuals. Decreases in peak aerobic power, muscle force and endurance, flexibility, and balance reduce overall functional capacity and progressively limit an elderly person's ability to undertake activities of daily living. Independence is thus compromised, with a corresponding deterioration in quality of life. A lifestyle that incorporates adequate amounts of physical activity is important at any age, but is particularly necessary in old age. Boosting physical activity will enhance overall health and mood-state, but has little, if any, effect on longevity in this age group. The most important benefit of increased physical activity is probably a substantial reversal of functional losses. The enhanced functional capacity extends the period of independent living and improves the individual's quality-adjusted life expectancy. Although detailed medical examination is needed for the person who wishes to engage in high-level athletic competition, the interpretation of findings is difficult, because test results often show features that would be regarded as abnormal in a younger individual. In contrast, a modest increase in physical activity (e.g., gentle walking) is safe, and even if it does not extend average life expectancy, it will increase the individual's quality-adjusted life expectancy. Such activity is best recommended in simple terms, without creating the potential barriers of detailed medical clearance, stress testing, and an elaborate exercise prescription.

DISCUSSION QUESTIONS

1 What are the most important arguments to advance when persuading an older person to become physically active?

2 What factors are likely to threaten the independence of the senior citizen? How does functional deterioration contribute to this picture?

3 What type of examination should be given to the senior citizen before he or she embarks on a program of light physical activity? How should the examination be modified if the individual expresses a desire to participate in Masters' competition?

CASE STUDY

Patient Information

Jim is a 69-year-old man who visits his family physician for a routine check-up. He was employed as a middle-grade civil servant with a desk job until 4 years ago. He stopped smoking 20 years ago, but has exercised little since high school. He responds favorably to suggestions that it might be a good idea to augment his physical activity; indeed, both he and his wife are contemplating joining the biweekly Seniors' Walking Club.

Assessments

Clinical examination shows that Jim is relatively healthy for his age. He is not taking any medication except a fairly heavy dose of Seldane during hay fever season. His body mass index of 28.5 kg/m² indicates some excess of body fat. Initial diastolic blood pressure reading was high (95 mm Hg), but after rest and reassurance, a reading of 140/85 mm Hg was obtained. There were no symptoms suggestive of diabetes mellitus, and a Lasix urine test was negative.

Questioning established that Jim could walk on level ground at a pace of 4.8 km/hr without shortness of breath. He admitted to some breathlessness if he attempted to maintain this pace on a slope, but even then he was able to continue chatting with his wife. He had no vision problems providing he wore his glasses, and no history of falling or loss of balance. The Seniors' Walking Club appears well organized. They walk at a moderate pace along well-maintained trails, usually for 1 hour. The climate of the town is mild and wet, and the walks proceed "rain or shine." The leader carries a cell-phone, and anyone who becomes tired can rest with the "rear guard" until the more vigorous members of the party have covered their intended distance and return.

Do not create iatrogenic disease when examining an elderly patient who expresses an interest in physical activity. Remember that the overall prognosis is better for the active than for the sedentary patient. In particular, it is important not to comment on a first blood pressure reading that appears high. About 20% of all patients have been told by their physician that they have a high blood pressure, but in a high proportion of cases the true diagnosis is "white-coat hypertension"—a transient increase of blood pressure as a reaction to anxiety in the setting of a doctor's office. Such pressures normalize with rest, reassurance, and relaxation.

Questions

1. What advice would you give Jim regarding his exercise plan?
2. What special investigations would you undertake?
3. What would you tell him about prognosis?
4. What follow-up would you propose?

REFERENCES

1. Blair SN, Franks AL, Shelton DM, Livengood JR, Hull FL, Breedlove B, eds. Physical Activity and Health: A Report of the Surgeon General. Atlanta, GA: U.S. Dept. of Health & Human Services, Centers for Disease Control and Prevention, National Center for Chronic Disease Prevention and Health Promotion; 1996.
2. Paffenbarger RS, Hyde RT, Wing AL, Lee I-M, Kampert JB. Some interrelations of physical activity, physiological fitness, health and longevity. In: Bouchard C, Shephard RJ, Stephens T, eds. Physical Activity, Fitness and Health. Champaign, IL: Human Kinetics; 1994:119–133.
3. Shephard RJ. Habitual physical activity and the quality of life. Quest 1996;48:354–365.
4. Paterson DH, Cunningham DA, Koval JJ, St. Croix C. Aerobic fitness in a population of independently living men and women aged 55–86 years. Med Sci Sports Exerc 1999;31:1813–1820.
5. Lakatta EG. Cardiovascular regulatory mechanisms in advanced age. Physiol Rev 1993;73:413–467.
6. Lakatta EG. Aging and cardiovascular structure and function in healthy sedentary humans. Aging (Milano) 1998;10:162–164.
7. Jackson AS, Beard EF, Wier LT, Ross RM, Stuteville JE, Blair SN. Changes in aerobic power of men ages 25–70 yr. Med Sci Sports Exerc 1995;27:113–120.
8. Fiatarone-Singh MA. Exercise, Nutrition and the Older Woman. Boca Raton, FL: CRC Publishing; 2000.
9. Fitness Canada. Fitness and Lifestyle in Canada. Ottawa, Ontario: Government of Canada; 1983.
10. Overstall PW, Downton JH. Gait, balance and falls. In: Pathy MSJ, ed. Principles and Practice of Geriatric Medicine. 3rd ed. Chichester, UK: John Wiley; 1998:1121–1132 (vol 2).
11. Drinkwater B. Physical activity, fitness and osteoporosis. In: Bouchard C, Shephard RJ, Stephens T, eds. Physical Activity, Fitness and Health. Champaign, IL: Human Kinetics, 1994:724–736.

12. Kasch FW, Boyer JL, Van Camp SP, Verity LS, Wallace JP. Effect of exercise on cardiovascular ageing. Age Ageing 1993;22:5–10.
13. Kasch FW, Boyer JL, Schmidt PK, et al. Ageing of the cardiovascular system during 33 years of aerobic exercise. Age Ageing 1999;28:531–536.
14. Shephard RJ, Kavanagh T, Mertens DJ. Personal health benefits of Masters athletic competition. Br J Sports Med 1995;29:35–40.
15. Shephard RJ. Aging, Physical Activity and Health. Champaign, IL: Human Kinetics; 1997.
16. Fiatarone M, O'Neill EF, Ryan ND, et al. Exercise training and nutritional supplementation for physical frailty in very elderly people. N Engl J Med 1994;330:1769–1775.
17. Cress ME, Thomas DP, Johnson J, et al. Effect of training on $\dot{V}_{O_{2max}}$, thigh strength and muscle morphology in septuagenarian women. Med Sci Sports Exerc 1991;23:752–758.
18. Morey MC, Cowper PA, Feussner JR, et al. Two-year trends in physical performance following supervised exercise among community-dwelling older veterans. J Am Geriatr Soc 1991;39:986–992.
19. Hopkins DR, Murrah B, Hoeger WWK, Rhodes RC. Effect of low impact aerobic dance on the functional fitness of elderly women. Gerontol 1990;30:189–192.
20. Jaglal SB, Kreger N, Darlington G. Past and recent physical activity and risk of hip fracture. Am J Epidemiol 1993;138:107–118.
21. MacRae PG, Feltner ME, Reinsch S. A 1-year exercise program for older women: effects on falls, injuries, and physical performance. J Aging Phys Activ 1994;2:127–142.
22. Montoye HJ, Van Huss WD, Olson HW, Pierson WO, Hudec AJ. The longevity and mortality of college athletes. Lansing, MI: Phi Epsilon Kappa Fraternity, Michigan State University; 1957.
23. Yamaji K, Shephard RJ. Longevity and causes of death of athletes: a review of the literature. J Hum Ergol 1977;6:13–25.
24. Karvonen MJ, Klemola H, Virkajarvi J, Kekkonen A. Longevity of endurance skiers. Med Sci Sports 1974;6:49–51.
25. Sarna S, Kaprio J. Life expectancy of former athletes. Sports Med 1994;17:149–151.
26. Robine JM, Ritchie K. Healthy life expectancy: evaluation of global indicator of change in population health. Br Med J 1991;302:457–460.
27. Paffenbarger RS, Lee I-M. Physical activity and fitness for health and longevity. Res Quart 1996;67 (suppl):S11–S28.
28. Pekkanen J, Marti B, Nissinen A, Tuomilehto J, Punsar S, Karvonen MJ. Reduction of premature mortality by high physical activity: a 20-year follow-up of middle-aged Finnish men. Lancet 1987;i:1473–1477.
29. Fries JF. Aging, natural death and the compression of morbidity. N Engl J Med 1980;303:130–135.
30. Linsted KD, Tonstad K, Kuzma J. Self-report of physical activity and patterns of mortality in Seventh-Day Adventist men. J Clin Epidemiol 1991;44:355–364.
31. Bouchard C, Shephard RJ. Physical activity, fitness and health: the model and key concepts. In: Bouchard C, Shephard RJ, Stephens T, eds. Physical Activity, Fitness and Health. Champaign, IL: Human Kinetics; 1994.
32. Shephard RJ, Montelpare WJ. Geriatric benefits of exercise as an adult. J Gerontol 1988;43:M86–M90.
33. Bassey EJ, Fiatarone MA, O'Neill EF, Kelly M, Evans WJ, Lipsitz LA. Leg extensor power and functional performance in very old men and women. Clin Sci 1992;82:321–327.
34. Tiidus P, Shephard RJ, Montelpare WJ. Overall intake of energy and key nutrients: data for middle-aged and older middle-class adults. Can J Sport Sci 1989;14:173–177.
35. North TC, McCullagh G, Todd IC, Tran ZV. Effect of exercise on depression. Exerc Sport Sci Rev 1990;18:379–416.
36. Ballor DL, Keesey RE. A meta-analysis of the factors affecting exercise-induced changes in body mass, fat mass and fat-free mass in males and females. Int J Obesity 1991;15:717–726.
37. Gudat U, Berger M, Lefèbvre P. Physical activity, fitness and non-insulin dependent (type 2) diabetes mellitus. In: Bouchard C, Shephard RJ, Stephens T, eds. Physical Activity, Fitness and Health. Champaign, IL: Human Kinetics; 1994:669–683.
38. Shephard RJ, Rode A. The Health Consequence of "Modernization": Evidence from Circumpolar Peoples. London, UK: Cambridge University Press, 1996.
39. Manson JE, Nathan DM, Krolewski AS, Stampfer MJ, Willett WC, Hennekens CH. A prospective study of exercise and incidence of diabetes among US male physicians. JAMA 1992;268:63–67.
40. Leon AS. Exercise in the prevention and management of diabetes mellitus and blood lipid disorders. In: Shephard RJ, Miller HS, eds. Exercise and the Heart in Health and Disease. New York, NY: Marcel Dekker; 1999:355–422.
41. Shephard RJ. Physical Activity, Training, and the Immune Response. Carmel, IN: Cooper Publications; 1997.
42. Shephard RJ. Exercise, aging, and immune resistance to infections and neoplasms. In: Huber G, ed. Healthy Aging, Activity and Sports. Hamburg, Germany: Health Promotion Publications; 1997:174–180.
43. Shinkai S, Konishi M, Shephard RJ. Aging and immune response to exercise. Can J Physiol Pharmacol 1998;76:562–572.
44. Shephard RJ, Futcher R. Physical activity and cancer: how may protection be maximized? Crit Rev Oncogen 1997;8:219–272.
45. Shephard RJ, Shek PN. Associations between physical activity and susceptibility to cancer: possible mechanisms. Sports Med 1998;26:293–315.
46. Kujala UM, Kaprio J, Sarna S. Osteoarthritis of weight-bearing joints of lower limbs in former elite male athletes. Br Med J 1994;308:231–234.
47. Lane N, Micheli B, Bjorkengren A, et al. The risk of osteoarthritis with running and aging: a 5-year longitudinal study. J Rhemumatol 1993;20:461–468.
48. Minor MA, Hewett JE, Webel RR, Anderson SK, Kay DR. Efficacy of physical conditioning exercise in patients with rheumatoid arthritis and osteoarthritis. Arthritis Rheum 1989;32:1396–1405.
49. Shephard RJ, Corey P, Renzland P, Cox M. The influence of an industrial fitness programme upon medical care costs. Can J Public Health 1982;73:259–263.
50. Mathews AM. Contributors to the loss of independence and the promotion of independence among seniors. Ottawa, Ontario: Community Health Division, Health & Welfare, Canada; 1989.
51. Cress ME, Buchner DM, Questad KA, Esselman PC, deLateur BJ, Schwartz RS. Exercise: effects on physical functional performance in independent older adults. J Gerontol 1999;54:M242–M248.
52. Evans WJ. Exercise training guidelines for the elderly. Med Sci Sports Exerc 1999;31:12–17.
53. Feigenbaum MS, Pollock ML. Prescription of resistance training for health and disease. Med Sci Sports Exerc 1999;31:38–45.
54. American College of Sports Medicine. Exercise and physical activity for older adults. Med Sci Sports Exerc 1998;30:992–1008.

SUGGESTED READINGS

Fiatarone-Singh MA. Exercise, Nutrition and the Older Woman. Boca Raton, FL: CRC Publishing; 2000.
Harris S, Harris WS, Harris JO. Lifelong Health and Fitness. Albany, NY: Center for the Study of Aging; 2000.
Huber G. Healthy Aging, Activity and Sports. Hamburg, Germany: Health Promotion Publications; 1997.
Shephard RJ. Aging, Physical Activity and Health. Champaign, IL: Human Kinetics; 1997.
Spirduso WW. Physical Dimensions of Aging. Champaign, IL: Human Kinetics; 1995.

CHAPTER 35

Eye Diseases in the Elderly

David A. Lightman, Andrew Schachat

Overview

Many eye diseases can affect the ability or willingness to engage in recreational or rehabilitative exercise; conversely, exercise can influence the course and prognosis of some eye diseases. This chapter describes the **epidemiology, pathophysiology**, and treatments of the 4 most prevalent sight-threatening eye disorders in the elderly: **cataract, glaucoma, diabetic retinopathy**, and **age-related macular degeneration**. Cataract and glaucoma are rarely seen before adulthood, but they increase in prevalence with advancing age. Vision loss from diabetes is common at any age after puberty, and is the major cause of blindness between the ages of 20 and 74 (1). Age-related macular degeneration (ARMD) is primarily a disease of the elderly, and is rarely seen before age 50 (2). After age 65, ARMD is the leading cause of irreversible legal blindness in the United States and other developed countries (3).

It is often said that the eye is the window of the body, and a physician can glean much about a person's general health by peering inside the eye. Indeed, in no other organ can blood vessels and nerves be examined noninvasively with such ease. Of the 4 conditions discussed in this chapter, only diabetic retinopathy is highly correlated with a person's general health. The other 3 ocular diseases can occur in otherwise healthy individuals. However, all of these conditions can cause visual impairment and affect well-being and ability to participate in exercise.

Basic Anatomy and Physiology of the Eye

The eye functions much like a camera (Figure 35.1). A powerful lens system is needed to focus light from the front of the eye to the back, a distance of merely 1 inch. Most of this refracting power comes from the spherical surface of the **cornea**. The remainder of the power is provided by the **crystalline lens**. The lens also has the remarkable capacity to change shape and focus at various distances (**accommodate**). It is suspended behind the iris by threadlike fibers called **zonules** that attach to the muscular **ciliary body**. When the eye focuses on something close, the ciliary body contracts and reduces zonular tension on the equator of the lens. The lens becomes more spherical and thereby stronger in power. With age, the lens becomes more rigid and eventually loses its facility to change shape, hence the need for reading glasses or bifocals.

The **pupil** is a hole in the muscular colored iris. It changes size in various lighting conditions (much like a camera f-stop) to regulate the amount of light reaching the **retina**, the "film" of the eye. In bright light, the pupil gets smaller, and in dim illumination it dilates.

The retina is a thin, transparent tissue that blankets the back of the eye. Its inner half (toward the **vitreous**) is nourished by the intrinsic retinal blood vessels. The outer half

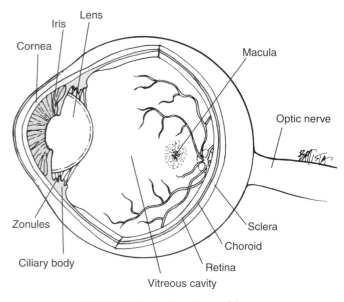

FIGURE 35.1. Basic anatomy of the eye.

(toward the **sclera**) contains the light-sensitive **photoreceptors** (rods and cones) and is nourished by the underlying richly vascular **choriocapillaris** of the **choroid**. The retina is separated from the choriocapillaris by a sheetlike condensation of collagen (**Bruch's membrane**) and a monolayer of hexagonal cells called the **retinal pigment epithelium** (**RPE**). The RPE is vitally important for the health and function of the retina because it facilitates the transport of metabolic supplies and wastes between the retina and choroid. The rods and cones are loosely apposed to the RPE, and contain the photoreactive chemicals that trigger the neural chain reaction resulting in vision.

The **macula** is the central portion of the retina with the highest density of photoreceptors (Figures 35.1, 35.2). It enables detailed visual discrimination for tasks like reading, driving, recognizing faces, and distinguishing colors. The

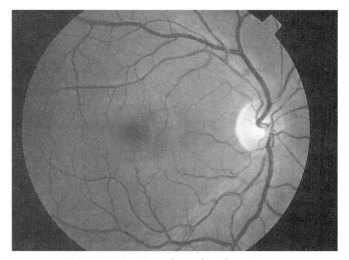

FIGURE 35.2. Normal macula and optic nerve.

retina outside the macula provides peripheral vision for detecting gross movements and shapes. The "image" from the retina is transmitted by the optic nerve through complex neural pathways to the back of the brain (occipital cortex) where vision is perceived.

Within the eye are 2 compartments, each filled with a unique fluid (or humor). The large vitreous cavity contains **vitreous humor**, a clear gelatinous substance that remains essentially constant throughout life. It is not produced after birth and never leaves the eye. However, it does liquefy with age and in later life separates from the retinal surface, occasionally leading to retinal tears and detachments. The **aqueous humor** that fills the small chamber between the cornea and the iris (**anterior chamber**), on the other hand, is in a constant state of turnover. This clear, watery fluid is continuously produced by the ciliary body throughout life. It bathes and nourishes the **avascular** structures in the front of the eye, notably the lens and cornea. The aqueous fluid constantly drains from the eye through the **trabecular meshwork** located in the "angle" between the iris and cornea. The equilibrium between the rate of aqueous production and the ease of aqueous drainage determines the **intraocular pressure (IOP)**. If outflow is impaired, the pressure will build up and damage the optic nerve, a disease known as glaucoma. In contrast, aqueous production can decline in some very diseased eyes, leading to low pressure, a shrunken eye, and poor vision.

The tough white outer wall of the eye is called the **sclera**, and serves as a protective vessel for the delicate intraocular structures. The eye is further protected by the lids and by its recessed location within the bony orbit of the skull. Six different muscles attach to the sclera for precise movement of the eyeball.

Cataract

Epidemiology and Risk Factors

Cataract is an opacification of the normal crystalline lens (Figure 35.3). It is the leading cause of blindness and impaired vision worldwide, accounting for approximately half the cases of blindness in the world. An estimated 25 million people worldwide are bilaterally blind (<20/400) from cataract and an estimated 110 million are severely visually impaired (<20/200) (4). Coupled with a growing global population and increasing median age, those numbers are expected to double by the year 2020 (4). Approximately 95% of individuals over age 60 have some degree of lens opacification, but most often these opacities are not visually significant. By age 75, diminished vision from cataract reaches nearly 50% of the population (5). Most often cataracts occur in both eyes, with variable rates of progression from eye to eye and individual to individual. In the United States, more than 2 million cataract procedures are performed annually; it is the most common surgical procedure among Americans age 65 and older (6, 7).

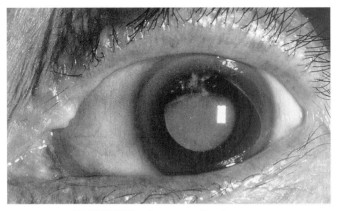

FIGURE 35.3. Dense age-related cataract.

Cataract has several causes (Box 35.1), but aging is by far the most common. Direct ocular trauma can cause immediate lens opacification; however, most cataracts grow slowly, taking years to develop. Nontraumatic cataracts are secondary to biochemical changes in the lens fibers that cause accumulation of large molecules, disruption of normal architecture, and loss of transparency.

Some risk factors for cataract formation are potentially modifiable. Smoking and exposure to ultraviolet light are established risk factors for cataract; however, the role of alcohol consumption remains controversial (8, 9). There are no proven medications or nutritional supplements to retard the progression of cataract. Some studies have suggested a beneficial role for antioxidant vitamins to prevent age-related cataract (10, 11). However, the Age-Related Eye Disease Study (AREDS) demonstrated no treatment benefit for patients taking antioxidant vitamins (vitamin C 500 mg, vitamin E 400 IU, and beta carotene 15 mg). In this double-blind, prospective clinical trial, more than 4,000 participants were randomized to either antioxidant therapy or placebo. At the end of 7 years, no statistically significant difference was seen between the 2 groups with respect to cataract progression (12).

BOX 35.1. Causes of Cataract

Congenital
1. Autosomal-dominant inheritance
2. Maternal infections, diseases, or medications
3. Prematurity

Traumatic

Senescent (aging)

Secondary
1. Drug therapy (e.g., corticosteroids)
2. Other eye diseases (e.g., retinitis pigmentosa, **uveitis**)
3. Metabolic diseases (e.g., diabetes mellitus)
4. Previous eye surgery (especially vitrectomy)

Treatment

The remarkable improvements in microsurgical techniques, instrumentation, and implant design have contributed to this procedure's excellent success rate and worldwide growth. Cataract surgery has evolved considerably over the millennia (13). It is thought that the first cataract procedures were performed more than 2,000 years ago in India before Hippocrates' time. Cataracts were "couched" or dislocated into the vitreous cavity with a sharp instrument. This technique was successful in clearing the visual axis and improving vision, but often resulted in late blinding complications. In the West, progress of cataract surgery may have been delayed by Aristotelian dogma that held sway for 1,500 years. The physiologic role of the lens and the anatomic location of cataract were poorly understood. According to Aristotle, the crystalline lens was the primary organ of vision. Johannes Kepler (1571–1630) determined by simple experiments and calculation that the retina was the sensory organ of vision and the lens a refracting body. In 1705 the French physician Pierre Brisseau recognized the lens as the anatomic site of a cataract. Modern cataract surgery with extraction of the opaque lens from the eye began with the French surgeon Jacques Daviel in 1750. However, it took more than a century for cataract extraction to replace couching as the method of choice.

Cataract surgery has improved dramatically over the past 150 years. Possibly the greatest contribution in the field of cataract surgery (and perhaps ophthalmology in general) came from Harold Ridley, a British ophthalmologist who was knighted in 2000 for his achievement (14). Shortly after World War II, Ridley noted that some injured RAF pilots tolerated intraocular fragments of Plexiglas (polymethylmethacrylate, PMMA) from their shattered cockpit canopies. He devised an **intraocular lens** from this material and performed the first implant in 1949 (15). Surgical implantation of intraocular lenses has been of immeasurable benefit to cataract patients, freeing them from contact lenses or the disturbing optical aberrations of thick cataract glasses. Intraocular lens design has evolved considerably over the past several decades to make them safer and better tolerated.

The second great technical advance in cataract surgery came from Charles Kelman in 1967 (7). He devised an ingenious **phakoemulsification** apparatus that uses ultrasound energy to break up and liquefy the cataract so that it can be suctioned from the eye through a small incision (Figure 35.4). Intraocular lenses are now made of pliable materials (e.g., acrylic or silicone). These lenses can be folded and inserted through a self-sealing corneal wound less than 3 mm long. Cataract surgery today is often performed without stitches under topical anesthesia (numbing drops). Patients can return to normal activity with good visual recovery within days or even hours of surgery. In contrast, only a few decades ago, large cataract wounds were

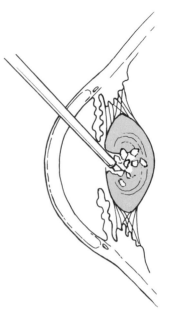

FIGURE 35.4.   Phakoemulsification.

closed with big stitches and patients' heads were immobilized with sandbags for days or weeks.

Cataract surgery is one of the most successful procedures performed in medicine today. It promises to enjoy continued improvement with the development of new instrumentation and techniques. Laser phakoemulsification (6) and a high-speed intraocular rotor are 2 such devices under investigation (7). There are hopes of implanting lenses that have the capacity to change shape and restore our ability to accommodate (6). Because of good access to medical care in the United States, there is little reason why anyone should be blind from cataract in this country. With modern techniques in cataract surgery, most people are able to resume unrestricted activity, including strenuous exercise, shortly after their surgery.

Exercise and Cataract

As noted earlier, trauma to the eye is one of the causes of cataract. These ocular injuries often occur in sports with high-speed balls or pucks (baseball, tennis, racquet ball, squash, hockey). Most of these injuries can be avoided with appropriate protective eyewear (Box 35.2). With modern small-incision cataract surgery, exercise may be resumed within days or weeks of surgery; however, patients should take special care to avoid direct eye trauma because the cataract wound takes months to heal completely.

Many sports, particularly high-speed racquet sports, require good depth perception for optimal performance. Patients with reduced vision in one or both eyes from cataract (or any other eye disease) will lose the ability for fine spatial discrimination. This may affect athletic performance, and should be considered when planning an exercise program.

Eye trauma during sports activities is a tragic and preventable cause of vision loss. It primarily affects young people, but can occur at any age. Of the 2.4 million eye injuries that occur annually in the United States, 100,000 are sports-related and severe enough to warrant a visit to a doctor or emergency room. High-risk sports involve one or more of the following:

1. A stick or a racquet (hockey, lacrosse, racquet sports)

2. High-speed balls or pucks (baseball, racquet sports, soccer, hockey)

3. Aggressive physical contact (basketball, football, wrestling)

Sports-related eye injuries could be virtually eliminated with proper use of sport-specific protective devices (e.g., full-face protectors or **polycarbonate** goggles). Some protective goggles can be made with prescription lenses.

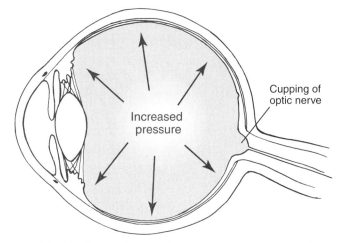

FIGURE 35.5. Increased intraocular pressure causes optic nerve damage (cupping).

Stereopsis is the remarkable ability to perceive 3-dimensionality. Fine spatial discrimination is possible in large part because our 2 eyes are horizontally separated, and each eye has a slightly different view of our surroundings. Our brain can fuse these 2 slightly disparate images to create a 3-dimensional picture. Many other animals, including all primates, also possess this specialized form of vision. To achieve optimum stereopsis, our 2 eyes must have excellent vision and be perfectly aligned. Any eye disease that causes ocular misalignment or reduced vision will degrade our ability to perceive depth. Because we also can use several monocular clues to gauge depth, stereopsis is helpful but not essential for most sports.

Glaucoma

Glaucoma is a major cause of visual impairment in the United States and worldwide. The hallmark of this disease is elevated **intraocular pressure** (IOP) that is of sufficient magnitude and duration to damage the optic nerve. The nerve enters the back of the eye and conjoins with the retina at the **optic disc** (see Figure 35.1). If the pressure is too high for too long, the optic nerve loses tissue, with concomitant loss of the field of vision. These "cupping" changes in the optic nerve can be detected visibly and monitored by an eye doctor (Figure 35.5). Pressure damage to the optic nerve initially causes loss of peripheral vision. If the disease is undetected or inadequately treated, it can eventually lead to loss of central vision and complete blindness.

Types

The many types of glaucoma can be broadly divided between primary and secondary. In **primary glaucoma**, the disease is strictly the result of ocular anatomic and physiologic factors. **Secondary glaucoma** is the result of other ocular or nonocular diseases that secondarily cause high pressure.

Primary open-angle glaucoma is by far the most common form in the United States. In this type of glaucoma, the drainage structure angle is anatomically "open," but there is abnormal resistance to aqueous outflow through the trabecular meshwork (Figure 35.6A). The degree of resistance roughly correlates with the increase of intraocular pressure. The prevalence of open-angle glaucoma increases after age 40, and approaches 3% of individuals over age 75. Men and woman are affected equally among blacks and whites, but blacks acquire the disease with greater frequency and earlier in life than whites. In fact, open-angle glaucoma is the leading cause of blindness in African Americans. The disease is familial, but the precise mode of inheritance is unknown. Other controversial risk factors for developing open-angle glaucoma include hypertension, diabetes, and myopia (nearsightedness) (16).

The second major category of primary glaucoma is angle-closure glaucoma. This is typically a crowding phenomenon of the front of the eye where the drainage angle is anatomically too narrow (Figure 35.6B). If the angle closes off, there can be a sudden, severe, and painful buildup of intraocular pressure. Without prompt treatment this condition can lead to blindness. The prevalence of acute angle-closure glaucoma increases with age and is more common in women than men. It also occurs more commonly in some ethnic groups, such as Eskimos (17).

Both open-angle and angle-closure glaucoma can occur secondary to other eye diseases or ocular insults. For example, the use of steroid-containing eye drops can cause the eye pressure to increase in some susceptible individuals. Severe blunt trauma to the eye can also lead to glaucoma months or years after the injury. Some diseases (e.g., diabetes or retinal vascular occlusion) can cause diminished blood flow to the retina. The eye may respond with formation of abnormal blood vessels on the iris that can obstruct

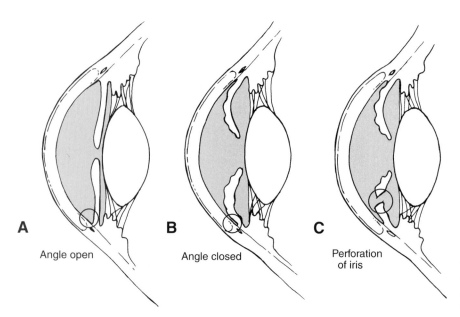

A Angle open   B Angle closed   C Perforation of iris

FIGURE 35.6. (A) Increased resistance to outflow in open-angle glaucoma. (B) Narrow-angle blocks outflow of aqueous. (C) Surgical hole in peripheral iris deepens angle and permits aqueous outflow.

or obliterate the normal drainage angle (**neovascular glaucoma**) (Figure 35.7). The intraocular pressure can mount to a painful level and be quite difficult to control.

Treatment

The principal goal of glaucoma treatment is to reduce the intraocular pressure enough to avoid optic nerve damage. Open-angle glaucoma is insidious in onset with no symptoms, not even pain or subjective visual disturbance. This is one reason why eye doctors recommend annual examinations in people over age 40. There is no absolute threshold for abnormal pressure, and every eye seems to have a unique susceptibility or resistance to pressure damage. Most normal people have eye pressures in the range of 10 to 20 mm Hg. If potentially damaging intraocular pressure is detected, there is a customary hierarchy of treatment options.

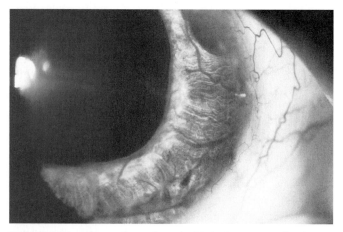

FIGURE 35.7. Abnormal vessels on the iris lead to neovascular glaucoma.

Most physicians in the United States first use one or more classes of glaucoma drops. Eye drops are absorbed into the bloodstream through the nasal **mucosa** and can have systemic side effects. Some of these theoretically could affect the ability to engage in exercise. For example, beta-blockers can cause asthma, low blood pressure, heart failure, and fatigue. Some adrenergic agents can cause high blood pressure, rapid heart rate, and abnormal heart rhythm.

If the pressure does not respond adequately to drops, laser treatment of the trabecular meshwork can often help lower the eye pressure. If the pressure is still too high, then a surgical procedure is performed to create an alternate outlet for aqueous drainage.

Primary angle-closure glaucoma has a relatively straightforward and anatomically elegant cure. A hole placed in the peripheral iris with laser or surgery will permit aqueous to flow from the ciliary body where it is secreted into the anterior chamber (see Figure 35.6C). The closed angle reopens and aqueous drainage resumes. If the trabecular meshwork is not permanently damaged, the pressure will promptly return to normal.

Secondary glaucoma treatment is first directed at treating the underlying condition. For example, steroids are used to suppress ocular inflammation in **uveitic** (inflammatory) glaucoma. **Panretinal photocoagulation** (**PRP**) with laser is used to treat neovascular glaucoma secondary to diabetes or vascular occlusion (see Diabetes section). The high pressure is concomitantly treated with the usual glaucoma medications. Severe cases may require surgical implantation of an artificial shunt for aqueous drainage.

Exercise and Glaucoma

In general, other than medical treatment, people can do little to modify their intraocular pressure. Intraocular pressure appears to be genetically determined as is, for example, the color of one's iris. However, lifestyle factors can influence the intraocular pressure somewhat. Caffeine may transiently lower the pressure 1 to 2 mm Hg, whereas cigarette smoking may increase it. Some drugs (alcohol, marijuana) lower the intraocular pressure. Chronic use of corticosteroids in any form (topical, oral, or inhaled) may cause a significant rise in intraocular pressure in some individuals, especially those with chronic open-angle glaucoma or a family history of this disease. Some systemic diseases are risk factors for the development of open-angle glaucoma including obesity, hypertension, and diabetes (18).

Exercise may play a useful adjunctive role in the management of glaucoma. Depending on the type of exercise, physical exertion may increase or lower the intraocular pressure. Several studies have demonstrated the pressure-lowering effect of exercise (19–24). This effect occurs despite differences in age, physical condition, blood pressure, initial IOP, or the presence of glaucoma (22). Pressure reduction with exercise can also be observed in many elderly patients (25). Harris has shown that acute dynamic exercise lowers IOP in a graded fashion proportional to exercise intensity (23). In glaucoma patients, the pressure can decline 7 to 13 mm Hg after intense aerobic exercise (18).

The physiologic mechanism of exercise-induced pressure reduction is unknown, but may be related to **hypocapnia**, increased blood lactate, or changes in **plasma osmolarity** (19, 23, 24). Other investigators have suggested that exercise increases **plasma colloid osmotic pressure**, resulting in ocular dehydration and pressure reduction (26). Hormonal factors released during exercise (e.g., vasopressin and epinephrine) that affect aqueous production might also play a role in pressure reduction (19). **Isokinetic** exercise is more effective in lowering intraocular pressure than **isotonic** exercise, given the same intensity and total energy consumption. The reason for this discrepancy may be due to the greater number of muscle fibers recruited during isokinetic exercise (27). There does not appear to be a significant difference in pressure lowering between aerobic and anaerobic exercise (19).

The acute pressure-lowering effect of exercise is transient, and the eye pressure returns to baseline in about 40 minutes (18, 24). However, Passo has demonstrated a long-term ocular hypotensive effect of exercise when physical fitness is maintained (21). In a group of glaucoma suspects, the resting intraocular pressure declined an average of 4.6 mm Hg within 3 months of exercise training, and the benefit persisted for 3 years. Once a person returned to a sedentary lifestyle, the eye pressure increased to baseline within 3 weeks (20).

Some exercise conditions can actually raise the intraocular pressure. **Isotonic** exertion with a **Valsalva maneuver** may acutely raise the pressure by 5 mm Hg. Total body inversion to a head-down position may increase the pressure 11 to 16 mm Hg above baseline in normal or glaucomatous individuals (18). Pigmentary glaucoma is an uncommon

form of glaucoma caused by pigment granules flaking off the back of the iris and clogging up the trabecular meshwork. Some exercises (e.g., jogging) may accelerate the dispersement of pigment and cause an acute increase in intraocular pressure. These patients should have their pressures checked before and after their routine exercise regimen to ensure they are not causing a dangerous increase in intraocular pressure (28).

Diabetic Retinopathy

Pathophysiology

Diabetes is a multifactorial disease that shares a common endpoint of altered glucose metabolism. Microvascular end-organ complications of diabetes include blinding retinal disease (**retinopathy**), end-stage **renal** disease, and lower extremity amputations. The mechanism by which **hyperglycemia** causes damage to various organs throughout the body (including the eye) is complex. The disease damages the small blood vessels in the retina with **microaneurysm** formation, damage or destruction of the capillary bed, and increased vascular permeability resulting in leakage. Microscopic examination of retinal tissue demonstrates selective loss of the capillary **pericytes** and thickening of the capillary **endothelial cell** basement membrane. The microaneurysms and damaged capillaries can leak blood components into the retina, resulting in **edema**. When blood, lipid, or fluid involves the center of the macula, visual acuity is impaired (Figure 35.8). Macular edema is the most common cause of visual impairment in diabetic patients and is the second most common cause of severe visual loss (29).

Diabetic retinal disease progresses from **background** or **nonproliferative diabetic retinopathy** to **proliferative di-**

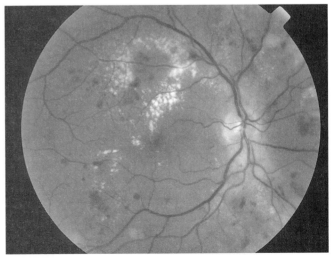

FIGURE 35.8. Diabetic macular edema with blood, lipid, and fluid in the macula.

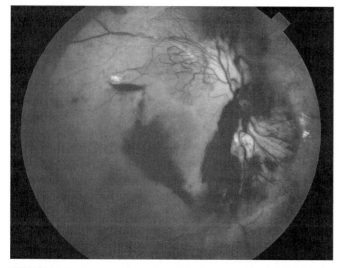

FIGURE 35.9. Neovascularization of the disc and retina with vitreous hemorrhage.

abetic retinopathy (PDR) as more and more capillaries and arterioles become occluded. The retina responds to this **ischemic** insult by producing abnormal (neovascular) blood vessels that sprout from the optic nerve or retinal surface like weeds, using the vitreous as scaffolding. These new vessels provide no nutritional or metabolic support for the retina. They are typically quite fragile and can bleed into the eye as it moves and the swirling vitreous humor tugs on the vessels (Figure 35.9). Severe vision loss may occur if the vitreous becomes clouded with blood. Sometimes the abnormal vessels develop associated contractile scar tissue that can distort or detach the retina, including the macula (Figure 35.10). In some severely ischemic eyes, abnormal blood vessels can even grow on the iris surface (see Figure 35.7). The neovascular tissue may obliterate the aqueous drainage structure, resulting in painful and potentially blinding neovascular glaucoma.

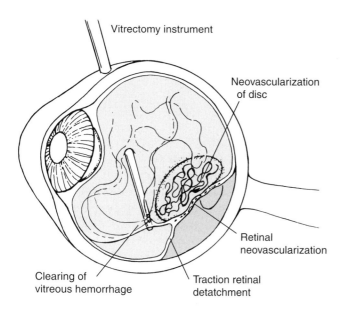

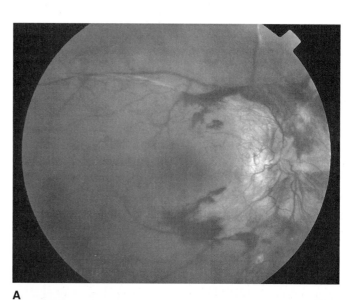

A

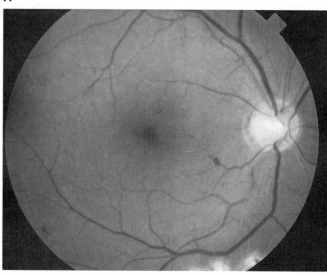

B

FIGURE 35.10.   Neovascularization of the optic nerve and retina cause vitreous hemorrhage and traction retinal detachment.

Epidemiology

The prevalence of diabetes is increasing in the United States and worldwide. In 1998 there were an estimated 10.5 million people in the United States with diabetes, compared to 1.5 million in 1958 (1). The rising prevalence may be partially due to better diabetic treatment and greater longevity of diabetic patients. However, socioeconomic and lifestyle factors, including diet and obesity, may also play a role in the epidemic of this disease. Men and women are affected equally, but there is a disproportionate prevalence among minority populations, including African Americans, Native Americans, and Mexican Americans. Type 1 diabetes represents approximately 10% of the cases. It occurs before age 30, often in early childhood, and requires insulin for control. An autoimmune process selectively destroys the insulin-producing beta cells of the pancreas. There is genetic susceptibility to this disease that appears to be triggered by environmental factors (e.g., viruses) (30, 31). Type 2 diabetes typically occurs in obese people who are often asymptomatic at the time of diagnosis. Type 2 patients can still secrete insulin, but it is less effective in regulating glucose metabolism at the cellular level in the liver and peripheral tissues. A third type of diabetes is secondary to other conditions, such as pancreatitis, pregnancy, hormonal disorders, and various drugs.

Diabetes is the most common cause of blindness in the United States in persons between ages 20 and 74 (1). According to the Wisconsin Epidemiologic Study of Diabetic Retinopathy (WESDR), 80% of patients with type 2 diabetes will develop retinopathy within 20 years, and 20% will have proliferative disease. Virtually all patients with type 1 diabetes will develop retinopathy, and 60% will have proliferative disease within 20 years of diagnosis (1).

Treatment

The treatment of diabetic retinopathy has evolved considerably over the past several decades with the development of laser and vitreous surgery. Blindness from diabetes can be largely prevented today with appropriate patient education; compulsive blood sugar, lipid, and pressure control; and timely laser and surgical intervention.

The Diabetic Control and Complications Trial (DCCT) definitively demonstrated that patients who maintain tight control of their diabetes have fewer retinal and renal complications compared to their more loosely controlled cohorts. Peripheral neuropathy is less common as well in patients with excellent control (32, 33). Tight control of diabetes can often be achieved with home blood glucose monitoring and multiple daily insulin injections. An insulin pump is also effective in maintaining more rigorous blood sugar control. Pancreas transplants or islet cell transplants (often in conjunction with kidney transplants) in people with type 1 diabetes are becoming more widespread (34,

35). Transplanted pancreas or islet cells can normalize blood sugar and eliminate the need for exogenous insulin.

Tight blood pressure control is also important in reducing microvascular and macrovascular complications of diabetes, including diabetic retinopathy and vision loss (36). Elevated serum lipid levels are associated with increased risk of visual impairment in patients with diabetes. Lipid lowering may be beneficial for vision as well as for cardiovascular health (37).

When patients develop vision-threatening macular leakage, laser **photocoagulation** of the leaky retinal microvasculature can reduce retinal thickening (edema) and improve vision. With timely and appropriate macular laser treatment, the frequency and severity of vision loss from diabetic macular edema can be minimized. Laser-treated patients with diabetic macular edema had less than half the risk of vision loss compared to a matched observation group (38, 39).

Laser photocoagulation is also the mainstay of treatment for proliferative diabetic retinopathy (PDR). Once neovascularization reaches a threshold level, panretinal photocoagulation is performed with laser burns scattered outside the macula. For poorly understood reasons, the laser burns cause the neovascular tissue to regress and, in some cases, disappear altogether (Figure 35.11). With timely and appropriate laser treatment, the risk of severe visual loss from complications of proliferative diabetic retinopathy is reduced 50% to 60% (40).

Even with early detection and timely laser treatment, many diabetic patients develop severe vitreous hemorrhage or traction retinal detachment, the first and third most common causes, respectively, of severe vision loss in diabetic patients (29). Vitreous surgery with modern instrumentation has been a boon to these patients, enabling many to regain their vision. Using microsurgical instrumentation, the vitreoretinal surgeon can now safely remove the hemorrhagic vitreous and dissect the fibrovascular membranes from the retinal surface (Figures 35.10, 35.12). The Diabetic Vitrectomy Study showed that early vitrectomy surgery for vitreous hemorrhage is helpful in restoring and preserving good vision, particularly in people with type 1 diabetes (41).

Exercise and Diabetic Retinopathy

Because of the propensity for retinal or vitreous hemorrhage, diabetic patients or their health care workers often raise the following questions: Is it safe to take aspirin or other medication that impairs clotting? Is it safe to engage in vigorous exercise?

It has been shown that treatment with aspirin does not significantly increase the risk of hemorrhagic complications or vision loss compared to **placebo**. There is no reason for diabetic patients not to take aspirin (650 mg/day) if needed for cardiovascular or other medical conditions (42, 43).

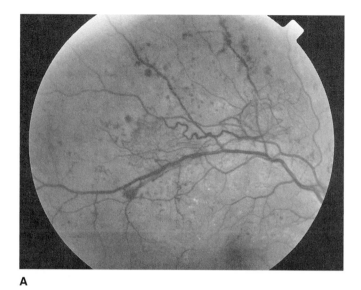

A

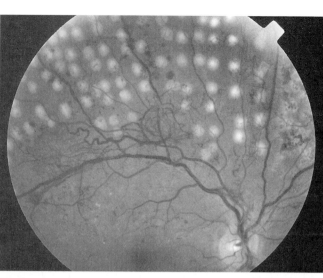

B

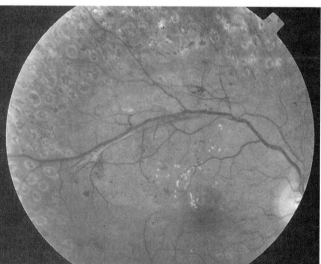

C

FIGURE 35.11. (A) Diabetic neovascularization of the retina. (B) Immediately after panretinal photocoagulation. (C) Regression of neovascular tissue 5 months after laser treatment.

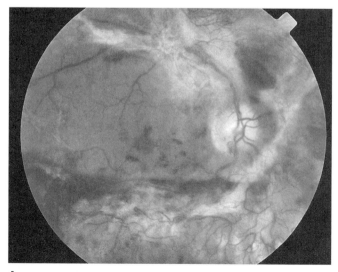

A

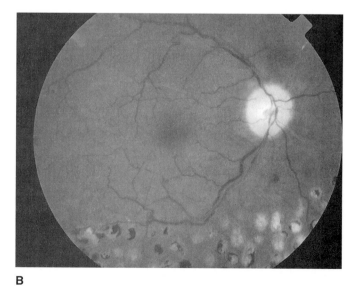

B

FIGURE 35.12. (A) Severe diabetic retinal neovascularization before vitreoretinal surgery. (B) Same eye after surgical removal of blood and scar tissue.

Prospective data analysis in the Wisconsin Epidemiologic Study of Diabetic Retinopathy showed no increased risk of retinopathy progression in type 1 diabetics engaging in regular physical activity (44). Another study suggests higher levels of physical activity may reduce the risk of proliferative diabetic retinopathy (PDR) in women (45). Physical activity may reduce the risk of PDR by its beneficial lowering effect on blood pressure and serum cholesterol (45).

Strenuous activities like coughing, lifting, straining at stool, or vomiting can cause vitreous and retinal hemorrhages, particularly in diabetic patients (46). However, Anderson studied a consecutive group of 72 diabetic patients presenting with vitreous hemorrhage and found that sleep was the most common associated activity (36%), followed closely by sitting or lying down (26%). Only 16% of the hemorrhages were associated with strenuous activity (47).

Hemorrhagic complications of proliferative diabetic retinopathy can now be routinely and safely managed with vitrectomy surgery. Because of the known beneficial effects of exercise, including reduced cardiovascular disease and early mortality as well as improved self-esteem, it is reasonable to advise diabetic patients to exercise regardless of the stage of retinal disease. However, it is imperative that a diabetic patient be under the care of an eye doctor and general physician before initiating an exercise program (Box 35.35).

Age-Related Macular Degeneration

Epidemiology and Risk Factors

Age-related macular degeneration (ARMD) is a chronic degenerative and **dystrophic** disease primarily affecting the choriocapillaris, Bruch's membrane, and the retinal pigment epithelium. Metabolic or neovascular changes within these structures secondarily damage the overlying macula and commonly cause visual impairment or blindness in the elderly. Approximately 200,000 Americans lose vision in an eye annually from this disease. It is the leading cause of irreversible legal blindness in people 65 years and older in the United States. This is the fastest growing segment of the U.S. population, and is expected to continue its rapid expansion, as baby boomers become senior citizens. Between the years 2000 and 2020, the number of persons in the United States age 65 and older is expected to grow from 35 to 53 million, a 53% increase. This age group will constitute 16.5% of the entire U.S. population (48). In the Beaver Dam, Wisconsin study, ARMD was found in 1.37% of people age 65 to 74. The prevalence increases with age, rising to nearly 7% in those 75 to 84 years old, and 14% in those older than 85. Similar prevalence rates are reported in other developed nations (49). Given the high prevalence rate of this visually devastating disorder, ARMD is a major public health concern.

Age-related macular degeneration appears to be a genetically inherited disease, with, perhaps, some modulating environmental factors. The condition is most commonly found in white individuals and vision loss is rarely seen in blacks. It tends to cluster in families. Several nongenetic risk factors have been implicated in the pathogenesis of this disease. Some have suggested dietary changes are responsible for the recent rise of ARMD in Japan and Great Britain (50–52). However, the increased prevalence may be simply the result of changing demographics and an aging population (51, 52). Many risk factors have been investigated with inconclusive results, including sedentary lifestyle, obesity, excessive alcohol, farsightedness, iris color, cardiovascular disease, high cholesterol levels, previous lung infection, and ultraviolet light (5, 48–50, 53–59). The risk of macular degeneration may increase with systemic hypertension (48, 60), but not all studies confirm this association (49).

Smoking appears to be the most important, consistent, and potentially modifiable risk factor for ARMD. There is ample epidemiological data demonstrating an association between cigarette smoking and visual loss from ARMD in both men and women (48, 49, 57–59, 61). The risk of vision loss increases with quantity and duration of smoking. Smokers have approximately 2.5 times the risk of vision loss from neovascular ARMD compared to nonsmokers. Furthermore, this risk persists after smoking cessation for 15 or more years (57).

Etiology and Clinical Features

The propensity of the disease to affect the central retina (macula) of older individuals provides the basis for its descriptive name. The hallmark of ARMD is the accumulation of metabolic degenerative debris (**drusen**) under the retinal pigment epithelium. They typically appear in the macular region and look like little yellow spots (Figure 35.13). Most people over age 50 have a few drusen (62), and there is no consensus on how many drusen are required to make a diagnosis of ARMD. Drusen alone cause little or no vision

---

BOX 35.3. Common-Sense Rules for Exercise in Diabetic Patients

1. The first rule of exercise prescription is that the benefits must outweigh the risks.

2. Patients with diabetic complications should undergo a thorough physical and eye examination prior to beginning an exercise program.

3. A program of daily, moderate aerobic exercise helps to maintain or improve cardiovascular functioning while improving insulin sensitivity and blood sugar control, which may be beneficial for diabetic retinopathy.

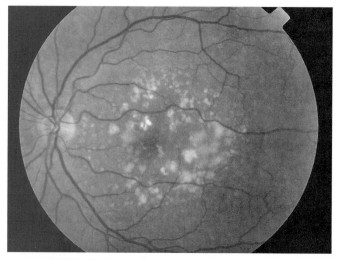

FIGURE 35.13.   Dry macular degeneration with drusen

tive cracks in the thin barrier (Bruch's membrane) between the retina and choroid. These abnormal vessels leak fluid, blood, or lipid under the retina, blurring or distorting central vision (Figure 35.14). They are most easily identified with a photographic technique called fluorescein angiography. An inert dye (fluorescein) is injected into an arm vein, and travels through the bloodstream to the eye. With a special camera and filters, the abnormal vessels "light up" (fluoresce) under the RPE and retina (Figure 35.15). Without treatment, the abnormal vessels often slowly evolve into scars (Figure 35.16). The photoreceptors over these scars eventually degenerate, leaving a blind spot in the central vision. Peripheral vision is spared in all but the most advanced cases. We can safely tell most patients they will never go completely blind from this disorder.

loss. The presence of drusen or pigmentary changes in the macula without leakage is termed "dry" ARMD. It accounts for 90% of the cases but only about 10% of severe visual loss from this disease. Unfortunately, about 10% of patients with ARMD develop the "wet" variety, usually with devastating visual consequences. Indeed, wet or exudative macular degeneration accounts for 90% of the cases of severe visual loss in this disease.

In wet macular degeneration, abnormal blood vessels from the choroid insinuate themselves through degenera-

Treatment

The plethora of treatments offered for ARMD over the years attests to the public health importance of this disease, the disappointing results of therapy, and the desperation of physicians and patients. There has been a huge interest in dietary supplements to prevent macular degeneration. Because of the association of white race, light iris color, and cigarette smoking, photo-oxidative stress may play a role in this disease. Some studies have suggested that antioxidant nutrients, like lutein and zeax-

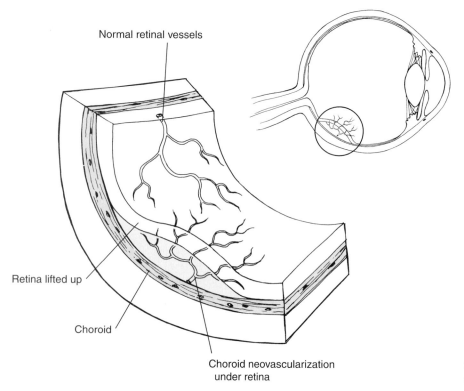

Normal retinal vessels

Retina lifted up

Choroid

Choroid neovascularization under retina

FIGURE 35.14.   Wet macular degeneration with abnormal vessels leaking under the retina.

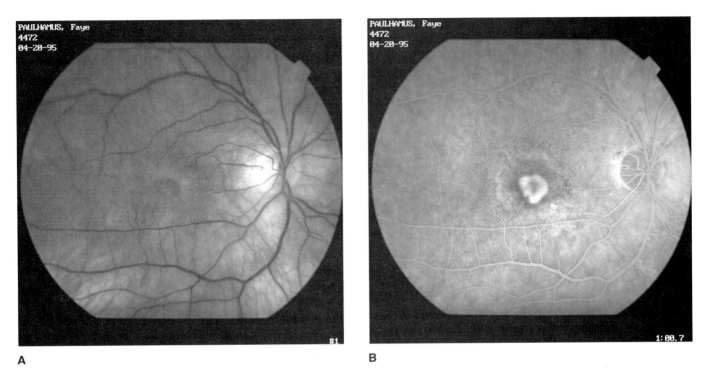

A   **B**

FIGURE 35.15.   (A) Neovascular membrane under the central macula before fluorescein injection. (B) Neovascular membrane enhanced by fluorescein.

anthin, reduce the risk of exudative ARMD (63), but this association was not supported in the Beaver Dam Eye Study (64). Zinc, a metallic cofactor for 2 antioxidant enzymes, is normally found in high concentrations in the retina. Investigations of the protective role of supplementary dietary zinc have been conflicting and inconclusive (53, 65–67). However, the Age-Related Eye Disease Study (AREDS) has provided credible evidence in a randomized, placebo-controlled, prospective trial that antioxidant vitamins and zinc reduce the risk of disease progression and visual loss in patients with ARMD. Those patients taking

daily vitamin C 500 mg, vitamin E 400 IU, and beta carotene 15 mg had 17% less risk of disease progression compared to placebo after 5 years. The group taking zinc 80 mg alone did even better, with a 21% risk reduction. The group taking vitamins plus zinc on a daily basis fared the best, with a 25% reduction in ARMD progression. This group also had 27% less visual loss compared to placebo after 5 years of treatment (68).

Alfa-interferon injections have been investigated with disappointing results (69). Low-dose radiation for neovascular complications of ARMD has been studied for years by numerous centers, with conflicting and inconclusive results. The National Eye Institute is launching a new study using a slightly higher dose of radiation (70). Filtration of the blood (much like hemodialysis) is a controversial treatment for macular degeneration practiced for years in Europe and the United States. So-called **rheotherapy** has limited medical justification for its popularity, but it is now being investigated by more rigorous, scientific methodology.

Some extraordinary surgical procedures are now being performed for neovascular ARMD. In one procedure, a small hole is made in the retina and the neovascular tissue is carefully extracted from the subretinal space. In another procedure, the retina is intentionally detached and then reattached so the macula overlies healthier tissue. These procedures have their advocates and successes, but they are expensive, labor intensive, and not without risk. The future role of surgery in the management of neovascular ARMD is undetermined.

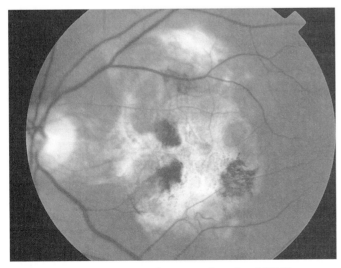

FIGURE 35.16.   Macular scarring from "wet" ARMD.

The first scientifically proven treatment for exudative macular degeneration is laser photocoagulation. In the 1980s and early 1990s a landmark series of randomized prospective clinical studies were performed by the Macular Photocoagulation Study (MPS) to determine if laser treatment to the abnormal subretinal vessels could improve the devastating natural history of this disease (71, 72). The MPS found that treatment was, indeed, beneficial in reducing the risk of severe visual loss even when the vessels were under the center of the macula. This was a major breakthrough in the treatment of macular degeneration, but by no means a cure. The treatment has 3 limitations: (1) Laser photocoagulation not only obliterates the abnormal vessels under the retina, but destroys the overlying retina as well. Wherever there is a laser burn, there is a blind spot in the field of vision. (2) The MPS treatment parameters only apply to about 15% of all cases of neovascular AMD that meet the study entry criteria. (3) Even with initially successful treatment, there is a 50% risk that the abnormal vessels will start growing and leaking again. Despite these limitations, laser photocoagulation remains prominent in treatment of neovascular ARMD.

Photodynamic therapy is a new and exciting treatment for neovascular ARMD. A **photosensitizing** drug (verteporfin) is infused into the bloodstream where it is preferentially absorbed by the neovascular tissue under the retina and RPE. The drug is exquisitely sensitive to a unique wavelength of light (689 nm), and the abnormal vessels can be obliterated with a low-energy laser that does not damage the overlying retina. In a specific subgroup of patients with neovascular ARMD, the risk of severe visual loss with verteporfin therapy was significantly reduced compared to placebo (41% versus 69%) (73). These results are encouraging, but fall far short of a cure. Many patients continue to lose vision despite treatment, and this therapy is recommended only for a select subgroup of patients with neovascular ARMD. Other photosensitizing drugs (SnET2 and Lutex) that may improve our results are undergoing clinical investigation.

Studies are also underway to see if laser treatment to drusen can prevent neovascular complications of ARMD. Other popular, but unproved, laser treatments for this disorder include transpupillary thermotherapy (TTT), in which the abnormal vessels are gently heated with low-energy laser; and feeder vessel treatment, in which the abnormal vessels are photocoagulated at their source in the choroid before they extend under the center of the macula.

A greater understanding of the hereditary and environmental factors that lead to ARMD may help prevent or cure this visually devastating ocular disorder. The greatest hope for curing "wet" macular degeneration lies in prevention or suppression of the neovascular process from the outset. New **antiangiogenic** drugs such as ancecortave acetate (an **angiostatic steroid**) that may one day accomplish this goal are under investigation.

BOX 35.4. Good Exercises for the Visually Impaired

1. Stationary exercise equipment (e.g., treadmills, rowers, ski machines, bicycles)
2. Walking with a guide wire or sighted assistant
3. Swimming or water walking with the aid of lane buoys and floats
4. Aerobics videos that include verbal descriptions of all movements
5. Outdoor activities (e.g., skiing, tandem bicycling, and in-line skating) with the assistance of sighted guides

Adapted from Scheiner G. Exercise options for people with diabetic eye complications. J Ophthalmic Nurs Technol 1994;13(6):267–269.

Exercise and Age-Related Macula Degeneration

There is no evidence that exercise or physical fitness alters the course of macular degeneration. Theoretical concerns exist that strenuous activity, including Valsalva maneuver, could increase the risk for bleeding under the retina. In reality, this does not seem to be the case, and macular degeneration patients should not be discouraged from engaging in an exercise program. However, many of them are visually impaired, a condition that may limit their exercise options (Box 35.4). Because hypertension is associated with ARMD, exercise could theoretically play an ameliorating role, at least with respect to this particular risk factor.

What We Know
About Exercise and Eye Disease in the Elderly

1 We have achieved remarkable success in diagnosing and treating the most prevalent eye diseases in the elderly.

2 Exercise does not need to be restricted in most patients with eye disorders, even after eye surgery.

3 Exercise may improve pressure control in glaucoma patients.

4 Although exercise may precipitate a vitreous hemorrhage in a patient with advanced diabetic retinopathy, the overall improvement in cardiovascular fitness may outweigh the risk of bleeding.

5 Antioxidant vitamins with zinc retard the progression of macular degeneration and vision loss, but do not seem to reduce the risk of cataract formation.

What We Would Like to Know
About Eye Disease in the Elderly

1 We are still a long way from a cure for age-related macular degeneration. We would like to be able tell more precisely which patients are at risk for macular degeneration, so we can prevent it altogether, or treat more effectively at its earliest stages.

2 The powerful tools of genetics and molecular biology may allow us to diagnose and treat some eye diseases that have a genetic basis. For example, healthy genes can be inserted into patients who have an unhealthy variant or absence of a particular gene or combination of genes.

3 Genetic testing may enable us to customize drug therapy and determine which patients are more likely to respond to various treatments.

4 A complete eye transplant is currently a remote medical possibility. However, exciting progress is being made for an artificial retinal implant. A miniscule array of electrodes can be implanted on the retinal surface to stimulate retinal nerve cells when the native photoreceptors no longer function.

Summary

The elderly population suffers from several visually disabling or blinding disorders, including cataract, glaucoma, diabetic retinopathy, and age-related macular degeneration. Modern cataract surgery is safe and effective, and most people with this condition can be rehabilitated rapidly with no eye-related activity restrictions. Glaucoma continues to be a "silent thief" of vision with a chronic, insidious course. It is imperative that older people have periodic eye examinations to monitor and treat this condition if it arises. Exercise may be beneficial for long-term pressure reduction in glaucoma patients. Diabetic retinopathy is the chief cause of severe visual impairment in people under age 65. With current therapy, including strict diabetic control, timely laser treatments, and vitreous surgery, most diabetic patients can avoid blindness. In general, diabetic patients should not shun exercise because of retinopathy concerns. Exercise theoretically might have a mitigating influence on diabetic retinopathy by improving blood pressure, blood sugar levels, or cholesterol control. Despite recent advances in the diagnosis and treatment of age-related macular degeneration, this condition continues to be the major cause of vision loss in the elderly population. It robs people of precious sight and independence during their "golden years." Exercise need not be avoided in patients with macular degeneration, and it may have a positive influence psychologically and physically. However, special considerations for appropriate exercise may be necessary, because many of these patients are legally blind.

DISCUSSION QUESTIONS

1 What kind of medical and social information would be helpful in recommending an exercise regimen for a visually impaired individual?

2 What do you think the world would look like to a person with dense cataract? Advanced glaucomatous visual field loss? Diabetic vitreous hemorrhage? Severe age-related macular degeneration?

3 How might various types of visual impairment affect activities of daily living?

4 How would various types of eye disease and visual impairment change your recommended exercise program?

CASE STUDY

Patient Information

Mr. Peters is an overweight 65-year-old white type 2 diabetic patient who smokes. In addition to diabetes, he is treated for hypercholesterolemia, hypertension, and heart disease. He is taking daily low-dose aspirin for heart disease. His internist has recommended a weight loss and exercise program to improve his physical fitness and help control his hypertension and diabetes. He has had multiple laser treatments by his ophthalmologist for proliferative diabetic retinopathy, but he continues to get vitreous hemorrhages from time to time. Mr. Peters is also treated for open-angle glaucoma with eye drops. His mother went blind from macular degeneration.

Discussion

Mr. Peters is an ideal candidate for an exercise program, particularly since he is already under the care of an internist and ophthalmologist. He should be encouraged to stop smoking, because smoking will limit his exercise capacity, worsen his cardiovascular condition, and increase his risk for cataract and macular degeneration. An exercise program may help lower his intraocular pressure and reduce his risk for glaucomatous optic nerve damage. Aspirin need not be discontinued if required for his cardiovascular health, and vigorous exercise need not be discouraged despite his history of ocular bleeding. Diabetic vitreous hemorrhages occur most commonly during sleep and are rarely precipitated by strenuous activity. The overall physical and psychological benefits of exercise and weight loss probably outweigh the slight increased risk for vitreous hemorrhage.

REFERENCES

1. Harris MI. Diabetes in America: epidemiology and scope of the problem. Diabetes Care 1998;21(suppl 3):C11–4.
2. Gass JDM. Stereoscopic Atlas of Macular Diseases: Diagnosis and Treatment. 4th ed. St. Louis, Mo: Mosby; 1997:72.
3. Klein R. Epidemiology. In: Berger JW, Fine SL, Maguire MG, eds. Age-Related Macular Degeneration. St. Louis, Mo: Mosby; 1999:31–55.
4. Apple DJ. Cataract: epidemiology and service delivery. Survey Ophthalmol 2000;45(suppl 1):S32–S44.
5. Schachat AP. Common problems associated with impaired vision. Cataracts and age-related macular degeneration. In: Barker LR, Burton JR, Zieve PD, Finucane TE, eds. Principles of Ambulatory Medicine, 5th ed. Baltimore, Md: Williams & Wilkins; 1999:1415–1422.
6. Kanellopoulos AJ, and the Photolysis Investigative Group. Laser cataract surgery. A prospective clinical evaluation of 1000 consecutive laser cataract procedures using the Dodick photolysis Nd:YAG system. Ophthalmology 2001;108:649–655.
7. Piccone MR, Sulewski ME. Cataract surgery update. Current Concepts in Ophthalmology 2000;8:25–30.
8. Bochow TW, West SK, Azar A, Munoz B, Sommer A, Taylor HR. Ultraviolet light exposure and risk of posterior subcapsular cataracts. Arch Ophthalmol 1989;107:369–372.
9. Cumming RG, Mitchell P. Alcohol, smoking, and cataracts. Arch Ophthalmol 1997;115:1296–1303.
10. Jacques PF, Chylack LT, Hankinson SE, et al. Long-term nutrient intake and early age-related nuclear lens opacities. Arch Ophthalmol 2001;119:1009–1019.
11. Leske MC, Chylack LT, He Q, et al. Antioxidant vitamins and nuclear opacities: the Longitudinal Study of Cataract. Ophthalmology. 1998;105:831–836.
12. Age-Related Eye Diseases Study Research Group. A randomized, placebo-controlled, clinical trial of high-dose supplementation with vitamins C and E and beta carotene for age-related cataract and vision loss. AREDS Report No. 9. Arch Ophthalmol 2001;119:1439–1452.
13. Blodi FC. Cataract Surgery. In: Albert DM, Edwards DD, eds. The History of Ophthalmology. Cambridge, Mass: Blackwell Science; 1996.
14. Apple DJ. Harold Ridley knighted. Opthalmology 2000;107:412–413.
15. Apple DJ, Mamalis N, Loftfield K, et al. Complications of intraocular lenses. A historical and histopathological review. Surv Ophthalmol 1984;29:1–54.
16. Schachat AP. Glaucoma. In: Barker LR, Burton JR, Zieve PD, Finucane TE, eds. Principles of Ambulatory Medicine, 5th ed. Baltimore, Md: Williams and Wilkins; 1999:1423–1428.
17. Congdon N, Wang F, Tielsch JM. Issues in the epidemiology and population-based screening of primary angle closure glaucoma. Surv Ophthalmol 1992;36:411–423.
18. Stewart WC. The effect of lifestyle on the relative risk to develop open-angle glaucoma. Curr Opin Ophthalmol 1995;6(2):3–9.
19. Ashkenazi I, Melamed S, Blumenthal M. The effect of continuous strenuous exercise on intraocular pressure. Invest Ophthalmol Vis Sci 1992;33:2874–2877.
20. Passo MS, Goldberg L, Elliot DL, Van Buskirk EM. Exercise training reduces intraocular pressure among subjects suspected of having glaucoma. Arch Ophthalmol 1991;109:1096–1098.
21. Passo MS, Elliot DL, Goldberg L. Long-term effects of exercise conditioning on intraocular pressure in glaucoma suspects. J Glaucoma 1992;1:39–41.
22. Lempert P, Cooper KH, Culver JF, Tredici TJ. The effects of exercise on intraocular pressure. Am J Ophthalmol 1967;63:1673–1676.
23. Harris A, Malinovsky V, Martin B. Correlates of acute exercise-induced ocular hypotension. Invest Ophthalmol Vis Sci 1994;35:3852–3857.
24. Stewart RH, LeBlanc R, Becker B. Effects of exercise on aqueous dynamics. Am J Ophthalmol 1970;69:245–248.
25. Era P, Pärssinen O, Kallinen M, Suominen H. Effect of bicycle ergometer test on intraocular pressure in elderly athletes and controls. Acta Ophthalmol 1993;71(3):301–307.
26. Martin B, Harris A, Hammel T, Malinovsky V. Mechanism of exercise-induced ocular hypotension. Invest Ophthalmol Vis Sci 1999;40(5):1011–1015.
27. Avunduk AM, Yılmaz B, Şahin N, Kapıcıoğlu Z, Dayanır V. The comparison of intraocular pressure reductions after isometric and isokinetic exercises in normal individuals. Ophthalmologica 1999;213:290–294.
28. Haynes WL, Johnson AT, Alward WLM. Effects of jogging exercise on patients with the pigmentary dispersion syndrome and pigmentary glaucoma. Ophthalmology 1992;99:1096–1103.
29. Fong DS, Ferris FL, Davis MD, Chew EY, for the Early Treatment Diabetic Retinopathy Study Research Group. Causes of severe vision loss in the early treatment diabetic retinopathy study: ETDRS Report No. 24. Am J Ophthalmol 1999;127:137–141.
30. Chowdhury TA, Mijovic CH, Barnett AH. The aetiology of type I diabetes. Baillieres Best Pract Res Clin Endocrinol Metab 1999;13:181–195.
31. Knip M, Akerblom HK. Environmental factors in the pathogenesis of type I diabetes mellitus. Exp Clin Endocrinol Diabetes 1999;107(suppl 3)S93–100.
32. The Diabetes Control and Complications Trial Research Group. The effect of intensive diabetes treatment on the progression of diabetic retinopathy in insulin-dependent diabetes mellitus. Arch Ophthalmol 1995;113:36–51.
33. Diabetes Control and Complications Trial/Epidemiology of Diabetes Interventions and Complications Research Group. Retinopathy and nephropathy in patients with type I diabetes four years after a trial of intensive therapy. N Engl J Med 2000;342:381–389.

34. Koznarova R, Saudek F, Sosna T, et al. Beneficial effect of pancreas and kidney transplantation on advanced diabetic retinopathy. Cell Transplant 2000;9:903–908.

35. Rosenberg L. Pancreatic and islet transplantation. Curr Gastroenterolog Rep 2000;2:165–72.

36. UK Prospective Diabetes Study Group. Tight blood pressure control and risk of macrovascular and microvascular complications in type 2 diabetes: UKPDS 38. BMJ 1998;317:703–713.

37. Chew EY, Klein ML, Ferris FL, et al, for the ETDRS Research Group. Association of elevated serum lipid levels with retinal hard exudates in diabetic retinopathy. Early Treatment Diabetic Retinopathy Study (ETDRS) Report 22. Arch Ophthalmol 1996;114:1079–1084.

38. Early Treatment Diabetic Retinopathy Study Group. Photocoagulation for diabetic macular edema (Early Treatment Diabetic Retinopathy Study Report No. 1). Arch Ophthalmol 1985;103:1796–1806.

39. Early Treatment Diabetic Retinopathy Study Group. Treatment techniques and clinical guidelines for photocoagulation of diabetic macular edema. Early Treatment Diabetic Retinopathy Study Report No. 2. Ophthalmology 1987;94:761–774.

40. Diabetic Retinopathy Study Group. Photocoagulation treatment of proliferative diabetic retinopathy. Clinical application of Diabetic Retinopathy Study (DRS) findings. Diabetic Retinopathy Study Report No. 8. Ophthalmology 1981;88:583–600.

41. Diabetic Retinopathy Vitrectomy Study Research Group. Early vitrectomy for severe vitreous hemorrhage in diabetic retinopathy. Arch Ophthalmol 1990;108:958–964.

42. Chew EY, Klein ML, Murphy RP, Remaley NA, Ferris FL, for the Early Treatment Diabetic Retinopathy Study Research Group. Effects of aspirin on vitreous/preretinal hemorrhage in patients with diabetes mellitus. Early Treatment Diabetic Retinopathy Study Report No. 20. Arch Ophthalmol 1995;113:52–55.

43. Schachat AP. Can aspirin be used safely for patients with proliferative diabetic retinopathy? Arch Ophthalmol 1992;110:180.

44. Cruickshanks KJ, Moss SE, Klein R, Klein BE. Physical activity and the risk of progression of retinopathy on the development of proliferative retinopathy. Ophthalmology 1995;102:1177–1182.

45. Cruickshanks KJ, Moss SE, Klein R, Klein BE. Physical activity and proliferative retinopathy in people diagnosed with diabetes before age 30 yr. Diabetes Care 1992;15:1267–1272.

46. Kassoff A, Catalano RA, Mehu M. Vitreous hemorrhage and the Valsalva maneuver. Retina 1988;8:174–176.

47. Anderson B. Activity and diabetic vitreous hemorrhages. Ophthalmology 1980;87:173–175.

48. Age-Related Eye Disease Study Research Group. Risk factors associated with age-related macular degeneration. A case-control study in the age-related eye disease study. Age-Related Eye Disease Study Report Number 3. Ophthalmology 2000;107:2224–2232.

49. Smith W, Assink J, Klein R, et al. Risk factors for age-related macular degeneration. Ophthalmology 2001;108:697–704.

50. Richer S. Part I: A protocol for the evaluation and treatment of atrophic age-related macular degeneration. J Am Optom Assoc 1999;70:13–23.

51. Maruo T, Ikebukuro N, Kawanabe K, Kubota N. Changes in causes of visual handicaps in Tokyo. Jpn J Ophthalmol 1991;35:268–272.

52. Evans J, Wormald R. Is the incidence of registrable age-related macular degeneration increasing? Br J Ophthalmol 1996;80:9–14.

53. Eye Disease Case-Control Study Group. Risk factors for neovascular age-related macular degeneration. Arch Ophthalmol 1992;110:1701–1708.

54. Hyman L, He O, Grimson R, et al, and the Age-related Macular Degeneration Study Group. Risk factors for age-related maculopathy. Invest Ophthalmol Vis Sci 1992;33(suppl):801.

55. Bressler NM, Bressler SB. Preventive ophthalmology. Age-related macular degeneration [review]. Opthalmology 1995;102(8):1206–1211.

56. Cruickshanks JK, Klein R, Klein BEK, Nondahl DM. Sunlight and the 5-year incidence of early age-related maculopathy. Beaver Dam Eye Study. Arch Ophthalmol 2001;119:246–250.

57. Seddon JM, Willett WC, Speizer FE, Hankinson SE. A prospective study of cigarette smoking and age-related macular degeneration in women. JAMA 1996;276:1141–1146.

58. Christen WG, Glynn RJ, Manson JE, Ajani UA, Buring JE. A prospective study of cigarette smoking and risk of age-related macular degeneration in men. JAMA 1996;276:1178.

59. Klein R, Klein BE, Moss SE. Relation of smoking to the incidence of age-related maculopathy. Beaver Dam Eye Study. Am J Epidemiol 1998;147:103–110.

60. Sperduto RD, Hiller R. Systemic hypertension and age-related maculopathy in the Framingham Study. Arch Ophthalmol 1986;104:216–219.

61. Vingerling JR, Hoffman A, Grobbee DE, de Jong PT. Age-related macular degeneration and smoking. Rotterdam Study. Arch Ophthalmol 1996;114:1193–1196.

62. Klein R, Klein B, Linton KLP. The prevalence of age-related maculopathy. Beaver Dam Eye Study. Opthalmology 1992;99:933–943.

63. Seddon JM, Ajani UA, Sperduto RD, et al. Dietary carotenoids, vitamins A, C, and E, and advanced age-related macular degeneration. JAMA 1994;272:1413–1420.

64. Mares-Perlman JA, Brady WE, Klein R, et al. Serum antioxidants and age-related macular degeneration in a population-based case-control study. Arch Ophthalmol 1995;113:1518–1523.

65. Newsome DA, Swartrz M, Leone NC, Elston RC, Miller E. Oral zinc in macular degeneration. Arch Ophthalmol 1988;106:192–198.

66. Stur M, Tittl M, Reitner A, Meisinger V. Oral zinc and the second eye in age-related macular degeneration. IOVS 1996;37:1225–1235.

67. Mares-Perlman JA, Klein R, Klein BEK, et al. Association of zinc and antioxidant nutrients with age-related maculopathy. Arch Ophthalmol 1996;114:991–997.

68. Age-Related Eye Diseases Study Research Group. A randomized, placebo-controlled, clinical trial of high-dose supplementation with vitamins C and E, beta-carotene, and zinc for age-related macular degeneration and vision loss. AREDS Report No. 8. Arch Ophthalmol 2001;119:1417–1436.

69. Pharmacological Therapy for Macular Degeneration Study Group. Interferon alfa-2a is ineffective for patients with choroidal neovascularization secondary to age-related macular degeneration. Results of a prospective randomized placebo-controlled clinical trial. Arch Ophthalmol 1997;115:915–916.

70. Fine SL, Maguire MG. It is not time to abandon radiotherapy for neovascular age-related macular degeneration. Arch Ophthalmol 2001;119:275–276.

71. Macular Photocoagulation Study Group. Argon laser photocoagulation for neovascular maculopathy. Five-year results from randomized clinical trials. Arch Ophthalmol 1991;109:1109–1114.

72. Macular Photocoagulation Study Group. Laser photocoagulation of subfoveal neovascular lesions of age-related macular degeneration. Updated findings from two clinical trials. Arch Ophthalmol 1993;111:1200–1209.

73. Treatment of Age-Related Macular Degeneration with Photodynamic Therapy (TAP) Study Group. Photodynamic therapy of subfoveal choroidal neovascularization in age-related macular degeneration with verteporfin. Two-year results of 2 randomized clinical trials. TAP Report 2. Arch Ophthalmol 2001;119:198–207.

SUGGESTED READINGS

Albert SG, Bernbaum M. Exercise for patients with diabetic retinopathy. Diabetes Care 1995;18:130–132.

Cassel GH, Billig MD, Randall HG. The Eye Book: A Complete Guide to Eye Disorders and Health. Baltimore, Md: Johns Hopkins University Press; 1998.

Graham C, Lasko-McCarthey P. Exercise options for persons with diabetic complications. Diabetes Educ 1990;16:212–220.

Scheiner G. Exercise options for people with diabetic eye complications. J Ophthalmic Nurs Technol 1994;13(6):267–269.

COGNITIVE AND EMOTIONAL DISORDERS

CHAPTER 36

Psychosocial Considerations in Injury Rehabilitation

Robert C. Eklund, Theresa Bianco

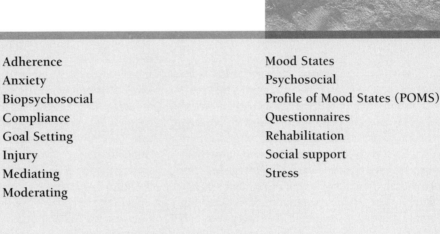

Overview

Injury is an event or process involving micro- or macro-trauma to one's physicality (1). Such traumas have social and psychological implications. The evidence indicates that this **biopsychosocial** complex interactively influences the processes and outcomes of **rehabilitation** (2).

In this chapter, we examine psychosocial issues associated with injury and rehabilitation and consider their relationship to treatment compliance. We begin by presenting a theoretical framework outlining the link between psychosocial issues and rehabilitation outcomes, and go on to discuss various factors that can influence responses to in-

jury. We then discuss different methods of assessing injured individuals to determine their psychosocial status and needs. Finally we conclude by offering suggestions as to how psychosocial considerations can be managed in clinical settings.

Psychosocial Issues Associated With Sports Injury

The clinical setting presents numerous challenges for injured athletes. In addition to coping with the pain and discomfort associated with injury and rehabilitation, injured athletes also must contend with feelings of distress, concerns about the consequences of their injury, isolation from their loved ones, and the need to develop trusting relationships with treatment providers (3–6). Confronting this multitude of challenges at once can take an emotional toll and have an adverse effect on their ability to cope with the physical and motivational challenges of rehabilitation (7–12).

Research shows that difficulties coping with injury and the demands of rehabilitation can give rise to problems with **compliance**, such as missing appointments, not doing prescribed exercises or doing them with suboptimal effort, not doing home exercises, and not taking medication as prescribed (7, 13–16). Behavior in clinical settings may be viewed as an index of an athlete's psychological and emotional adjustment to injury and the process of rehabilitation (6, 14, 17).

Noncompliance behaviors are of concern for several reasons. Noncompliance can slow recovery and interfere with the healing process, leaving the injured area vulnerable to further injury (18–21). For example, Gould and Udry (20) have noted that the failure to do exercises designed to prevent scar tissue build-up following knee injuries can result in reduced knee mobility, thereby increasing the risk of reinjury.

Another difficulty with treatment noncompliance is that disappointing rehabilitative progress can aggravate an athlete's distress and perpetuate or further exacerbate noncompliance (9, 12–14). Several studies have shown that rehabilitative mood and behavior vary according to perceptions of progress (16, 22–24). In general, athletes are more compliant when they believe in the efficacy of the treatment and are achieving favorable results. Compliance, however, may waver considerably when athletes are faced with rehabilitation setbacks and plateaus. In a series of interviews conducted with downhill skiers who had experienced complicated recoveries, Bianco (25) reported that several of the skiers claimed to have experienced motivational difficulties during periods of little or no improvement.

Noncompliance also can affect the patient–practitioner relationship and the quality of care extended to the injured athlete (26). Health care providers can view noncompliers as "problem patients" (27–29). Unfortunately, this perception has been associated with withdrawal of empathy and a minimization of patient contact. The withdrawal of attention and support from individuals who do not take active measures to resolve their problems is well documented in the literature (30, 31). Care providers (e.g., physical therapists) prefer treating individuals who take responsibility for their recovery and adhere to treatment protocols over those who do not (32).

There are compelling reasons to want to improve coping with injury and rehabilitation processes (i.e., treatment compliance). Improved coping and **adherence** are likely to contribute to a more efficacious recovery and produce re-

sults that can relieve the patient's distress and foster further treatment compliance. Moreover, compliance can contribute to the development of a positive working alliance between the patient and the health care provider. Treatment providers have a significant influence on how athletes cope with injury and rehabilitation (14, 26). Thus, fostering a positive relationship between the health care provider and the patient is extremely important.

Responses to Sports Injury and Rehabilitation

Contemporary approaches to explaining injury and rehabilitation processes typically are grounded in cognitive appraisal theories of **stress** and **coping**. Lazarus and Folkman (33, 34), for example, conceptualize stress as a dynamic process that involves a transaction between the environment and personal factors. They contend that when faced with environmental changes, individuals engage in two types of cognitive appraisals. The event first is assessed in terms of the amount of disruption it is likely to cause. The second assessment involves a determination of whether sufficient resources are available to manage the demands posed by the event. The perception that demands exceed coping resources has emotional and behavioral consequences. In general, greater perceived discrepancies between demands and coping resources contribute to greater emotional and behavioral disruption, which may be expressed as depression and poor treatment compliance.

Lazarus and Folkman's (33) theory also addresses how individuals cope with events appraised as being stressful. They describe coping (or stress management) as "a process of constantly changing cognitive and behavioral efforts to manage specific external and/or internal demands or conflicts appraised as taxing or exceeding the resources of the person" (p.141). Coping involves drawing on one's personal and social resources and, in broad terms, can be classified as either emotion-focused or problem-focused in nature. Emotion-focused coping is aimed at regulating emotions resulting from the stressful encounter. In instances of injury and rehabilitation, emotion-focused coping can manifest itself as cognitive restructuring and positive self-talk. This coping strategy is most appropriate for dealing with the uncontrollable aspects of the stressful environment. Problem-focused coping is, by contrast, aimed at actively managing the problem that is causing the individual to feel distressed. It can include activities such as goal-setting, seeking **social support**, and participation in rehabilitative protocols. Problem-focused coping is most rational when aimed at dealing with or resolving controllable factors.

In general, individuals engage in both emotion- and problem-focused strategies to cope with stress. The outcomes of these coping efforts are constantly monitored and appraised in terms of their success in meeting desired goals and their appropriateness to dealing with the ever-changing environment. The results of these appraisals influence subsequent emotions, behaviors, and coping efforts. Take, for example, an athlete who obtains positive results (e.g., favorable progress) from his problem-focused efforts in rehabilitation (e.g., adhering to prescribed treatment protocol). This positive reinforcement is likely to lift his spirits and motivate him to persevere with his problem-focused approach to injury recovery. Consider, in contrast, the athlete who also adopts a problem-focused approach effort (e.g., adhering to prescribed treatment protocol) that fails to produce positive results (e.g., no improvement). The negative feedback may leave this athlete feeling despondent and amotivated. Her coping efforts may be redirected to regulating emotions, and problem-focused efforts may falter until her distress is under control.

According to Lazarus and Folkman (33), the stress and coping process continues in this cyclical fashion until the stressor is no longer present. Furthermore, because the process of stress appraisal and coping is tied to perceptions of the person–environment relationship, it is necessarily influenced both by characteristics of the individual (e.g., personality, coping skills) and the environment (e.g., injury severity, social resources available).

Several conceptual models of the rehabilitative process based on extensive reviews of the sports injury literature have been developed (2, 12, 35). These models have considerable heuristic utility. Brewer and colleagues (2), for example, recently presented a biopsychosocial model outlining important interactions among biologic, psychologic, and sociologic factors within the rehabilitation process. In this chapter we focus on the model posited by Wiese-Bjornstal and colleagues (12, 35) because it not only builds on issues highlighted in the sports injury literature but also incorporates stress-process principles outlined by Lazarus and Folkman (33, 34).

In the model presented by Wiese-Bjornstal and colleagues (12, 35), injury is conceptualized as a stressful event wherein cognitive appraisals are central mediators of psychological and behavioral responses to the injury itself and to associated rehabilitation efforts. In line with the propositions of Lazarus and Folkman (33, 34), it is postulated that behavior in rehabilitation (e.g., compliance) influences outcomes (e.g., recovery) and that these outcomes determine subsequent cognitions, emotions, and behaviors. In addition to outlining issues relevant to the rehabilitative process, this model has heuristic utility as a framework for identifying problem areas and targeting intervention efforts.

The remainder of this chapter highlights research on issues identified in this model and discusses relevant implications for efforts in clinical settings. A full discussion of the model is available in the work of Wiese-Bjornstal and her colleagues (12, 35).

The Psychosocial Stresses of Injury

Wiese-Bjornstal and coworkers' model (12, 35) is based on viewing injury as a stressful event. It is, therefore, worth considering why being injured might be stressful for athletes. The challenges presented by injury and rehabilitation are numerous (see Table 36.1). At the physical level, athletes have to contend with the pain and discomfort associated with injury and rehabilitation. It is not unusual to find concomitant symptoms, such as sleep disturbance, loss of appetite, and a lack of energy (6). Depending on the type of injury incurred, mobility and physical activity may be quite restricted. In such instances it is not surprising to find that feelings of boredom and frustration as well as a loss of independence are prevalent (3).

Injury also can be psychologically disruptive. Not only do substantial injuries interfere with or terminate current athletic involvement, but they also can raise doubts about dreams and ambitions for the future—particularly when

TABLE 36.1. STRESSORS ASSOCIATED WITH INJURY REHABILITATION

Physical Stressors
Injury-related symptoms
Pain
Physical rigors of treatment
Restricted physical activity
Permanent physical changes

Stressors Related to Rehabilitation Environment
Lack of personal attention
Inaccessibility of services
Motivational demands of rehabilitation
"Rehabbing" alone
New relationships with treatment providers
Necessity of depending on medical team
Poor quality of information

Emotional Stressors
Psychological trauma of injury
Feelings of loss and grief
Slow progress and rehabilitation setbacks

Cognitive Stressors
Threats to future performance
Threats to life goals and values
Sports career concerns
Loss of sense of control
Threats to self-concept
Decision-making under stress

Financial Stressors
Loss of income
Loss of athletic scholarship support

Social Stressors
Isolation
Loss of important social roles
Lack of social support
Pressure from others
Overinvolvement of others

the diagnosis and prognosis are uncertain. Injured athletes tend to worry, and apprehensions over whether they will fully recover, how their playing ability will be affected, whether they will retain their spot on the team, and so on all become salient (3, 5, 36). Typically, serious injuries produce greater uncertainty and more distressed appraisals. Athletes who have been seriously injured can come to feel they lack control over their futures, and the thought of not participating in their sport can be particularly distressing for athletes whose sense of self-worth and identity are substantially invested in their athletic pursuits (37). These athletes are at the greatest risk of drops in self-esteem (16, 38, 39) and altered athletic identity (40, 41).

People who are injured often have to rely on others (often in new relationships with strangers) for several types of assistance—for medical care, to get around, and for social support, among other things. It is not uncommon for this reliance to be associated with a decreased sense of independence, self-esteem, and personal control (42). Being injured can also result in the loss or disruption of valued and (from a mental health perspective) valuable social relationships (6, 11, 43). For example, injured athletes can find themselves separated from the athletic environment, where they normally benefit from the camaraderie of teammates and the interaction with their coaches. The resulting feelings of isolation and loneliness are not surprising (e.g., 3, 6, 11, 44).

Cognitive Appraisals of Injury

Perceptions are not always accurate, particularly when people are under stress and emotional turmoil (6, 45). Depressed individuals, for example, are extremely prone to cognitive distortions and flawed interpretations of events (45). The issue of cognitive distortions among injured athletes has not been directly investigated but it has enjoyed speculation (6). There is anecdotal evidence, however, suggesting that injured athletes do experience exaggerated interpretations of events, at least during the initial stages of their injury. In Bianco and coworkers' (3) interviews with formerly injured skiers, injury distortions were evident. These included catastrophization (e.g., "my career is over"), incident personalization (e.g., "Why me?") and dichotomous thinking (e.g., feeling worthless because they were injured).

Emotional Responses to Injury and Rehabilitation

The emotional responses of athletes to injury typically range from mild disappointment to severe depression. For example, evidence indicates that injured athletes characteristically show elevated levels of tension, anger, depression,

confusion, and fatigue, and lower levels of vigor (4, 16, 22, 38, 46–48). These responses generally are transient in nature and tend to proceed from negative to positive affect over time (16, 47–49).

Some authors (6, 17, 50) have suggested that athletes can experience injury as a loss and hence show emotional responses similar to the grieving response described by Kubler-Ross (51). Based on her work with terminally ill cancer patients, Kubler-Ross claimed that grief-stricken individuals progress through a sequence of stages as they adjust to the reality of their situation. The stages she identified, in order, included shock, denial, anger, bargaining, depression, and acceptance. Grove and Gordon (17) argued that shock is a reasonably typical response following a significant athletic injury and that the associated denial (a sense of disbelief) can range from negligible to an outright inability to accept the severity of the injury. Denial may serve an adaptive function during the early stages of injury in that it can attenuate the initial emotional onslaught and thus allow for slower and more systematic processing of the event (6). Prolonged periods of denial, however, can actually interfere with the work of emotional recovery, and hence, are counterproductive and maladaptive.

A period of heightened emotionality is likely to follow the initial period of denial as the injured athlete begins to appreciate the reality of the situation (17). This period can be characterized by feelings of anger, depression, frustration, and loneliness. As the athlete begins to come to terms with the injury, he or she may engage in bargaining behavior. Bargaining can include making irrational pacts with oneself (e.g., "If I am nice to everyone, I will heal more quickly") or unrealistic deals with physical therapists (e.g., "If I work really hard on my exercises this week, promise me that I won't have to do any next week"). This behavior is indicative of the individual's failure to fully accept the injury and its ramifications. Bargaining might provide momentary relief (because the athlete sees a possible "out"), but it typically results in disappointment and depressed moods. Eventually, sadness and depressed moods are thought to give way to varying degrees of general acceptance as the athlete becomes resigned to the limitations imposed by the injury and begins to take an active role in the rehabilitation process.

Kubler-Ross's (51) conceptualization of the grieving process has intuitive appeal, and it has demonstrated heuristic value. Nonetheless, many contemporary loss theorists believe that the very notion of stages may, in and of itself, be problematic for providing a full understanding of psychological responses during recovery from injury. Injury can elicit a wide variety of psychological reactions depending on the characteristics of the person who is injured and the context in which injury (and rehabilitation) occur (52–54). It certainly is possible to grieve in ways that are more complex than stage models can accommodate or explain.

Behavioral Responses to Injury and Rehabilitation

An individual's behavior in clinical settings is a good indicator of how he or she is coping with the stresses of injury and rehabilitation, because behavioral responses tend to be consistent with psychological adjustment (55, 56). Indicators of positive adjustment include treatment adherence, high motivation, taking responsibility for rehabilitation, asking a lot of questions, and a positive attitude. Conversely, indicators of poor psychological adjustment to injury include treatment noncompliance (or overcompliance), lack of motivation, failure to take responsibility for rehabilitation, and absenteeism.

Other signs of poor adjustment can include unusual pain complaints, sleep disturbance, fatigue, moodiness, situational anxiety, excessive or awkward optimism, and a poor understanding of the rehabilitation process. Heil (6) termed this cluster of symptoms the "subclinical syndrome," because they are the types of symptoms that are not extreme but can over time be quite disruptive to the individual. According to Heil, the subclinical syndrome is most likely to occur in cases where the injury is severe, requires surgery or a long period of rehabilitation, or is perceived as a threat to the athlete's career. The subclinical syndrome also can lead to compliance difficulties.

As for the actual extent of compliance difficulties, "hard" numbers are difficult to pin down. Research shows that treatment noncompliance rates among injured athletes—a relatively motivated rehabilitation subpopulation—can range from 10% to 60% (7). The research is difficult to interpret because studies in the area employ vastly different populations (i.e., recreational versus elite athletes) with no consistency in injury examination or classification. This research also is confounded by the number of behaviors that make up compliance (e.g., attendance at clinical sessions, degree of effort exerted, and completion of home exercises) and the variety of ways in which it is assessed (e.g., patient self-reports, attendance records, and practitioner ratings). Adherence has proven to be a thorny issue in a variety of areas (57) and research on injury rehabilitation seems to offer similar challenges.

Although the patient's rehabilitative behavior can be indicative of psychological adjustment to injury, considerable variation in behavioral responses to distress is possible (29, 58, 59). Some people are outspoken about their distress, whereas others exhibit few outward signs of discomfort or unease. An absence of clear signs of distress (e.g., crying, frustration, anger) should not be assumed to indicate an absence of suffering. Conversely, individuals who are most effusive in their expressions of distress should not be assumed to be struggling the most with the rehabilitative process. Cultural (social) and individual differences are tremendously influential on these accounts, and accurate interpretation of these signals is difficult.

Factors Influencing the Injury and Rehabilitation Process

The response to injury and rehabilitation is influenced by a variety of personal and situational factors (Figure 36.1). In their model, Wiese-Bjornstal and colleagues (12, 35) highlight the influence of mediator and moderator variables. Mediator variables are variables that exert influence as part of a causal chain in producing outcomes in causal relationships. Athlete's responses to injury and rehabilitation are mediated by factors such as personality and personal history of stressors, coping resources, and the intervention itself. Moderator variables, by contrast, are variables thought to influence the strength of the cause–effect relationships. For example, it is reasonable to wonder if the relation between injury and negative affective responses (e.g., depression) is equally strong for season-ending injuries (with hope of future return to competition) and career-ending injuries (no hope of future return). A variety of personal and situational factors (e.g., the severity of the injury, sport-specific situational factors, interactions with the sports medicine team, and individual differences) are thought to influence post-injury responses.

As Smith, Smoll, and Ptacek (60) point out, **mediating** and **moderating** variables merit consideration because the presence of variables such as, for example, pre-injury stress and impaired coping is likely to amplify post-injury mood disturbance. The extent to which many relevant variables act in mediating or moderating capacities is unclear and requires further empirical examination. Certainly the roles played by mediating and moderating variables in the injury appraisal process are complex. Indeed, some variables (e.g., interaction with the sports medicine team) probably serve both mediating and moderating roles in producing rehabilitative outcomes (61).

Personal Factors

Personal and personality factors have been identified as influencing the ways in which people appraise their injuries as well as their emotional and behavioral responses to the injuries. These individual difference variables include age (62), medical history and experience with injury (12), self-esteem (16, 38), optimism (63, 64), hardiness (63, 64), explanatory style (64), athletic identity (40, 41), and coping skills (10, 24, 65).

Grove, Stewart, and Gordon (66), for example, collected mood and personality data (hardiness, optimism, and explanatory style) from athletes during the first 3 months following knee reconstruction surgery. Results were consistent with theoretical contentions. Negative moods (e.g., tension, depression, anger) were positively associated with explanatory pessimism and negatively associated with hardiness and opti-

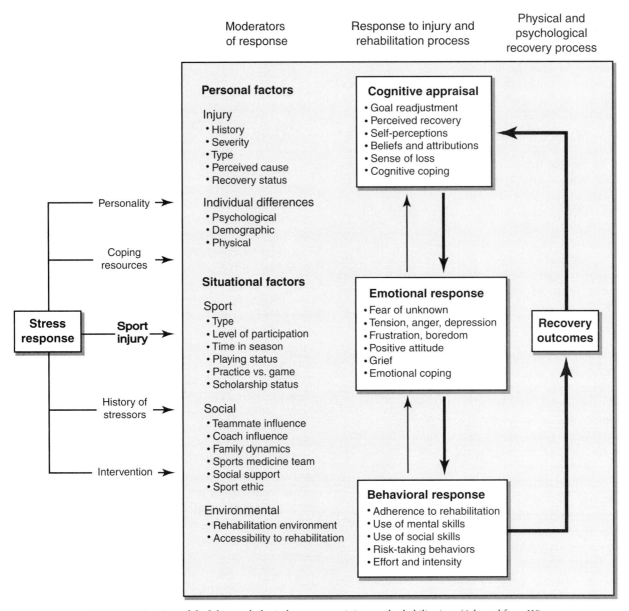

FIGURE 36.1. A model of the psychological response to injury and rehabilitation. (Adapted from Wiese-Bjornstal DM, Smith AM, LaMott EE. A model of psychologic response to athletic injury and rehabilitation. Athletic Training 1995;1:17–30.)

mism. Positive emotions (e.g., vigor, esteem-related affect), on the other hand, were positively related to hardiness and optimism and negatively related to explanatory pessimism. In a separate study by Grove, Bahnsen, and Eklund (65) neuroticism scores correlated strongly with coping strategies that were emotion-focused or avoidant in nature (e.g., venting, denial, mental disengagement, alcohol and drug use).

Injury severity is an important individual difference variable to consider because it dictates, in large degree, how long the athlete will be absent from his or her sport. Longer absences from the sport provide greater opportunity for niggling concerns to escalate into major distress (e.g., concern about being dropped from the team). Also,

the more serious the injury, the greater the possibility of permanent impairment to functioning. Research has shown that the athlete's mood is influenced by injury severity and that more serious injuries tend to be more disruptive (6, 47, 62, 67). Personal factors also have been linked with rehabilitation adherence. Most individual differences associated with clinical compliance in the extant literature are not surprising. Specifically, greater compliance has been associated with higher self-motivation (68); greater athletic competitive accomplishment (13–15); higher self-esteem (69); greater pain tolerance (13, 15); greater rehabilitation self-efficacy (68, 70); and better understanding of the rehabilitation process (12).

Situational Factors

Situational factors influencing athlete response to injury and the rehabilitative process are manifold. Sport-related factors include competitive level, player status, and the time in the season at which the injury occurred. It is easy to appreciate how being injured can be devastating for athletes whose livelihoods are contingent upon their ability to perform. It also is not difficult to imagine how an athlete could regard a last-minute injury precluding Olympic involvement as more distressing than the occurrence of the same injury after a long, successful, and fulfilling career.

Social factors that may influence athletes' responses to injury and rehabilitation include social support received from their coaches, team mates, and loved ones, and their interactions with the treatment team (71). There is a growing body of literature (44, 63, 72–75) indicating that social support has an important impact on how injured athletes cope with injury and rehabilitation. Generally, these studies indicate that injured athletes need and want social support from a variety of sources (e.g., coaches, teammates, significant others, health care providers) and that the absence of support is disruptive because it adds to their distress. Additional studies focusing specifically on adherence to rehabilitation show that the presence of supportive others can have a positive impact on adherence (15, 68, 76).

The treatment provider plays a significant role in the rehabilitation of injured athletes, particularly with regard to providing relevant information and offering guidance and encouragement (28). Not surprisingly, adherence behaviors are, to some degree, the product of patient–provider interactions (15). The growing recognition of the role of psychosocial factors in rehabilitation has been highlighted by the recent implementation by the United States National Athletic Trainers' Association (NATA) of a psychosocial intervention and referral competency requirement for accreditation for athletic trainer educational programs (77).

Finally, environmental factors that may influence athletes' responses to injury and rehabilitation include characteristics of and accessibility to the treatment clinic (12, 14, 35, 71). Bianco (25), for example, noted that elite downhill skiers preferred sports medicine clinics to centers that had more diverse patient populations, for several specific reasons. First, they viewed sports medicine clinics as providing opportunities to interact with other injured athletes. This interaction was regarded as motivating because the athletes could "rehab" together and support and push each other. Second, the skiers believed that the treatment offered in sports medicine centers was more "aggressive" and appropriate for the needs of athletes. They had a sense that sports physical therapists had a better understanding of the sports experience and were more tuned in to their physical and emotional needs. Johnston and Carroll (44) encountered similar beliefs in their interviews with athletes.

Incorporating Psychosocial Issues Into Injury Management

The growing awareness of the importance of psychosocial issues in injury and rehabilitation has been manifested in an emerging trend toward more holistic approaches to injury management (29). It is increasingly acknowledged that successful management of injuries requires more than just attention to a patient's physical needs. It is now understood that successful management of injuries also requires consideration of psychosocial needs if the rehabilitative process is to proceed optimally (6, 10, 20, 58, 73). Recent findings demonstrate that a comprehensive plan that interfaces rehabilitation procedures with psychological states enhances preventive and rehabilitative outcomes (78–80).

Responses to injury and the rehabilitative process are complex. Although discussion of injury issues in reductive isolation serves to facilitate communication and comprehension, it is important to remember that injuries are experienced holistically. Injuries cannot be experientially reduced to situational, personal, cognitive, emotional, and behavioral "subexperiences." All of the components discussed earlier influence one another to some degree. To address psychosocial issues in the management of injury effectively, it is useful to consider as many of these factors as possible. Examining the "big picture" in this manner will provide insight into how the athlete is experiencing injury and rehabilitation, and will help identify problem areas that can be targeted for intervention. Issues requiring consideration, then, are methods of assessing the injured athlete's psychosocial needs and a conceptual model for intervention.

Assessment of Psychosocial Needs

Appreciation of the range and extent of individual needs is integral to the success of psychosocial interventions (6). Several methods, ranging from very simple and quick to more in-depth approaches, can be used to assess the psychosocial needs of injured athletes. Obviously, the choice is a matter of convenience—keeping in mind that the more in-depth the information obtained, the better the understanding of the patient's needs. The methods also differ in terms of the expertise needed to conduct the assessments. We have restricted our discussion to assessment methods that can be used by people with a basic understanding of the psychosocial issues surrounding rehabilitation (if you understood the preceding discussion, you can probably use the tools we discuss subsequently without too much difficulty).

Regardless of the method used, the overall aim of the assessment is to obtain an indication of how much distress the athlete is experiencing and how well he or she is mobilizing his or her coping resources (6). The point is not to look for pathology (e.g., clinical depression) per se—the identification and treatment of pathology extends far beyond anything this chapter is intended to pursue or advocate—but to determine whether a person is having difficulty coping. Identification of such difficulties can be useful in facilitating rehabilitative efforts and, in certain instances, for referring the client for more in-depth clinical assistance. Also, because stress and coping are dynamic processes that vary across time, assessment should be systematic and should be repeated throughout the course of recovery if it is to provide useful information for the rehabilitative process. Many things can change over the course of recovery that can affect a person's perceptions of stress and coping ability (e.g., changes in social environment, such as pressure from the coach to hurry up and get better, or changes in rehabilitation, such as setbacks and plateaus). Failure to take these changes into consideration can jeopardize the effectiveness of the intervention (6, 7, 12, 58).

Diagnostic Interviews

The heart of assessment is the personal interview. It may vary from highly structured to open-ended—again, the choice will depend on the amount of time available to conduct the interview and the competencies of the practitioner conducting the interview. The diagnostic interview is useful for several reasons. It elicits information from both self-report and nonverbal behavior and, perhaps more importantly, it provides an opportunity to sow the seeds for a trusting treatment relationship (6, 29). By showing interest in the athlete's overall situation and responding with empathy to his or her distress, the health care provider can pave the way for acceptance of the rehabilitative activities.

The model outlined in Figure 36.1 can serve as a guide in terms of the types of issues to explore in the diagnostic interview. Issues relating to the personal costs of injury, the individual's understanding of injury and rehabilitation, beliefs about his or her ability to cope with stress, and availability of various types of social support are all relevant areas for exploration. Other matters worth noting can include signs of cognitive distortions, unrealistic expectations, and the presence of extreme emotional responses and noncompliance. Finally, secondary gain issues—benefits the athlete seems to derive from the injury—may emerge in diagnostic interviews (e.g., valued extra attention, undue relief from expectations, avoidance of training). These issues can easily warrant referral to a person with relevant specialized training (58), and the diagnostic interview also may serve to ensure that the injured patient is introduced to people with appropriate expertise. Symptom checklists such as that provided in Box 36.1 also can facilitate monitoring of psychosocial rehabilitative states and any potential emergence of a subclinical adjustment syndrome.

BOX 36.1. Symptom Checklist to Monitor Psychosocial Rehabilitative States

- Unusual pain complaints
- Sleep disturbance
- Fatigue
- Moodiness
- Situational anxiety
- Compliance problems
- Rehabilitation setbacks
- Excessive or awkward optimism
- Poor understanding of rehabilitation

Because interviewing is an interactive process, the success of the interview depends not only on the patient's candor but also on the interviewer's skill in eliciting the desired information (81, 82). Box 36.2 provides a few general interviewing tips to maximize the potential for success in diagnostic interviews.

The information obtained from the interviews can be supplemented by paper and pencil questionnaires and interviews with other people in the athlete's treatment team and support network. When interviewing network members, the degree to which they support the athlete and understand her situation is of interest. Expectations and the provision of social support within social networks exert a substantial influence on the patient's cognitive, emotional, and behavioral responses to the rehabilitative process (44, 72, 73, 83, 84).

Paper and Pencil Questionnaires

There is a plethora of questionnaires that can be used to measure various aspects of personality (e.g., neuroticism, dispositional optimism, explanatory style), psychological functioning (e.g., **mood states**, coping style), and social resources (e.g., social support). Each of these instruments varies in length, type and depth of information obtained, and expertise required to interpret the results. Although the

---

BOX 36.2. General Tips for Diagnostic Interviews

- Maintain good eye contact
- Listen carefully and attentively
- Pay attention to nonverbal cues (e.g., wincing and shifting indicate pain and discomfort)
- Encourage person to ask questions and reply to them in great detail
- Respect the person's wishes to explore or avoid certain topics (i.e., don't "push")

use of questionnaires has several advantages, such as ease of administration, efficient use of time, and reliance on objective measures of functioning, there are some disadvantages. The patient might see the exercise as unnecessarily time-consuming and impersonal. If such inventories are to be used, it is important to explain the purpose of the tests before administration to allay the athlete's anxieties about whole process (6).

When using questionnaires, it is important to understand what is being measured and the limitations of the instruments employed. If unfamiliar with the underlying principles associated with the specific instruments and constructs being measured, it is best to seek advice from someone with relevant expertise and training (e.g., a psychologist) to make sure the results are interpreted properly. As Heil (6) explains, diagnostic methods and measures are gateways to effective treatment only if they are used correctly. Instruments developed for idiographic clinical purposes are more suitable than instruments developed for nomothetic research purposes. Validity and reliability are always important considerations in instrument selection.

Several inventories have demonstrated utility in rehabilitative settings. For example, the Millon Behavioral Health Inventory (MBHI) (85), developed specifically for use with ill or injured people, is designed to measure coping styles, identify factors that may precipitate or complicate physical illness, and assess the extent to which emotional factors are likely to complicate responses to specific medical problems. The instrument is unique in that it makes specific predictions about the way in which patients are likely to relate to health personnel and various treatment regimens. For example, high levels of somatic anxiety indicated on the MBHI have been found to correlate with poor compliance in injured athletes (6).

The **Profile of Mood States (POMS)** (86) is a widely used instrument with face validity for clinical settings. The POMS assesses mood states on six subscales to characterize the psychological functioning of the individual in terms of vigor, tension, depression, anger, fatigue, and confusion. In general, injury states have been associated with decreased levels of vigor and increased negative affect, particularly in the initial stages (16, 22, 47, 48) and tend to proceed to more positive levels over time (16, 22, 47, 48). Idiographic profiling can be suggestive in terms of changes in mood states over the course of rehabilitation, and the availability of norms can be useful for contextualizing patient responses.

Another questionnaire that has clinical application is the Emotional Responses of Athletes to Injury Questionnaire (ERAIQ) developed by Smith, Scott, and Wiese (23). The ERAIQ (see Figure 36.2) was based on interviews with hundreds of injured athletes. It provides a quick way of assessing injury-relevant factors such as the importance of sports in the athlete's life, the emotional impact of injury, the social support available to the athlete, and the athlete's understanding of injury and rehabilitation. The ERAIQ can be administered as a questionnaire or used as an interview guide.

There is likely to be considerable pain associated with injury and rehabilitation. Pain is, in some degree, both biological and emotional in that it results from the interplay of physiological and psychological factors (6). It is a complex and individual experience that merits important consideration in patient assessment. Inventories can prove quite useful in assessing the pain experience. The McGill Pain Questionnaire (MPQ) (87), for example, has demonstrated relevance in rehabilitative settings. It is a widely used (outside of sports psychology) multidimensional pain index consisting of 78 terms commonly used to describe pain. The descriptors assess sensory (e.g., sharp, burning, aching) and affective-evaluative (e.g., fearful, agonizing, exhaustive) attributes of the experience. The questionnaire can facilitate the qualitative description of pain, and the results can be used to determine whether pain responses are normal with respect to the type of injury incurred. If responses deviate significantly from typical patterns, it is likely the patient will have difficulties adapting to injury and the rigors of rehabilitation.

Computer-Based Assessment and Monitoring

It has been argued that computer-based instrumentation has considerable clinical potential for assessing and monitoring injury adjustment over the course of rehabilitation (Heil, personal communication, 2002). For example, the Sport Injury Management (SIM) system (88) allows patients to enter data directly into their personal database in providing their responses to computer-based versions of questionnaires discussed earlier in this chapter (e.g., ERAIQ, a short version of the POMS, the Affective subscale of the MPQ). These data are almost simultaneously available for processing or graphic representation. In addition to providing information on psychosocial adjustment, the SIM program has a feature that provides for the generation of handouts for distribution to patients after each therapy session. Therapists and patients provided favorable assessments of the tool in initial clinical evaluations of the SIM program (88).

The Psychosocial Intervention

The goals of the psychosocial intervention should be to facilitate the recovery process, help the athlete maintain emotional equilibrium, help the athlete mobilize existing coping resources, and promote a sense of self-efficacy and control (6, 80). Three methods that can be particularly effective in achieving these goals are education, goal-setting, and social support (6, 89). The focus of such interventions is not necessarily on speeding recovery but on promoting treatment compliance, which, in turn, may contribute to a quicker recovery (1).

Emotional Responses of Athletes to Injury Questionnaire (ERAIQ)

- If you could be anything you wanted in life, what would your dream be? _____

- List in order of preference the sports and activities you participate in:

  1 _____ 3 _____

  2 _____ 4 _____

- Why do you participate in sport?
  (rank in order: 10=high, 0=low)

  _____ Self-discipline _____ Stress management
  _____ Competition _____ Personal improvement
  _____ Socialization _____ Outlet for aggression
  _____ Fitness _____ Weight management
  _____ Fun _____ Other (e.g., well-being)

- Would you describe yourself as an athlete? (circle)

  1   2   3   4   5

  (absolutely not)   (absolutely yes)

- When did your injury occur? _____

  Before   mid   end   of season? (circle)

- What is the nature of your injury? _____
  _____

- What sport were you injured in? _____
- How did it happen? _____

- What specific goals do you have in sports? _____
  _____

- Have they changed since the injury?   Y   N   (circle)

  If yes, how? _____

- Are you encouraged in sports by your significant others?   Y   N   (circle)
- Is their support pressure, or just right? _____

- Who exerts the most pressure?   (circle)

  Self   Mother   Father   Coach   Other _____

- What are the major sources of stress in your life now?

  1 _____ 3 _____

  2 _____ 4 _____

- Were you under any recent stress (life changes) before the injury?   Y   N   (circle)
- If yes, describe: _____
  _____

- Do you have a strong family support system or close friends who know about your injury?   Y   N   (circle)

- If yes, who are they? (e.g., coach, friends, parents)
  _____
  _____

- How have you been feeling emotionally since the injury?
  _____

- Please rank how the following emotions describe how you are feeling because of the injury. (10=high, 0=low)

  _____ Helpless _____ Depressed
  _____ Bored _____ Frustrated
  _____ Angry _____ Discouraged
  _____ Shocked _____ Optimistic
  _____ Frightened _____ Relieved
  _____ In pain _____ Other
  _____ Tense

- If 0% is no recovery, what % recovery have you made to your preinjury status? _____ %

- When is your estimated date of return to sports?
  _____

- Do you have fears about returning to sports? Y N (circle)
- If yes, what are they? _____
  _____

- Are you a motivated person toward exercise? (circle)

  1   2   3   4   5   6   7   8   9   10

  (not at all)   (extremely)

- How well do you handle pain? (circle)

  1   2   3   4   5

  (not at all)   (very well)

- What do you think is the most important thing necessary for a successful recovery? _____
  _____

- Is the most important thing something you have power over? (circle)

  1   2   3   4   5

  (not at all)   (very well)

- How optimistic are you about fully recovering from your injury/surgery? (circle)

  1   2   3   4   5

  (not at all)   (very well)

FIGURE 36.2.   Emotional Responses of Athletes to Injury Questionnaire (ERAIQ). Adapted from Smith (1996).

Education

Injury and rehabilitation are complex processes. The primary goal of education is to help the injured person understand underlying processes. Danish (8) pointed out that one of the major barriers to effective rehabilitation was a lack of knowledge about the process. Rationally speaking, it is difficult to apply effort to something one does not understand. Even if one were motivated and enthusiastic, the lack of a framework to guide one's efforts could substantially compromise the success of one's actions. Surveys of athletic trainers (90) and sports physical therapists (73) reveal a belief that patient education on the nature of injury and the recovery process contributes greatly to rehabilitation success.

Several benefits are available when the patient is more knowledgeable about the anatomy of injury, the significance of pain ("good pain" versus "bad pain"), and the importance of adhering to rehabilitation prescriptions. By understanding that periods of little or no improvement nearly always occur during rehabilitation, patients are less likely to panic when they hit a plateau. Also, patients are more likely to do their home exercises and cryotherapy if they understand that doing so will make their rehabilitation sessions less painful. It is important for patients to be able to distinguish between "good pain" (e.g., discomfort associated with the fatigue) and "bad pain" (e.g., tender soreness indicating additional injury). Such an understanding allows patients to make decisions on whether they are appropriately (and productively) tolerating discomfort in their rehabilitative efforts or further aggravating the injury that landed them in rehabilitation in the first place.

Sometimes, patients can be overmotivated in the sense that they can exhibit a tendency to overdo rehabilitation. Instances have been noted where injured athletes eager to return to their sport have taken on extra exercises outside of the prescribed regimen in counterproductive efforts to speed their recovery. Bianco (25) reported an extreme example of this sort of behavior. One downhill skier she interviewed admitted to seeing three physical therapists at the same time in hopes that it would help him recover more quickly. Education is a useful tool for encouraging smart rehabilitation practices and for underscoring that more rehabilitation is not necessarily good rehabilitation.

Educating athletes about injury and the process of recovery can help them have more realistic expectations for recovery. They are better able to plan for the future better, and the opportunities for disappointment (and, therefore, distress) are minimized. Because progress in rehabilitation has such a big impact on adherence behaviors, it is important to help patients interpret their progress correctly. Other components of the educational process can include teaching mental skills such as relaxation training for coping with pain and stress, mental imagery to visualize healing processes and to see oneself taking charge of recovery efforts (see oneself in a mastery role), and cog-

nitive restructuring to change negative thoughts into positive self-affirmations (i.e., focus on "controllables" and see oneself as competently mastering the environment). Heil (6) has recommended a variety of topics as relevant in the educational component of a psychosocial intervention (see Box 36.3).

Videotape modeling is one technique that can be effective for conveying information about injury and rehabilitation (1). This procedure involves having patients view a videotape of people—either similar others or models—in similar situations discussing relevant experiences. Fear and a perceived lack of control can compromise recovery (91). Videotape modeling can afford patients opportunities for vicarious experiences that can serve to attenuate such fears and anxieties. Further, information can be conveyed to enhance the patients' sense of control and mastery in the rehabilitative process.

Two aspects of the videotape that will determine its success are the similarity between the model and the patient/viewer, and the informational content. The greater the similarity between the model and the patient/viewer, the greater the likelihood is that the patient/viewer will be motivated to pay attention to the message conveyed (92). Model characteristics that are likely to be salient to a patient/viewer in the sports injury setting may include age, gender, sport type, level of competition, injury type, and type of medical procedure involved.

As mentioned earlier, the aim of using the modeling videotape often is to reduce fear and increase the patient's sense of mastery in the rehabilitation process. Discussion of the following issues can prove quite effective: the physical and emotional effects of injury and surgery; the process of

---

BOX 36.3. Relevant Educational Components of a Psychosocial Intervention (Heil, 1993)

- Basic anatomy of the injured area
- Changes caused by injury
- Active and passive rehabilitation methods
- Mechanisms by which rehabilitation methods work (e.g., how "icing" works)
- Potential problems and how to deal with them
- Distinguishing between "good" pain and "bad" pain
- Anticipated rehabilitation timeline (broken down into milestones)
- Possibility of treatment plateaus
- Rationale for limiting physical activity
- Rehabilitation as a collaborative learning process
- Methods of assessing readiness to return to play
- Deciding when to hold back and when to go all out
- Long-term maintenance and care of healing injury

From Heil J (6).

healing; obstacles to be expected; strategies for dealing with challenging or threatening situations in rehabilitation; and realistic expectations for recovery. The videotape also can be used to demonstrate the correct execution of exercises.

Using videotape modelling has several potential benefits. If carefully thought out, the videotape can provide much of the information appropriate for patient education and thereby free the practitioner from spending time on matters not unique or specific to a given patient. Also, it is a resource that the patient can consult as often as needed and at times when it is needed the most, such as when setbacks occur. Patients receiving too much information on medical technicalities can be overwhelmed and hence they may misunderstand or miss the intended message (93). Development of these videotapes can be time-consuming but, if appropriate resources are available, the investment should save time in the long run.

Goal Setting

Goal setting provides a means of structuring and measuring one's efforts over time; hence, it can be an effective technique for motivating individuals in rehabilitation (94–96). By identifying objectives at various points in time, individuals can determine what they need to do to achieve those objectives. Goals can be long- or short-term. Long-term goals typically refer to the end goal (e.g., increased mobility); short-term goals describe the steps necessary to achieve the end goal (e.g., doing 20 minutes of stretching every day for 2 weeks). Goal setting is a means of linking motivation to action and encourages athletes to take an active role in their recovery rather than being passive recipients of medical care (6, 95).

For goal setting to be successful, the patient should be involved in the goal setting process (6, 97, 98). Although it is true that shared decision-making can be more time-consuming, this approach to goal setting fosters a sense of commitment to the program. There is no point in treatment providers spending time developing programs to which patients are not going to adhere. By the same token, it makes no sense to have patients or athletes doing goal setting in the absence of relevant clinical expertise and guidance. It is easy to imagine resultant goals that are too easy, totally unrealistic, or even completely irrelevant to the rehabilitative process. Collaborative goal setting allows for informed guidance of the process and provides a sense of accountability for the athlete (99). The process of setting, monitoring, and refining goals also clarifies communication between the injured person and the treatment team—everyone has the same expectations. The effectiveness of this communication will influence the quality of the treatment relationship and will most likely influence treatment effectiveness (6, 26).

The goals identified in the goal setting plan should parallel the treatment plan (94, 95). Weinberg (96) provides a variety of observations on desirable attributes for effective goal setting. The goals identified should be specific and measurable (e.g., a goal of increasing range of motion should specifically target the desired range of motion in degrees). They are typically best stated in positive rather than negative terms (e.g., statements such as "I will remember to..." are preferable to statements such as "Don't forget to...."). Goals must be challenging but realistic—the point is to encourage, not discourage, the individual. Setting unrealistic goals, or those beyond any reasonable prospect for the patient, can result in disappointment and withdrawal of effort. The goals should help focus the patient's efforts on the rehabilitative *process*—that is, what they need to do to achieve a specific outcome. The focus should be on factors that are within the athlete's control, and a time line for achieving the goals ought to be laid out. This time line should include short-, medium- and long-term goals. For example, the plan can include goals related to both in-hospital/clinic and posttreatment activities to maintain fitness and enhance healing.

Goal setting is a flexible, not a rigid, process (96). It is a plan, not a contract. Goals must be monitored and readjusted on a regular basis in accordance with changes in the environment and the patient. Many things can change along the way, and goal setting must accommodate these changes, otherwise it will be ineffective. The acronym SMARTER is a useful reminder of the principles of goal setting (Box 36.4). Goal setting also can be used to develop a plan for dealing with rehabilitation setbacks. The goals can be geared to managing cognitive, emotional, and behavioral responses to such situations. By identifying potential problems and having a coping plan in place, athletes are likely to feel less distraught and more in control should these events arise (6, 94, 95).

Social Support

Social support refers to a process in which individuals communicate their concern for one another, and provide each other with resources that are intended to alleviate distress and facilitate coping (100, 101). Social support is communicated or provided through a variety of behaviors, such as expressing affection, showing empathy, offering advice, giving feedback, and providing practical assistance (102). Building on the work of Pines, Aronson, and Kafry

---

BOX 36.4. SMARTER Goal Setting Principles

S—specific
M—measurable
A—acceptable
R—realistic
T—time-based
E—evaluated on a regular basis
R—readjusted as needed

TABLE 36.2. TYPES OF SOCIAL SUPPORT

Dimension	Definition
Emotional Support	
Listening support	Behaviors that indicate people listen to you without giving advice or being judgmental
Emotional comfort	Behaviors that comfort you and indicate that people are on your side and care for you
Emotional challenge	Behaviors that challenge you to evaluate your attitudes, values, and feelings
Informational Support	
Reality confirmation	Behaviors that indicate that people are similar to you—see things the way you do—helps you confirm your perceptions and perspectives of the world and helps you keep things in focus
Task appreciation	Behaviors that acknowledge your efforts and express appreciation for the work you do
Task challenge	Behaviors that challenge your way of thinking about your work in order to stretch you, motivate you, and lead you to greater creativity, excitement, and involvement in your work
Tangible Support	
Material assistance	Behaviors that provide you with financial assistance, products, or gifts
Personal assistance	Behaviors that indicate a giving of time, skills, knowledge, and/or expertise to help you accomplish your tasks

From Hardy and Crace (1993)

(103), Hardy and Crace (104) proposed eight categories of social support (Table 36.2). Together, these categories represent the three major dimensions of social support—that is, emotional support, informational support, and tangible support. Emotional support is intended to facilitate emotion-focused forms of coping and involves activities such as listening and showing empathy and understanding. Informational support encourages the adoption of problem-focused coping strategies and includes activities such as providing information, offering guidance, and acknowledgment of effort. Tangible support can facilitate both emotion-focused and problem-focused coping and involves activities such as the provision of material goods or services.

Research conducted across a variety of medical populations has shown that social support can greatly enhance the process of recovery (6, 105). In sports injury settings, the presence of social support has been linked with improved coping (4, 44, 72, 73), faster recovery (106), and better treatment adherence (15, 68, 107). Findings such as these have led a number of authors (6, 10, 18, 89, 108) to conclude that social support is critical in the rehabilitation of the injured athlete and should, therefore, be a concern of those who are directly involved in the care and treatment of injured athletes.

Social support can be provided by a variety of individuals, including loved ones, family members, friends, teammates, coaches and treatment providers. In general, those closest to the person in need are best suited to providing emotional support (e.g., reassurance of self-worth), whereas those with relevant expertise are best equipped to provide informational support (e.g., feedback of effort) (109). Studies show that athletes tend to receive emotional support from family and friends and informational support from individuals with relevant expertise, such as coaches or medical professionals (44, 72, 73, 75, 110).

Although certain individuals tend to be associated with specific support types, that does not mean that they do not or cannot provide other types of social support. Research shows that in addition to being sources of informational support, treatment providers can be important sources of emotional support to injured athletes (44, 72). For example, injured skiers in Bianco's (72) study explained that they looked to sports physical therapists for emotional support when they wanted to speak to someone who understood (1) what being injured meant to them; (2) their need to do as much as they could to recover quickly; (3) the frustrations connected with the rehabilitation process; and (4) their concerns about no longer being able to ski at the elite level.

The role of the treatment provider in providing social support to injured athletes has been highlighted by several authors (14, 15, 26, 28, 73, 89). Heil (6) claims that the relation between the patient and his or her treatment providers is the cornerstone of support for the injured athlete. Injured athletes benefit from knowing that their treatment providers understand and support them. The research shows that (1) the provision of understanding, compassion and reassurance can help alleviate the patient's distress; (2) the provision of encouragement and relevant information can keep the athlete positive and motivated; and (3) showing a willingness to help and to "be there" for the athlete can reduce feelings of isolation and improve mood (14, 15, 26, 72).

By providing social support, treatment providers can establish rapport with their patients and cultivate a climate of trust and open communication—the foundations of a good therapeutic relationship. Providing effective support involves being attentive to the athlete's needs and using what Burleson (111) termed "sophisticated support messages." These types of messages acknowledge, elaborate, legitimize, and contextualize the feelings and perspectives of distressed others, and have been rated helpful by support recipients. The following is an example of a sophisticated support message: "I see that you are frustrated (acknowledgment) because you are working so hard and not getting the results you want (elaboration). That's perfectly understandable (legitimization). Just remember that plateaus are to be expected in rehabilitation (contextualization). The good news is that they don't last—they are temporary—so don't give up hope (reassurance)."

Emotional Support

- Be an attentive and patient listener.
- Focus on both the feeling and content of what person says.
- Allow patients to express themselves, without cutting them off.
- Reflect back what you've heard and observed.
- Show appropriate empathy.
- Present alternative interpretations of events (if appropriate), but don't argue with the patient.

Informational Support

- Share anecdotes of athletes who have been in similar situations.
- Acknowledge both effort and mastery.
- Balance the use of technical appreciation and technical challenge.
- Provide feedback in a sincere, sensitive, and respectful manner.
- Sandwich technical instruction between affirming and encouraging statements.
- Critique the activity, not the person.

Tangible Support

- Be clear about what your boundaries are.
- Let athletes know what you are and are not able to do.
- Deliver on your promises—and on time.

Specific recommendations for providing social support to injured athletes are provided in Box 36.5.

It is important for the treatment provider to be aware that other members of the individual's support network also can provide social support, including family, friends, and others with similar injuries. Part of the treatment provider's mandate is to help mobilize these social resources (89). For example, setting up a buddy system or arranging for people in similar situations to do their rehabilitation together can be a useful way of mobilizing support for the injured person. They can share their experiences with that person, motivate and encourage each other, use the other person as a basis for comparison, and just have some company through what is often a lonely and isolating time.

With regard to mobilizing support from members of the athlete's support network, remember that not all close relationships are supportive. Support provided through close relationships marked by high degrees of conflict can exacerbate rather than relieve distress (112–114). Although it is true that the support provided through close relationships may not always be beneficial, it is evident that close relationships are essential to health and well-being. In fact, re-search shows that support from more distant ties cannot compensate for a lack of support from close intimates (115).

What We Know
About Psychosocial Aspects of Injury and Injury Rehabilitation

1 Injury is an event or process that extends beyond micro- or macro-trauma to one's physicality. Injury does have social and psychological implications. Injury appraisals are central mediators (i.e., determinants) of cognitive, affective, and behavioral responses to the event.

2 Treatment compliance tends to fall far short of optimal. Research indicates that adherence difficulties commonly stem from psychosocial (rather than physical) issues related to injury and rehabilitation.

3 Cognitive distortions of injuries are not uncommon. These distortions can involve catastrophization, overgeneralization, selective abstraction of event irrelevancies, and absolutistic interpretations.

4 Injury can elicit a wide variety of psychological reactions depending on the characteristics of the person who is injured and the context in which the injury (and rehabilitation) occurs. Some heightened emotionality should be expected, and grieving associated with the injury can be complex. Stereotypical affective responses tend to be negative in valance and range from mild disappointment to severe depression. Extended periods of depression or denial are likely to be counterproductive and maladaptive.

5 Evidence indicates that rehabilitative noncompliance can to be a substantive problem. Reported compliance rates range from 10% to 60%. Compliance is difficult to measure because of the number of different behaviors involved (e.g., attendance, rehabilitative exertion, exercise completion), and compliance rates are difficult to interpret because of the variety of ways they can be assessed (e.g., self-report, attendance records, practitioner ratings).

6 Injury and rehabilitation are biopsychosocial processes. Recommendations for the integration of psychosocial factors into rehabilitative programs are based on this realization. The assessment of individual needs can facilitate psychosocial interventions by identifying psychoeducational needs, laying the groundwork for appropriate goal setting programs, and ensuring that appropriate social support resources are made available.

What We Would Like to Know
About Psychosocial Aspects of Injury and Injury Rehabilitation

1 Although research on psychosocial factors influencing injury recovery has grown considerably in recent years, there have been few prospective investigations of the injury adjustment process (2). This lack makes it difficult to understand fully the processes of change operating in the transition across preinjured, injured, and rehabilitated states. Carefully controlled, repeated measure design investigations involving prospective biopsychosocial data are warranted and would contribute substantively to understanding in this area.

2 A greater understanding of relational effects of social support during the rehabilitative process is needed (71). The ways in which provision (or receipt) of social support over the course of injury affects qualitative aspects of interpersonal relationships has not been extensively examined. Because relational aspects of social support (e.g., between practitioners and patients) are assumed to affect instrumental outcomes (e.g., treatment adherence, rehabilitative outcomes), a greater understanding in this area may prove revealing. Evaluation of social support manipulations in clinical trials could provide important information.

3 Given that evidence suggests that social support exchanges play an important role in the rehabilitative process, variables moderating social support interaction and effectiveness must be better understood (71). Sociocultural norms and attitudes, for example, tend to dictate the appropriateness of social support provision (e.g., by treatment providers) and acceptance (e.g., by patient recipients) in specific situations, and among certain age, gender, and relationship groups. Examination of factors affecting palliative social support exchanges in rehabilitative settings may prove revealing.

4 Research efforts on the rehabilitation and recovery of athletes is limited by its largely correlational nature and hampered by construct ambiguity and poor operationalization of key variables (e.g., injury types, injury severity, adherence, recovery). Conceptualizations of key variables must be refined. Research evaluating the implications of various operationalizations is warranted to facilitate a greater understanding of extant data. Greater reliance on experimental and clinical investigation would be desirable.

Summary

Evidence indicates that injury is a psychosocial as well as a physical event. Optimal treatment should, therefore, engender a holistic approach. Rehabilitation should not be aimed simply at the injury. It must acknowledge and accommodate the person who has been injured, because the stresses of injury influence cognitive-emotional states and rehabilitative behaviors. Holistic injury management requires an awareness and understanding of the psychosocial needs and experiences of injured athletes.

Assessment of psychosocial needs is an important starting point in injury rehabilitation. Once needs are identified, psychosocial interventions involving educational, goal setting, and social support strategies can be developed to optimize rehabilitative efforts. Much of injury recovery or rehabilitation requires affective "work," but cognitive awareness of relevant issues can make the affective work easier. As a consequence, educational processes offer important intervention possibilities. Videotape modeling, for example, has been effective for conveying information suitable for alleviating affective states that can compromise recovery (e.g., reducing fear and anxiety and increasing perceptions of control and mastery). Goal setting strategies often are useful motivational tools for structuring and monitoring rehabilitative efforts over time. Finally, social support processes have been consistently associated with rehabilitative and recovery benefits. The role of the treatment provider in providing social support rehabilitative settings has become increasingly evident. Treatment providers typically have the expertise and proximity to acknowledge, elaborate, legitimize, and contextualize the feelings and perspectives of distressed others, and these acts have been regularly identified as helpful by support recipients.

Treatment adherence is important to ensuring effective recovery from injury states. Unfortunately, treatment adherence is not always optimal. Injury is a psychosocial insult as well as a physical trauma to the injured individual. Effective treatment of injury, therefore, acknowledges the complex of interactions inherent in this biopsychosocial event.

DISCUSSION QUESTIONS

1 What does it mean to adopt a biopsychosocial view of injury? What are the implications of adopting this view?

2 What potential psychosocial issues may be associated with injury? Why should these be considered a concern in the rehabilitation process?

3 What are the implications of adopting the view that injury and rehabilitation are best understood within the context of stress process appraisals? How does this conceptualization clarify injury (or rehabilitation)-related cognition, affect, and behavior?

4 What sorts of cognitive distortions may be encountered when working in clinical settings?

5 Why has Kubler-Ross's (51) conceptualization of the grieving process been characterized as having intuitive appeal and heuristic value? What limitations does it appear to have as a conceptual model?

6 What personal factors appear to influence the injury response and the rehabilitation process?

7 Discuss sports-related, social, and environmental factors moderating the injury adjustment process.

8 Why is assessment one of the most important phases for the success of psychosocial interventions? Which assessment type is most useful? Why?

9 What psychosocial modules are likely to be important for successful intervention? Why?

CASE STUDY

Patient Information

Like many athletes, Pete had Olympic dreams. His Olympic goals had been set years ago, and he had been diligently pursuing them ever since. He was determined to win a spot on the national team in Olympic trials so he could compete in the Olympic tournament. Once in that tournament, he had every intention of collecting Olympic gold. It appeared that the dedication and hard work was paying off—and he would participate in an Olympiad sooner than he'd hoped! He had only to win a single match against an opponent whom he had regularly vanquished in earlier qualifying tournaments.

Pete crashed from intoxicating heights of anticipation into abject misery with a single misstep on a light training run. He initially refused to believe the surgeon's assessment that the knee had to be completely reconstructed. He was certain he could win the final match to make the Olympic team even with his damaged knee and that proper rest and care over the intervening month to the Olympic tournament would leave him ready to take on the world. A couple of weeks of failed treatment shattered those illusions. He withdrew from the final qualifying trial and underwent surgery on the knee.

The surgery went well and the prognosis was good. In the months following surgery, however, Pete sat at home in the recliner watching movies. His compliance with his physical therapist's recommendations was nonexistent. He adamantly asserted to visitors (progressively fewer over the months) that his Olympic debut was "postponed but not canceled." Aside from angry outbursts, Pete could only be described as listless in the months following surgery.

Assessment and Treatment

At a postoperative follow-up visit to his orthopaedic surgeon, Pete "unloaded" his frustration on his lack of progress toward a return to competition. She found his frustrated outburst unsettling and puzzling. Her examination revealed nothing organically inappropriate in his surgical recovery given the postoperative time frame—and especially in light of his rehabilitative noncompliance. She reiterated her earlier admonitions about the importance of the rehabilitative treatment program. Believing that things were physically satisfactory, she nonetheless gave him a referral letter to consult with a psychologist who specialized in postoperative rehabilitation.

The psychologist explained to Pete that biological, psychological, and social factors interact to produce rehabilitative outcomes. They discussed a variety of issues ranging from the injured knee itself, thoughts and feelings about the circumstances, future athletic plans, and so on. They then worked together on a goal setting program to facilitate his recovery. The first goals were primarily educational in nature (e.g., goals about developing Pete's working knowledge of the anatomy of *his* knee and *his* injury, the surgery *he* underwent, the rehabilitative protocol for *his* knee and to find and talk to other athletes who faced similar challenges). His subsequent goals were grounded in his rehabilitative program and his determination to return to elite level competition.

Pete is still adamant that he'll make the next Olympic team. For the most part he seems to have shaken off his listless, moody state. He is showing signs of adjustment to his circumstances. His rehabilitative compliance is not perfect, but his occasional deviations seem reasonable and justifiable. He does appear to be on track for a return to competition. Whether or not he will return to pre-injury form is anyone's guess—but it seems that he's now doing the things that could make it possible.

It is important for all health professionals to recognize the limits of their training and to develop a referral network of practitioners in related fields. In this instance, no organic problems were evident in Pete's regularly scheduled postoperative checkup. His surgeon felt that there was potential for psychosocial issues to complicate matters—something outside a surgeon's training—and so she referred Pete to another professional with relevant competence.

Questions

1. What are the cognitive, affective, and behavioral symptoms suggesting that focusing solely upon an organic "fix" of Pete's injured knee might be misguided? How certain can you be that these symptoms signal psychological difficulties of clinical significance?

2. What psychosocial strategies and methods did the psychologist employ in working with Pete? What important information would you need to know to evaluate whether the SMARTER principles had been employed?

3. What *personal* factors may have made Pete's adjustment to his knee injury more difficult? What *situational* factors may have made Pete's adjustment to his knee injury more difficult?

REFERENCES

1. Flint FA. Integrating sport psychology and sports medicine in research: the dilemmas. J Appl Sport Psychol 1998;10:83–102.
2. Brewer BW, Andersen MB, Van Raalte JL. Psychological aspects of sport injury rehabilitation: toward a biopsychosocial approach. In: Mostofsky DI, Zaichkowsky LD, eds. Medical and Psychological Aspects of Sport and Exercise. Morgantown, WV: Fitness Information Technology, 2002.
3. Bianco T, Malo S, Orlick T. Sport injury and illness: elite skiers describe their experiences. Res Q Exerc Sport 1999;70:1–13.
4. Gordon S, Lindgren S. Psycho-physical rehabilitation from a serious sport injury: case study of an elite fast-bowler. Aust J Sci Med Sport 1990;22:71–76.
5. Gould D, Udry E, Bridges D, Beck L. Stress sources encountered when rehabilitating from season-ending ski injuries. The Sport Psychologist 1997;11:361–387.
6. Heil J. Psychology of Sport Injury. Champaign, IL: Human Kinetics Publishers, 1993:338.
7. Brewer BW. Adherence to sport injury rehabilitation programs. J Appl Sport Psychol 1998;10:70–82.
8. Danish SJ. Psychological aspects in the care and treatment of athletic injuries. In: Vinger PF, Hoerner EF, eds. Sports Injuries: The Unthwarted Epidemic. Littleton, MA: PSG Publishing, 1986:345–353.
9. Daly JM, Brewer BW, Van Raalte JL, et al. Cognitive appraisal, emotional adjustment, and adherence to rehabilitation following knee surgery. J Sport Rehabilitation 1995;4:23–30.
10. Rotella RJ, Heyman SR. Stress, injury, and the psychological rehabilitation of athletes. In: Williams JM, ed. Applied Sport Psychology: Personal Growth to Peak Performance. Mountain View, CA: Mayfield, 1993:338–355.
11. Shelley GA. The psychological ramifications of sport injuries. In: Henschen KPS, W. F., eds. Sport Psychology: An Analysis of Athlete Behavior. Longmeadow, MA: Mouvement, 1995:315–330.
12. Wiese-Bjornstal DM, Smith AM, Shaffer SM, Morrey MA. An integrated model of the response to sport injury: Psychological and sociological dynamics. J Appl Sport Psychol 1998;10:46–69.
13. Fields J, Murphey M, Horodyski M, Stopka C. Factors associated with adherence to sport injury rehabilitation in college-age recreational athletes. J Sport Rehabilitation 1995;4:172–180.
14. Fisher CA. Adherence to sports injury rehabilitation programmes. Sports Med 1990;9:151–158.
15. Fisher CA, Domm MA, Wuest DA. Adherence to sports-injury rehabilitation programs. Physician and Sportsmedicine 1988;16:47–49.
16. Leddy M, Lambert M, Ogles B. Psychological consequences of athletic injury among high-level competitors. Res Q Exerc Sport 1994;65:347–354.
17. Grove JR, Gordon AMD. The psychological aspects of injury in sport. In: Bloomfield J, Fricker PA, Fitch KD, eds. Textbook of Science and Medicine in Sport. Melbourne: Blackwell, 1995:194–205.
18. Crossman J. Psychological rehabilitation from sports injuries. Sports Med 1997;23:333–339.
19. Doyle J, Gleeson NP, Rees D. Psychobiology and the athlete with anterior cruciate ligament (ACL) injury. Sports Med 1998;26:379–393.
20. Gould D, Udry E. The psychology of knee injuries and injury rehabilitation. In: Griffin LY, ed. Rehabilitation of the Injured Knee. St. Louis: Mosby, 1995:86–98.
21. Steadman JR. A physician's approach to the psychology of injury. In: Heil J, ed. Psychology of Sport Injury. Champaign, IL: Human Kinetics, 1993:25–32.
22. McDonald SA, Hardy CJ. Affective response patterns of the injured athlete: an exploratory analysis. The Sport Psychologist 1990;4:261–274.
23. Smith AM, Scott SG, Wiese DM. The psychological effects of sports injuries: coping. Sports Med 1990;9:352–369.
24. Weiss MR, Troxel RK. Psychology of the injured athlete. Athletic Training 1986;21:104–109.
25. Bianco T. Social support influences on recovery from sport injury. 1996, University of Ottawa: Ottawa, Canada.

26. Brewer BW, Van Raalte JL, Petitpas AJ. Patient-practitioner interactions in sport injury rehabilitation. In: D., P, eds. Psychological Bases of Sport Injury. Morgantown, WV: Fitness Information Technology, 1999:157–174.

27. Fisher CA, Mullins SA, Frye A. Athletic trainers' attitudes and judgements of injured athletes' rehabilitation adherence. J Athletic Training 1993;28:43–47.

28. Gordon S, Potter MA, Ford IW. Toward a psych-educational curriculum for training sport-injury rehabilitation personnel. J Appl Sport Psychol 1998;10:140–156.

29. Miller R. Managing Difficult Patients. London: Faber & Faber, 1990.

30. Hall JA, Roter DL, Katz NR. Meta-analysis of correlates of provider behavior in medical encounters. Med Care 1988;26:1–19.

31. Silver RC, Wortman CB, Crofton C. The role of coping in support provision: the self-presentational dilemma of victims of life crises. In: Sarason BR, Sarason IG, Pierce GR, eds. Social Support: An Interactional View. New York: Wiley, 1990:397–426.

32. Ford IW, Gordon S. Perspectives of sport physiotherapists on the frequency and significance of psychological factors in professional practice: Implications for curriculum design in professional training. Aust J Sci Med Sport 1997;29:34–40.

33. Lazarus RS, Folkman S. Stress, Appraisal, and Coping. New York: Springer, 1984.

34. Lazarus RS, Folkman S. The concept of coping. In: Monat A, Lazarus RS, eds. Stress and Coping: An Anthology. New York: Columbia University Press, 1991:189–206.

35. Wiese-Bjornstal DM, Smith AM, LaMott EE. A model of psychologic response to athletic injury and rehabilitation. Athletic Training 1995;1:17–30.

36. Gould D, Udry E, Bridges D, Beck L. Coping with season-ending injuries. The Sport Psychologist 1997;11:379–399.

37. Thomas CE, Rintala JA. Injury as alienation in sport. J Philos Sport 1989;16:44–58.

38. Chan CS, Grossman HY. Psychological effects of running loss on consistent runners. Percept Mot Skills 1988;66:875–883.

39. McGowan RW, Pierce EF, Williams M, Eastman NW. Athletic injury and self-diminution. J Sports Med Phys Fitness 1994;34:299–304.

40. Young K, White P. Sport, physical danger, and injury: the experiences of elite women athletes. J Sport Soc Issues 1995;19:

41. Young K, White P, McTeer W. Body talk: male athletes reflect on sport, injury, and pain. Soc Sport J 1994;11:175–194.

42. Pellegrino ED. Toward a reconstruction of medical morality: the primacy of the act of profession and the fact of illness. J Med Philos 1979;4:32–56.

43. Henderson J. Suicide in sport: Are athletes at risk? In: Pargman D, ed. Psychological bases of sport injuries. Morgantown, WV: Fitness Information Technology, 1999:287–302.

44. Johnston LH, Carroll D. The context of emotional responses to athletic injury: a qualitative analysis. J Sport Rehabilitation 1998;7:206–220.

45. Beck AT, Rush AJ, Shaw BP, Emory G. Cognitive Therapy of Depression. New York: Guilford Press, 1979.

46. Pearson L, Jones G. Emotional effects of sports injuries: implications for physiotherapists. Physiother 1992;78:762–770.

47. Smith AM, Scott SG, O'Fallon WM, Young ML. Emotional responses of athletes to injury. Mayo Clin Proc 1990;65:38–50.

48. Smith AM, Stuart MJ, Wiese-Bjornstal DM, et al. Competitive athletes: Preinjury and postinjury mood state and self-esteem. Mayo Clin Proc 1993;68:939–947.

49. Quackenbush N, Crossman J. Injured athletes: a study of emotional responses. J Sport Behav 1994;17:178–187.

50. Astle SJ. The experience of loss in athletes. J Sports Med Phys Fitness 1986;26:279–284.

51. Kubler-Ross E. On Death and Dying. London: Tavistock, 1969.

52. Archer J, Rhodes V. The grief process and job loss: a cross-sectional study. Br J Psychol 1993;8:395–410.

53. Brewer BW. Review and critique of models of psychological adjustment to athletic injury. J Appl Sport Psychol 1994;6:87–100.

54. Evans L, Hardy L. Sport injury and grief responses: a review. J Sport Exerc Psychol 1995;17:227–245.

55. Larson GA, Starkey C, Zaichkowsky L. Psychological aspects of athletic injuries as perceived by athletic trainers. The Sport Psychologist 1994;37–47.

56. Gordon S, Milios D, Grove JR. Psychological adjustment to sport injuries: implications for therapists and trainers. Sport Health 1991;10:13–15.

57. Dishman RK. Increasing and maintaining exercise and physical activity. In: Morgan WP, Goldston SE, eds. Exercise and Mental Health. Washington, DC: Hemisphere Publishing, 1987:57–83.

58. Petitpas A, Danish S. Caring for injured athletes. In: Murphy S, ed. Sport Psychology Interventions. Champaign, IL: Human Kinetics, 1995:255–281.

59. Rotella RJ, Ogilvie BC, Perrin DH. The malingering athlete: psychological considerations. In: Pargman D, ed. Psychological Bases of Sport Injuries. Morgantown, WV: Fitness Information Technology, 1999:111–122.

60. Smith RE, Smoll FL, Ptacek JT. Conjunctive moderator variables in vulnerability and resiliency research: Life stress, social support and coping skills, and adolescent sport injuries. J Pers Soc Psychol 1990;58:360–370.

61. Baron RM, Kenny DA. The moderator-mediator variable distinction in social psychological research: Conceptual, strategic and statistical considerations. J Pers Soc Psychol 1986;51:1173–1182.

62. Brewer BW, Linder DE, Phelps CM. Situational correlates of emotional adjustment to athletic injury. Clin J Sport Med 1995;5:241–245.

63. Ford IW, Eklund RC, Gordon S. An examination of psychosocial variables moderating the relationship between life stress and injury time-loss among athletes of a high standard. J Sports Sci 2000;5:301–312.

64. Grove JR, Bianco T. Personality of correlates of psychological processes during injury rehabilitation. In: Pargman D, ed. Psychological Bases of Sport Injuries. Morgantown, WV: Fitness Information Technology, 1999:89–110.

65. Grove JR, Bahnsen A, Eklund RC. Neuroticism, injury severity, and coping with rehabilitation. In IX World Congress of Sport Psychology. 1997. Netanya, Israal: Ministry of Education, Culture, and Sport, 1997.

66. Grove JR, Stewart RML, Gordon S. Emotional reactions of athletes to knee rehabilitation. In Australian Sports Medicine Federation. 1990. Alice Springs, AUS.

67. Smith AM, Milliner EK. Injured athletes and the risk of suicide. J Athletic Training 1994;29:337–341.

68. Duda JL, Smart AE, Tappe MK. Predictors of adherence in the rehabilitation of athletic injuries: An application of personal investment theory. J Sport Exerc Psychol 1989;11:367–381.

69. Lampton CC, Lambert ME, Yost R. The effects of psychological factors in sports medicine rehabilitation adherence. J Sports Med Phys Fitness 1993;33:292–299.

70. Taylor AH, May S. Threat and coping appraisal as determinants of compliance with sports injury rehabilitation: an application of Protection Motivation Theory. J Sports Sci 1996;14:471–482.

71. Bianco T, Eklund RC. Conceptual considerations for social support research in sport and exercise settings: the case of sport injury. J Sport Exerc Psychol 2001;23:85–107.

72. Bianco T. Social support and recovery from sport injury: elite skiers share their experiences. Res Q Exerc Sport 2001;72:376–388.

73. Ford IW. Psychosocial processes in sport injury occurrence and rehabilitation. In Human Movement and Exercise Science. Crawley, WA: University of Western Australia, 1999.

74. Udry E. Social support: exploring its role in the context of athletic injuries. J Sport Rehabilitation 1996;5:151–163.

75. Udry E. Coping and social support among injured athletes following surgery. J Sport Exerc Psychol 1997;19:71–90.

76. Oldridge NG, Donner A, Buck CW, et al. Predictive indices for dropout: the Ontario exercise heart collaborative study experience. Am J Cardiol 1983;51:70–74.

77. National Athletic Trainers Association. Competencies in Athletic Training: Curriculum 2001. *http://www.caahep.org/standards/at_01.htm.*

78. Green LB. The use of imagery in the rehabilitation of injured athletes. In: Pargman D, ed. Psychological Bases of Sport Injuries. Morgantown, WV: Fitness Information Technology, 1999:235–251.

79. Kerr G, Goss J. The effects of a stress management program on injuries and stress levels. J Appl Sport Psychol 1996;8:109–117.

80. Ross MJ, Berger RS. Effects of stress inoculation training on athletes' postsurgical pain and rehabilitation after orthopedic injury. J Consult Clin Psychol 1996;64:406–410.

81. Marshall C, Rossman GB. Designing Qualitative Research. Newbury Park, CA: Sage, 1989.

82. Fontana A, Frey JH. Interviewing: the art of science. In: Denzin NK, Lincoln YS, eds. Handbook of Qualitative Research. Thousand Oaks, CA: Sage, 1994:361–376.

83. Udry E, Gould D, Bridges D, Beck L. Down but not out: athlete responses to season-ending injuries. J Sport Exerc Psychol 1997;19:229–248.

84. Wills TA. Supportive functions of interpersonal relationships. In: Cohen S, Syme SL, eds. Social Support and Health. San Diego, CA: Academic Press, 1985:61–82.

85. Millon T, Green CJ, Meagher RB. Millon Behavioral Health Inventory Manual. Vol. 3. Minneapolis: NCS Interpretive Scoring Systems, 1982.

86. McNair DM, Lorr M, Droppleman LF. Profile of Mood States Manual. San Diego, CA: Educational and Industrial Testing Service, 1971.

87. Melzack R. The McGill pain questionnaire: major properties and scoring methods. Pain 1975;1:277–299.

88. Van Heerden JC. The implementation of a model for the rehabilitation of sports injuries. 2000, University of Stellenbosch: South Africa.

89. Hardy CJ, Burke KL, Crace RK. Social support and injury: a framework for support-based interventions with injured athletes. In: Pargman D, eds. Psychological Bases of Sport Injuries. Morgantown, WV: Fitness Information Technology, 1999:175–198.

90. Wiese DM, Weiss MR, Yukelson DP. Sport psychology in the training room: a survey of athletic trainers. The Sport Psychologist 1991;5:15–24.

91. Kulik JA, Mahler HIM. Emotional support as a moderator of adjustment and compliance after coronary artery bypass surgery: a longitudinal study. J Behav Med 1993;16:45–63.

92. McCullaugh P, Weiss MR, Ross D. Modeling considerations in motor skill acquisition and performance: an integrated approach. In: Pandolf KB, ed. Exercise and Sport Sciences Reviews. Baltimore: Williams & Wilkins, 1989:475–513.

93. Samples P. Mind over muscle: Returning the injured athlete to play. Physician and Sportsmedicine 1987;15:172–180.

94. Gilbourne D. Goal-setting during rehabilitation. In: Reilly T, ed. Science and Soccer. London: Chapman & Hall, 1996:185–200.

95. Gilbourne D, Taylor AH. From theory to practice: the integration of goal perspective theory and life development approaches within an injury-specific goal-setting program. J Appl Sport Psychol 1998;10:124–139.

96. Weinberg R. Goal-setting and performance in sport and exercise settings: a synthesis and critique. Med Sci Sports Exerc 1994;4:469–477.

97. Beggs WDA. Goal setting in sport. In: Jones JG, Hardy L, eds. Stress and performance in sport. New York: John Wiley & Sons, 1990:135–170.

98. Gould D, Petlichkoff L, Hodge K, Simons J. Evaluating the effectiveness of a psychological skills educational workshop. The Sport Psychologist 1990;4:249–260.

99. Danish SJ, Petitpas AJ, Hale BD. A developmental-educational intervention model of sport psychology. The Sport Psychologist 1992;6:403–415.

100. Hobfoll SE, Stokes JP. The processes and mechanics of social support. In: Duck S, ed. Handbook of Personal Relationships. New York: Wiley, 1988:497–517.

101. Shumaker SA, Brownell A. Toward a theory of social support: closing conceptual gaps. J Soc Issues 1984;40:11–36.

102. Albrecht TL, Adelman MB. Social support and life stress: new directions for communications research. Hum Communication Res 1984;11:3–22.

103. Pines A, Aronson E, Kafry D. Burnout. New York: The Free Press, 1981.

104. Hardy CJ, Crace RK. Social support within sport. Sport Psychology Training Bulletin 1991;3:1–8.

105. Sarason BR, Pierce GR, Sarason IG. Social support: the sense of acceptance and the role of relationships. In: Sarason BR, Sarason IG, Pierce GR, eds. Social Support: An Interactional View. New York: Wiley, 1990:97–128.

106. Ievleva L, Orlick T. Mental links to enhanced healing: an exploratory study. The Sport Psychologist 1991;5:25–40.

107. Byerly PN, Worrell T, Gahimer J, Domholdt E. Rehabilitation compliance in an athletic training environment. J Athletic Training 1994;29:352–355.

108. Silva JM, Hardy CJ. The sport psychologist: psychological aspects of injury in sport. In: Mueller FO, Ryan A, eds. The Sports Medicine Team and Athlete Injury Prevention. Philadelphia: FA Davis, 1991:114–132.

109. Lin N. Conceptualizing social support. In: Lin N, Dean A, Ensel WM, eds. Social support, life events, and depression. Orlando, FL: Academic Press, 1986:17–30.

110. Rosenfeld LB, Richman JM, Hardy CJ. Examining social support networks among athletes: Description and relationship to stress. The Sport Psychologist 1989;3:23–33.

111. Burleson BR. Comforting messages: features, functions, and outcomes. In: Daly JA, Wortman JM, eds. Strategic Interpersonal Communication. Hillsdale, NJ: Lawrence Erlbaum, 1994:135–161.

112. Dakof GA, Taylor SE. Victims' perceptions of social support: what is helpful from whom? J Pers Soc Psychol 1990;58:80–89.

113. Pierce GR, Sarason IG, Sarason BR. Integrating social support perspectives: working models, personal relationships, and situational factors. In: Duck S, ed. Personal Relationships and Social Support. Newbury Park, CA: Sage, 1990:173–189.

114. Rook KS. Detrimental aspects of social relationships: taking stock of an emerging literature. In: Veiel HOF, Baumann U, eds. The Meaning and Measurement of Social Support. New York: Hemisphere Publishing, 1992:157–169.

115. Coyne JC, Ellard JH, Smith DAF. Social support, interdependence, and the dilemmas of helping. In: Sarason BR, Sarason IG, Pierce GR, eds. Social Support: An Interactional View. New York: Wiley, 1990:129–149.

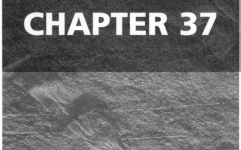

CHAPTER 37

Exercise and Anxiety

J. Robert Grove, Robert C. Eklund

Overview

Anxiety is an emotional reaction characterized by physiological arousal, muscular tension, and feelings of apprehension or dread. It typically occurs in response to real or imagined threats to one's well being; however, it sometimes can occur without an identifiable cause. Cognitive correlates of anxiety include pessimistic rumination, feelings of helplessness, and/or a loss of confidence. Although everyone experiences anxiety from time to time, some individuals have a tendency to react with high levels of **state anxiety** in a variety of situations. These individuals are deemed to be high in **trait anxiety**.

Anxiety is a normal human response, and when not persistent or severe, can have functional value. Specifically, it not only "fires-up" the system, but also tends to make one more vigilant and therefore can facilitate coping. On the other hand, persistent and/or severe anxiety reactions can interfere with coping efforts by "paralyzing" one's behavior. These negative consequences are readily observable among sufferers of clinical **anxiety disorders** (e.g., agoraphobia; panic attack), but they are also problematic for many individuals who suffer from subclinical anxiety (i.e., anxiety that is severe but not of sufficient magnitude or duration to justify a formal diagnosis).

Formal estimates from a study commissioned by the World Health Organization indicate that approximately 10% of the world's population suffers from some form of clinical anxiety disorder, and that roughly another 4% experiences significant symptoms at a subclinical level (1). In the United States, anxiety disorders are the most common form of mental illness, affecting close to 20 million people and costing over $45 billion per year (2). The identification of cost-effective methods for reducing anxiety is therefore an important undertaking, and a substantial body of research has emerged in which exercise has been examined in this regard.

In this chapter, we review the evidence for the **anxiolytic** effects of exercise from 2 perspectives. First, we examine findings from studies where state or trait anxiety has been assessed following participation in either a single bout of exercise or in an exercise program consisting of multiple sessions. Second, we examine findings from studies in which anxiety levels have been assessed after regular exercise has been discontinued. Evidence for the impact of any treatment can be obtained by noting the consequences when exercise is either added or withdrawn, but prior reviews of the effects of exercise on anxiety have focused almost exclusively on the changes produced by adding the exercise stimulus. An examination of the **exercise deprivation** literature suggests that removal of the exercise stimulus also influences anxiety, and we believe consideration of these complementary effects is important for a thorough understanding of the relationship between exercise and anxiety. Potential mechanisms for the observed effects are also discussed, along with intensity and measurement issues that have received increasing attention recently. We conclude by offering some guidelines for exercise prescription based on the collective findings in this area of research.

Effects of Exercise Involvement on Anxiety

The effect of exercise involvement on anxiety has greatly interested researchers for several decades. Hundreds of studies involving thousands of subjects have been conducted, and many reviews have been published. In this section, we discuss findings and conclusions from 5 reviews that appeared in the literature during the past 12 years. In one review, McDonald and Hodgdon (3) conducted a **meta-analysis** of 22 anxiety studies reported between 1973 and 1989. These studies included aerobic exercise protocols that ranged from recreational walking and jogging to high-intensity training regimens characteristic of elite runners and military personnel. Results from the meta-analysis revealed that exercise had statistically significant beneficial effects on state and trait anxiety, and that these effects were not dependent on the aerobic exercise undertaken. More specifically, the average **effect size** across 13 assessments of state anxiety was 0.28, and the average effect size across 20 assessments of trait anxiety was 0.25. According to conventional guidelines for interpreting effect sizes in the behavioral sciences (4), these findings suggest a small-to-moderate beneficial effect of exercise on anxiety levels. However, there was an indication that certain personal factors also influenced the degree to which exercise decreased anxiety. That is, the beneficial effects of exercise were more regularly observed in studies using male participants than in studies using female participants. In addition, exercise-related reductions in anxiety were more evident for young and middle-aged adults than for older adults. Better evidence of anxiety reduction was seen in studies that used the State-Trait Anxiety Inventory

(5) to measure anxiety rather than the Manifest Anxiety Scale (6).

Petruzzello and coworkers (7) conducted separate meta-analyses of the effects of exercise on self-reported state anxiety, self-reported trait anxiety, and the physiological correlates of anxiety. These analyses included data from 104 studies that appeared in the literature between 1960 and 1989, and they included more than 400 effect sizes based on responses from over 3000 participants. Distinctions were made between aerobic and nonaerobic exercise as well as between different frequencies, intensities, and durations of exercise activity. The time between exercise cessation and anxiety assessment was also taken into account. Findings for self-reported state anxiety indicated that aerobic exercise had a small-to-moderate beneficial impact on anxiety responses (average effect size = 0.26), but that nonaerobic exercise did not influence anxiety responses. The reductions in state anxiety produced by aerobic exercise occurred for both acute and chronic exercise activities, and they were independent of exercise intensity, exercise duration, the specific anxiety measure employed, and the timing of assessment (0 to 30 minutes post-exercise). In addition, exercise-mediated reductions in state anxiety were found to be comparable to the reductions produced by more traditional therapies (e.g., meditation and relaxation training).

All of the trait anxiety studies reviewed by Petruzzello and coworkers (7) involved chronic exercise, and more than 95% of them involved aerobic exercise activities. Within these parameters, there was additional evidence for the anxiety-reducing effects of exercise. Specifically, an overall average effect size of 0.34 indicated that exercise had a significant and beneficial effect on trait anxiety. Moreover, effects of roughly this magnitude were observed regardless of the participant's age or health status, and regardless of the exercise intensity or the anxiety scale employed. Factors that did appear to influence the impact of chronic aerobic exercise on trait anxiety, however, were the length of the training program and the duration of the exercise sessions. The average effect size for exercise programs lasting 10 weeks or more was 0.47, whereas the average effect size for programs lasting 9 weeks or less was 0.16. Similarly, the average effect size for exercise programs containing sessions of more than 20 minutes was 0.38, whereas the average effect size for exercise programs containing sessions of 20 minutes or less was not significantly different than zero. Petruzzello and coworkers (7) advised, however, that this duration finding required **cross-validation** because most of the studies using sessions of 20 minutes or less also involved exercise programs of less than 10 weeks' duration.

The studies reviewed by Petruzzello and coworkers (7) that included **psychophysiological** measures also employed aerobic exercise protocols. The overall mean effect size for these studies was 0.56, indicating a significant reduction in the psychophysiological correlates of anxiety in response to exercise. Effects of this magnitude were observed regardless of the participant's age and health status, and the effects were also independent of exercise intensity, the length (in weeks) of the exercise program, and the time at which the measures were taken (0 to 30 minutes or more). Although there was some indication that blood pressure and heart rate measures were less influenced by exercise than **electroencephalogram** (EEG), **electromyogram** (EMG), and **skin conductance**, all of these measures produced effect sizes that were significantly greater than zero. At the same time, larger effects were observed on psychophysiological parameters for exercise regimes lasting 30 minutes or less (n = 72; weighted average effect size = 0.77) than for exercise regimes lasting more than 30 minutes (n = 54; weighted average effect size = 0.29).

Schlicht conducted a meta-analysis of the effects of exercise on anxiety in 22 independent samples containing over 1,300 subjects (8). The exercise protocols in these studies ranged from aerobic fitness activities (e.g., running; swimming) to less aerobically demanding activities (e.g., strength training; calisthenics). Aerobic protocols were over-represented among the studies, however. On the basis of his findings, Schlicht concluded that there was only limited evidence for anxiety-reducing effects from exercise. Specifically, he suggested that evidence existed for "marginal" anxiolytic effects among persons 30 to 50 years of age, but that these effects were probably mediated by expectancies for reduced health risk. Petruzzello (9) criticized these conclusions, arguing that restricted sampling of the available research undermined the validity of Schlicht's findings and conclusions. A close inspection of the effect sizes reported by Schlicht suggests that this criticism may be warranted. That is, the overall population effect size reported by Schlicht was $r = 0.15$, which corresponds to a **Cohen's** d of approximately 0.30. This value is very similar to the average effect sizes of 0.26 for state anxiety and 0.34 for trait anxiety reported by Petruzzello and coworkers (7). It is also similar to the effect sizes of 0.28 for state anxiety and 0.25 for trait anxiety reported by McDonald and Hodgdon (3). Moreover, Schlicht noted an effect size of $r = 0.22$ ($d = 0.42$) for male exercisers and an effect size of $r = 0.12$ ($d = 0.23$) for female exercisers, which was consistent with McDonald and Hodgdon's observation of greater anxiolytic effects for males than for females.

Further positive evidence for the anxiety-reducing effects of exercise was obtained in a **meta-analytic review** conducted by Long and van Stavel (10). This analysis included 40 studies in which adults over the age of 18 participated in at least 20 minutes of aerobic or nonaerobic exercise on multiple occasions each week for a minimum of 5 weeks. Clinical samples were excluded from the analysis, but some high-stress samples from nonclinical populations were included. Consistent with earlier quantitative reviews, findings from this study revealed weighted average effect sizes of 0.31 for state anxiety and 0.34 for trait anxiety. No differences were observed in the effect sizes for males (0.38) and females (0.34), and there were not enough studies involving nonaerobic exercise to make meaningful comparisons between aerobic and nonaerobic protocols. However, significant differences in effect sizes were noted between studies involving highly stressed and minimally stressed participants. More specifically, the anxiolytic effects of exercise were found to be greater within the high-stress samples ($d = 0.51$) than within the low-stress samples ($d = 0.28$).

Raglin (11) reviewed findings from studies examining the effects of acute exercise on state anxiety and the effects of chronic exercise on trait anxiety. Within the acute exercise category, a further distinction was made between activities that were primarily aerobic and those that were resistance-oriented. Raglin concluded that there is considerable evidence for reductions in state anxiety following acute aerobic exercise. He also concluded that these reductions may persist for several hours, and that their magnitude compares favorably to passive anxiety management strategies (e.g., quiet rest; meditation). Although some researchers have suggested that high-intensity aerobic exercise might undermine these anxiolytic effects, Raglin cites evidence for reductions in state anxiety following cycling and running activities at intensities ranging from 70% of $\dot{V}O_2$ peak to voluntary exhaustion (12–14). However, he notes that acute bouts of resistance exercise may not exert the same effects on anxiety as acute bouts of aerobic exercise. More specifically, significant *increases* in systolic blood pressure have been observed following resistance exercise at both self-selected intensities and controlled intensities of 70–80% of $\dot{V}O_2$ max (15, 16). Self-report measures of state anxiety are also elevated following resistance training at these intensities, although they appear to return to baseline in less than 30 minutes (16).

Raglin (11) acknowledges that chronic exercise has been associated with reduced trait anxiety in several studies, and he notes that these reductions are comparable to those produced by **cognitive-behavioral therapy** such as stress inoculation training. In opposition to the views of Schlicht (8), he also cites research suggesting that these exercise-induced reductions in trait anxiety cannot be explained in terms of expectancy effects (17) or the perceived importance of exercise (18). However, he calls attention to 2 issues that need to be examined further in connection with trait anxiety effects. Specifically, it appears that initial levels of trait anxiety need to be considered because the benefits of chronic exercise may be greater for individuals with high baseline levels of trait anxiety (19). In addition, the effects of various exercise intensities needs closer scrutiny because of the well-documented negative effects of chronic high-intensity exercise on emotional state (20).

Effects of Exercise Deprivation on Anxiety

Restriction of physical activity has been shown to produce several psychological symptoms in regular exercisers. Some common symptoms are guilt, depression, irritability, and increases in tension and anxiety (21). The fact that exercise deprivation is associated with increased tension and anxiety is noteworthy because it complements the findings reviewed above. In other words, there is considerable evidence that adding the exercise stimulus decreases anxiety levels, and there is also considerable evidence that removing the exercise stimulus increases anxiety and anxiety-related emotions.

Baekeland (22) was one of the first to call attention to the possible anxiety-producing effects of exercise deprivation. In his study, undergraduate students who were accustomed to regular exercise were prohibited from exercising for a month. Analysis of their sleep patterns and self-report data suggested that tension and anxiety increased considerably during the deprivation period. Subsequent studies have corroborated these findings, and have shown that deprivation periods as short as 24 hours can produce anxiety symptoms in habitual exercisers. Sachs and Pargman (23), for example, interviewed highly committed runners and discovered that many of them experienced withdrawal symptoms within 24 to 36 hours of a missed run. The most frequently cited symptoms included restlessness, irritability, tension, and anxiety. Thaxton (24) provided quantitative verification that such effects can occur within 24 hours in a study examining self-reported mood and **galvanic skin response** (GSR) among habitual runners. Participants in her study either continued their regular training regimen or voluntarily abstained from running for 1 day. Although self-reports of anxiety were not significantly different between these groups, GSR readings were significantly lower in the running group than in the abstinence group. Thaxton interpreted these differences in GSR scores as evidence of increased somatic anxiety for the abstainers (24).

Results from several questionnaire studies conducted with runners reinforce these findings by documenting increases in anxiety as a common withdrawal symptom when training sessions are missed. For example, Harris (25) surveyed 156 women runners to determine why they participated in the activity and how they reacted if they were not able to run. Their responses indicated that feelings of relaxation were perceived as an important psychological benefit of involvement, and that increases in tension frequently occurred when they did not run. In a larger study of 345 male and female runners who averaged 20 to 25 miles per week, Robbins and Joseph (26) observed that descriptions of the sensations experienced following a missed workout typically fell into 3 categories: anxiousness, feelings of loss, and fatigue. Specific responses within the anxiousness category included feeling edgy, nervous, and unable to cope. Similar findings were obtained in studies of runners conducted by Blumenthal and coworkers (27) and by Acevedo and coworkers (28). More specifically, Blumenthal and coworkers found that highly dedicated runners cited tension and irritability as 2 of the most frequently experienced side effects of missing a planned workout, and Acevedo and coworkers found that marathon runners reported increased anxiety when they did not run.

Experimental studies in which exercise involvement has been manipulated provide the strongest evidence for increases in anxiety as a function of withdrawing the exercise stimulus. Morris and coworkers (29) examined anxiety and other negative mood states in a study involving middle-aged male runners. This study lasted for 6 weeks, with a 2-week baseline followed by a 2-week experimental phase in which the participants were randomly assigned to exercise deprivation or control groups. The deprivation group abstained from regular exercise during the experimental phase of the study, but the control group maintained their normal training schedule. Results revealed that runners who stopped exercising experienced increases in both perceived stress and anxiety during the deprivation period. Mondin and coworkers (30) obtained similar findings in a quasi-experimental study that employed an **ABA design**. Participants in that study were 10 individuals who engaged in aerobic activities such as jogging, cycling, or swimming for a minimum of 45 minutes per day on 6 days each week. These regular exercisers completed daily assessments of anxiety and other mood states over a 5-day period during which their exercise involvement was manipulated. They engaged in their normal exercise activities on days 1 (baseline) and 5 (follow-up) but remained sedentary on days 2, 3, and 4 (deprivation phase). Significant changes over time were noted for measures of tension and anxiety, with both measures peaking on the second day of exercise withdrawal and then returning toward baseline at follow-up. Effect sizes for tension were 0.50 after 24 hours of exercise deprivation and 1.30 after 48 hours of exercise deprivation, whereas effect sizes for state anxiety were 1.00 and 1.32 after 24 and 48 hours, respectively.

Effects Within Groups Characterized by High Anxiety

Anxiety experiences can range from mild, transitory episodes of heightened concern to extremely intense and debilitating symptoms that persist for an extended period. When the symptoms are extreme and/or persistent, an anxiety disorder may exist. Anxiety disorders are clusters of identifiable symptoms that disrupt day-to-day functioning enough to be considered clinically significant. Several types of anxiety disorders have been identified (31), including the following:

- Stress disorders
- Generalized anxiety disorder
- Phobias
- Panic disorder
- Obsessive-compulsive disorder

Distinguishing features for variants of these clinical anxiety disorders are summarized in Table 37.1

It is not unusual for anxiety disorders to accompany eating disorders, substance abuse, depression, or serious

TABLE 37.1. DISTINGUISHING FEATURES OF CLINICAL ANXIETY DISORDERS

Type of Disorder	Distinguishing Features
Acute Stress Disorder	Exposure to a traumatic event produces anxiety symptoms, re-experiencing of the event, and avoidance of stimuli related to the event for less than 4 weeks.
Posttraumatic Stress Disorder	Same as above, but symptoms persist for more than 4 weeks.
Generalized Anxiety Disorder	Constant, exaggerated worrisome thoughts and tension about routine life events and activities that last for at least 6 months. Usually accompanied by physical symptoms such as fatigue, insomnia, and impaired concentration.
Specific Phobia	Excessive, unreasonable, and persistent fear related to the presence or anticipated presence of a specific object or situation. Avoidance of these situations or objects whenever possible. Examples include claustrophobia (small spaces), acrophobia (heights), and arachnophobia (spiders).
Social Phobia	Marked and persistent fear of social or performance situations where there is exposure to unfamiliar people or to possible scrutiny by others. The individual fears that he or she will behave in a way that will be humiliating or embarrassing, and therefore avoids such situations whenever possible.
Agoraphobia	Excessive anxiety and avoidance behavior associated with open spaces or any place outside of one's home or a personal "safe zone."
Panic Disorder	Recurrent episodes of intense anxiety with sudden onset and brief duration. At least one of these "panic attacks" has been followed by a month or more of (a) persistent concern about having additional attacks, or (b) worry about the implications of the attack or its consequences (e.g., losing control, having a heart attack, "going crazy"), or (c) a significant change in behavior related to the attacks.
Obsessive-Compulsive Disorder	Repetitive thoughts (obsessions) or behaviors (compulsions) that the person feels compelled to continue despite awareness that they may be excessive or inappropriate. Feelings of distress are experienced when these thoughts or behaviors are stopped or blocked.
Anxiety Disorder due to Medical Condition	Persistent anxiety symptoms (including panic attacks, obsessions, and/or compulsions) that have arisen out of a general medical condition.

medical conditions. Treatment for anxiety disorders generally needs to be separated from treatment for these accompanying conditions, but some medications used for treating depression have also been found to be effective for anxiety disorders. **Selective serotonin reuptake inhibitors** (SSRIs) are an example of this type of medication; other anti-anxiety medications include **benzodiazepines** and beta-blockers. Forms of psychotherapy used to treat anxiety disorders include behavior therapy and cognitive-behavioral therapy. Behavior therapy focuses on changing specific reactions via reinforcement and conditioning, whereas cognitive-behavioral techniques focus on changing thought processes (and therefore reactions) toward situations that cause anxiety.

Given the documented anxiolytic effects of exercise and the anxiety-producing effects of exercise withdrawal, it is not surprising that there has been considerable speculation about the potential therapeutic uses of exercise for individuals with atypically high levels of anxiety. Such speculation has involved both the use of exercise in clinical settings (32), and the use of exercise in nonclinical settings by individuals experiencing transitory but substantial increases in anxiety (33). Recent studies suggest that such applications have merit, and that the anxiolytic effects of exercise may be especially potent in this context. For example, Breus and O'Connor (34) screened female university students for elevated trait anxiety scores and then exposed them to 20 minutes of low-intensity cycling. Twenty minutes after completing the exercise, these women exhibited reductions in state anxiety that were considerably larger than those typically observed in exercisers who are not characterized by high pre-exercise anxiety scores. In another study, Youngstedt and coworkers (35) used caffeine ingestion to artificially increase anxiety levels immediately before exercise. Participants in this study undertook 60 minutes of moderate-intensity cycling exercise after ingesting either 800 mg of caffeine or a placebo. Administration of the caffeine produced elevations in pre-exercise state anxiety, and subsequent reductions following exercise were substantially larger than those typically observed in studies without such elevations.

Such findings imply that exercise might be an effective anxiety management strategy within clinical populations characterized by chronically high levels of anxiety. Although an early study by Pitts and McClure (36) suggested that exercise might be contraindicated for individuals with clinically relevant levels of anxiety, the bulk of the evidence indicates otherwise (37). Indeed, investigations conducted in both medical and psychological populations have shown that exercise is associated with beneficial effects in clinical groups with elevated anxiety scores.

Kugler and coworkers (38) reviewed the evidence along these lines from a medical perspective. They conducted a meta-analytic review of studies examining the effects of exercise on anxiety in coronary rehabilitation settings where emotional disturbances such as anxiety and depression are commonly observed. Their review encompassed 13 studies conducted between 1965 and 1990 involving more than 1800 coronary patients and exercise programs of sufficient intensity and duration to produce training effects. Studies in which exercise was combined with other treatments (e.g., psychotherapy; counseling) were consciously excluded. The findings indicated that exercise participation led to reductions in anxiety among coronary patients, and that the average effect size (Cohen's *d*) was 0.31. Moreover, these beneficial effects were independent of methodological variables such as the duration of the exercise program or the time at which anxiety was assessed post-exercise. Kugler and coworkers concluded that, although exercise should not be considered the only treatment for emotional disturbances in coronary patients, it could operate effectively as an adjunct to other therapies. Similar conclusions have been drawn in more recent studies of cardiac patients as well as studies of other medical groups (39–42).

O'Connor and coworkers (43) reached a similar conclusion in a review of studies conducted with patients undergoing psychological treatment for anxiety disorders. Work by Martinsen and coworkers, for example, has suggested that participation in exercise programs consisting of brisk walking, jogging, or strength and flexibility training is associated with anxiety reductions in psychiatric inpatients hospitalized for a variety of anxiety disorders (44, 45). Similarly, Broocks and coworkers have shown that participation in 10 weeks of aerobic exercise training can produce decreases in anxiety among **panic disorder** patients that, although not as sudden as the decreases produced by drug treatment, are nevertheless significantly greater than placebo effects (46, 47). At least one study of the effects of acute exercise on anxiety symptoms in panic disorder patients reinforces these findings. O'Connor and Davis (48) found that state anxiety was significantly reduced in panic disorder sufferers after 20 minutes of treadmill exercise at 70% of $\dot{V}O_2$ peak, and that the reduction was greater than that produced by a control condition involving 20 minutes of quiet rest.

Mechanisms for Exercise and Anxiety Relationships

The prevalence of anxiety symptoms and anxiety disorders has prompted speculation about its etiology from psychodynamic, sociogenic, neurobiologic, genetic, and cognitive-behavioral perspectives (37, 43). Although quite disparate, each explanation has implications for understanding the anxiolytic effects of exercise. For example, O'Connor and coworkers (37, 43) argue that although clear evidence exists to indicate at least a moderate degree of genetic predisposition for anxiety disorders, there is also evidence that anxiety disorders and co-morbid states (e.g., depression) are influenced by behavioral, environmental, and cognitive factors. Thus, it is not surprising that psychological mechanisms such as distraction or "time-out" have been proposed as potential explanations for the anxiolytic effects of exercise. In brief, these explanations propose that being distracted from stressful stimuli is responsible for the anxiety reduction associated with certain forms of exercise, and

there is research evidence supporting them (34, 49). Similarly, cognitive theories of anxiety that focus on appraisal (i.e., personal evaluation) of external or internal events have also been proposed. Consistent with these models, cognitive-behavioral treatments employing re-interpretations of the somatic symptoms of anxiety as normal responses to physical exertion have proven successful (37, 43).

Despite such findings, however, no single theory or model appears capable of adequately explaining exercise-related reductions in anxiety. In other words, evidence that psychological mechanisms (e.g., distraction or cognitive restructuring) can attenuate anxiety does not vitiate the likelihood that physiological mechanisms are at the core of the anxiolytic effects of exercise (50). Indeed, investigators have recently been focusing more intently upon neurotransmitters and **thermogenic** effects as potential mechanisms for the observed relationship between exercise and anxiety reduction (37, 43, 51–53), and evidence has emerged suggesting that this interest is warranted.

Some investigators believe that exercise may exert anxiolytic effects through mechanisms associated with neurotransmitter systems (37, 43). Implicated neurotransmitters or neurotransmitter systems known to be involved in anxiety include the serotonergic system, the noradrenergic system, adenosine, and gamma-aminobutyric acid (GABA). Examination of these specific agents and biochemical systems has been stimulated by a variety of research findings, including the observation that SSRIs have been successfully employed in treating various anxiety disorders (54). Additional documentation of exercise effects on the neurotransmitter systems has been forthcoming (55), although well-controlled experiments focusing specifically on understanding the anxiolytic effects of exercise through these mechanisms have been limited.

Other investigators (7, 56) have hypothesized that thermogenic changes may play an important role in the anxiolytic effects of exercise. However, available evidence related to this view (i.e., that the anxiolytic effects of exercise are a consequence of increases in core temperature associated with physical exertion) is somewhat mixed. Specifically, although several studies have found that increases in core temperature are associated with reductions in state anxiety (57, 58), other studies have produced contrary findings (59, 60). Methodological inconsistencies (i.e., different measures of core temperature, modes and intensities of physical activity, and measures of anxiety) must be considered when evaluating these results. Nevertheless, it appears that currently only indirect support exists for the thermogenic hypothesis; although it remains a tenable explanation for the anxiolytic effects of exercise, it requires further evaluation (7, 53). In particular, the possibility that neurotransmitter and thermogenic mechanisms may operate interactively and/or redundantly as mediators of anxiety reduction deserves consideration (53).

Mode, Intensity, and Measurement Considerations

Additional issues deserve attention in future research related to the effects of exercise on anxiety. These issues include the effects of different exercise modes and intensities on post-exercise anxiety responses as well as the timing of assessment and the instruments used. With respect to exercise mode, it is clear from the literature reviewed above that the anxiolytic effects of exercise have been most clearly documented for aerobic activities. These activities have been shown repeatedly to reduce anxiety. However, findings from studies examining the effects of other forms of exercise (e.g., strength training) are not so clear-cut. For example, Raglin and coworkers (16) found that a 30-minute session of high-intensity cycling produced steady declines in systolic blood pressure (SBP) and state anxiety for 60 minutes after exercise, but 30 minutes of weight training at the same intensity did not. In fact, the weight training led to significant increases in both SBP and state anxiety that dissipated over a 60-minute post-exercise measurement period but did not move below baseline. Similarly, Koltyn and coworkers (15) measured state anxiety and SBP immediately before and after 50 minutes of weight training at self-selected intensities, and found that SBP increased but state anxiety did not change.

Findings from other studies suggest that exercise intensity and timing of assessment are important considerations when evaluating the effects of resistance exercise on anxiety. O'Connor and coworkers (61) found that state anxiety was reduced when resistance exercise was performed at 60% of 10-repetition maximum, but these declines were not significant until 90 minutes post-exercise. On the other hand, resistance exercise performed at 40% or 80% of the 10-repetition maximum did not have an anxiolytic effect at any time. Bartholomew and Linder (62) also found intensity-related effects in a study where intensity was defined as a percentage of each participant's 1-repetition maximum. In their study, both males and females reported increases in anxiety following 20 minutes of high-intensity resistance exercise (75–85% of 1-repetition maximum), but significant decreases in anxiety following 20 minutes of low-intensity exercise (40–50% of 1 repetition maximum). In a subsequent study, Bartholomew (63) observed significant increases in state anxiety and anger 5 minutes after high-intensity resistance exercise. However, anger returned to baseline after 15 minutes, and state anxiety was significantly below baseline within 30 minutes. Significant reductions in state anxiety were also reported 120 and 180 minutes after moderate-intensity resistance exercise in a study by Focht and coworkers (64).

Interpretation of intensity-related effects is also complicated by the structure of the questionnaires typically used to assess state anxiety. For example, Rejeski and coworkers (65) noted that ratings on activation-oriented items in the frequently used State Anxiety Inventory (SAI) (5) increased during exercise performed at 75% of age-predicted maximum heart rate reserve, but ratings on cognition-oriented items decreased. When these items were combined (as they typically are when state anxiety is assessed with the SAI), the net result was no change in the total score during exercise followed by a significant reduction after 10 minutes of recovery. McAuley and coworkers (66) obtained similar results in 2 additional studies where SAI items were analyzed in addition to total scores. In one of these investigations, SAI totals were no different from baseline when assessed immediately after 20 minutes of exercise performed at a level of 14 to 16 ("hard") on Borg's Ratings of Perceived Exertion (RPE) Scale (66). However, analyses of individual items revealed decreases for cognitive items, but increases for arousal-oriented items on the immediate post-exercise assessment. Subsequent decreases in ratings on all items produced significant reductions in total anxiety scores after 15 minutes of recovery. In the other investigation, low-intensity exercise led to decreased ratings on arousal-oriented items and cognitively oriented items as well as decreases in total SAI scores, whereas high-intensity exercise led to decreased ratings on cognitive items but increases on arousal-oriented items and SAI totals (67).

Ekkekakis and coworkers (68) have provided additional evidence that instrument properties can interact with timing of assessment and exercise intensity to influence self-reports of anxiety. In an initial study, they assessed state anxiety with the SAI before, during, and immediately after an aerobics class where participants exercised for 50 minutes at approximately 60% of age-predicted maximum heart rate reserve. Total SAI scores did not change from baseline to during exercise, but this lack of change in the total score was a result of divergent patterns of change for individual items. Specifically, items related to activation (e.g., not calm, not relaxed) tended to increase during exercise and then return to baseline immediately after exercise. On the other hand, items related to cognitive anxiety (e.g., upset, worried, confused) tended to decline during exercise and then either remain low or decline further after exercise. In a second study, participants completed the SAI immediately before, immediately after, and 10 minutes after 22 minutes of treadmill exercise at 75% of $\dot{V}O_2$ max. Findings revealed a significant increase in total scores from before to immediately after exercise, but no difference between pre-exercise scores and the 10-minute post-exercise scores. Consistent with the findings from the prior study, however, persistent increases in ratings for activation- and tension-related items (e.g., jittery, not calm) were responsible for the increased SAI totals immediately after exercise as well as the maintenance of relatively high totals at 10 minutes post-exercise. Examination of the ratings for items related to cognitive apprehension (e.g., nervous, worrying) revealed that they decreased significantly during exercise and remained low over the 10-minute recovery period. Thus, it appears that the arousal component of anxiety should be distinguished from the cognitive component of anxiety when evaluating the anxiolytic effects of high-intensity exercise. Many investigators have not done so, and conclusions based on composite scores should therefore be scrutinized carefully.

Summary

Given the prevalence of anxiety symptoms in the general population and the public health costs associated with anxiety disorders, it is important to identify effective and inexpensive protocols for both prevention and treatment. Exercise offers promise as one such protocol. Despite some suggestions to the contrary (8), there is a great deal of evidence that exercise has beneficial effects on anxiety symptoms, and that these benefits can be achieved within both clinical and nonclinical populations. Although the precise mechanisms responsible for the anxiolytic effects of exercise have not been determined, it is likely that multiple physiological and psychological processes play a role. At this time, moderate-intensity, aerobic exercise has the most consistent research support as a method for reducing anxiety symptoms. Other modes of exercise (e.g., strength training) and higher-intensity exercise may also have beneficial effects, but firm conclusions must await further research in which the components of anxiety and the timing of post-exercise anxiety assessments are examined more systematically. Therefore, until additional research findings are forthcoming, the following recommendations are offered for practitioners who wish to prescribe exercise for the purpose of preventing and/or reducing anxiety symptoms (Box 37.1; 69, 70).

First, it is important that the activity is freely chosen and matched to the participant's perceived level of skill. Activities undertaken because one "must" do so, or at a level that is well above or below one's perceived ability, will produce negative effect and undermine the potential for anxiolytic effects. Second, based on the findings reviewed here, the activity should have a substantial aerobic component. If there is a strong preference for nonaerobic activities (e.g., weight training), then it may be advisable to include an aerobic component (e.g., circuit training). Third, the activity should be undertaken at moderate intensity for 35 ± 15 minutes on 3 to 5 occasions per week.

What We Know
About Exercise and Anxiety

1 Aerobic exercise has a statistically significant and clinically meaningful impact on state and trait anxiety.

2 Acute bouts of aerobic exercise produce small-to-moderate reductions in state anxiety, and regular sessions of aerobic exercise reduce trait anxiety by approximately the same amount.

3 The anxiolytic effects of aerobic exercise have been documented using both self-report and psychophysiological measures.

4 Among regular exercisers, an inability to exercise is often associated with an increase in negative mood states (e.g., tension; anxiety).

5 The anxiolytic effects of exercise may be especially pronounced for individuals with higher-than-normal levels of anxiety (e.g., people who are under stress or suffering from an anxiety disorder).

6 The available evidence suggests that exercise activities are most likely to have anxiety-reducing effects if they include a substantial aerobic component and have a repetitive/rhythmical quality. It is also important that these activities are freely chosen, matched to existing skills and abilities, and undertaken at moderate intensity for at least 20 minutes on a regular basis.

What We Would Like to Know
About Exercise and Anxiety

1 How do the proposed mechanisms for the anxiolytic effects of exercise dovetail with each other? Do they operate simultaneously, or do certain mechanisms assume priority for certain forms of exercise?

2 What is the nature of the post-exercise anxiety response for nonaerobic exercise activities (e.g., strength training)?

3 How do exercise mode, exercise intensity, and timing of assessment interact to influence the profile of the post-exercise anxiety response?

4 Is it necessary or desirable to independently assess the arousal and cognitive components of anxiety in order to adequately understand the impact of exercise on anxiety?

BOX 37.1. Prescribing Exercise for Anxiety Reduction: Guidelines for Practitioners

- Freely chosen activities
- Matched to participant's perceived skills and abilities
- Activities include a substantial aerobic component
- Undertaken at a moderate intensity
- Last for 35 ± 15 minutes
- Take place 3–5 times per week
- Have repetitive and rhythmical qualities
- Weight-bearing and non-weight-bearing options are available

The guidelines for intensity, duration, and frequency are similar to those recommended for producing fitness effects in healthy adults (71). At the same time, they are flexible enough to encourage a noncompulsive attitude toward the exercise program. Fourth, activities with a closed-loop, repetitive quality (e.g., swimming, cycling, jogging, brisk walking) are recommended because they may foster dissociation and thereby provide more opportunity for distraction or "time-out" mechanisms to operate. The rhythmical nature of these activities may also have a dampening effect on the central nervous system via afferent feedback mechanisms (7). Finally, we recommend experimentation with both weight-bearing and non-weight-bearing activities. This recommendation is based on the assumption that, at some point, most active people will suffer minor injuries (e.g., strains; sprains) that will temporarily limit their ability to perform weight-bearing exercise. Cultivation of non-weight-bearing options could promote exercise adherence during these periods, and thereby prevent the anxiety-producing consequences of forced deprivation from a regular exercise regimen.

DISCUSSION QUESTIONS

1 Are anxiety-related problems "meaningful" from a public health perspective? If so, why? If not, why not?

2 What are meta-analyses, and what conclusions can we draw from meta-analytic reviews that have focused on the effects of exercise on anxiety?

3 What happens when regular exercisers are deprived of physical activity for an extended period?

4 What are anxiety disorders, and what forms do they take?

5 What mechanisms have been proposed to account for the anxiolytic effects of exercise?

6 Do aerobic exercise and resistance exercise have similar effects on anxiety responses?

7 What "structural features" of exercise seem to be important for producing reductions in anxiety?

CASE STUDY

Patient Information

Like most people, Joe was horrified by the events that took place in New York City on September 11, 2001. The tragic events of that day had a particularly strong impact on him, however, because he was about to embark on a long-awaited overseas trip. Joe had dreamed about international travel since he was young, and had been planning this trip for years. He desperately wanted to take the trip now, because he feared that the circumstances might never be right for him to do it again. After the 9/11 tragedy, however, he became increasingly worried about whether it would be safe to travel at this time. He kept seeing images of the disaster in his mind, and he thought constantly about what he should do. His preoccupation was so complete that he couldn't study effectively or perform his part-time job productively. He felt "spaced-out" most of the time, had great difficulty making decisions, withdrew from many of his normal activities, began losing weight, and suffered from insomnia.

Assessment and Treatment

Joe consulted his family doctor, who conducted a routine physical and found no obvious organic cause for Joe's loss of appetite, weight loss, and insomnia. During the examination, Joe's doctor asked if there were any unusual stressors in his life at the moment, and Joe commented that he had been "hit very hard" by the terrorist incident. He also told his doctor about the impending trip, and noted that he was "scared to death" about it and was "thinking about it 24 hours a day." Upon hearing Joe's description of his symptoms, his doctor wrote him a nonrefillable prescription for a benzodiazepine, and gave him a referral letter for a consultation with a psychologist who specialized in treating anxiety disorders.

The psychologist used a cognitive-behavioral approach to help Joe reduce his anxiety. This approach involved discussions about the strong impact that thoughts have on emotions and the use of exercises designed to help Joe distinguish between realistic (rational) concerns for safety and unrealistic (irrational) concerns. It also involved deliberate listing and evaluation of the pros and cons associated with the planned trip and its possible alternatives. The psychologist did not ask Joe to stop taking the benzodiazepine that his doctor had prescribed, but she did request that he keep a journal of how much medication he was using and when he used it. She also encouraged him to get at least 30 minutes of moderate-intensity exercise every second day, and she helped him to learn coping skills for anxiety management. These coping skills included abdominal breathing, mental imagery, an abbreviated form of progressive muscular relaxation, and a strategy for blocking intrusive thoughts and refocusing attention. Over a period of weeks, the combined impact of this cognitive-behavioral therapy program was a reduction in Joe's level of anxiety and a rational assessment of his options. In the end, Joe took his trip, but not before he postponed it for 6 months "in order to let things settle down." It proved to be a wise decision, because he no longer felt as much anxiety, and he enjoyed the experience immensely.

It is important for all health professionals to recognize the limits of their training and to develop a referral network of practitioners in related fields. The symptoms that prompt an initial visit to the clinic (in this case, Joe's loss of weight and insomnia) may be secondary to other problems. A single-minded focus on dealing with the presenting symptoms and/or a reluctance to utilize the expertise of colleagues in other professions is counterproductive and potentially dangerous.

Questions

1 What are the primary symptoms that Joe is experiencing? Use the information in the "Patient Information" section of the case study to answer this question.

2 Do you believe Joe had an anxiety disorder? If so, which of the disorders summarized in Table 37.1 best fits his symptoms, and why?

3 Joe's treatment program contained medical, behavioral, and cognitive elements. Can you identify the components of his treatment program that fall under each of these headings?

REFERENCES

1. Üstün TB, Sartorius N. Mental Illness in General Health Care: An International Study. London: John Wiley & Sons; 1995.
2. National Institute of Mental Health. Quick facts about anxiety disorders. Available at: http://www.thebody.com/nimh/anxiety_facts.html. Accessed April 15, 2001.
3. McDonald DG, Hodgdon JA. Psychological Effects of Aerobic Fitness Training: Research and Theory. New York: Springer-Verlag; 1991.
4. Cohen J. A power primer. Psychol Bull 1992;112:155–159.
5. Speilberger CD. Manual for the State-Trait Anxiety Inventory (Form Y. Self-evaluation Questionnaire). Palo Alto, CA: Consulting Psychologists Press; 1983.
6. Taylor JA. A personality scale of manifest anxiety. J Abnorm Soc Psychol 1953;48:285–290.
7. Petruzzello SJ, Landers DM., Hatfield BD, Kubitz KA, Salazar W. A meta-analysis on the anxiety-reducing effects of acute and chronic exercise: outcomes and mechanisms. Sports Med 1991;11:143–182.
8. Schlicht W. Does physical exercise reduce anxious emotions? A meta-analysis. Anxiety Stress Coping 1994;6:275–288.
9. Petruzzello SJ. Does physical exercise reduce anxious emotions? A reply to W. Schlicht's meta-analysis. Anxiety Stress Coping 1995;8:353–356.
10. Long BC, van Stavel R. Effects of exercise training on anxiety: a meta-analysis. J Appl Sport Psychol 1995;7:167–189.
11. Raglin JS. Anxiolytic effects of physical activity. In: Morgan WP, ed. Physical Activity and Mental Health. Washington, DC: Taylor & Francis; 1997:107–126.
12. O'Connor PJ, Carda RD, Graf BK. Anxiety and intense running exercise in the presence and absence of interpersonal competition. Int J Sports Med 1991;12:423–426.
13. O'Connor PJ, Petruzzello SJ, Kubitz KA, Robinson TL. Anxiety responses to maximal exercise testing. Br J Sports Med 1995;29:97–102.
14. Raglin JS, Wilson M. State anxiety following 20-min of leg ergometry at differing intensities. Int J Sports Med 1996;17:467–471.
15. Koltyn KF, Raglin JS, O'Connor PJ, Morgan WP. Influence of weight training on state anxiety, body awareness, and blood pressure. Int J Sports Med 1995;16:266–269.
16. Raglin JS, Turner PE, Eksten F. State anxiety and blood pressure following 30 min of leg ergometry or weight training. Med Sci Sports Exerc 1993;25:1044–1048.
17. Steptoe A, Edwards S, Moses J, Mathews A. The effects of exercise training on mood and perceived coping ability in anxious adults from the general population. J Psychosom Res 1989;33:537–547.
18. Simons CW, Birkimer JC. An exploration of factors predicting the effects of aerobic conditioning on mood state. J Psychosom Res 1988;32:63–75.
19. De Gues EJC, Van Doornen LJP, Orlebeke JF. Regular exercise and aerobic fitness in relation to psychological make-up and physiological stress reactivity. Psychosom Med 1993;55:347–363.
20. Raglin JS, Wilson GS. Overtraining in athletes. In: Hanin Y, ed. Emotions in Sport. Champaign, IL: Human Kinetics; 2000:191–207.
21. Szabo A. The impact of exercise deprivation on well-being of habitual exercisers. Aust J Sci Med Sport 1995;27:68–75.
22. Baekeland F. Exercise deprivation: sleep and psychological reactions. Arch Gen Psychiatry 1970;22:365–369.

23. Sachs ML, Pargman D. Running addiction: a depth interview examination. J Sport Beh 1979;2:143–155.

24. Thaxton L. Physiological and psychological effects of short-term exercise addiction on habitual runners. J Sport Psychol 1982;4:73–80.

25. Harris DV. Women runners' views of running. Percept Mot Skills 1981;53:395–402.

26. Robbins JM, Joseph P. Experiencing exercise withdrawal: possible consequences of therapeutic and mastery running. J Sport Psychol 1985;5:314–331.

27. Blumenthal JA, O'Toole LC, Chang JL. Is running an analogue of anorexia nervosa? An empirical study of obligatory running and anorexia nervosa. JAMA 1984;252:520–523.

28. Acevedo EO, Dzewaltowski DA, Gill DL, Noble JM. Cognitive orientations of ultramarathoners. Sport Psychol 1992;6:242–252.

29. Morris M, Steinberg H, Sykes EA, Salmon P. Effects of temporary withdrawal from regular running. J Psychosom Research 1990;34:493–500.

30. Mondin GW, Morgan WP, Piering PD, et al. Psychological consequences of exercise deprivation in habitual exercisers. Med Sci Sports Exerc 1996;28:1199–1203.

31. American Psychiatric Association. Diagnostic and Statistical Manual of Mental Disorders. 4th ed. Text revision. Washington, DC: Author; 2000.

32. Tkachuk GA, Martin GL. Exercise therapy for patients with psychiatric disorders: research and clinical implications. Prof Psychol Res Prac 1999;30:275–282.

33. Plante TG, Marcotte D, Manuel G, Willemsen E. The influence of brief episodes of aerobic exercise activity, soothing music-nature scenes condition, and suggestion on coping with test-taking anxiety. Int J Stress Manage 1996;3:155–166.

34. Breus MJ, O'Connor PJ. Exercise-induced anxiolysis: a test of the "time-out" hypothesis in high anxious females. Med Sci Sports Exerc 1998;30:1107–1112.

35. Youngstedt SD, O'Connor PJ, Crabbe JB, Dishman RK. Acute exercise reduces caffeine-induced anxiogenesis. Med Sci Sports Exerc 1998;30:740–745.

36. Pitts FN, McClure JN. Lactate metabolism in anxiety neurosis. N Engl J Med 1967;277:1329–1336.

37. O'Connor PJ, Smith JC, Morgan WP. Physical activity does not provoke panic attacks in patients with panic disorder: a review of the evidence. Anxiety Stress Coping 2000;13:333–353.

38. Kugler J, Seelbach H, Krüskemper GM. Effects of rehabilitation exercise programmes on anxiety and depression in coronary patients: a meta-analysis. Br J Clin Psychol 1994;33:401–410.

39. Emery CF, Schein RL, Hauck ER, McIntyre NR. Psychological and cognitive outcomes of a randomized trial of exercise among patients with chronic obstructive pulmonary disease. Health Psychol 1998;17:232–240.

40. Courneya, KS, Keats MR, Turner AR. Physical exercise and quality of life in cancer patients following high dose chemotherapy and autologous bone marrow transplantation. Psychooncology 2000;9:127–136.

41. Peters ML, Turner SM, Blanchard EB. The effects of aerobic exercise on chronic tension-type headache. Headache Q 1996;7:330–334.

42. Tanco S, Linden W, Earle T. Well-being and morbid obesity in women: a controlled therapy evaluation. Int J Eat Disord 1998;23:325–339.

43. O'Connor PJ, Raglin JS, Martinsen EW. Physical activity, anxiety, and anxiety disorders. Int J Sport Psychol 2000;31:136–155.

44. Martinsen EW, Hoffart A, Solberg ØY. Aerobic and non-aerobic forms of exercise in the treatment of anxiety disorders. Stress Med 1989;5:115–120.

45. Martinsen EW, Sandvik L, Kolbjørnsrud OB. Aerobic exercise in the treatment of nonpsychotic mental disorders: an exploratory study. Nord J Psychiatry 1989;43:521–529.

46. Bandelow B, Broocks A, Pekrun G, et al. The use of the Panic and Agoraphobia Scale (P & A) in a controlled clinical trial. Pharmacopsychiatry 2000;33:174–181.

47. Broocks A, Bandelow B, Pekrun G, et al. Comparison of aerobic exercise, clomipramine, and placebo in the treatment of panic disorder. Am J Psychiatry 1998;155:603–609.

48. O'Connor PJ, Davis JC. Anxiety reduction following intense exercise in individuals with panic attacks. Paper presented at: Annual Meeting of the American Psychological Association; August 1992; Washington, DC.

49. Bahrke MS, Morgan WP. Anxiety reduction following exercise and meditation. Cognit Ther Res 1978;2:323–333.

50. Morgan WP, O'Connor PJ. Exercise and mental health. In: Dishman RK, ed. Exercise Adherence: Its Impact on Public Health. Champaign, IL: Human Kinetics; 1988:91–121.

51. Chaouloff F. The serotonin hypothesis. In: Morgan WP, ed. Physical Activity and Mental Health. Washington, DC: Taylor & Francis; 1997:179–198.

52. Dishman RK. The norepinephrine hypothesis. In: Morgan WP, ed. Physical Activity and Mental Health. Washington, DC: Taylor & Francis; 1997;199–212.

53. Koltyn KF. The thermogenic hypothesis. In: Morgan WP, ed. Physical Activity and Mental Health. Washington, DC: Taylor & Francis; 1997:213–226.

54. Goddard AW, Charney DS. SSRIs in the treatment of panic disorder. Depress Anxiety 1998;8(suppl 1):114–120.

55. Dishman RK. Brain monoamines, exercise, and behavioral stress: animal models. Med Sci Sports Exerc 1997b;29:63–74.

56. deVries HA. Tension reduction with exercise. In: Morgan WP, Goldston SE, eds. Exercise and Mental Health. Washington, DC: Hemisphere; 1987:99–104.

57. Petruzzello SJ, Landers DM, Salazar W. Exercise and anxiety reduction: examination of temperature as an explanation for affective change. J Sport Exerc Psychol 1993;15:63–76.

58. Raglin JS, Morgan WP. Influence of vigorous exercise on mood states. Behav Therapist 1985;8:179–183.

59. Reeves DL, Levinson DM, Justesen DR, Lubin B. Endogenous hyperthermia in normal human subjects: experimental study of emotional states (II). Int J Psychosomatics 1985;32:18–23.

60. Youngstedt SD, Dishman RK, Cureton KJ, Peacock LJ. Does body temperature mediate anxiolytic effect of acute exercise? J Appl Physiol 1993;74:825–831.

61. O'Connor PJ, Bryant CX, Veltri JP, Gebhardt SM. State anxiety and ambulatory blood pressure following resistance exercise in females. Med Sci Sports Exerc 1993;25:516–521.

62. Bartholomew JB, Linder DE. State anxiety following resistance exercise: the role of gender and exercise intensity. J Behav Med 1998;21:205–219.

63. Bartholomew JB. The effect of resistance exercise on manipulated pre-exercise mood states for male exercisers. J Sport Exerc Psychol 1999;21:39–51.

64. Focht BC, Koltyn KF, Bouchard LJ. State anxiety and blood pressure responses following different resistance exercise sessions. Int J Sport Psychol 2000;31:376–390.

65. Rejeski WJ, Hardy CJ, Shaw J. Psychometric confounds of assessing state anxiety in conjunction with acute bouts of vigorous exercise. J Sport Exerc Psychol 1991;13:65–74.

66. McAuley E, Mihalko SL, Bane SM. Acute exercise and anxiety reduction: does the environment matter? J Sport Exerc Psychol 1996;18:408–419.

67. Katula JA, Blissmer BJ, McAuley E. Exercise and self-efficacy effects on anxiety reduction in healthy, older adults. J Behav Med 1999;22:233–247.

68. Ekkekakis P, Hall EE, Petruzzello SJ. Measuring state anxiety in the context of acute exercise using the State Anxiety Inventory: an attempt to resolve the brouhaha. J Sport Exerc Psychol 1999;21:205–229.

69. Berger BG, Owen DR. Stress reduction and mood enhancement in four exercise modes: swimming, body conditioning, hatha yoga, and fencing. Res Q Exerc Sport 1988;59:148–159.

70. Csikszentmihalyi M. Flow: The Psychology of Optimal Experience. New York: Harper & Row; 1990.

71. American College of Sports Medicine. Guidelines for Exercise Testing and Prescription. 5th ed. Baltimore, MD: Williams & Wilkins; 1995.

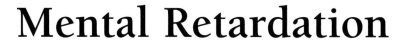

CHAPTER 38

Mental Retardation

Bo Fernhall

Overview

Mental retardation (MR) is the most common developmental disorder in industrialized society, with an estimated prevalence of 3% of the total population (1). Traditionally, an individual's **IQ scores** constituted the sole definition of MR. By this definition, 4 classifications typically were used: mild (IQ scores between 50 and 70), moderate (IQ scores between 35 and 40), severe (IQ scores between 25 and 40) and profound (IQ scores below 25) (2). Although these classifications are still widely used, a new classification system has been adopted by the Association for Retarded Citizens (ARC) (formerly the American Association on Mental Retardation). According to the ARC, MR should be defined in the following manner:

> MR is manifested by significantly subaverage intellectual functioning, existing concurrently with related

limitations in two or more of the following adaptive skills areas: communication, self-care, home living, social skills, community use, self direction, health and safety, functional academics, leisure and work. In addition, MR must be evident before age 18 (3).

Significant subaverage intellectual function is usually defined as an IQ of 2 standard deviations below the mean, thus an individual must have an IQ below 70, plus adaptive skill deficits, to meet the initial classification for MR. However, even though MR is developmental in nature, it is no longer considered a static, nonchangeable condition. Instead, it is now recognized that MR is a fluid condition, and with early intervention, some individuals may progress to the point where they would no longer be classified as having MR (4).

Under the new definition, there are 2 levels of MR—mild and severe—instead of the traditional 4 levels. Classification is based primarily on how well an individual can function in the adaptive skill areas and the level of support the individual requires (1). There are 4 designated levels of support: intermittent (on an as-needed basis, either high or low intensity; limited (support needed consistently over time, but of lesser intensity); extensive (regular involvement in at least some environments); and pervasive (constant high-intensity support across environments—constant care). In general, persons with mild MR have IQs between 35 and 70, need adaptive schooling, have minimal reading, writing, and math capabilities, but can be productive in unskilled or semi-skilled jobs; they may manage independent living, or group living in the community. It is estimated that over 90% of all persons with MR would be classified with mild MR (1, 4). Individuals with severe MR usually would have an IQ below 35 and typically depend on others for care. It is not unusual to find gross motor deficits, anatomical deformities, and sensory deficits in this population. Most individuals with severe MR will have substantial problems with simple self-care skills (4). Only 10% or less of the population with MR would be considered to have severe MR.

Over the past 30 years, there has been a movement to de-institutionalize persons with MR. As a result, most large institutions have been closed, and the individuals formerly housed in them have been placed in community settings. Today the great majority of persons with MR live in the community, either at home with their parents or guardians, in group homes, or in assisted-living situations. Coupled with mainstreaming children with MR in the public schools, individuals with MR are gradually becoming more integrated in the community. This also increases the likelihood of contact with **exercise** professionals in school physical education programs, health clubs, YMCAs, or special community-based exercise programs (5).

Pathophysiology

Although mental retardation has many potential causes, frequently there is no specifically known cause. Some identified contributing factors to MR include genetic and maternal disorders, birth trauma, and infectious diseases. It is also believed that behavioral or societal factors such as poverty, malnutrition, maternal drug and alcohol use, and severe stimulus deprivation can contribute to MR. In general, the contributing factors fall into the following groups: (1) **chromosomal abnormalities**, of which **Down syndrome** (DS) and fragile X syndrome are the most common; (2) genetic disorders such as phenylketonuria, Tay-Sachs disease, and neurofibromatosis; (3) maternal infections during pregnancy, such as rubella and herpes simplex; (4) maternal drug use during pregnancy, including alcohol, cocaine, and prescription medications; (5) other perinatal factors such as low birth weight, prematurity, and CNS bleed-

ing; (6) postnatal factors including malnutrition, lead poisoning, severe infections accompanied by high fever, and asphyxia (1, 4).

The most common known cause of MR is maternal drug abuse, with fetal alcohol syndrome being the most common form. The incidence of fetal alcohol syndrome may be as high as 1 in 100 births (3, 4). When maternal drug or alcohol use is more severe, so is the resulting developmental disability. Fetal alcohol syndrome can be accompanied by physical modifications such as growth deficiencies, changed facial features, poor motor coordination, and hypotonia (4). However, the most common characteristics are behavioral, such as attention deficit disorders, poor organizational skills, and poor judgment.

The second leading known cause of MR is Down syndrome (DS), with an incidence rate of approximately 1 in 800 births. Maternal age is a definite risk factor, as the incidence of DS increases to 1 in 400 births in women older than age 35, and increases further with maternal age. The risk of having a child with DS at age 45 is 1 in 35 (6). Down syndrome is caused by an extra chromosome 21, leading to 47 chromosomes instead of 46, in over 90% of cases. Hence, DS is also known as trisomy 21. Other causes of DS include disjunction (24 chromosomes in one haploid cell and 22 in the other) and translocation (2 chromosomes grown together as 1, but containing the genetic material of both) (6).

Down syndrome is often associated with physical and physiological characteristics that could impact the exercise response. These include small stature, short limbs and digits, digital malformations (especially malformations of the feet and toes causing difficulties with walking or running), small mouth and nasal cavities with a large protruding tongue (can impact breathing), and slanted eyes. Also associated with DS is joint laxity, which is especially important because of the common occurrence of atlantoaxial instability, skeletal muscle hypotonia, and pulmonary hypoplasia. In addition, up to 40% of individuals born with DS have congenital heart disease. Most individuals with DS exhibit reduced immune function, are at much higher risk than normal of developing leukemia, and most develop Alzheimer's disease as they age (1, 6, 7).

Individuals with MR have much higher mortality rates compared to their peers without MR (from 1.7 to 4 times higher) (8). Mortality rates are associated with lower IQ and poor self-care skills. The highest mortality rates are found in persons with DS, whose average life expectancy is only 55 years if they survive past age 1 and do not have congenital heart disease (9, 10). Coupled with the high mortality rate is an increased rate of medical problems in populations with MR (11). The most common medical problems of persons with MR are cardiovascular and pulmonary disorders, and for persons with DS, infections, leukemia, and early development of Alzheimer's disease (11). It has been suggested that low levels of physical activity further exacerbate the mortality and morbidity of persons with MR (8, 11). Consequently, a major challenge for exercise professionals is to improve physical activity habits of individuals with MR.

Potential Medications

It is not unusual for individuals with MR to take various psychotropic medications, with antidepressants being fairly common. Many persons with MR also take anticonvulsive agents. These medications do not affect MR per se, but help control inappropriate behavior and physiological symptoms caused by MR. Some medications such as hypnotics are used to control psychotic behavior, but only in more severe cases. Use of beta-blockers is common, particularly in persons without DS (1).

Hypothyroidism is a common condition in individuals with DS. This condition is often diagnosed during adolescence or in early adulthood. Thus, many individuals will be receiving thyroxine replacement therapy. It is not unusual to observe large weight gains in persons with DS during late adolescence, which may indicate hypothyroidism or poor lifestyle choices. However, large weight gains should be evaluated in this population, even in persons who have already been diagnosed, because dose titration of the thyroxine replacement therapy is often necessary as the individual matures.

Although psychotropic medications can have minor influences on heart rate and blood pressure, in general, they do not substantially alter the response to acute or chronic exercise. They may produce inappropriate "false positive or negative" stress test results, but it is more likely that they affect the individual's ability to understand and follow directions, and motivation to perform during high-intensity exercise (1, 12). Thyroid medications increase both heart rate and blood pressure and may provoke arrhythmias. Thyroxine increases cardiac contractility and may provoke anginal episodes until the dose has been appropriately titrated. Beta-blockers will reduce heart rate and blood pressure both at rest and in response to exercise. It is also possible that beta-blockers may reduce work capacity in individuals not limited by angina (13).

The Exercise Response

Cardiovascular Exercise Responses

Cardiovascular fitness is usually evaluated by treadmill or cycle ergometry **exercise testing**, with or without metabolic measurements. Typically, terms such as *aerobic capacity*, *work capacity* and *peak oxygen uptake* are used interchangeably. The most common findings in persons with MR are low work capacity and peak oxygen uptake ($\dot{V}O_2$ peak) values (Box 38.1). Most studies report values considerably below expected norms in nondisabled populations regardless of age (1, 11). In children, $\dot{V}O_2$ peak values are generally between 25 and 41 ml/kg/min (11, 14–16), which is

---

BOX 38.1. Peak Cardiovascular Exercise Responses in Individuals With MR

- Low work capacity
- Low $\dot{V}O_2$ peak (usually between 25–35 ml/kg/min in young adults
- Low maximal heart rates—usually 15–30 bpm below predicted levels
- Low peak exercise ventilation
- Normal respiratory exchange ratios
- Normal blood pressure responses
- May have problems with motivation to perform maximal exercise

---

considerably below expected $\dot{V}O_2$ peak levels of 45 to 55 ml/kg/min (17). However, some children show normal values, and $\dot{V}O_2$ peak as high as 56 ml/kg/min has been reported. A recent study (18) showed that boys with MR exhibited similar $\dot{V}O_2$ peak values to their nondisabled peers, whereas girls with MR showed much lower values compared to their nondisabled peers. Consequently, the available data are highly variable, and work capacity of children with MR may be low or in the normal range.

Adults with MR also have very low $\dot{V}O_2$ peak values and reported $\dot{V}O_2$ peak is typically between 25 and 35 ml/kg/min for young adults below 30 years of age (19–23). However, individual values over 50 ml/kg/min have been reported (24). A recent investigation of runners with MR (25) also showed that in this select, but highly active group, $\dot{V}O_2$ peak averaged 56 ml/kg/min, suggesting that aerobic capacity can be above average in well-trained persons with MR. At this time, no data are available on older individuals with MR, as the research to date has included only persons younger than age 45 years.

Both children and adults with DS have even lower $\dot{V}O_2$ peak values compared to their peers with MR but without DS. Findings in persons with DS are much more uniform than in persons without DS. In general children, adolescents, and young adults with DS show $\dot{V}O_2$ peak values of 18 to 25 ml/kg/min, with little influence of age (20, 23, 26, 27). However, there are no data on persons with DS over age 40. A recent study showed that trained young adults with DS exhibited higher aerobic capacity than their untrained counterparts, but their $\dot{V}O_2$ peak values were still below 40 ml/kg/min, even though some trained as much as 10 hours per week (28). Thus, DS appears to negatively affect aerobic capacity.

In addition to low aerobic capacity, most individuals with MR also have low maximal heart rates. Persons with MR without DS exhibit maximal heart rates of 12–15 beats per minute below predicted values. Children with MR but without DS may exhibit normal maximal heart rates. Individuals with DS have even lower maximal heart rates, often

30 to 35 beats per minute below predicted values (29). It is likely that the low maximal heart rates contribute to the low V̇O₂ peak values because of limitations to cardiac output. Both children and adults exhibit low maximal heart rates, but maximal heart rates are more consistently low in persons with DS regardless of age.

Consistent with low aerobic capacity, peak exercise ventilation is also low in persons with MR, and is extremely low in persons with DS (23). It is unknown if ventilation limits exercise performance in this population, or if exercise ventilatory capacity is reduced in conjunction with low aerobic capacity. In persons with DS, exercise ventilation may be limited because of anatomical characteristics, such as small mouth and nasal cavities, protruding tongue, and pulmonary hypoplasia (11). Although maximal ventilation is reduced, the respiratory exchange ratio (RER) is typically in a normal range, suggesting effort during the test is not a limitation in persons with MR. Individuals with DS typically exhibit slightly lower RER than their peers without DS, but this does not appear to be the reason for their lower aerobic capacity (23).

Field Testing

Cardiorespiratory fitness in persons with MR is usually evaluated by means of exercise testing using various field tests. Field tests are attractive because they provide information on work capacity and V̇O₂ peak without the need for expensive laboratory-based testing, and many field tests tend to be submaximal in nature. The most commonly used field tests in persons with MR are the 300-yard run/walk, 1-mile run/walk, 1.5-mile run/walk, the 1-mile Rockport walk fitness test (RWFT), the 20-m shuttle run, step testing, and submaximal cycle ergometry. However, it is important to realize that only some of these tests have been validated for use in persons with MR. Based on available research, the 600-yard run/walk, 1-mile RWFT, and the 20-m shuttle run are valid and reliable tests for children with MR (16, 30, 31). For adults with MR, the 1-mile RWFT and the 1.5-mile run/walk have been validated (24, 30, 32, 33). The other tests are either not valid as indicators of aerobic capacity in persons with MR, or they have not yet been validated; therefore, they should not be used (Box 38.2).

Field-testing of persons with MR yields similar results as laboratory tests, showing that work capacity and run performance are reduced in this population. Valid formulas for predicting V̇O₂ peak are available for each of the recommended tests (16, 24, 30–34), although the formulas differ from those used in nondisabled populations. Children and adolescents with MR differ from their nondisabled peers in that run performance does not improve with maturation (35). Furthermore, run performance is dependent on **muscle strength**, aerobic capacity, and body composition in children with MR, whereas run performance is primarily a function of aerobic capacity and body composition in nondisabled children (17, 36).

BOX 38.2. Field Tests for Evaluating Cardiovascular Fitness in Individuals With MR

Validated Field Tests for Adults With MR
- 1.5-mile run/walk
- 1-mile Rockport Walk Fitness Test

Validated Field Tests for Children With MR
- 20-m shuttle run (FITNESSGRAM shuttle run)
- 600-yard run/walk
- 1-mile Rockport Walk Fitness Test

Tests NOT Valid for Use With Persons With MR
- 1-mile run/walk
- 0.5-mile run/walk
- 300-yard run/walk
- Step testing
- Submaximal cycle ergometer testing (YMCA or Astrand protocols)

Muscle Strength

Muscle strength has been extensively evaluated in persons with MR using a variety of measurement tools including exercise machines, hand-grip dynamometry, hand-held dynamometry, leg and back dynamometry, and isokinetic dynamometry (15, 28, 36–42). Regardless of the type of measurement, the results are very uniform. Individuals with MR have very low levels of strength; typically a reduction of 30% to 50% compared to values of nondisabled individuals is seen (37, 39, 41, 42). Individuals with DS exhibit even lower levels of muscle strength, typically exhibiting between 30% and 40% of strength levels expected of nondisabled individuals (39, 40). These low levels of muscle strength are present in childhood (15, 36, 41) and persist into adulthood (38–40, 42). Interestingly, in individuals with MR who were extremely active and exhibited very high aerobic capacity, muscle strength was still below expected levels and about 25% below the strength values of age and activity matched subjects without MR (25).

The low strength levels of individuals with MR may have several important implications. Muscle strength is important for performing recreational activities and activities of daily living (40, 43) and may be a prerequisite for vocational activities (1). More importantly, muscle strength has been shown to be related to work productivity in persons with MR (44) and may be related to level of independence (11). In addition, leg strength has been shown to contribute to V̇O₂ peak in persons with MR, suggesting that poor muscle strength may limit aerobic capacity in this population (15, 37). Consequently, low levels of muscle strength are of considerable concern for individuals with MR.

Exercise Test Recommendations

Pre-test Considerations

Testing individuals with MR can be challenging because of this population's unique characteristics. Since many persons with MR may have difficulty with task understanding, understanding directions, motivation to perform, short attention spans, and possibly a variety of behavioral problems (11), it is essential to conduct an appropriate familiarization process. The familiarization process allows the individual to become accustomed to the laboratory setting and test personnel, practice the test protocols, and try the various pieces of equipment. Depending on the person being tested and the testing to be conducted, an individual may need 1 to 3 familiarization sessions. The person is ready to be tested when he/she can readily perform the beginning stages of the tests without undue stress and behavioral problems.

One of the main aspects of the familiarization session(s) is to establish the correct protocol for testing. That may involve establishing the appropriate walking or running speed or work rate increments and evaluating the person for possible ambulatory or coordination problems that may impact test results. Allowing the individual appropriate familiarization will increase the likelihood of appropriate test performance and decrease the chances of early test termination due to fear rather than fatigue (1).

Pre-test screening is also important when testing individuals with MR. Although the literature offers no information regarding untoward responses in persons with MR, relatively few persons older than age 40 have been tested. Considering the high prevalence of obesity, inactivity, and low work capacity in this population, pre-screening for signs of premature cardiovascular disease is indicated in persons over age 30. Furthermore, it is important to obtain information on other common co-morbidities such as diabetes, neuromuscular conditions, hypertension, musculoskeletal disorders, pulmonary problems, and coordination problems. It is also important to evaluate medications that may impact the exercise response. Part of this information can be obtained from the individual with MR being tested, but often, most of the pre-screening information must be obtained from the parent or guardian.

Individuals with DS present a unique challenge, and pre-screening is especially important in this population. Up to 40% of individuals with DS have some form of congenital heart disease, such as septal or valvular defects, tetralogy of Fallot, or aortic arch defects (1). In addition, up to 17% of individuals with DS have atlantoaxial instability (laxity of ligaments between C1 and C2), which makes them susceptible to spinal cord injury. It is often recommended that running and jumping activities should be avoided in these individuals, but there is little evidence for the efficacy of this recommendation. Tumbling activities are contraindicated in individuals with atlantoaxial instability. Furthermore, persons with DS may also exhibit skeletal muscle hypotonia and/or pulmonary problems. Because persons with DS often have reduced immune function, it is not unusual for these individuals to present with infections.

Protocol Selection

Cardiovascular Exercise Testing

Treadmill testing has been the most common form of testing used in persons with MR. A variety of protocols have been used and validated for this population. Many studies have used an individualized approach (5, 23), where the walking speed is determined based on the walking ability of the subject. Most commonly, walking speeds of 2.0 to 3.5 mph have been selected. Walking speed is kept constant and grade is typically increased 2.5% to 4.0% every 2 to 3 minutes. In protocols that use a grade ceiling, after grade reaches 12.5%, the treadmill speed is gradually increased, with the subject finishing the test jogging (5, 45). In addition to individualized protocols, modified versions of Balke and Naughton protocols have been suggested (1).

Standard cycle ergometry has not been used successfully for exercise testing of persons with MR (5). This is probably related to problems associated with keeping constant pedaling rates during the test using mechanically braked cycle ergometers. It is unknown if using electronically braked ergometers will solve this problem in persons with MR. However, combined arm and leg ergometry using the Schwinn Air-Dyne has been successfully used and validated for persons with MR (1, 45). This form of ergometry appears to yield similar results to treadmill testing. The validated protocol starts at 25 watts and increases work rate by 25 watts every 2 minutes (5).

Muscular Strength Testing

Protocols for testing muscular strength in persons with MR vary by the type of strength testing. Isokinetic testing is well validated and reproducible in this population (15, 37, 41). Testing is typically conducted at 60 and 90 degrees/second, but 30 degrees/second has also been used (37, 41, 45). It is suggested that a 10-minute general warm up (e.g., treadmill walking or cycle ergometry) be conducted prior to the strength tests, followed by 1 or 2 isokinetic practice trials of 6 to 8 repetitions (46). For both 60- and 90-degree/second isokinetic testing, 2 trials of 6 repetitions are used, and the highest value produced during any one muscular contraction is considered peak torque (15, 37, 41).

Isometric strength can be evaluated by hand grip testing, leg and back dynamometry, and hand-held dynamometry using a Nicholas Manual Muscle Tester (28, 45, 47, 48). A warm up may not be as crucial for these tests, and the research is unclear whether warm up is useful. Several practice trials are allowed after familiarization. Usually 2 or 3 test trials are performed, and the highest value produced is used as peak isometric strength for the muscle group tested.

Exercise Programming Options

Endurance-Training Programs

Although many exercise-training studies aimed at improving cardiovascular fitness have been conducted, few have employed appropriate methodologies (5, 49). The major weakness in most studies is failure to use validated tests or lack of control groups. Very few studies have used a randomized controlled trial approach. Nevertheless, the information in the literature is remarkably uniform. Box 38.3 summarizes the expected outcomes of exercise training in persons with MR. Several studies have shown that both children and adults with MR can improve field test or submaximal exercise performance following an **endurance-training** program (50–53). Unfortunately, none of these studies used appropriately validated test protocols.

Several studies have shown substantial improvements in $\dot{V}O_2$ peak in response to endurance training in persons with MR (54–56). However, Kasch and Zasueta (55) only tested $\dot{V}O_2$ peak in 6 of 41 children with MR and did not include a control group. Shurrer and coworkers (54) reported a 43% increase in $\dot{V}O_2$ peak following a 23-week walk-jog program in adults with MR. Unfortunately, they included only a

small number of subjects, without a control group. More recently, Pitetti and Tan (56) showed a 16% increase in $\dot{V}O_2$ peak in adults with MR following a 16-week aerobic-training program using the Schwinn Air-Dyne. They did not use a control group; however, in a follow-up almost 7 months after the conclusion of the training program, they found that all subjects had reverted to their pre-training $\dot{V}O_2$ peak. This cross-over design provides strong evidence for the effectiveness of endurance training in improving $\dot{V}O_2$ peak in persons with MR. This study also provided detailed information on the exercise prescription used, showing that a standard training program (3 times/week, 60–70% of $\dot{V}O_2$ peak, 25 minutes per session) is effective in improving cardiorespiratory endurance in this population. Furthermore, the longitudinal studies are supported by cross-sectional information (25), showing that $\dot{V}O_2$ peak can be very high in highly trained adults with MR.

All of the above studies included only persons with MR without DS. The response to endurance training in persons with DS appears to be substantially different. Only 2 studies have measured the response of $\dot{V}O_2$ peak to endurance training in persons with DS, but both studies found similar results. Millar and coworkers (27) reported no change in $\dot{V}O_2$ peak following 10 weeks of endurance training, but the training group improved their work capacity as shown by treadmill time, whereas the control group did not change either $\dot{V}O_2$ peak or work capacity. Varela and coworkers (57) showed similar results following a rowing program, where the exercise group improved the amount of work done on the rowing ergometer, but not $\dot{V}O_2$ peak. These investigations suggest that $\dot{V}O_2$ peak is immutable to change in response to a standard endurance program. Since work capacity is improved even in the absence of change in $\dot{V}O_2$ peak, endurance training still provides an important benefit to persons with DS, but suggests that the mechanism of adaptation is different in this population.

Potential Mechanisms of Adaptation to Endurance Training

There are no specific data on mechanisms of adaptation to exercise training in persons with MR. No studies to date have measured variables such as stroke volume, cardiac output, or specific muscle metabolism in response to exercise training. Based on available data, it is possible to speculate on the following:

1. Persons with MR without DS most likely will exhibit standard improvements in central circulation, such as small improvements in stroke volume and cardiac output. Maximal heart rate does not change with exercise training in this population, but reductions in submaximal heart rate have been reported (52, 53, 56). This would suggest that stroke volume has increased, because submaximal cardiac output does not usually change with exercise training. If stroke vol-

---

BOX 38.3. Expected Outcomes of Exercise Training in Persons With MR

Cardiovascular Endurance Training Outcomes
- Improved work capacity as measured by treadmill time or exercise work
- Improved $\dot{V}O_2$ peak in persons without DS
- Improved peak exercise ventilation
- Improved run performance
- No change in maximal heart rate or respiratory exchange ratio
- No change in $\dot{V}O_2$ peak in individuals with DS
- Some evidence for improved behavior

Resistance Training Outcomes
- Improved muscle strength as measured by 1-RM, isometric contractions, or isokinetic measures.
- Improved ability of muscle work
- Improved muscle endurance
- Possible improvements in run performance
- Possible improvements in vocational performance

ume were then maintained at its highest level up to maximal exercise intensity increased (which is the normal exercise response in nondisabled populations), maximal cardiac output would also be increased in response to training, because there was no change in maximal heart rate.

2. Persons with MR without DS probably exhibit standard improvements in muscle metabolism in response to endurance-based exercise training. Many studies have shown improved run performance following endurance training, and run performance is usually improved through a combination of central and peripheral changes. In nondisabled athletes, run performance can be improved without changes in $\dot{V}O_2$ peak, as a result of changes in peripheral muscle metabolism (36).

3. In persons with DS, it is unlikely that central adaptations occur, because no changes in $\dot{V}O_2$ peak have been reported. However, because work capacity is improved, muscle metabolism may be improved in persons with DS. It is also possible that anaerobic capability may be improved, because the last part of maximal exercise testing is dependent on anaerobic metabolism, and this could contribute to improved maximal treadmill time.

Endurance-Training Exercise Prescription

The focus of the exercise-training program should be daily involvement and enjoyment. Because persons with MR have a very high incidence of obesity and inactive lifestyles (11, 49), it is important to encourage this population to become active first, and focus on specific exercise prescription later. Box 38.4 summarizes the exercise prescription guidelines. A very important distinction for any exercise program for persons with MR is program supervision. Because motivation, task understanding, and behavioral problems can create problems with exercise adherence, supervision is paramount. It has been shown that even when provided the opportunity, but without supervision and encouragement, persons with MR do not generally exercise on their own (56). Motivational techniques (e.g., tokens and rewards) may also be needed.

The exercise intensity should be between 60% and 80% of $\dot{V}O_2$ peak to ensure improvements in $\dot{V}O_2$ peak (1). However, because this becomes a very intense exercise regimen, particularly if the goal is daily exercise, this intensity should be used only 3 or 4 days per week, especially when beginning a program. Exercise on the other days should focus on comfort and enjoyment. It is important to exercise most days of the week. The duration should be 20 to 60 minutes per session, depending on the exercise intensity and the conditioning of the participant. Although walking, jogging, and cycling are used most commonly, exercise programs set to music appear to enhance enjoyment of the session and may improve adherence.

BOX 38.4. Suggested Exercise Prescription Guidelines for Persons With MR

Cardiovascular Exercise Prescription Suggestions
- Focus on daily activity
- Ignore exercise intensity in the beginning and on most days—focus on participation
- For improvements in $\dot{V}O_2$ peak: 3–4 days per week, 50%–80% of measured $\dot{V}O_2$ peak; 30–40 minutes per session; aerobic activities such as walking, cycling, jogging or swimming—exercise to music is recommended
- Do not base exercise prescriptions on predicted maximal heart rate, because maximal heart rates are lower than predicted in this population.
- Encourage participation in Special Olympics or other organized sport programs

Resistance Training Prescription Suggestions
- Use weight machines for training; free weights may not be safe
- 2–3 days per week
- 8–12 RM (75%–80% of 1-RM)
- 2–3 sets
- 1–2 minutes rest between sets
- Closely supervise the program for the first 3 months
- Provide feedback on improvement as a form of motivation

Muscular Strength and Endurance Training

The results of muscular strength and endurance training in persons with MR are remarkably uniform. Early work used primarily school-based muscular endurance programs, and measured muscular performance through chin-up and sit-up performance (49). Typically, such programs lasted from 3 to 10 weeks and found improvements between 33% and 180% (49). The methods varied considerably, but all showed considerable improvements in muscle performance, regardless of the program used. More recent information also shows that an exercise program based on exercises performed with surgical tubing provided substantial improvements in muscle performance (44).

Relatively few studies on the effect of traditional resistance-training programs have been conducted in persons with MR. Rimmer and Kelly (58) showed that a 9-week program of 2 sessions per week using variable-resistance machines improved muscle strength in all 8 exercises used. Also, the weight-training group scored significantly better than a control group on 5 of the 8 exercises, showing the efficacy of more traditional resistance-training for individuals with MR. Two other **randomized controlled trials** also showed that a variable resistance-training program improved muscle strength in persons with MR (38, 46). In the first study, subject trained 3 times per week for 12 weeks using up to 5 sets of exercises for each muscle group. Muscle strength was improved between 8% and 83%, and the total amount of work performed improved between 25% and 177% (46). In a follow-up investigation (38), subjects improved strength between 19% and 36% after 12 weeks of training, and the control group showed a general decline in strength. The initial 12 weeks consisted of a traditional supervised resistance-training program. For the next 9 months, the exercise group continued the program in an unsupervised setting, and maintained their strength exercising 2 times per week. The strength level of the control group continued to decline.

Clearly, muscular strength and endurance-training programs are very effective in improving muscle performance in persons with MR. Considering the relationship between muscle strength and vocational productivity (5, 49) and the contribution of muscle strength to $\dot{V}O_2$ peak and run performance in this population, strength and endurance programs should be a high priority for individuals with MR. It is also important to realize, however, that to date no information is available on the effectiveness of resistance training for individuals with DS.

Potential Mechanisms of Adaptation to Resistance Training in Persons With MR

No information is available on mechanisms of adaptation to resistance training in individuals with MR; however, considering the limited number of investigations, this is not surprising. Because these programs provided exercise training aimed at improving muscle performance for only a short time (the 1-year program was 12 weeks of improvement and 9 months of maintenance), it is unlikely that significant amounts of muscle hypertrophy were elicited. The improvements observed were most likely due to neurological adaptations, because in nondisabled populations neurological changes account for initial improvements in muscle strength (59). However, this is pure speculation because no data are available.

Resistance Training Exercise Prescription

Although little information is available on the specifics of exercise prescription for resistance training in individuals with MR, it appears that persons with MR do not differ from the nondisabled populations in response to resistance training. Thus, standard exercise guidelines can be used. In general, individuals with MR should perform resistance training 2 to 3 times per week at an exercise intensity of 6% to 80% of 1 maximum repetition (RM). The focus should be on an overall program, including 8 to 12 exercises for all major muscle groups. Ideally, the program would not have a finite ending point, but should be integrated into the weekly routine of each individual. Re-testing of the 1 RM should be done in 4- to 6-week intervals to optimize performance gains. Significant improvements should be expected after 4 to 12 weeks.

What We Know
About Individuals With Mental Retardation

1 Mental retardation is the most common developmental disability in industrialized society, with an estimated prevalence of 3%.

2 The cause of MR is often unknown, but the most common known cause is fetal alcohol syndrome. Down syndrome is the most common genetic cause of MR.

3 There are 2 levels of MR, mild and severe. Classification depends on IQ and adaptive skills.

4 Individuals with MR have shortened life expectancy. Lack of self-care skills and physical mobility contribute to lower life expectancy. Low levels of physical activity in general may also contribute.

5 Individuals with MR have very low levels of work capacity and $\dot{V}O_2$ peak. In persons without DS, this appears to be related to sedentary living and poor lifestyle choices.

6 Individuals with DS have extremely low levels of work capacity and $\dot{V}O_2$ peak. This appears to be a function of DS, possibly related to low maximal heart rate.

7 Maximal heart rate is low in persons with MR, and even lower in persons with DS.

8 Muscle strength and endurance is low in persons with MR. Improving muscle strength and endurance may be very important in this population, because muscle strength is related to aerobic capacity and run performance in persons with MR. Muscle strength is related to vocational performance in this population.

9 Standard endurance training improves aerobic capacity in persons with MR but without DS. Endurance training does not appear to improve aerobic capacity in individuals with DS.

10 Resistance-training programs improve muscle strength and endurance in persons with MR. There is no information on the effect of such programs on persons with DS.

11 Standard exercise prescriptions appear to be effective in producing desirable results in persons without DS; however, in persons with DS, standard exercise prescriptions do not improve aerobic capacity.

What We Would Like to Know **About Persons With MR**

1 What can be done to decrease the incidence of MR?

2 What are the mechanisms of adaptation to exercise training in persons with MR?

3 Why does $\dot{V}o_2$ peak appear to be immutable to change in persons with DS?

4 Can resistance training improve $\dot{V}o_2$ peak and independence in persons with MR?

5 What can we do to increase physical activity levels in persons with MR?

6 Will an increase in physical activity levels of persons with MR lead to improved $\dot{V}o_2$ peak? Will increased physical activity lead to improved health outcomes in this population?

7 Will an increase in physical activity levels of persons with MR decrease the incidence of obesity in this population?

8 What is the effect of aging on physiological development and physical performance in persons with MR?

9 What is the relationship between physical activity and functional level?

Summary

An increasing number of individuals with MR are now living and functioning as contributing members in society. The number of persons with MR in the community is expected to increase due to improved life expectancy and the process of deinstitutionalization. Sedentary lifestyles are the norm among persons with MR, and aerobic capacity is very low. Individuals with DS have even lower aerobic capacity than their peers without DS. Low aerobic capacity appears to be linked to low maximal heart rates and poor leg strength.

Individuals with MR, but without DS, respond normally to exercise training. Substantial improvements in run performance, $\dot{V}o_2$ peak, and work capacity have been documented. Similarly, resistance training improves muscle strength and performance in persons with MR. Standard exercise prescriptions appear to yield noted improvements. It appears individuals with MR need supervision and motivation to adhere to an aerobic endurance program, but may be able to participate successfully in an independent resistance-training program. Persons with DS do not improve $\dot{V}o_2$ peak with aerobic endurance training, but still show improvements in work capacity. The response to resistance training in persons with DS is unknown at this time.

CASE STUDY

Patient Information

Jane is a 22-year-old woman with mild MR but without DS. She lives at home with her parents, and she has just completed public schooling. She is now working part time at a local fast-food restaurant. Since leaving school, Jane has gained a substantial amount of weight and she no longer participates in physical education classes. However, she does participate in Special Olympics, and she attends swim-training sessions once a week for 10 weeks during a year. Her favorite activity is watching TV, and she enjoys eating popcorn while watching movies. Her parents have noted she gets out of breath walking up the stairs to her bedroom. This is a change that has occurred during the past year. Although her parents try to encourage her to be more active, she has not participated in any physical activity on her own.

Assessments

During her last doctor's appointment, Jane weighed 155 pounds and she was 5 feet 2 inches tall. With a BMI of approximately 28, she is considered overweight, and she had gained 12 pounds over the past year. She had a maximal treadmill test in a university laboratory (as part of a research study), which showed she had $\dot{V}o_2$ peak of 25 mL/kg/min with a maximal heart rate of 179 bpm. Her blood pressure and cholesterol levels were normal, and she had no health complaints. A body composition test (skin folds) measured her at 39% body fat. She was not taking any medications at the time of testing.

REFERENCES

1. Fernhall B. Mental retardation. In: American College of Sports Medicine, ed. Exercise Management for Persons With Chronic Disease and Disability. Champaign, IL: Human Kinetics; 1997:221–226.
2. Rimmer J. Fitness and Rehabilitation Programs for Special Populations. Dubuque, IA: Brown and Benchmark; 1994.
3. American Association on Mental Retardation: Classification in Mental Retardation. Washington DC, 2002.
4. Auxter D, Pfyfer J, Huettig C. Principles and Methods of Adapted Physical Education and Recreation. New York, NY: McGraw-Hill; 2001.
5. Pitetti K, Rimmer J, Fernhall B. Physical fitness and adults with mental retardation: an overview of current research and future directions. Sports Med 1993;16:23–56.
6. Krebs P. Mental retardation. In: Winnick J, ed. Adapted Physical Education and Sport. Champaign, IL: Human Kinetics; 1990:153–176.
7. Lever A, Boushel R. Hypertension. In: Saltin B, Boushel R, Secher N, Mitchell J, eds. Exercise and Circulation in Health and Disease. Champaign, IL: Human Kinetics; 2000:296–297.
8. Pitetti K, Campbell K. Mentally retarded individuals: a population at risk? Med Sci Sports Exerc 1991;23:586–593.
9. Hayden M. Mortality among people with mental retardation living in the United States: research review and policy application. Ment Retard 1998;36:345–359.
10. Eyman R, Call T. Life expectancy of persons with Down syndrome. Am J Ment Retard 1991;95:603–612.
11. Fernhall B, Pitetti K. Limitations to work capacity in persons with mental retardation. Clin Exerc Physiol 2001;3:176–185.
12. American College of Sports Medicine. Guidelines for Exercise Testing and Exercise Prescription. 6th ed. Philadelphia, PA: Lippincott Williams & Wilkins; 2000.
13. Fernhall B, Szymanski L, Gorman P, Kamimoir G. Both atenolol and propanolol blunt and fibrinolytic response to exercise but not resting fibrinolytic potential. Am J Cardiol 2000;86:1398–1400.
14. Fernhall B, Pitetti K, Stubbs N, Stadler L. Validity and reliability of the 1/2-mile run-walk as an indicator of aerobic fitness in children with mental retardation. Pediatr Exerc Sci 1996;8:130–142.
15. Pitetti K, Fernhall B. Aerobic capacity as related to leg strength in youths with mental retardation. Pediatr Exerc Sci 1997;9:223–236.
16. Teo-Koh S, McCubbin J. Relationship between peak $\dot{V}O_2$ and 1-mile walk test performance of adolescents with mental retardation. Pediatr Exerc Sci 1999;11:144–157.
17. Cureton J, Sloniger M, O'Bannon J, Black D, McCormack W. A generalized equation for prediction of $\dot{V}O_2$ peak from 1-mile run/walk performance. Med Sci Sports Exerc 1995;27:445–451.
18. Pitetti K, Millar A, Fernhall B. Reliability of peak performance treadmill test for children and adolescents with and without mental retardation. Adapted Phys Activity Q 2000;17:322–332.
19. Fernhall B, Tymeson G. Graded exercise testing of mentally retarded adults; a study of feasibility. Arch Phys Med Rehabil 1987;63:363–365.
20. Fernhall B, Tymeson G, Millar A, Burkett L. Cardiovascular fitness testing and fitness levels of adolescents and adults with mental retardation including Down syndrome. Educ Training Ment Retard 1989;68:363–365.
21. Fernhall B, Tymeson G, Webster G. Cardiovascular fitness of mentally retarded adults. Adapted Phys Activity Q 1988;5:12–28.
22. Fernhall B, Millar A, Tymeson G, Burkett L. Maximal exercise testing of mentally retarded adolescents and adults: reliability study. Arch Phys Med Rehabil 1990;71:1065–1068.
23. Fernhall B, Pitetti K, Rimmer J, et al. Cardiorespiratory capacity of individuals with mental retardation including Down syndrome. Med Sci Sports Exerc 1996;28:366–371.
24. Rintala P, Dunn J, McCubbin J, Quinn C. Validity of cardiovascular fitness test for men with mental retardation. Med Sci Sports Exerc 1992;24:941–945.
25. Frey G, McCubbin J, Hannigan-Downs S, Kasser S, Skaggs S. Physical fitness of trained runners with and without mild mental retardation. Adapted Phys Activity Q 1999;16:126–137.
26. Pitetti K, Climstein M, Campbell K, Barrett P, Jackson J. The cardiovascular capacities of adults with Down syndrome: a comparative study. Med Sci Sports Exerc 1992;24:13–19.
27. Millar A, Fernhall B, Burkett L, Tymeson G. Effect of aerobic training in adolescents with Down syndrome. Med Sci Sports Exerc 1993;25:260–264.
28. Guerra M, Roman B, Geronimo C, Violan M, Cuadrado E, Fernhall B. Physical fitness levels of sedentary and active individuals with Down syndrome. Adapted Phys Activity Q 2000;17:310–321.
29. Fernhall B, McCubbin J, Rintala P, et al. Predicting maximal heart rate in individuals with mental retardation including Down syndrome. Med Sci Sports Exerc 2001;33:1655–1660.
30. Fernhall B, Pitetti K, Vukovich M, et al. Validation of cardiovascular fitness field tests in children with mental retardation. Am J Ment Retard 1998;102:602–612.
31. Fernhall B, Pitetti K, Millar A, Hensen T, Vukovich M. Cross validation of the 20 m shuttle run in children with mental retardation. Adapted Phys Activity Q 2000;17:402–412.
32. Rintala P, McCubbin J, Downs S, Fox S. Cross validation of the 1-mile walking test for men with mental retardation. Med Sci Sports Exerc 1997;29:133–137.
33. Kittredge J, Rimmer J, Looney M. Validation of the Rockport fitness walking test for adults with mental retardation. Med Sci Sports Exerc 1994;26:95–102.
34. Fernhall B, Tymeson G. Validation of cardiovascular fitness field tests for persons with mental retardation. Adapted Phys Activity Q 1988;5:49–59.
35. Pitetti K, Yarmer D, Fernhall B. Cardiovascular fitness and body composition of youth with and without mental retardation. Adapted Phys Activity Q 2001;18:127–141.
36. Fernhall B, Pitetti K. Leg strength is related to endurance run performance in children and adolescents with mental retardation. Pediatr Exerc Sci. 2000;12:324–333.
37. Pitetti K, Boneh S. Cardiovascular fitness as related to leg strength in adults with mental retardation. Med Sci Sports Exerc 1995;27:423–428.

38. Suomi R. Self directed strength training: its effect on leg strength in men with mental retardation. Arch Phys Med Rehabil 1998;79:323–328.

39. Pitetti K, Climstein M, Mays M, Barret P. Isokinetic arm and leg strength of adults with Down syndrome: a comparative study. Arch Phys Med Rehabil 1992;73:847–850.

40. Croce R, Pitetti K, Horvat M, Miller J. Peak torque, average power, and hamstring/quadriceps ratios in non-disabled adults and adults with mental retardation. Arch Phys Med Rehabil 1996;77:369–372.

41. Horvat M, Croce R, Pitetti K, Fernhall B. Comparison of isokinetic peak force and work parameters in youth with and without mental retardation. Med Sci Sports Exerc 1999;31:1190–1195.

42. Horvat M, Pitetti K, Corce R. Isokinetic torque, average power, and flexion/extension ratios in nondisabled adults and adults with mental retardation. J Orthop Sports Phys Ther 1997;6:395–399.

43. Horvat M, Croce R. Physical rehabilitation of individuals with mental retardation; physical fitness and information processing. Crit Rev Phys Rehabil Med 1995;7:233–252.

44. Croce R, Horvat M. Effects of reinforcement based exercise on fitness and work productivity in adults with mental retardation. Adapted Phys Activity Q 1992;9:148–178.

45. Suomi R, Surburg P, Lecius P. Reliability of isokinetic and isometric measurements of leg strength on men with mental retardation. Arch Phys Med Rehabil 1993;74:848–852.

46. Suomi R, Surburg P, Lecius P. Effects of hydraulic resistance strength training on isokinetic measures of leg strength in men with mental retardation. Adapted Phys Activity Q 1995;12:377–387.

47. Horvat M, Croce R, Roswal G, Seagraves F. Single trial versus maximal or mean values for evaluating strength in individuals with mental retardation. Adapted Phys Activity Q 1995;12:52–59.

48. Morris A, Vaughan S, Vaccaro P. Measurement of neuromuscular tone and strength in Down's syndrome children. J Ment Defic 1982;26:41–46.

49. Fernhall B. Physical fitness and exercise training of individuals with mental retardation. Med Sci Sports Exerc 1993;25:442–450.

50. Bundschuh E, Cureton K. Effect of bicycle ergometer conditioning on the physical work capacity of mentally retarded adolescents. Am Corrective Ther J 1982;36:159–163.

51. Beasley C. Effects of a jogging program on cardiovascular fitness and work performances of mentally retarded persons. Am J Ment Defic 1982;86:609–613.

52. Tomporowski P, Ellis N. Effects of exercise on the physical fitness, intelligence, and adaptive behavior of institutionalized mentally retarded adults. Appl Res Ment Retard 1985;5:329–337.

53. Tomporowski P, Jameson L. Effects of a physical training program on the exercise behavior of institutionalized mentally retarded adults. Adapted Phys Activity Q 1985;2:197–205.

54. Schurrer R, Weltman A, Brammel H. Effects of physical training on cardiovascular fitness and behavior patterns of mentally retarded adults. Am J Ment Defic 1985;90:167–170.

55. Kasch F, Zasueta S. Physical capacities of mentally retarded children. Acta Paediatr Scand 1971;217:217–218.

56. Pitetti K, Tan D. Effects of a minimally supervised exercise program for mentally retarded adults. Med Sci Sports Exerc 1991;23:594–601.

57. Varela A, Sardinha L, Pitetti K. Effects of aerobic rowing training in adults with Down syndrome. Am J Ment Retard. 2001;106:135–144.

58. Rimmer J, Kelly L. Effects of a resistance training program on adults with mental retardation. Adapted Phys Activity Q 1991;8:146–153.

59. Tanaka H, Swensen T. Impact of resistance training on endurance performance: a new form of cross training? Sports Med 1998;25:191–200.

GLOSSARY

-A-

ABA design a quasi-experimental research design where assessments occur at baseline (A), after the introduction of a treatment (B), and following the removal of the treatment (A); often used in single-group or single-subject research where it is impractical to use control groups for comparison purposes

acanthosis nigricans an eruption of velvet, warty benign growths and hyperpigmentation occurring in the skin of the axillae, neck, anogenital area, and groin. It usually is associated with endocrine disorders or obesity.

accelerated graft coronary disease (graft vessel disease) the development of obstructive lesions in the arteries and veins of transplant recipients. It is the major cause of late mortality.

accelerometry measurement of energy expenditure with an accelerometer, a portable measurement device; single plane reflects movement in the vertical plane only; triaxial reflects three-dimensional movement

accommodate to focus at varying distances by contracting or relaxing the ciliary body muscle to change the shape and power of the crystalline lens

acetaminophen a pain reliever that belongs to a class of drugs called analgesics (pain reliever) and antipyretics (fever reducer). Acetaminophen relieves pain by elevating the pain threshold. It reduces fever through its action on the heat-regulating center of the brain.

acquired immunodeficiency syndrome (AIDS) CD4$^+$ T cell count <200 cells/mm^3 or the presence of an AIDS-defining illness

active living an approach to increase of habitual physical activity sponsored by Health Canada, whereby the population is encouraged to incorporate the physical activity needed for health into the pattern of daily life—for example, walking or cycling to work

activities of daily living (ADLs) any daily activity a person performs for self-care (e.g., feeding, grooming, bathing, dressing), work, mobility, homemaking, and leisure. The ability to undertake such activities unaided is needed for continued independent living in old age.

acute having rapid onset, usually with recovery; not chronic or long-lasting

acute rejection the immune response of a transplant recipient against the donor heart manifested by infiltration of mononuclear cells (T-lymphocytes) that may destroy the myocardium

adherence a state of complying with, adhering to or completing the requirements of a treatment protocol or regimen

adipocyte hyperplasia an increase in the number of fat cells

adipocyte hypertrophy an increase in the size of fat cells

adipocytes cells whose functions include triglyceride synthesis for energy storage, triglyceride degradation for energy release, and signal transmissions to the brain concerning energy storage in the form of leptin

adjuvant therapy treatment given after the primary treatment to increase the chances of curing the disease or keeping it in check. Adjuvant therapy may include chemotherapy, radiation therapy, or hormonal therapy.

adrenergic describes nerve fibers that release norepinephrine as a neurotransmitter

age-related macular degeneration (ARMD) a chronic degenerative disease of the choroid, Bruch's membrane, and retinal pigment epithelium which secondarily affects the macula, typically occurring in older individuals

AIDS see acquired immunodeficiency syndrome

airway obstruction a process by which the airways are narrowed through one or more of several mechanisms, including (1) contraction of the airway smooth muscle, (2) accumulation of mucus in the airway, (3) swelling of the airway wall, or (4) loss of support structure surrounding the airway.

airway resistance resistance to airflow caused by airway obstruction

akinesia impairment in starting movements

alveolar ventilation volume of air moving into and out of the alveoli during each respiratory cycle

alveoli the part of the lung where gas exchange takes place

amenorrhea   absence of menstrual periods

anabolic therapy   use of testosterone and testosterone analogs to build lean body mass

anaphylaxis   an abnormal reaction to a particular antigen, in which histamine is released from tissues and causes either local or widespread symptoms. In severe cases, swelling, constriction of bronchioles, heart failure, circulatory collapse, and even death may occur.

androgens   endogenous or exogenous hormones that control male secondary sex characteristics and facilitate protein synthesis in both skeletal and cardiac muscle

anemia   low red blood cell count

angioedema   an allergic condition producing transient or persistent swelling of areas of skin accompanied by itching, which may be severe. Caused by allergy to food substances, drugs, or other allergens or it may be precipitated by heat, cold, or emotional factors.

annulus fibrosus   the ring of fibrocartilage and fibrous tissue forming the circumference of the intervertebral disc; surrounds the nucleus pulposus, which is prone to herniation when the annulus fibrosus is compromised

anovulation   the absence of a follicle maturing and being released in a menstrual cycle

anterior chamber   the small, domed compartment in the front of the eye between the cornea and the iris that is filled with aqueous humor

antiangiogenic   the quality of something that suppresses the formation of new vessels

antibiotics   drugs used in the therapy of bacterial infections

anticholinergic   inhibiting the action of acetylcholine

antigen   any substance that the body regards as foreign or potentially dangerous and against which it produces an antibody or allergic response. Antigens usually are proteins, but simple substances, even metals, may become antigenic by combining with and modifying the body's own proteins.

antihyperlipidemic drugs   agents that are used in the prevention or control of elevated blood lipid concentrations.

anxiety   an affective experience characterized by physiologic arousal, muscular tension, and feelings of apprehension or dread

anxiety disorders   identifiable clusters of extreme anxiety symptoms that cause great distress and disrupt family or social relationships as well as impairing one's ability to undertake routine activities such as work or study. General categories of anxiety disorders include stress disorders, generalized anxiety disorder, phobias, panic disorder, and obsessive-compulsive disorder.

anxiolytic   anxiety-reducing

aortic valve   the semilunar valve that separates the left ventricle from the ascending aorta and prevents the regurgitation of blood into the left ventricle during ventricular diastole

aphakia   the absence of the crystalline lens, typically the result of cataract surgery without an implant

apolipoproteins   proteins associated with lipoproteins. These proteins act to stabilize the lipid portion of the lipoprotein in transit, as ligands for cell-receptor binding, and as cofactors in enzyme reactions.

aqueous humor   the watery fluid constantly produced by the ciliary body that fills the anterior chamber in the front of the eye

arousal   an increased neural activity in the reticular formation of the brain; associated with increases in heart rate, blood pressure, sweating, muscle tone, and reaction speed. Some increase in arousal enhances performance, but an excessive level of arousal leads to a deterioration in performance and difficulty in sleeping.

arrhythmia   any deviation from the normal rhythm of the heart

arterial blood gases (Pao_2, $Paco_2$)   the partial pressure of oxygen (O_2) or carbon dioxide (CO_2) in the arterial blood

arterial hypertension   higher than normal arterial blood pressure (i.e., resting blood pressure greater than 140/90 mm Hg)

arteriovenous oxygen difference (A-Vo_2 diff)   the average difference between the oxygen content of arterial and mixed blood and oxygen uptake

arthralgia   pain in a joint, without swelling or other signs of arthritis

arthroplasty   surgery of a joint (as the hip or knee); the operative formation or restoration of a joint

articular cartilage   cartilage that covers the articular surfaces of bones

asthenia   the lack or loss of strength and energy, weakness

asthma   a disease process that is characterized by narrowing of the bronchi, making breathing difficult.

ataxia   failure of muscular coordination; irregularity of muscular action; most often caused by disease activity in the cerebellum. The lack of coordination and unsteadiness that result from the brain's failure to regulate the body's posture and the strength and direction of limb movements.

atherogenesis   formation of atherosclerotic lesions in the walls of arteries

atherosclerosis   a common degenerative condition of the arteries, marked by the accumulation of cholesterol plaques beneath the endothelial lining of the vessels; the most common form of arteriosclerosis

atherosclerotic lesion   fatty degeneration or thickening of the arterial walls; lesions also may include necrotic tissue, calcification, and clot debris

athlete's heart   the morphologic and functional cardiac changes induced by regular, intensive athletic conditioning in healthy individuals

atrioventricular synchrony   Normally, atrial impulses are generated by sinoatrial node and transmitted through the conduction system to the ventricles. The atrioventricular node modulates this transmission and determines a physiological delay that is represented by the PR interval on surface ECG. In cardiac pacing, a pacemaker stimulus is synchronous when it is emitted in response to a sensed event after an appropriate delay. The maintenance of AV synchrony is associated with improvements in cardiocirculatory hemodynamics

atrioventricular valves the cardiac valves that separate the atria from the ventricles and prevent blood from regurgitating into the atria during ventricular systole. (See entries for mitral and tricuspid valves)

atrophy reduction and decrease in size of tissue

autoimmune abnormal function of the immune system that causes the production of antibodies against one's own tissues

autosomal dominant a pattern of inheritance, carried on one of the non–sex chromosomes, in which the gene's effect is shown in the individual regardless of whether its corresponding allele is the same or different

avascular having no blood supply.

-B-

background diabetic retinopathy (BDR) an older term for diabetic retinal disease characterized by retinal hemorrhages, microaneurysms, or edema *without* neovascularization tissue (*see* nonproliferative diabetic retinopathy, proliferative diabetic retinopathy)

balance ability to maintain a postural position, usually standing

basal metabolic rate the minimal level of energy required to sustain the body's vital functions in the waking state

benign used to define abnormal growths that are not cancerous, do not invade nearby tissue or spread to other parts of the body

benzodiazepines a group of prescription medications that operate as tranquilizers on the central nervous system; frequently prescribed for the purpose of relieving anxiety or promoting sleep. Commonly used variants include alprazolam (Xanax), chlordiazepoxide (Librium), diazepam (Valium), and lorazepam (Ativan).

beta-3 adrenergic agonists agents that augment daily caloric output by elevating basal metabolic rate

beta-oxidation modification of free fatty acids by cleaving two carbon atoms to form acetyl CoA to be used in the Krebs cycle

bile acid–binding resins drugs that bind bile acids in the intestine, preventing reabsorption of bile acids by the liver

bile acids complex acids that occur as salts in the bile and may be reabsorbed by the liver. These acids are important for digestion of fats in the intestine

bioelectrical impedance a method of measuring body composition based on the concept that the electrical impedance of an object is influenced by the volume of conducting tissue

biological age the age of an individual expressed in terms of his or her functional abilities. An adverse lifestyle will cause a biological age that exceeds the calendar age, a discrepancy that can be reduced by a training program.

biological therapy treatment to stimulate or restore the ability of the immune system to fight infection and disease; also used to lessen side effects that may be caused by some cancer treatments

biopsychosocial conceptualization positing that outcomes are a consequence of interacting biological, psychological, and social causal influences

blood shunting blood diverted from one organ or tissue mass to another controlled by central nervous system and metabolic demands. Alterations in blood flow are evident during exercise, posture changes, and heat to maximize function and system maintenance.

body mass index (BMI) body weight in kilograms (kg) divided by the square of height in meters, or, kg/m^2

Bohr effect alteration of hemoglobin's binding affinity for oxygen by changing temperature or pH of the blood

bone marrow/peripheral blood stem cell transplant a complex treatment that may be used to treat certain solid tumors or hematologic cancers. The bone marrow transplant makes it possible to use very high doses of chemotherapy that would otherwise be impossible. In autologous bone marrow transplant, the patient's own bone marrow is used. An allogeneic bone marrow transplant uses marrow from a donor whose tissue type closely matches the patient's.

bone scan a tracer element (technetium-99) is injected into the patient's blood which is then imaged with a collimator to differentiate uptake typically in three phases: blood, tissue, and bone. The tracer localizes to areas of increased metabolic activity such as fracture, inflammation, infection, and cancer.

bradycardia slow heartbeat, usually <60 beats per minute

bradykinesia slowing down of movements

brain stem auditory evoked potential a test in which the brain's electrical activity in response to auditory stimuli (e.g., clicking sounds) is recorded by an electroencephalograph and analyzed by a computer. Demyelination such as that seen in multiple sclerosis results in a slowed response.

breast reconstruction surgery to rebuild a breast shape after a mastectomy

bronchioles the divisions of the conducting airways less than 1 mm in diameter

bronchodilator drugs that either directly or indirectly cause relaxation of the airway smooth muscle (bronchodilation)

Bruch's membrane the thin, transparent membrane that forms the innermost layer of the choroid. The retinal pigment epithelium is adherent to Bruch's membrane; Bruch's membrane forms a protective barrier between the choroid and the retinal pigment epithelium.

-C-

cachexia a profound and marked state of constitutional disorder, general ill health and weight loss and wasting occurring in the course of a chronic disease or emotional disturbance

calcitonin hormone responsible for controlling blood calcium when the level is high

caloric equivalent number of kilocalories produced per liter of oxygen consumed

calorimetry measurement of heat dissipation. When heat dissipation is estimated from other measures it is termed *indirect calorimetry.*

cancer a general term for more than 100 diseases in which abnormal cells divide out of control; a malignant tumor

cancer stage the extent to which cancer has spread from its original site to other parts of the body; usually denoted by a number from Stage 1 (least severe) to Stage 4 (more advanced)

cardiac amyloid accumulation of insoluble fibrillar proteins in the myocardium that leads to poor cardiac function and heart failure

cardiac denervation interruption of direct nervous system connections to the heart at the time of harvesting the donor organ.

cardiac output volume of blood pumped from the left ventricle in 1 minute; the product of stroke volume and the heart rate

cardiac reinnervation reestablishment through growth of direct nervous system connections to the heart after transplantation

cardiac sarcomere the functional unit of the myocytes, consisting of thick (myosin) and thin (actin) myofilaments, which allow the sarcomere to shorten when activated by calcium ions

cardiopulmonary exercise testing integrative physiologic test that measures oxygen uptake, lactic acidosis threshold, ventilation, heart rate, 12-lead ECG, work performed, and oxygen saturation continuously during exercise.

cardiorespiratory fitness/capacity a health-related component of physical fitness that relates to the ability of the circulatory and respiratory systems to supply oxygen during sustained physical activity.

cardiovascular diseases diseases of the heart and blood vessels

cardiovascular reflexes response of the heart and vascular system to external stimuli mediated by the sympathetic and parasympathetic nervous system

catabolism breakdown of energy-yielding substances

cataract clouding or opacification of the crystalline lens

catecholamines hormones (epinephrine and norepinephrine) secreted by the nerve endings and the adrenal medulla, involved in the "fight-or-flight" reaction that prepares the heart for exercise and other forms of stress.

category RPE scale a rating of perceived exertion (RPE) that ranges from 6 (very, very light) to 20 (very, very hard).

category-ratio RPE scale another type of RPE that ranges from 0 (nothing at all) to 10 (very, very strong)

cauda equina syndrome compression of the spinal nerve roots by a large bulging central disc; generally associated with saddle anesthesia in the perineal region and bowel or bladder dysfunction. Immediate neurosurgical consultation indicated.

causality a set of criteria useful in establishing whether a cause-and-effect relation is supported by the scientific literature

CBT cognitive-behavioral therapy

chemotherapy the use of drugs to destroy cancer cells. Chemotherapy often is used with surgery or radiation to treat cancer when the cancer has spread, when it has come back (recurred), or when there is a strong chance that it could recur.

cholecystokinin a hormone that stimulates enzyme release from the pancreas and bile release from the gallbladder

cholesterol a sterol that is widely distributed in animal tissues occurring in cell membranes and nerve tissue of the brain and spinal chord, and as precursors for various hormones.

cholesterol ester transfer protein (CETP) protein in the circulation that transfers nonpolar lipids (triglycerides and cholesterol esters) between lipoproteins

cholesterol esters cholesterol that is attached to a fatty acid by an ester bond

cholinergic nervous system nerve fibers that release acetylcholine as a neurotransmitter

chondroitin sulfate any of several sulfated forms of chondroitin found in various tissues (e.g., cartilage, adult bone, and tendons)

chordae tendineae thin, very strong cords of connective tissue that anchor the edges of the atrioventricular valve leaflets to the papillary muscles

choriocapillaris the innermost layer of the choroid, directly beneath the retinal pigment epithelium, composed on an interconnecting network of capillaries. It provides the major source of nutrition for the RPE and outer retinal layers.

choroid the richly vascular layer of the eye sandwiched between the sclera and the retinal pigment epithelium. In the macula it has the highest rate of blood flow of any tissue in the body.

chronic bronchitis a chronic inflammatory disease of the airways

chronic obstructive pulmonary disease (COPD) chronic lung disease that results in narrowing of the airways; emphysema and chronic bronchitis

chronic pulmonary disease the result of abnormal mucus, airway obstruction, recurrent infection, and inflammation in cystic fibrosis, leading to progressive loss of lung tissue and lung function

chronotropic incompetence the failure of heart rate to increase in response to exercise or catecholamines. The upper limit of heart rate response to cycle ergometer or treadmill exercise stress testing is below 100 beats/min. Chronotropic incompetence suggests sinoatrial node disease, more common in patients with a history of hypertension or coronary artery disease with involvement of sinoatrial branch of the right coronary artery.

chronotropic reserve the difference between the heart rate at rest and the highest heart rate during graded exercise.

chylomicrons relatively large, triglyceride-rich lipoprotein secreted by the intestine after digestion and absorption of food

ciliary body a muscular ring of tissue behind the iris that secretes aqueous and contracts to change the shape and focusing power of the lens

clonus a sign of spasticity in which involuntary shaking or jerking of the leg occurs when the toe is placed on the floor with the knee slightly bent. The shaking is caused by repeated, rhythmic, reflex muscle contractions.

cognitive-behavioral therapy a psychological intervention approach that combines elements of cognitive therapy (i.e., modifying patterns of thinking) and behavior therapy (i.e., modifying behavior through the use of reinforcement techniques). Forms used to treat anxiety conditions include stress inoculation training and stress management training.

Cohen's *d* a frequently used measure of effect size; defined as the difference between the means of two groups divided by the standard deviation of one of the groups (or the pooled standard deviation of both groups

cohort studies a design that identifies a group based on some predefined exposure criteria and then, over time, compares subgroups of the population on an outcome of interest. Also called concurrent, follow-up, incidence, longitudinal, or prospective studies.

collagen an insoluble fibrous protein of vertebrates that is the chief constituent of the fibrils of connective tissue (e.g., skin and tendons) and of the organic substance of bones and yields gelatin and glue on prolonged heating with water

complementary alternative medicine (CAM) combination of a nontraditional therapy (i.e., alternative therapy) with a traditional medical treatment

complementary therapy

compliance a state of adhering to or completing the requirements of a treatment protocol or regimen

computed tomography a composite radiographic study that obtains multiple image slices through the body, which are then computer oriented to allow differentiation of various body structures

confounder a confusing item

contracture a permanent shortening of the muscles and tendons adjacent to a joint, which can result from severe, untreated spasticity and interferes with normal movement around the affected joint

cornea the transparent convex structure that forms the anterior wall of the eye and allows light to enter the eye.

coronary artery disease narrowing of the coronary arteries to the extent that blood flow to the myocardium is inadequate to meet metabolic needs of the heart tissue

coronary heart disease decreased flow of blood to the heart muscle to the extent that oxygen supply is insufficient to meet the metabolic needs of the heart; most commonly caused by atherosclerosis in the coronary arteries

corticosteroids drugs used in therapy of inflammation and immunosuppression

COX-2 inhibitors a recently developed class of nonsteroidal anti-inflammatory drugs that are more selective in their analgesic and anti-inflammatory actions (selective inhibition of the cyclooxygenase-2 pathway), and have a reduced risk of causing gastrointestinal and renal problems (associated with indiscriminant COX-1 inhibition).

creatine kinase muscle enzyme that when detected in serum indicates some degree of muscle fiber overexertion and damage

cross-sectional studies a design in which subjects are identified and classified as to the exposure and outcome at the same time; also called prevalence study

cross-validation a technique used to assess the generalizability of a treatment or a research finding. It involves applying the same procedures to a person or group *not* involved in the original study and noting whether the same results are obtained

crystalline lens the transparent biconvex structure behind the iris that focuses light on the retina.

cue trigger or signal. *Example of an internal cue:* Neurons of the basal ganglia discharge phasically. The phasic discharge interacts with movement preparatory activity in the sensory motor cortex and turns off the preparatory movement, which allows the movement to be executed. *Example of an external cue:* use of light signals or auditory signals to prompt walking or touching leg of patient to support continuation of walking.

Cushing syndrome a state of excess cortisol resulting from either iatrogenic causes, pituitary tumors, or tumors of the adrenal gland

cyclosporine a cyclosporin $C_{62}H_{111}N_{11}O_{12}$ used as an immunosuppressive drug, especially to prevent rejection of transplanted organs

-D-

dead space (Vd) part of the lung where air is moved in and out, but no exchange of gas occurs

deconditioning the process of losing muscle strength and neuromuscular coordination, which occurs with inactivity or excessive rest

degenerative disc disease a natural process of aging that results in decreased water content in the disc and degenerative bony changes of the vertebral bodies. There is no causal relationship between these changes and pain.

degranulation the process in which mast cells or other cell types release stored substances into the extracellular fluid

demyelination a loss of myelin in the white matter of the central nervous system (brain, spinal cord).

dermis the thick layer of tissue that lies directly beneath the epidermis. It consists mainly of loose connective tissue containing capillaries, lymph vessels, nerve endings, sweat glands and ducts, hair follicles, sebaceous glands, and smooth muscle fibers.

diastolic dysfunction inability of the heart to fill with blood during diastole at a normal filling pressure

diabetes mellitus metabolic disease characterized by hyperglycemia resulting from defects in insulin secretion, insulin action, or both

differentiated rate of perceived exertion cues and sensations of exertion and effort from one particular body part or area. Often used to distinguish exertion of a certain muscle group or limb.

dilated cardiomyopathy the most common form of cardiomyopathy, characterized by cardiac enlargement and impaired systolic function of one or both ventricles

discectomy removal of a portion of the intervertebral disc (*see* microdiscectomy.)

discogenic of, or pertaining to, an intervertebral disc

disordered eating condition in which an individual is not consuming the necessary calories to sustain the body's energy demands. This includes not eating, binging, purging, and other eating-related disruptions.

dopamine a catecholamine produced in the body that acts as a neurotransmitter in the central nervous system. The transmitter is directly involved in pathways that mediate movements

dopaminergic neurons Dopamine is produced in the pars compacta of substantia nigra. Axon terminals of these pars compacta neurons are located in caudate nucleus where dopamine when produced can be excitatory or inhibitory depending upon whether interaction is with direct (excitatory) or indirect (inhibitory) pathways.

doubly-labeled water a measurement method of energy expenditure. A quantity of water with a known concentration of isotopes of hydrogen and oxygen is ingested. From the difference in the elimination rates of the two isotopes from urine, sweat, and respiration, oxygen consumption and caloric expenditure can be calculated.

drusen nodular yellow deposits between Bruch's membrane and the retinal pigment epithelium composed of metabolic byproducts of the retina, retinal pigment epithelium, and choroid

dual energy x-ray absorptiometry (DEXA) a method of body composition analysis used to provide regional estimates of fat mass with minimal radiation exposure. DEXA measures the differential attenuation of two main x-ray photon energies as they pass through the body. Total tissue mass is separated into fat, bone mineral, and lean according to measured x-ray attenuation.

ductal carcinoma in situ (DCIS) abnormal cells that involve only the lining of a duct; the cells have not spread outside the duct to other tissues in the breast

dynamic stabilizers muscles and fascia that provide active support to the spine and generate force vectors to allow locomotion

dyslipidemia plasma lipid disorder resulting in abnormal lipid profile

dyspepsia abnormal or painful digestion that may be characterized by abdominal discomfort, heartburn, nausea, vomiting, and loss of appetite

dyspnea A sensation of breathlessness; shortness of breath; difficult or labored breathing

dystrophic pertaining to a disorder that arises from defective or faulty nutrition

-E-

ecological studies a study design in which exposure characteristics of an area are compared to outcome data from the same area; also called correlational studies

economy the energy cost of work

ectomorphic one of three basic types of body build, characterized by long limbs, limited muscle development, and a low content of body fat

edema swelling of a tissue due to excessive fluid accumulation outside the cells

EEG electroencephalogram

effect size an estimate of treatment impact that (unlike statistical significance) is independent of group size; frequently used as an indicator of the "meaningfulness" of a treatment

efficiency the relationship of the mechanical energy produced to the metabolic energy used to produce the mechanical movement

elastin a protein involved in connective tissue

electroencephalogram a recording of the electrical activity in the cerebral cortex that is sometimes used as an index of arousal or anxiety; obtained by placing surface electrodes on the scalp; relaxation is associated with slow, steady, high-amplitude impulses; arousal and agitation are associated with rapid, irregular, low-amplitude impulses

electromyogram a recording of the electrical activity in the muscles that sometimes is used as an index of tension and anxiety; most often obtained by placing surface electrodes on the skin

electromyography recording of skeletal muscle action potentials by either noninvasive (electrodes on skin) or invasive (needle-type wires inserted into skin) means to assess normality of contraction

EMG electromyogram

emphysema a chronic obstructive pulmonary disease (COPD) involving chronic inflammation and destruction of the lung

endocrine therapy treatment with hormones, with drugs to interfere with hormone production or hormone action, or the surgical removal of hormone-producing glands. Endocrine therapy may kill cancer cells or slow their growth.

endogenous   arising within or derived from the body

endomyocardial biopsy   the technique of obtaining a tissue sample from the right ventricle by insertion of a catheter through the jugular vein for the analysis of acute rejection after heart transplantation

end-stage heart failure   the last stage of severe, symptomatic chronic heart failure with a very high probability of death within weeks to months

end-tidal CO$_2$ (P$_{ET}$CO$_2$)   carbon dioxide measured in exhaled air at the end of the exhalation

eosinophil   a type of white blood cell that has coarse granules within its cytoplasm. The numbers of eosinophils in blood often rise when there is an allergic reaction in progress.

ephedrine   plant-derived, indirect-acting sympathomimetic amine that stimulates the release of norepinephrine from sympathetic nerve endings

epidemiology   the study of the relation among various factors that determine the frequency and distribution of diseases in a population

epidural anesthesia   injection of an analgesic and (usually) a soluble corticosteroid into the epidural space, where the fluid diffuses across the dura into the subarachnoid space to act on nerve roots as an anesthetic

Epstein-Barr virus   a herpesvirus that causes infectious mononucleosis and is associated with Burkitt lymphoma and nasopharyngeal carcinoma

estradiol (E$_2$)   a steroid hormone that maintains the secondary sex characteristics and helps to prepare the ovary for ovulation

estrogens   endogenous and synthetic forms of female sex hormones

eumenorrhea   infrequent or irregular menstrual periods

eumenorrhea   is the regular or normal menstrual cycle pattern of more than 10 menstrual cycles that occur in a year. The cycle length usually ranges from 28 to 32 days, with the follicular phase lasting 10 to 20 days and the luteal phase lasting 14 days.

exacerbation   the appearance of new symptoms or the aggravation of old ones, lasting at least 24 hours (synonymous with attack, relapse, flare-up, or worsening); usually associated with inflammation and demyelination in the brain or spinal cord

exercise   physical activity undertaken with a specific purpose, such as enhancing health or increasing performance

exercise deprivation   abstinence from exercise; may be voluntary or involuntary (e.g., because of injury); depriving regular exercisers of physical activity appears to increase their anxiety levels

exercise-induced (arterial) hypoxemia (EIH)   decreases in arterial partial pressure of oxygen (Pa$_{O_2}$) and oxyhemoglobin saturation (Hb$_{O_2}$) during or after exercise; e.g., Pa$_{O_2}$ <75 mm Hg or an Sa$_{O_2}$ <92%

exercise-induced bronchoconstriction/bronchospasm   airflow obstruction during or after exercise; e.g., FEV1%

decreases by more than 10% to 15% from preexercise measurements

exercise-induced hypercapnia   increased arterial partial pressure of carbon dioxide (Pa$_{CO_2}$) during or after exercise; e.g., Pa$_{CO_2}$ >45 mm Hg

exercise-induced hypotension   blood pressure drop that occurs at the end of an exercise session or during recovery period

exercise testing   the performance of a controlled physical task with increasing workload to examine a person's maximal physical capacity

exercise training   physical activity that is planned, structured, and repetitive and aims to improve or maintain physical fitness

exocrine pancreatic insufficiency   inadequate secretion of digestive enzymes from pancreatic tissue into the intestine, causing malabsorption

exogenous   originating outside the body

expectoration   expulsion of mucus from the airways by coughing and spitting

extracellular matrix   a structure situated or occurring outside a cell

-F-

5-year relative survival rate   the likelihood that a cancer patient will still be alive in 5 years. It excludes from the calculations patients dying of other diseases, and is considered to be a more accurate way to describe the prognosis for patients with a particular type and stage of cancer

facultative thermogenesis   heat produced in excess of that required to maintain basal metabolic rate due to purposeful exercise, shivering, and fidgeting

familial aggregation   characteristics affecting more members of the same family than can be accounted for by chance

familial dyslipidemia   plasma lipid disorders that have a genetic origin

fatty acids   a hydrocarbon chain in which one of the hydrogen atoms has been replaced with a carboxyl group

female triad   a trio of disorders that are believed to be interrelated although they may not all manifest at the same time; includes amenorrhea, eating disorders, and osteoporosis

FEV$_1$ measure of lung function obtained from simple spirometry: forced expiratory volume in 1 second expressed as percentage predicted from reference value; used to classify disease severity

fibric acid derivatives   drugs that reduce the liver production of triglycerides and also reduce the existing triglyceride in the circulation; may slow the progression of graft vessel disease and improve survival after transplantation. Also known as fibrates.

fibrillation   (1) an act or process of forming fibers or fibrils; (2) a muscular twitching involving individual muscle fibers acting without coordination or very rapid irregular contractions of the muscle fibers of the heart resulting in a lack of synchronism between heartbeat and pulse

flaccid paralysis absence of reflex and voluntary movements resulting in muscle laxity and lack of resistance to stretch; usually caused from destruction of majority of peripheral motor fibers supplying a muscle

flushing sudden redness of the skin

foam cell type of cell with an abundance of intracellular lipid; found in atherosclerotic lesions

follicle-stimulating hormone (FSH) a peptide hormone produced in the anterior pituitary gland that signals the ovaries to mature a follicle

foot drop a condition of weakness in the muscles of the foot and ankle, caused by poor nerve conduction, which interferes with a person's ability to flex the ankle and walk with a normal heel-toe pattern. The toes touch the ground before the heel, causing the person to trip or lose balance.

force plate device for measuring the forces generated by body movements in each of three planes of movement

forward cholesterol transport the transport of cholesterol, from exogenous or endogenous sources, to various extrahepatic tissues of the body

free cholesterol unesterified cholesterol

functional foods foods that impart a medicinal or health benefit beyond what would occur with basic nutrition

functional restoration a rehabilitation philosophy that focuses on returning to functional daily activity rather than on elimination of pain symptoms before returning to activity

fusion bony union of two adjacent vertebrae, typically using instrumentation (screws, plates, or wires) and bone fragments when removal of damaged intervertebral disc has made the segment unstable or to reduce pain as the result of instability or degenerative change

-G-

galvanic skin response a recording of electrical resistance across the surface of the skin; sometimes used as an index of arousal or anxiety. High arousal or anxiety decreases skin resistance; low arousal or relaxation increases skin resistance.

glaucoma a group of diseases characterized by optic nerve damage and visual field loss, most commonly caused by abnormally high intraocular pressure

glucocorticoid hormone that affects predominantly the metabolism of carbohydrates and, to a lesser extent, fats and proteins. Glucocorticoids are made in the outside portion (the cortex) of the adrenal gland and chemically classed as steroids. Cortisol is the major natural glucocorticoid. The term *glucocorticoid* also applies to equivalent hormones synthesized in the laboratory.

gluconeogenesis the conversion of a substance other than carbohydrate into glucose.

glutamine the most abundant amino acid in the body, with a large pool originating in skeletal muscle. Required by lymphocytes as a substrate and for DNA replication.

glycogen principal form in which carbohydrates are stored in the body, primarily in the liver and muscle. Readily broken down into glucose when needed by the body.

goal-setting a cognitively based planning, organizational, and evaluation process involving explicit identification of performance objectives, standards, or aims of action to facilitate task accomplishment.

goblet cells specialized cells that produce mucus in the airways

goniometer device for measuring the range of motion at a joint

graded progressive incremental exercise test (GXT) exercise test with increasingly greater intensity

GSR galvanic skin response

-H-

healthy life expectancy the number of years of life anticipated for an individual free of major chronic disease

heart attack may reflect either a blockage of a coronary artery, leading to myocardial infarction, or the sudden and usually fatal disruption of the normal cardiac rhythm

hemochromatosis a disease of iron deposition in the myocardium that may result in poor cardiac performance and chronic heart failure

hepatic lipase (HL) lipase that is produced in the liver; hydrolyzes triglycerides and phospholipids of very-low-density lipoproteins and high-density lipoproteins, resulting in the hepatic uptake of fatty acids; also contributes to hepatic uptake of cholesterol

herniated disc bulging, protrusion, extrusion, or sequestration of the nucleus pulposus outside of the annulus fibrosus; "slipped disc"

heterotopic heart transplant attachment of the donor heart to the recipient heart in parallel, resulting in the patient having "piggyback" hearts; rarely performed

high-density lipoprotein (HDL) a classification of lipoproteins containing various apo A, C, and E isoforms and a relatively small amount of lipid relative to protein. These lipoproteins are central to reverse cholesterol transport. High-density lipoproteins protect against coronary heart disease by taking up excess cholesterol from peripheral tissues, scavenging cholesterol and other lipids in the circulation and serving as an antioxidant.

histamine substance that plays a major role in many allergic and anaphylactic reactions. Histamine dilates blood vessels and makes the vessel walls abnormally permeable. It is an important mediator of inflammation, and causes dilation of blood vessels and contraction of smooth muscle (in the lungs, for example).

HIV human immunodeficiency virus, an RNA retrovirus that is the cause of AIDS

hives urticaria

HLA haplotype inherited human leukocyte antigen (HLA) system that codes for polymorphic proteins on the surface of most nucleated cells. A haplotype is a complete set of HLA antigens inherited from either parent.

HMG-CoA reductase inhibitors statin drugs. HMG-CoA reductase inhibitors are used to reduce blood cholesterol, particularly LDL-cholesterol, by blocking the biosynthesis of cholesterol in the liver.

homeostasis maintenance of a constant or unchanging internal state of the body

homocysteine an amino acid formed during the breakdown of methionine. Homocysteine is thought to promote cardiovascular disease by damaging the endothelial lining of arteries.

hormone therapy an oral systemic treatment of cancer that interferes with the estrogen or progesterone receptors responsible for the growth of breast cancer cells

hydrodensitometry a method of measuring body composition based on the concept that the density of the body, or body mass divided by body volume, reflects the body's fat content. Body density can be estimated by dividing its mass in air by a volume obtained by weighing a subject both in the air and under water.

hypercholesterolemia elevated blood cholesterol concentrations

hyperglycemia abnormally increased content of sugar in the blood

hyperinflation a condition in which the lungs are inflated more than normal; the end expiratory lung volume is above normal

hyperlipidemia elevated blood lipid levels that include elevated cholesterol and triglyceride concentrations; abnormally high concentration of lipids (cholesterol or triglycerides) in the circulating blood

hypertension high blood pressure, defined as values $\geq 140/90$ mm Hg

hypertriglyceridemia elevated blood triglyceride concentrations

hypertrophic cardiomyopathy a type of cardiomyopathy characterized by inappropriate left ventricular hypertrophy, often with asymmetrical involvement of the interventricular septum and with preserved or enhanced contractile function

hyperuricemia enhanced blood concentrations of uric acid

hyperventilation breathing in excess of the need to expel CO_2 such that arterial CO_2 is reduced

hypocapnia deficiency of carbon dioxide in the blood

hypoglycemia low level of blood glucose, exercise-induced hypoglycemia is a common problem experienced by exercising diabetics who take exogenous insulin

hypokinesia movement sequences that are too short in amplitude

hypotension a condition in which the arterial blood pressure is abnormally low

hypothalamic nuclei centerpiece of the limbic system in the cerebral cortex. Links subcortical structures of the limbic system (amygdala, hippocampus), and nuclei (accumbens, septal, and anterior nuclei of thalamus). Influential in the integration and expression of emotional behavior.

hypothalamus region at the base of the brain that contains cells that play a role in the regulation of hunger, respiration, body temperature, and other body functions

hypothyroidism a deficiency in activity or secretion of thyroid hormones T3 or T4 (or both) leading to a decreased metabolic rate and possible subsequent weight gain

hypoventilation breathing that is inadequate for the CO_2 produced such that arterial CO_2 is elevated.

hypoxia low oxygen levels

-I-

idiopathic denoting a disease or condition the cause of which is not known or that arises spontaneously

idiopathic dilated cardiomyopathy the process of myocardial weakening and cardiac chamber enlargement that results in poor cardiac output and the syndrome of chronic heart failure

IgA immunoglobulin A, one of five classes of immunoglobulin; the most prevalent Ig found in mucosal secretions of the upper and lower respiratory tracts. An important effector of host defense against viral pathogens causing upper respiratory tract infection.

IgE one of a group of five structurally related protein classes that act as antibodies; plays a major role in allergy and anaphylaxis

immune function The immune system defends the body against foreign proteins, whether in viruses, bacteria, or cancer cells. Key features of immune function include the counts for certain subsets of leukocytes and tissue levels of various substances such as immunoglobulins.

immune suppression blocking or lowering of some aspects of immune function

immunoglobulin (Ig) family of glycoproteins produced and expressed on cell surfaces of B cells, serving as antigen receptors; also found in bodily fluids such as mucosal secretions and serum

immunosuppressants drugs with the property of reducing the ability of the recipient's immune response to damage the donor organ

implantable cardioverter-defibrillator a subcutaneous implantable device that monitors the heart rhythm and is activated when rapid ventricular arrhythmias occur, restoring the normal heart rhythm through electrical shock

incidence the number of new cases with a given outcome at a specified point in time.

inflammation a response to injury or irritation involving the body's attempt to heal the injury or remove the irritation through cellular or chemical reactions; key features are redness, warmth, swelling, and pain.

injury trauma to the body

insufficiency leakage through a valve when closed due to incomplete coaptation of the leaflets, or prolapse of a valve leaflet; regurgitation

insulin the glucose-regulating hormone secreted by the islet cells of the pancreas

intense exercise training regular exercise performed on a daily or more frequent basis by athletes as part of their preparation for competition. Exercise intensity is high, generally over 75% maximum capacity, either continuously or in intervals over several hours each day.

intensity the energy cost of performing an activity, usually expressed in metabolic equivalents (METs)

interleukin-1 an interleukin produced especially by monocytes and macrophages that regulates cell-mediated and humoral immune responses by activating lymphocytes and mediates other biological processes (e.g., the onset of fever) usually associated with infection and inflammation; IL-1

intermediate-density lipoproteins (IDL) lipoproteins resulting from the metabolism of very-low-density lipoproteins in the circulation

intertrigo a form of cutaneous candidiasis occurring between the folds or surfaces of the skin, caused by friction, sweat retention, moisture, warmth, and concomitant overgrowth of resident microorganisms

intervertebral disc resilient fibrocartilaginous shock absorber that forms the center of the motion segment of the spine

intraocular lens an artificial lens, typically made of plastic or silicone, that is surgically implanted into the eye to correct vision

intraocular pressure (IOP) the pressure within the eye

invasive cancer cancer that has spread beyond the layer of tissue in which it developed and is growing into surrounding healthy tissues

ischemia decreased blood supply to a body organ or part, usually caused by atherosclerosis

ischemic pertaining to deficient blood supply

ischemic left ventricular dysfunction the process of development of heart failure by the weakening of pump function due to myocardial infarction or myocardial ischemia

isokinetic exercise in which the muscle generates force against a variable resistance and the speed of movement is maintained at a constant level by a preset rate controlling device

isometric exercise in which the muscle generates force, but there is no observable movement, e.g. pushing against a building

isotonic exercise in which the muscle generates force against constant resistance and movement results

-J-

jejunoileal bypass anastomosis of the upper jejunum to the terminal ileum; one of the original surgical treatments of morbid obesity

-K-

kilocalorie (kcal) the quantity of heat necessary to raise the temperature of 1 kg of water 1° Celsius

kinetic chain the concept of the interrelatedness of the appendicular skeleton, both upper and lower limbs, via the axial musculature

kyphosis hunchback, or "dowager's hump"; with the convexity of the curvature (of the spine) being posterior; typically an abnormal prominence of the thoracic spine as the result of anterior wedging compression fractures (often seen in osteoporosis), from postural abnormalities, or other bony deformity or disease

-L-

lactate product of the reduction of pyruvate by the addition of two hydrogen ions

lactic acidosis threshold the oxygen uptake ($\dot{V}O_2$) during exercise at which net lactate accumulation occurs

laminectomy removal of the bony laminae or expansion of the interlaminar space for access to the nerve root and offending disc fragments

laminotomy removal of the bony laminae or expansion of the interlaminar space for access to the nerve root and offending disc fragments

latency period the time from an exposure to a causal agent to the development of disease

lean tissue mass includes muscle, other body tissues, body fluids and bone; usually calculated as total body mass minus fat mass

left ventricular diastolic function the ability of the heart to accept the flow of blood during diastole

left ventricular end-diastolic dimension an increase in venous return causing greater ventricular filling during the diastolic phase of the cardiac cycle

left ventricular filling the pattern of the transmitral flow into the left ventricle during diastole, which is clinically assessed by Doppler echocardiography

left ventricular systolic function the ability of the heart to contract during systole and eject blood

legal blindness a federal definition of blindness specifying best corrected binocular vision of 20/200 or worse in the better eye or binocular visual field less than 20 degrees

leptin a body-fat-signaling, hormone-like protein secreted in the bloodstream. It is transported to the satiety center in the hypothalamus, and blunts the appetite when caloric intake is sufficient to maintain ideal fat stores.

lesion an area of inflamed or demyelinated central nervous system tissue

leukocytes white blood cells found in the blood and various lymphoid tissues and organs. Leukocytes include lymphocytes, monocytes, polymorphonuclear leukocytes, and natural killer cells.

leukocytosis an increase in the number of white blood cells in the blood

leukotrienes a group of hormones that are thought to mediate the allergic response that causes lung constriction and muscle contraction in asthma

l'Hermitte's sign an abnormal sensation of electricity or "pins and needles" going down the spine into the arms and legs that occurs when the neck is bent forward so that the chin touches the chest

lipolysis metabolic breakdown of fats for energy

lipoprotein complex of proteins, phospholipids, cholesterol, and triglycerides that serves to transport lipids in aqueous mediums found in the blood, interstitium, and lymph

lipoprotein lipase an enzyme found in extrahepatic tissues, such as muscle and adipose tissue, that hydrolyzes triglycerides. The breakdown of triglycerides results in fatty acids, which are taken up by these tissues for energy use or storage.

lipoprotein receptors various forms of cell receptors that bind with lipoproteins, signaling the breakdown of the lipoprotein or internalization of the lipoprotein by endocytosis

lipoprotein(a) [Lp(a)] a lipoprotein similar to LDL, but linked to an apoprotein (a) by a disulfide bridge. Apolipoprotein(a) is structurally similar to plasminogen, which functions to break down clots. Lp(a) is thought to contribute to cardiovascular disease by inhibiting the activity of plasminogen.

lobular carcinoma in situ (LCIS) a very early type of breast cancer that develops within the lobules (milk-producing glands) of the breast and does not penetrate through the wall of the lobules; places a woman at increased risk of developing an invasive breast cancer later in life

local injection therapy may include trigger point injections, iliolumbar injections, acupuncture, or intradiscal injections

logistic regression statistical analysis used to model the effect of one or several independent or explanatory variables on a dichotomous outcome

lordosis condition in which the normal posterior concavity of the lumbar and cervical spines is balanced by the thoracic and (to a lesser degree) sacral kyphoses

low back pain pain in the lumbar region of the spine and lower back extending from the posterior iliac spines, superiorly to the thoracolumbar articulation, and inferiorly to the tip of the coccyx.

low-density lipoproteins (LDL) lipoproteins that contain apolipoprotein B-100 and are responsible for transporting about 70% of the cholesterol found in the circulation; deliver cholesterol to various tissues throughout the body via receptor-mediated endocytosis

lumbago pain in the lower or lumbar region of the back or loins, especially chronic or recurring pain

lumbar extensor strengthening focused exercise program designed to strengthen the back extensors selectively, particularly the erector spinae groups

lumpectomy surgery to remove breast tumor and a small amount of surrounding normal tissue

lung compliance a measure of the elasticity of the lung

lung dysfunction a decrease in lung function as measured by pulmonary function tests

luteinizing hormone a peptide hormone produced in the anterior pituitary gland; signals the ovary to have the biggest follicle to release its egg

lymphedema a complication that may occur after breast cancer treatments in which swelling in the arm is caused by excess lymph fluid that collects after lymph nodes and vessels are removed by surgery or treated by radiation

lymph node dissection surgery to remove lymph nodes found in the armpit region

lymphocyte a type of leukocyte; includes B cells and T cells (and various T cell subsets)

-M-

macrophage a monocyte that has left the circulation and settled in a tissue; a type of white blood cell that ingests foreign material. Macrophages are key players in the immune response to foreign invaders such as infectious microorganisms.

macule a flat, non-raised spot, discoloration, or thickening of the skin that forms an area distinct from the surrounding normal surface

magnetic resonance imaging (MRI) a diagnostic procedure that produces visual images of the body's tissue compartments without the use of x-rays. Nuclei of atoms are influenced by a high-frequency electromagnetic impulse inside a strong magnetic field. The nuclei then give off resonating signals that can produce pictures of parts of the body. By "weighting" the images in different ways, tissues with high water or fat content can be selectively differentiated.

malnutrition poor nutritional status; may result from starvation, exocrine pancreatic insufficiency, malabsorption, deficiency of nutrients, and catabolism associated with other chronic disease aspects (e.g,. inflammation, infection)

manual muscle testing isometric assessment of skeletal muscle strength of upper or lower extremity or trunk through application of resistance with hands and arms of another person

mast cell a connective tissue cell whose normal function is unknown, the mast cell is frequently injured during allergic reactions, releasing strong chemicals including histamine into the tissues and blood that are very irritating and cause itching, swelling, and fluid leaking from cells. These allergic chemicals can also cause muscle spasm and lead to lung and throat tightening as is found in asthma and loss of voice.

mastectomy a surgery to remove all or part of the breast and sometimes other tissue

matching pairs   collection of persons or things more or less exactly like or corresponding to another

maximal heart rate   heart rate attained in the final minute of a progressive treadmill test, carried to exhaustion. (In fact, the body can reach higher heart rates during brief physical efforts such as a tight ski turn.)

maximal oxygen uptake   the greatest oxygen uptake observed at peak exercise in an exercising subject; related to cardiac output and arteriovenous oxygen content differences

maximum heart rate   greatest heart rate attained in a maximal exercise test

McKenzie technique   McKenzie popularized the concept of "centralization" when treating patients with low back pain as a sign of having reduced the "derangement" of the spine and improvement, whereas "peripheralization" of symptoms had a less favorable prognosis.

mechanostat   theory posited by Frost to explain how bone mass and strength are regulated by mechanical loads

mediating variables   variables that exert influence as part of a causal chain in producing outcomes in causal relationships (e.g., Y is a mediator between X and Z in the XYZ causal chain)

menarche   the age at which the first menstrual cycle occurs (mean age is 12.2 years)

METs   metabolic equivalents; the intensity of physical activity, expressed as a ratio of the observed oxygen consumption to resting metabolism

meta-analysis   a statistical synthesis of the results of a systematic review of scientific studies of a particular exposure–outcome relationship; allows an appropriately weighted combination of data from several similar studies which each, individually, may be statistically insignificant

metabolic syndrome   a multitude of lipid and non-lipid risk factors that exist as a result of metabolic disorder(s). Metabolic syndrome often occurs as a result of insulin resistance and is characterized by excess body fat, abdominal obesity, elevated blood glucose, cholesterol and triglycerides, low high-density lipoproteins, and elevated blood pressure.

metastasis   the spread of cancer cells to distant areas of the body by way of the lymph system or bloodstream

methacholine   a substance related to the neurotransmitter acetylcholine, used in provocative testing for several conditions, including cholinergic urticaria

methotrexate   a toxic anticancer drug ($C_{20}H_{22}N_8O_5$) that is an analog of folic acid and an antimetabolite; also called amethopterin

micelle   a lipid vesicle

microaneurysm   microscopic outpouching of the capillary wall, typically occurring where there is loss of the pericytes

microdiscectomy   removal of a small portion of the disc, often only 5% to 8%, and usually limited to the offending, herniated portion. This surgical procedure is done using a microscope through a small access incision rather than requiring a complete laminectomy. Recovery is usually accelerated, and the success rate is high (>90%).

minute ventilation (V_E)   the volume of air breathed each minute (L/min)

mitochondria   site of cellular respiration, and the principal energy source of the cell. Contain the cytochrome enzymes of terminal electron transport and the enzymes of the citric acid cycle, fatty acid oxidation, and oxidative phosphorylation.

mitogenic   protein substances that, when secreted, stimulate cells to divide

mitral valve   the atrioventricular valve that separates the left atrium from the left ventricle and prevents the regurgitation of blood into the left atrium during ventricular systole

mm Hg   millimeters of mercury, a unit for measuring pressure (e.g., intraocular pressure)

moderating variables   variables thought to influence the strength of cause–effect relationships (e.g., gender would be a moderating variable if the relationship between X and Y differed for males and females)

monilial dermatitis   a skin condition characterized by fungal growth

monounsaturated fatty acids   fatty acids with one double or triple bond in the carbon chain

mood state   an affective condition that endures for some time but, nonetheless, is much more transitory than a personality disposition

morbidity   the number of cases of disease in a population

morbilliform   describing a skin rash resembling that of measles, with many small red papules

mortality   the number of deaths in a population

motion segment (couple)   the functional three-structure unit of vertebral motion, consisting of an intervertebral disc and the vertebra above and vertebra below

motor cortex   striplike column located in the frontal lobe of the cerebral cortex which refines the control of physical activity

motor neuron   nerve that is part of the motor unit, which transmits impulses to muscle fibers

mucolytics   drugs used in the therapy of abnormal, highly adherent, viscous mucus (effect is to increase sputum amount, increase expectoration rate)

mucosa   mucous membrane

muscle fasciculations   spontaneously discharge of motor unit potentials from a few motor units or from bundles of muscle fibers; usually seen with pathology. May be normal or polyphasic and have increased or decreased duration and amplitude.

muscle tremor   rhythmic oscillating movement of skeletal muscle frequently observed in fingers, hands, and wrists at rest and during physical activity. Also evident in weakened and atrophied muscle, especially if there is a central nervous system lesion.

mutation a change in the chemistry of a gene that is perpetuated in subsequent divisions of the cell in which it occurs

myalgia tenderness or pain in or arising from the muscles and connective tissue

myocardial contractility sum of forces that increase ventricular contraction and amount of blood ejected. Forces include sympathetic stimulation by catecholamines, greater venous return or diastolic volume, and resistance in cardiac outflow vessels.

myocardial infarction irreversible necrosis or death of the heart tissue that results from prolonged ischemia

myocarditis inflammation of the myocardium that may result in a poorly contracting heart and heart failure

myocardium cardiac muscle

myocyte necrosis death of myocardial cells

myoglobin oxygen-binding pigment in muscle cell, with particularly good storage in type I fibers. Also facilitates favorable oxygen intracellular transport and diffusion from cell membrane to mitochondria where it is utilized.

myopathy any disease or abnormal condition of muscle tissue

-N-

natural killer (NK) cells a subset of leukocyte involved in the first line of defense against invading micro-organisms. Characterized by intracellular granules and specific cell surface antigens; capable of recognizing and killing certain tumor and virally infected cells without prior exposure.

neoadjuvant therapy treatment given before the primary treatment

neovascular glaucoma glaucoma caused by abnormal vessels blocking the drainage angle

nerve conduction velocity electrical conductivity of motor and sensory nerves; generally measured from one site of nerve or muscle to another portion of same nerve or muscle by application of external electrical stimulus

neuropathy any abnormal condition characterized by inflammation and degeneration of the peripheral nerves

neuropeptide Y a small protein that increases food intake and reduces energy expenditure when injected into the brain of experimental animals

neurotransmitter a chemical substance released from nerve endings to transmit impulses across synapses to other nerves, muscles, or glands

neutropenia leukopenia in which the decrease in white blood cells is chiefly in neutrophils

neutrophil the major class of leukocyte in peripheral blood. Neutrophils play an important role in the early defense against bacterial and viral pathogens. Neutrophils also migrate to sites of tissue injury, as part of the inflammatory response.

nonalcoholic steatohepatitis disorder marked by elevated liver enzymes, hypertriglyceridemia, hepatomegaly, and hepatic histologic changes similar to alcoholic hepatitis

nonpolar lipid lipid that is completely insoluble in water

nonproliferative diabetic retinopathy *see* background diabetic retinopathy

nonsteroidal anti-inflammatory agents commonly prescribed medications for the inflammation of arthritis and other body tissues, such as in tendinitis and bursitis. e.g., aspirin, indomethacin, ibuprofen, naproxen, piroxicam, and nabumetone.

nonsustained ventricular tachycardia an abnormal accelerated rhythm originating in the left or right ventricle, defined as nonsustained if it lasts <30 seconds

noradrenergic agents substances that induce anorexia through a centrally mediated pathway in the hypothalamus

NSAIDs nonsteroidal anti-inflammatory agents/drugs

nucleus pulposus the central core of the collagenous intervertebral disc, which normally has a high water and proteoglycan content. It is this portion of the disc that usually is extruded or "herniates" through a tear in the surrounding annulus fibrosus.

-O-

obesity excess body fat accumulation, defined by a body mass index (BMI) ≥30 or weight 20% or more above desirable body weight

obligatory thermogenesis minimal heat produced to maintain a basal metabolic rate in a thermoneutral environment

odds ratio the ratio of the odds of exposure among those with the disease divided by the odds of exposure among those without the disease

oligomenorrhea <10 menstrual cycles per year. The menstrual cycle length usually is longer than 36 days and shorter than 60 days.

open chain distal segment of body moves freely in space

optic disc the surface of the optic nerve where it enters the back of the eye and conjoins to the retina

orthotic a mechanical appliance such as a leg brace or splint that is specially designed to control, correct, or compensate for impaired limb function (e.g., ankle-foot orthosis); also called orthosis.

orthotopic heart transplant the procedure of excision of the failing recipient heart and implantation of the donor heart

osteoarthritis a degenerative condition of the joints characterized by a loss of articular cartilage; also called degenerative arthritis, degenerative joint disease, hypertrophic arthritis

osteoblasts bone-forming cells located on bone surfaces

osteoclasts multinucleated cells that remove bone

osteocyte the mature bone cell responsible for maintaining bone tissue. Once the osteoblast surrounds itself with matrix it differentiates into an osteocyte and remains embedded in bone.

osteogenic sarcoma a malignant bone tumor

osteopenia decrease in bone volume to below normal levels, especially due to inadequate replacement of bone lost to normal lysis

osteophytes a pathological bony outgrowth

osteoporosis reduced bone mineral density seen most commonly in postmenopausal women which predisposes them to fractures of the wrist, hip, and spine

osteotomy surgical procedure in which a bone is divided or a piece of bone is excised (as to correct a deformity)

Oswestry Low Back Pain Questionnaire a functional disability scale frequently used to measure outcomes in longitudinal "pre-post" studies of low back pain

outcome all possible results that stem from exposure to a causal factor

overload principle in order for adaptations to occur, a threshold stress level must be exceeded

overtraining excessive training in an athlete. If left unchecked, may result in symptoms of overtraining syndrome, characterized by poor performance, persistent fatigue, disturbed sleep patterns, neuroendocrine changes, alterations in mood state, and frequent illness

oxidation the process of a substance combining with oxygen

oxidative phosphorylation the formation of ATP and water via the electron transport chain

oxygen saturation (SaO_2) the amount of hemoglobin (Hb) that is associated with oxygen, expressed as a percent.

oxygen supplementation enrichment of the inspired air with oxygen to maintain or increase a patient's arterial oxygen levels

-P-

panic disorder an anxiety disorder characterized by sudden, brief, and recurrent episodes of intense anxiety

pannus (1) a vascular tissue causing a superficial opacity of the cornea and occurring especially in trachoma; (2) a sheet of inflammatory granulation tissue that spreads from the synovial membrane and invades the joint in rheumatoid arthritis, ultimately leading to fibrous ankylosis

panretinal photocoagulation treatment of the retina with a laser that burns through all of the retina except the macular region

papule a small superficial raised abnormality or spot on the skin; usually forms part of a rash

parathyroid hormone (PTH) hormone responsible for maintaining adequate serum calcium levels

pars interarticularis the posterior elements of the vertebra connecting the vertebral body to the spinous process. Fractures through this portion of the vertebra may be either "congenital" or traumatic, and are more common in adolescent athletes.

passive modalities therapeutic techniques that do not require the patient's active participation

passive stabilizers The ligaments provide passive stabilization of the otherwise unstable spinal column. Ligaments are static and, unlike muscles, do not contract or lengthen.

pathophysiology the basic processes underlying a disease condition of an organ or organism.

peak aerobic capacity ($\dot{V}O_2$ peak) the highest value of oxygen uptake measured during a maximal oxygen test

peak aerobic power the maximum power output or peak oxygen intake that the individual can attain safely when performing a large-muscle activity such as treadmill walking or cycle ergometry

peak heart rate The highest heart rate observed under specific conditions (e.g., a symptom-limited treadmill stress test)

pelvic stabilization immobilization of the pelvis to prevent hip flexion and extension from compensating for lumbar range of motion

peptic ulcer an ulcer occurring in the lower esophagus

percent heart rate reserve Heart rate reserve is determined by subtracting resting heart rate from maximal heart rate.

pericytes elongated cells that wrap around retinal capillaries and have contractile properties that help to regulate blood flow through the capillary bed

phakoemulsification a surgical technique using ultrasound energy for liquefying and removing cataracts

phospholipids lipids containing phosphorus, fatty acids and a nitrogenous base

photocoagulation condensation of protein material by the controlled use of light rays, typically laser

photoreceptor type of nerve cell in the retina (rods and cones) that is sensitive to light.

photosensitizing pertaining to abnormally heightened reactivity of a tissue to the influence of light

physical activity any form of movement that induces a significant increase over resting energy expenditure; may include exercise, sport, occupational activity, and domestic chores

plant stanol fully saturated form of sterol

plant sterol a cholesterol-like chemical compound made up of carbon and alcohol and derived from plants such as pine trees, soybeans, rice, and various nuts

plasma colloid osmotic pressure the osmotic pressure induced by larger, complex organic substances (proteins) in the fluid portion of the blood (plasma)

plasma osmolarity the concentration of osmotically active particles in the fluid portion of the blood

pneumothorax condition in which air enters the intrapleural space, causing collapse of the lung

polar lipid lipids that are partially soluble in water

polycarbonate the strongest plastic material available that is clear enough to see through; 20 times stronger than everyday streetwear lenses

polycystic ovarian syndrome dysregulation of the pituitary-gonadal axis in which increased luteinizing hormone secretion increases ovarian production of androstenedione and adipose production of estrone;

characterized by infertility, abnormal vaginal bleeding, and hirsutism

polyphasic motor unit motor unit consisting of a greater number of muscle fibers than originally given. The increased number of fibers most likely are orphaned fibers, which are reinnervated by a healthy motor neuron. The EMG generally shows larger, abnormal action potentials compared to motor units with fewer innervated muscle fibers.

polyunsaturated fatty acid fatty acids with multiple double or triple bonds in the carbon chain.

population attributable risk a measure used to assess the public health impact of an exposure–outcome relationship that takes into account the prevalence of the exposure in the population; an estimate of the deaths that would not occur in a population if a risk factor or disease did not exist

population-based pertaining to a general population defined by geopolitical boundaries; this population is the denominator or the sampling frame.

postprandial following a meal

power work divided by time, usually expressed as watts (W) or preferably kilojoules (kJ) where 16.67 W = 1 kJ = 4.19 calories

power position the position of optimal body mechanics for lifting in which the knees are bent slightly forward, with little bend at the hips and no bending of the back

premature death death during the period when a person would normally be a healthy and productive member of society

premotor corticol part of the frontal lobe directly interconnected with the motor cortex. Interconnected with other cortices in the motor cortex such as prefrontal and primary motor; receives information from motor cortex but has a higher movement threshold stimulation than the motor cortex

pressure overload excessive work created by increased resistance to the outflow of blood from the ventricle during systole; a feature of aortic or pulmonic stenosis

prevalence the number of existing cases with a given outcome at a point in time

primary dyslipidemia dyslipidemia that results from a genetic or environmental condition

primary glaucoma an ocular disease characterized by elevated intraocular pressure resulting primarily from anatomic or pathophysiologic factors affecting aqueous drainage

primary-progressive a clinical course of multiple sclerosis characterized from the beginning by progressive disease, with no plateaus or remissions, or an occasional plateau and very short-lived, minor improvements

progesterone a steroid hormone secreted by the corpus luteum and placenta; its values are low in the follicular phase and high during the luteal phase

progressive-relapsing a clinical course of multiple sclerosis that shows disease progression from the beginning, but with clear, acute relapses, with or without full recovery from those relapses along the way

progressive resistance exercises gradual but incremental increase in load on a biologic system to promote increased strength and muscle mass via mitochondrial stimulation; progressive strengthening results from overload exercise.

progressive resistance training training program that uses progressive resistance (flexion/extension) to build lean body mass and strength

proliferative diabetic retinopathy ocular disease caused by diabetes characterized by the presence of abnormal (neovascular) tissue on the optic nerve, retina, or iris

proprioception a sense or perception, usually at a subconscious level, of the movements and position of the body and especially its limbs, independent of vision

prospective study a design that identifies a group based on some predefined exposure criteria and then, over time, compares subgroups of the population on an outcome of interest; also called concurrent, follow-up, incidence, longitudinal, or cohort studies

prostaglandins a group of biologically active substances involved in inflammatory reactions, and countered by nonsteroidal anti-inflammatory agents such as aspirin and ibuprofen

prosthesis artificial replacement for a part of the body

protoporphyrin IX the type of porphyrin most commonly found in nature; a constituent of hemoglobin, myoglobin, most of the cytochromes, and the more common chlorophylls

pruritus severe itching

psychophysiological measurement of physiological processes in an effort to draw conclusions about psychological states

psychosocial intervention comprehensive treatment processes involving emotional, mental, and behavioral efforts to return an injured person to preinjury status

pulmonary reserve the difference between the maximum possible capacity to exchange gas based on lung morphology and that actually used

pulmonic valve the semilunar valve that separates the pulmonary artery from the right ventricle and prevents the regurgitation of blood into the right ventricle during ventricular diastole

pulse oximeter a device used to measure arterial oxygen saturation noninvasively

pupil the circular opening in the iris that can dilate or constrict to regulate the amount of light entering the eye

pyrogen any substance or agent producing fever

-Q-

quality of life the individual's perception of the pleasure derived from his or her life; current quality of life may be measured on an arbitrary scale, extending (for example) from 0 to 1.0

quality-adjusted life expectancy the individual's calendar life-expectancy, multiplied by the integral of multiple quality of life assessments covering the remainder of his or her lifespan

quasi-experimental a research design that does not involve random assignment but incorporates other control features in an effort to eliminate as many threats to internal validity as possible

questionnaire a series of questions dealing with a topic (e.g., psychological, social, behavioral, educational) with the object of obtaining data (e.g., diagnostic, evaluative)

-R-

radiation therapy treatment with high-energy rays such as x-rays to kill or shrink cancer cells. The radiation may come from outside of the body (external radiation) or from radioactive materials placed directly in the tumor (internal or implant radiation). Radiation therapy may be used to reduce the size of a cancer before surgery, to destroy any remaining cancer cells after surgery, or, in some cases, as the main treatment.

radiculopathy/radiculitis irritation or inflammation of a nerve root (can be of either mechanical or chemical etiology) producing paresthesias or sensory or motor changes in a characteristic dermatomal pattern, depending on the spinal level affected

randomized without a particular principle

randomized controlled trials a study design in which subjects are assigned randomly to treatment or control groups, then followed to assess disease occurrence

rates the number of persons with the outcome (or exposure) of interest divided by the population

rating of perceived exertion (RPE) numerical rating assigned to the perceived effort associated with performance of an exercise task

reaction speed rate of response to an external signal (e.g., braking at a red light).

recurrent cancer return of cancer in spite of apparently successful initial treatment, usually within the first 2 or 3 years after treatment

red flags signs or symptoms that may alert the examiner to the possibility of medical disease which may require further evaluation

refractory period a period after an event or reaction in which there is unresponsiveness or a decreased likelihood of the event repeating itself

rehabilitation the process of seeking to restore (at a minimum) preinjury capacities, capabilities, or condition to an injured person

relative risk the ratio of the risk of disease in an exposed cohort over a defined time interval to the risk of disease in an unexposed cohort over the same time interval. Relative risk can be estimated from cohort studies and, for rare diseases, from case-control studies.

renal pertaining to the kidney

residual volume volume of air in the lungs that cannot be expelled

resistance exercise muscle contraction where the shortening of the muscle is opposed by an external force such as weights

respiratory exchange ratio (RER) the ratio of oxygen uptake to carbon dioxide output at rest and during exercise

respiratory failure insufficient alveolar ventilation, with resulting hypoxemia and hypercapnia

respiratory quotient the exchange of oxygen and carbon dioxide measured at the lung that reflects the actual gas exchange from nutrient catabolism in the cell.

resting metabolic rate (RMR) minimal amount of energy expended to support basic physiological processes

restrictive reduced effective lung volume

reticular formation a part of the brain stem (midbrain, pons, tegmentum of medulla) that is formed by many nuclei scattered throughout central part of brain stem

retina the thin, transparent, light-sensitive membrane lining the inner eyeball and connected by the optic nerve to the brain

retinal pigment epithelium the monolayer of pigmented, hexagonal cells beneath the retina that provide metabolic and structural support for the photoreceptors

retinopathy any noninflammatory disease of the retina

reverse cholesterol transport the transport of cholesterol from peripheral tissues to the liver

rheotherapy a process of removing unwanted compounds from the blood using a series of filters

rheumatoid arthritis a usually chronic disease that is considered an autoimmune disease, characterized especially by pain, stiffness, inflammation, swelling, and sometimes destruction of joints; also called atrophic arthritis

rigidity increased muscle tone in Parkinson disease

risk factor a behavior, trait, condition or genetic alteration that increases a person's chance of developing a disease

Roland Disability Scale the back pain scale most frequently cited in the medical literature

Roux-en-Y gastric bypass procedure alternative procedure to reverse obesity in which a loop of proximal jejunum is attached to the stomach

RPE rating of perceived exertion

-S-

saturated fatty acid fatty acid that has no double or triple bonds in the carbon chain

sciatica low back pain accompanied by radicular symptoms, typically pain along the course of the sciatic nerve due to irritation or inflammation of the nerve itself or the contributing roots. May be due to disc herniation with pain, numbness, tingling; occasionally leads to loss of sensation or tendon reflex

scintigraphy a method of examining the blood supply of the heart based on the intravascular injection of a radioactive marker

secondary dyslipidemia dyslipidemia resulting indirectly from another condition, such as the use of medications, metabolic disorders, and liver or kidney disease

secondary glaucoma an ocular disease characterized by elevated intraocular pressure resulting from other ocular or nonocular diseases

secondary progressive multiple sclerosis a clinical course of multiple sclerosis that initially is relapsing-remitting and then becomes progressive at a variable rate, possibly with an occasional relapse and minor remission

selective serotonin reuptake inhibitor a prescription medication that blocks re-entry of the neurotransmitter serotonin into the nerve cells, thus allowing it to accumulate; originally used to treat depression but also found to be effective for treating some anxiety disorders; examples include fluoxetine (Prozac), paroxetine (Paxil), sertraline (Zoloft), and fluvoxamine (Luvox)

semilunar valves the cardiac valves that separate the great arteries from the ventricles and prevent regurgitation of arterial blood into the ventricles during diastole; called "semilunar" because the valves have three leaflets that resemble the half moon

sentinel node biopsy procedure in which a dye or radioactive substance is injected near the tumor and flows into the sentinel lymph nodes (first lymph nodes that cancer is likely to spread to from the primary tumor). The surgeon removes the sentinel nodes to check for the presence of tumor cells.

serotonergic agents substances that enhance presynaptal release of serotonin and increase its concentration at the synapse

signal-averaged electrocardiogram (SAECG) recording of the averaged electrocardiographic complexes that may identify the presence of late potentials; expression of a delayed (or abnormal) myocardial activation, usually associated with a pathologic heart condition

sit and reach test a simple test of flexibility at the hip and lower back in which the subject reaches forward along a board placed immediately above the toes

skin conductance the ability of the skin to transmit electrical impulses; *see* galvanic skin response

sleep apnea bouts of breathing cessation during sleep due to the upper airway closing; often associated with obesity due to increased fat deposition around the neck and upper chest

social support activities in which individuals engage with the intention of helping one another

soluble fiber edible fiber that is soluble in water

somatosensory evoked potential a test that measures the brain's electrical activity in response to repeated (mild) electrical stimulation of different parts of the body; extremely important in the diagnosis of multiple sclerosis because it can confirm the presence of a suspected lesion (demyelination) or identify the presence of an unsuspected lesion that has produced no symptoms

spasticity abnormal increase in muscle tone, manifested as a spring-like resistance to moving or being moved

sphygmomanometer inflatable cuff and pressure measuring device for determining blood pressure

spina bifida failure of the posterior elements of the spinous process to form completely, resulting in an unroofed vertebral canal. Often occult (asymptomatic), but may be a cause of neurologic problems, depending on degree.

spinal stenosis narrowing of the spinal canal; may be congenital, due to trauma, or due to encroachment of degenerative bony spurs or osteophytes

spondylolisthesis forward displacement of the superior vertebral body on the one below due to bilateral defects of the pars interarticularis, excessive wear of the facets, or abnormal length of the pars structure; most commonly seen at the level of L5-S1 and L4-L5

spondylolysis a fracture or defect in the pars interarticularis of the vertebra which may be either congenital or acquired. May be unilateral or bilateral; the latter may allow vertebral body slippage, i.e., spondylolisthesis.

sputum mixture of bronchial secretions

SSRI selective serotonin reuptake inhibitor

stabilimeter device for measuring the ability to maintain balance as the subject stands on a balanced beam

stage the extent of a cancer, especially whether a cancer has spread from the original site to other parts of the body

state anxiety a temporary emotional response that is characterized by an increase in physiological arousal and muscular tension as well as feelings of concern, apprehension, or fear

statin medications blood lipid–improving drugs that may reduce the incidence of acute rejection, slow the progression of graft vessel disease, and improve survival after heart transplantation

statins *see* HMG-CoA reductase inhibitors

steady state state in which certain body systems achieve a consistent level and are able to maintain that level for an extended period of time

stenosis a narrowing of the valve orifice that increases the resistance of blood flow across the valve. The stenosis may be congenital, due to a developmental abnormality, or may be acquired and secondary to sclerosis and calcification of the leaflets

stereopsis the ability to perceive three-dimensionality

stress a dynamic appraisal process involving an assessment of the potential disruption caused by an event and the balance (or imbalance) of demands and response capacity

stridor the noise heard on breathing when the trachea or larynx is obstructed. It tends to be louder and harsher than wheezing.

stroke volume the volume of blood pumped from the heart with each beat

subaortic stenosis narrowing of the outflow tract of the left ventricle below the aortic valve by a ridge of muscle or discrete membrane

supravalvular (aortic) stenosis narrowing of the aorta above the aortic valve by a ridge of tissue

sustained ventricular tachycardia Ventricular tachycardia is an abnormal accelerated rhythm originated in the left or right ventricle; defined as sustained according to the time duration and hemodynamic consequences.

sympathetic activity activity of the sympathetic nervous system

sympathetic nervous system the part of the nervous system that regulates involuntary vital functions, including the activity of the heart, smooth muscles, and adrenal glands

syncope fainting; a temporary loss of consciousness

synergistic the effect seen when two drugs given together increase activity so that it is greater than the sum of the effects of the two drugs given separately

synovectomy surgical removal of a synovial membrane

synovitis inflammation of a synovial membrane, usually with pain and swelling of the joint

systemic therapy treatment that reaches and affects cells throughout the body (e.g., chemotherapy)

-T-

tachycardia an increase in the heart rate above normal

teratogenic agent any substance that interferes with normal prenatal development, causing formation of one or more developmental abnormalities in the fetus

terminal sprouting axon from healthy motor neuron reinnervating abandoned muscle fibers, resulting in smaller number of motor units but larger fiber mass per motor unit

thalamic nuclei nuclei located in the thalamus which act as a relay in processing information from the spinal cord, cerebellum, and basal ganglia and report to the cerebral cortex with transmission between the cerebellum and cerebrum

thermic effect of activity (TEA) energy expended above the resting metabolic rate to perform physical activity and muscular movement

thermic effect of food (TEF) the increase in metabolism that occurs during the digestion, absorption, and metabolism of energy-yielding nutrients

thermogenic a process that creates heat; in the exercise science area, the term typically is used in connection with increases in core temperature

thrombocytopenia a decrease in the number of platelets in the blood; can be a side effect of chemotherapy

tidal volume (Vt) volume of gas moved in the lungs during each respiratory cycle

T lymphocytes small white blood cells (leukocytes) that play a large role in defending the body against disease; also can destroy myocardial cells of the donor heart during acute rejection orchestrated by the immune system

TNM system a staging system used to indicate whether cancer has spread and if so, how far. T, the size of the tumor; N, how far the cancer has spread to nearby nodes; M, whether the cancer has spread (metastasized) to other organs of the body.

tolerance a reduction in or loss of the normal response to a drug or other inciting event that usually provokes a response; may occur with repeated exposure to the drug or provocation

tomography Computed tomography is a radiologic technique used to assess cross-sectional areas of muscle, fat, and bone at various body sites.

total body potassium a method of measuring body composition based on the principle that the concentration of potassium in the body represents a constant proportion of fat-free mass

trabecular bone the same material as cortical bone, but with a "spongy" appearance. It is composed of rods, struts, and sheets of bone tissue surrounded by marrow cells. It is located in the proximal and distal ends of long bones and in the axial skeleton (i.e., vertebrae).

trabecular meshwork the fenestrated tissue in the anterior chamber angle that permits drainage of aqueous from the eye

training in the physiological context, an increase of the individual's functional capacity by an appropriate intensity, frequency, and duration of physical activity

trait anxiety a predisposition to perceive circumstances as threatening and a resulting tendency to respond with heightened levels of state anxiety in a variety of situations

tricuspid valve the atrioventricular valve that separates the right atrium from the right ventricle and prevents the regurgitation of blood into the right atrium during ventricular systole. The tricuspid valve has three leaflets.

triglyceride the major form of lipid in the body and in food

tumor an abnormal lump or mass of tissue; may be benign (not cancerous) or malignant (cancerous)

tumor necrosis factor a protein that is produced by monocytes and macrophages in response especially to endotoxins and that activates white blood cells and has anticancer activity; TNF

type 2 diabetes mellitus (NIDDM) A form of diabetes in which ketosis is not commonly seen. Insulin therapy can be used but often is not required; often associated with obesity or advanced age. The primary problem is a development of cellular resistance to insulin.

type I muscle fiber skeletal fiber with high aerobic capacity and slow reaction time

type II muscle fiber skeletal fiber with high anaerobic capacity and fast reaction time; the fast-twitch muscle fibers responsible for rapid, forceful muscle contractions

-U-

UPDRS Unified Parkinson's Disease Rating Scale; has 6 subscores

upper respiratory tract infection infection of the oral, nasal and pharyngeal surfaces causing symptoms such as sneezing, runny or congested nose, irritated or "sore" throat, and cough

urticaria   an allergic reaction in which red round wheals develop on the skin, ranging in size from small spots to several inches across. They itch intensely and may last for hours to days; also called hives.

uveitis   any inflammatory condition of uveal tissue (e.g., iris, ciliary body, or choroid)

-V-

Valsalva maneuver   any forced expiratory effort against a closed airway, as when an individual holds his breath and tightens his muscles in a concerted strenuous effort to move a heavy object

valvotomy   a surgical or balloon catheter procedure during which the leaflets of a stenotic valve are cut or ruptured to provide a larger orifice

valvuloplasty   a surgical procedure that reconstructs a diseased valve with the goal of restoring normal function

vasoactive   affecting the diameter of blood vessels, especially arteries

venous return   amount of blood returning to the right atrium of the heart; influenced by intrathoracic and intra-abdominal pressure, constriction of veins, dynamic activity of skeletal musculature, and body position changes

ventilation   the amount of air pumped in and out of the chest at rest, or during exercise

ventilation and perfusion matching   a ratio of the amount of alveolar ventilation (V_A) and the blood flow or perfusion (Q) in part or all of the lung (V_A/Q)

very-low-density lipoproteins (VLDL)   lipoproteins that contain a large amount of lipid relative to protein. VLDL are synthesized in the liver, are rich in triglyceride, and give rise to low-density lipoproteins as they are broken down in the circulation.

visual evoked potential   a test in which the brain's electrical activity in response to visual stimuli (e.g., a flashing checkerboard) is recorded by an electroencephalograph and analyzed by computer. Demyelination results in a slowing of response time.

vitamins   organic substances, present in food in small quantities and essential for normal growth and health

vitreous humor   the clear gelatinous fluid that fills the vitreous cavity of the eye

$\dot{V}O_{2max}$ highest oxygen consumption during a maximal exercise test

$\dot{V}O_{2peak}$ maximal oxygen uptake during exercise that is sub- or maximal.

-WXYZ-

Waddell signs   five tests that may help to identify nonorganic factors which may be contributing to a patient's back pain

wallerian degeneration   the biochemical and morphologic alterations following trauma that occur in a nerve due to loss of axonal continuity

wheal   a temporary red or pale raised area of the skin, often accompanied by severe itching; often a sign of local or generalized allergy (*see* urticaria, hives)

work   force times distance, usually reported as keg or footpounds

yellow flags   biopsychosocial factors which may explain a patient's failure to heal or progression to a chronic disorder

zonules   the suspensory fibers extending between the ciliary body and the equator of the lens that hold the lens in position behind the iris

Index

Page numbers in *italics* denote figures; those followed by a t denote tables.